P9-BJP-980

MAGILL'S

MEDICAL GUIDE

MAGILL'S

MEDICAL GUIDE

Fourth Revised Edition

Volume I

Abdomen — Corns and calluses

Medical Consultants

Anne Lynn S. Chang, M.D.
Stanford University

Laurence M. Katz, M.D.
University of North Carolina, Chapel Hill

H. Bradford Hawley, M.D.
Wright State University

Nancy A. Piotrowski, Ph.D.
University of California, Berkeley

Connie Rizzo, M.D., Ph.D.
Columbia University

Project Editor

Tracy Irons-Georges

SALEM PRESS, INC.
Pasadena, California Hackensack, New Jersey

Magill's Medical Guide: Health and Illness, 1995
Supplement, 1996
Magill's Medical Guide, revised edition, 1998
Second revised edition, 2002
Third revised edition, 2005
Fourth revised edition, 2008

∞ The paper used in these volumes conforms to the American National Standard for Permanence of Paper for Printed Library Materials, Z39.48-1992 (R1997).

Note to Readers

The material presented in *Magill's Medical Guide* is intended for broad informational and educational purposes. Readers who suspect that they suffer from any of the physical or psychological disorders, diseases, or conditions described in this set should contact a physician without delay; this work should not be used as a substitute for professional medical diagnosis or treatment. This set is not to be considered definitive on the covered topics, and readers should remember that the field of health care is characterized by a diversity of medical opinions and constant expansion in knowledge and understanding.

Library of Congress Cataloging-in-Publication Data

Magill's medical guide. — 4th rev. ed. / medical consultants, Anne Lynn S. Chang . . . [et al.] ; project editor, Tracy Irons-Georges.

p. ; cm.
Includes bibliographical references and index.
ISBN 978-1-58765-384-1 (set : alk. paper)
ISBN 978-1-58765-385-8 (vol. 1 : alk. paper)
ISBN 978-1-58765-386-5 (vol. 2 : alk. paper)
ISBN 978-1-58765-387-2 (vol. 3 : alk. paper)
ISBN 978-1-58765-388-9 (vol. 4 : alk. paper)
ISBN 978-1-58765-407-7 (vol. 5 : alk. paper)

1. Medicine—Encyclopedias. I. Chang, Anne. II. Title: Medical guide.
[DNLM: 1. Medicine — Encyclopedias — English. W 13 M194 2008]

RC41.M34 2008
610.3—dc22

2007033818

First Printing

PRINTED IN THE UNITED STATES OF AMERICA

Publisher's Note

Since 1995, *Magill's Medical Guide* has had a reputation for providing general readers with the most authoritative yet accessible reference source that helps bridge the gap between medical encyclopedias and dictionaries for professionals and popular self-help guides. This *Fourth Revised Edition*, expanded to five volumes, continues to build on this value.

New to This Edition

This edition of *Magill's Medical Guide* is unlike any reference work Salem Press has published. The difference is simple, but significant: The purchase of the printed set entitles the buyer to free online access to the *Guide*'s content until December 31, 2010. Use of the content is unlimited within a school or library—regardless of whether the purchaser is a single site or a system. This online version is made available through Salem's new reference platform, Salem Health. It features all the text of the print version and most of the illustrations. Users can search the full text or browse the contents by demographic (men, women, children, elderly) and through subject categories (Anatomy & Physiology; Diagnosis & Testing; Diseases, Disorders, & Symptoms; Mental Health; Prevention & Lifestyle; Social Issues; Specialties & Health Care Providers; Treatment & Therapy), which are further divided into numerous subcategories. Information about how to activate online access to Salem Health can be found at the end of this "Publisher's Note."

To the entries in the previous encyclopedia, 58 completely new topics have been added, bringing the total number of entries to 1,017. Some of these essays fill gaps in the table of contents—such as *Sleep*, *Cardiac arrest*, and *Brain damage*—while others address new and emerging concerns and procedures, such as *Avian influenza* (bird flu) and *Facial transplantation*. Overviews of the health issues and statistics for women, men, African Americans, American Indians, and Asian Americans are included for the first time. In addition, 37 newly commissioned essays have replaced those from the previous edition, and another 167 have been updated by medical experts.

This edition includes 44 "In the News" sidebars that evaluate recent media stories about ongoing research and experimental treatments. These boxes both highlight the latest information and provide readers with a critical view of popular reports that may (or may not) prove crucial to the future understanding and treatment of certain medical conditions. The topics covered include the side effects of Ambien and other sleep aids, methicillin-resistant staphylococci, the dangers of COX-2 inhibitors, new treatments for Alzheimer's disease and breast cancer, and Iraq War-related diseases.

Every entry from the previous edition has been evaluated by the panel of Medical Consultants and then updated by experts or reedited to ensure its currency and accuracy, as needed. All cross-references to other relevant entries in *Magill's Medical Guide* have been revised. Every bibliography has been updated with the latest editions and sources, and entry bibliographies include Web sites for relevant organizations. All appendixes from the previous edition have been updated and checked for accuracy, and two new ones have been added: a list of "Symptoms and Warning Signs," listing possible causes, and a "Pharmaceutical List" surveying brand name and generic drugs and their main uses.

Scope of Coverage

The 1,017 entries in this encyclopedia describe major diseases and disorders of the human body, the basics of human anatomy and physiology, specializations in medical practice, and common surgical and nonsurgical procedures. The *Fourth Revised Edition* offers entries by 330 writers from the fields of life science and medicine. Every essay is signed by the original author, including medical or other advanced degrees, and each updated entry is also signed by the revising author. These writers examine various diseases and disorders, both genetic and acquired, the detailed knowledge of human bodily systems and structures that medical practice requires, and the medical professions and procedures that apply this knowledge. More than 400 photographs and medical drawings provide invaluable visual context for entries about diseases, research, surgery, and human anatomy.

For each disease and disorder, a concise information box lists causes, symptoms, duration, and treatments, acting as a quick reference tool. Readers will find topics focusing on specific disorders, as well as those surveying the range of afflictions attacking a particular system. The majority of entries treat physical disorders:

- bacterial and viral infections
- cancers of various types
- genetic defects
- heart and circulatory disorders
- abdominal and gastrointestinal disorders
- bone and muscle defects
- brain and nervous system problems
- dental diseases
- eating and nutritional disorders
- endocrine disorders
- reproductive system disorders of both men and women
- immune disorders
- kidney and urinary system disorders
- liver disorders
- respiratory diseases
- sexually transmitted diseases
- skin disorders
- sleep disorders
- trauma-related disorders
- vector-borne diseases
- visual disorders

Other entries consider psychic-emotional and learning disorders that originate in or have significant impact on the physical health of the body. Some basic conditions that are often the object of medical attention are covered, including *Aging*, *Pregnancy and gestation*, *Childbirth* and its complications, *Puberty and adolescence*, *Menopause*, and *Sexuality*.

Entries on anatomy and biology include overviews of anatomical organs and systems and of biological components and processes. A broad view of medical practice—its areas of specialization and health care provision—is offered by entries on such topics as *Emergency medicine*, *Nursing*, and *Orthopedics*. Diagnostic and imaging techniques as well as nonsurgical and surgical procedures, both major and minor, are covered. In addition, other areas of medical science are represented: alternative medicine, ethical issues, genetics, organizations, procedures in the field of psychiatry, testing and examinations, and various types of transplantation.

ENTRY LENGTH AND FORMAT

The essays in the *Fourth Revised Edition* are arranged in an encyclopedic format—alphabetically from *Abdomen* through *Zoonoses*. The lengths of the entries vary from shorter entries of 500 words to medium-length entries of 1,000 words to full, essay-length treatments of 2,500 to 3,500 words. All entries begin with standard information about the type of entry, the anatomy or bodily system affected, the specialties involved, and a brief definition of the topic. For essays of 1,000 words or more, next comes a list of key terms with brief definitions. Several main subsections of text follow and depend on the type of entry.

- Entries on Diseases or Disorders: "Causes and Symptoms" defines the condition and describes its cause and its possible manifestations in patients, and "Treatment and Therapy" explores the various treatments available to alleviate symptoms or effect a cure.

- Entries on Anatomy or Biology: "Structure and Functions" defines the physiological or biological system, including its components and role, and "Disorders and Diseases" describes the medical conditions that can result from malfunction of and injury to this physiological system.

- Entries on Development: "Physical and Psychological Factors" charts the stages of development and analyzes the underlying physiological and emotional/psychological components, and "Disorders and Effects" addresses the overall impact of the developmental process.

- Entries on Procedures: "Indications and Procedures" relates the circumstances under which the procedure is usually performed, identifying the condition it is intended to correct and detailing the basic steps involved, and "Uses and Complications" discusses the various applications and possible risks and complicating factors.

- Entries on Specialties: "Science and Profession" addresses the training and responsibilities of various specialists and "Diagnostic and Treatment Techniques" outlines the means by which they counsel patients, diagnose conditions, perform operations or procedures, and otherwise treat medical problems.

Topics that do not fall into these categories depart from these standard subheadings but follow a similar format style.

The last section of all longer entries is "Perspective and Prospects," which places the topic in a larger context within medicine—past, present, and future. For example, an entry on a disease may cover the earliest known investigation into the condition, the evolution of its treatment over time, and promising areas of research for a greater understanding of its causes and cure. An entry on a procedure may address the innovations that led to contemporary technology, improvements or changes that have been made in the procedure, and where this medical technique may be headed. Every entry ends with the author's byline and a listing of cross-references to other entries of interest in the encyclopedia. All essays conclude with the section "For Further Information," which lists general bibliographic works for the reader to consult; bibliographies for entries of 2,500 or 3,500 words provide brief annotations evaluating the features, contents, and value of the sources.

Special Features

Several special features in the *Fourth Revised Edition* assist readers in locating topics of interest. The "Complete List of Contents," found at the beginning of each volume, allows the scope of the encyclopedia to be seen in its entirety. At the back of every volume are the lists "Entries by Specialties and Related Fields" and "Entries by Anatomy or System Affected," which can direct the reader to essays by category; for example, a reader looking up "Oncology" on the specialty list will find entries on diseases (such as *Cancer*, *Malignancy and metastasis*, and *Sarcoma*), specialties (such as *Cytology* and *Pathology*), diagnostic procedures (such as *Mammography* and *Screening*), and treatments (such as *Chemotherapy*, *Radiation therapy*, and *Tumor removal*).

At the back of volume 5 are a number of valuable features: a thorough glossary of medical terms; definitions of almost 900 "Diseases and Other Medical Conditions"; an appendix detailing the training, degrees, and duties of various health care professionals; a list of medical journals; a general bibliography arranged by category; a Web site directory; a helpful resources list of organizations and support groups, with full contact information; the new "Symptoms and Warning Signs" and "Pharmaceutical List" appendixes; and a comprehensive subject index.

The Editors and Contributors

The contributors to this work are academicians from a variety of disciplines in the life sciences, as well as health care professionals and faculty members at medical teaching institutions; their names, degrees, and affiliations are listed in the front matter to volume 1. We thank them for generously sharing their expertise. Special acknowledgment is extended to the panel of Medical Consultants for *Magill's Medical Guide, Fourth Revised Edition*: Anne Lynn S. Chang, M.D., from Stanford University; H. Bradford Hawley, M.D., from Wright State University; Laurence M. Katz, M.D., from the University of North Carolina, Chapel Hill; Nancy A. Piotrowski, Ph.D., from the University of California, Berkeley; and Connie Rizzo, M.D., Ph.D., from Columbia University. Their efforts ensured a thorough revision.

Salem Health Database

Activating online access to Salem Health is easy. Every purchaser of *Magill's Medical Guide* should determine an Administrator to manage access to the database. This person can easily activate Salem Health and manage its use within a library or school. Volume 1 of every set of *Magill's Medical Guide* includes an Activation Number attached to the inside back cover. This number is used to activate your Salem Health online account. The Activation Number is unique to each printed set and can be used by only one school, college, or library.

Purchasers of the set should go to www.health.salempress.com and click on the "Salem Health Activation" button there. Doing so will take the Administrator first to a simple registration page and then to an activation area where the Activation Number is input. Once this is done, the Administrator will provide information about his or her library so that all the Internet-connected computers in the institution will have access to the database.

For help with this process, please call (800) 221-1592 and our Customer Service department will assist you.

Contents

List of Contributors

Richard Adler, Ph.D.
University of Michigan—Dearborn

E. Victor Adlin, M.D.
Temple University School of Medicine

Patricia A. Ainsa, M.P.H., Ph.D.
University of Texas, El Paso

Saeed Akhter, M.D.
Texas Technological University Health Science Center

Bruce Ambuel, Ph.D.
Medical College of Wisconsin

John J. B. Anderson, Ph.D.
University of North Carolina, Chapel Hill

Earl R. Andresen, Ph.D.
University of Texas, Arlington

Walter Appleton
Grosse Pointe Woods, Michigan

Michele Arduengo, Ph.D.
Milton, Wisconsin

Bryan C. Auday, Ph.D.
Gordon College

Gloria Reyes Báez, M.D.
University of Puerto Rico School of Medicine

Pamela J. Baker, Ph.D.
Bates College

Anita Baker-Blocker, M.P.H., Ph.D.
Ann Arbor, Michigan

Iona C. Baldridge
Lubbock Christian University

Veronica N. Baptista, M.D.
Stanford Medical Group

Lawrence W. Bassett, M.D.
University of California, Los Angeles, School of Medicine

Robert J. Baumann, M.D.
University of Kentucky

John A. Bavaro, Ed.D., R.N.
Slippery Rock University

Barbara C. Beattie
Sarasota, Florida

Tanja Bekhuis, Ph.D.
TCB Research

Paul F. Bell, Ph.D.
Heritage Valley Health System

Alvin K. Benson, Ph.D.
Utah Valley State College

Cynthia Breslin Beres
Glendale, California

Carol D. Berkowitz, M.D.
Harbor-UCLA Medical Center

Leonard Berkowitz, D.O.
South Nassau Communities Hospital

Milton Berman, Ph.D.
University of Rochester

Matthew Berria, Ph.D.
Weber State University

Silvia M. Berry, M.Sc., R.V.T.
Englewood Hospital and Medical Center, New Jersey

Massimo D. Bezoari, M.D.
Huntingdon College

Virginiae Blackmon
Fort Worth, Texas

Robert W. Block, M.D.
University of Oklahoma

Jane Blood-Siegfried, R.N., D.N.Sc., C.P.N.P.
Duke University School of Nursing

Paul R. Boehlke, Ph.D.
Wisconsin Lutheran College
Dr. Martin Luther College

Prodromos G. Borboroglu, M.D.
Navy Medical Center, San Diego

Wanda Bradshaw, R.N.C., M.S.N., N.N.P./P.N.P.
Duke University School of Nursing

Barbara Brennessel, Ph.D.
Wheaton College

Peter N. Bretan, M.D.
University of California Medical Center, San Francisco

Kenneth H. Brown, Ph.D.
Northwestern Oklahoma State University

Thomas L. Brown, Ph.D.
Wright State University School of Medicine

Mitzie L. Bryant, B.S.N., M.Ed.
St. Louis Board of Education

Faith Hickman Brynie, Ph.D.
Bigfork, Montana

Fred Buchstein
John Carrol University

Amy Webb Bull, D.S.N., A.P.N.
Tennessee State University School of Nursing

Michael A. Buratovich, Ph.D.
Spring Arbor University

Edmund C. Burke, M.D.
University of California Medical Center, San Francisco

John T. Burns, Ph.D.
Bethany College

Rosslynn S. Byous, D.P.A., PA-C
University of Southern California, Keck School of Medicine

Jeffrey R. Bytomski, D.O.
Duke University Medical Center

Lauren M. Cagen, Ph.D.
University of Tennessee, Memphis

James J. Campanella, Ph.D.
Montclair State University

Edmund J. Campion, Ph.D.
University of Tennessee

Louis A. Cancellaro, M.D.
Veterans Affairs Medical Center, Mountain Home, Tennessee

Byron D. Cannon, Ph.D.
University of Utah

Mary Allen Carey, Ph.D.
University of Oklahoma

Culley C. Carson III, M.D.
University of North Carolina School of Medicine

Anne Lynn S. Chang, M.D.
Stanford University

Karen Chapman-Novakofski, R.D., L.D., Ph.D.
University of Illinois

Kathleen A. Chara, M.S.
Roseville, Minnesota

Paul J. Chara, Jr., Ph.D.
Northwestern College

Kerry L. Cheesman, Ph.D.
Capital University

Richard W. Cheney, Jr., Ph.D.
Christopher Newport University

David L. Chesemore, Ph.D.
California State University, Fresno

Francis P. Chinard, M.D.
New Jersey Medical School

Leland J. Chinn, Ph.D.
Biola University

David A. Clark, M.D.
Louisiana State University Medical School, New Orleans

Nancy Handshaw Clark, Ph.D.
American University of the Caribbean School of Medicine/ Kingston Hospital, Surrey, England

Julien M. Cobert
Duke University

Jaime S. Colomé, Ph.D.
California Polytechnic, San Luis Obispo

Arlene R. Courtney, Ph.D.
Western Oregon State College

Sarah Crawford, Ph.D.
Southern Connecticut State University

LeAnna DeAngelo, Ph.D.
Arizona State University

Roy L. DeHart, M.D., M.P.H.
University of Oklahoma

Patrick J. DeLuca, Ph.D.
Mount St. Mary College

Thomas E. DeWolfe, Ph.D.
Hampden-Sydney College

Shawkat Dhanani, M.D., M.P.H.
VA Greater Los Angeles Healthcare System

Kenneth Dill, M.D.
South Nassau Communities Hospital

Katherine Hoffman Doman
Greene County, Tennessee

Mark R. Doman, M.D.
Veterans Affairs Medical Center, Mountain Home, Tennessee

Cherie H. Dunphy, M.D.
University of North Carolina, Chapel Hill

Miriam Ehrenberg, Ph.D.
City University of New York, John Jay College

Ebrahim Elahi, M.D.
Mount Sinai School of Medicine

Benjamin Estrada, M.D.
University of South Alabama

C. Richard Falcon
Roberts and Raymond Associates, Philadelphia

L. Fleming Fallon, Jr., M.D., Ph.D., M.P.H.
Bowling Green State University

Meika A. Fang, M.D.
Veterans Affairs Medical Center, West Los Angeles

Phillip A. Farber, Ph.D.
Bloomsburg University

Frank J. Fedel
Henry Ford Hospital, Detroit

Mary C. Fields, M.D.
Collin County Community College

K. Thomas Finley, Ph.D.
State University of New York, Brockport

Kimberly Y. Z. Forrest, Ph.D.
Slippery Rock University of Pennsylvania

Ronald B. France, Ph.D.
LDS Hospital, Salt Lake City

Katherine B. Frederich, Ph.D.
Eastern Nazarene College

Paul Freudigman, Jr., M.D.
Pennsylvania State University, Hershey Medical Center

Paul J. Frisch
Nanuet, New York

Frances García, M.D.
Universidad Central del Caribe School of Medicine

Keith Garebian, Ph.D.
Mississauga, Ontario

Jason Georges
Glendale, California

Soraya Ghayourmanesh, Ph.D.
City University of New York

Lenela Glass-Godwin, M.WS.
Texas A&M University
Auburn University

Wallace A. Gleason, Jr., M.D.
University of Texas, Houston

James S. Godde, Ph.D.
Monmouth College

Daniel G. Graetzer, Ph.D.
University of Montana

Hans G. Graetzer, Ph.D.
South Dakota State University

David A. Gremse, M.D.
University of South Alabama College of Medicine

Frank Guerra, M.D.
University of Colorado School of Medicine

Lonnie J. Guralnick, Ph.D.
Western Oregon State College

L. Kevin Hamberger, Ph.D.
Medical College of Wisconsin

Ronald C. Hamdy, M.D.
James H. Quillen College of Medicine

Robert J. Harmon, M.D.
University of Colorado School of Medicine

Linda Hart, M.S., M.A.
University of Wisconsin—Madison

Peter M. Hartmann, M.D.
York Hospital, Pennsylvania

Robin Hasslen, Ph.D.
St. Cloud State University

H. Bradford Hawley, M.D.
Wright State University

Robert M. Hawthorne, Jr., Ph.D.
Marlboro, Vermont

Carol A. Heintzelman, D.S.W.
Millersville University of Pennsylvania

Peter B. Heller, Ph.D.
Manhattan College

Diane Andrews Henningfeld, Ph.D.
Adrian College

Martha M. Henze, M.S., R.D.
Boulder Community Hospital, Colorado

Jane F. Hill, Ph.D.
Bethesda, Maryland

Carl W. Hoagstrom, Ph.D.
Ohio Northern University

David Wason Hollar, Jr., Ph.D.
Rockingham Community College

Carol A. Holloway
Grosse Point Woods, Michigan

Ryan C. Horst
Eastern Mennonite University

Howard L. Hosick, Ph.D.
Washington State University

Katherine H. Houp, Ph.D.
Midway College

Shih-Wen Huang, M.D.
University of Florida

Jason A. Hubbart, M.S.
University of Idaho, Moscow

Larry Hudgins, M.D.
Veterans Affairs Medical Center, Mountain Home, Tennessee

Mary Hurd
East Tennessee State University

Tracy Irons-Georges
Glendale, California

Vicki J. Isola, Ph.D.
Hope College

Louis B. Jacques, M.D.
Wayne State University School of Medicine

Thomas C. Jefferson, M.D.
University of Arkansas for Medical Sciences

Albert C. Jensen, M.S.
Central Florida Community College

Karen E. Kalumuck, Ph.D.
The Exploratorium, San Francisco

Ahmad Kamal, M.D.
Stanford University Medical School

Susan J. Karcher, Ph.D.
Purdue University

Armand M. Karow, Ph.D.
Xytex Corporation

Laurence Katz, M.D.
University of North Carolina, Chapel Hill

Mara Kelly-Zukowski, Ph.D.
Felician College

Michael R. King, Ph.D.
University of Rochester

Cassandra Kircher, Ph.D.
Elon University

Vernon N. Kisling, Jr., Ph.D.
University of Florida

Samuel V. A. Kisseadoo, Ph.D.
Hampton University

Hillar Klandorf, Ph.D.
West Virginia University

Robert T. Klose, Ph.D.
University College of Bangor

Jeffrey A. Knight, Ph.D.
Mount Holyoke College

Steven A. Kuhl, Ph.D.
Lander University

David J. Ladouceur, Ph.D.
University of Notre Dame

Nicholas Lanzieri
Pace University
New York University

Victor R. Lavis, M.D.
University of Texas, Houston

David M. Lawrence
J. Sargeant Reynolds Community College

Charles T. Leonard, Ph.D., P.T.
University of Montana

Lorraine Lica, Ph.D.
San Diego, California

Stan Liu, M.D.
University of California, Los Angeles, School of Medicine

Martha Oehmke Loustaunau, Ph.D.
New Mexico State University

Eric v. d. Luft, Ph.D., M.L.S.
SUNY, Upstate Medical University

Courtney H. Lyder, M.D.
Yale University School of Nursing

Maura S. McAuliffe
Austin, Texas

Nancy E. Macdonald, Ph.D.
University of South Carolina, Sumter

Jeffrey A. McGowan
West Virginia University

Mary Beth McGranaghan
Chestnut Hill College

James P. McKenna, M.D.
Heritage Valley Health System

Wayne R. McKinny, M.D.
University of Hawaii School of Medicine

Janet Mahoney, R.N., Ph.D., A.P.R.N.
Monmouth University

Laura Gray Malloy, Ph.D.
Bates College

Nancy Farm Mannikko, Ph.D.
National Park Service

Debra Ellen Margolis, D.O.
St. Joseph's Hospital and Medical Center, Paterson, New Jersey

Bonita L. Marks, Ph.D.
University of North Carolina, Chapel Hill

Charles C. Marsh, Pharm.D.
University of Arkansas for Medical Sciences

Robert L. Martone
Wyeth Neuroscience

Karen A. Mattern
Visiting Nurse Association Home Health Services

Grace D. Matzen
Molloy College

Ralph R. Meyer, Ph.D.
University of Cincinnati

Robert D. Meyer, Ph.D.
Chestnut Hill College

Elva B. Miller, O.D.
Harrisonburg, Virginia

Roman J. Miller, Ph.D.
Eastern Mennonite College

Randall L. Milstein, Ph.D.
Oregon State University

Eli C. Minkoff, Ph.D.
Bates College

Paul Moglia, Ph.D.
South Nassau Communities Hospital

Robin Kamienny Montvilo, Ph.D.
Rhode Island College

Sharon Moore, M.D.
Veterans Affairs Medical Center, Mountain Home, Tennessee

George A. Morgan, Ph.D.
Colorado State University

Sheila J. Mosee, M.D.
Howard University

Rodney C. Mowbray, Ph.D.
University of Wisconsin, LaCrosse

William L. Muhlach, Ph.D.
Southern Illinois University

John Panos Najarian, Ph.D.
William Patterson College

Donald J. Nash, Ph.D.
Colorado State University

Victor H. Nassar, M.D.
Emory University

Mary A. Nastuk, Ph.D.
Wellesley College

Elizabeth Marie McGhee Nelson, Ph.D.
Christian Brothers University

Cindy Nesci, D.C.
East Pointe, Michigan

Bryan Ness, Ph.D.
Pacific Union College

Marsha M. Neumyer
Pennsylvania State University College of Medicine

William D. Niemi, Ph.D.
Russell Sage College

Jane C. Norman, R.N., Ph.D.
Tennessee State University

Kathleen O'Boyle
Wayne State University

Annette O'Connor, Ph.D.
La Salle University

Oladele A. Ogunseitan, Ph.D., M.P.H.
University of California, Irvine

Colm A. Ó'Moráin, M.A., M.D., M.Sc., D.Sc.
University of Dublin, Trinity College

Gwenelle S. O'Neal, D.S.W.
Rutgers University

J. Timothy O'Neill, Ph.D.
Uniformed Services University of the Health Sciences

Oliver Oyama, Ph.D.
Duke/Fayetteville Area Health Education Center

Maria Pacheco, Ph.D.
Buffalo State College

Robert J. Paradowski, Ph.D.
Rochester Institute of Technology

Gowri Parameswaran
Southwest Missouri State University

RoseMarie Pasmantier, M.D.
State University of New York Health Science Center, Brooklyn

Paul M. Paulman, M.D.
University of Nebraska Medical Center

Cheryl Pawlowski, Ph.D.
University of Northern Colorado

Joseph G. Pelliccia, Ph.D.
Bates College

Fortunato Perez-Benavides, M.D.
Texas Tech University

Carol Moore Pfaffly, Ph.D.
Fort Collins Family Medicine Center

Kenneth A. Pidcock, Ph.D.
Wilkes University

Heather E. Pierce, L.S.W.
Unison Behavioral Health Group, Toledo, Ohio

Linda L. Pierce, Ph.D, R.N.
Medical College of Ohio

Scott W. Pierce, L.S.W.
Firelands Counseling and Recovery Services, Sandusky, Ohio

Nancy A. Piotrowski, Ph.D.
University of California, Berkeley

George R. Plitnik, Ph.D.
Frostburg State University

Darleen Powars, M.D.
Los Angeles County-USC Medical Center

Frank J. Prerost, Ph.D.
Midwestern University

Layne A. Prest, Ph.D.
University of Nebraska Medical Center

Victoria Price, Ph.D.
Lamar University

Rashmi Ramasubbaiah, M.D.
Western Kentucky University

Lillian M. Range, Ph.D.
University of Southern Mississippi

Dandamudi V. Rao, Ph.D.
University of Medicine and Dentistry of New Jersey

C. Mervyn Rasmussen, M.D.
Bremerton Naval Hospital, Washington

Diane C. Rein, Ph.D., M.L.S.
Purdue University

Douglas Reinhart, M.D.
University of Utah

Wendy E. S. Repovich, Ph.D.
Eastern Washington University

Peter D. Reuman, M.D., M.P.H.
University of Florida

Betty Richardson, Ph.D.
Southern Illinois University, Edwardsville

John L. Rittenhouse
Eastern Mennonite College

Connie Rizzo, M.D., Ph.D.
Columbia University

Jeffrey B. Roberts, M.D.
Duke University Medical Center

Larry M. Roberts, J.D.
Pasadena, California

James L. Robinson, Ph.D.
University of Illinois, Urbana-Champaign

Hilda Velez Rodriguez, M.S.
San Juan, Puerto Rico

Charles W. Rogers, Ph.D.
Southwestern Oklahoma State University

Eugene J. Rogers, M.D.
Chicago Medical School

John Alan Ross, Ph.D.
Eastern Washington University

Lynne T. Roy
Cedars-Sinai Medical Center, Los Angeles

Irene Struthers Rush
Boise, Idaho

Virginia L. Salmon
Northeast State Community College

Susan L. Sandel, Ph.D.
MidState Behavioral Health System

Robert Sandlin, Ph.D.
San Diego State University

Alexander Sandra, M.D.
University of Iowa, Carver College of Medicine

Tulsi B. Saral, Ph.D.
University of Houston, Clear Lake

Lisa M. Sardinia, Ph.D.
Pacific University

David K. Saunders, Ph.D.
Emporia State University

Elaine M. Schaefer, D.O.
South Nassau Communities Hospital

Elizabeth D. Schafer, Ph.D.
Loachapoka, Alabama

Rosemary Scheirer, Ed.D.
Chestnut Hill College

Steven A. Schonefeld, Ph.D.
Tri-State University

Kathleen Schongar, M.S., M.A.
The May School

John Richard Schrock, Ph.D.
Emporia State University

Jay D. Schvaneveldt, Ph.D.
Utah State University

Jason J. Schwartz, Ph.D., J.D.
Los Angeles, California

Miriam E. Schwartz, M.D., M.A., Ph.D.
University of California, Los Angeles

Rebecca Lovell Scott, Ph.D., PA-C
Sandwich, Massachusetts

Rose Secrest
Chattanooga, Tennessee

John J. Seidl, M.D.
Medical College of Wisconsin

Gregory B. Seymann, M.D.
University of California, San Diego School of Medicine

Frank E. Shafer, M.D.
Allegheny University of the Health Sciences

Christopher D. Sharp, M.D.
Stanford University School of Medicine

John M. Shaw
Education Systems

Martha Sherwood-Pike, Ph.D.
University of Oregon

George C. Shields, Ph.D.
Lake Forest College

R. Baird Shuman, Ph.D.
University of Illinois, Urbana-Champaign

Mel Siegel, M.A.
Fordham University

Sanford S. Singer, Ph.D.
University of Dayton

Virginia Slaughter, Ph.D.
University of Queensland, Australia

Jane A. Slezak, Ph.D.
Fulton Montgomery Community College

Julie M. Slocum, R.N., M.S., C.D.E.
Women and Infants' Hospital
Brown University School of Medicine

Genevieve Slomski, Ph.D.
New Britain, Connecticut

Caroline M. Small
Silver Spring, Maryland

Dwight G. Smith, Ph.D.
Southern Connecticut State University

H. David Smith, Ph.D.
University of Michigan

Jane Marie Smith
Butler County Community College

Roger Smith, Ph.D.
Linfield College

Lisa Levin Sobczak, R.N.C.
Santa Barbara, California

Angela Spano
Huntingdon College

Sharon W. Stark, R.N., A.P.R.N., D.N.Sc.
Monmouth University

William D. Stark, D.D.S.
Monrovia, California

Toby R. Stewart, Ph.D.
University of Nebraska Medical Center, Omaha

Glenn Ellen Starr Stilling, M.A., M.L.S.
Appalachian State University

James R. Stubbs, M.D.
University of South Alabama

Wendy L. Stuhldreher, Ph.D, R.D.
Slippery Rock University

Giri Sulur, Ph.D.
University of California, Los Angeles

Pavel Svilenov
Wisconsin Lutheran College

Steven R. Talbot, R.V.T.
University of Utah Vascular Laboratory

Sue Tarjan
Santa Cruz, California

Billie M. Taylor, M.S.E., M.L.S.
Arkadelphia, Arkansas

William F. Taylor
Detroit, Michigan

Gerald T. Terlep, Ph.D.
Wayne State University

Susan E. Thomas, M.L.S.
Indiana University South Bend

Roberta Tierney, M.S.N., J.D., A.P.N.
Indiana University
Purdue University

Venkat Raghavan Tirumala, M.D., M.H.A.
Western Kentucky University

Leslie V. Tischauser, Ph.D.
Prairie State College

Winona Tse, M.D.
Mount Sinai School of Medicine

Mary S. Tyler, Ph.D.
University of Maine

John V. Urbas, Ph.D.
Kennesaw State College

Maxine M. Urton, Ph.D.
Xavier University

Anju Varanasi, M.D.
South Nassau Communities Hospital

Charles L. Vigue, Ph.D.
University of New Haven

James Waddell, Ph.D.
University of Minnesota

Peter J. Waddell, Ph.D.
University of South Carolina

Anthony J. Wagner, Ph.D.
Medical University of South Carolina

Edith K. Wallace, Ph.D.
Heartland Community College

Peter J. Walsh, Ph.D.
Fairleigh Dickinson University

Marc H. Walters, M.D.
Portland Community College

Annita Marie Ward, Ed.D.
Salem-Teikyo University

John F. Ward, M.D.
Navy Medical Center, San Diego

Marcia Watson-Whitmyre, Ph.D.
University of Delaware

Marcia J. Weiss, M.A., J.D.
Point Park College

Barry A. Weissman, O.D., Ph.D.
University of California, Los Angeles, School of Medicine

David J. Wells, Jr., Ph.D.
University of South Alabama Medical Center

Mark Wengrovitz, M.D.
Pennsylvania State University, Hershey Medical Center

Lee Williams
New York City, New York

Russell Williams, M.S.W.
University of Arkansas for Medical Sciences

Bradley R. A. Wilson, Ph.D.
University of Cincinnati

Michael Windelspecht, Ph.D.
Appalachian State University

Stephen L. Wolfe, Ph.D.
University of California, Davis

Bonnie L. Wolff
Pacific Coast Cardiac and Vascular Surgeons

Paul Y. K. Wu, M.D.
University of Southern California

Daniel L. Yazak, D.E.D.
Montana State University, Billings

Kathleen Zanolli, Ph.D.
University of Kansas

W. Michael Zawada, Ph.D.
University of Colorado Health Sciences Center

Ming Y. Zheng, Ph.D.
Gordon College

Nillofur Zobairi, Ph.D.
Southern Illinois University

Complete List of Contents

Volume 1

VOLUME 2

Volume 3

Volume 4

VOLUME 5

MAGILL'S
MEDICAL GUIDE

Abdomen

Anatomy

Anatomy or system affected: Bladder, gastrointestinal system, intestines, kidneys, liver, reproductive system, stomach, urinary system, uterus

Specialties and related fields: Gastroenterology, gynecology, internal medicine, nephrology, urology

Definition: The cavity in the central portion of the trunk that contains the vital organs most closely associated with the digestive process and the elimination of waste material.

Key terms:

chyme: the semiliquid state of foods that have gone through the first stage of digestion in the stomach

Kupffer cells: specialized cells in the liver that perform the function of removing bacterial debris from the blood that has circulated throughout the body

urea: the major waste product produced in the kidneys that, when gathered in sufficient quantity and liquefied, flows into the bladder for elimination as urine

Structure and Functions

The abdomen is the portion of the body's trunk that begins immediately below the diaphragm, which is the main respiratory muscle in the chest cavity, and extends to the lower pelvic region. The abdominal area is defined by a muscular wall made up of fatty tissue and skin, which determines the general shape of the body from the chest to the lower pelvis. The entire abdominal cavity is lined by a membrane called the peritoneum. This membrane encloses the essential organs of the abdomen: the stomach, small and large intestines, liver, gallbladder, bladder, pancreas, and kidneys. In females, the abdominal casing also contains the uterus, ovaries, and Fallopian tubes. At the front of the abdomen is the navel, essentially a scar which forms following the cutting of the umbilical cord after birth.

Any overview of the abdomen requires a composite view of the functions performed by each of the organs contained in it. With the exception of the female reproductive organs, all the organs contained in the abdominal cavity serve in one way or another in the process of food digestion, the transfer of diverse essential food byproducts to the rest of the body, and the disposal of waste products via the urinary tract and the anal passage.

The esophagus is the tube through which all solid and liquid foods enter the stomach, which is the topmost organ in the abdominal cavity. Because it is essentially a bag, the stomach can assume different shapes and adjust in size to accommodate different volumes of food that reach it through the esophagus. In adult humans, the average capacity of the stomach is about one quart. The essential digestive function of the stomach is to convert foods from their original states to a general semiliquid state referred to as chyme.

This first stage of digestion is carried out by the chemical action of some thirty-five thousand gastric glands which make up the inner folds of the inner layer of the stomach, the gastric mucosa. As the gastric glands actively secrete gastric juice, the second layer of the stomach wall, which is muscle tissue, contracts and expands, providing the physical movement that is necessary for the gastric juice and food material to come into full contact.

Gastric juice actually begins to flow from the inner lining of the stomach even before food is present. This may occur when one smells food or even when one imagines the flavor of food. Among the component parts of gastric juice are the enzymes pepsin and rennin, hydrochloric acid, and mucus, which protects the lining of the stomach from the effects of high acidity. Pepsin and rennin begin to break down different types of proteins when an optimum acid environment (a pH between 1 and 3) exists.

Once the initial stage of digestion has occurred, food passes from the stomach into the upper portion of the small intestine, or duodenum, via the pyloric sphincter. This passageway will not allow food to enter the small intestine until it is suitably modified by the action of the stomach.

In the small and large intestines, partially broken-down food is reduced further by the action of gastric juices that are either secreted into the intestines from other abdominal organs (the pancreas and liver, most notably) or secreted by the mucous membranes of the intestines themselves. It is in the small intestine that most of the breaking-down digestive work of gastric juices takes place. Food particles reach a certain level of decomposition so that they may be absorbed into the bloodstream through the mucous membranes of the intestine. The bulk of what is left is allowed to pass, through a gatelike passageway called the cecum, from the small to the large intestine, or colon.

The function of the colon and the component juices that it contains is to separate out the three essential components that remain following the absorptive work of the small intestine: water, undigested foodstuff, and bacteria. Most of the water passes back into the body through the walls of the colon, while undigested food and bacteria are propelled farther down the gastrointestinal tract for eventual elimination as feces.

The importance of other organs in the abdomen—the liver, kidneys, pancreas, gallbladder, and bladder—is as complex as that of the intestines and in several cases goes beyond the basic function of digestion. Closest to the stomach and the digestive process itself, perhaps, is the action of the pancreas. The pancreas is the glandular organ located directly beneath the stomach. It is connected to the duodenum, to which it provides pancreatic juice containing three digestive enzymes: trypsin, amylase, and lipase. These agents join the secretions of the small intestine, as well as bile flowing from the liver, to complete the digestive process that breaks down proteins, carbohydrates, and fats. They can then be absorbed through the walls of the intestine for the general nourishment of the body. In addition to its role in the digestive process, the pancreas possesses endocrine cells, called the islets of Langerhans, that secrete two hormones, insulin and glucagon, directly into the bloodstream. These two hormones work together to influence the level of sugar in the blood. When the insulin-secreting cells of the pancreas fail to function effectively, then diabetes mellitus may result.

Like the pancreas, the liver, which is the largest glandular organ of the body, shares in the digestive process by producing bile, a fluid essential for the emulsification of fats passing through the small intestine. Bile salts, as they are called, are stored in the gallbladder until they are released into the small intestine. This contribution to the digestive process, however, represents only a minimal part of the liver's functions, many of which have vital effects on body functions far beyond the abdominal cavity. Because blood filled with oxygen flows into the liver from the aorta through the hepatic artery, on one hand, and blood containing digested food enters the liver from the small intestine via the portal vein, on the other, the relationship between "harmonizing" liver functions and the content of the blood is absolutely critical.

The metabolic cells that make up liver tissue, known as hepatic cells, are highly specialized. According to their specialized function, the hepatic cells in the four unequal-sized lobes of the liver may affect several factors: the amount of glycogen (converted and stored glucose) that should be reconverted to glucose and passed (for added energy) into the bloodstream; the conversion of excess carbohydrates and protein into fat; the

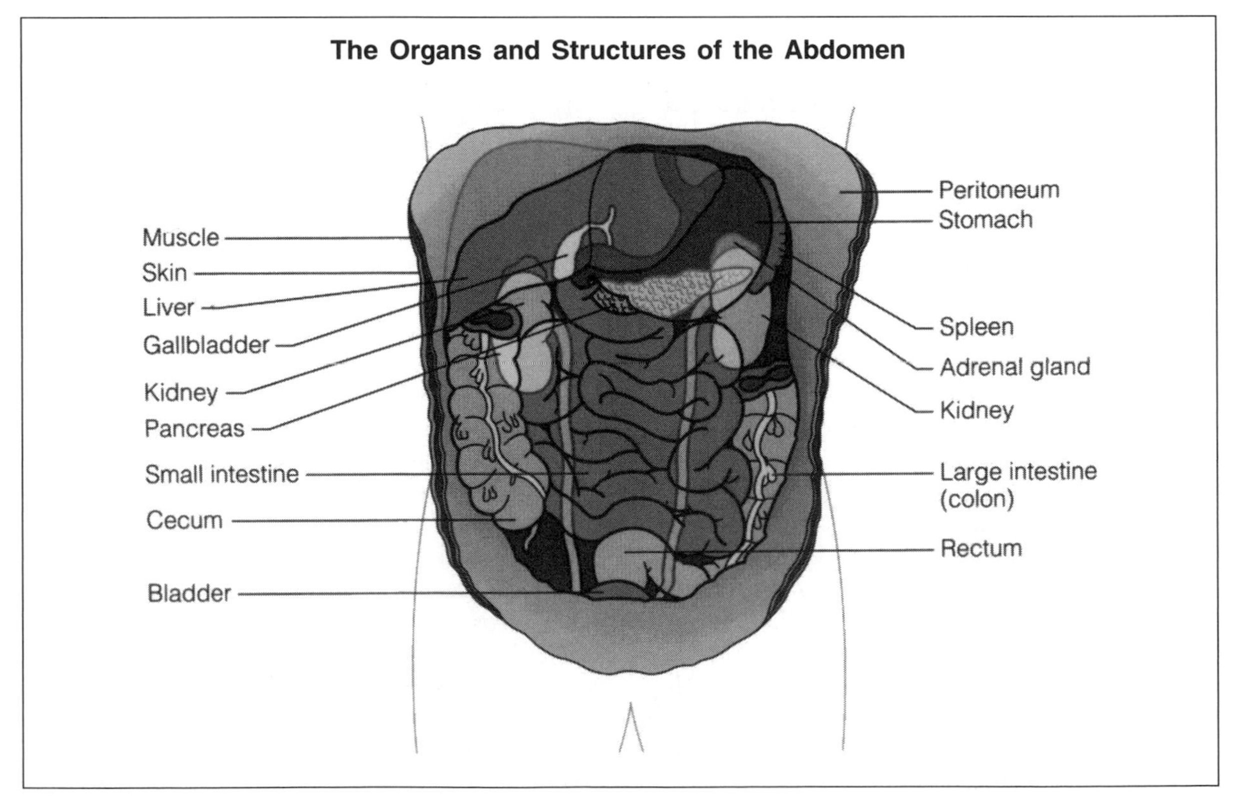

Abdominal organs and structures are those located between the rib cage and the pelvic bone.

counteraction of the harmful ammonia by-product of protein breakdown by the production of urea; the production of several essential components of blood, including plasma proteins and blood-clotting agents; the storing of key vitamins and minerals such as vitamins A, D, K, and B_{12}; and the removal of bacteria and other debris that collect in the blood itself—a function of the phagocytic, or Kupffer, cells in particular.

It is the next pair of vital abdominal organs, the kidneys, that separates many of the waste products associated with the liver's metabolic functions, including urea and mineral salts, out of the blood and removes them from the body in the form of urine. This separation is performed by millions of tiny filtering agents called nephrons. Blood penetrates the interior of the kidney by way of an incoming arteriole that branches off from the main renal artery. After the filtering process has been completed, cleansed blood flows back into the main bloodstream via an outgoing arteriole and a system of blood vessels leading to the main renal vein. Waste materials remain, after filtering, in a tube-like extension of each nephron until they can be concentrated, in the form of urine, in a chamber in the middle of the kidney, the kidney pelvis. From this chamber, urine is propelled by muscular compression through the ureter tubes leading to the bladder, the last organ (in males) contained within the lower abdominal cavity. In addition to removing waste products from the blood, the kidneys can adjust the level in the blood of other substances, such as sodium, potassium, and calcium, that are needed by the body but that may exist in excess at certain times. Because the two kidneys perform exactly the same functions, it is possible for the organism to survive as long as one of the two is healthy.

Although obviously essential for temporary storage of urine and final elimination of liquid waste through the process of urination, the bladder is the least complicated organ in the abdominal cavity. The bladder is essentially a sac with a liquid capacity of about one pint. Its functions are governed by varied tension in, and loosening of, muscles in the walls of the sac and the external sphincter. When the pressure of collected urine reaches a certain point, nervous impulses cause the external sphincter to relax. Urine flow out of the bladder into the urethra tube can be controlled, up to a certain point, in humans and most mammals by conscious thought.

DISORDERS AND DISEASES

Given the concentration in the abdomen of vital regulatory organs, much medical research has focused on the pathology of this area of the body. Although there are a number of specific diseases that attack individual abdominal organs, the entire region is vulnerable to cancerous tumors. Medical science has tended to associate cancers in certain abdominal organs with dietary habits that are either of recent origin (consumption of highly processed foodstuffs in industrialized Western societies, for example) or geographically or ethnically distinctive—the East Asian, specifically Japanese, vulnerability to certain types of stomach cancer, for example. The latter vulnerability may, however, also be tied to dietary or other environmental considerations that vary in different populated areas of the globe.

Although cancers may strike any of the vital abdominal organs, chances of successful surgical intervention to remove tumors vary greatly according to the location of the cancer. Liver cancer, for example, is essentially untreatable through surgery, while the treatment of cancer of the colon has a significant success rate. This variation is partially attributable to the fact that the vital processes performed by the intestines may not be seriously threatened when a portion of the organ is removed in cancer surgery.

The most important specific diseases associated with the abdomen include peritonitis, hepatitis, and diabetes. Among these diseases, diabetes has received the most attention, both for its widespread impact on all sectors of the population and for the amount of research that has gone into the task of finding a cure. Diabetes occurs when the pancreas fails to produce enough insulin to metabolize the sugar substance glucose. A breakdown in this function impairs proper cell nourishment and results in excessive sugar in the blood and urine. This state, referred to as hyperglycemia, can affect a number of body functions outside the abdominal cavity, leading, for example, to atherosclerosis and vascular degeneration in general. Because many diabetes patients must inject insulin into their bodies to counteract malfunctioning of the pancreas, an opposite, equally dangerous side effect, hyperinsulinism, may also occur. The most serious degenerative effect that menaces patients suffering from diabetes, however, occurs when the chemical and hormonal imbalance originating in the pancreas brings negative reactions to the kidneys, causing the latter to fail. Medical science has perfected various technical means for addressing this problem, most connected with the mechanical process called dialysis.

Hepatitis is an inflammation that attacks the liver. The two common forms are hepatitis A (formerly called infectious hepatitis) and hepatitis B (formerly called serum hepatitis). Both are transmitted as a result of unsanitary conditions, the first in food and water supplies and the second when unsterile hypodermic needles or infected blood come into contact with the victim's own bloodstream. Unlike most other diseases associated with the abdominal organs, hepatitis is extremely contagious. Hepatitis B can present dangers in using plasma supplied by donors, as there can be an incubation period from six weeks to six months before external signs of the disease occur.

Perhaps the most common abdominal disease, curable through the use of antibiotics if treated in time, is peritonitis. This is an acute inflammation of the peritoneum, the membrane that lines the entire abdominal cavity. It can occur as a result of direct bacterial invasion from outside the body or as a side effect of ruptures occurring in one of the organs contained in the abdomen. Peritonitis typically develops as a result of complications from appendicitis, bleeding ulcers, or a ruptured gallbladder.

Perspective and Prospects

The history of medical analysis of disorders of the abdominal area goes back as far as written history itself, ranging from simple indigestion and painful (and possibly fatal) gallstones to very serious and only recently understood diseases such as diabetes.

Perhaps the most noteworthy advancement in medical knowledge affecting the organs of the abdominal region has been the development of more sophisticated means to counteract the effects of kidney disorders. While there were some striking advances (but not full levels of success) in organ transplant surgery beginning in the 1970's, a technique called dialysis made remarkable strides. First used shortly after World War II as an effective but costly and physically limiting treatment, dialysis involves the use of a machine that receives blood pumped directly from the patient's heart and processes this blood in place of the kidney. This involves filtering out excretory products, adding essential components that "refresh" blood needs (such as heparin, to combat clotting, and proper amounts of saline fluid), and then returning the blood to resume its vital function within the circulatory system.

Although the essential principles of dialysis did not change drastically in the last quarter of the twentieth century, levels of efficiency in a process that had to be repeated over a ten-hour period several times a week definitely did. Development of much smaller, portable dialysis devices made it possible for patients to follow their doctors' instructions in carrying out their own treatment between hospital or office visits, thus lessening the chances of very dangerous crises at the outset of kidney failure.

The most notable hope for patients afflicted with kidney disorders is successful transplant from a healthy or recently deceased donor. By the early twenty-first century, transplants had also become foreseeable for those suffering from diseases that strike other organs in the abdominal cavity, especially the liver. Thus, healthy organ transplant technology can be said to represent one of the most important domains of future research, involving specialists of all the subsections of medicine relating to the abdominal cavity.

—*Byron D. Cannon, Ph.D.*

See also Abdominal disorders; Adrenalectomy; Amniocentesis; Anatomy; Appendectomy; Appendicitis; Bariatric surgery; Bladder removal; Bypass surgery; Cesarean section; Cholecystectomy; Colitis; Colon and rectal polyp removal; Colon and rectal surgery; Colon cancer; Colon therapy; Colonoscopy and sigmoidoscopy; Constipation; Crohn's disease; Dialysis; Diarrhea and dysentery; Digestion; Diverticulitis and diverticulosis; Endoscopy; Enemas; Fistula repair; Gallbladder diseases; Gastrectomy; Gastroenterology; Gastroenterology, pediatric; Gastrointestinal disorders; Gastrointestinal system; Gastrostomy; Hernia; Hernia repair; Ileostomy and colostomy; Incontinence; Indigestion; Internal medicine; Intestinal disorders; Intestines; Irritable bowel syndrome (IBS); Kidney transplantation; Kidneys; Laparoscopy; Liposuction; Lithotripsy; Liver; Liver transplantation; Nephrectomy; Nephritis; Nephrology; Nephrology, pediatric; Obstruction; Pancreas; Pancreatitis; Peristalsis; Peritonitis; Pregnancy and gestation; Prostate gland; Reproductive system; Roundworms; Splenectomy; Sterilization; Stomach, intestinal, and pancreatic cancers; Stone removal; Stones; Tubal ligation; Ultrasonography; Urethritis; Urinary disorders; Urinary system; Urology; Urology, pediatric; Worms.

For Further Information:

Bernard, Claude. *Memoir on the Pancreas and on the Role of Pancreatic Juice in Digestive Processes.* Translated by John Henderon. New York: Academic Press, 1985. An English translation of a classic mid-nineteenth century study, published by a physiologist concerned with the main organs of the abdominal cavity. Illustrated.

De Wardener, H. E. *The Kidney: An Outline of Normal and Abnormal Function*. 5th ed. New York: Churchill Livingstone, 1985. Although this text on the functions and pathology of the kidney predates the impressive advances made in kidney transplant techniques, it is extremely comprehensive and comprehensible for the general, educated reader.

Feldman, Mark, Lawrence S. Friedman, and Lawrence J. Brandt, eds. *Sleisenger and Fordtran's Gastrointestinal and Liver Disease: Pathophysiology, Diagnosis, Management*. 8th ed. 2 vols. Philadelphia: W. B. Saunders, 2006. A comprehensive textbook of gastrointestinal diseases and physiology. Contains excellent chapters on abdominal disorders.

Marieb, Elaine N. *Essentials of Human Anatomy and Physiology*. 8th ed. San Francisco: Pearson/Benjamin Cummings, 2006. This introductory anatomy and physiology textbook, easily accessible to those with little science background, is richly illustrated with diagrams and photographs, which help to illuminate body systems and processes.

Palmer, Melissa. *Dr. Melissa Palmer's Guide to Hepatitis and Liver Disease*. Garden City Park, N.Y.: Avery, 2000. Palmer, a nationally recognized hepatologist, divides her text into four units: "The Basics," "Understanding and Treating Viral Hepatitis," "Understanding and Treating Other Liver Diseases," and "Treatment Options and Lifestyle Changes."

Ronco, Claudio, and Rinaldo Bellomo, eds. *Critical Care Nephrology*. Boston: Kluwer Academic, 1998. This text provides an overview of the treatment of critically ill patients with renal failure and multiple organ dysfunction syndrome.

Tortora, Gerard J., and Bryan Derrickson. *Principles of Anatomy and Physiology*. 11th ed. Hoboken, N.J.: John Wiley & Sons, 2006. An outstanding textbook of human anatomy and physiology.

Abdominal disorders

Disease/disorder

Anatomy or system affected: Abdomen, bladder, gastrointestinal system, intestines, kidneys, liver, stomach, urinary system

Specialties and related fields: Emergency medicine, family medicine, gastroenterology, internal medicine

Definition: Disorders affecting the wide range of organs found in the torso of the body, including diseases of the stomach, intestines, liver, and pancreas.

Key terms:

gastrointestinal: referring to the small and large intestines

pathogen: any microorganism that can cause infectious disease, such as bacteria, viruses, fungi, or other parasites

peritoneum: a membrane enclosing most of the organs in the abdomen

Causes and Symptoms

The main trunk, or torso, of the body includes three major structures: the chest cavity, contained within the ribs and housing the lungs and heart; the abdomen, containing the stomach, kidneys, liver, spleen, pancreas, and intestines; and the pelvic cavity, housing the sexual organs, organs of elimination, and related structures.

The abdomen is, for the most part, contained within a membrane called the peritoneum. The stomach lies immediately below the chest cavity and connects directly with the small intestine, a long tube. It fills the bulk of the abdominal cavity, winding around and down to the pelvic bones in the hips. The small intestine then connects to the large intestine, which extends upward and crosses the abdomen just below the stomach and then turns down to connect with the rectum. Other vital organs within the abdominal cavity include the liver, kidneys, spleen, pancreas, and adrenal glands. All these structures are subject to infection by viruses, bacteria, and other infective agents; to cancer; and to a wide range of conditions specific to individual organs and systems.

Diseases in the abdominal cavity are usually signaled by pain. Identifying the exact cause of abdominal pain is one of the most difficult and important tasks that the physician faces. The familiar stomachache may be simple indigestion, or it may be caused by spoiled, toxic foods or by infection, inflammation, cancer, obstruction, or tissue erosion, among other causes. It may arise in the stomach, the intestines, or other organs contained within the abdominal cavity. In addition, pain felt in the abdomen may be referred from other sources outside the abdominal cavity. A good example would be a heart attack, which arises in the chest cavity but is often felt by the patient as indigestion. Another example is the abdominal cramping that is often associated with menstruation and premenstrual syndrome (PMS). Because abdominal pain could mean that the patient is in great danger, the physician must decide quickly what is causing the pain and what to do about it.

Information on Abdominal Disorders

Causes: Appendicitis, cancer, cirrhosis, colitis, constipation, Crohn's disease, diabetes mellitus, diverticulitis, food poisoning, gastritis, gastroenteritis, hepatitis, obstruction, pancreatitis, peritonitis, stones, ulcers, etc.
Symptoms: Pain
Duration: Acute or chronic
Treatments: Lifestyle changes, acid-neutralizing drugs, surgery

By far the most common cause of stomach pain is indigestion, but this term is so broad as to be almost meaningless. Indigestion can be brought on by eating too much, eating the wrong foods or tainted foods, alcohol, smoking, poisons, infection, certain medications such as aspirin, and a host of other causes. It may be merely an annoyance, or it may indicate a more serious condition, such as gastritis, gastroenteritis, ulcers, or cancer.

The stomach contains powerful chemicals to help digest foods. These include hydrochloric acid and chemicals called pepsins (digestive enzymes). In order to protect itself from being digested, the stomach mounts a defense system that allows the chemical modification of foods while keeping acid and pepsin away from the stomach walls. In certain people, however, the defense mechanisms break down and bring the corrosive stomach chemicals into direct contact with the stomach walls. The result can be irritation of the stomach lining, called gastritis. Gastritis may progress to a peptic ulcer, identified as a gastric ulcer if the inflammation occurs in the stomach wall or a duodenal ulcer if it occurs in the wall of the duodenum, the first section of the small intestine. In most cases, the ulcer is limited to the surface of the tissue. In severe cases, the ulcer can perforate the entire wall and can be life-threatening.

A common cause of stomach pain is the medications used to treat arthritis and rheumatism. These drugs include aspirin and a group of related drugs called nonsteroidal anti-inflammatory drugs (NSAIDs). As part of their activity in reducing bone and joint inflammation and pain, they interfere with part of the stomach's network of self-protective devices and allow acids to attack stomach and duodenal walls.

Bacterial and viral infections often result in abdominal distress. Foods that sit too long unrefrigerated can be infected by bacteria, or they can become infected by pathogens on the hands of people who prepare and serve them. The bacteria release toxins into the food. Once eaten, these poisons can cause pain and diarrhea. This can be a mere annoyance, a debilitating illness, or a deadly infection, depending upon the organism involved. Salmonella and staphylococcus are two of the many bacteria that can cause food poisoning. *Clostridium botulinum* is occasionally found in canned or preserved foods. It is probably the most serious infective agent in food; victims often do not recover.

Bacterial and viral infections of the gastrointestinal tract are also common causes of abdominal disease. Viral gastroenteritis is the second most common disease in the United States (after upper respiratory tract infections) and a leading cause of death in infants and the elderly.

Appendicitis (inflammation of the appendix) is frequently seen. The appendix is a tiny organ at the end of the small intestine. It has no purpose in the physiology of modern humans, but occasionally it becomes infected. If the infection is not treated quickly, the appendix can burst and spread infection throughout the abdominal area, a condition that can be life-threatening.

Diarrhea, with or without accompanying abdominal pain, is a major symptom of gastrointestinal disease. It is commonly associated with bacterial or viral infection but may also be attributable to the antibiotics used to treat bacterial infections.

Other gastrointestinal diseases are peritonitis (inflammation of the membrane that covers the abdominal organs), diverticulitis, constipation, Crohn's disease, obstruction, colitis, and the various cancers that can afflict the gastrointestinal system, such as stomach and colon cancers.

The liver is the largest internal organ in the human body and perhaps the most complicated; it is subject to a wide range of disorders. It is the body's main chemical workshop and is responsible for a large number of activities that are vital to body function. The liver absorbs nutrients from the intestinal tract and metabolizes them, that is, modifies them so that they can be used by the cells. The liver introduces nutrients into the bloodstream, supplying it with the glucose, protein, and other substances that the body needs. The liver detoxifies the blood and allows poisons, drugs, and other harmful agents to be eliminated. The liver also manufactures and stores many important substances, such as vitamin A and cholesterol.

Chief among liver disorders are the various forms of

hepatitis and cirrhosis. Hepatitis can be caused by a viral infection, can be related to the use of alcohol or drugs, or can result from poisoning. There are many forms of viral hepatitis; the two most significant are hepatitis A and hepatitis B.

Hepatitis A is the most common form; it is caused by a virus that is transmitted through contaminated food or water. Hepatitis B is a blood-borne disease; that is, the virus is carried in the blood and other body fluids of the victim, such as semen and saliva. It can be transmitted only when infected body fluids are transferred from one person to another. The disease is commonly spread by sexual contact and bites, through the use of contaminated needles, and during surgical and dental procedures. Nurses and other staff members in health care facilities are constantly exposed to hepatitis B when taking and handling infected blood samples. Pregnant women who are infected can pass the disease on to their children.

Cirrhosis develops when the liver is damaged by some substance such as alcohol. Liver cells are destroyed, and as the liver attempts to regenerate, scar tissue is formed. The steady flow of blood through the organ is impeded, as are vital functions such as the removal of waste materials from the blood.

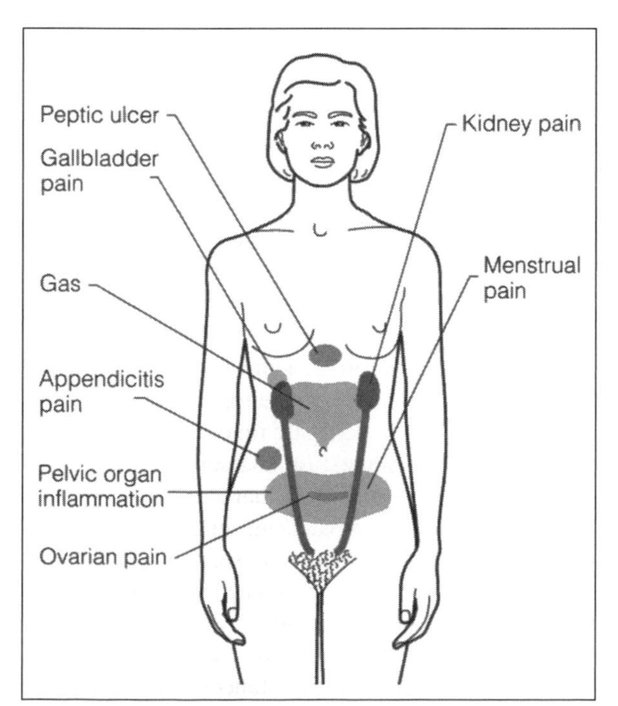

Abdominal disorders are many and varied; some common disorders and their sites are shown here.

The liver is also subject to a number of cancers. Cancer cells can spread to liver tissue from other parts of the body, or they can originate there as a result of hepatitis B or other chronic liver diseases such as cirrhosis.

The gallbladder is a small sac connected to the liver. The liver manufactures bile, a substance that aids in the digestion of fats. Bile is stored in the gallbladder and passes through the bile duct into the small intestine. A common disorder of the gallbladder is the formation of gallstones, crystalline growths that can be as fine as sand or as large as a golf ball. If the stones clog the passage to the bile duct, severe pain may result.

The pancreas, a vital gland situated near the liver, is subject to a number of disorders. The most prominent is diabetes mellitus, a condition in which the pancreas ceases to produce insulin or produces defective insulin. Pancreatitis is a disorder characterized by inflammation of the pancreas.

The other major organ system in the abdomen comprises the kidneys and the urinary tract. The system includes the two kidneys, which sit in the middle of the back on either side of the spine; the two ureters, which transport urine from the kidneys; the bladder, a pouchlike organ that collects the urine; and the urethra, which expels urine from the body. The kidneys and related organs are subject to several disorders, some inborn and some caused by infection, illnesses in other organs and systems, or cancer.

TREATMENT AND THERAPY

Many abdominal disorders are related to the overproduction of stomach acids, which damage the intestinal walls; the treatment of such conditions is often associated with changes in lifestyle. In treating gastrointestinal reflux disease, in which stomach acid backs up into the throat, physicians may suggest that the patient change habits that may be contributing to the condition, perhaps by stopping smoking, reducing the intake of alcohol, losing weight, and avoiding certain foods and medications. Preparations to neutralize stomach acids are used, as well as drugs that reduce the amount of stomach acid produced. Surgery is rarely indicated.

Hiatal hernia, the protrusion of part of the stomach through the diaphragm, usually produces no symptoms. There may be reflux of stomach acids into the esophagus, which can be treated by the same methods used in treating gastrointestinal reflux disease. Surgery is sometimes indicated.

Gastritis is commonly treated with agents that neutralize stomach acid or others that reduce the production of stomach acid. When gastritis appears to be caused by drugs taken for arthritis or rheumatism (for example, aspirin or NSAIDs), the physician may change the drug or the dosage to reduce stomach irritation.

In treating gastric and duodenal ulcers, the physician seeks to heal the ulcers and prevent their recurrence. Acid-neutralizing agents are sometimes helpful, but more often agents that reduce the flow of stomach acids are used. It has been suggested that gastritis and ulcers are associated with certain bacteria. Consequently, some physicians add an antibiotic to the antacid regimen in order to destroy the pathogens. Surgery is sometimes required to heal ulcers.

Bacterial infections in the gastrointestinal tract are, as a rule, self-limiting. They run their course, and the patient recovers. Sometimes, however, appropriate antibiotics are needed. For viral infections, few medications are useful in eradicating the pathogens.

Appendicitis is usually treated surgically. Peritonitis, whether resulting from appendicitis or from other gastrointestinal infection, is also treated surgically in order to remove infected tissue. In addition, antibiotic therapy is often used.

For two of the major liver diseases, hepatitis A and hepatitis B, there is no treatment once the person has become infected. For the most part, the diseases resolve without incident. Bed rest, dietary measures, and general support procedures are the only steps that can be taken. In a small percentage of patients, however, hepatitis B can progress to chronic active hepatitis, which may lead to liver failure, cirrhosis, liver cancer, and death. The main defense against hepatitis B is immunization. A vaccine is available and is recommended for all children and all adults who are at high risk. There is no treatment for cirrhosis, although physicians may be able to treat some of its complications.

Perspective and Prospects

Medical science has made great progress in the treatment of disorders arising in the abdominal cavity, but there is much to be done. Most important is the identification of agents to treat or immunize against various viral diseases, particularly those that occur in the gastrointestinal tract and the liver.

A vaccine against hepatitis A is being sought. The vaccine against hepatitis B has been in use for years, but the incidence of the disease has remained relatively constant. In the United States, the practice now is to vaccinate all young children. If this immunization approach is successful, the rate of hepatitis B infection among American children should drop.

New treatment modalities are being developed for many of the diseases that occur in the abdominal cavity. One of the most significant successes has been in the treatment of peptic ulcers. The new drugs being used not only neutralize acid in the stomach but also cut off the secretion of acid into the stomach. One of these agents was the most-prescribed drug in the world for many years, indicating the importance of this therapeutic approach.

Innovations are also occurring in the treatment of diabetes mellitus, the disease caused by malfunction in the pancreas. Medications have been found that promise to treat and prevent some of the potentially fatal diseases that diabetes can cause.

Because the abdominal area contains so many vital organ systems, it is the seat of perhaps the widest range of diseases that afflict the human body—and hence, the target for the greatest amount of research and, potentially, the greatest advances in medicine.

—C. Richard Falcon

See also Abdomen; Appendectomy; Appendicitis; Bladder cancer; Bladder removal; Cholecystectomy; Colitis; Colon and rectal polyp removal; Colon and rectal surgery; Colon cancer; Colon therapy; Colonoscopy and sigmoidoscopy; Constipation; Crohn's disease; Diabetes mellitus; Dialysis; Diarrhea and dysentery; Digestion; Diverticulitis and diverticulosis; Endoscopy; Gallbladder diseases; Gastroenterology; Gastroenterology, pediatric; Gastrointestinal disorders; Gastrointestinal system; Gastrostomy; Hernia; Hernia repair; Incontinence; Indigestion; Internal medicine; Intestinal disorders; Irritable bowel syndrome (IBS); Kidney cancer; Kidney transplantation; Kidneys; Laparoscopy; Lithotripsy; Liver; Liver transplantation; Nephrectomy; Nephritis; Nephrology; Nephrology, pediatric; Nonalcoholic steatohepatitis (NASH); Obstruction; Peristalsis; Peritonitis; Prostate cancer; Prostate enlargement; Shunts; Splenectomy; Stomach, intestinal, and pancreatic cancers; Stone removal; Stones; Ultrasonography; Urethritis; Urinary disorders; Urinary system; Urology; Urology, pediatric.

For Further Information:

Guillory, Gerard. *IBS: A Doctor's Plan for Chronic Digestive Disorders*. 3d ed. Point Roberts, Wash.: Hartley & Marks, 2001. Guillory includes both preventive and treatment recommendations for people suffering from chronic gastrointestinal problems, often referred to as irritable bowel syndrome.

Janowitz, Henry D. *Indigestion: Living Better with Upper Intestinal Problems from Heartburn to Ulcers and Gallstones*. New York: Oxford University Press, 1994. This book covers upper intestinal problems, such as heartburn, stomach disorders, ulcers, and gallstones. Designed for the lay reader.

Kapadia, Cyrus R., James M. Crawford, and Caroline Taylor. *An Atlas of Gastroenterology: A Guide to Diagnosis and Differential Diagnosis*. Boca Raton, Fla.: Parthenon, 2003. Provides a fully illustrated, nonspecialist understanding of myriad gastrointestinal diseases, including heartburn, dyspepsia, diarrhea, irritable bowel syndrome, and pancreatitis. Includes bibliographic references and index.

Litin, Scott C., ed. *Mayo Clinic Family Health Book*. 3d ed. New York: HarperResource, 2003. Diseases of the abdominal cavity are discussed in sections titled "Diseases and Disorders" and "Tests and Treatments."

ABORTION

PROCEDURE

ANATOMY OR SYSTEM AFFECTED: Reproductive system, uterus

SPECIALTIES AND RELATED FIELDS: Ethics, gynecology

DEFINITION: The induced termination of pregnancy, which usually is legal only before the fetus is viable.

KEY TERMS:

dilation: making something wider or larger

embryo: the unborn young from conception to about eight weeks

fetus: the unborn young from about eight weeks to birth

quickening: the point at which a fetus first begins to move in the uterus

uterus: a hollow, muscular organ located in the pelvic cavity of females, in which a fertilized egg develops

viability: the point at which a fetus is able to survive outside the uterus

THE CONTROVERSY SURROUNDING ABORTION

Abortion is the deliberate ending of a pregnancy before the fetus is viable, or capable of surviving outside a woman's body. It has been practiced in every culture since the beginning of civilization. It has also been controversial. The first law designating it as a crime dates to ancient Assyria, where, in the fourteenth century B.C.E., women who were convicted of abortion were impaled on a stake and left to die. Early Hebrew law also condemned abortion, except when necessary to save the woman's life. The Greeks allowed abortion, but the famous physician Hippocrates (c. 460-c. 370 B.C.E.) denounced the procedure and said that it violated a doctor's responsibility to heal. Roman law said that a fetus was part of a woman and that abortion was her decision, although a husband could divorce his wife if she had an abortion without his consent. Most abortions in ancient times seemed to be related to unwanted pregnancies.

The Christian church called abortion a sin in the first century. In the fifth century, however, Saint Augustine argued that the fetus did not have a soul before "quickening," that point during a pregnancy, usually between the fourth and sixth months, at which the woman first senses movement in her womb. Until 1869, abortion until quickening was legal in most areas of Europe. In that year, however, Pope Pius IX declared abortion at any point outright murder. This position has been upheld by all subsequent popes.

In Protestant countries, the principle of legality until quickening held true until around 1860. In that year, the British parliament declared abortion a felony; that law remained on the books for more than one hundred years. In 1968, the Abortion Act passed by Parliament radically reduced the restrictions, allowing abortions in cases in which doctors determined that the pregnancy threatened the physical or mental health of the woman.

In the United States, abortion before quickening was legal until the 1840's. By 1841, ten states had declared abortion to be a criminal act, but punishments were weak and the laws frequently ignored. The movement against abortion was led by the American Medical Association (AMA), founded in 1847. Doctors were becoming increasingly aware that the "first sign of life" took place well before the fetus actually moved. By this time, scientists had established that fetal development actually began with the union of sperm and egg. In 1859, the AMA passed a resolution condemning abortion as a criminal act. Within a few years, every state declared abortion a felony. Not until 1950 did the AMA reverse its position, when it began a new campaign to liberalize abortion laws. Many doctors were concerned about the thousands of women suffering from complications and even death from illegal abortions. Consequently, seventeen states, including California, passed laws providing for legal abortions under certain conditions. The remaining states, however, continued to prohibit abortions. In 1973, the Supreme Court of the United States ruled in *Roe v. Wade* that abortions in all states were generally legal. That ruling made abortions in the United States available on the request of the pregnant woman.

More than fifty countries, with about 25 percent of the world's population, continue to make abortions illegal. Most other nations authorize abortions under various conditions. The World Health Organization (WHO) estimates that more than 50 million abortions occur per year throughout the world and that about 20 million of these are illegal.

Before 1970, statistics on abortions in the United States were generally not kept or reported, and they can only be estimated. In the nineteenth century, it is believed that there was one abortion for every four live births, a rate only a bit lower than that in the latter part of the twentieth century. The number of abortions in any year varied from 500,000 to 1 million, most of them illegal. In 1969, the Centers for Disease Control (CDC), a branch of the U.S. Department of Health and Human Services, began an annual abortion count. Legal abortions in 1970 numbered about 200,000. The number of illegal abortions is unknown. Ten years later, legal abortions reached 1,200,000, and by 1990 they had increased to 1,600,000; they have dropped slightly but steadily since 1990. The CDC estimated that there were about 325 abortions for every 1,000 live births in the 1980's, a number consistent with findings for the 1990's. The number of abortions in any year rarely fluctuated by more or less than 3 percent from these figures.

Ireland, which has the most stringent abortion laws, performs 139 abortions per 1,000 live births. Eastern European countries, with more abortions than live births, have abortion rates three to four times higher than Western European countries. Nearly 60 percent of all abortions occur in Asia, with Vietnam and China having the highest rates of abortion.

In *Roe v. Wade*, the Supreme Court ruled that abortions were legal under certain conditions. Those conditions included the welfare of the woman and the viability of the fetus. During the first three months of pregnancy, according to the Court, the government had no legitimate interest in regulating abortions. The only exception was that states could require that abortions be performed by a licensed physician in a "medical setting." Otherwise, the decision to abort was strictly that of the pregnant woman as a constitutional right of privacy. During the second trimester, abortions were more restricted. They would be legal only if the woman's health needed to be protected, and they would require the consent of a doctor. The interest of the fetus would be protected during the third trimester, when it became able to survive on its own outside the woman's body, with or without artificial life support. States, at this point, could prohibit abortions except in cases where the life or health of the mother was threatened. In the companion case *Doe v. Bolton*, health was defined as "all factors—physical, emotional, psychological, familial, and the woman's age." This broad definition of health effectively made it possible for a woman to have an abortion throughout all nine months of the pregnancy, circumventing state restrictions. The determination of viability would be made by doctors, not by legal authorities. This ruling effectively struck down all antiabortion laws across the United States.

In the aftermath of *Roe v. Wade*, abortion became an intensely emotional political issue in the United States. The Hyde Amendment of 1976 eliminated federal funding for abortions, and other legislation blocked foreign aid to family planning programs, which members of Congress who were opposed to abortion saw as "pro-abortion." In *Webster v. Reproductive Health Services* (1989), the Supreme Court upheld its ruling in *Roe v. Wade*, but it also sustained a rule forbidding the use of public facilities or public employees for carrying out abortions. The Court also supported a requirement that a test for viability be done before any late-term abortion and said states could ban funding for abortion counseling. The issue continued to divide North Americans, with opponents arguing that abortion at any point during the pregnancy constituted murder.

A 2000 survey of women who had abortions, conducted by the Alan Guttmacher Institute, revealed the most common reasons for making that decision. Seventy-five percent said that having a baby would interfere with work or going to school. About two-thirds said they could not afford a child. Half of the women said that they did not want to be a single parent or were having problems with their husbands. This same survey revealed that almost 60 percent of the women seeking abortions were experiencing their first pregnancy. Women beneath the poverty level, regardless of race, religion, or ethnic background, were more likely to have an abortion than middle-class women. African American and Hispanic women had higher rates of abortion than did white women (three and two times as likely, respectively). Fifty-two percent of abortions are performed on women under the age of twenty-five.

Religion appears to be a factor in the decision to seek an abortion: The percentage of Catholic women having abortions was 29 percent higher than the percentage of Protestant women. The lowest percentage of abortions was found among Evangelical, "born-again" Christians. Nonreligious women have abortions at four times the rate of religious women. Teenagers under fifteen and women over forty had the highest rates of abortion of any age group. Thirty-three percent of all abortions occur before the fetal period of development. Fifty-five percent of abortions are performed between eight and twelve weeks into the pregnancy. The risk of death associated with abortion increases from one death for every 530,000 abortions at eight weeks or fewer to one death per 6,000 abortions performed at twenty-one or more weeks of gestation.

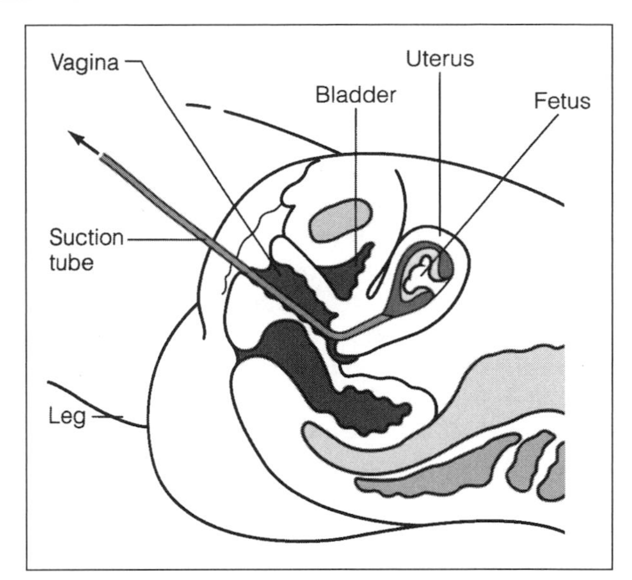

Elective or induced abortions can be performed in the first trimester using a simple suction technique; after the third month, much riskier and more complex methods are required.

Techniques and Procedures

A variety of techniques can be used to perform abortions. They vary according to the length of the pregnancy, which is usually measured by the number of weeks since the last menstrual period (LMP). Instrumental techniques are usually used very early in a pregnancy. They include a procedure called menstrual extraction, in which the entire contents of the uterus are removed. It can be done as early as fourteen days after the expected onset of a period. A major problem with this method is a high risk of error; the human embryo may still be so small at this age that it can be missed. It is also true that a high proportion of women undergoing this procedure are in fact not pregnant. Nevertheless, this method is easy and very safe. Death rates from this technique average less than 1 in 100,000.

The majority of abortions in the United States are done by a procedure known as vacuum aspiration, or suction curettage. This technique can be used up to about fourteen weeks after the LMP. It can be performed with local anesthesia and follows several steps. First, the cervix is expanded with metal rods that are inserted one at a time, with each rod being slightly larger than the previous one. When the cervix is expanded to the right size, a transparent, hollow tube called the vacuum cannula is placed into the uterine cavity. This instrument is attached to a suction device, which looks something like a drinking straw. An electric or hand-operated vacuum pump then empties the uterus of its contents. Finally, a spoon-shaped device called a curette is used to check for any leftover tissue in the uterus. The entire procedure takes less than five minutes. This method, first used in China in 1958, is among the safest procedures in medicine. There are about six times more maternal deaths during regular birth than during vacuum aspiration.

An older method, dilation and curettage (D & C), was common up to the 1970's, but it has largely been replaced by vacuum aspiration. In a D & C, the cervix is expanded or dilated and a curette used to scrape out the contents of the uterus. The biggest difference is the use of general anesthesia during the process. Since most abortion-related deaths result from complications from anesthesia, a method that requires only local anesthesia, such as aspiration, greatly reduces the dangers of the procedure.

For the period from thirteen to twenty weeks, a method called dilation and evacuation (D & E) is usually preferred. The cervix is expanded with tubes of laminaria (a type of seaweed), and the fetus is removed with the placenta, the part of the uterus by which the fetus is nourished. Forceps, suction, or a sharp curette is sometimes used. The procedure is usually safe, but sometimes if the fetus is large, it must be crushed and dismembered in order to remove it through the cervix. One variation of this procedure, the controversial partial-birth abortion, involves delivering the fetus breech, except for the head, and then inserting a suction tube through an incision made in the head. The brain is then sucked out, which collapses the skull, and the fetus is then easily removed. In October, 2003, legislation banning this procedure, called the Partial-Birth Abortion Ban Act of 2003, was passed by Congress and signed into law by President George W. Bush.

Along with these methods of menstrual extraction, physicians can use "medical induction" techniques when required. Amnioinfusion is an old example of this method that was used on fetuses from sixteen to twenty weeks old. This process has largely been replaced by D & E, which has proven far less dangerous.

Amnioinfusion usually requires hospitalization, local anesthesia, and the insertion of a large needle into the uterus. Between 100 and 200 milliliters of fluid is withdrawn and a similar amount of hypertonic saline solution infused into the uterine cavity. Within ninety minutes, the fetal heart stops. The woman then goes into labor and delivers a dead fetus within twenty-four to seventy-two hours. These kinds of abortions generally have much higher risk of complications than did D & E. On rare occasions, a fetus has been born alive, but the main risks are infection, hemorrhage, and cervical injuries to the woman. The psychological difficulties associated with this procedure can be severe, especially the knowledge that the fetus delivered would be dead.

Another method uses prostaglandins, naturally occurring hormones that cause uterine contractions and expulsion of the fetus, rather than a saline solution. The hormones can be given to the patient in several different ways: intravenously, intramuscularly, through vaginal suppositories, or directly into the amniotic sac. Prostaglandins are used for inducing second-trimester abortions and are as safe as saline solutions. Their major advantage is to reduce the duration of the abortion, but they also have severe side effects. They cause intense stomach cramps and other gastrointestinal discomfort, and about 7 percent of the fetuses expelled show some sign of life.

Surgical techniques for abortion are very rare, although sometimes they prove necessary in special cases. Hysterotomy resembles a cesarean section. An incision is made in the abdomen, and the fetus is removed. Hysterotomy is usually used in the second trimester, but only in cases where other methods have failed. The risk of death is much higher in this procedure than in most others. Even more rare is a hysterectomy, the removal of the uterus. This is done only in cases in which a malignant tumor threatens the life of the pregnant woman.

In the late 1980's, the French "abortion pill," RU-486, was approved for use in many parts of Europe. By the mid-1990's, it had been used in more than fifty thousand abortions. Progesterone is a hormone which causes the uterus to develop the lining that can be used to house a fertilized egg. If the egg is not fertilized, the production of progesterone stops, and the uterine lining is discarded during menstruation. RU-486 contains an antiprogesterone, which means that it prevents the production of progesterone. The pill has proven to be effective about 90 percent of the time if used in early pregnancy.

A few serious side effects sometimes occur with RU-486, the major one being sustained bleeding. About one in one thousand users bleeds so much that a transfusion is required. Cramps and nausea are also reported in a number of cases. There is apparently no effect on subsequent pregnancies. The drug must be taken under medical supervision and requires, under French law, at least three visits to a doctor's office. The first visit is for testing and counseling. On the second visit, the patient is given the drug. On the third, she receives an injection of prostaglandin. RU-486 was approved for legal use in the United States in 2000.

By the late 1990's, there was growing interest and usage in what is commonly termed "emergency contraception" or "morning after pills"—pills that contain high doses of the hormones found in ordinary birth control pills and prevent ovulation, fertilization, or implantation before a pregnancy can occur. In 1998, the Food and Drug Administration (FDA) approved the public sale and marketing of emergency contraception pills to the United States market. They must be taken within seventy-two hours of unprotected intercourse to work correctly, and efficacy rates of the pills range from 75 to 89 percent. By 2003, the pills were available only by prescription except in Alaska, California, and Washington, where women could obtain them from pharmacists who were authorized to dispense prescription drugs.

PERSPECTIVE AND PROSPECTS

Abortion is the most frequently performed surgical procedure in the United States. As long as women have unwanted pregnancies, that will continue to be the case. Abortion is a very safe procedure, although there can be complications. Generally, the earlier the procedure is performed, the less severe the risk. The lowest chance of medical complications occurs during the first eight weeks of pregnancy. After eight weeks, the risk of complications increases by 30 percent for each week of delay. Nevertheless, the death rate per case is very low, about half that for tonsillectomy. These statistics apply only to those areas of the world where abortion is legal, since women in those places tend to have earlier abortions.

In parts of the world where it remains against the law, abortion is a leading cause of death for women. WHO estimates that as many as 500,000 women a year die during abortions. About 200,000 of these deaths result from complications following abortions performed by unqualified medical personnel. About half of the total deaths take place in Southeast Asia and Africa. Before the *Roe v. Wade* decision, it was estimated that anywhere from a few hundred to several thousand American women died every year from the procedure. The best estimate was that in the 1960's about 290 women died every year as a result of complications from abortions. In the 1980's, the average was 12 per year, mostly from anesthesia complications. In 1998, the Centers for Disease Control identified 22 maternal deaths with some indication of abortion on the death certificate. How many women suffer from the psychological effects of having an abortion is a question that has not been fully researched.

—Leslie V. Tischauser, Ph.D.; updated by Paul J. Chara, Jr., Ph.D.

See also Amniocentesis; Cervical, ovarian, and uterine cancers; Childbirth; Childbirth complications; Contraception; Embryology; Ethics; Fetal tissue transplantation; Genetic counseling; Genetics and inheritance; Gynecology; Hippocratic oath; Hysterectomy; Law and medicine; Pregnancy and gestation; Reproductive system; Sterilization; Women's health.

For Further Information:

Baer, Judith A. *Historical and Multicultural Encyclopedia of Women's Reproductive Rights in the United States*. Westport, Conn.: Greenwood Press, 2002. Examines the nexus of birth control, abortion, and government policy with race, ethnicity, age, class, education, religion, and sexual preference. Also includes articles on laws, court cases, political attitudes, prominent activists, and technological advances as they relate to reproductive rights in the United States.

Denney, Myron K. *A Matter of Choice: An Essential Guide to Every Aspect of Abortion*. New York: Simon & Schuster, 1983. A good overview of the subject which presents both pro-choice and antiabortion views. Discusses the medical and psychological problems involved and also presents alternatives to abortion.

Greer, Germaine. *Sex and Destiny: The Politics of Human Fertility*. New York: Harper & Row, 1984. Greer describes the attitudes of people in various cultures around the world toward questions about children, birth control, abortion, infanticide, and the family.

Hull, N. E. H., and Peter Charles Hoffer. *Roe v. Wade: The Abortion Rights Controversy in American History*. Lawrence: University Press of Kansas, 2001. A balanced view of the opposing sides of the abortion debate and the constitutional response, placed in the context of social movements and women's history.

McFarlane, Deborah R. *The Politics of Fertility Control: Family Planning and Abortion Policies in the American States*. New York: Chatham House, 2001. Reviews and analyzes policies and practices in the last three decades of the twentieth century in each of the fifty states.

Mohr, James C. *Abortion in America: The Origins and Evolution of National Policy, 1800-1900*. New York: Oxford University Press, 1979. A scholarly examination of American abortion policy in the nineteenth century.

National Abortion Rights Action League. http://www.naral.org/. Site offers information about reproductive health issues, including daily news items, publications, organized links, and Act Now opportunities.

National Right to Life Organization. http://www.nrlc.org/. Site offers sources of information on pro-life issues in relation to abortion, RU-486, organization support, euthanasia, and federal legislation.

Riddle, John M. *Contraception and Abortion from the Ancient World to the Renaissance*. Cambridge, Mass.: Harvard University Press, 1994. The various contraceptive methods used from antiquity to the Middle Ages are discussed in this scholarly book.

Sachdev, Paul, ed. *International Handbook on Abortion*. Westport, Conn.: Greenwood Press, 1988. An extensive collection of data from thirty-three nations covering the legal status of abortion, abortion rates, and the availability of services.

Sciarra, John J., et al. *Gynecology and Obstetrics*. Vol. 6. Philadelphia: Harper & Row, 1991. A textbook that discusses methods, demographics, health concerns, and the psychological and medical consequences of abortions.

Abscess drainage

Procedure

Anatomy or system affected: Brain, breasts, gallbladder, glands, gums, kidneys, liver, lungs, nervous system, pancreas, respiratory system, skin, spleen, stomach, urinary system

Specialties and related fields: Dermatology, emergency medicine, family medicine, general surgery

Definition: The removal of a collection of pus in tissue through an opening in the skin.

Indications and Procedures

When bacteria infect tissue, the body's defense systems attempt to isolate them and destroy the infective agents. An abscess develops when the bacteria become walled off from surrounding noninfected tissues and white blood cells enter the area to rid the body of the pathogens. The ensuing battle between the white blood cells and bacteria causes the death of these cells as well as of surrounding tissue. These dead cells form pus.

Staphylococci bacteria are the most common pathogens that cause abscesses to form, resulting in pain, swelling, and fever. If the abscess is near the skin, it is easily detected. The presence of abscesses in deeper tissues, however, may need to be confirmed using computed tomography (CT) scanning or magnetic resonance imaging (MRI).

The physician will usually prescribe antibiotics to help destroy the bacteria. Unfortunately, the antibiotics may not have access to the site of infection since the abscess is usually encapsulated by tissue. If this is the case, the physician must drain the abscess cavity. He or she will make an incision into the cavity to allow the pus to drain. Occasionally, a tube will be inserted to maintain the opening for continued drainage of the cavity. The tube can be removed once the infection is gone.

The patient will be asked to watch for signs of recurrent infection after the abscess is removed, because some bacteria may remain. The abscess can reappear if these bacteria are not destroyed by the body's immune system or by antibiotics.

Uses and Complications

Abscesses can develop in any organ. Common sites, however, are under the skin, in the breasts, and around the teeth and gums. In rare cases, abscesses are found in the liver or brain. Fungi and protozoans are important pathogens in liver abscesses.

Most abscesses dissipate after they are drained and/or the patient is treated with antibiotics. Occasionally, antibiotic treatment alone will cause the abscess to subside. The rapid detection and treatment of abscesses in the liver and brain are musts because the damage to these vital organs is irreparable.

—*Matthew Berria, Ph.D., and Douglas Reinhart, M.D.*

See also Abscesses; Antibiotics; Bacterial infections; Biopsy; Breast biopsy; Breast disorders; Breasts, female; Culdocentesis; Cyst removal; Cysts; Cytology; Cytopathology; Dermatology; Ganglion removal; Hydrocelectomy; Infection; Otorhinolaryngology; Periodontal surgery; Periodontitis; Quinsy; Root canal treatment; Skin; Skin disorders; Staphylococcal infections; Testicular surgery.

For Further Information:

Ariel, Irving M., and Kirk K. Kazarian. *Diagnosis and Treatment of Abdominal Abscesses*. Baltimore: Williams & Wilkins, 1971.

Balasegaram, M. *Management of Hepatic Abscess*. Chicago: Year Book Medical, 1981.

Hau, T., J. R. Haaga, and M. I. Aeder. *Pathophysiology, Diagnosis, and Treatment of Abdominal Abscesses*. Chicago: Year Book Medical, 1984.

Icon Health. *Abscess: A Medical Dictionary, Bibliography, and Annotated Research Guide to Internet References*. San Diego, Calif.: Author, 2004.

Abscesses

Disease/disorder

Anatomy or system affected: All

Specialties and related fields: All

Definition: Any enclosed collection of pus, whether sterile or infected.

Causes and Symptoms

When bacteria enter the body's tissue, white blood cells migrate to the site to fight infection. As they fight off the bacteria, they subsequently die. These dead white blood cells, and the enzymes that they produce as they decay, accumulate as fluid. It is this fluid that forms what is commonly known as pus. An enclosed collection of pus is called an abscess. Abscesses may occur at various sites within the body. Because bacteria often enter the body through the skin, abscesses commonly occur at sites just under the skin. Perhaps the most common abscesses are staph infections, which are caused by the bacterium *Staphylococcus aureus*.

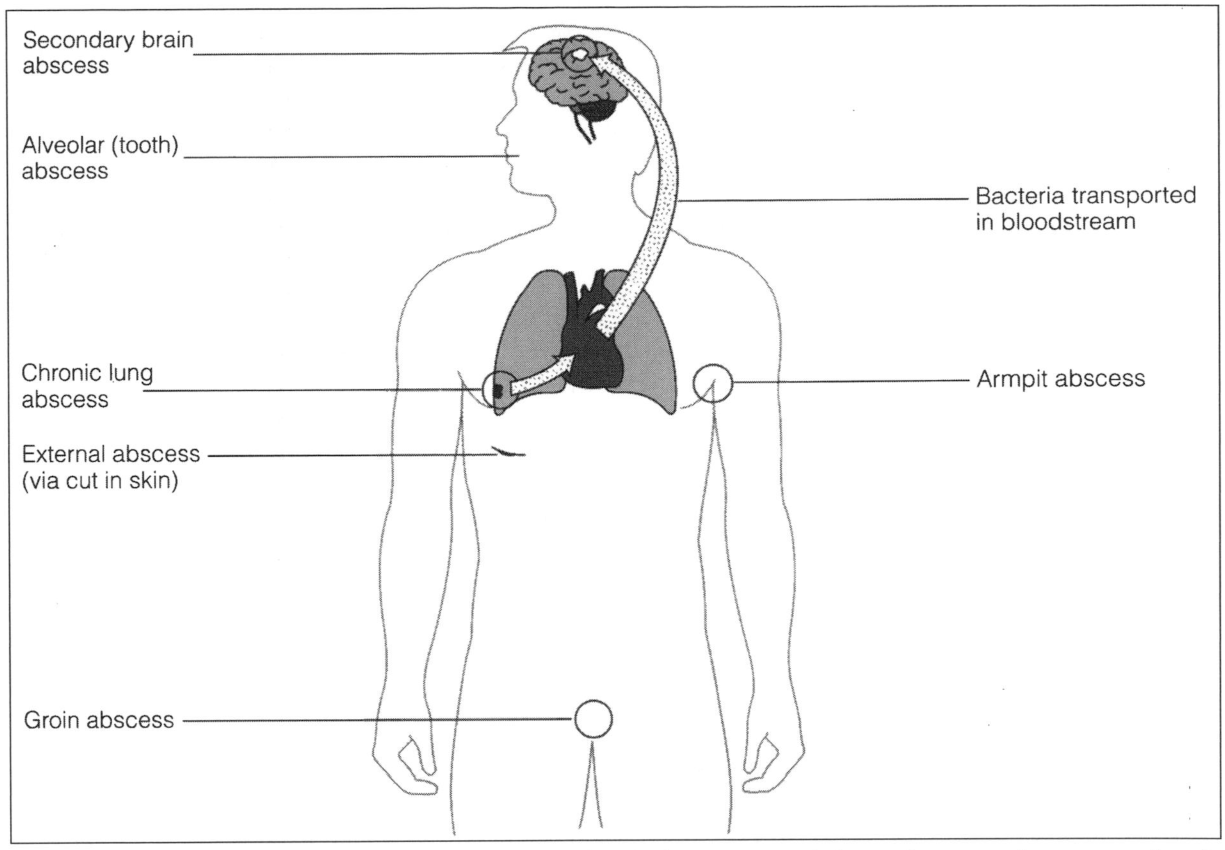

Abscesses are commonly located in soft tissues and near lymph nodes but may appear in internal organs and may cause other abscesses via bacterial migration.

Abscesses can occur in the abdomen, pelvis, kidneys, spleen, pancreas, liver, or prostate gland, or in the area behind the abdominal cavity (the retroperitoneal space). Abscesses can also occur in the head, neck, or hands, or in any of the muscles throughout the body. Throat abscesses are more likely to develop in children than in adults, often as a result of an infection such as strep throat. Though most commonly under the skin, where they are readily discernible, abscesses can also form deep within the body, where they are undetectable unless a diagnostic procedure such as computed tomography (CT) scanning or magnetic resonance imaging (MRI) is used. Signs aiding in the diagnosis of an abscess include heat, swelling, tenderness, and redness at the site. Bodywide, or systemic, symptoms such as fever or weight loss can also accompany abscesses, often when they are deeper.

Because people with weakened immune systems have a decreased ability to ward off infection, they are more likely to develop abscesses than are people with healthy immune systems. Abscess formation is frequently seen in patients with diabetes, sickle cell disease, and acquired immunodeficiency syndrome (AIDS) or in patients on steroid therapy.

Abscesses can foster processes that infect the blood, causing sepsis, which can spread infection to distant sites within the body. A locally spread abscess can cause bleeding in nearby vessels or impair the functioning of a major organ.

TREATMENT AND THERAPY

Patients often will not seek medical attention for an abscess until it has become painful or inconvenient. The abscess may come to a point, or "head," and rupture spontaneously. If the abscess does not rupture, then it may require drainage. The site is numbed with an anesthetic; the abscess is cut open and drained. The pus is manually expressed. When the abscess is large enough, packing may be inserted to minimize bleeding and help prevent reaccumulation of pus. The packing is often removed the following day. Usually, antibiotics are not needed, but they may be prescribed to prevent reinfec-

> **Information on Abscesses**
>
> **Causes:** An enclosed collection of pus following bacterial infection
> **Symptoms:** Heat, swelling, tenderness, redness at the site; when systemic, fever or weight loss
> **Duration:** Acute
> **Treatments:** Drainage

tion. Deep abscesses sometimes require CT-guided drainage. Analyzing the pus in a laboratory can often help to guide treatment.

Prompt treatment of infections will often prevent the development of abscesses. Patients should be instructed to take care of injuries of any type, particularly bites and puncture wounds. The prognosis after treatment is good, as most abscesses should heal well.

—Leonard Berkowitz, D.O., and Paul Moglia, Ph.D.

See also Abscess drainage; Acne; Bacterial infections; Cyst removal; Cysts; Infection; Lymphatic system; Quinsy; Septicemia; Skin; Skin disorders; Staphylococcal infections; Tumor removal; Tumors; Wounds.

For Further Information:

"Abscess." In *Ferri's Clinical Advisor: Instant Diagnosis and Treatment*, edited by Fred F. Ferri. Philadelphia: Mosby, 2003.

"Abscesses." In *The Merck Manual of Medical Information: Second Home Edition*, edited by Mark H. Beers. Whitehouse Station, N.J.: Merck Research Laboratories, 2003.

Hau, T., J. R. Haaga, and M. I. Aeder. *Pathophysiology, Diagnosis, and Treatment of Abdominal Abscesses*. Chicago: Year Book Medical, 1984.

Icon Health. *Abscess: A Medical Dictionary, Bibliography, and Annotated Research Guide to Internet References*. San Diego, Calif.: Author, 2004.

Accidents

Disease/disorder

Anatomy or system affected: All

Specialties and related fields: All

Definition: An occurrence in a sequence of events that produces unintended injury, death, or property damage. "Accident" refers to the event, not the result of the event. "Unintentional injury" refers to the result of an accident and is the preferred term in the health community for accidental injury.

Key terms:

autograft: a thin layer of skin taken from an unburned area on the patient's body and placed over the burned area

comminuted fracture: a bone broken into fragments

compound fracture: a bone break that breaks the skin

compression fracture: a break of a short bone in which its soft tissue is damaged

computed tomography (CT) scanning: a technique for producing cross-sectional images of the body in which X rays pass through at different angles and are computer analyzed

concussion: disturbance of electrical activity in the brain due to a blow to the head or neck

contusion: a bruise; injury to tissue without breaking the skin

corrosives: having a burning (caustic) and locally destructive effect

emetic: something that causes vomiting (emesis)

magnetic resonance imaging (MRI): a technique that uses magnetic fields and radio waves to create high-quality cross-sectional images without using radiation

mucous membrane: the soft, pink layer of cells that produce mucus to keep body structures lubricated; found in eyelids and respiratory and urinary tracts

whiplash injury: injury to the ligaments, joints, and soft tissues of the neck region of the spine due to a sudden, violent jerking motion

Causes and Symptoms

Unintentional injury continued to be the fifth leading cause of death in the United States as of 2000, exceeded by heart disease, cancer, stroke, and chronic obstructive pulmonary diseases (asthma, pneumonia, and influenza). In 2000, injuries had a financial impact on the average American household of approximately $4,600. Individuals and households sustain this loss by paying higher prices for goods and services and higher taxes or through direct, out-of-pocket loss. The leading cause of unintentional injury and death remains motor vehicle accidents, followed by poisoning, falls, drowning, and burns. Other injuries and deaths result from air transportation accidents, weather, and major disasters.

As of 2000, motor vehicle unintentional injuries, including those from automobile and motorcycle accidents, remained the leading cause of injury and death in the United States in individuals aged one to thirty-eight. Males between fifteen and twenty-one accounted for 60 percent of the deaths from automobile crashes.

Not wearing seat belts in automobiles and not wearing helmets while operating other vehicles can lead to serious head trauma and death. Falls are a serious problem for seniors and the leading cause of death in people sixty-five and older.

Broken bones, cuts, bruises, and whiplash are the most common injuries in accidents involving one or more vehicles. More serious injuries from vehicles, sports, and falls include trauma to the head and neck; spinal cord injuries; knee injuries; eye injuries and blindness; comminuted, compression, and compound fractures; hip fractures; severed limbs; and severe burns.

Vehicle accidents are those caused by automobiles and motorcycles and cause more serious injuries, such as head trauma, spinal cord injuries, blindness, and burns. Self-propelled vehicles, bicycles, scooters, skateboards, and in-line skates are also included in this group and produce less serious injuries, such as cuts, bruises, and simple fractures.

Head injuries are always considered serious. They cause more deaths and disabilities than any other neurologic condition before the age of fifty and occur in 70 percent of all unintentional injuries. They are the leading cause of death in men and boys up to thirty-five years of age. Motorcycle head injuries are most serious in those who do not wear helmets. Upon impact, the rider is thrown toward the ground at accelerated speeds, causing severe blunt force trauma, especially to the head.

The brain fits loosely within the skull so that blunt force to the skull or violent shaking of the head back and forth causes the brain to bounce off the skull. This violent brain movement causes bruising, tearing, and bleeding between the brain tissue and the skull.

There are two types of brain injury, diffuse and focal. Diffuse is most common and includes concussion. One-third of those who die from brain injury die from diffuse brain injury. An injury victim can have a concussion without losing consciousness and have no visible signs of trauma on the head, such as a bump or cut. If signs of amnesia, impaired attention, distractibility, and changes in cognitive functioning (knowing information such as one's immediate location) are temporary after concussion, this may imply the patient has had no structural damage. This does not, however, indicate the severity of the injury. A CT (computed tomography) scan or MRI (magnetic resonance imaging) is used to diagnose the extent of diffuse and focal brain injuries. Careful examination by a neurosurgeon is necessary.

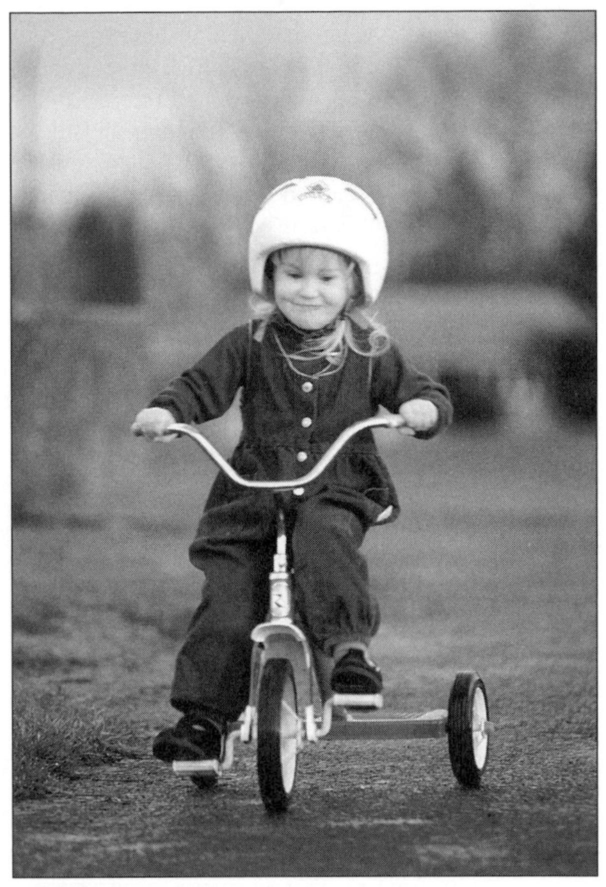

Children and adults should wear helmets to guard against head injuries when cycling, even with stable vehicles such as tricycles. (PhotoDisc)

Focal brain injury involves a specific area of the brain. This includes brain contusions that occur from a direct blow to the head (and are similar to other external bruises); ischemia, which is damage to the brain tissue due to a reduction in the flow of blood to the brain; infarction, which causes affected brain tissue to die from lack of blood supply; and pressure which is caused by the brain tissue swelling from the trauma.

A direct blow to the head can cause an epidural hematoma, which is bleeding between the skull and the brain membranes. This occurs quickly and causes unconsciousness at the time of injury, perhaps a lucid interval, and then coma. Subdural hematomas cause bleeding that occurs slowly within the brain tissue, are frequently complicated by contusions of the brain tissue, and carry a significant risk of death even with surgery. A favorable outcome with any brain injury depends on rapid and careful transportation to a hospital for diagnosis and treatment.

Bicycle, scooter, skateboard, and in-line skate injuries are sustained in falls. About half of these occur to hands and arms, one-third to head and face, and one-third to legs and feet, including fractures and dislocations. Other injuries include lacerations requiring stitches, cuts and bruises, and strains and sprains. Fatalities may occur when a victim collides with an automobile.

Sports injuries are generally to ligaments, muscles, and joints. More serious sports injuries include concussions, broken bones, and spinal cord injuries. Knee injuries can be sustained in vehicular and sports accidents and falls. Most severe knee injuries occur in competitive sports accidents, particularly football. The most common are ligament or cartilage tears and traumatic arthritis. A "blown out knee" is a tear of the anterior cruciate ligament, one of four principal ligaments in the knee and most important for stability of the knee.

Unintentional injuries from falls are most common in patients aged fifty-five to seventy-five and are the primary cause of fatal injury for people aged sixty-five and older. Approximately 60 percent of fatal falls occur in the home, 30 percent in public places, and 10 percent in institutions. Hip fractures are the most serious injury sustained from falls. The impact on the injured individual's quality of life can be devastating. Most patients cannot return home or live independently after a hip fracture. A seriously injured patient requires a caregiver on duty twenty-four hours a day, which can be costly. Lack of mobility causes severe depression, especially for someone who had been active. Climbing to reach an object is not the cause of most falls in older adults, but rather vision problems, poor lighting, slippery surfaces, wearing house shoes with soft soles, balance problems resulting from disease or medication, and clutter such as papers or magazines on the floor.

Poison is any substance that produces disease conditions or tissue injury, or otherwise interrupts natural life processes when in contact with or absorbed into the body. Most poisons taken in sufficient quantity are lethal. A poison, depending on the type, may attack the surface of the body or, more seriously, internal organs or the central nervous system.

Poisoning is a leading cause of accidents resulting in unintentional injury and death. These agents include illicit drugs (street drugs and those not prescribed by a physician), medicines (over-the-counter and prescribed drugs), mushrooms, eggs, shellfish, and gases or vapors. Poisons are usually classified by effects as corrosives, irritants, or systemic or nerve poisons (narcotics).

The American Association of Poison Control Centers estimates that 2.5 million poison cases, fatal and nonfatal, were reported during 2000. These incidents have nearly tripled in the last thirty years. This may be due to the increase in the use of illegal street drugs.

Common results of poisoning include burns to the skin or eye tissue, or to mucous membranes of the mouth, throat, esophagus, stomach, and other parts of the body with which a caustic poison might come in contact when swallowed or inhaled; central nervous stimulation or depression; cerebral edema; renal (kidney) and/or hepatic (liver) failure; brain damage; and death.

Corrosives are strong acids or alkalies that, when swallowed, burn the skin or lining of the mouth, throat, and stomach, causing bloody vomiting. Ammonia is an example of a common household corrosive. Irritants (such as iodine, arsenic, and laxatives) act directly on the mucous membrane, causing inflammation and gastrointestinal upset with pain and vomiting. Irritants can be absorbed slowly and become cumulative until they take effect suddenly, causing serious illness or death. Central nervous system poisons (narcotics) affect the heart, liver, lungs, and kidneys, as well as the respiratory and circulatory systems. Examples of household narcotics include alcohol, turpentine, cyanide, and strychnine (found in some pesticides). Botulin toxin, the bacteria that causes botulism (food poisoning), is one of the most dangerous poisons known and is included in this group. Asphyxiants include gas poisons such as carbon monoxide. Gases, when inhaled, get into the bloodstream and prohibit the body from properly absorbing oxygen. Blood poisoning, or septicemia, is included in this category. Microorganisms get into the bloodstream through a wound or infection, also preventing, in advanced stages, proper oxygen absorption. Smoke from house fires is an asphyxiant and causes most fire-related deaths.

Deaths from residential fires are second only to those occurring as the result of automobile accidents. In 2000 alone, five thousand people were killed in house fires. Most accidents causing burns can be avoided by preventing the cause. Burns are the most devastating of all unintentional injuries, causing red and painful areas on skin with blisters, scarring, contractions of skin resulting in a decrease in motion, dehydration, shock, damage to lungs from inhalation of smoke and hot air, and loss of skin that can be traumatic and life-threatening.

Treatment and Therapy

Simple fractures, those bones broken with little or no displacement, can be set in the hospital emergency room or clinic by a general or orthopedic surgeon. A cast is applied to hold the bones in place until they grow together again. The patient is usually asked to come back in six weeks for new X rays and probable cast removal. Comminuted fractures (bone broken into fragments), compression fractures (damage to soft tissue at site), and compound fractures (bone protruding through skin) require surgery. These fractures may cause deformity of the limbs if extensive and if surgical intervention cannot return the bone fragments to proper alignment. In some compression or comminuted fractures, a steel plate is attached with screws through healthy bone above and below the fractured area, and a cast is applied. Traction may be required and the patient kept hospitalized and immobile for several weeks. Physical therapy may be required to regain strength and mobility in the legs or motion in the joints of the upper extremities.

Skull fractures are easier to diagnose and treat. A simple linear skull fracture, depending on the location, often requires no intervention except hospitalization for observation. A skull fracture that goes deeper than the thickness of the skull requires surgical evaluation.

Any foreign objects or objects impaled in a victim's head will be removed only in the operating room by a neurosurgeon, with the patient being kept for at least a twenty-four-hour observation. Patients who have had severe head wounds often require extensive physical and psychological therapy. Personality changes can occur, causing the patient to exhibit agitated behaviors, anger, and the inability to cope with everyday activities. Relearning normal bodily functions, such as speech, walking, and writing, becomes a series of frustrating, monumental tasks. Behaviors can be so uncontrolled that confinement is necessary so that there is no danger to the patient or others. Medications combined with psychotherapy and physical therapy can typify the long road back to normalcy. Some patients never fully recover.

Repair to an injured knee is done under general anesthesia. Instruments are inserted into the knee joint through several small punctures. While viewing the ligaments through the arthroscope, the surgeon can repair or remove damaged tissue. If torn, the anterior cruciate ligament can be rebuilt. Most arthroscopic surgery is performed on an outpatient basis. Meniscal cartilages are the "shock absorbers" between the femur (thighbone) and the tibia (large leg bone) at the knee joint. A tear in the meniscal cartilage is the most common knee injury requiring surgical intervention. Arthroscopic surgery is done on an outpatient basis, and the patient is allowed to walk on the affected leg as soon as it feels comfortable. Physical therapy may be recommended for both anterior cruciate ligament and meniscal cartilage tears. Chances of returning to competitive sports are quite good, even for those who play professionally.

Poisoning should be treated immediately but with the direction of a health care professional. Most poison cases can be handled in the home after consulting a poison control center. In most cases of poisoning, ingestion of large quantities of water or milk (dilution) is called for. Sometimes an emetic is administered. Some common household emetics include a tablespoon of salt dissolved in warm water or two tablespoons of mustard dissolved in a pint of warm water. Vomiting must never be induced in a person who has swallowed a corrosive poison. An antidote is given for ingestion of corrosives, which neutralizes the chemical, absorbs it, or prevents it from being absorbed. Transport to a local hospital is always necessary.

The first forty-eight hours are important in burn treatment. When admitted to the hospital for severe burns, patients require stabilization of breathing and replacement of fluids to prevent dehydration and shock. Wounds are debrided in surgery to promote blood flow to healthy tissue underneath the wound. Grafts may be required. Surgical dressings soaked in antibiotics are applied to prevent infection. Many surgeries may be required until the grafts cover all the burned areas. Medical staff work to develop pain management strategies specific to each person's suffering. Physical and occupational therapy, though painful, must not be avoided. Burn injury places the patient at risk for severe loss of motion. Exercise, nutrition, and emotional support are important factors in helping the burn patient to heal.

Perspective and Prospects

There are three major ways to prevent accidents: education, making the home and workplace safer, and banning dangerous activities and equipment. Air bags have helped tremendously to eliminate many types of injuries in automobiles, and many lives have been saved. Whiplash, head and neck trauma, and eye injuries have been less serious since air bags have been installed in automobiles. With bicycle riders especially, wearing a helmet is the single most effective safety device available to reduce fatal injury to the brain and disfiguring injury to the face from crashes. The best investment against bicycle, scooter, skateboard, and in-line skate injuries is protective gear.

New technologies and advanced training in sports medicine for health care professionals have greatly advanced complete recovery for unintentional injuries received in competitive sports. Artificial turf, though easier to care for, causes many knee and back injuries from slipping. Biotechnology has made great advances in providing safer equipment for sports participants, more effective imaging technology (such as magnetic resonance imaging, or MRI, and computed tomography, or CT, scanning equipment) for diagnosing all injuries, and physical therapy techniques and equipment to help those who have disabling injuries such as those involving the spinal cord. New materials and designs for limb prostheses are aiding those who have lost limbs to lead normal lives, even in competitive sports. There have been several examples of runners being competitive despite a leg or foot prosthesis. Pharmaceutical research is making advances in medications that can control pain without being addictive, for those with behavior problems and depression resulting from severe head trauma.

For seniors, a simple screening test can accurately identify those who are most likely to fall. Constant review and adjustment of medications by a physician are musts for preventing side effects such as dizziness, drowsiness, or disorientation. Installing grab bars in the shower and around the toilet, installing rails on both sides of the stairs, increasing lighting throughout the home and encouraging its use, and removing tripping hazards have been very effective in preventing falls. Most important for seniors is the encouragement of regular exercise to improve strength and balance.

Measures to prevent poisoning include labeling of household products, elimination of lead from gasoline, use of carbon monoxide detectors, and improved monitoring of exposure to toxic elements within industry and throughout the environment. The telephone number of a poison control center should be posted at home and in the workplace. More than 50 percent of accidental poisonings in 2000 happened in the home and involved such products as aspirin, barbiturates, insecticides, and cosmetics. Awareness, safety, and education are the keys to preventing accidents involving poisons.

Improvements in burn care have resulted in fewer deaths and better infection control. Technological advances in the provision of skin substitutes, improved monitoring techniques, surgical instrumentation, and better understanding of the underlying metabolic changes have all contributed to successful therapy.

—*Virginiae Blackmon*

See also Asphyxiation; Balance disorders; Bleeding; Brain damage; Brain disorders; Bruises; Burns and scalds; Choking; Coma; Concussion; Critical care; Critical care, pediatric; Death and dying; Drowning; Electrical shock; Emergency medicine; Emergency medicine, pediatric; Food poisoning; Fracture and dislocation; Fracture repair; Frostbite; Hip fracture repair; Hip replacement; Hyperbaric oxygen therapy; Laceration repair; Lead poisoning; Mercury poisoning; Paramedics; Poisoning; Poisonous plants; Prostheses; Radiation sickness; Resuscitation; Safety issues for children; Safety issues for the elderly; Shock; Snakebites; Spinal cord disorders; Sunburn; Unconsciousness; Whiplash; Wounds; Zoonoses.

For Further Information:

Beers, Mark H., et al. *The Merck Manual of Diagnosis and Therapy*. 18th ed. Whitehouse Station, N.J.: Merck Research Laboratories, 2006. The sections on burns, poisoning, and bites and stings are very complete and informative resources for the lay reader, if a bit technical. Includes pictures, charts, and grafts.

English, Peter. *Old Paint: A Medical History of Childhood Lead-Paint Poisoning in the United States to 1980*. New Brunswick, N.J.: Rutgers University Press, 2001. Chapters include "Lead Poisoning Before 1920," "The Scientific Study of the American Workplace," "Peeling and Flaking Paint. A 1950's Transformation," and "New Therapies: Industry and Public Health Responses."

Gronwall, Dorothy, Philip Wrightson, and Peter Waddell. *Head Injuries: The Facts—A Guide for Families and Care-Givers*. New York: Oxford University Press, 1998. Examines common wounds and injuries of the brain and the process of rehabilitation.

Matthews, Dawn D., ed. *Household Safety Sourcebook: Basic Consumer Health Information About Household Safety*. Detroit: Omnigraphics, 2001. A comprehensive and accessible handbook detailing the prevention and treatment of common household accidents, including those caused by fire, chemicals, water, electricity, and home equipment and appliances.

Monafo, W. W. "Initial Management of Burns." *New England Journal of Medicine* 335 (1996): 1581-

1586. A technical article but accessible to the lay reader with some medical knowledge.

National Center for Emergency Medicine Informatics. http://ncemi.org. Site provides Web links, frequently asked questions, automatic e-mail list subscriber, bibliographies, and articles.

National Safety Council. *Injury Facts 2005-2006*. Itasca, Ill.: Author, 2006. Complete injury statistics without much text, offering good facts and topic organization.

Nestle, Marion. *Safe Food: Bacteria, Biotechnology, and Bioterrorism*. Berkeley: University of California Press, 2003. Examines food-borne microbial illnesses that plague American consumers as part of its range of topics, arguing that the food industry acts in its own economic self-interest rather than out of concern for the public welfare.

Roberts, Anthony H. N. "Burn Prevention: Where Now?" *Burns* 26, no. 6 (August, 2000). Accessible to the lay reader and includes applicable information.

ACID-BASE CHEMISTRY

BIOLOGY

ANATOMY OR SYSTEM AFFECTED: Cells

SPECIALTIES AND RELATED FIELDS: Biochemistry, cytology, hematology, pharmacology

DEFINITION: The interaction between acids and bases in the cells of the body, the proper functioning of which is crucial in digestive metabolism, respiration, and the buffering capacity of body fluids.

KEY TERMS:

acidosis: condition of high blood carbon dioxide levels and low pH that results from such diseases as emphysema and pneumonia

alkalosis: a condition of abnormally low carbon dioxide levels that results from hyperventilation (rapid breathing)

Brønsted-Lowry definition (of an acid and a base): an acid is a substance that can donate protons, while a base is a proton acceptor

buffer: a solution which contains components that enable a solution to resist large changes in pH when small quantities of acids and bases are added

cellular respiration: the chemical utilization of oxygen and the production of carbon dioxide in the cell itself

extracellular respiration: the process of oxygen transport from the lungs to the cells and carbon dioxide transport from cells back to the lungs

general acid (or base) catalysis: the process in which a partial transfer of a proton from a Brønsted acid (or partial proton abstraction by a Brønsted base) lowers the free energy of a reaction's transition state

pH: a measure of acidity in a solution, which is equal to the negative logarithm of the hydrogen ion concentration; a neutral solution has a pH of 7, an acidic solution has a pH less than 7, and a basic solution has a pH greater than 7

STRUCTURE AND FUNCTIONS

The existence of acids and bases is critical to the functioning of the human body. An acid is a compound that contains hydrogen, can accept unshared electron pairs, has a pH that is less than 7, and is water-soluble. A base is a compound that contains a hydroxyl (OH) group, can give up unshared pairs of electrons, can accept protons, has a pH that is greater than 7, and is water-soluble. An acid and a base can react together to form a salt.

Both acids and bases can be classified further as either "hard" or "soft." Bases are classified as soft if they have high polarizability and low electronegativity, are easily oxidized, or have low-energy, empty orbitals. Opposite properties tend to classify them as hard bases. Hard acids are those that have low polarizability, small size, and a high oxidation state (valence) and that do not have easily removed outer electrons. Soft acids possess reversed properties. Generally, a hard acid always reacts with a hard base and a soft acid always reacts with a soft base. The reaction of a hard acid (or base) with a soft base (or acid) is always unfavorable (absorbs energy). The hard-and-soft concept of acids and bases is used only as a way to classify and predict reactions. In the acid-base reactions of a living being, however, one must consider acids as proton donors and bases as proton acceptors.

A neutral solution is defined as one whose proton (hydrogen ion) and hydroxyl concentrations are equal. A solution that has more protons than hydroxyl groups is acidic, while a solution with more hydroxyl ions than protons is basic. Expressing the hydrogen ion concentration in moles per liter is rather complex. Instead, the pH of a solution is used. The pH is the negative logarithm of the hydrogen ion concentration. Neutral solutions have a pH of 7, acidic solutions have a pH that is less than 7, and basic solutions have a pH that is higher than 7. Thus, a pH of zero is strongly acidic and a pH of 14 is strongly basic.

Buffers are solutions whose contents allow very small changes in pH upon the addition of small quantities of acids and bases. Usually, buffers are solutions of a weak acid and one of its salts, or solutions of a weak base and one of its salts. A buffer becomes ineffective when there are no more anions (if a weak acid is part of the buffer) or cations (if a weak base is involved). At this point, the buffer capacity of the solution is said to be exceeded.

General acid catalysis is a process in which partial proton transfer from an acid lowers the free energy of a reaction's transition state. A reaction can also be accomplished by a general base catalysis, in which a base enhances the rate by partially stealing a proton. Such reactions often have such a high activation energy that they cannot take place unless the specific catalysis is involved.

Many well-known substances encountered in everyday life are weak acids or bases. Aspirin (acetylsalicylic acid, a headache remedy), phenobarbital (a sedative), niacin (nicotinic acid, vitamin B), and saccharin (an artificial sweetener) are weak acids. The majority of drugs and narcotics (such as heroin, cocaine, and morphine) in their free-base states are weak bases. Among the components of deoxyribonucleic acid (DNA), which is a polymer of deoxyribonucleotide units, are nitrogenous bases, the purines and pyrimidines. An amino acid is either neutral, acidic, or basic, depending on the chemical group found in its side chain.

The normal metabolic processes of the body result in the continuous production of acids, such as carbonic acid (H_2CO_3), phosphoric acid (H_3PO_4), lactic acid, and pyruvic acid. In cellular oxidations, the main acid end product is carbonic acid, with 10 to 20 moles formed per day. In terms of acidity, this amount is equivalent to 1 to 2 liters of concentrated hydrochloric acid. Although some alkaline end products are also formed, the acid type predominates, and the body is faced with the necessity of continually removing the large quantities of acids that are formed within cells. The greatest restriction is that these products should be transported to the organs of excretion (via the extracellular fluids) with a minimal change in the hydrogen ion concentration.

Most biochemical processes are extremely sensitive to the level of hydrogen ions. The enzymes and other proteins involved in biological reactions, as well as many of the smaller molecules, are weak electrolytes whose state of ionization is a function of the hydrogen ion concentration. Most enzymes are active only within a narrow pH range, usually from 5 to 9. At a pH other than the optimum one, the binding of substrates to enzymes, the catalytic activity of enzymes, and changes in protein structure are seriously affected. Since the catalytic properties of enzymes are dependent on their state of ionization, it is not surprising that living cells cannot tolerate more than very minor changes in hydrogen ion levels. As a result, biological fluids are in general strongly buffered, so that their pH is maintained within narrow limits under physiological conditions.

Blood is buffered by plasma proteins and by hemoglobin, which can either accept or donate protons. The role of buffers can be understood by the following example. The addition of 0.01 mole hydrochloric acid in 1 liter of blood lowers the pH only from 7.4 to 7.2. When added to an isotonic saline (sodium chloride) solution, the same amount of hydrochloric acid lowers the pH from 7.0 to 2.0, since the saline solution has no buffering capacity. Another example of the effectiveness of the blood plasma indicates that 1.3 liters of concentrated hydrochloric acid are needed to drop the pH of the whole 5.5 liters of blood of an average human being from 7.4 to 7.0.

Metabolism in tissues leads to the production of carbon dioxide (CO_2), which, when dissolved in water, forms carbonic acid and the following equilibrium:

$$\underset{\text{carbon dioxide}}{CO_2} + \underset{\text{water}}{H_2O} \rightleftharpoons \underset{\text{carbonic acid}}{H_2CO_3} \rightleftharpoons H^+ + \underset{\text{bicarbonate anion}}{HCO_3^-}$$

Carbon dioxide enters the bloodstream from tissues and is exchanged in the lungs for oxygen, which is then transported throughout the body by the hemoglobin in the blood. The fact that the ratio of bicarbonate to carbonic acid is relatively high (10:1) seems to put this buffer well outside its maximum capacity. Nevertheless, the system is appropriate, because the need to neutralize excess acid (such as lactic acid, which is produced during exercise) is much greater than the need to neutralize excess base. The excess bicarbonate serves this purpose. Strenuous exercise also leads to an increased formation of carbon dioxide by body tissues, which is accumulated in the air spaces of the lungs. Under normal circumstances, the bicarbonate in the blood buffer will lead to a shifting in the equilibrium toward the optimum 7.4 value. Should excess alkalinity take place, carbon dioxide from the lungs can be reabsorbed to form carbonic acid, which will help the neutralization process.

Many biochemically important reactions take place because of either acid or base catalysis, including the hydrolysis of peptides and esters, the reactions of phosphate groups, tautomerizations (ketoenol equilibria), and condensations of carbonyl groups. Sometimes, the side chains of several amino acid residues in aspartic acid, glutamic acid, histidine, cysteine, tyrosine, and lysine act in the enzymatic capacity of general acid and/or base catalysis.

The kidneys, which are usually seen as the organs of excretion, also act as regulators in water, electrolyte, and acid-base balance. Acid-base balance takes place in the tubules of the kidneys through the exchange of sodium ions and hydrogen ions. It is regulated by the pH of blood plasma and the ability of the tubular cells to acidify the urine through proton and ammonia formation. The glomerular filtrate contains the electrolytes, acids, and bases present in the blood plasma. The cations are mostly sodium ions, while the anions are either chloride, phosphate, or bicarbonate. At a pH of 7.4, 95 percent of the carbon dioxide is in the form of sodium bicarbonate, while 83 percent of the phosphate is disodium hydrogen phosphate. Normally, most of the sodium ions are taken up by the tubular cells in exchange for the protons formed there. The sodium ions are then returned to the plasma after associating with the bicarbonate anions. The role of the kidneys is to stabilize the bicarbonate concentration and to neutralize the nonvolatile sulfuric and phosphoric acids. Base conservation by the kidneys takes place with the aid of ammonia formed by the decomposition of glutamine (via the enzyme glutaminase) and the amino acids (via amino acid oxidase).

Disorders and Diseases

Acids and bases are among the most important chemicals of the living being. Life depends on pH and acid-base reactions. The presence of buffers is also important for the optimum function of enzymes. Thus, in metabolic reactions enzymes have pH optima that allow the maximum catalysis of the substrate reactions. The means of maintaining a steady pH of 7.4 in the blood involve a mechanism for the regulation of acid-base balance, which includes water and electrolyte balance, hemoglobin, and blood buffers, as well as the action of lungs and kidneys.

The pH of different body fluids in human beings varies greatly. For example, the pH range of gastric juices is 1 to 2, while that of intestinal juices is 8 to 9. If the blood plasma pH of 7.4 for a healthy individual varies by 0.2 or more units, then serious medical conditions arise; if not corrected, they may lead to death. Such reactions occur primarily because the functioning of enzymes is sharply pH-dependent.

Life can be described as a continuous fight against pH change. Nature has equipped the body with the buffers and the various mechanisms that keep organs functioning. The kidneys, lungs, and skin all share the common role of controlling the ionic balance of the organism, and thus controlling the bicarbonate concentration and pH. Cell pH regulation is complicated, however, because of the heterogeneous nature of the cell contents. For example, mitochondrial fluid is more alkaline than that of the cytoplasm, which allows the establishing of a hydrogen ion gradient between these two compartments of the cell. Basic functions such as oxidative phosphorylation, which is the transfer of metabolic energy to adenosine triphosphate (ATP), are believed to depend on this hydrogen ion gradient.

When the blood pH is lower than 7.4, acidosis results. Most forms of acidosis are metabolic or respiratory in origin. Metabolic acidosis is caused by a decrease in bicarbonate and occurs with uncontrolled diabetes mellitus (as a result of ketosis, the excessive production of ketone bodies such as acetone), with certain kidney diseases, with poisoning by an acid salt, and in cases of vomiting when nonacid fluids are lost. Respiratory acidosis may occur with diseases that impair respiration, such as emphysema, asthma, and pneumonia. Under these conditions, carbon dioxide is not properly expired and, as a result, carbonic acid levels increase relative to those of bicarbonate.

Alkalosis results when bicarbonate becomes favored in the buffer ratio. Metabolic alkalosis is observed when excessive vomiting (loss of acid, in the form of hydrochloric acid) takes place, while respiratory alkalosis occurs with hyperventilation (such as that brought on by a high altitude). Mountain climbers reaching the summit of Mount Everest without supplemental oxygen were found to have pH increases to 7.7 or 7.8.

The chief cause of dental decay is lactic acid, which is formed in the mouth by the action of specific bacteria, such as *Streptococcus mutans*, on the carbohydrates (and their by-products) that are attached to tooth surfaces in a sticky plaque. The normal pH of plaque is 6.8, but lactic acid lowers it to 5.5 or less, which speeds up the corrosion of enamel and leads to tooth decay. The application of fluoride-containing substances directly to the teeth or the drinking of fluoride-containing water changes the composition of teeth and forms a new substance called fluorapatite, which forms a new enamel that is much more resistant to acidity.

Perspective and Prospects

Acids and bases have been known to human beings since ancient times. The word "acid" is derived from the Latin *acidus* (sour) and has been redefined several times over the centuries. Alchemists have considered an acid as a substance with a sour taste which dissolved many metals and reacted with alkalies to form salts. The French scientist Antoine-Laurent Lavoisier (1743-1794) insisted that an acid should involve the presence of oxygen. In 1810, the English chemist Sir Humphry Davy (1778-1829) showed that hydrogen is the element that all acids have in common. In 1840, German Justus von Liebig (1803-1873) redefined an acid as a compound that contains hydrogen and produces hydrogen gas upon reaction with metals. His definition coincided with the theories postulated separately by the Swedish chemist Svante A. Arrhenius (1859-1927) and the German chemist Carl W. Ostwald (1883-1943), who also pointed out that bases were substances that carried a hydroxyl group.

In 1909, the Danish chemist Søren Peter Lauritz Sørensen (1868-1939) proposed the pH system, which has become the standard measure of acidity. In separate works announced in 1923, Johannes N. Brønsted (1879-1947) and Thomas M. Lowry supported the Arrhenius-Ostwald theory and went further to postulate that the hydrogen ion is never found in the free state but instead exists in combination with another base (for example with water, when the hydrogen is in an aqueous solution). As a result, their work broadened the definition of a base, which according to them would include any compound that was a proton (hydrogen ion) acceptor. In 1938, American Gilbert N. Lewis (1875-1946) broadened even further the acid-base concept: An acid is an electron pair acceptor, while a base is an electron pair donor. In 1963, Ralph Gottfrid Pearson proposed the simple and effective way of classifying acids and bases as hard or soft.

—*Soraya Ghayourmanesh, Ph.D.*

See also Cells; Cytology; Enzymes; Fluids and electrolytes; Food biochemistry; Kidneys; Metabolism; Respiration.

For Further Information:

Berg, Jeremy M., John L. Tymoczko, and Lubert Stryer. *Biochemistry*. 6th ed. New York: W. H. Freeman, 2007. An advanced text in biochemistry. Acids and bases are discussed in "Part I: Molecular Design of Life."

Bishop, Michael L., Edward P. Fody, and Larry Schoeff, eds. *Clinical Chemistry: Principles, Procedures, Correlations*. 5th ed. Philadelphia: Lippincott Williams & Wilkins, 2005. An advanced text on clinical chemistry. Discusses acid-base balance and ways of measuring the oxygen and carbon dioxide pressures. Also provides case studies.

Caret, Robert L., Joseph J. Topping, and Katherine J. Denniston. *Principles and Applications of Organic and Biological Chemistry*. 2d ed. Dubuque, Iowa: Wm. C. Brown, 1997. A simple introductory text for the health sciences. Chapter 2, "Chemical Change," describes acid-base chemistry and its applications.

Petrucci, Ralph H., William S. Harwood, and F. Geoffrey Herring. *General Chemistry: Principles and Modern Applications*. 8th ed. Upper Saddle River, N.J.: Prentice Hall, 2002. A general chemistry text for undergraduates that covers acids and bases.

Sackheim, George I., and Dennis D. Lehman. *Chemistry for the Health Sciences*. 8th ed. Upper Saddle River, N.J.: Prentice-Hall, 1998. An accessible guide to the chemical processes involved in human health. Stresses the relationship between inorganic chemistry and the life processes, with a focus on acids and bases.

Voet, Donald, and Judith G. Voet. *Biochemistry*. 3d ed. Hoboken, N.J.: John Wiley & Sons, 2004. A text that approaches biochemistry via organic chemistry reactions.

Acid reflux disease

Disease/disorder

Also known as: Gastroesophageal reflux disease (GERD)

Anatomy or system affected: Gastrointestinal system, mouth, stomach, throat

Specialties and related fields: Gastroenterology

Definition: A chronic digestive disorder in which the lower esophageal sphincter (LES), designed to keep digestive juices in the stomach, relaxes and permits gastric acid to rise into the esophagus, causing a burning sensation.

Key terms:

barium study: a medical procedure in which the patient drinks a liquid barium sulfate mixture prior to undergoing an X-ray examination of the chest and abdomen; used to identify problems in the upper gastrointestinal tract

esophagus: the gullet and beginning of the digestive tract

heartburn: a burning sensation generally felt in the chest and below the breastbone, often extending from the neck into the chest, in which acid and pepsin rise from the stomach into the esophagus

hiatal hernia: a condition in which a portion of the stomach protrudes into the chest cavity through an opening in the diaphragm

upper endoscopy: a medical procedure in which the physician inserts a flexible tube down the throat to inspect and examine the lining of the esophagus, stomach, and small intestine; to assess injuries; and to take biopsies (tissue samples)

CAUSES AND SYMPTOMS

Approximately one-third of Americans experience heartburn at least once a month, and 10 percent experience the sensation daily. Heartburn reportedly affects sufferers during the day and at night, impacting their job performance as well as their sleep. Heartburn is the major symptom of acid reflux disease, also called gastroesophageal reflux disease (GERD). A burning sensation radiating up through the middle of the chest behind the sternum (breastbone) characterizes heartburn, which can be aggravated by a variety of foods; alcohol; emotions such as anger, fear, or stress; and even particular positions such as reclining, lifting, or bending forward. Abdominal exercises, girdles, and tight belts can increase abdominal pressure and trigger reflux. Many women experience heartburn during pregnancy, especially in the later stages. Overweight people and smokers are also commonly affected.

Common foods and beverages implicated in acid reflux disease include coffee, tea, cocoa, cola drinks, mints, chocolate, fried and fatty foods, onions, garlic, citrus fruits, tomato products, and spicy foods. This list is not exhaustive, and certain people may be troubled by substances not included. Medications can exacerbate heartburn and reflux, including, but not limited to, oral contraceptives; aspirin; medications used to treat asthma, rheumatoid arthritis, and osteoporosis; antidepressants; and tranquilizers. Additionally, medical conditions such as asthma, diabetes, peptic ulcers, and some cancers may contribute to acid reflux disease, as can treatments such as chemotherapy or narcotic use for pain management.

The lower esophageal sphincter (LES), which connects the esophagus to the stomach, acts as a barrier to protect the esophagus from the backflow of acid from the stomach. Normally, it works like a dam, opening to allow food to pass into the stomach and closing to prevent food and acid from flowing back into the esophagus. If the sphincter weakens or relaxes, the contents of the stomach flow up into the esophagus. The reason for this occurrence is uncertain, but it is known that sphincter function can be impaired by diet, medications, and nervous system factors. Other factors that can also contribute to acid reflux disease include impaired stomach motility or an inability of the stomach muscles to contract normally, resulting in a delayed emptying of the contents. The acid remains at the top of the stomach near the LES rather than moving downward, creating pressure and reflux. Failure of contractions to clear the acid or a shortage of saliva to neutralize the acid may also contribute to heartburn.

Hiatal hernia, a condition in which a portion of the stomach protrudes into the chest cavity through an opening (hiatus) in the diaphragm (the muscle separating the chest and abdomen), exists to some degree in about 30 percent of Americans. In cases of hiatal hernias so large that they risk strangulation (becoming twisted and cutting off blood supply), complicated by severe GERD or esophagitis, surgery may be performed. Otherwise, medication in the form of a histamine blocker, which suppresses the secretion of stomach acids, is used.

TREATMENT AND THERAPY

Medical tests often used to evaluate the presence and severity of acid reflux disease include barium studies and upper endoscopy. Other tests performed less frequently include pH monitoring (to measure reflux over a twenty-four-hour period), the Bernstein test, and esophageal manometry. In the Bernstein test, which is performed after heart problems are ruled out, saline and

INFORMATION ON ACID REFLUX DISEASE

CAUSES: Relaxation of the lower esophageal sphincter, allowing gastric acid into the esophagus; aggravated by some foods, alcohol, some medications, stress, certain positions, late-stage pregnancy

SYMPTOMS: Burning sensation in chest and throat

DURATION: Chronic, with acute episodes

TREATMENTS: Diet and lifestyle changes (smaller meals, avoidance of some foods, etc.), antacids, histamine blockers, acid-pump inhibitors, surgery

diluted hydrochloric acid are infused into the esophagus to determine whether chest pain is related to reflux. Esophageal manometry measures pressure in the esophagus and LES.

Counseling patients to modify their diet and lifestyle is the basic treatment for reflux symptoms. Generally, patients should eat smaller meals more often and more slowly, avoiding spicy foods and those that increase acid production. They should not have bedtime snacks. Patients should relax both while eating and between meals. They should remain upright after eating and should not bend, strain, or lift for the following three hours. Those who are overweight should try to lose excess pounds, and patients should not smoke or chew gum. They should exercise on an empty stomach and avoid tight, constricting clothing which may put pressure on the stomach. Patients with GERD should elevate the head of their beds by placing blocks under the legs.

Over-the-counter antacids (Tums, Rolaids, and Mylanta, for example) can be effective in reducing or neutralizing acid in mild cases of heartburn. In chronic cases, however, histamine blockers may be prescribed. These medications act directly on the acid-secreting cells in the stomach to stop them from producing hydrochloric acid that can wash into the esophagus. Several of these medications (Tagamet, Zantac, and Pepcid) are available over the counter. Prokinetics or gastrokinetics are a group of medications that increase the speed at which the stomach empties food, acid, and fluids. In severe cases of GERD, they may be used instead of histamine blockers. Another class of medication is the proton-pump inhibitor or acid-pump inhibitor, which suppresses acid secretion in the stomach by inactivating the enzyme responsible for acid release in the stomach. These medications include Prevacid, Aciphex, Protonix, Nexium, and Prilosec (the latter is available over the counter). Additionally, chamomile, ginger, licorice, catnip, papaya, pineapple, marshmallow root, and fennel have all been said to aid in digestion.

Approximately 95 percent of GERD cases are controlled by medication; the remainder require surgery (fundoplication) to tighten the LES. Another technique is radiofrequency ablation, which applies controlled radiofrequency energy to the LES and upper part of the stomach, causing the lining to expand slightly as the valve tightens. The Bard endoscopic suturing system places stitches on either side of the sphincter; as the physician ties the sutures together, the valve tightens.

—Marcia J. Weiss, M.A., J.D.

See also Gastroenterology; Gastroenterology, pediatric; Gastrointestinal disorders; Gastrointestinal system; Heartburn; Hernia; Hernia repair; Indigestion; Over-the-counter medications; Stress; Stress reduction; Vagotomy.

For Further Information:

Lasalandra, Michael. *The Sensitive Gut*. New York: Fireside, 2000.

Rosenthal, M. Sara. *Fifty Ways to Relieve Heartburn, Reflux, and Ulcers*. Chicago: Contemporary Books, 2001.

Sachar, David B., Jerome D. Waye, and Blair S. Lewis, eds. *Pocket Guide to Gastroenterology*. Baltimore: Williams & Wilkins, 1991.

Acne

Disease/disorder

Anatomy or system affected: Skin

Specialties and related fields: Dermatology, family medicine, pediatrics

Definition: A group of skin disorders, the most common of which, acne vulgaris, usually affects teenagers; another form, acne rosacea, usually afflicts older people.

Key terms:

acne rosacea: a skin eruption that usually appears between the ages of thirty and fifty; unlike acne vulgaris, it is not characterized by comedones

acne vulgaris: a skin eruption that usually occurs in puberty and is characterized by the development of comedones, which may be inflamed

comedo (pl. *comedos, comedones):* the major lesion in acne vulgaris; it occurs when a hair follicle fills with keratin, sebum, and other matter, and may become infected

pilosebaceous: referring to hair follicles and the sebaceous glands

sebaceous glands: glands in the skin that usually open into the hair follicles

sebum: a semifluid, fatty substance secreted by the sebaceous glands into the hair follicles

testosterone: the most potent male hormone, which exists in both sexes; it starts the chain of events that leads to acne vulgaris

Causes and Symptoms

Many skin disorders are grouped together as acne. The two most common are acne vulgaris and acne rosacea. Other acne diseases include neonatal acne and infantile acne, seen respectively in newborn babies and infants. Drug acne is a consequence of the administration of such medications as corticosteroids, iodides, bromides, anticonvulsants, lithium preparations, and oral contraceptives, to name some of the more common agents that are sometimes involved in acne outbreaks. Pomade acne and acne cosmetica are associated with the use of greasy or sensitizing substances on the skin, such as hair oil, suntan lotions, cosmetics, soap, and shampoo. They may be the sole cause of acne in some individuals or may aggravate existing outbreaks of acne vulgaris. Occupational acne, as the name implies, is associated with exposure to skin irritants in the workplace. Chemicals, waxes, greases, and other substances may be involved. Acné excoriée des jeunes filles, or acne in young girls, is thought to be associated with emotional distress. In spite of the name, it can occur in boys as well. Two forms of acne are seen in young women. One is pyoderma faciale, a skin eruption that always occurs on the face. The other is perioral dermatitis (*peri*, around; *ora*, the mouth), characterized by redness, pimples, and pustules. Acne conglobata is a rare but severe skin disorder that is seen in men between the ages of eighteen and thirty.

In acne vulgaris, a disruption occurs in the normal activity of the pilosebaceous units of the dermis, the layer of the skin that contains the blood vessels, nerves and nerve endings, glands, and hair follicles. Ordinarily, the sebaceous glands secrete sebum into the hair follicles, where it travels up hair shafts and onto the outer surface of the skin, to maintain proper hydration of the hair and skin and prevent loss of moisture. In acne vulgaris, the amount of sebum increases greatly, and the hair shaft that allows it to escape becomes plugged, holding in the sebum.

Acne vulgaris usually occurs during puberty and is the result of some of the hormones released at that time to help the child become an adult. One of the major hormones is testosterone, an androgen (*andros*, man or manhood; *gen*, generating or causing), so called because it brings about bodily changes that convert a boy into a man. In boys, testosterone and other male hormones cause sexual organs to mature. Hair begins to grow on the chest and face and in pubic areas and armpits. Musculature is increased, and the larynx (voice box) is enlarged, so the voice deepens. In males, testosterone and other male hormones are produced primarily in the testicles. In girls, estrogens and other female hormones are released during puberty, directing the passage of the child from girlhood to womanhood. Testosterone is also produced, mostly in the ovaries and the adrenal glands.

In both sexes during puberty, testosterone is taken up by the pilosebaceous glands and converted to dihydrotestosterone, a substance that causes an increase in the

Development of Acne

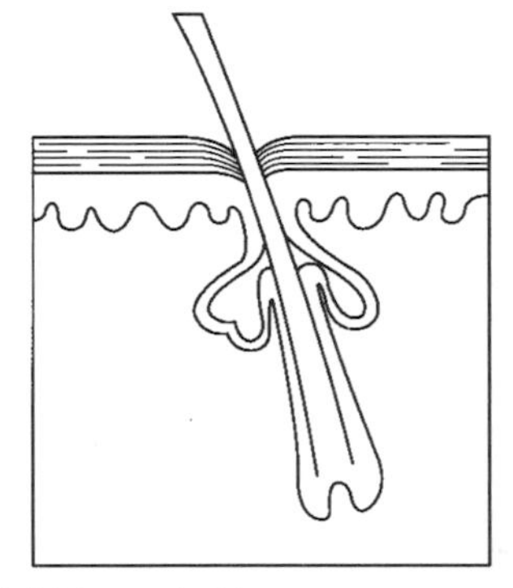

(1) Normal skin

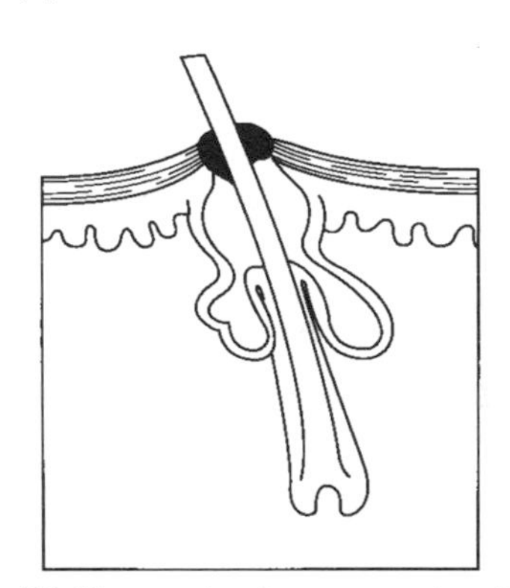

(2) Clogged sebaceous gland

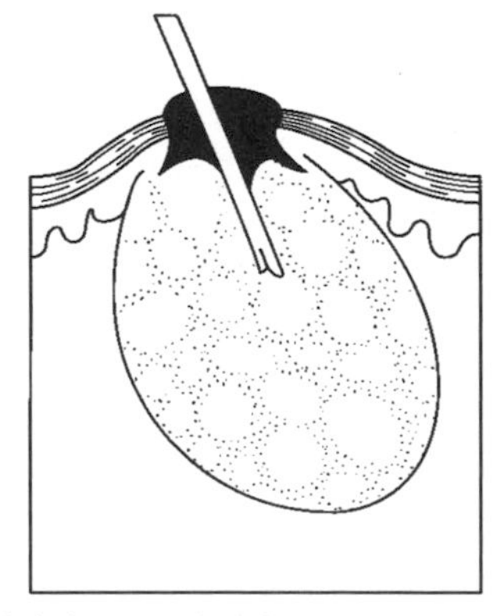

(3) Acne vulgaris

INFORMATION ON ACNE

CAUSES: Medications, greasy substances or irritants, hormones
SYMPTOMS: Skin lesions, inflammation
DURATION: Often chronic
TREATMENTS: Drying agents (resorcinol, salicylic acid, sulfur); vitamin A acid (Retin A, tretinoin); topical antibiotics (benzoyl peroxide, tetracycline, clindamycin, erythromycin); oral antibiotics (tetracycline)

size of the glands and increased secretion of the fatty substance sebum into hair follicles. At the same time, a process occurs that closes off the hair follicle, allowing sebum, keratin, and other matter to collect. This process is called intrafollicular hyperkeratosis (from *intra*, inside, *follicular*, referring to the follicle, *hyper*, excessive, and *keratosis*, production of keratin). Keratin buildup creates a plug that blocks the follicle opening and permits the accumulation of sebum, causing the formation of a closed comedo. As more and more material collects, the comedo becomes visible as a white-capped pimple, or whitehead. Closed comedones are the precursors of the papules, pustules, nodules, and cysts characteristic of acne vulgaris. *Papula* means "pimple," a pustule is a pimple containing pus, *nodus* means a small knot, and the word "cyst" comes from *kystis*, meaning "bladder," or in this case a sac filled with semisolid material. Sometimes cysts are referred to generically as sebaceous cysts, but the material inside is usually keratin.

Another lesion in acne vulgaris, called an open comedo, occurs when a sac in the outer layer of the skin fills with keratin, sebum, and other matter. Unlike the closed comedo, it is open to the surface of the skin and the material inside appears black—hence the term "blackhead." Blackheads are unsightly, make the skin look dirty, and suggest that they are caused by bad hygienic habits. This is not true, but exactly why the material in the sac turns black is not fully understood. Some believe that the natural skin pigment melanin is involved.

Blackheads are usually easily managed and rarely become inflamed. It is the closed comedo, or whitehead, that causes the disfiguring lesions of acne vulgaris. As the closed comedo fills with keratin and sebum, colonies of bacteria, usually *Propionibacterium acnes*, develop at the site. The bacteria secrete enzymes that break down the sebum, forming free fatty acids that inflame and irritate the follicle wall. With inflammation, white blood cells are drawn to the area to fight off the bacteria.

The comedo enlarges with further accumulation of white blood cells, keratin, and sebum until the follicle wall ruptures, spreading inflammation. If the inflammation is close to the surface of the skin, the lesion will usually be a pustule. If the inflammation is deeper, a larger papule, nodule, or cyst may form.

Clothing, cosmetics, and other factors may exacerbate acne vulgaris. Headbands, chin straps, and other items can cause trauma that ruptures closed comedones and spreads infection. Ingredients in cosmetics, soaps, and other preparations used on the skin can contribute to the formation of comedones in acne vulgaris. Lanolin, petrolatum, laurel alcohol, and oleic acid are among the chemicals commonly found in skin creams, cosmetics, soaps, shampoos, and other preparations applied to the skin. They have been shown to aggravate existing acne in some people and to bring on acne eruptions in others.

It was long thought that fatty foods—such as chocolate, ice cream, desserts, and peanut butter—contributed to acne, perhaps because teenagers eat so much of them. This theory has been largely discarded. Except for specific allergic sensitivities, foods do not appear to cause or in any other way affect the eruptions of acne vulgaris.

Cases of acne vulgaris are classified as mild, moderate, or severe. In mild and moderate acne vulgaris, the number of lesions ranges from a few to many, appearing regularly or sporadically and occurring mostly in the top layer of the skin. Consequently, these cases are sometimes called "superficial acne." In severe cases, the acne lesions are deep, extending down into the skin, and characterized by inflamed papules and pustules.

Superficial acne, or mild-to-moderate acne vulgaris, is easily managed with the therapies available. The teenager goes through a year to two dealing with "zits." The problem may be irritating and may cause inconvenience and discomfort, but it is common among teenagers, and little lasting harm is done. With time and treatment, the skin clears and the problem is over.

With deep or severe acne, however, the condition can be devastating, physically and psychologically. In these cases, the lesions may come in massive eruptions that cover the face and extend to the neck, chest, and back. The lesions can be large and deep, frequently causing disfiguring pits and craters that become lifelong scars. The victims of severe acne can suffer profound psychological damage. The disease strikes at a time when most teenagers are especially concerned with being gregarious, popular, and well liked. The chronic, constant disfigurement effectively isolates the individual, however, often making him or her unwilling to risk social contact.

The other common form of acne is acne rosacea, so called because of the "rosy" color that appears on the face. Unlike acne vulgaris, it rarely strikes people under thirty years of age and is not characterized by comedones, although papules and pustules are common. It is predominantly seen in women, although its most serious manifestations are seen in men. The cause of acne rosacea is unknown, but it is more likely to strike people with fair complexions. It is usually limited to the center of the face, but eruptions may occur on other parts of the body.

Acne rosacea is progressive; that is, it gets worse as the patient grows older. It seems to occur most often in people who have a tendency to redden or blush easily. The blushing, whether it is caused by emotional distress, such as shame or embarrassment, or by heat, food, or drink, may be the precursor of acne rosacea. The individual finds that episodes of blushing last longer and longer until, eventually, the redness becomes permanent. Papules and pustules break out, and surface blood vessels become dilated, causing further redness. As the disease progresses, tissue overgrowth may cause the nose to swell and become red and bulbous. Inflammation may develop in and around the eyes and threaten vision. These severe symptoms occur more often in men than in women.

TREATMENT AND THERAPY

The majority of acne patients are treated at home with over-the-counter preparations applied topically (that is, on the skin). For years, many of the agents recommended for acne contained sulfur, and some still do. Sulfur is useful for reducing comedones, but it has been suggested that sulfur by itself may also cause comedones; however, sulfur compounds, such as zinc sulfate, are not suspected of causing comedones. Resorcinol and salicylic acid are commonly included in topical over-the-counter preparations to promote scaling and reduce comedones. Sometimes sulfur, resorcinol, and salicylic acid are used singly, sometimes together, and sometimes combined with topical antiseptics or other agents.

While most patients will be helped by the available over-the-counter agents, many will not respond adequately to such home therapy. These patients must be seen by a doctor, such as a family practitioner or dermatologist. The physician attempts to eliminate existing lesions, prevent the formation of new lesions, destroy microorganisms, relieve inflammation, and prevent the occurrence of cysts, papules, and pustules. If the patient's skin is oily, the physician may advise washing the face and other affected areas several times a day. This has little effect on the development of comedones, but it may improve the patient's appearance and self-esteem. The physician will also use medications that are similar to over-the-counter antiacne agents but more powerful. These include drying agents, topical antibiotic preparations, and agents to abrade the skin, such as exfoliants or desquamating (scale-removing) agents.

Various topical antibiotics have been developed for use in acne vulgaris, such as topical tetracycline, clindamycin, and erythromycin. One that is often used is benzoyl peroxide, a topical antibiotic that can penetrate the skin and reach the sites of infection in the hair follicles. It is also a powerful irritant that increases the growth rate of epithelial cells and promotes sloughing, which helps clear the surface of the skin. It is effective in resolving comedones and seems to suppress the release of sebum. Because it has a high potential for skin irritation, benzoyl peroxide must be used carefully. Physicians generally start with the weaker formulations of the drug and increase the strength as tolerance develops.

Vitamin A has been given orally to patients with acne vulgaris in the hope of preventing the formation of comedones. The effective oral dose of the vitamin for this purpose is so high, however, that it could be toxic. Therefore, a topical form of vitamin A was developed called vitamin A acid, retinoic acid, or tretinoin (marketed as Retin A). Applied directly to the skin, it has proved highly beneficial in the treatment of acne vulgaris. It clears comedones from the hair follicles and suppresses the formation of new comedones. It reduces inflammation and facilitates the transdermal (through-the-skin) penetration of medications such as benzoyl peroxide and other topical antibiotics. Like benzoyl peroxide, vitamin A acid can be irritating to the skin, so it must be used carefully. When benzoyl peroxide and vitamin A acid are used in combination in the treatment of acne vulgaris, their therapeutic effectiveness is significantly increased. The physician generally prescribes a morning application of one and an evening application of the other.

When large comedones, pustules, or cysts form, the physician may elect to remove them surgically. The procedure is quite effective in improving appearance, but it does nothing to affect the course of the disease. Furthermore, it demands great skill on the part of the physician to avoid causing damage and irritating the surrounding skin, rupturing the comedo wall, and allowing inflammation to spread. The patient should be advised not to try to duplicate the process at home: Picking at pimples could create open lesions that may take weeks to heal and may produce deep scars. Sometimes, the physician will insert a needle into a deep lesion in order to drain the material from it. Sometimes, the physician tries to avoid surgery by injecting a minute quantity of corticosteroid, such as triamcinolone acetonide, into a deep lesion to reduce its size.

The physician may wish to add the benefits of sunlight to medical therapy. Sunlight helps dry the skin and promotes scaling and clearing of the skin, which is probably why acne improves in summer. The physician may suggest sunbathing, but an overzealous patient could become sunburned or chronically overexposed to the sun, thereby risking skin cancer. The beneficial effects of natural sunlight are not necessarily achievable with a sunlamp and, over a long period of exposure, the ultraviolet light produced by some lamps may actually increase sebum production and promote intrafollicular hyperkeratosis.

About 12 percent of patients with acne vulgaris develop severe or deep acne. In devising a treatment regime for these cases, the physician has many options to help clear the patient's skin, reduce the number and occurrence of lesions, and prevent the scarring that can disfigure the patient for life. Both the topical medications benzoyl peroxide and vitamin A acid are used, singly and in combination, as well as many other topical preparations. Nevertheless, these patients often also require oral antibiotics to fight their infection from within.

It may take weeks for oral antibiotic therapy to achieve results, and it may even be necessary for the patient to continue the therapy for years. Therefore, the physician looks for an antibiotic that is effective and safe for long-term use. Oral tetracycline is often the physician's choice because it has been proven effective against *Propionibacterium acnes*, and it seems to suppress the formation of comedones. Oral tetracycline is usually safe for long-term therapy, and it is economical. Other

In the News: Registry for Women Using Accutane

On March 1, 2006, the Food and Drug Administration (FDA) started iPledge, a registry designed to control use of the powerful acne medicine isotretinoin, sold under the brand name Accutane and also under the trade names Amnestreem, Claravis, and Sotret. The registry had been recommended by FDA advisory committees in 2000 and 2004 to help prevent birth defects in children born to women using isotretinoin and to collect information on the incidence of suicide among users. The manufacturer of Accutane, Roche Pharmaceuticals, had always strongly warned women of the dangers that Accutane use during pregnancy posed for developing fetuses. Even so, Roche reported that between 1982, when the FDA first approved sale of isotretinoin, and 2000 there had been 383 live births among women taking the drug; 162 of the infants (42 percent) were born with brain or heart defects or mental retardation.

Women of childbearing age registering with iPledge have to submit two negative pregnancy tests before receiving a prescription, have another test before each monthly refill, and agree to take two forms of birth control while using the drug—or else promise to abstain from sex for one month before treatment, while under treatment, and for one month afterward. Women have to sign a document acknowledging that they understand isotretinoin increases the risk of birth defects, depression, and suicide. Men desiring the drug are required to sign the document as well, to ensure that they knew why they should not share pills with female friends. Physicians prescribing isotretinoin and wholesalers and pharmacists who distributed it were also required to register with iPledge and agree to enforce the restrictions.

Many dermatologists were uncomfortable with the iPledge regulations. Although aware of the drug's dangers, they considered isotretinoin indispensable in treating severe cases of acne resistant to less powerful medications and were afraid that onerous conditions for access to the drug might discourage patients from obtaining medication that they really needed.

—Milton Berman, Ph.D.

oral antibiotics used to treat acne vulgaris are erythromycin, clindamycin, and minocycline.

Yet in long-term therapy with any broad-spectrum antibiotic, there is always the possibility that the agent being used will not only kill the offending organism but also destroy "friendly" bacteria that aid in bodily processes and help protect the body from other microorganisms. When this happens, disease-causing pathogens may be allowed to flourish and cause infection. For example, prolonged use of antibiotics in women may allow the growth of a yeastlike fungus, *Candida*, which can cause vaginitis. Prolonged use of clindamycin may allow the proliferation of *Clostridium difficile*, which could result in ulcerative colitis, a severe disorder of the lower gastrointestinal tract.

If, for any reason, the physician believes that oral antibiotics are not working or must be discontinued, there are other therapeutic agents and other procedures that may be helpful in treating severe, deep acne vulgaris. One medication that is highly effective, but also potentially very harmful, is isotretinoin. As the name implies, isotretinoin (meaning "similar to tretinoin") is derived from vitamin A, but it is both more effective and more difficult to use. Unlike the topical vitamin A acid preparations, isotretinoin is taken orally. It is highly effective in inhibiting the function of sebaceous glands and preventing the formation of closed comedones by reducing keratinization, but isotretinoin also produces a wide range of side effects. The majority of these are skin disorders, but the bones and joints, the eyes, and other organs can be affected. Perhaps the most serious adverse effect of isotretinoin is that it can cause severe abnormalities in the fetuses of pregnant women. Therefore, pregnancy is an absolute contraindication for isotretinoin. Before they take this drug, women of childbearing age are checked to ensure that they are not pregnant. They are advised to use strict contraceptive measures one month before therapy, during the entire course of therapy, and for at least one month after therapy has been discontinued.

Estrogens, female hormones, have been used to treat severe acne in women who are more than sixteen years of age. The aim of this therapy is to counteract the sebum-stimulating activity of circulating testosterone and to reduce the formation of comedones by reducing the amount of sebum produced. Estrogens cannot be used in males because the dose required to reduce sebum production could produce feminizing side effects.

Persistent lesions can be treated with cryotherapy. In this procedure, an extremely cold substance such as dry ice or liquid nitrogen is carefully applied to the lesion. This technique is effective in reducing both small pustules and deeper cysts. For patients whose skin has been deeply scarred by acne, a procedure called dermabrasion, in which the top layer of skin is removed, may help improve the appearance.

Although its cause is unknown, acne rosacea can be treated. The topical antiparasitic drug metronidazole, applied in a cream, and oral broad-spectrum antibiotics such as tetracycline have been found effective. It may be necessary to continue antibiotic therapy for a long period of time, but the treatment is usually effective. Surgery may be required to correct the bulbous nose that sometimes occurs with this condition.

PERSPECTIVE AND PROSPECTS

Most acne vulgaris (about 60 percent) is treated at home. There has been significant improvement in the treatment of mild-to-moderate acne vulgaris, so for most of these patients, the condition can be limited to an annoyance or an inconvenience of the teen years. Only recalcitrant cases of acne vulgaris are seen by physicians. Of those cases treated by doctors, the majority are seen by family physicians, general practitioners, and other primary care workers. Severe acne is usually referred to the dermatologist, who is skilled in the use of the more serious medications and the more exacting techniques that are required in treatment.

For at least 85 percent of those experiencing puberty, acne vulgaris is a fact of life. It is a natural consequence of the hormonal changes that occur at this time. It is not likely that any drugs or techniques will be found to avoid acne in the teenage years, as this would involve tampering with a fundamental growth process. It can be expected, however, that in this condition, as in so many others, progress will continue to be made, and newer, more effective, and safer agents will be developed.

—C. Richard Falcon

See also Abscesses; Blisters; Boils; Cysts; Dermatology; Puberty and adolescence; Rosacea; Skin disorders.

FOR FURTHER INFORMATION:

Ceaser, Jennifer. *Everything You Need to Know About Acne*. Rev. ed. New York: Rosen, 2003. Covers the different forms of acne, their causes, and treatment forms in an approachable manner.

Chu, Anthony C., and Anne Lovell. *The Good Skin Doctor: A Leading Dermatologist's Guide to Beat-*

ing Acne. New York: HarperCollins, 1999. Explores causes and treatments of acne, includes case histories, and discusses the emotional impact of acne.

Litin, Scott C., ed. *Mayo Clinic Family Health Book*. 3d ed. New York: HarperResource, 2003. One of the most thorough and accessible medical texts for the layperson.

Parker, James N., and Philip M. Parker, eds. *The Official Patient's Sourcebook on Acne Rosacea*. San Diego, Calif.: Icon Health, 2002. Draws from public, academic, government, and peer-reviewed research to provide a wide-ranging handbook for patients with rosacea.

Webster, Guy F., and Anthony V. Rawlings, eds. *Acne and Its Therapy*. New York: Informa Healthcare, 2007. Intended for dermatologists. Analyzes the physiology, diagnosis, clinical features, and control of acne.

Acquired immunodeficiency syndrome (AIDS)

Disease/disorder

Anatomy or system affected: Blood, brain, eyes, gastrointestinal system, immune system, intestines, liver, lungs, lymphatic system, mouth, psychic-emotional system, reproductive system, respiratory system, skin, throat

Specialties and related fields: Bacteriology, dermatology, epidemiology, gastroenterology, gynecology, hematology, immunology, internal medicine, microbiology, neurology, oncology, ophthalmology, osteopathic medicine, otorhinolaryngology, pathology, pharmacology, proctology, psychiatry, public health, pulmonary medicine, virology

Definition: A disease state caused by infection with human immunodeficiency virus (HIV), leading to a progressive deterioration of the immune system and characterized by development of any of a large number of opportunistic infections.

Key terms:

highly active antiretroviral therapy (HAART): the use of a combination of three or four anti-HIV drugs in an HIV-positive individual to suppress replication of new HIV particles and slow the progression to full-blown AIDS

Kaposi's sarcoma: a form of blood vessel tumor that produces pink to purple splotches or plaques on the skin in about 25 percent of AIDS patients and may also affect internal organs; caused by sexual transmission of human herpes virus 8 (HHV8)

lentivirus: a classification of retroviruses characterized by a very long incubation period (ten to twenty years) before symptoms of a disease appear

opportunistic infection: an infection caused by any type of pathogen in individuals who have an impaired immune system

Pneumocystis pneumonia: a form of pneumonia caused by the fungus *Pneumocystis carinii* and commonly seen in AIDS patients

protease inhibitors: any of a number of drugs that inhibit the assembly of HIV

retrovirus: a virus with ribonucleic acid (RNA) as its genetic material that produces a deoxyribonucleic acid (DNA) copy of the RNA to be integrated into a chromosome of the host cell, from which it will make new infectious copies of the RNA during the viral life cycle

seroconversion: the detection of anti-HIV antibodies in the blood of an HIV-infected person, who is then said to be HIV-positive

syndrome: a collection of symptoms associated with a particular disease state; an individual patient may show some, but not necessarily all, of these symptoms

T4 cells: also called CD4 cells or T-helper cells; a specific type of white blood cell (lymphocyte) which regulates the entire immune system and is the preferred target for HIV infection, resulting in immunodeficiency

viral load: a measurement of the amount of HIV present in the blood; often used to monitor the effectiveness of anti-HIV therapy

Causes and Symptoms

AIDS is caused by the human immunodeficiency virus (HIV), a member of the lentivirus family of retroviruses. This virus is thought to have arisen in Africa sometime in the early to mid-twentieth century from related viruses in the chimpanzee and the sooty mangabey monkey. The virus cannot survive long in the air and cannot be transmitted by casual contact. Individuals can be infected only by the exchange of certain body fluids, including semen, vaginal fluid, blood, and human milk. Other body fluids such as sweat, tears, saliva, urine, and feces may contain HIV, but the virus exists in such low concentrations that these fluids are completely ineffective in transmitting an infection. The most common mode of transmission is through sexual contact in which semen or vaginal fluid is exchanged. The presence of another sexually transmitted disease

(STD), such as gonorrhea, syphilis, chlamydia, genital herpes, or human papillomavirus, increases dramatically the risk of acquiring an HIV infection through sexual contact.

The second most common mode of transmission is through the sharing of needles contaminated with HIV-positive blood by intravenous (IV) drug users. A pregnant HIV-positive woman may transmit the virus to her child in utero, or more commonly during childbirth. Mother-to-child transmission may also occur through breast-feeding in which the virus is present in the milk. Early in the AIDS epidemic and before a blood test for HIV was available, blood and blood products from blood banks were sometimes contaminated with HIV that subsequently infected recipients. Indeed, more than 90 percent of hemophiliacs became HIV-positive through injections of HIV-contaminated clotting factor VIII. Because of the development of a heat treatment for clotting factor VIII and the screening of the blood supply, hemophiliacs are no longer at high risk for HIV infection. Although the blood supply is relatively safe today, a very low probability of acquiring HIV through a transfusion of contaminated blood still exists, as a recently infected donor may not yet test positive for HIV.

Although HIV can infect virtually all cells of the body, it has a strong affinity for cells of the immune system. The virus uses a cell surface receptor called CD4 to bind to the membrane of a cell. The CD4 receptor is found on many cells in the body but is in relatively high concentrations on the surface of a class of T lymphocytes called T4 or CD4 cells. The virus uses a coreceptor called CXCKR4, also found on the membrane, that promotes the fusion of the membrane of the virus particle with the membrane of the cell, thereby allowing entry of the virus. Persons who lack the coreceptor on their cells appear to resist infection by the virus. The T4 cells are also known as T-helper cells, as they produce a series of chemical signals called lymphokines that are needed for the development and maintenance of the entire immune system. While the body constantly makes new T4 cells, HIV has a very small edge in the rate at which these T4 cells are infected and destroyed. Thus, there is a slow but progressive decrease in T4 lymphocytes in the body and loss of immune function. This process may take ten or more years.

The clinical course of infection occurs in three stages. Initially upon infection, HIV produces an acute retroviral syndrome referred to as the prodromal stage, beginning about three to four weeks after initial infection and lasting for two to three weeks. During a retroviral syndrome, the patient experiences flulike or mononucleosis-like symptoms. The patient will believe that he or she simply has a moderate-to-severe case of influenza or, if the symptoms are prolonged, mononucleosis. During this period, HIV is rapidly proliferating, disseminating throughout the body and infecting lymphoid tissues. Viral load is high at this stage, and the patient is highly infectious. At the same time, the T4 cell count, which normally is about 1,000 per cubic millimeter, drops by about half. The patient's immune system will mount an antibody response against HIV, but these antibodies are ineffective in stopping the infection. When such antibodies are detectable, the patient is then said to have seroconverted. Anti-HIV antibody detection by a simple blood test is the basis for assigning HIV-positive status. In most cases, seroconversion occurs between six to eighteen weeks after initial infection, although, in rare cases, antibodies may not be detectable until later. By three months, 95 percent of patients will have seroconverted; by six months, more than 99 percent will have detectable circulating antibodies to HIV.

The second stage is called the clinical latency period or asymptomatic stage. Without anti-HIV therapy, this period may last ten or more years. It is during this time that the patient usually has no AIDS symptoms. Early in the latent period, T4 cell counts usually recover somewhat during the first year of infection, averaging approximately 700 per cubic millimeter. After that, there is a very slow decline. In the meantime, viral loads, which were high during the acute retroviral syndrome stage, drop by several orders of magnitude as the T4 count rises. At about one year into the infection, the viral load very slowly increases as the latent period progresses.

The third phase is full-blown AIDS. This usually occurs when the T4 count drops below 200 per cubic millimeter. Opportunistic infections and cancers become common, and patients may have several infections simultaneously. Many of these diseases are rare in normal, healthy individuals. Most common is *Pneumocystis carinii* pneumonia, a form caused by a fungus that is virtually unseen in individuals with a normal immune system. Indeed, the fungus is present in a majority of the population yet almost never causes pneumonia unless the immune system is compromised. As one of the functions of the immune system is to destroy cancer cells when they arise, immune impairment leads to development of cancer in about 40 percent of AIDS pa-

Information on Acquired Immunodeficiency Syndrome (AIDS)

Causes: HIV infection through the exchange of certain body fluids, then destruction of T lymphocytes of the immune system

Symptoms: Initially, flulike or mononucleosis-like symptoms, then none until opportunistic infections (candidiasis, cytomegalovirus, ulcers, *Pneumocyctis carinii* pneumonia, histoplasmosis, toxoplasmosis) and cancers (Kaposi's sarcoma, Burkitt's lymphoma) become common

Duration: Chronic, eventually fatal

Treatments: Surgery, chemotherapy, and radiation for cancers; antibiotics for bacterial and fungal infections; anti-HIV drugs (nucleoside analogues, reverse transcriptase inhibitors, protease inhibitors, fusion inhibitors)

tients. One of these cancers is Kaposi's sarcoma, a normally very rare tumor of blood vessels characterized by pink to purple spots or slightly raised areas on the skin. These lesions may also arise on internal organs, where they can impair function. Kaposi's sarcoma is caused by human herpes virus 8 (HHV8) and is sexually transmitted. It is primarily found in gay men with AIDS and not often seen in IV drug users or female AIDS patients. Other common cancers associated with AIDS include non-Hodgkin's lymphoma, leukemia, and brain tumors.

In 1987, the Centers for Disease Control (CDC) published the criteria for the diagnosis of AIDS, including the appearance of one or more opportunistic infections or cancers. Twenty-three different conditions were listed in the definition: candidiasis of the bronchi, trachea, or lungs; esophageal candidiasis; disseminated or extrapulmonary coccidiomycosis; extrapulmonary cryptococcosis; chronic intestinal cryptosporidosis (greater than one month in duration); cytomegalovirus disease (other than liver, spleen, or lymph nodes); cytomegalovirus retinitis (with loss of vision); HIV encephalopathy; herpes simplex causing chronic ulcers (greater than one month in duration) or bronchitis, pneumonitis, or esophagitis; disseminated or extrapulmonary histoplasmosis; chronic intestinal isosporiasis (greater than one month in duration); Kaposi's sarcoma; Burkitt's lymphoma; immunoblastic lymphoma; primary lymphoma of the brain; *Mycobacterium avium* complex or *M. kansasii*; *Mycobacterium tuberculosis*; other or unidentified *Mycobacterium* species; *Pneumocystis carinii* pneumonia; progressive multifocal leukoencephalopathy (PML); recurrent *Salmonella* septicemia; toxoplasmosis of the brain; and wasting syndrome caused by HIV. In 1993, three conditions were added to the criteria: pulmonary tuberculosis, recurrent pneumonia, and invasive cervical carcinoma. Moreover, the definition was expanded to include any HIV-positive person whose T4 count had dropped to 200 per cubic millimeter or lower or whose level of T4 lymphocytes had fallen to 14 percent or less of total lymphocytes.

Treatment and Therapy

As of 2006, no effective vaccine had yet been developed to prevent HIV infection. While a number of candidate vaccines have been under development and in clinical trials, none has proven successful. The usual strategies used with most antiviral vaccines in the past, immunization with attenuated or inactivated viruses, have so far proven ineffective for HIV given its significant rate of mutation. Control of the epidemic has shifted significantly toward prevention.

AIDS treatment and therapy fall into two categories: treatment of opportunistic infections and treatment of HIV disease to slow progression to full-blown AIDS. Treatment of opportunistic infections must follow established guidelines for the individual disease. Thus, in the treatment of Kaposi's sarcoma, surgery, chemotherapy, and radiation treatment singly or in combination are utilized. Bacterial and yeast or other fungal infections are treated with antibiotics. Although some medications may reduce the severity of viral infections, such infections are not easily treated. Because an AIDS patient may suffer from more than one opportunistic infection and/or cancer at the same time, simultaneous treatments often take a severe toll on the patient. The life expectancy for an individual who has progressed to full-blown AIDS is about two years. Death results from an opportunistic infection or cancer.

The second strategy for HIV treatment involves interfering with the viral life cycle with the aim of slowing viral replication. Anti-HIV drugs target several steps in the life cycle, primarily at the levels of reverse transcription or assembly. In 1987, the first generation of drugs was developed to treat HIV. The first effective treatment utilized zidovudine (ZDV), commonly called azidothymidine (AZT), a drug originally developed for chemotherapy of cancer. ZDV inhibits the viral encoded enzyme, reverse transcriptase, involved in copying the RNA viral genome into a DNA copy. As a result, a nucleoside analogue is inserted into the growing DNA, which stops further synthesis of the DNA copy. Other nucleoside analogues that have a similar effect included ddI, ddC, d4T, and 3TC. In a similar manner, the nucleotide analogue Tenofor blocks DNA replication. Nevirapine, delaviridine, and efavirenz are non-nucleoside drugs that bind directly to and inhibit reverse transcriptase. Although this group of drugs inhibits reverse transcriptase, their mode of action is different from nucleoside or nucleotide analogues.

The final step in HIV replication involves the cleavage of a large precursor protein into smaller structural proteins, an event taking place at the cell surface and followed by release of the completed virus. The cleaving enzyme is called a protease and is encoded by the virus. The second generation of anti-HIV drugs, which were developed in the 1990's, were protease inhibitors, drugs that interfere with cleavage of the precursor and prevent viral assembly. As a result, functional virions cannot be made. Saquinavir, ritonavir, indinavir, nefinavir, amprenavir, and ABT-378 are approved drugs in this class. Other types of anti-HIV drugs called fusion inhibitors interfere with entry of the virus into a cell. In addition, integrase inhibitors, a new class of drugs, have been in clinical trials. These drugs prevent the DNA copy of the virus from inserting itself into one of the cell's chromosomes. Thus the anti-HIV arsenal includes drugs that act at different sites or stages in the HIV life cycle.

The HIV reverse transcriptase makes numerous mutations during the synthesis of DNA. Consequently, resistance to individual anti-HIV drugs arises easily and frequently. Beginning in 1995, a new strategy for anti-HIV therapy called highly active antiretroviral therapy (HAART), also also known as "AIDS cocktail" therapy, was developed. HAART consists of using a combination of three or more anti-HIV drugs, including two reverse transcriptase inhibitors and at least one protease inhibitor. HAART therapy is very effective, as it has been estimated that it prolongs the life expectancy of an AIDS patient by three to ten years. Moreover, many patients with full-blown AIDS and in terminal stages of the disease have made remarkable recoveries when placed on HAART. In many cases, viral loads were dramatically reduced, T4 cells made some recovery, and the incidence of opportunistic infections was reduced. Another advantage of multiple drug therapy is that the probability of HIV developing simultaneous resistance to three or four different drugs is very low, extending the useful therapeutic life of the individual drugs.

The long-term effectiveness of HAART is underscored by an examination of the AIDS deaths in the United States. In 1981, the CDC began to track the number of AIDS deaths. Each year, the number of deaths climbed steadily, reaching a peak of 50,610 in 1995. In 1996, the first full year of widespread HAART therapy, AIDS deaths dropped by 25 percent, and they have continued to drop every year since. By 2003, annual AIDS deaths had decreased by 73 percent. While these statistics are very encouraging, about half of AIDS patients cannot tolerate the drugs. Moreover, those taking anti-HIV drugs often experience mild-to-serious side effects.

PERSPECTIVE AND PROSPECTS

AIDS was first recognized as a new disease in the United States in late 1980. Dr. Michael Gottlieb at the University of California at Los Angeles (UCLA) diagnosed gay men with *Pneumocystis carinii* pneumonia and Kaposi's sarcoma, diseases that in the past were extremely rare. In June, 1981, the CDC alerted doctors in a report on this new epidemic for the first time in the *CDC Weekly Morbidity and Mortality Report*. Shortly thereafter, *The New York Times* reported on the new "gay cancer." At first, the disease was called gay-related immunodeficiency (GRID). The name was changed to acquired immunodeficiency syndrome, or AIDS, in an August 8, 1982, article in *The New York Times*, representing the first time that the term was used in a publication. The change reflected the fact that this new disease was not restricted to gay men; cases involving intravenous drug users, hemophiliacs, and infants were being diagnosed. In January, 1983, Luc Montagnier and colleagues at the Pasteur Institute in Paris were the first to isolate the virus causing AIDS. It was given the name human immunodeficiency virus, or HIV, in 1985; previously, the virus had been given several names by different researchers. With the isolation of the virus, a blood test could be developed. Testing of blood and blood products started in March, 1985. A test called enzyme-linked immunosorbent assay (ELISA) screens for the presence of anti-HIV antibodies. Results once took weeks, but the test is now automated and is performed in less than four hours at a cost of less than ten dollars at publicly supported laboratories.

HIV has been confirmed in the United States since at least 1969. At that time, a physician in St. Louis had a young male patient with a variety of AIDS symptoms. After the patient died, the pathologist took samples of his tissues and froze them. Later, when tests to detect HIV became available, the tissue samples were tested and found positive for HIV. The oldest positively identified HIV sample came from blood collected from a male patient by a Belgian physician in Kinshasa, Democratic Republic of the Congo. The doctor had saved many blood samples taken between 1959 and 1982; thus, the earliest confirmation of HIV infection in Africa dates from 1959. The virus has probably been present in the human population for much longer, but without blood or tissue samples, this cannot be positively confirmed.

Two major classes of HIV have been identified: HIV-1, which arose in Central Africa, and HIV-2, which arose in Western Africa. HIV-1 and HIV-2 have long been known to be genetically similar to viruses know as simian immunodeficiency viruses (SIV) in chimpanzees (SIVcmp) and the sooty mangabey monkey (SIVsm). In 2006, scientists determined that in all likelihood, HIV-1 originated in chimpanzees from regions of the nation of Cameroon; as many as one-third of chimpanzees from some colonies were found to carry SIV. The first confirmed human infection was that of a man from the nearby Congo, who developed AIDS in 1959. However, evidence suggests that HIV may have emerged in humans as early as 1930.

The statistics associated with the AIDS epidemic are startling. In the United States at the end of 2005, an estimated 950,000 persons were living with AIDS; approximately 14,000 persons died from AIDS during the year. Worldwide numbers only begin to illustrate the extent of the epidemic. The World Health Organization (WHO) estimates that in 2005, over 4 million persons became infected with the virus, with nearly 3 million deaths. Nearly half of newly infected persons were in the fifteen-to-twenty-four age group. Nearly 40 million persons worldwide were estimated to be living with AIDS. In the absence of effective treatment, most of those persons will die, often after infecting others with the virus, and leave behind a generation of orphans.

It is hoped that several new medications in development will enlarge the arsenal of anti-HIV drugs. The success of HAART promises to extend the life of AIDS patients by many years. Current studies are testing whether it is better to start HAART therapy early after infection or to wait until T4 counts are declining. Additional studies will determine whether the therapy may be interrupted for varying periods of time. A significant issue is the high financial burden of such therapy. A typical HAART regimen may cost $1,500 to $2,000 per month. Although many people in affluent countries can purchase these drugs through insurance providers or government subsidy, this financial burden precludes the use of HAART or indeed almost any anti-HIV drug in Third World countries where HIV prevalence is so high. Thus effective prevention of HIV infections, through vigorous public education about HIV and AIDS, is absolutely critical. Such a program in Uganda dramatically reduced the incidence of HIV infections, showing the effectiveness of public education campaigns.

—Ralph R. Meyer, Ph.D.; updated by Richard Adler, Ph.D.

See also Epidemiology; Gates Foundation; Human immunodeficiency virus (HIV); Immune system; Immunodeficiency disorders; Immunology; Kaposi's sarcoma; Sexually transmitted diseases (STDs); Terminally ill: Extended care; Viral infections.

For Further Information:

Behrman, Greg. *The Invisible People: How the U.S. Has Slept Through the Global AIDS Pandemic.* New York: Simon & Schuster, 2004. The author addresses the effect of the AIDS outbreak on social and economic conditions both in the United States and in other regions of the world.

Ezzell, Carol. "Hope in a Vial: Will There Be an AIDS Vaccine Anytime Soon?" *Scientific American* 186 (June, 2002): 38-45. This article explores the failure of candidate vaccines and discusses the prospects for a future anti-HIV vaccine.

Fan, Hung, Ross F. Conner, and Luis P. Villarreal. *The Biology of AIDS.* 4th ed. Sudbury, Mass.: Jones & Bartlett, 2000. This small text covers the biomedical aspects of HIV and AIDS. It is written at a level understandable by a layperson.

Friedman-Kien, Alvin, and Clay J. Cockerell. *Color Atlas of AIDS.* 2d ed. Philadelphia: Elsevier Health Sciences, 1996. A collection of photographs depicting many of the opportunistic diseases associated with AIDS, such as Kaposi's sarcoma (including a photograph of Moritz Kaposi) and *Pneumocystis pneumonia.*

Keele, Brandon, et al. "Chimpanzee Reservoirs of Pandemic and Nonpandemic HIV-1." *Science* 313 (July 28, 2006): 523-525. A demonstration of the likely origin of HIV-1 in the primate populations of Cameroon.

Matthews, Dawn D., ed. *AIDS Sourcebook*. 3d ed. Detroit: Omnigraphics, 2003. This large volume is written for the layperson and covers all aspects of HIV and AIDS. Includes updated statistics and information on current research.

Stine, Gerald J. *AIDS Update 2007*. Upper Saddle River, N.J.: Prentice Hall, 2007. Each year, the author provides an update on all aspects of HIV and AIDS. Very useful for the latest information on the subject.

Acupressure

Treatment

Also known as: Shiatsu

Anatomy or system affected: Muscles, musculoskeletal system, nervous system, skin

Specialties and related fields: Alternative medicine, preventive medicine, sports medicine

Definition: A specialized form of massage used to stimulate the body's energy pathways.

Indications and Procedures

Acupressure is an ancient Chinese procedure which uses pressure from the fingertips, knuckles, or a blunt-tipped instrument called a *tei shin* to stimulate points on the body. (The Japanese version is known as shiatsu.) The rhythmic, moderately deep massage is used to treat muscular pain, migraines, insomnia, backaches, and gastrointestinal and gynecological problems. The procedure can be performed by the patient and is beneficial for relieving chronic pain and increasing the range of motion by loosening tight muscles. Practitioners claim that acupressure can alleviate fatigue because it opens blocked energy pathways.

Uses and Complications

Acupressure works on the body's organ, glandular, and muscular systems. Like acupuncture, acupressure targets designated points on the body along lines called meridians. Meridians are not nerve pathways; rather, they correspond to energy pathways through which healthy Ch'i (pronounced "chee") energy flows. (Ch'i is comparable to the Western idea of vitality or life force.) These body points are believed to correspond to various organs and body functions. Practitioners believe that when these points are stimulated, the balance of energy in the body is restored and the patient finds relief from physical illness or disease.

Muscle tension causes the large muscle groups to contract and so restricts the flow of Ch'i. The body is then out of balance, and the ability of the patient's body to deal with a physical problem is inhibited. Acupressure massage seeks to increase blood circulation, relieve muscle tension, and unblock energy pathways.

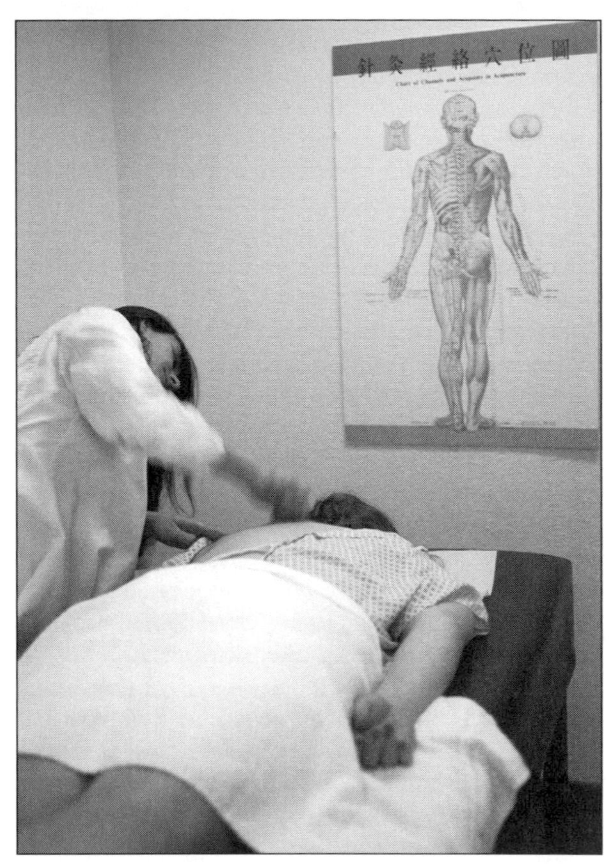

A patient receiving acupressure treatment. (PhotoDisc)

Practitioners of traditional Western medicine believe that acupressure stimulates the release of endorphins, the body's own chemicals that act as pain-blockers. Other benefits of acupressure have been recognized and accepted by traditional medicine. Acupressure is used in sports medicine to relieve muscle spasms and pain. The increased blood flow and muscle relaxation help to minimize possible or further injury to the body. Acupressure is often used in connection with other traditional Western medical treatments because no known risks are associated with the procedure.

—*Virginia L. Salmon*

See also Acupuncture; Alternative medicine; Anxiety; Circulation; Holistic medicine; Massage; Motion sickness; Muscle sprains, spasms, and disorders; Muscles; Pain; Pain management; Sports medicine; Stress; Stress reduction; Touch.

For Further Information:

Bauer, Cathryn. *Acupressure for Everybody: Gentle, Effective Relief for More than One Hundred Common Ailments.* New York: Henry Holt, 1991. Safer and easier to administer than acupuncture, this ancient form of massage can be used to relieve a multitude of physical and psychological discomforts from backaches and bee stings to anxiety and insomnia. Fully illustrated with charts and diagrams.

Cross, John R. *Acupressure and Reflextherapy in the Treatment of Medical Conditions.* Boston: Butterworth-Heinemann, 2001. Explores the methods and efficacy of acupressure and reflextherapy.

Gach, Michael R. *Acupressure's Potent Points: A Guide to Self-Care for Common Ailments.* New York: Bantam Books, 1990. Outlines the various acupressure points for treatment of various pain sites. The instructions for self-administration of acupressure techniques are specific and outlined in a steplike manner. The author also includes tips on proper eating and lifestyles.

Meeus, Cathy. *Secrets of Shiatsu.* New York: Dorling Kindersley, 2000. A handbook that provides shiatsu terminology, details the therapeutic value of the practice, and gives instructions on performing the technique on oneself.

Saul, Helen. *Healing with Acupressure.* New York: McGraw-Hill, 2001. Using diagrams and charts, demonstrates how acupressure can be used for relaxation and rejuvenation of muscles and joints, where the various acupressure points in the body are located, and how each point can be used to alleviate particular disorders.

Teeguarden, Iona Marsaa. *A Complete Guide to Acupressure: Jin Shin Do.* Tokyo: Japan Publications, 2002. Examines mind-body relations in the context of the practice of acupressure.

Acupuncture

Treatment

Anatomy or system affected: All

Specialties and related fields: Alternative medicine, anesthesiology, preventive medicine

Definition: An ancient therapy developed in China in which designated points on the skin are stimulated by the insertion of needles, the application of heat, massage, or a combination of these techniques in order to treat impaired body functions or to induce anesthesia.

Key terms:

Ch'i: Chinese concept of the vital essence; when Ch'i is unbalanced, disease results

meridians: designated pathways in the body with points that react to acupuncture stimulation

yang: Chinese concept of the positive, male element of the universe

yin: Chinese concept of the negative, female element of the universe

Indications and Procedures

The theory and practice of acupuncture are rooted in the Chinese concept of life—the Ch'i or qi (both are pronounced "chee")—which, according to ancient writings, is the beginning and the end, life and death. The belief, which has been handed down for thousands of years, is that all things, animate and inanimate, have an internal source of energy. This energy stabilizes the chemical composition of matter, and when this matter is broken down, energy is released. The Chinese view differs from the Western view of life in its adherence to the belief that human beings are all one with the cosmos, obeying the rhythms of the natural order. This oneness with the entire universe is represented by two forces: yin and yang.

Yang, the positive force in human beings and nature, is exemplified by powerful elements such as heat, energy, vitality, the lush growing period of summer, and the sun. Yin, on the other hand, is the passive, almost negative force that is most obvious during winter, when plant growth almost comes to a standstill and certain animals hibernate. The yin force is believed to be at work nightly in humans when they sleep. People who suffer from rheumatic pains frequently claim that they can forecast a change in the weather by noting the onset of those pains, and many people respond emotionally to the flow of energy in their bodies. They can feel either full of life or deeply depressed for no apparent reason.

According to the ancient Chinese system of medicine, two categories of organs are associated with the Ch'i: the Tsang and the Fou. The Fou is the group of organs that absorb food, digest it, and expel the waste products. They are all hollow organs such as the stomach, the large and small intestines, the bladder, and the gallbladder, and all are yang by nature. Tsang organs are all associated with the blood—the heart, which circulates the blood around the body; the lungs, which oxygenate the blood; the spleen, which controls the red corpuscles; and the liver and the kidneys. These organs are yin by nature. For the flow of energy to remain steady, it must pass unimpeded from one organ to another. If the organ is weak, the resultant energy that is passed on to the next organ is weakened. Acupuncture stimulates specifically designated points found on pathways in the body (called meridians) and corrects the problem.

According to the Chinese system, the human "circuit" of energy is made up of twelve meridians, which stretch along the limbs from the toes and the fingers to the face and chest. There are six meridians in the upper limbs and six in the lower. Ten meridians are connected to a main organ by branches from the sympathetic nervous system, and each of these meridians contains the Ch'i, which varies in strength and is governed by the nerve impulses arising from the organs. The meridians and their attendant vessels contain the flow of energy that enables the body to function efficiently.

The meridian points that proved to be effective for certain ailments were organized, and specific names were given to each. Later, the meridian line concept was hypothesized in order to explain the effectiveness of the points. These meridian points were selected by observing the effects of stimulation on particular signs and symptoms.

According to modern medical concepts, some of these points are thought to be relating points at which the autonomic nervous system is stimulated by a specific visceral disorder. Anatomically, some of the meridian points appear to correspond to areas where a nerve appears to surface from a muscle or areas where vessels and nerves are relatively superficially located, such as areas between a muscle and a bone or between a bone and a joint. These areas are generally composed of connective tissue.

The meridians are stimulated by the insertion of needles. The needles that are commonly used range in size from the diameter of a hair to that of a sewing needle. In China, round and cutting needles are commonly used. In Europe, the needles are slightly shorter and slightly wider in diameter.

The needles are made of gold, silver, iron, platinum, or stainless steel. Stainless steel needles are most commonly used. Infection caused by needle puncture is said to be extremely rare. This may be the case because the minor injury created by the needle is controlled by biological reaction. It is routine to wipe the skin with alcohol before inserting the sterilized needle. The needle itself may be wiped with alcohol sponges before each insertion on the same patient. Needles are discarded after being used in patients with a history of jaundice or hepatitis.

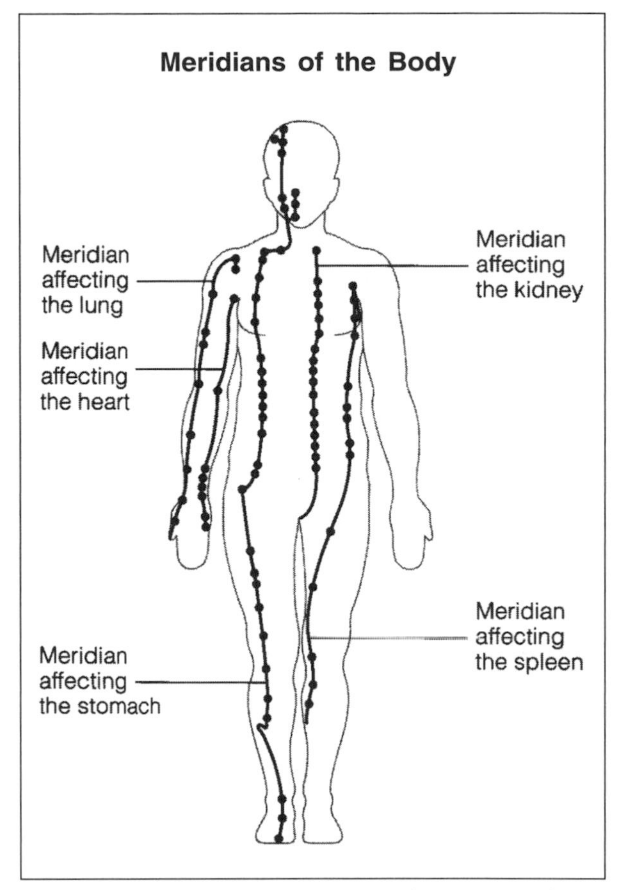

Acupuncture is an ancient Chinese medical practice based on the concept of meridians, channels in the body through which flows the life force called Ch'i; acupuncture involves the insertion and manipulation of tiny needles along these meridians.

Insertion of a needle requires great skill and much practice. There are three different angles of penetration into the skin: perpendicular, oblique, and horizontal. These angles correspond to 90 degrees, 45 degrees, and a minimum angle, respectively. The angles may be chosen on the basis of the thickness of the skin and the proximity to muscle or bone at the desired puncture point. The depth of penetration will vary.

Tapping (the tube method) is one method of insertion: When the diameter of the needle is small, this method is extremely effective. The needle is placed into the tube from either direction, and the tube is shorter than the needle. Gentle tapping of the needle handle with the right index finger introduces the needle easily. The tapping finger must be removed from the needle head immediately; otherwise, it causes pain. The tube is removed gently with the right index finger and thumb.

In the twirling method (the freehand method), the left thumb and index finger make contact at the acupuncture point. The left hand is called the pushing hand. Next, the skin is cut with the needle tip, after which the needle is inserted by pushing and twirling it with the right hand.

The objective of the advancement of the needle and the needle motion is to create a needle feeling in the patient. This is a dull, aching, paralyzing, or compressing feeling or a combination of these sensations that radiates to a distal or proximal portion of the body. When the patient notices the needle feeling, the operator increases the feeling by using various needle motions. Numerous motions are available, such as the single-stick, twirling, vibration, intermittent, and retention motions.

Light skin and muscle massage is recommended in order to prepare the body to accept needle stimulation. Prepuncture massage makes skin cutting easier and helps the patient relax. In addition to these advantages, massage may make it possible to detect pathologies such as nodules, spasms, pain, and depression. Postpuncture massage helps to confirm muscle hypersensitivity and the disappearance of pain or hard nodules that existed before the acupuncture was performed.

The amount of stimulation equals the strength of stimulation multiplied by the number of treatments; this is dependent on the sensitivity of the patient. Gradual increases of stimulation are essential. In general, for acute disease, treatment is usually given once a day for ten days and then terminated for three to seven days. For chronic ailments, treatment is administered once every two to three days for ten treatments and then terminated for seven days. The patient is placed in a supine, sitting, prone, or side position—the position that is most convenient for the patient and physician. A special position, however, may be needed in order to relax the painful area.

One of the most important factors to be considered in effective acupuncture is the accurate selection of acupuncture points. These points must be selected according to the specific ailment. The precise location of acupuncture points is crucial for obtaining the maximum therapeutic effect. This is difficult because of the different sizes and shapes of patients' bodies. Each acupuncture point is considered to be only about 3 millimeters in diameter.

Uses and Complications

Excluding pain caused by cerebral pathology, certain mechanisms of pain are universally recognized. These are causal factors (stimuli), such as inflammation or trauma, the peripheral nervous system, and the brain. Acupuncture, which is one mode of stimulation therapy, works by changing the pattern of passage of stimulation from the peripheral nerves to the central nervous system. Stimulation treatments such as hot soaks and the management of certain pain problems with physical therapy have long been in existence. Chinese medicine has accumulated experiences, analyzed the quality of stimulation, and organized its findings into a medical system.

The basic approach of modern medicine involves removing the causal factor of disease. In this approach, the pain associated with disease or with a surgical procedure may not be eradicated instantaneously, however, and the management of pain becomes an issue until the disease is cured or until the surgery and recuperation are complete. Controlling chemical receptors and reducing the sensitivity of those receptors is one way of treating pain. Intensive studies of the stimulation that causes pain have indicated that intrinsic chemical substances (polypeptides) such as histamine and serotonin, which stimulate the receptors, are essential for pain. Therefore, an antagonistic drug for these chemicals is often effective in controlling pain.

Although acupuncture is used to treat conditions as diverse as allergies, circulatory disorders, dermatologic disorders, gastrointestinal disorders, genital disorders, musculoskeletal disorders, neurologic disorders, and psychiatric and emotional disorders, the use of acupuncture for pain control (analgesia) can be described as the most basic level of treatment.

The English words "anesthesia" and "analgesia" are misleading when used to describe the freedom from surgical or obstetrical pain that can be produced by acupuncture. If "analgesia" is described as insensibility to pain without loss of consciousness, it is a more appropriate word than "anesthesia," which is described as an insensibility, general or local, induced by anesthetic agents, and a loss of sensation of neurogenic or psychogenic origin.

Acupuncture can produce numbness in any part of the body. The patient under acupuncture analgesia remains able to converse and cooperate with the surgical or obstetrical team. Obstetric patients are aware of uterine contractions and are able to use their muscles to bring forth the fetus. Surgical patients can tell when incisions are made but do not perceive them as painful. There is no loss of memory, as in hypnosis or general anesthesia, and no paresthesia (abnormal sensations) comparable to the sensations following local anesthesia.

Most operating room deaths and cases of cardiac arrest in the United States are caused by chemical anesthesia rather than by surgery. Patients who are poor anesthetic risks because of heart, liver, or kidney disease tolerate acupuncture analgesia well. Acupuncture is contraindicated for children under the age of seven, hemophiliacs, pregnant women, and people who have a fear of needles.

Acupuncture can be used to induce a feeling of well-being and calmness to allay the fear and apprehension most patients feel before surgery. It also appears to reduce both bleeding during surgical procedures and the incidence of shock. Postoperative acupuncture analgesia patients are spared nausea and the difficulties with urinating and defecating that frequently follow chemical anesthesia. Acupuncture analgesia does not mask symptoms as chemical anesthetics and analgesics do. The patient remains aware of his or her symptoms, but acupuncture diminishes those symptoms to a tolerable level.

Postoperative pain does not usually occur for several hours after acupuncture analgesia has been terminated. When it does occur, acupuncture can be used again instead of narcotics, and the treatment seldom needs to be repeated more than once or twice. Some acupuncturists leave small needles superficially inserted for several days to give postoperative pain relief. Others give regular acupuncture treatments, leaving the needles in place for twenty minutes per day for as many days as are necessary.

The main disadvantage of acupuncture analgesia is that it is less reliable than chemical analgesia or anesthesia. In some cases, acupuncture analgesia cannot be induced or becomes inadequate during a surgical procedure. It may not produce the relaxation desirable for some abdominal surgery. For this reason, backup chemical anesthetics and analgesics are also available in most cases.

The actual induction of acupuncture analgesia takes about twenty minutes—slightly longer than chemical anesthesia. In most cases, electroacupuncture instruments must remain attached to all acupuncture needles during the entire procedure, but these can usually be kept away from the surgical field. The more skilled the acupuncturist, the fewer the needles required. In China, major surgical procedures have been performed with only one acupuncture needle as analgesia and without electric supplementation.

The same type of thin (usually 30-gauge) stainless steel needles that are used for acupuncture treatments are used for acupuncture analgesia. In general, the points that are used to relieve chronic pain in a specific area are the points of choice for analgesia. To obtain enough analgesia for surgery, it is usually necessary to heighten the effect of the acupuncture needles by twirling them continually or by attaching electronic instruments to them to deliver a current of about two hundred microamperes, with a pulsating wave at a frequency of two hundred per minute during the entire procedure. The use of electronic instruments will usually increase the depth of analgesia or prolong an analgesic effect that is beginning to wear off.

Besides the acupuncture points for analgesia of specific areas of the body, points are often used to relieve anxiety and promote a feeling of well-being. Needles are usually inserted for twenty minutes the evening before surgery as well as for at least twenty minutes before the actual surgery begins.

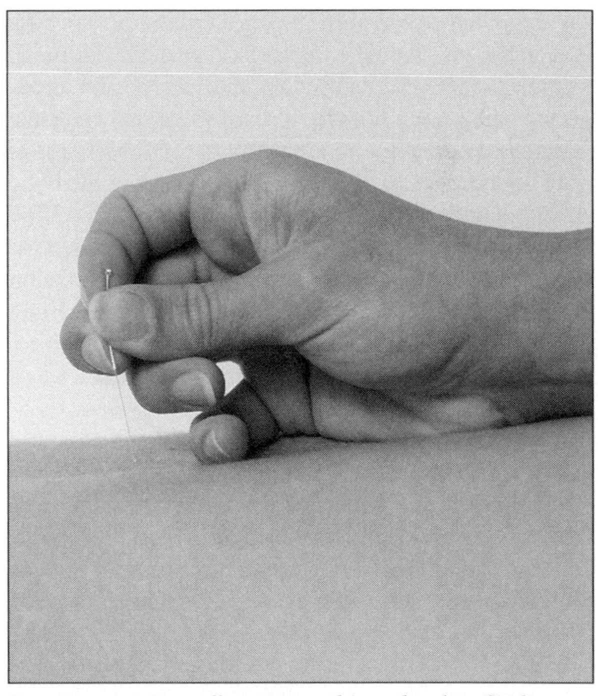

An acupuncture needle is inserted into the skin. Such treatment has gained in acceptance among Western health care providers, and many insurance companies now provide coverage for it. (PhotoDisc)

The theoretical principles of vital energy transmission are used in determining which acupuncture points should be effective for the anticipated surgery. Acupuncture points on meridians passing directly through, or in the vicinity of, the surgical area are usually selected. An attempt is made to use points on these meridians that are as far away from the surgical field as possible.

Perspective and Prospects

According to most reports, acupuncture appears to have been developed in the northernmost area of the middle region of China around 300 B.C.E. People in this area were primarily nomads, moving from one area to another in an attempt to avoid cold weather. They were peace-loving people but from time to time were forced to fight, either to repel invaders or to recover territory that had been occupied. The weapons they normally used were spears and bows and arrows, which inflicted grotesque wounds.

The high priests of China, like the high priests of biblical times in the Middle East, were also the society's physicians. These Chinese priests observed that men who were wounded in combat often reported the sudden disappearance of illnesses from which they had suffered for years. For example, a wound in a specific area of the foot would reduce blood pressure or relieve a headache or toothache, or an injury on the dorsal aspect of the knee joint would cure migraine. Over the years, the high priests recorded numerous observations of the phenomenon of a wound in one part of the body curing a long-standing complaint at another point. They discovered that it was the location of the wound that was significant. A pinprick in the correct location was enough to effect relief. It was noted that certain points of the body responded more noticeably to stimulation than other points and that frequently there was a direct correlation between the points that were responsive and a particular ailment. They were subsequently named meridian points.

At a later time, when metal was introduced to the culture, needles were used as an irritant at meridian points, and it was thought that pain from a specific ailment was diverted in a linear fashion through the meridian points to the surface of the body. Thus the concept of the "meridian line" was developed, and thus acupuncture was discovered.

At first, the surgeon-priests used fish bones and sharpened splinters of bamboo to effect the pricks. Later came finely honed needles. The warlords and nobles were treated with needles forged from gold and silver. As the science of acupuncture developed, it was discovered that the needles needed only to be inserted in a point of skin measuring about one-tenth of an inch.

The earliest book describing acupuncture was written in 50 B.C.E. It described the clinical applications of acupuncture with anatomical physiological references that were based principally on the concept of the meridian lines of the body.

In 1911, Yüan Shih-K'ai, who had trained in a modern Western culture, formed the Republic of China. Under his rule, old Chinese medicine—including acupuncture—which had developed from tradition and experience was unable to survive except in outlying areas of China. In 1949, however, when Mao Zedong formed the People's Republic of China, he tried to repopularize the old methods of Chinese medicine, which had been helpful to him. In the 1930's, when Mao and his followers were retreating to the north, he was forced to depend mainly on these traditional methods for medical treatment.

In 1955, Shyuken, a follower of Mao, stated his belief that acupuncture was effective in the management of illness. He wished to study the ancient Chinese way of medicine more systematically, comparing it to Western medicine, which he believed to be too analytical. Thus, a new medical movement began that united Western and Chinese medical practices.

Stimulation therapy using local heat, massage, and pressure has been known since ancient times. Long periods of observations and analysis by Chinese physicians of the effects on signs and symptoms of irritation of varying degrees at particular points on the body surface made it possible to relate specific points on the body (meridian points) to specific conditions.

According to ancient Chinese clinical concepts, the meridian points served as peeping holes into the body and passing holes for energy. The total number of meridian points was believed to be 365. Each was named according to its effect, anatomical location, appearance, and relation to the meridian line. These meridian points were selected initially according to measurements based on the patient's own unique anatomical standard (using the length between certain anatomical points; for example, between the shoulders). The exact location of a meridian point was then selected by the examiner, who felt with his or her fingertips the areas chosen by the initial measurement and observed the patient's response.

Acupuncture's popularity, like that of most techniques and discoveries, has waxed and waned throughout the years; for the most part, however, the Chinese have remained faithful to the five-thousand-year-old practice. The laws and methods of acupuncture have endured, although these methods have been increasingly combined with Western medical techniques. Gradually, the practice of acupuncture has spread throughout the world, particularly in France, Russia, Japan, Switzerland, Germany, and the United States.

In 1997, the National Institutes of Health (NIH) concluded that the efficacy of acupuncture is very promising and a worthwhile research endeavor, especially in treating postoperative chemotherapy nausea and vomiting and dental pain. It was noted that acupuncture could be useful in asthma and addiction treatment and in stroke rehabilitation. Research has identified many of the mechanisms of action in acupuncture, most notably the release of opioids and other peptides and the corresponding changes of neuroendocrine functioning.

In 2002, the National Health Interview Survey found that 8.2 million adults in the United States had used acupuncture and that 2.1 million had used it within the last year. Although the number of people who use acupuncture is significant, the Food and Drug Administration (FDA) reports exceedingly few complications.

A review of government-funded research studies on acupuncture in the years 2005-2006 finds numerous uses being evaluated, including labor stimulation, postsurgical wound healing, control of chemotherapy-induced vomiting, and the treatment of substance abuse, incontinence, autism, cerebral palsy, and depression.

—Genevieve Slomski, Ph.D.;
updated by LeAnna DeAngelo, Ph.D.

See also Acupressure; Addiction; Alternative medicine; Anesthesia; Anesthesiology; Anxiety; Circulation; Holistic medicine; Motion sickness; Muscle sprains, spasms, and disorders; Muscles; Pain; Pain management; Sports medicine; Stress; Stress reduction.

For Further Information:

Cassidy, Claire Monod. *Contemporary Chinese Medicine and Acupuncture*. New York: Churchill Livingstone, 2002. A good introduction to the history, theory, and practice of Oriental medicine. Includes pertinent discussions of acupuncture's effectiveness in pain management, HIV, women's issues, substance abuse, asthma, digestive disorders, and depression.

Ernst, Edzard, and Adrian White, eds. *Acupuncture: A Scientific Appraisal*. Boston: Butterworth-Heinemann, 1999. Examines acupuncture's possible mechanisms of action. Contains chapters on both Eastern and Western approaches. Reviews the evidence for the effectiveness of acupuncture and provides in-depth coverage of safety aspects.

Kidson, Ruth. *Acupuncture for Everyone: What It Is, Why It Works, and How It Can Help You*. Rochester, Vt.: Inner Traditions International, 2001. A good introduction guide to the principles of Chinese medicine that underlie acupuncture, on how to find a good doctor, and for what to expect from this form of treatment.

Manaka, Yoshio, Kazuko Itaya, and Stephen Birch. *Chasing the Dragon's Tail: The Theory and Practice of Acupuncture in the Work of Yoshio Manaka*. Brookline, Mass.: Paradigm, 1997. The definitive text by Manaka, one of the most famous acupuncturists of the twentieth century. Explains his treatment approach and his research in and understanding of acupuncture.

Mann, Felix. *Reinventing Acupuncture: A New Concept of Ancient Medicine*. Boston: Butterworth Heinemann, 2000. A practicing acupuncture therapist introduces the theory and practice of acupuncture.

National Center for Complementary and Alternative Medicine at the National Institutes of Health. http://www.nccam.nih.gov/. A search for "acupuncture" directs one to a plethora of information.

Stux, Gabriel, and Bruce Pomeranz. *Basics of Acupuncture*. Rev. ed. New York: Springer-Verlag, 2003. An updated reference on acupuncture that provides details about the procedure and explores Western science and medicine in the context of traditional Chinese concepts.

Addiction

Disease/disorder

Anatomy or system affected: Brain, nervous system, psychic-emotional system

Specialties and related fields: Psychiatry, psychology

Definition: A process whereby an organism comes to depend on a substance psychologically and/or physiologically. Physiological dependence is marked tolerance and/or withdrawal from the specific substance.

KEY TERMS:

abstinence: complete refrainment from the use of a substance of abuse

compulsion: a persistent, irresistible urge to perform a stereotyped behavior or irrational act, often accompanied by repetitious thoughts (obsessions) about the behavior

pharmacodynamics: changes in tissue sensitivity or physiologic systems in response to pharmacological substances

pharmacokinetics: the action of pharmacological substances within a biological system; pharmacologic substance absorption, distribution, metabolism, and elimination by an organism

physiological dependence: a state of tissue adaptation to a substance of abuse marked by tolerance and/or withdrawal

psychological dependence: need for a substance provided by its reinforcing properties, causing persistent desire to cut down or control use, use across varied situations to the exclusion of other behavior, use despite other worsening physical or psychological conditions, and/or great amounts of time spent finding, using, or recovering from substance effects

reinforcement: a process that increases the frequency or probability of a response

substance abuse: the continued use of a psychoactive substance despite repeated impairment, within a twelve-month period, of social, occupational, or legal functioning or continued exposure to physical hazards

tolerance: a condition in which the same dose achieves a lesser effect, or in which successively greater doses of a substance are required to achieve the same desired effect

withdrawal: a physical and mental condition following decreased intake of an abusable substance, with symptoms ranging from anxiety to convulsions and seizures

CAUSES AND SYMPTOMS

Addiction is a disorder that can affect any animal and may result from the use of a variety of psychoactive substances. Typically, it involves both psychological and physiological dependence.

Tolerance involves pharmacokinetics, pharmacodynamics, and environmental or behavioral conditioning. Pharmacokinetics refers to the way in which a biological system, such as a human body, processes a drug. Substances are subject to adsorption into the bloodstream, distribution to different organs (such as the brain and liver), metabolization by these organs, and then elimination. Over time, the processes of distribution and metabolism may change, such that the body eliminates the substance more efficiently. Thus, the substance has less opportunity to affect the system than it did initially, reducing any desired effects. As a result, dose increases are needed to achieve the initial or desired effect.

Pharmacodynamics refer to changes in the body as a result of a pharmacologic agent being present. Tissue within the body responds differently to the substance at the primary sites of action. For example, changes in sensitivity may occur at specific sites within the brain, with direct or indirect impact on the primary action site. Direct changes at the primary sites of action denote tissue sensitivity. An example might be an increase in the number of receptors in the brain for that particular substance. Indirect changes in tissue remote from the primary action sites denote tissue tolerance, or functional tolerance. In functional tolerance, physiologic systems that oppose the action of the drug compensate by increasing their effect. Once either type of tolerance develops, the only way for the desired effect to be achieved is for the dose of the substance to be increased.

Finally, environmental or behavioral conditioning is involved in the development of tolerance. Organisms associate the reinforcing properties of substances with the contexts in which the drugs are experienced. Such contexts may be physical environments, such as places, or emotional contexts, such as when the individual is depressed or anxious. Over the course of repeated administrations in the same context, the tolerance that develops is associated with that specific context. Thus, an organism may experience tolerance to a drug in one situation, but not another. Greater doses of the reinforcing substance would be needed to achieve the same effect in the former situation, but not in the latter.

Tolerance develops differently depending on the type of substance taken, the dose ingested, and the routes of administration used. Larger doses may contribute to quicker development of tolerance. Similarly, routes of administration that produce more rapid and efficient absorption of a substance into the bloodstream tend to increase the likelihood of an escalating pattern of substance use leading to dependence. For many drugs, intravenous injection and inhalation are two of the fastest routes of administration, while oral ingestion is one of the slowest. Other routes include intranasal, transdermal, rectal, sublingual, intramuscular, subcutaneous, and intraocular administration.

For some substances, the development of tolerance also depends on the pattern of substance use. For example, even though two individuals might use the same amount of alcohol, it is possible for tolerance to develop more quickly in one person than in the other. Two individuals might each drink fourteen drinks per week, but they would develop tolerance at different rates if one consumes two drinks on each of seven nights and the other consumes seven drinks on each of two nights in a week. Because of their patterns of use, the first drinker would develop tolerance much more slowly than the second, all other things being equal.

Withdrawal occurs when use of the substance significantly decreases or ceases. Withdrawal varies by the substance of abuse and ranges from being minor or nonexistent with some drugs (such as hallucinogens) to quite pronounced with other drugs (such as alcohol). Mild symptoms include anxiety, tension, restlessness, insomnia, impaired attention, and irritability. Severe symptoms include seizures, convulsions, perceptual distortions, irregular tremors, high blood pressure, and rapid heartbeat. Typically, withdrawal symptoms can be alleviated or extinguished by readministration of the substance of abuse. Thus, a compounding problem is that the addicted individual often learns to resume drug use in order to avoid the withdrawal symptoms.

Addiction occurs with both legal and illegal drugs. Alcohol and nicotine are two of the most widely abused legal addictive drugs.Over-the-counter drugs, such as sleeping aids and high doses of antihistamines and cough medicines, also have abuse potential. Similarly, prescription drugs, such as tranquilizers (for example, sedative-hypnotics) and antianxiety agents, have abuse and addiction potential. Common illegal addictive drugs include cocaine, marijuana, hallucinogens, heroin, and methamphetamine.

Not everyone who uses these substances will automatically become addicted. In the United States, for example, surveys have shown that approximately 65 percent of adults drink alcohol each year. In contrast, less than 13 percent of the population goes on to develop alcohol problems serious enough to warrant a medical diagnosis of alcohol abuse or dependence. Similarly, despite the fact that large numbers of individuals are prescribed opiates or sedative-hypnotics for pain while hospitalized, roughly 0.7 percent of the adult population is addicted to opiates and 1.1 percent is addicted to sedative-hypnotics or antianxiety drugs. Thus, the development of addiction often requires repeated substance administration, as well as other biological and environmental factors. This does not mean that anyone is immune to addiction; any person can become addicted to a drug given enough dosage and exposure.

When addiction is present, the consequences are multiple and complex. Substance abuse, for instance, is distinct from substance dependence. Substance abuse involves repeated use in hazardous situations or repeated use resulting in deteriorated performance in social, occupational, or legal functioning. Substance dependence usually involves a pattern of problems that have persisted for a year or longer. These problems are characterized by tolerance, withdrawal, unsuccessful quit attempts or repeated desire to quit, continued use despite psychological or physical problems caused or exacerbated by the substance use, increasing amounts of time spent on the substance, decreasing amounts of time spent on other activities, and loss of control over one's use of the substance. Loss of control occurs when a person uses the substance in greater amounts or for longer periods of time than intended.

In terms of health, there are many acute and chronic effects of addiction. With cocaine, for example, acute cardiac functioning may be affected, such that the risk of heart attacks may be increased. Similarly, individuals addicted to opiates, alcohol, and sedative-hypnotics must contend with such risks as falling into a coma or experiencing depressed respiratory functioning. Finally, the acute effects of any of these drugs can impair judgment and contribute to careless behavior and social problems. As a result, accidents, severe trauma, and habitually dangerous behavior, such as risky sex-

INFORMATION ON ADDICTION

CAUSES: Repeated use of psychoactive substances
SYMPTOMS: Tolerance; withdrawal (anxiety, convulsions, seizures); associated health risks (heart attacks, breathing difficulties, coma, cancer, cirrhosis, ulcers)
DURATION: Chronic
TREATMENTS: Cognitive and behavioral therapies; replacement drugs (methadone for heroin, nicotine patches for smoking); antagonists (naltrexone for opiates); metabolic inhibitors (Antabuse for alcohol)

ual behavior, may be associated with substance use disorders such as abuse and dependence.

Chronic health consequences are common. Smoking and exposure to secondhand smoke are associated with cancers of the mouth, throat, and lungs, as well as premature deterioration of the skin. Chew tobacco products have similar associations with cancers of the throat and mouth. Alcohol is associated with cancers of the mouth, throat, and stomach, as well as ulcers and liver problems. General malnutrition is a risk for heroin and alcohol users, since they often fail to eat properly. Injected drugs such as heroin and cocaine are associated with problems such as abscesses, hepatitis, and acquired immunodeficiency syndrome (AIDS), since shared needles may transmit blood-borne diseases. Finally, substance use contributes to health problems during pregnancy. Problems such as low birth weight in the children of smokers, fetal alcohol syndrome in the children of female drinkers, and withdrawal difficulties in children born to other types of substance users are well documented.

An emerging area of "new" addiction has been the phenomenon of Internet addiction, or compulsive use of on-line services such as e-mail and chat rooms. Such problems (such as gambling, compulsive sexual behavior, compulsive shopping, eating disorders, and workaholism) share features with other addictive behaviors involving substance use and are often studied together. Additionally, these behaviors may often coexist in persons who have use substances of abuse, so there is a clear need to study them simultaneously.

TREATMENT AND THERAPY

Because of the potential combination of psychological and physiological addiction processes, dependence is a type of disorder that often demands both psychological and pharmacological treatments. Typically, interventions focus on decreasing or stopping the substance use and reestablishing normal psychological, social, occupational, and physical functioning in the addicted individual. Though the length and type of treatments may vary with the particular addictive drug and the duration of the addiction problem, similar principles are involved in the treatment of all addictions. Similar strategies are used for problems of abuse. Because abuse is limited to problems that are more social in nature, however, pharmacological treatments often are not used for abuse problems alone.

Psychological treatments focus primarily on extinguishing psychological dependence, as well as on facilitating more effective functioning by the addicted individual in other areas of life. Attempts to change the behavior and thinking of the addicted individual usually involve some combination of individual, group, and family therapy. Adjunctive training in new occupational skills and healthier lifestyle habits is also common.

In general, treatment focuses on understanding how the addictive behavior developed, how it was maintained, and how it can be removed from the person's daily life. Assessments of the situations in which the drug was used, the needs for which the drug was used, and alternative means of addressing those needs are primary to this understanding. Once these issues are identified, a therapist then works with the client to break habitual behavior patterns that were contributing to the addiction. For example, a client would learn not to drive through neighborhoods where drugs might be sold, go to business meetings at restaurants that serve alcohol, or maintain relationships with drug-using friends. Concurrently, the therapist helps the client design new behavior patterns that will decrease the odds of continued problems with addiction. Problems related to the drug use would then be addressed in some combination of individual, family, or group therapy. Drug education is also important to help clients and family members learn about the dangers of continued use.

The therapy or therapies selected depend on the problems related to drug use. For example, family therapy might be more appropriate in cases in which family conflicts are related to drug use. In contrast, individual therapy might be more appropriate for someone whose drug use is linked to thinking distortions or mood problems. Similarly, group therapy might be most appropriate for individuals lacking social support to deal with stress, or whose social interactions are contributing to their drug use. Regardless of the type of therapy, however, the basic goal remains: facilitating the client's solving of his or her specific problems. Additionally, the development of new ways of coping with intractable problems, rather than relying on drug use as a means of coping, would be critical.

Cognitive and behavioral therapies have been quite useful for breaking the conditioned effects of addiction. Some psychological dependence, for example, is based on placebo effects. A placebo effect occurs as a result of what people believe a drug is doing for them, rather than from anything that the drug actually has the power to accomplish. In addition, the practice of using addictive drugs within certain contexts is associated with drug tolerance, such that certain situations trigger compulsions leading to drug use. In this way, cognitive therapy can be used to challenge any faulty thinking associations that individuals have made about what the drugs do for them in different situations. This may involve increasing patients' awareness of the negative consequences of their drug use and challenging what they perceive to be its positive consequences. As a complement, such therapies correct distorted thinking that is related to coping with stressful situations or situations in which drug use might be especially tempting. In such situations, individuals might actually have the skill to handle the stress or temptation without using drugs. Without the confidence that they can successfully manage these situations, however, they may not even try, and instead revert to drug use. As such, therapy facilitating realistic thinking about stress and coping abilities can be quite beneficial.

The first nationwide study examining the effects of matching treatments to clients with alcohol problems has concluded its initial phase. The United States-based study, Project MATCH, initiated in 1989, was supported by the National Institute on Alcohol Abuse and Alcoholism. It was designed to examine the effect of matching clients to one of three individual treatment approaches—cognitive-behavioral, twelve-step facilitation, or motivational enhancement—based on the psychosocial characteristics of the participants, such as severity of problems or the presence of other mental health problems. Results of this study suggested that all clients gain benefits from participating in assessment and treatment. Additionally, the data suggested that clients without other severe psychiatric symptoms do better in twelve-step facilitation treatment than clients with more severe problems, relative to the other two treatments.

Similarly, behavioral therapies are used to break down conditioned associations between situations and drug use. For example, smokers are sometimes made to smoke not in accordance with their desire to smoke, but according to a schedule over which they have no con-

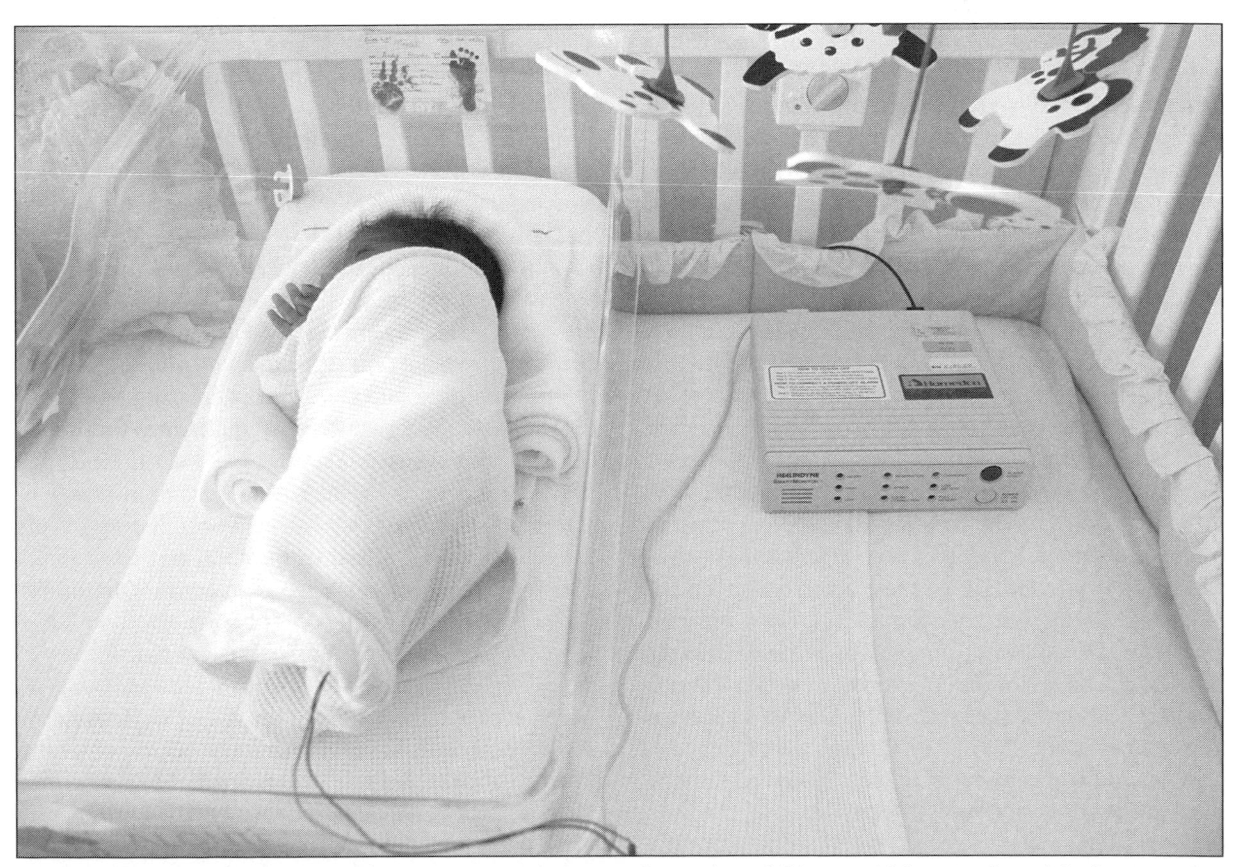

A baby born addicted to cocaine is monitored closely; women put their unborn children at risk by using harmful substances during pregnancy. (PhotoDisc)

trol. As a result, they are made to smoke at times or in situations where it is inconvenient, leading to an association between unpleasant feelings and smoking. While such assigned drug use would not be used with illegal drugs, the basic principles of increasing negative or unpleasant feelings with drug use in specific situations can be used. Rewarding abstinence has also been a successful approach to treatment. In this way, positive reinforcement is associated with abstinence and may contribute to behaviors related to abstinence being more common than behaviors related to drug use.

Pharmacological treatments concentrate on decreasing physical dependence on the substance of abuse. They rely on behavioral principles and on five primary strategies. The first strategy, based on positive reinforcement, is pharmacological replacement. Prescribed drugs with effects at the sites of action similar to those of the addictive drug are used. These prescribed drugs, however, usually fail to have reinforcing properties as powerful as the addictive drug and focus mainly on preventing the occurrence of withdrawal symptoms. Nicotine patches for smokers and methadone for heroin users are examples of replacement therapies.

A second strategy involves the use of both reinforcement and extinction, the behavioral process of decreasing and eventually extinguishing the drug-taking behavior. Partially reinforcing and partially antagonistic drugs are prescribed. The net effect is that the prescribed drug staves off withdrawal symptoms but yields less reinforcement than drug replacement therapy, serving to facilitate the process of extinction for the drug taking.

Antagonists, or drugs that completely block the receptors responsible for the reinforcing effects of the drug action, are prescribed alone as a third strategy. With this strategy, extinction is the primary behavioral principle in effect. The prescribed drug blocks the primary receptor sites and does not yield positively reinforcing drug effects. Even if the addictive drug is taken in addition to the antagonist, no positively reinforcing effects are experienced. Thus, without reinforcement, drug-taking behavior should eventually cease. Naltrexone, typically used for opiate addiction, is a good example of this strategy.

Punishment is another behavioral principle used in pharmacological therapy. Metabolic inhibitors, or drugs that make the effects of the addictive substance more toxic, are often used to discourage drug use. Antabuse, a drug often given for problems with alcohol, is such a substance. When metabolic inhibitors are prescribed, individuals using these drugs in combination with their substance of abuse experience toxic and unpleasant effects. Thus, they begin to associate use of the addictive substance with very noxious results and are discouraged from continuing their drug use.

Symptomatic treatment of withdrawal effects is used as a fifth strategy. Based on reinforcement, this strategy simply encourages the use of drugs likely to reduce withdrawal effects. Unfortunately, these drugs may also have abuse potential. For example, when benzodiazepines are given to individuals with alcohol or opiate dependence, one dependency may be traded for another. As such, symptomatic treatment is helpful but is not a treatment of choice by itself. In fact, none of these pharmacological treatments is recommended for use in isolation; they are recommended for use with complementary psychological treatments.

An exciting development has been the discovery of the utility of naltrexone, a drug commonly used in the treatment of opioid addiction, in the early phases of successful response to treatment for alcohol dependence when it is combined with psychosocial therapies. In addition, investigators have been studying how alternative medicine might be of use for substance use problems. Examples are the use of acupuncture and massage in the treatment of illicit substance use, such as stimulant use. While results in this area are promising, it is important to note that none of these treatments should be used alone but rather as an adjunct to traditional treatment approaches.

Finally, vaccines are being designed to help immunize people against addiction to such drugs as amphetamines, cocaine, nicotine, and phencyclidine (PCP). Vaccines are designed to create antibodies that attack the drug once it is inside the body but before it has reached the brain; proteins bind to the drug and prevent it from having its effects. The benefit is that it prevents individuals who use the drug from feeling the drug's effects, thereby decreasing the cravings for the drug.

PERSPECTIVE AND PROSPECTS

The use of substances to alter the mind or bodily experiences is a practice that has been a part of human cultures for centuries. Time and again, even through legislated acts such as Prohibition, drug and alcohol use have persisted. The continued use of drugs for recreational and medicinal practices seems virtually inevitable, and it is unlikely that substance abuse and dependence will disappear from the world's societies.

Consequently, an understanding of substance use, how it leads to addiction, ways to minimize the development of addiction problems, and strategies for improving addiction treatments will be critical.

At different times in history, addiction has been viewed as strictly a moral, medical, spiritual, or behavioral problem. As the science of understanding and treating addiction has progressed, the variety of ways in which these aspects of addiction combine has been noted. Modern treatments and theories no longer view addiction from one strict point of view, but instead recognize the heterogeneity of paths leading to addiction. Such an approach has been helpful not only in treating addiction but also in preventing it. Efforts to curb the biological, social, and environmental forces contributing to addiction have become increasingly important.

Addiction remains a disorder with no completely effective treatment. Of individuals seeking treatment across all addictive disorders, fewer than 20 percent succeed the first time that they attempt to achieve long-term abstinence. As a result, individuals suffering from addiction often undergo multiple treatments over several occasions, with some individuals experiencing significant problems throughout their lives. Many people, however, do make gains in treatment, so treatment should be pursued.

While no real treatment exists for addiction, researchers have made important strides in understanding some of the biological underpinnings of it. For example, in studies on cocaine addiction, it has been shown that hormonal fluctuations play an important role in women's responses to drugs. It appears that women have decreased sensitivity to cocaine, relative to men, and that this effect varies depending on a woman's stage of her menstrual cycle.

Researchers are also examining whether circadian rhythms may also be related to addiction. Moreover, since fruit flies and humans share genetic similarities, the flies are often used for the study of human conditions, such as addiction. New research on fruit flies suggests that sensitivity to cocaine appears to be related to the genes that control what is commonly called the "biological clock." In experiments using flies missing several biological clock genes, the flies did not become sensitized to cocaine. This suggests that biological clocks may be related to the development or maintenance of addiction to cocaine.

In this context, the challenges ahead are not to prevent all substance use, but rather to decrease the odds that a person will abuse substances or become addicted and to reduce harm for those already experiencing problems by getting them to treatment. Improved pharmacological and psychological treatments will be important. Finding new ways of tailoring treatment for addiction to the needs and backgrounds of the different individuals affected will be one critical task for health professionals, particularly as ethnic, racial, and cultural differences are better understood. Continued exploration of new pharmacological treatments to combat withdrawal, decrease cravings, and facilitate abstinence is necessary. Additionally, further research into the relationship among use, abuse, and dependence will be helpful in making diagnoses in this area of work even more useful.

—*Nancy A. Piotrowski, Ph.D.*

See also Alcoholism; Caffeine; Club drugs; Eating disorders; Ergogenic aids; Marijuana; Mouth and throat cancer; Narcotics; Nicotine; Obsessive-compulsive disorder; Psychiatry; Psychology; Steroid abuse; Stress; Weight loss medications.

For Further Information:

American Psychiatric Association. *Diagnostic and Statistical Manual of Mental Disorders: DSM-IV-TR*. 4th rev. ed. Washington, D.C.: Author, 2000. This manual provides detailed descriptions of the behaviors and types of symptoms used to describe and diagnose different addictive disorders. It is written by mental health professionals from psychiatric, psychological, and social work backgrounds.

Brickman, Philip, et al. "Models of Helping and Coping." *American Psychologist* 37 (April, 1982): 368-384. This article describes a four-model perspective on helping and coping with problems related to addiction. A classic in the addiction field, providing a good review of historical factors influencing different treatment models.

Dupont, Robert L. *The Selfish Brain: Learning from Addiction*. Center City, Minn.: Hazelton, 2000. Discusses the commonalities across different types of addiction in an easy-to-understand manner.

Julien, Robert M. *A Primer of Drug Action: A Concise, Nontechnical Guide to the Actions, Uses, and Side Effects of Psychoactive Drugs*. 10th ed. New York: Worth, 2005. A nontechnical guide to drugs, written by a medical professional. Describes the different classes of drugs, their actions in the body, their uses, and their side effects. Basic pharmacologic principles, classifications, and terms are defined and discussed.

Miller, William R., and Nick Heather, eds. *Treating Addictive Behaviors*. 2d ed. New York: Plenum Press, 1998. This book, written by medical and psychological scientists, is an overview of treatment strategies for problems ranging from nicotine to opiate addiction. Psychological, behavioral, interpersonal, familial, and medical approaches are outlined and discussed.

Schlaadt, Richard G., and Peter T. Shannon. *Drugs: Use, Misuse, and Abuse*. 4th ed. Needham Heights, Mass.: Allyn & Bacon, 1994. A good introduction to the complex issues surrounding addiction and drug use. Describes different drugs of abuse, legal and social issues, the differences between illegal and legal drugs, and continuing controversies.

Weil, Andrew, and Winifred Rosen. *From Chocolate to Morphine: Everything You Need to Know About Mind-Altering Drugs*. Rev. and updated ed. New York: Houghton Mifflin, 2004. This book on psychoactive substances provides basic information to the general reader. Psychoactive substances are identified and defined. Also outlines the relationships between different types of drugs, the motivations to use drugs, and associated problems. As the title suggests, the discussion ranges from legal, caffeinated substances to illegal and prescription drugs.

Addison's disease

Disease/disorder

Also known as: Chronic adrenal insufficiency, hypoadrenocorticism

Anatomy or system affected: Endocrine system, glands, kidneys

Specialties and related fields: Endocrinology, nephrology

Definition: A failure of adrenal cortex function in which production of any or all of the hormones synthesized by the cortex is decreased.

Key terms:

adrenal cortex: the outer portion of adrenal gland; produces a wide variety of regulatory hormones

adrenal gland: the gland located on top of each of the kidneys

androgenic hormones: any of several hormones that regulate the expression of male characteristics

corticosteroid: an adrenal cortex hormone that controls processes such as protein and carbohydrate metabolism and electrolyte balance

cortisol: a steroid hormone that regulates inflammation

glucorticoid: an adrenal cortex hormone that regulates a variety of bodily functions, such as inflammation and the mobilization of fat

mineralocorticoid: an adrenal cortex hormone that regulates the retention of minerals such as potassium and sodium

Causes and Symptoms

Anything that results in damage to the adrenal gland has the potential to cause the development of Addison's disease. Most commonly, the disorder is the result of an autoimmune malfunction, in which the body begins to react against its own tissue. The disorder may also result from adrenal cancers or infections. The prevalence rate is approximately 1 per 100,000 people.

The specific cause of the adrenal insufficiency may be either primary or secondary. In the case of primary adrenal insufficiency, the disorder arises directly within the outer region of the adrenal gland, called the adrenal cortex. Most of the time, the disorder is associated with an autoimmune dysfunction in which the body produces antibodies against adrenal tissue. Over time, the adrenal cortex is destroyed and the secretion of glucorticoid, mineralocorticoid, and adrenogenic hormones, the products of the adrenal cortex, ceases. Another cause of primary adrenal insufficiency is bacterial infections, particularly those associated with tuberculosis. The first identification of the disease, described by Thomas Addison in 1855, was associated with a tuberculosis infection in his patient. Other less common causes include fungal infections and malignancies.

Secondary adrenal insufficiency does not originate with the adrenal glands but rather is associated with abnormal regulation of adrenal hormone production, a function of the pituitary gland. Among the hormones produced within the pituitary gland is adrenocorticotropic hormone (ACTH), which stimulates glucocorticoid production by the adrenal cortex. Insufficient ACTH production results in a decrease in corticoid secretion. Any damage to the pituitary (or the hypothalamus, which actually regulates ACTH production by the pituitary) has the potential to affect ACTH production indirectly.

With Addison's disease, the onset of symptoms is gradual and can easily be overlooked or misdiagnosed during the early stages of the disease. Initially, the person may exhibit extreme fatigue, low blood pressure, and loss of appetite. The person may faint upon standing. Severe diarrhea and vomiting are also common. As a result of salt loss, the person may crave salty foods.

INFORMATION ON ADDISON'S DISEASE

CAUSES: Lack of hormone production by adrenal cortex from autoimmune dysfunction, cancer, or infection; abnormal regulation of adrenal hormone production by pituitary gland
SYMPTOMS: Extreme fatigue, low blood pressure, appetite loss, fainting, severe diarrhea and vomiting, craving of salty foods, skin darkening
DURATION: Chronic, with acute episodes (Addisonian crises)
TREATMENTS: Hormone replacement, dietary changes (such as increased salt content)

Severe expression of such symptoms is referred to as an Addisonian crisis; if untreated, it may be life-threatening. Because the production of ACTH itself is regulated by corticosteroid production in a feedback mechanism, reduced adrenal function results in increased levels of ACTH. This in turn can produce skin changes, particularly a darkening which mimics that of deep tanning. The presence of darkening equally over both exposed and unexposed skin can be indicative of Addison's disease, particularly if other symptoms are also present.

A definitive diagnosis of Addison's disease is based upon a series of blood and urine tests. Patients may exhibit abnormally high levels of potassium, a potentially life-threatening situation, or a low level of sodium. More definitive tests measure the concentration of corticol hormones in the urine. Because ACTH production is controlled by corticosteroid concentrations, an increase in blood ACTH may also be observed. The definitive test begins with the intravenous injection of ACTH. Cortisol levels in the blood are then measured over a one-hour period. If cortisol levels do not change, this result is indicative of a likely adrenal insufficiency.

TREATMENT AND THERAPY

The treatment of Addison's disease generally involves replacing the hormones that the adrenal cortex is no longer manufacturing. Oral medication is available for most of these hormones, though dietary changes may also be necessary. For example, if the mineralocorticoid aldosterone is insufficient, resulting in a salt imbalance, then patients taking aldosterone supplements may also be advised to increase the salt content of their food.

Other forms of treatment may be symptomatic. If the patient suffers from low blood pressure or severe salt imbalances, conditions that are potentially life-threatening, then intravenous medication may be necessary.

As the monitoring of potassium and sodium levels is critical, it is generally recommended that patients routinely visit their physicians. It is important that a patient exhibiting symptoms of an Addisonian crisis (vomiting, diarrhea) receive immediate salt replacement and probably hydrocortisone as well.

Because secondary adrenal deficiency most often originates in the pituitary gland, the primary result is a decrease in ACTH production. In turn, the adrenal cortex is deficient only in the production of cortisol. Treatment generally involves the oral replacement of cortisol, often in the form of synthetic prednisone.

PERSPECTIVE AND PROSPECTS

Addison's disease is a lifelong, chronic condition. While in the past it was often a life-threatening disorder, proper monitoring and hormone replacement can allow most people with the disease to live relatively normal lives with no restrictions. Because in most individuals the immediate cause is an autoimmune disorder, it is possible that eventually stem cell research, along with improved methods of controlling autoimmune phenomena, will provide a means for replacing adrenal tissue.

—Richard Adler, Ph.D.

See also Adrenalectomy; Autoimmune disorders; Corticosteroids; Endocrine disorders; Endocrinology; Endocrinology, pediatric; Glands; Hormones.

FOR FURTHER INFORMATION:

Bar, Robert, ed. *Early Diagnosis and Treatment of Endocrine Disorders*. Totowa, N.J.: Humana Press, 2003.

Besser, G. Michael, and Michael Thorner, eds. *Clinical Endocrinology*. 2d ed. St. Louis: Gower-Mosby, 1994.

Greenspan, Francis S., and David G. Gardner, eds. *Basic and Clinical Endocrinology*. 7th ed. New York: McGraw-Hill, 2003.

Larsen, P. Reed, et al., eds. *Williams Textbook of Endocrinology*. 10th ed. Philadelphia: W. B. Saunders, 2003.

Parker, James N., and Philip M. Parker, eds. *The Official Patient's Sourcebook on Addison's Disease*. San Diego, Calif.: Icon Health, 2002.

Adenoid removal. *See* Tonsillectomy and adenoid removal.

Adolescence. *See* Puberty and adolescence.

Adrenal disorders. *See* Addison's disease; Cushing's syndrome.

Adrenalectomy

Procedure

Anatomy or system affected: Abdomen, endocrine system, glands, kidneys, urinary system

Specialties and related fields: Endocrinology, general surgery

Definition: The surgical removal of one or both of the adrenal glands.

Indications and Procedures

The adrenal glands produce chemical substances which regulate the body's responses to stress, including the fight-or-flight response. Occasionally, if the adrenal glands become diseased (for example, with cancer) or the hormones that they produce aggravate another condition (such as breast cancer), a physician may determine that they must be surgically removed. Benign tumors of the adrenal gland may sometimes produce additional hormones that disrupt body functions. The tumors, and possibly the adrenal glands, must be removed to rectify the condition.

Depending on the type of tumor, adrenalectomy may require a major surgery or a less invasive laparoscopic surgery. Candidates for laproscopic surgery include patients whose tumors are less than 10 centimeters in diameter and have no malignant characteristics. In the laparoscopic procedure, the surgeon makes three to four small incisions, then inserts small telescopes on long instruments into the abdominal cavity. The abdomen is inflated with gas, and a camera on an instrument displays images on a monitor. The surgeon uses these images to navigate to the tumor and, with fine instruments, ties off blood vessels and disconnects the adrenal gland. The gland is placed into a small plastic bag inserted into the abdomen and then removed through the incision.

An open adrenalectomy is performed on large or cancerous tumors. It requires a large incision under the rib cage along the middle of the abdomen, or along the side of the body. This more invasive procedure allows the surgeon to explore the organs of the abdominal cavity for disease. The colon and a portion of the small intestine are moved to expose the kidneys. After the adrenal veins and arteries are sealed, each gland is dissected from its position at the top of each kidney. Internal organs are replaced, drains are brought out through the incisions, and the incisions are closed. The procedure may also be performed by a posterior approach through the rib cage.

Uses and Complications

Open adrenalectomies require four to five days of hospitalization, whereas laparoscopic procedures require two to three days. Complications of abdominal surgery are possible, including infection and internal bleeding, as are other potential complications of major surgery, including negative reaction to anesthesia. The risks of the surgery are small in comparison to the risk of doing nothing about the adrenal tumor. The patient is monitored closely postsurgery and given oral supplements for the hormones normally provided by the adrenal glands.

—*Karen E. Kalumuck, Ph.D.*

See also Abdomen; Abdominal disorders; Cancer; Corticosteroids; Cushing's syndrome; Endocrinology; Glands; Hormones; Kidneys; Nephrectomy; Tumor removal; Tumors.

For Further Information:

Beldegrum, Arie, et al., eds. *Renal and Adrenal Tumors*. New York: Oxford University Press, 2002.

Ernest, Ingrid. *Adrenalectomy in Cushing's Disease: A Long-Term Follow-up*. Copenhagen: Periodica, 1972.

Hunt, Thomas K., et al. *Adrenalectomy*. Boston: Little, Brown, 1978.

Libertino, John A., and Andrew C. Novick, eds. *Adrenal Surgery*. Philadelphia: W. B. Saunders, 1989.

African American health

Overview

Anatomy or system affected: All

Specialties and related fields: All

Definition: Statistical information and the most common disease processes that affect the African American community.

Key terms:

African Americans: a group of individuals whose origins are from any of the black racial groups of Africa

autoimmune disease: a disorder in which the body destroys or alters its own normal tissues

cancer: uncontrolled growth of the body's cells, which invade local cells or distant sites
cessation: stopping of an activity
diabetes: a disease in which the pancreas is unable to produce enough insulin to remove glucose (sugar) from the bloodstream
hypertension: an elevation of blood pressure above the normal range
morbidity: a term used when a person has a disease, usually a chronic one
mortality: a term used when researchers or clinicians are discussing death
obesity: an unhealthy accumulation of body fat; strictly defined as having a BMI greater than 30
screening: a process used to detect diseases before they cause damage to the body
sexually transmitted diseases (STDs): diseases that are spread by sexual or intimate contact, such as herpes, human immunodeficiency virus (HIV), chlamydia, and syphilis

Population and Statistics

African Americans have a rich cultural history in the United States. According to the 2000 census, they represent more than 12 percent of the nation's population. In order to address the diversity that exists within the African American population, it is imperative to understand how they, and society, define their cultural heritage, which has a direct impact on their health beliefs and practices. When defining who are considered to be African Americans, the United States, encyclopedias, and dictionaries use "individuals whose origins are from any of the black racial groups of Africa." This category also includes people who self-report their ethnicities as "Black, African American, or Negro" or who describe themselves on written documents as African American, Afro American, Angolan, Negro, West Indian, Afro Caribbean, Nigerian, Haitian, Gullah, Creole, West African, Afro Latin, Afro Brazilian, Congolese, Americo-Liberian, Bantu, Guinean, Moor, Pygmy, or Liberian. Therefore, the African American population in the United States comprises all these individuals.

African Americans primarily live in the Southern region of the United States, and their number continues to grow. African Americans are returning to the South largely in the hope of achieving financial and social success. It is currently noted that 1 out of 10 African Americans who live in the South is considered to be a "newcomer." At the same time, the Northeast has experienced a decline in the African American population. The top metropolitan areas with the most significant growth in the African American population are New York City, Washington, D.C., and Atlanta. The African Americans who are making the decision to return to the South or to make New York City, Washington, D.C., and Atlanta their homes are usually educated and considered to be middle to upper class in terms of their financial status. In spite of these gains, African Americans overall have a lower median household income than the rest of the U.S. population. It is this financial chasm that has led to the disparities in African American health care.

The country as a whole has benefited from an extended life span. The average life expectancy was 49.2 years in the nineteenth century. By the twenty-first century, the current average life expectancy had increased to 71.1 years. However, this increase in life expectancy is not as high in the African American community. The average life expectancy of African Americans is 65.1, which is six years less than the national average. In order to explain this phenomenon, one must take a closer look at the disease processes that affect African Americans throughout their life span.

Major Health Concerns

The life span can be classified into life cycles with four stages: infant/child, adolescent, adult, and elder. Each of these stages has specific diseases or illnesses that increase the possibility of mortality (death). Infant and child mortality rates in the African American community are two to three times higher than the national average. The reason for this is linked directly to the fact that African American infant birth weights tend to be lower than the national average; 3.306 pounds is termed very low birth weight (VLBW), and 5.5 pounds is termed low birth weight (LBW). Even African American infants who are born at normal birth weights (approximately 6 pounds) and at thirty-six to forty weeks (the normal length of pregnancy) still have a threefold greater likelihood of dying from infections and a twofold likelihood of dying from sudden infant death syndrome (SIDS).

Several theories are associated with why African American infants generally weigh less. One theory involves the quality and type of prenatal care that African American women received during their pregnancies. African American mothers often do not participate in prenatal care until they are in their third trimester. Therefore, they do not have access to appropriate screening tests, nutritional information, and dietary supplementation (such as iron and vitamins) which can significantly improve the health of their babies. Additionally, studies have shown that African American mothers do not always receive the educational information that is needed to prevent low birth weights when they do take advantage of prenatal care. Information about not smoking (substance abuse), eating a well-balanced diet, and seeking out early prenatal care is often not a part of their medical encounters. Various studies have identified the following behaviors and attitudes as risk factors for LBW and VLBW births among African American mothers: teenaged, unmarried (regardless of age), did not graduate from high school, smoked cigarettes or used alcohol or drugs during pregnancy, and began prenatal care in the third trimester.

In order to improve the health status of African American infants, there must be a concerted effort to increase community awareness regarding this issue. Mothers must be given information regarding state and federal programs that are directed at improving the health care of the mothers, which will ultimately lead to increasing the survival rates of the babies. Mothers should undergo the appropriate screening tests: sickle cell disease, glucose, and alpha fetoprotein (indicative of Down syndrome). They should receive prenatal vitamins and information regarding a balanced diet and exercise, and regular prenatal visits should be emphasized. They should also be educated on how substance abuse and issues pertaining to domestic violence and sexually transmitted diseases (STDs) can lead to premature births and complications after birth, which may lead to infant death. All pregnant females should have an initial prenatal visit that consists of a history, physical, and screening tests. They should see their health care team (provider, nurse, and educational support staff) at four-week intervals to ensure that the fetus is growing and developing at a rate that increases the likelihood of an uneventful delivery.

In adults, hypertension, diabetes, end-stage renal disease (ERSD), cardiovascular disease, cerebrovascular disease, and cancer are several of the diseases that most commonly affect African Americans. The American Heart Association states that high blood pressure (hypertension) is the leading preventable cause of excess deaths yearly among African Americans. The incidence or prevalence of hypertension among African Americans is among the highest in the world. Compared to Caucasians, African Americans develop hypertension at an earlier age, and their average blood pressure readings tend to be much higher. The specific risk factors that have been linked to hypertension among blacks are high salt intake, higher rates of overweight and obesity, higher incidence of cigarette smoking over the age of thirty-five, and a familial sensitivity to salt. It is also common for African Americans to have diabetes mellitus along with the hypertension. The two diseases combined increase the morbidity (illness/disease) and mortality (death) associated with hypertension.

African Americans who have a family history of hypertension should monitor their blood pressures monthly and should begin monitoring as early as adolescence. They should undergo regular physical examinations and laboratory tests. These tests should routinely include a complete blood count, a fasting lipid profile and glucose test, an electrocardiogram, and other laboratory tests depending on the medications they are taking. African Americans should make sure that they follow a diet that is low in fat and salt. They should also exercise daily. The goal is to prevent the development of other diseases, such as stroke, and to improve the overall quality of life by taking part in physical activity. Additionally, anyone who smokes should be warned about the effects that smoking has on increasing the chance of stroke, heart attack, cancer, and death.

The American Diabetes Association (ADA) estimates that approximately 2.3 million African Americans, or 11 percent of the African American community, have a diagnosis of diabetes. Diabetes mellitus is considered to be an autoimmune disease, which means that the body has turned against itself. The pancreas normally produces insulin. In diabetes, for various reasons, it does not make insulin at all (Type I diabetes) or it makes very little insulin (Type II diabetes). Insulin is important because it controls the body's blood sugar (glucose) levels. Diabetes occurs when the blood sugar levels increase and there is no way for the body to bring them down. The most common type of diabetes that African Americans have is Type II, which means that the body makes some insulin but not enough to control blood sugar. People who have Type II diabetes usually do not have to take insulin shots. This type of diabetes, depending on blood sugar levels, can be controlled with weight loss, diet, and exercise. One of the most common reasons that Type II diabetes is high among African Americans is obesity. The common age at diagnosis is forty-five to sixty-four, and it is more likely to be diagnosed in women.

Diabetes affects every organ in the body. Therefore, it is important that people who have diabetes see an eye doctor on a regular basis, monitor their blood pressure, and make sure that their feet are checked for sores or cuts. Diabetes affects a person's ability to heal, so a simple cold, flu, sore, or cut can cause blood sugar levels to go out of control, which can be life-threatening. The rule of thumb is to have fasting blood sugar tests on a regular basis (no food after a certain time), monitor the hemoglobin A1C levels (a test that tells how well blood sugar is controlled), watch dietary intake, and exercise regularly. Major complications of diabetes are hypertension, stroke, coronary artery disease, amputation, and kidney failure.

African Americans have a high rate of end-stage renal disease (ESRD), also known as kidney failure. This is largely attributable to the numbers of African Americans who have diabetes. ESRD has been closely associated with hypertension. It has also been implied that the increased rate is of ESRD is directly related to African Americans' lack of access to health care, which leads to the disease being identified at a more advanced stage. As a result, African Americans tend to have a much greater chance of having a poorer health outcome. The average age of an African American diagnosed with ESRD is fifty-nine, in comparison to whites, who are at an average age of seventy when they are diagnosed. The effects of hypertensive ESRD occur in all age groups and can be detected as early as fifteen. It is important that all African Americans who have diabetes and/or cardiovascular disease see their health care provider at regular intervals of every six to twelve weeks, depending upon their provider's recommendations and their ability to adhere to their medications and diets. They should also undergo laboratory tests that monitor how well their kidneys are functioning.

The American Heart Association states that more than sixty-one million Americans have cardiovascular disease, which includes high blood pressure, coronary artery disease, stroke, and congestive heart failure. African Americans have a higher death rate as a result of all these diseases. In 1999, statistics showed that Afri-

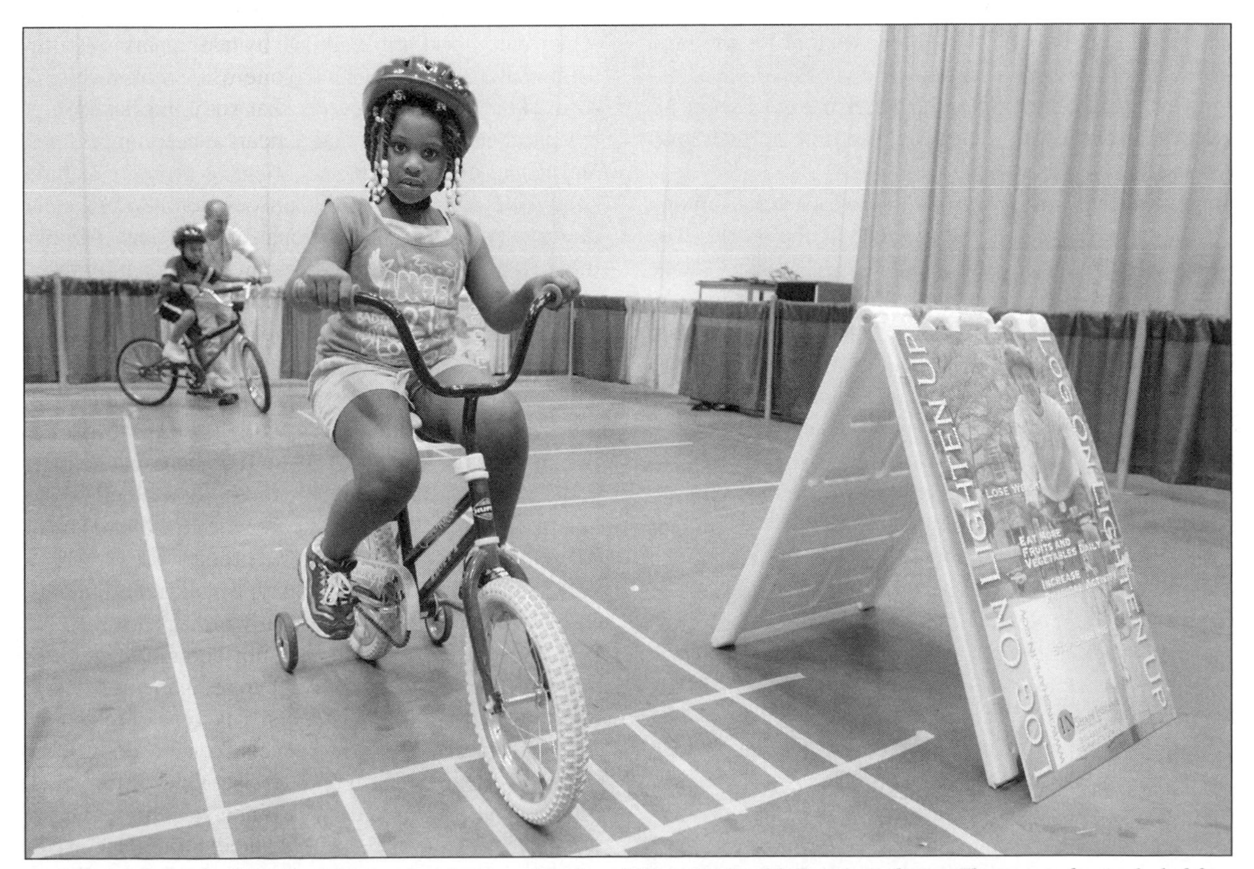

A girl goes through a bicycle safety course during a Black and Minority Health Fair in Indiana. The event also included free screenings for cholesterol, blood pressure, sickle cell disease, and HIV. (AP/Wide World Photos)

can American males have a 28 percent higher death rate and African American females have a 36 percent higher death rate from cardiovascular disease when compared to their white counterparts. African American women have a 71 percent higher death rate from coronary artery disease when compared to white females. It has also been documented that African Americans are more likely to die in out-of-hospital situations. This has been attributed to biases that exist in regard to African Americans receiving the necessary treatment to prevent deaths associated with cardiovascular disease. Whites undergo one-third more coronary angiographies (tests that are used to identify blockages in the vessels of the heart) and more than twice as many coronary bypass graft procedures. In addition to health care inequities, African Americans are at risk to develop such conditions as high blood pressure, diabetes, stroke, overweight, and obesity. All these diseases have been documented as precursors for the development of cardiovascular disease. Lifestyle is a major factor in the development of cardiovascular disease. The two most significant factors are physical inactivity and smoking. Other contributing factors for the high death rate is that African Americans often delay seeking treatment or care, which makes the chance for recovery and return to their previous state of health unlikely.

Death from cerebrovascular disease, or stroke, among African Americans is the highest in the world. The southeastern United States is referred to the "stroke belt." African American deaths from stroke tend to be higher in this region of the country. Recent studies from the Centers for Disease Control and Prevention have indicated that the stroke belt is expanding to include Texas and Arkansas. U.S. Census data estimate that 60 percent of African Americans reside in the stroke belt. The death rates of stroke in every age group are higher for African Americans, and death occurs at a younger age. The increased likelihood of stroke is related to the following: severity of hypertension (including age at onset), diabetes, elevated cholesterol (hypercholesterolemia), smoking, and high rates of physical inactivity.

The American Cancer Society reports that prostate, lung, and colorectal cancer in African American men and breast, colorectal, and lung cancer among African American women are the leading causes of cancer in the African American population. When these cancers are identified in African Americans, they are often very aggressive in terms of their growth and devastation of surrounding tissues. African Americans have an overall higher cancer rate than any other racial or ethnic group, and a higher mortality rate. Survival rates for African Americans are 44 percent, compared with 60 percent for whites. African Americans are more likely to be diagnosed with cancer later in the disease process, which leads to an increased likelihood of death. Southern-born African Americans have the highest cancer-related death rate.

African Americans are more likely to suffer from chronic obstructive pulmonary disease (COPD), sarcoidosis, pneumonia, and influenza. Traditionally, pulmonary diseases are associated with low socioeconomic status, less education, and residence in urban communities. African Americans are also more likely to participate in jobs that are hazardous, including those involving exposure to cotton, hemp, or grain dust. Asthma and allergy are included in the pulmonary disease class. The prevalence of asthma among African Americans is almost twice as high as for whites. In 1998, there were an estimated 1.7 million cases of asthma among African Americans. Approximately 24 percent of asthma-related deaths occur in the African American population. African Americans develop asthma at an earlier age and experience a more severe form of the disease. Factors commonly associated with the number of asthma cases are socioeconomic level and living in urban areas. Patients who have asthma should be educated on the preventive measures that they can take to prevent asthma attacks, such as smoking cessation, control of allergies, and use of medications as directed.

Perspective and Prospects

This section on African American health concerns only touches the tip of the health and disease iceberg. Key factors that are necessary to improve the health outcomes of African Americans begin with access to health care that is culturally appropriate and culturally sensitive. This simply means that the current health care system must educate, train, and prepare a health care workforce that is intimately aware of the health issues that dominate the African American patient population and be sensitive to the perceptions, concerns, and fears that may exist.

A concerted effort also must be made to educate African Americans regarding the role that they play in improving their own health. They must understand the importance of health care screenings, weight control and reduction, and regular physical examinations at every stage of their life cycle. The majority of the diseases that are prevalent in African Americans are associated with lifestyle choices. From hypertension to infectious diseases, an informed and educated African American population can become empowered to take control of their health by seizing every opportunity to improve it.

Other health concerns of the African American community that should be addressed are the increase rate of HIV among African American women, violence, substance abuse (such as alcohol and marijuana), and obesity.

—*Rosslynn S. Byous, D.P.A., PA-C*

See also Acquired immunodeficiency syndrome (AIDS); American Indian health; Asian American health; Asthma; Cancer; Diabetes mellitus; Heart disease; Hypertension; Men's health; Obesity; Pulmonary diseases; Renal failure; Screening; Strokes; Sudden infant death syndrome (SIDS); Women's health.

For Further Information:

African American Task Force for the Unity in Health, Diversity in Culture Conference. *African American Task Force Report on the Year 2000: Health Promotion Objectives and Recommendations for California*. Sacramento: California Department of Health Services, 1992.

American Diabetes Association. *African Americans and Diabetes*. http://www.diabetes.org/community programs-and-localevents/africanamericans.jsp. Provides health information and community support.

Blackhealthcare.com. http://www.blackhealthcare.com/. A private, for-profit online resource that provides health information on a variety of health issues including sickle cell, prostate cancer, and diabetes.

Braithwaite, Ronald, and Sandra F. Taylor, eds. *Health Issues in the Black Community*. 2d ed. San Francisco: Jossey-Bass, 2001. Examines the most pressing health problems affecting African Americans.

Closing the Health Gap. http://www.omhrc.gov/healthgap/. Provides health information ranging form cardiovascular disease to diabetes affecting African American communities.

MedlinePlus. *African-American Health*. http://www.nlm.nih.gov/medlineplus/africanamericanhealth.html. Provides online health information on African American health issues ranging from depression to glaucoma.

Sisters Network. http://www.sistersnetworkinc.org/. A national breast cancer network that provides online health information, support and referrals to African American survivors of breast cancer.

Age spots

Disease/disorder

Also known as: Liver spots, solar lentigo

Anatomy or system affected: Skin

Specialties and related fields: Dermatology

Definition: Benign lesions, also known as liver spots or solar lentigo, found on sun-exposed skin. Age spots are seen in more than 90 percent of Caucasians sixty-five years of age and older; they typically represent no immediate danger.

Causes and Symptoms

Age spots are flat tan or brown spots with well-defined borders between 2 millimeters and 30 millimeters in size. Occasionally, they can be slightly scaly or have a rough surface. Age spots are caused by a proliferation of normal melanocytes (the cells that produce melanin) in the epidermis as the result of chronic sun exposure. These lesions are commonly found on the face, especially the forehead and temples, the backs of the forearms and hands, and the shoulders and back. They are less commonly found on the trunk and legs. Age spots have no malignant potential.

Treatment and Therapy

No treatment is needed for age spots. Sunscreens and sun protection are usually advised because they help to decrease the rate of appearance and darkening of these lesions. Some older adults may seek treatment for cosmetic reasons. When treatment is sought, liquid nitrogen cryotherapy is usually used to lighten or remove the spots. This therapy is usually effective because melanocytes are more sensitive to cold than epidermal cells are. Trichloracetic acid may also be used to lighten or remove age spots. Bleaching agents such as tretinoin (Retin A) or hydroquinone may lighten age spots slowly, usually over three to four months. The color will return, however, if the use of the bleaching cream is discontinued. Aesthetic laser therapy is also becoming another option for treatment. It works by di-

Information on Age Spots

Causes: Sun exposure
Symptoms: Skin lesions, often scaly or rough
Duration: Chronic
Treatments: Cryotherapy, trichloracetic acid, bleaching agents (Retin A, hydroquinone)

recting a specific wavelength of light that passes through the skin but is absorbed by the discolored area. The rapid absorption of light energy causes the lesion to retract. It is then removed by the body's natural filter system. The procedure is performed on an outpatient basis and typically without local anesthesia.

—*Courtney H. Lyder, M.D.*

See also Aging; Plastic surgery; Skin; Skin cancer; Skin disorders; Stretch marks; Wrinkles.

For Further Information:

Baumann, Leslie, and Edmund Weisberg. *Cosmetic Dermatology*. New York: McGraw-Hill, 2002.

Graham-Brown, Robin, and Tony Burns. *Lecture Notes on Dermatology*. 8th ed. Boston: Blackwell Scientific, 2002.

Lamberg, Lynne. *Skin Disorders*. Philadelphia: Chelsea House, 2001.

Paslin, David. *The Hide Guide: Skin Problems and How to Deal with Them*. Millbrae, Calif.: Celestial Arts, 1981.

Sams, W. Mitchell, Jr., and Peter J. Lynch, eds. *Principles and Practice of Dermatology*. 2d ed. London: Churchill Livingstone, 1996.

Turkington, Carol, and Jeffrey S. Dover. *The Encyclopedia of Skin and Skin Disorders*. New York: Facts On File, 2002.

Aging

Development

Anatomy or system affected: All

Specialties and related fields: Geriatrics, gerontology, psychology

Definition: A series of time-dependent anatomical, physiological, and psychological changes that diminish physiological reserve and functional capacity and that produce emotional transformations. Some changes can also signal positive processes of maturation.

Key terms:

ageism: a negative or prejudiced view of aging endorsed by an individual or society

geriatrics: the medical specialty focusing on the treatment of elderly patients

gerontology: the formal study of the phenomena of aging from maturity to old age

normative age-graded: biological and environmental factors affecting aging that are correlated with chronological age

normative history-graded: events affecting aging that are widely experienced within a particular culture at a given time

non-normative aging: significant factors that affect aging that are person-specific

primary aging: aging intrinsic to a person as determined by inherent or hereditary influences

secondary aging: changes in a person caused by hostile factors in the environment, which could include trauma, pollution, and acquired disease

Physical and Psychological Factors

Aging takes place over the course of life, and the rate of change varies between individuals and groups. Differences in aging are genetically determined in part, but there is also a substantial environmental component. These environmental factors can include nutrition, lifestyle choices, and toxins in the environment. Primary aging relates to the genetic components of aging, while secondary aging focuses on environmental factors.

Aging is influenced by a number of normative age-graded factors that typically take place at a particular chronological time. These factors can be biological, as reflected in puberty and menopause, as well as environmental, having an impact on the socialization of the individual, such as the changes needed to enter school or to assume a work role. Normative history-graded factors refer to events that are shared by a society and have an impact, either positive or negative, on the aging process. The Great Depression in the 1930's, World War II, and the Vietnam War are examples of normative history-graded events. When a major event has an impact on a single generation in a society, it is known as a cohort effect. When an event affects the entire population, it is termed a period effect. The Great Depression is considered to be a period effect, while the Vietnam War is labeled a cohort effect. Normative age-graded factors are considered to be most important during childhood and in old age, while normative history-graded events are considered to have their greatest impact on aging in the early and middle adulthood periods of life. Non-normative factors recognize that each individual experiences unique factors that influence the personal aging process. A natural disaster, a divorce, and winning the lottery are considered to be non-normative factors.

A multitude of age-related changes are typically benign and permit an individual to function, perform daily functions, and remain active in society. With increasing age, however, a number of biological changes lead to a decline in efficiency of function and performance. Some general signs of bodily aging include decreases in physical stature and loss of bone mineral density. A quantitative loss of cells in the body results in a decrease in overall muscle mass, perhaps as high as 80 percent. A loss of fat beneath the skin results in an increased sensitivity to temperature extremes. In general, the skin of the aging person atrophies with shrinking of the sweat and sebaceous glands, leading to dry and itchy skin. A decline in blood vessels causes a slowing of healing, and a loss of skin elasticity occurs with the breakdown of elastin.

Age-related changes in the cardiovascular system include narrowing of the blood vessels due to the thickening of the endothelial lining and a decline in smooth muscle mass. The blood vessels become rigid and contribute to a gradual elevation of blood pressure. Changes in the heart include thickening of the myocardium, a reduction in size of the ventricular cavities, and a decrease in volume of blood pumped per contraction. Heart rate may slow with age, as the cells in the sinus node can decline up to 90 percent. Consequently, elderly people may show limited heart rate increases when experiencing stress or trying to increase activity level. Changes in the respiratory system show a number of functional declines. Smooth muscle in the bronchi, diaphragm, and chest wall becomes weakened as a result of an increase of collagen deposits, contributing to a diminished work capacity in late life. Reductions in the lung surface area, decreased maximum ventilatory volume of the lungs, and limitations on maximum oxygen utilization can produce senile emphysema. This age-related condition limits the amount of exercise and energy that an older person can expend at any given time. By age sixty-five, an individual cannot fully expand the chest when seated. Secondary aging factors can contribute significantly to the diminished function of the respiratory system, as pollutants in the environment and smoking have been found to exaggerate these changes.

Musculoskeletal changes caused by aging include a loss of muscle mass, with striated musculature diminishing by approximately 50 percent by age eighty. As these cells are lost, they are replaced by fat cells. With age, the mineralization of bone declines for both men and women, but women experience osteoporosis at an accelerated rate after menopause. Both older men and older women are at increasing risk of fractures with age, but women experience this enhanced risk ten years sooner than do men.

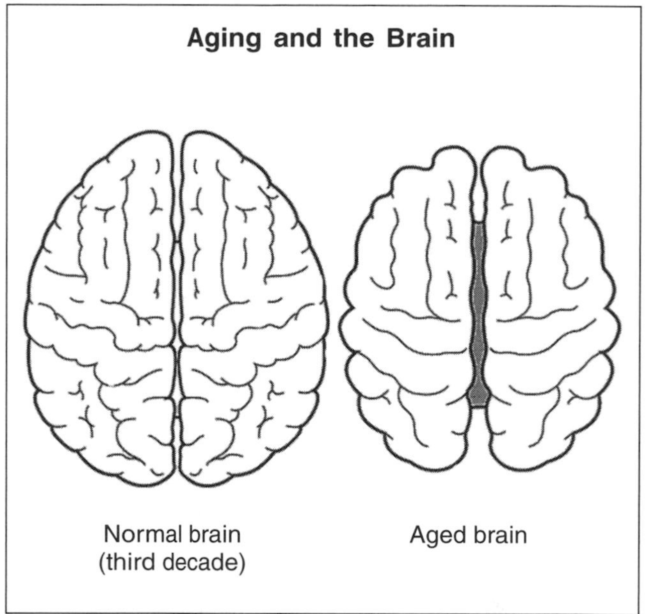

The human brain shrinks with age as nerve cells are lost and brain tissue atrophies.

In the nervous system, the brain shows a number of normative changes with age. In general, the brain decreases in size, primarily due to loss of mass in the white matter. Gray matter loss contributes significantly to this decrease after age seventy-five. Brain weight also diminishes beginning at age forty. The somatosensory system provides information from nerve endings located in the skin, joints, and muscles. As people age, the ability of the somatosensory system to detect stimuli in the environment and to provide accurate sensory information declines. Older adults have difficulty perceiving joint movement and position; this decline places them at an increased risk for falls.

Significant changes take place in the gastrointestinal system, with impaired gastric acid production in the stomach, slowing of the transit time in the large intestine, and decreased absorptive surface areas in the small intestine. The liver decreases in size and weight and shows a reduction in function. Other significant age-related changes to biological function include decreased renal blood flow; impaired function of the immune system; diminished levels of estrogen, progesterone, and testosterone; and decline in thyroid hormone levels.

Most noticeable to many older adults are the age-related changes to the sensory systems, as visual and auditory losses can routinely have an adverse effect on the performance of daily activities. With age, the lens and cornea of the eye thicken and show a yellowing. The lens is less flexible and increases in opaqueness, making focus more difficult. Production of the aqueous humor, the clear liquid that fills the anterior chamber of the eye, is reduced, leading to the increase in intraocular pressure associated with glaucoma. The ability to track moving objects declines as smooth pursuit eye movements show decrements. With advancing age, the auditory system shows a diminished capacity for sensitivity to higher frequencies, a condition known as presbycusis. According to the National Center for Health Statistics, 25 to 40 percent of adults over age sixty-five report concerns about a decline in speech perception. The problem is worsened in noisy environments. Taste and smell decrease in sensitivity with age to a degree that eating experiences become less pleasurable.

Although one unifying biological theory of aging does not exist, the National Institute on Aging has proposed two categories of aging theories: program theories and error theories. The program theories suggest that aging is due to a switching on and off of specific genes. When defects develop in the switching process, people experience the biological changes and functional declines associated with primary aging. The genetic nature of aging is shown in the maximal life spans that are found in all species. These species-specific differences in life span suggest an underlying genetic basis for aging. Since aging involves a complex array of normative age-related changes, it is expected that many interacting genes are involved in the overall process of growing old. One example of a program theory is the deliberate biological programming theory. This theory evolved from the research of Leonard Hayflick, who identified a limit for cell duplication. The theory holds that within a normal cell is a store of memory that dictates its life expectancy.

In contrast, the error theory approach maintains that aging is due in part to the wear and tear process that takes place over time. This approach posits that important components in the biological makeup of individuals wear out and cannot be repaired or replaced. Toxins in the environment and free radicals may contribute to the reduction in function of various systems as a result of wear and tear. Free radicals are chemical molecules with an odd number of electrons that makes them highly reactive with other chemical compounds. Free radicals are produced through normal metabolic processes as well as by exposure to ionizing radiation, ozone, and chemical toxins. Research has shown that free radicals are associated with deoxyribonucleic acid (DNA) damage, cross-linkage with collagen to alter the characteristics of connective tissue, and cancer.

Psychological theories of aging usually are concerned with explaining the differences in behavior, changes in behavior, and patterns of action shown among persons of various ages. The psychological theories can be divided into three major categories: stability template, orderly change, and random change. The stability template approach emphasizes that the primary factors associated with development take place during infancy and childhood. It is during the early years of life that one's personality is formed, and this provides a template for all future behaviors. As the aging individual faces new situations or challenges from the environment, behavior can be predicted based on the outcomes of early childhood experiences. From the stability template perspective, the older adult often demonstrates regressive behaviors, acting in childlike fashion, when normative age-related biological changes produce excessive stress. The resulting anxiety causes the older person to seek behaviors that were rewarding or comforting in the past. The theories of Sigmund Freud are an example of the stability template approach and promote the idea that the essentials of personality development are concluded at age five or six.

The orderly change theories suggest that aging takes place in a predictable pattern throughout the life span. This pattern is defined by specific stages that accompany the progression through life. Orderly change theorists believe that each stage of life—adolescence, young adulthood, middle age, and late life—presents specific challenges or tasks that must be completed in order to experience successful aging and avoid negative emotions such as depression. The eight stages of development described by Erik Erikson are an example of an orderly change theory.

The random change perspective emphasizes the non-normative factors of aging and suggests that development takes place as a result of a variety of events that may or may not have an impact on individuals at different points in life. This approach is highlighted by the work of Paul B. Baltes, who concludes that a wide variation occurs in the behavior of people as they age dependent upon each individual's particular circumstances.

In addition to general developmental theories, the psychological factors of aging focus on the changes in mental processes. Psychology differentiates between fluid intelligence and crystallized intelligence. Fluid intelligence is considered to be the basic abilities and cognitive skills found in a person. It reflects on the quality of one's brain and how quickly information is perceived and processed, how well associations and patterns are recognized, and the efficiency of memory function. This is analogous to a computer's hardware structure. Crystallized intelligence refers to culturally based and acquired cognitive functions. Development is dependent on experience with the world and the formal education system. The computer analogy would be its software. Development of cognitive ability is usually viewed as a stage phenomenon that begins during infancy, when the child interacts with the surrounding environment through his or her reflexes, and continues throughout life. Exposure to an enriched environment facilitates the development of crystallized intelligence. As a person reaches old age, tests of intelligence requiring speed or reaction time typically show a decline in ability. The developmental theory of Jean Piaget is an example of a well-known and highly researched approach to explain cognitive development from infancy onward.

Another significant approach to explain aging has been through the formation of social theories focusing on activity level throughout the life span. Disengagement theory suggests that aging inevitably requires a process of separating or disengaging oneself from physical, social, and psychological efforts. This disengagement is needed in response to the biological changes associated with old age. Activity theory was designed as an alternative view of aging and holds that normative aging requires remaining active throughout life. High activity levels are seen as positively related to good health, longevity, and life satisfaction. Most recently, continuity theory has been proposed as a compromise position between disengagement and activity theories. The continuity approach promotes the notion that older adults must maintain behavior according to the pattern of life that had been established before old age.

DISORDERS AND EFFECTS

Hutchinson-Gilford syndrome and Werner's syndrome are two forms of accelerated aging called progeria. The person with Hutchinson-Gilford syndrome experiences dwarfism and pseudosenility. Individuals with this genetic form of accelerated aging appear like very old small humans. They usually die in their teenage years of coronary heart disease. Werner's syndrome, also caused by genetic factors, affects persons in their late twenties and thirties and produces a shortened life span. The afflicted person ages very rapidly and develops a pinched facial expression, cataracts, diabetes, hypogonadism, a beaklike nose, prominent teeth, and a recessive chin.

Dementia is a fairly common condition that increases in frequency with age. It involves deficits in two or more areas of cognition that have a negative impact on daily functioning. Dementia produces impairment of memory and orientation and disruption in the ability to plan, organize, sequence, and make decisions. The majority of persons in old age who experience dementia have Alzheimer's disease. Current estimates suggest that between 2.5 and 4 million people have this disease. With the expanding size of the elderly population, however, the number of persons with Alzheimer's disease should increase to 9 million by the year 2025. The risk for Alzheimer's disease increases by approximately 1 percent with each year of life after age sixty-five. It is a progressive deteriorating disorder that attacks memory first before progressing through wandering, aggressiveness, and confusion of time and space to an eventual loss of self-awareness and a total inability to assume self-care. The characteristic brain pathology of Alzheimer's disease includes cell loss, neurofibrillary tangles, and senile plaques found throughout the neocortex of the brain but concentrated in the hippocampus, frontal, parietal, and temporal lobes. Persons with Alzheimer's disease can experience loss of approximately 40 percent of their brain mass. Four different chromosomes have been identified that heighten risk for the development of Alzheimer's disease. Currently, there is no cure for the disorder and treatment is primarily supportive. Cholinesterase inhibitors, which improve the naturally occurring neural transmitter acetylcholine in the brain, have been the medication of choice in treatment. Vascular dementia is caused by underlying cerebrovascular disease and has a more abrupt onset compared to Alzheimer's disease.

Many of the age-related changes experienced among older adults have been suggested as contributing to the development of late life depression. Depression is the most common emotional disturbance found in the elderly population. The prevalence of depression is highest among those older adults experiencing some medical illness or functional impairment. Suicide rates are high among older adults and highest among white men over the age of eighty-five. Many older adults experience "chronic suicide," a slow steady decline in health and function caused by personal neglect of one's needs.

One of the major effects of age-related changes is the need to compensate for functional declines. In order for many older adults to live independently, they often require some degree of home care. According to the U.S. Census Bureau, approximately 18 percent of all elderly adults trying to live independently are moderately or severely impaired. Impairments are measured in terms of the activities of daily living. which include eating, bathing, toileting, and moving in and out of chairs and bed. Remaining in the home can take on a significant level of psychological importance, since it is part of an older person's identity and helps to maintain a sense of autonomy and control in one's life.

Perspective and Prospects

Historically, the ancient Greeks provided some of the first writings on aging in discussing how old age brings increased anxiety about death. During the Roman era, Cicero suggested ways for elderly people to make themselves useful in advisory and administrative roles. He emphasized the importance of a developed mind and enhanced character as compensations for physical decline. The first manual to describe the problems associated with aging was published in the fifteenth century. Overall, however, historical writers had little to say about the positive attributes of aging.

Many common beliefs about aging have often resulted in oversimplified and biased stereotypes about older adults. These stereotypes may portray elderly persons as uninterested, weak, unattractive, undesirable, rigid, incapable of sexual activity, conservative, and lacking in intellectual acuity. This perspective encourages discrimination against older persons and is termed ageism. Senility is not a medical term but is commonly used in U.S. society. It implies that old people lose the intellectual capacity to make intelligent decisions. As the number of older adults has increased and the importance of scientific investigations of aging has been expanded, positive counterpoints to aging have emerged. A new realistic image of older adults portrays the healthy elderly population as resourceful, optimistic, intelligent, flexible, and sexual beings. The study of aging has increased in importance as the geriatric population continues to grow in number and proportion of the population. According to the U.S. Census Bureau, persons over age sixty-five constitute one of the fastest-growing segments of the American population. People are living longer than ever as a result of the control of infectious diseases, improvements in health care, sanitation, and nutrition. The segment of the population aged sixty-five and older grew from 5 percent of the population in 1900 to 13 percent in 2000, and it is projected to increase to 22.9 percent by the year 2050. In 2000, there were approximately 35 million Americans over the age of sixty-five, and this number is projected to increase to 70 million in 2030. Life expectancy at birth increased from forty-nine years in 1900 to more than seventy-nine years for women and seventy-four years for men in 2000. Women outlive men because of higher male mortality caused by heart disease, lung cancer, and emphysema.

Despite the increases in the older population, aging is a relatively young topic of study. Initially, the pioneers in the fields of development focused on describing, explaining, and understanding the infancy and childhood periods of life. Researchers next moved to the study of adolescence, and they considered old age as a period of deterioration with a focus on chronic disease. Gerontology, the formal study of the phenomena of aging from maturity to old age, began producing significant research only in the 1950's. Geriatrics, the medical treatment of elderly patients, was proposed as an academic discipline in 1987 by the National Institute of Medicine.

—*Frank J. Prerost, Ph.D.*

See also Age spots; Aging: Extended care; Alzheimer's disease; Arteriosclerosis; Arthritis; Deafness; Death and dying; Dementias; Depression; Diabetes mellitus; Geriatrics and gerontology; Gray hair; Hearing aids; Hearing loss; Heart disease; Hip replacement; Hormone replacement therapy (HRT); Hot flashes; Kyphosis; Memory loss; Menopause; Midlife crisis; Osteoarthritis; Osteoporosis; Parkinson's disease; Polypharmacy; Progeria; Prostate enlargement; Psychiatry, geriatric; Safety issues for the elderly; Sense organs; Stress; Strokes; Supplements; Vitamins and minerals; Wrinkles.

For Further Information:

Arking, Robert. *The Biology of Aging: Observations and Principles.* Boston: Oxford University Press, 2006. This is a comprehensive review of the age-related changes in all biological systems. The author provides the most up to date research findings and clinical observations related to aging processes.

Cohen, Gene D. *The Mature Mind: The Positive Power of the Aging Brain.* New York: Basic Books, 2005. The author provides a counterargument to the contention that the aging brain only experiences declines in function. He suggests that there are positive changes that are often ignored or not identified by researchers.

Eaton, William W., ed. *Medical and Psychiatric Comorbidity Over the Course of Life*. Washington, D.C.: American Psychiatric Publishing, 2006. The author provides a comprehensive review of the psychiatric and medical conditions common to old age. The book is written for the health care professional to understand how the processes of aging impact on physical and mental health.

Hill, Robert D. *Positive Aging: A Guide for Mental Health Professionals and Consumers*. New York: W. W. Norton and Company, 2006. Argues that even with the diminished physical and mental capacities associated with aging, the older adult can experience positive aging. The author provides specific strategies to overcome the age-related declines of late life.

Markut, Lynda A., and Anatole Crane. *Dementia Caregivers Share Their Stories: A Support Group in a Book*. Nashville: Vanderbilt University Press, 2005. This is an excellent resource book that describes the experience of dementia from a first-person perspective that can be useful for professionals and those affected by a family member with dementia.

AGING: EXTENDED CARE

SPECIALTY

ANATOMY OR SYSTEM AFFECTED: All

SPECIALTIES AND RELATED FIELDS: Audiology, cardiology, critical care, dentistry, geriatrics and gerontology, neurology, nursing, nutrition, oncology, ophthalmology, optometry, pharmacology, physical therapy, psychiatry, psychology, public health, rheumatology

DEFINITION: The management of the health, personal care, and social needs of elderly people as they experience decreases in physical, mental, and/or emotional abilities.

KEY TERMS:

ageism: discrimination against individuals based on their age or the overlooking of individuals' abilities to make positive contributions to society because of their age

case management: an interdisciplinary approach to medical care characterized by the inclusion of physical, psychological, social, emotional, familial, financial, and historical data in patient treatment

cognitive functioning: a general term describing mental processes such as awareness, knowing, reasoning, problem solving, judging, and imagining

malnutrition: a physical state characterized by an imbalance of dietary proteins, carbohydrates, fats, vitamins, and minerals, given an individual's physical activity and health needs

mental status exam: a comprehensive evaluation assessing general health, appearance, mood, speech, sociability, cooperativeness, motor activity, orientation to time and reality, memory, general intelligence, and other cognitive functioning

organic brain syndromes: clusters of behavioral and psychological symptoms involving impaired brain function, where etiology is unknown; includes delirium, delusions, amnesia, intoxication, and dementias

organic mental disorders: mental and emotional disturbances from transient or permanent brain dysfunction, with known organic etiology; includes drug or alcohol ingestion, infection, trauma, and cardiovascular disease

psychosocial interventions: treatments that enhance individual psychological and social functioning by assisting with the development of the skills, attitudes, or behaviors necessary to function as independently as possible

THE PROBLEMS ASSOCIATED WITH AGING

The process of aging is inevitable. In the earlier stages of life, aging involves the acquisition and development of new skills and abilities, facilitated by the guidance and assistance of others. Later, the middle stages involve the challenges of maintaining and applying those skills and abilities in a manner that is primarily self-sufficient. Finally, in the end stages of life, aging involves the deterioration and loss of skills and abilities, with adequate functioning again being somewhat dependent on the assistance of others.

For many individuals, the final stages are brief, allowing them to live independently right up to their time of death. Thus, many experience little loss of their abilities to function independently. Others, however, endure more extended stages of later life and require greater care. For these individuals, losses in physical, emotional, and/or cognitive functioning frequently result in a need for specialized care. Such care involves whatever is necessary so that these individuals may live as comfortably, productively, and independently as possible.

The conditions leading to a need for long-term care are as varied as the elderly themselves are. Special needs for elders requiring extended care often include the management of physical, health, emotional, and cognitive problems. Physical problems dictating lifestyle adjustments include decreased speed, dexterity, and strength, as well as increased fragility. Changes to the five senses are also common. Visual changes include the development of hyperopia (farsightedness) and sometimes decreased visual acuity. Hearing loss is also common, such that softer sounds cannot be heard when background noise is present or sounds need to be louder in order to be perceived. Particularly noteworthy is that paranoia, depression, and social isolation often result as side effects of visual and hearing impairments in elders; they are not always signs of mental deterioration. Similarly, one's sense of touch may also be affected, such that the nerves are either more or less sensitive to changes in temperatures or textures. Consequently, injuries attributable to a lack of awareness of potential hazards or supersensitivities to temperature or texture may result. One example would be an elderly woman overdressing or underdressing for the weather because of an inability to judge the outside temperature properly. Another would be an elderly man cutting or wounding himself out of a lack of awareness of the sharpness of an object. Finally, both taste and smell may change, creating a situation in which subtle tastes and odors become imperceptible or in which tastes and smells that were once pleasant become either bland or unpleasant.

Health problems among the aged often demand increased management as well. Coordination of drug therapies and other medical interventions by a case manager is critical, as a result of increasing sensitivities in elders to physical interventions. Typical health conditions bringing elderly people into long-term care settings may include heart disease and stroke, hypertension, diabetes mellitus, arthritis, osteoporosis, chronic pain, prostate disease, and cancers of the digestive tract and other vital organs. Estimates are that approximately 86 percent of the aged are affected by chronic illnesses. Long-term care addresses both the medical management of these chronic illnesses and their impact on the individual.

An issue related to health and physical problems in the aged is malnutrition. For a variety of reasons, elders often fall victim to malnutrition, which can contribute to additional health problems. For example, calcium deficiency can increase both the severity of heart disease and the likelihood of osteoporosis and tooth loss. Thus, a vicious cycle of medical problems can be put into motion. Factors contributing to malnutrition are multifaceted. Poverty, social isolation, decreased taste sensitivity, and tooth loss combine with lifelong dietary habits that can sometimes predispose certain elders to malnutrition. As such, attention to the maintenance of healthy dietary habits in the elderly is critical to successful long-term care, regardless of the type of setting in which the care is being given.

Along with these physical aspects of aging come emotional and cognitive changes. Depression, anxiety, and paranoia over health concerns, for example, are not uncommon. Additionally, concerns about the threat of losing one's independence, friends, and former lifestyle may contribute to acute or chronic mood disorders. Suicide is a particular danger with the elderly when mood disorders such as depression are present. Elderly people are one of the fastest growing groups among those who commit suicide. The stresses accompanying losing a spouse or enduring a chronic health problem can often be triggers to suicide for depressed elders. One should note, however, that elders are not particularly prone to depression or suicide because of their age but that they are more likely to experience significant stressors that lead to depression.

More common, less lethal problems associated with conditions such as depression, anxiety, and paranoia are weight change, insomnia, and other sleep problems. Distractibility, decreased ability to maintain attention and concentration, and rumination over distressing concerns are also common. Finally, some elders may be observed as socially isolated and prone to avoidance behavior. As a result, some become functionally incapacitated because of distressing emotions.

What is critical to remember, in addition to these signs, is that some elders may not describe their problems as emotional at all, even though that is the primary cause of their discomfort. Individual differences in how people express themselves must be taken into account. Thus, while some elders may report being depressed or anxious, others may instead report feeling tired. Reports of low-level health problems that are vague in nature, such as aches and pains, are also common in elders who are depressed. It is not uncommon for emotional problems to be expressed or described indirectly as physical complaints.

Decreased cognitive functioning may result from more serious problems than depression, such as organic brain syndromes. These typically include problems such as dementias from Alzheimer's disease, Pick's disease, Huntington's chorea, alcohol-related deterioration, or stroke-related problems. Other causes may be brain tumors or thyroid dysfunction. With all dementias, however, the hallmark signs are a deterioration of intellectual function and emotional response. Memory, judgment, understanding, and the experience and control of emotional responses are affected. Functionally, these conditions reveal themselves as a combination of symptoms, including increased forgetfulness, decreased ability to plan and complete tasks, difficulties finding names or words, decreased abilities for abstract thinking, impaired judgment, inappropriate sexual behavior, and sometimes severe personality changes. In some cases, affected individuals are aware of these difficulties, usually in the earlier stages of the disease processes. Later, however, even though their behavior and abilities may be quite disturbed, they may be completely unaware of the severity of their problems. In these cases, long-term care often begins as a result of outside intervention by concerned friends and family members.

Options for Long-Term Care

Extended care for the aged requires an interdisciplinary effort that usually involves a team of physicians, psychologists, nurses, social workers, and other rehabilitative specialists. Depending on the nature of the problems requiring care and management, any of these professionals may take part in the care process. Additionally, the involvement of concerned individuals who are close to the elder needing care is critical. Family members (including the spouse, children, and extended family) and close friends are invaluable sources of information and of emotional and instrumental support. Their ability to assist an elder with instrumental tasks such as cooking, housecleaning, shopping, and money and medication management is crucial to the successful implementation of a long-term care plan.

In all cases, long-term care for the aged involves the design of a comprehensive plan to address the multifaceted needs of the elder. Just as younger persons have psychological, social, intellectual, and physical needs, so do elders. As such, thorough assessment of an elder's abilities, goals, expectations, and functioning in each of these areas is required. A mental status exam and a thorough physical exam are usually the primary methods of evaluation. Once needs are identified, a plan can then be designed by the team of health care professionals, family and friends assisting with care, and, whenever possible, the elder. In general, the overarching goal is to design a case management plan that maximizes the independent functioning of the aged person, given certain physical, psychiatric, social, and other needs.

Specific management strategies are designed for the problems that need to be addressed. Physical, health, nutritional, emotional, and cognitive problems all demand different management settings and strategies. Additionally, care settings may vary depending on the severity of the problems that are identified. In general, the more severe the problems, the more structured the long-term care setting and the more intense the psychosocial interventions.

For less severe problems, adequate management settings may include the elder's own home, the home of a family member or friend, a shared housing setting, or a seniors' apartment complex. Shared housing is sometimes called group-shared, supportive, or matched housing. Typically, it refers to residences organized by agencies where up to twenty people share a house and its expenses, chores, and management. Ideal candidates for this type of setting include elders who want some daily assistance or companionship but who are still basically independent. Senior apartments, also called retirement housing, are usually "elderly-only" complexes that range from garden-style apartments to high-rises. Ideal candidates for this type of setting include nearly independent elders who want privacy, but who no longer desire or can manage a single-family home. In either of these types of settings, the use of periodic or regular at-home nursing assistance for medical problems, or "home-helpers" for more instrumental tasks, might be a successful adjunct to regular consultation with a case manager or physician.

Problems of moderate severity may demand a more structured setting or a setting in which help is more readily available. Such settings might include continuing care retirement communities or assisted-living facilities. Continuing care retirement communities, also called life-care communities, are large complexes offering lifelong care. Residents are healthy, live independently in apartments, and are able to use cafeteria services as necessary. Additionally, residents have the option of being moved to an assisted-living unit or an infirmary as health needs dictate. Assisted-living facilities—also called board-and-care, institutional living, adult foster care, and personal care settings—offer care that is less intense than that received in a medical setting or nursing home. These facilities may be as small as a home where one person cares for a small group of elders or as large as a converted hotel with several caregivers, a nurse, and shared dining facilities. Such set-

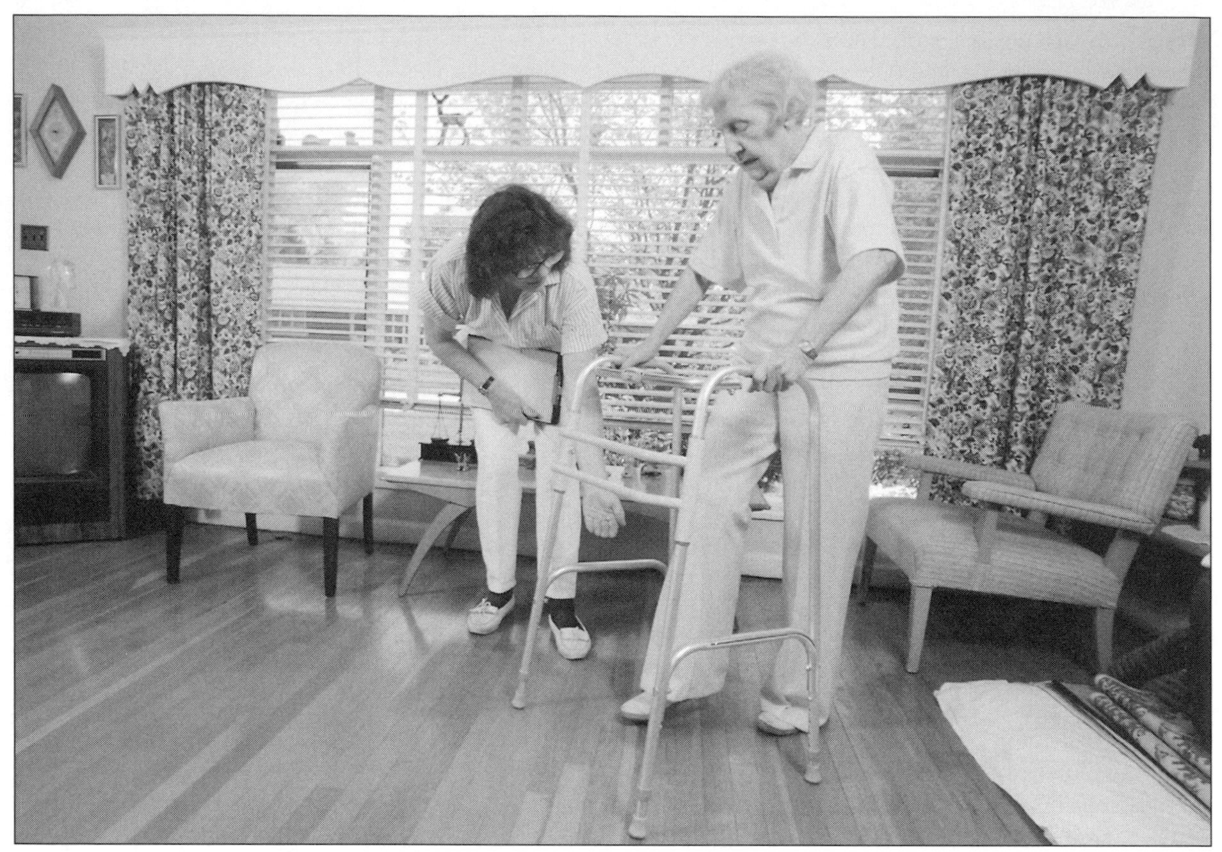

A home care professional helps an elderly woman use a walker for support. Such services allow many older people to have a more active and independent lifestyle. (Digital Stock)

tings are ideal for persons needing instrumental care but not round-the-clock skilled medical or nursing care.

When more severe conditions such as incontinence, dementia, or an inability to move independently are present, nursing, convalescent, or extended care homes are more appropriate settings. Intense attention is delivered in a hospital-like setting where all medical and instrumental needs are addressed. Typical nursing homes serve a hundred clients at a time, utilizing semiprivate rooms for personal living space and providing community areas for social, community, and family activities. Often, the decision to place an elder in this type of facility is difficult to make. The decision, however, is frequently based on the knowledge that these types of facilities provide the best possible setting for the overall care of the elder's medical, health, and social needs. In fact, appropriate use of these facilities discourages the overtaxing of the elder's emotional and familial resources, allowing the elder to gain maximum benefit. An elder's placement into this type of facility does not mean that the family's job is over; rather, it simply changes shape. Incorporation of family resources into long-term care in a nursing home setting is critical to the adjustment of the elder and family members to the elder's increased need for care and attention. Visits and other family involvement in the elder's daily activities remain quite valuable.

Regardless of the management setting, some basic caveats exist with regard to determining management strategies. First and foremost is that the aged individuals should, whenever possible, be encouraged to maintain independent functioning. For example, even though physical deterioration such as decreased visual or hearing abilities may be present, there is no need to take decision-making authority away from the elder. Decreased abilities to hear or see do not necessarily mean a decreased ability to make decisions or think. Second, it is crucial to ask elders to identify their needs and how they might desire assistance. Some elders may wish for help with acquiring basic living supplies from outside the home, such as foods and toiletries, but desire privacy and no assistance within the home. In contrast, others may desire independence outside the home with regard to social matters but need more instrumental assistance within the home. Finally, it is important to recognize that even the smallest amount of assistance can make a significant difference in the lifestyle of the elder. A prime example is availability of transportation. The loss of a driver's license or independent transportation signifies a major loss of independence for any elder. Similarly, the challenges posed by public transit may seem insurmountable because of a lack of familiarity or experience. As such, simple and small interventions such as a ride to a store or a doctor's office may provide great relief for elders by assisting their efforts to meet their own needs.

Special management strategies may be required for specific problem areas. For physical deterioration, adequate assessment of strengths and weaknesses is important, as are referrals to medical, rehabilitative, and home-help professionals. Hearing and visual or other devices to make lifting, mobility, and day-to-day tasks easier are helpful. Similarly, assisting the aged with developing alternative strategies for dealing with diminished sensory abilities can be valuable. Examples would be checking a thermometer for outdoor temperature to determine proper dress, rather than relying purely on sensory information, or having a phone that lights up when it rings. Health conditions also demand particular management strategies, varying greatly with the type of problem experienced. In all cases, however, medical intervention, drug therapies, and behavior modification therapies are commonly employed. Dietary problems (such as malnutrition or diabetes), cardiovascular problems (such as heart attacks), and emotional problems (such as depression) often require all three approaches. Finally, cognitive problems, particularly those related to depression, are sometimes alleviated with drug therapies. Others related to organic brain syndromes or organic mental disorders require both medical interventions and significant behavior modification therapies and/or psychosocial interventions for elders and their families.

PERSPECTIVE AND PROSPECTS

Advances in modern medicine are continually extending the human life span. Cures for dread diseases, improved management of chronic health problems, and new technologies to replace diseased organs are facilitating this evolution. For many, these advances translate into greater longevity, the maintenance of a high quality of life, and fewer obstacles related to ageism. For others, however, the trade-off for longevity is some loss of independence and a need for extended care and management. Thus, the medical field is also affected by the trade-off of extending life, while experiencing an increasing need to improve strategies for long-term care for those who are able to live longer and longer despite health conditions.

As a result of this evolution, long-term care for the aged presents special challenges to the medical field. Over time, medicine has been a field specializing in the understanding of particular organ systems and the treatment of related diseases. While an understanding of how each system affects the functioning of the whole body is necessary, health care providers must struggle to understand the complexities in the case management required for high-quality long-term care for the aged. Care must be interdisciplinary, addressing the physical, mental, emotional, social, and family needs of the aged individual. Failure to address any of these areas may ultimately sabotage the successful long-term management of elderly individuals and of their problems. In this way, medical, psychiatric, social work, and rehabilitative specialists need to work together with elders and their families for the best possible results.

Integrated case management with a team leader is increasingly the trend so that a variety of services can be provided in an orchestrated manner. While specialty providers still play a role, managers (usually primary care physicians) ensure that complementary drug therapies as well as psychiatric and other medical treatments are administered. Additionally, they are key in bringing forth family resources for emotional and instrumental support whenever possible, as well as community and social services when needed.

What was once viewed as helping a person to die with dignity is now viewed as helping a person to live as long and as productive a life as possible. Increasing awareness that old age is not simply a dying time has facilitated an integrated approach to long-term care. The news that elders can be as social, physical, sexual, intellectual, and productive as their younger counterparts has greatly stimulated improved long-term care strategies. No longer is old age seen as a time for casting elders aside or as a time when a nursing home is an inescapable solution in the face of health problems affecting the aged. Alternatives to care exist and are proliferating, with improved outcomes for both patients and care providers.

—*Nancy A. Piotrowski, Ph.D.*

See also Aging; Alzheimer's disease; Arthritis; Audiology; Brain; Brain disorders; Critical care; Death and dying; Dementias; Depression; Endocrinology; Ethics; Euthanasia; Geriatrics and gerontology; Hearing loss; Hospitals; Incontinence; Malnutrition; Nursing; Nutrition; Ophthalmology; Optometry; Orthopedics; Osteoporosis; Pharmacology; Polypharmacy; Psychiatry, geriatric; Rheumatology; Safety issues for the elderly; Sense organs; Terminally ill: Extended care; Vision disorders.

For Further Information:

American Psychiatric Association. *Diagnostic and Statistical Manual of Mental Disorders: DSM-IV-TR*. 4th rev. ed. Washington, D.C.: Author, 2000. This manual provides detailed descriptions of the behavior symptoms used to diagnose psychiatric disorders, such as organic brain syndromes and affective disorders. Written by mental health professionals, this manual covers issues related to psychiatry, psychology, and social work.

Cassel, Christine K., ed. *Geriatric Medicine*. 4th ed. New York: Springer-Verlag, 2003. Examines topics such as changing contexts of care in geriatric medicine, clinical approaches to the geriatric patient, palliative and medical care, and organ system diseases and disorders.

Ham, Richard, et al., eds. *Primary Care Geriatrics: A Case-Based Approach*. 5th ed. St. Louis: Mosby Elsevier, 2007. Divided into three parts: a discussion of the principles of geriatric primary care and the characteristics of older persons, an exploration of case-based approaches to major geriatric syndromes, and a presentation of common conditions and situations.

Katz, Paul R., Robert L. Kane, and Mathy D. Mezey. *Advances in Long-Term Care*. Vol. 1. New York: Springer, 1991. One volume in an ongoing series covering issues related to the long-term care of elders by caregivers, both professional and nonprofessional. Written by medical, psychiatric, and nursing professionals.

Levin, Mora Jean. *How to Care for Your Parents: A Practical Guide to Eldercare*. New York: W. W. Norton, 1997. This book may be of practical use to individuals anticipating a need to care for disabled elders.

Namazi, Kevan H., and Paul K. Chaftez, eds. *Assisted Living: Current Issues in Facility Management and Resident Care*. Westport, Conn.: Auburn House, 2001. Topics include understanding the context of assisted living, medical problems and care needs of older adults in assisted living facilities, developing dementia care units in assisted living facilities, and improving function and independence for elderly persons.

Weisstub, David N. *Aging: Caring for Our Elders*. Boston: Kluwer Academic, 2001. Multidisciplinary chapters include topics such as "Across the Generations: Family Care Dynamics into the New Millennium," "Financing Long-Term Care in the United States: Who Should Pay for Mom and Dad?," and "Appropriate Housing for the Elderly of the United States: An Integral Component of Their Health Care."

AIDS. *See* Acquired immunodeficiency syndrome (AIDS).

Albinos

Disease/disorder

Anatomy or system affected: Eyes, hair, skin

Specialties and related fields: Biochemistry, genetics

Definition: People who lack the normal amount of melanin pigment in hair, skin, and/or eyes.

Causes and Symptoms

Albinism is a group of inherited conditions caused by alteration, or mutation, of one of the genes that affect normal pigment production. Mutation in any one of several genes involved in melanin production can produce individuals with less than the normal amounts of melanin. Lack of melanin can lead to many problems. When melanin is absent from the skin, the skin has no protection against ultraviolet (UV) light and burns easily in the sun. The skin cancer risk for albinos is quite high. Lack of melanin in the retina leads to lessened visual acuity. Albinism is classified into two main types, oculocutaneous albinism (OCA) and ocular albinism (OA). The former affects the skin, hair, and eyes, while the latter affects only the eyes.

One form of OCA is called tyrosinase-related OCA. It is an autosomal recessive characteristic; thus, affected individuals must inherit a mutated gene from both of their parents. The parents may themselves be albinos or, more usually, may be normal-appearing heterozygous carriers of this mutation. The enzyme coded by the normal gene, tyrosinase, converts tyrosine to dopa, the first step in the production of melanin. Most commonly, individuals with two copies of the mutated

> **Information on Albinos**
>
> **Causes:** Mutation of a gene affecting melanin production
> **Symptoms:** Pale, unpigmented skin and hair, pale blue/gray or reddish irises, severely decreased visual acuity
> **Duration:** Lifelong
> **Treatments:** Limited sun exposure and sunscreens to protect against ultraviolet radiation, eyeglasses

gene lack this enzyme and are unable to produce any melanin. These individuals exhibit classic albino traits, which may include pale, unpigmented skin and hair, pale blue/gray or even reddish irises, and severely decreased visual acuity. Less commonly, the mutation in the gene leads to lowered amounts of the enzyme, so that the affected person produces some melanin. The amount of melanin produced determines how severely affected the individual will be. These albinos have very little pigment at birth but accumulate more as they age.

Other autosomal recessive OCAs are caused by mutations in the P gene, TRP1 gene, Hermansky-Pudlak syndrome (HPS) gene, and Chediak Higashi syndrome (CHS) gene. In all the above, some pigment is present at birth but individuals appear less pigmented when compared to siblings.

OA is an X-linked recessive disorder; therefore, it is more often seen in males. Skin, hair, and even iris color are in the normal range for the family, but examination shows a complete lack of pigment in the retina. Visual acuity is less than normal. Female heterozygous carriers show mosaicism, with some parts of the retina pigmented and other parts not.

Treatment and Therapy

Although no cure exists for albinism, some symptoms can be alleviated. Sunscreens of at least SPF 20 offer some protection from harmful UV radiation. Even with sunscreens, however, albinos should refrain from sun exposure between 10 A.M. and 3 P.M. Various types of eyeglasses can improve the vision of albinos, although visual acuity is rarely corrected completely. Albinos usually live a normal life span and have normal mental development.

—Richard W. Cheney, Jr., Ph.D.

See also Myopia; Pigmentation; Skin; Skin cancer; Skin disorders; Vision disorders.

For Further Information:

Icon Health. *Albinism: A Medical Dictionary, Bibliography, and Annotated Research Guide to Internet References*. San Diego, Calif.: Author, 2003.

Levine, Norman, ed. *Pigmentation and Pigmentary Disorders*. Boca Raton, Fla.: CRC Press, 1993.

Nordlund, James J., et al., eds. *The Pigmentary System: Physiology and Pathophysiology*. New York: Oxford University Press, 1998.

Scriver, Charles R., et al., eds. *The Metabolic and Molecular Bases of Inherited Disease*. New York: McGraw-Hill, 2001.

Alcoholism

Disease/disorder

Anatomy or system affected: Brain, liver, nervous system, psychic-emotional system

Specialties and related fields: Family medicine, internal medicine, psychiatry, psychology

Definition: The psychological and physiological process of dependency on beverages containing alcohol.

Key terms:

cirrhosis: chronic liver disease; its symptoms include nonfunctional tissue, blocked blood circulation, liver failure, and death

delirium tremens: severe alcohol withdrawal syndrome, with symptoms including confusion, delirium, terrifying hallucinations, and severe tremors

distillation: the use of heat to separate mixtures of liquid chemicals that boil at different temperatures by vaporization and cooling back into the liquid state

Korsakoff's psychosis: brain damage that may require hospitalization because of disorientation and impaired or false memory

metabolism: the chemical and physical processes involved in absorbing and using foods to convert them to energy and other nutrients

proof: a designation of beverage alcohol content; divided by two, it approximates the percentage of alcohol present

psychosis: a severe mental state characterized by loss of normal social function and being either withdrawn from or unable to accurately perceive reality

Causes and Symptoms

The basis for alcoholism is physical dependence on alcoholic beverages and consequent problems in behavior and health. Problems related to alcohol probably developed soon after prehistoric humans discovered that

Information on Alcoholism

Causes: Repeated and excessive use of alcohol
Symptoms: Lack of coordination, slurred speech, stupor, breathing difficulties, coma; tolerance; withdrawal (confusion, delirium, hallucinations, tremor); associated health risks (cirrhosis, fetal alcohol syndrome)
Duration: Chronic
Treatments: Cognitive and behavioral therapies, metabolic inhibitors disulfiram (Antabuse) and citrated calcium carbonate (Abstem)

fruit or grain, mashed and suspended in water, fermented into beverages that produced euphoria in users. The first recorded production of fermented beverages was of beer and wine in ancient Babylon and Egypt, respectively.

The active ingredient in fermented beverages is ethyl alcohol (alcohol), a colorless, mild-smelling liquid that boils at 79 degrees Celsius. Alcohol content in such beverages is indicated as "proof." If divided by two, the proof number indicates the approximate percentage of alcohol present. For example, 20-proof wine contains about 10 percent alcohol. In contrast, 80-proof brandy and vodka, beverages known as hard liquors, contain about 40 percent alcohol, because such liquors have been "fortified" by adding pure alcohol prepared via distillation. Other beverages known as hard liquors include whiskey, scotch, and rye. They typically are discussed separately from beer and wine.

Abuse of alcoholic beverages first became epidemic during the Middle Ages, when development of widespread alcohol distillation produced hard liquors and made it easy to attain alcoholic euphoria and stupor. In 2000, 62 percent of Americans over the age of eighteen used alcohol, 32 percent of current drinkers had five or more drinks on the same occasion at least once in the prior year, and more than 110,000 people died in alcohol-related deaths.

Some deaths attributable to alcohol result from alcohol poisoning, which is excessive consumption in a short time period. The drug primarily depresses the action of the central nervous system, creating the desired euphoric effects of alcohol consumption. Given a drink or two, a drinker may become relaxed and uninhibited. A few more drinks, however, may increase blood alcohol levels above .10 and further depress the central nervous system, causing lack of coordination, slurred speech, and stuporlike sleep. If just a little more alcohol is imbibed before stupor occurs and blood alcohol levels rise much above .25, further depression of the central nervous system stops breathing and kills.

People engaged in the problematic use of alcohol are sometimes called alcoholics. Many professionals, however, prefer to refer to these persons as individuals with alcohol problems or alcohol dependence. This is in keeping with the goal of not reducing a person to his or her behavior and engendering stigma. While it is true that some persons with alcohol dependence will use alcohol to the point of compulsive use, seriously disrupting their health and ability to survive, others may become physiologically dependent on alcohol and remain functional for a long time. If the problem worsens, however, then they may experience very serious results. It is not uncommon, for instance, for persons with severe alcohol dependence to suffer accidents, life-threatening withdrawal and other health problems, violence, and even suicide.

Chronic alcoholism damages many body organs. Best known is liver disease, or cirrhosis of the liver. Another common problem is brain damage. Mental disorders caused by injury to the cerebral hemispheres may include delirium tremens (the D.T.'s) and Korsakoff's psychosis. Both the D.T.'s, characterized by hallucination and other psychotic symptoms, and Korsakoff's psychosis, which is characterized by short-term memory loss and confabulation, or stories to cover this loss, may be accompanied by severe physical debility requiring hospitalization.

In addition, alcohol dependence can damage the kidneys, the heart, and the pancreas. In fact, a large number of instances of diseases of other organs are thought to arise from alcohol dependence. Also, much evidence suggests that alcoholism greatly enhances the incidence of mouth and throat cancer resulting from smoking tobacco.

Severe effects in the liver occur because most ingested alcohol is metabolized there. In the presence of alcohol, most other substances normally metabolized by the liver are not changed into useful and essential forms. One example has to do with fat, a major dietary source of energy. Decreased fat metabolism in the livers of individuals with alcohol dependence results in the fat accumulation, called a fatty liver, that precedes cirrhosis of the liver. Cirrhosis results in the replacement of liver cells with nonfunctional fibrous tissue. It should be noted, however, that not all fatty liver disease results from alcohol use. There are other causes, such as nonalcoholic fatty liver disease or nonalcoholic steatohepatitis (NFLD/NASH), which may result from many different types of health conditions.

Another problem that results from excessive alcohol metabolism is that the liver no longer destroys the many other toxic chemicals that are consumed. This defect adds to problems seen in cirrhosis and leads to dissemination of such chemicals through the body, where they can damage other body parts. In addition, resistance to the flow of blood through the alcoholic liver develops, which can burst blood vessels and cause dangerous internal bleeding. As a consequence of these problems, alcoholic liver disease, or cirrhosis, has become a major, worldwide cause of death from disease.

There is no one clear physical explanation for the development of alcoholism. It is a condition that varies from individual to individual and also has many different causes. Often, it is viewed as the result of a biological predisposition to addiction and/or social problems and psychological stresses. Those in cultures where consumption of alcoholic beverages is equated with manliness or sophistication may be at greater risk. Those under great psychological or social stress are also at risk, as drinking may be an inexpensive and easy way to experience some relief. Other proposed causes of behaviors that lead to alcoholism include, but are not limited to, habitual drinking, other mental health problems, domineering parents, adolescent peer pressure, exposure to deviant peer groups, personal feelings of inadequacy, loneliness, job pressures, marital discord, and cultural pressures to drink.

The fact that 20 percent of children of alcoholics tend to develop the disease, compared to 4 percent of the children of nonalcoholics, has led to investigations of the genetic proclivity for alcoholism. The fact that 80 percent of the progeny of alcoholic parents escape alcoholism, however, diminishes support for such theories. On the other hand, there are clearer indications that genetic factors are important to distaste for alcohol, precluding the development of alcoholism in some ethnic and national groups.

Another disease attributable to alcoholism is fetal alcohol syndrome, which occurs in many children of mothers who drank heavily during pregnancy. Such children may be hyperactive, mentally retarded, and facially disfigured, and they may exhibit marked growth retardation. Fetal alcohol syndrome is becoming more frequent as alcohol consumption increases worldwide.

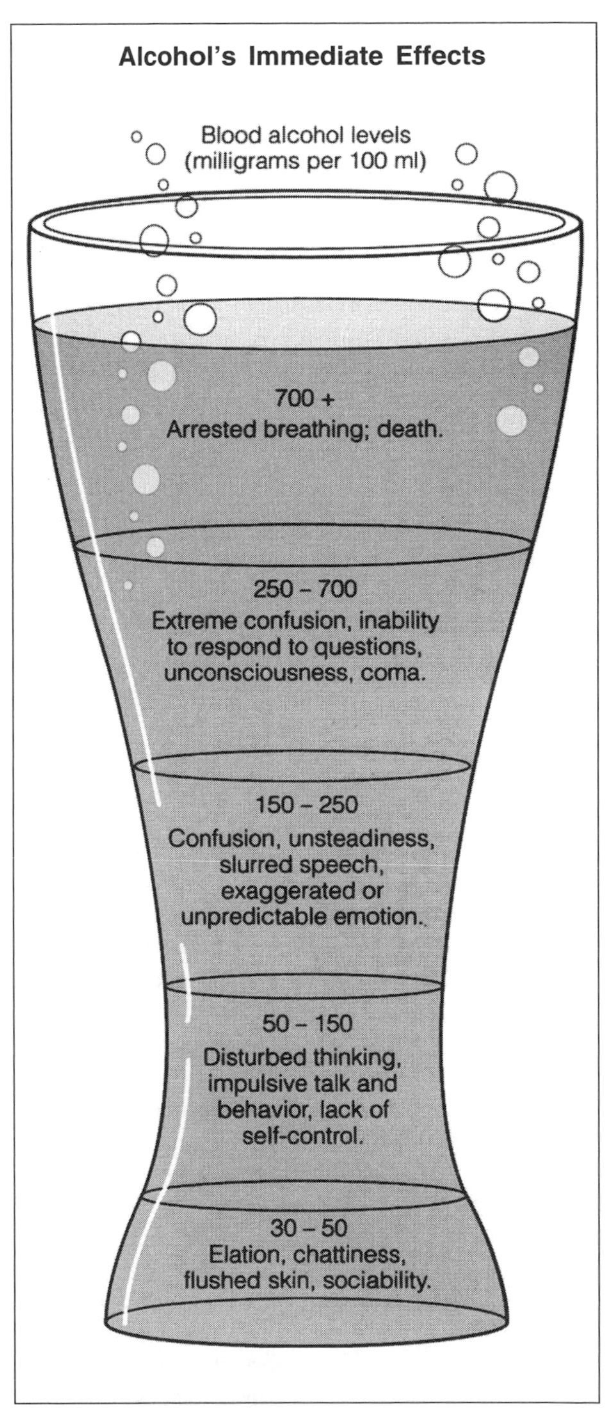

The presence of 30-50 milligrams of alcohol per every 100 milliliters of blood, which represents the effects of an average drink (a glass of beer, wine, or an ounce of hard liquor), has immediate effects; as the amount increases, effects progress toward death.

Commonly observed symptoms of alcoholism are physical dependence, as evidenced by signs such as tremors, shakes, other physical discomfort when not drinking, and excitability reversed only by alcohol intake; blackout and accompanying memory loss; diminished cognitive ability, exhibited as an inability to understand verbal instructions or to memorize simple series of numbers; and relaxed social inhibitions. These symptoms are attributable to the destruction of tissues of the central nervous system. Diminished sexual activity and sexual desire may also result from excessive alcohol consumption. A high level of alcohol appears to cause diminished libido and impotence.

Treatment and Therapy

In the mid-1930's, alcoholism, previously viewed as criminal and immoral behavior, was first conceived to be a disease.

There is no known immediate, miracle cure for alcoholism. Treatments with demonstrated effectiveness for alcohol problems, however, do exist. Treatments involving a combined biological, psychological, and social approach, complete with follow-up, often appear most helpful. For most individuals, however, an important phase—or possibly even a permanent feature—of treatment involves total abstinence from alcoholic beverages, all medications that contain alcohol, and any other potential sources of alcohol in the diet.

The recognition of alcoholism as a medical problem has led to the establishment of alcohol rehabilitation centers, where psychiatric treatment, medication, and other therapies are used in widely different combinations. The supportive programs of the organization Alcoholics Anonymous are also viewed as effective deterrents to a return to alcohol problems. Another well-known medical treatment aimed at encouraging sobriety is the drug disulfiram, more popularly known as Antabuse. This drug is given when individuals who wish to avoid all use of alcoholic beverages require a deterrent to drinking in order to achieve this goal. It is important to note, however, that no drug should ever be given secretly to someone by well-meaning family or friends. This is especially important with Antabuse because of the serious physical consequences that will be suffered if the person drinks alcohol.

These dangers are the result of the biochemistry of alcohol utilization via the two enzymes (biological protein catalysts) alcohol dehydrogenase and aldehyde dehydrogenase. Normally, alcohol dehydrogenase converts alcohol to the toxic chemical acetaldehyde, and aldehyde dehydrogenase quickly converts the acetaldehyde to acetic acid, the main biological fuel on which the body runs. Antabuse will turn off aldehyde dehydrogenase and cause acetaldehyde levels to build up in the body when alcohol is consumed. The presence of acetaldehyde in the body then quickly leads to violent headache, great dizziness, heart palpitation, nausea, and vertigo. When the amount of alcohol found in a drink or two (or even the amount taken in cough medicine) is consumed in the presence of Antabuse, these symptoms can escalate to the extent that they become fatal.

An interesting sidelight is the view of many researchers that abstinence from alcohol may be genetically related to the presence of too much alcohol dehydrogenase and/or too little aldehyde dehydrogenase in the body. Either of these unbalanced conditions is thought to produce enough acetaldehyde from a small amount of any alcohol source to cause aversion to all alcohol consumption. This is viewed as particularly relevant in Japan, where about 50 percent of the population lacks aldehyde dehydrogenase, and this lack correlates well with the low predisposition of many Japanese to become alcohol dependent. It must be remembered, however, that no one is immune from developing problems with alcohol. Even someone who belongs to a group known to lack these particular enzymes does not merit a license to use alcohol without care.

As a result of the symptoms of alcohol withdrawal common during detoxification and the presence of other mental health disorders in nearly half of all individuals diagnosed with alcohol dependence, other therapeutic drugs are often used in treatment. Examples include lithium (more often given when mood problems are present), tranquilizers, and sedative hypnotics. The function of these psychoactive drugs is to diminish the discomfort of alcohol withdrawal and stabilize the individual.

Tranquilizers and the related sedative hypnotics must also be used with great care, under close supervision of a physician. Many such drugs are addictive. In addition, some of these drugs have strong synergistic (additive) effects when mixed with alcohol, and such synergism can be fatal. Detailed information on the uses and dangers of these different drugs in the treatment of alcohol problems can be found in *The Merck Manual of Diagnosis and Therapy.*

It is believed that the advent of Alcoholics Anonymous in the 1930's has been crucial to the perception of alcoholism as a disease to be treated, rather than as immoral behavior to be condemned. This organization operates on the premise that abstinence is the best course of treatment for alcoholism. The methodology of the organization is psychosocial. First, individuals who wish to stop drinking are brought to the realization that they can never use alcoholic beverages without succumbing to serious problems. Then, the need for help from a "higher power" is identified as crucial to abstinence. In addition, the organization develops a support group of people in the same situation. It is this support group feature of Alcoholics Anonymous that is coming to be seen as more and more valuable to facilitating change.

An estimate of the membership of Alcoholics Anonymous in 2001 was two million. These people, ranging widely in age, achieve results varying from periods of sobriety (lasting longer and longer as membership in the organization continues) to lifelong sobriety. While valuable, it is important to remember that Alcoholics Anonymous is not a formal medical treatment for alcohol problems. It is not necessarily treatment managed by medical, psychiatric, and other formally trained counselors. The results of the operation, however, are viewed by most as beneficial to all parties who seek help from the organization.

Alcohol rehabilitation centers apply varied combinations of drug therapy, psychiatric counseling, and social counseling, depending on the treatment approach for the individual center. Group therapy, however, is the dominant mode of treatment in the United States.

Perspective and Prospects

Modern efforts to deal with alcohol problems are often considered to have begun in the early twentieth century, with the activities of the American temperance movement and the Anti-Saloon League. These activities culminated in the period called Prohibition after Congress passed the 1919 Volstead Act, proposed by Minnesota congressman Andrew J. Volstead. The idea behind the act was that making intoxicating beverages impossible to obtain would force sobriety on Americans. Prohibition turned out to be self-defeating, however, and it increased the incidence of alcohol and related problems. Subsequently, the act was repealed in 1933, ending Prohibition.

The next, and much more useful, effort to combat alcoholism was the psychosocial Alcoholics Anonymous organization, started in 1935 by William Griffith Wilson and Robert Holbrook Smith. Because that organization does not reach the majority of individuals with alcohol problems, other efforts have evolved as treatment methodologies. Among these have been psychiatric counseling, alcohol rehabilitation centers, family counseling, and alcohol management programs in the workplace. Treatment efforts have even taken to the Internet, with different types of meetings and resources posted online for individuals to find and use. These endeavors, funded by the federal government and private industry, reached workable levels in the last quarter of the twentieth century and remain an ongoing effort.

—Sanford S. Singer, Ph.D.;
updated by Nancy A. Piotrowski, Ph.D.

See also Addiction; American Indian health; Cirrhosis; Dementias; Fetal alcohol syndrome; Intoxication; Jaundice; Liver disorders; Osteonecrosis; Psychosis.

For Further Information:

Alcoholics Anonymous. http://www.alcoholics-anonymous.org/. A group whose primary purpose is to help members stay sober and help other alcoholics to achieve sobriety.

Alcoholics Anonymous World Service. *Alcoholics Anonymous*. 4th rev. ed. New York: Author, 2001. Offers steps to recovery and personal stories of rehabilitation.

Beers, Mark H., et al. *The Merck Manual of Diagnosis and Therapy*. 18th ed. Whitehouse Station, N.J.: Merck Research Laboratories, 2006. This book contains a compendium of data on the etiology, diagnosis, and treatment of alcoholism. Contains good cross-references to the psychopathology related to the disease, drug rehabilitation, and Alcoholics Anonymous.

Collins, R. Lorraine, Kenneth E. Leonard, and John R. Searles, eds. *Alcohol and the Family: Research and Clinical Perspectives*. New York: Guilford Press, 1990. Reprinted in 2005, this book addresses genetics, family processes, and family-oriented treatment. Aspects of genetic testing and markers are covered, along with adolescent drinking, children of alcoholics, and alcoholism's effect on a marriage.

Dwyer, Frank. *Annotated AA Handbook: A Companion to the Big Book*. Rev. ed. Ft. Lee, N.J.: Barricade Books, 2000. The entire text of the first edition of *Alcoholics Anonymous* is supplemented here with comprehensive explanatory notations and cross-references, as well as a history of the book and the AA treatment approach.

Goodwin, Donald D. *Alcoholism: The Facts*. New York: Oxford University Press, 2000. Accessible discussions of the range of social, psychological, and medical aspects of alcohol problems.

Hester, Reid K., and William R. Miller. *Handbook of Alcoholism Treatment Approaches*. 3d ed. Boston: Allyn & Bacon, 2002. A comprehensive guide to alcohol treatment methods designed for both practitioners and researchers.

Torr, James D. *Alcoholism*. San Diego, Calif.: Greenhaven Press, 2000. This well-balanced selection of primary source materials is designed for children in grades six through twelve. A lengthy bibliography and a list of organizations to contact are appended.

Allergies

Disease/disorder

Anatomy or system affected: Gastrointestinal system, immune system, lungs, nose, skin, stomach

Specialties and related fields: Dermatology, family medicine, immunology, internal medicine, otorhinolaryngology, pediatrics, pharmacology

Definition: Exaggerated immune reactions to materials that are intrinsically harmless; the body's release of pharmacologically active chemicals during allergic reactions may result in discomfort, tissue damage, or, in severe responses, death.

Key terms:

allergen: any substance that induces an allergic reaction

anaphylaxis: an immediate immune reaction, triggered by mediators that cause vasodilation and the contraction of smooth muscle

basophil: a type of white blood cell which contains mediators associated with allergic reactions; represents 1 percent or less of total white cells

histamine: a compound released during allergic reactions which causes many of the symptoms of allergies

IgE: a type of antibody associated with the release of granules from basophils and mast cells

mast cell: a tissue cell with granules containing vasoactive mediators such as histamine, serotonin, and bradykinin; the tissue equivalent of basophil

Information on Allergies

Causes: Antigens such as pollen, mold, certain foods (nuts, eggs, seafood), drugs (penicillin), bee or wasp venom, animal dander, dust mites, etc.

Symptoms: Sneezing, runny nose, coughing, itching, breathing difficulties, hives, inflammation, vomiting, diarrhea, shock

Duration: Chronic, with acute episodes

Treatments: Antihistamines, mast cell stabilizers, steroids (cortisone), desensitization

Causes and Symptoms

Allergies represent inappropriate immune responses to intrinsically harmless materials, or antigens. Most allergens are common environmental antigens. Approximately one in every six Americans is allergic to material such as dust, molds, dust mites, animal dander, or pollen. The effects range from a mere nuisance, such as the rhinitis associated with hay fever allergies or the itching of poison ivy, to the life-threatening anaphylactic shock that may follow a bee sting. Allergies are most often found in children, but they may affect any age group.

Allergy is one of the hypersensitivity reactions generally classified according to the types of effector molecules that mediate their symptoms and according to the time delay that follows exposure to the allergen. P. G. H. Gell and Robin Coombs defined four types of hypersensitivities. Three of these, Types I through III, follow minutes to hours after the exposure to an allergen. Type IV, or delayed-type hypersensitivity (DTH), may occur anywhere from twenty-four to seventy-two hours after exposure. People are most familiar with two of these forms of allergies: Type I, or immediate hypersensitivity, commonly seen as hay fever or asthma; and Type IV, most often following an encounter with poison ivy or poison oak.

Type I hypersensitivities have much in common with any normal immune response. A foreign material, an allergen, comes in contact with the host's immune system, and an antibody response is the result. The response differs according to the type of molecule produced. A special class of antibody, IgE, is secreted by the B lymphocytes. IgE, when complexed with the specific allergen, is capable of binding to any of several types of mediator cells, mainly basophils and mast cells.

Mast cells are found throughout the skin and tissue. The mucous membranes of the respiratory and gastrointestinal tract in particular have high concentrations of these cells, as many as ten thousand cells per cubic millimeter. Basophils, the blood cell equivalents of the mast cells, represent 1 percent or less of the total white-cell count. Though the cells are not identical, they do possess features related to the role that they play in an allergic response. Both basophils and mast cells contain large numbers of granules composed of pharmacologically active chemicals. Both also contain surface receptors for IgE molecules. The binding of IgE/allergen complexes to these cells triggers the release of the granules.

A large number of common antigens can be associated with allergies. These include plant pollens (as are found in rye grass or ragweed), foods such as nuts or eggs, bee or wasp venom, mold, or animal dander. A square mile of ragweed may produce as much as 16 tons of pollen in a single season. In fact, almost any food or environmental substance could serve as an allergen. The most important defining factor as to whether an individual is allergic to any particular substance is the extent and type of IgE production against that substance.

Type I allergic reactions begin as soon as the sensitized person is exposed to the allergen. In the case of hay fever, this results when the person inhales the pollen particle. The shell of the particle is enzymatically dissolved, and the specific allergens are released in the vicinity of the mucous membranes in the respiratory system. If the person has had prior sensitization to the materials, IgE molecules secreted by localized lymphocytes bind to the allergens, forming an antibody/antigen complex.

Events commonly associated with allergies to pollen—a runny nose and itchy, watery eyes—result from the formation of such complexes. A sequence of events is set in place when the immune complexes bind to the surface of the mast cell or basophil. The reactions begin with a cross-linking of the IgE receptors on the cell. Such cross-linking is necessary because, in its absence, no granules are released. On the other hand, artificial cross-linking of the receptors in laboratory experiments, even in the absence of IgE, results in the release of vasoactive granules.

Following the activation of the cell surface, a series of biochemical events occurs, the key being an influx of calcium into the cell. Two events rapidly follow: The cell begins production of prostaglandins and leukotrienes, two mediators that play key roles in allergic reactions, and preexisting granules begin moving toward the cell surface. When they reach the cell surface, the

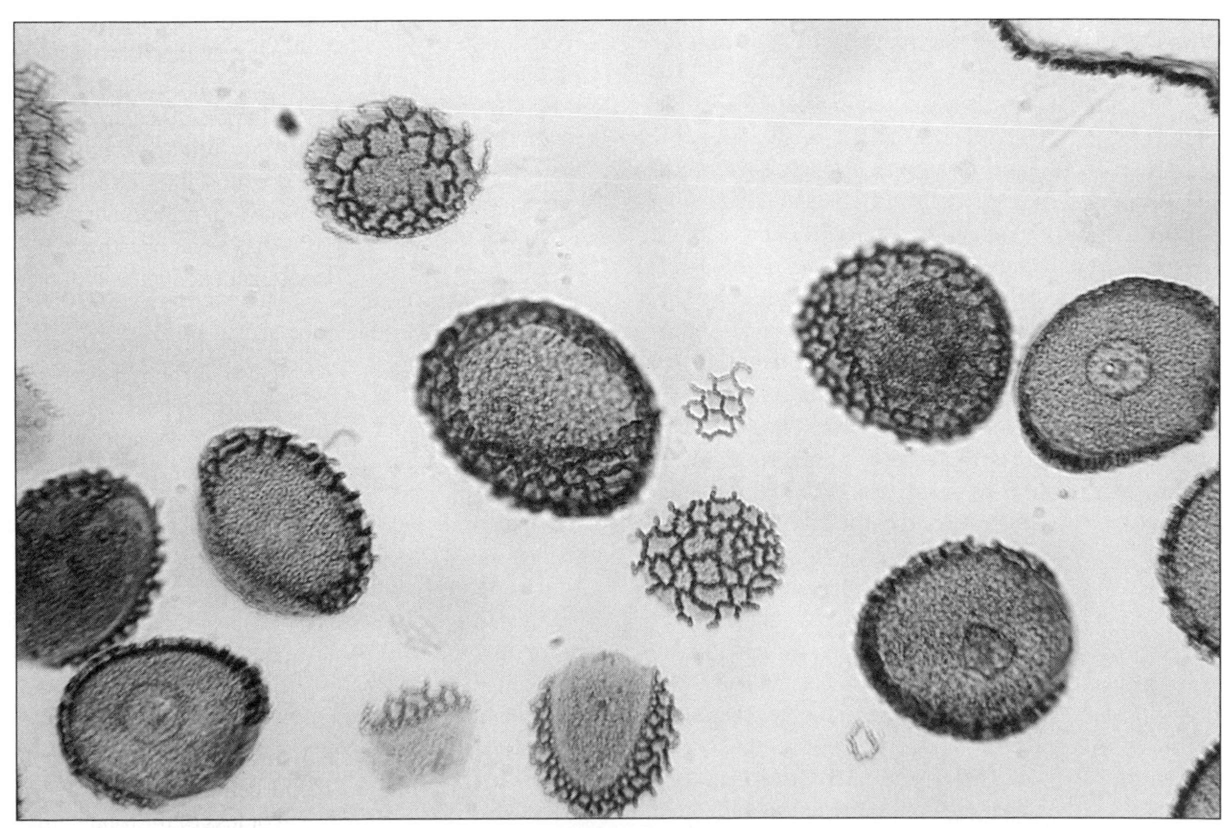

Microscopic pollens, which are responsible for many allergic reactions. (PhotoDisc)

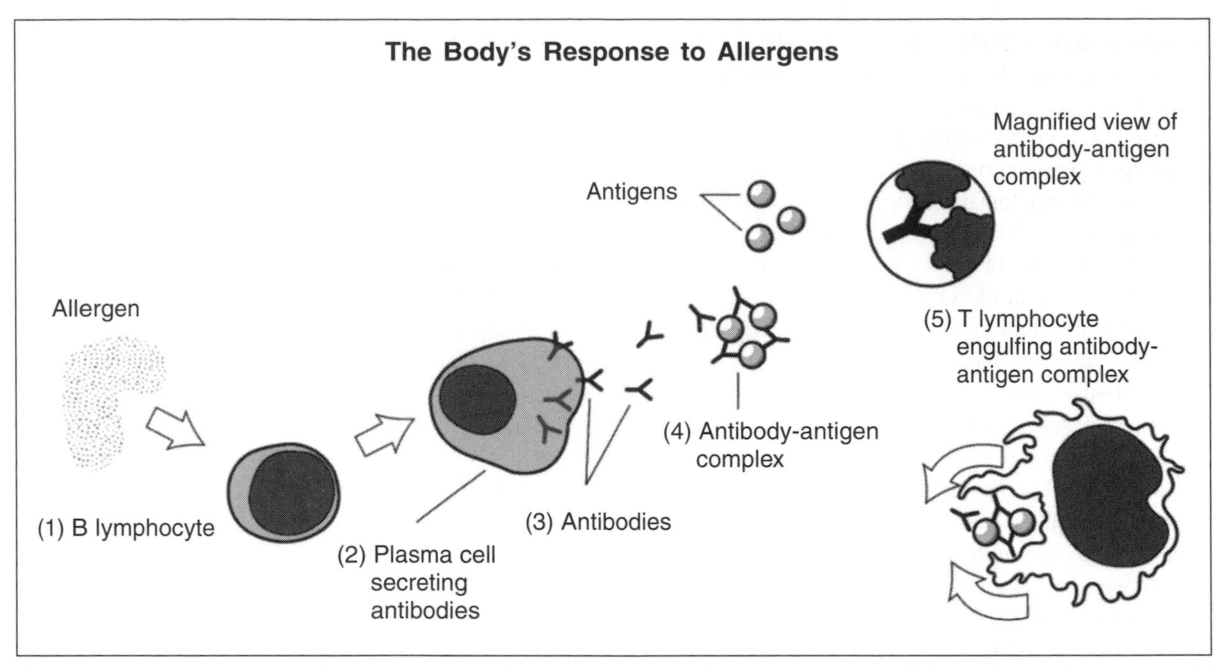

An allergic reaction is caused when foreign material, or antigens, enter the immune system, which produces B lymphocytes (1) that cause blood plasma cells to secrete antibodies (2). The antibodies (3) link with antigens to form antigen-antibody complexes (4), which then are engulfed and destroyed by a T lymphocyte (5).

granules fuse with the cell membrane, releasing their contents into the tissue.

The contents of the granules mediate the clinical manifestations of allergies. These mediators can be classified as either primary or secondary. Thus, clinical responses are divided into immediate and late-phase reactions. Primary mediators are those found in preexisting granules and that are released initially following the activities at the cell surface. They include substances such as histamine and serotonin, associated with increased vascular permeability and smooth muscle contraction. Histamine itself may constitute 10 percent of the weight of the granules in these cells. The results are the runny nose, irritated eyes, and bronchial congestion with which so many are familiar. Secondary mediators, which are released in the late phase, are synthesized following the binding of the immune complexes to the cell surface. These substances include the leukotrienes (also called slow reactive substances of anaphylaxis, or SRS-A) and prostaglandins. Pharmacological effects from these chemicals include vasodilation, increased capillary permeability, contraction of smooth muscles in the bronchioles, and, more important, a group of chemotactic activities that attract many different white cells in the site to magnify the inflammatory reaction. This is why an allergic reaction is divided into two phases and the late reaction may last for days.

Foods to which one is allergic may trigger similar reactions in the gut. Mast cells in the gastrointestinal tract also contain receptors for IgE, and contact with food allergens results in the release of mediators similar to those in the respiratory passages. The result may be vomiting or diarrhea. The allergen may also pass from the gut into the circulatory system or other tissues, triggering asthmatic attacks or urticaria (hives).

In severe allergic reactions, the response may be swift and deadly. The venom released during a bee sting may trigger a systemic response from circulating basophils or mast cells, resulting in the contraction of pulmonary muscles and rapid suffocation, a condition known as anaphylactic shock. The leukotrienes, platelet-activating factor, and prostaglandins play key roles in these reactions.

Delayed-type hypersensitivities, also known as contact dermatitis reactions, are most commonly manifested following the presentation of a topical allergen. These may include the catechol-containing oils of poison oak, the constituents of hair dyes or cosmetics, environmental contaminants such as nickel or turpentine, or any of a wide variety of environmental agents. Rather than being mediated by antibodies, as are the other types of hypersensitivities, DTH is mediated through a specific cellular response. These cells appear to be a special class of T (for thymus-derived) lymphocytes.

DTH reactions are initiated following the exposure to the appropriate antigen. Antigen-presenting cells in the skin bind and "present" the allergen to the specific T lymphocytes. This results in the secretion by these T cells of a variety of chemicals mediating inflammation. These mediators, or cytokines, include gamma interferon, interleukin-2, and tumor necrosis factor. The result, developing over a period of twenty-four to seventy-two hours, is a significant inflammatory response with subsequent localized damage to tissue.

The other classes of hypersensitivity reactions, Types II and III, are less commonly associated with what most people consider to be allergies. Yet they do have much in common with Type I, immediate hypersensitivity. Type II reactions are mediated by a type of antibody called IgG. Clinical manifestations result from the antibody-mediated destruction of target cells, rather than through the release of mediators. One of the most common forms of reaction is blood transfusion reactions, either against the A or B blood group antigen or as a result of an Rh incompatibility. For example, if a person with type O blood is accidentally transfused with type A, an immune reaction will occur. The eventual result is destruction of the incompatible blood cells. Rh incompatibilities are most commonly associated with a pregnant woman who is lacking the Rh protein in her blood (that is, Rh negative) carrying a child who is Rh positive (a blood type obtained from the father's genes). The production of IgG directed against the Rh protein in the child's blood can set in motion events that result in the destruction of the baby's red blood cells, a condition known as erythroblastosis fetalis.

Type III reactions are known as immune complex diseases. In this case, sensitivity to antigens results in formation of IgG/antigen complexes, which can lodge in the kidney or other sites in the body. The complexes activate what is known as the complement system, a series of proteins which include vasoactive chemicals and lipolytic compounds. The result can be a significant inflammation that can lead to kidney damage. Type III reactions can include autoimmune diseases such as arthritis or lupus, or drug reactions such as penicillin allergies.

It should be kept in mind, however, that none of these reactions is inherently abnormal. Under normal circumstances, these same reactions mediate an inflammatory defense against foreign pathogens. For example, the normal role of IgE appears to be associated with the destruction of parasites such as are found in helminthic infections (such as parasitic worms). The release of mediators under these conditions is important as a defensive reaction leading to the expulsion or destruction of worms. It is only when these same mediators are released inappropriately that one observes the symptoms of allergies.

Most individuals are familiar with immediate hypersensitivities as reactions involving a localized area. The most common form of allergy is rhinitis, known as hay fever, which affects approximately 10 percent of the population. When a person inhales an environmental allergen such as ragweed pollen, the result is a release of pharmacologically active mediators from mast cells located in the upper respiratory tract. If the release occurs in the lower respiratory tract, the condition is known as asthma. In both instances, the eyes and nose are subject to inflammation and the release of secretions. In mild cases, the person suffers from watery discharges, coughing, and sneezing. In more severe asthma attacks, the bronchioles may become constricted and obstruct the air passages.

TREATMENT AND THERAPY

Three methods for dealing with allergies exist: avoidance of the allergen, palliative treatments, and desensitization. Ideally, one can attempt to avoid the allergen. For example, cow's milk, a common allergen, should not be given to a child at too young an age, and one can stay away from patches of poison ivy or avoid eating strawberries if one is allergic to them.

Yet avoidance is not always possible or desirable, as the problem may be the fur from the family cat. In any event, it is sometimes difficult to identify the specific substance causing the symptoms. This is particularly true when dealing with foods. Various procedures exist to identify the irritating substance, skin testing being the most common. In this procedure, the patient's skin is exposed to small amounts of suspected allergens. A positive test is indicated by formation of hives or reddening within about twenty to thirty minutes. If the person is hypersensitive to a suspected allergen and finds a skin test too risky, then a blood test (RAST) may be substituted. In addition to running a battery of tests, a patient's allergy history (including family history, since allergies are in part genetic) or environment may give clues as to the identity of the culprit.

The most commonly used method of dealing with allergies is a palliative treatment—that is, treatment of

In the News: Peanut Allergies

In the United States alone, fifty to one hundred people die each year from serious allergic reactions to peanuts. One and a half million Americans have a demonstrated allergic sensitivity that puts them at risk for life-threatening reactions to peanut protein exposure. Reactions can be so severe to minute amounts of airborne peanut protein that some schoolchildren must eat lunch in peanut-free rooms, and many airlines have stopped serving peanuts to passengers. Because peanuts and peanut oil can be ingredients in a divcrse range of food items such as chili, potato chips, and egg rolls, peanut allergy sufferers live under a constant threat of having an adverse reaction despite their best efforts to avoid the allergen.

In the March 13, 2003, issue of the *New England Journal of Medicine* Dr. Hugh A. Sampson and his colleagues of Mount Sinai School of Medicine in New York reported the results of a study that shows the first successful preventive treatment for peanut allergy. In a double-blind study, eighty-four volunteers with peanut allergy were given either placebo shots or injections of various doses of the experimental drug TNX-901 once a month over a four-month period. At the end of the study, participants were given capsules of peanut flour in increasing amounts until they exhibited an allergic reaction. The results showed that those given placebos reacted when given the equivalent of half a peanut. People who received low doses of the drug could ingest a bit more before reacting. Those receiving the highest doses could ingest, on average, the equivalent of nine peanuts (and for some, twenty-four peanuts) before developing an allergic response.

TNX-901 is a genetically engineered antibody that prevents allergic response by binding to potentially harmful immune cells that are produced in response to allergen exposure. Binding these immune cells interrupts the series of events that lead to an allergic reaction.

While TNX-901 is not a cure for peanut allergy, its preventive potential makes the required monthly shot appealing to those afflicted with the disorder. Since accidental exposure to peanut protein is estimated to be equivalent to one or two peanuts, TNX-901 could provide sufferers with confidence that accidental peanut exposure would not lead to a life-threatening reaction. Legal disputes have hampered its development, however, and a similar drug called Xolair is being researched.

—Karen E. Kalumuck, Ph.D.

the symptoms. Antihistamines act by binding to histamine receptors on target cells, interfering with the binding of histamine. Two types of histamine receptors exist: H-1 and H-2. Histamine binding to H-1 receptors results in contractions of smooth muscles and increased mucus secretion. Binding to H-2 receptors results in increased vasopermeability and swelling. Antihistamines that act at the level of the H-1 receptor include alkylamines and ethanolamines and are effective in treating symptoms of acute allergies such as hay fever. Histamine II blockers such as cimetidine are effective in the symptomatic treatment of duodenal ulcers through the control of gastric secretions.

Many antihistamines can be obtained without a prescription. If they are not used properly, however, the side effects can be serious. Overuse may result in toxicity, particularly in children; overdoses in children can be fatal. Because antihistamines can depress the central nervous system, side effects include drowsiness, nausea, constipation, and drying of the throat or respiratory passage. This is particularly true of histamine 1 blockers. A new generation of H-1 antihistamines is available on the market. They are long-acting and are free of the sedative effect of other antihistamines.

Other symptomatic treatments include the use of cromolyn sodium, which blocks the influx of calcium into the mast cell, and thus is called a mast cell stabilizer. It acts to block steps leading to degranulation and the release of mediators. In more severe cases, the administration of steroids (cortisone) may prove useful in limiting symptoms of allergies.

Anaphylaxis is the most severe form of immediate hypersensitivity, and unless treated promptly, it may be fatal. It is often triggered in susceptible persons by common environmental substances: bee or wasp venom, drugs such as penicillin, foods such as peanuts and seafood, or latex protein in rubber. Symptoms include labored breathing, rapid loss of blood pressure, itching, hives, and/or loss of bladder control. The symptoms are triggered by a sudden and massive release of mast cell or basophil mediators such as histamine, leukotrienes, or prostaglandin derivatives. Treatment consists of an immediate injection of epinephrine and the maintenance of an open air passage into the lungs. If cardiac arrest occurs, cardiopulmonary resuscitation must be undertaken. Persons in known danger of encountering such a triggering allergen often carry with them an emergency kit containing epinephrine and antihistamines.

Contact dermatitis is a form of delayed-type hypersensitivity, developing several days after exposure to the sensitizing allergen. Rather than resulting from the presence of IgE antibody, the symptoms of contact dermatitis result from a series of chemicals released by sensitized T lymphocytes in the area of the skin on which the allergen (often poison ivy or poison oak) is found. Treatments generally involve the application of topical corticosteroids and soothing or drying agents. In more severe cases, systemic use of corticosteroids may be necessary.

In some persons, the relief of allergy symptoms may be achieved through desensitization. This form of immunotherapy involves the repeated subcutaneous injection of increasing doses of the allergen. In a significant number of persons, such therapy leads to a decrease in symptoms. The idea behind such therapy is that repeated injections of the allergen may lead to production of another class of antibody, the more systemic IgG. These molecules can serve as blocking antibodies, competing with IgE in binding to the allergen. Because IgG/allergen complexes can be phagocytosed (destroyed by phagocytes) and do not bind receptors on mast cells or basophils, they should not trigger the symptoms of allergies. Unfortunately, for reasons that remain unclear, not all persons or all allergies respond to such therapy.

The Type I immediate hypersensitivity reactions commonly run in families. This is not so surprising if one realizes that the regulation of IgE production is genetically determined. Thus, if both parents have allergies, there is little chance that their offspring will escape the problem. On the other hand, if one or both parents are allergy-free, the odds are at least even that the offspring will also be free from such reactions.

Perspective and Prospects

Though allergies in humans have probably existed since humans first evolved from ancestral primates, it was only in the nineteenth century that an understanding of the process began to develop. Type I hypersensitivity reaction was first described in 1839 through experiments in which dogs were repeatedly injected with

In the News: "Big 8" Allergens on Food Labels

On December 20, 2005, the Food and Drug Administration (FDA) announced that on January 1, 2006, it would put into effect regulations enforcing the Food Allergen Labeling and Consumer Protection Act of 2004. The FDA edict required manufacturers to list in clear language on product labels the presence of any of the eight most important food allergens—milk, eggs, fish, crustacean shellfish such as shrimp, tree nuts, peanuts, wheat, and soybeans—and protein derived from them. Thus, if a product contained casein, a milk-derived protein, then the label would have to say "contains milk," in addition to listing casein among the ingredients.

The FDA estimated that these eight allergens were responsible for 90 percent of all allergic reactions to food, requiring complete avoidance of the allergy-producing substances to prevent severe or even life-threatening reactions. The clear language provisions were expected to be particularly useful to children and teenagers who could not be expected to recognize technical names of all possible derivatives of allergens that they needed to avoid. About 11 million Americans—2 percent of adults and 5 percent of infants and young children—are affected by food allergies. Some 300,000 people end up in emergency rooms each year, and 150 die as a result of extreme reactions.

Consumer advocates welcomed the new rules, but, by the summer of 2006, they were complaining that some manufacturers confused purchasers by using "may contain" declarations on their labels rather than the specific language preferred by the FDA and customers. Larger food companies rarely used "may contain" statements, but smaller manufacturers, either uncertain about the regulations or fearful of product liability lawsuits, were major offenders. Ambiguous language was particularly perplexing to teenagers, unsure how seriously to take the warnings, who might either risk severe reactions or unnecessarily limit their choice of food.

—*Milton Berman, Ph.D.*

egg albumin and developed an immediate fatal shock. The term "anaphylaxis" was coined for this phenomenon in 1902, when Paul Portier and Charles Richet observed that dogs repeatedly immunized with extracts of sea anemone tentacles suffered a similar fate. Richet was awarded the 1913 Nobel Prize in Physiology or Medicine for his work on anaphylaxis.

In the 1920's, Sir Henry Dale established that at least some of the phenomena associated with immediate hypersensitivity were caused by the chemical histamine. Dale sensitized guinea pigs against various antigens. He then observed that, when the muscles from the uterus were removed and exposed to the same antigen, histamine was released and the muscles underwent contraction (known as the Schultz-Dale reaction).

The existence of a component in human serum which mediates hypersensitive reactions was demonstrated by Otto Prausnitz, a Polish bacteriologist, and Heinz Kustner, a Polish gynecologist, in 1921. Kustner had a strong allergy to fish. Prausnitz removed a sample of serum from his colleague and injected it under his own skin. The next day, Prausnitz injected fish extract in that same region. Hives immediately appeared, indicating that the serum contained components that mediated the allergy. For some time, the Prausnitz-Kustner test, or P-K test, remained a means of testing for allergens under circumstances in which a person could be tested for sensitivity. (It is no longer in use because of safety concerns.) In this test, a serum sample from the test subject was injected under the skin of a surrogate (usually a relative) and later followed with test allergens. The presence of a wheal and flare reaction (hives) indicated sensitivity to the allergen. The serum component responsible for this sensitivity was later identified as the antibody IgE by K. and T. Ishizaka and S. G. O. Johansson in 1967. The target cells to which the IgE bound were later identified as mast cells and basophils.

The discovery of IgE allowed scientists to develop a blood test called a radioallergosorbent test (RAST) that could measure a specific IgE antibody to an allergic substance. RAST is fully as sensitive as a skin test and thus can be a substitute in some clinical circumstances. Furthermore, discoveries of numerous mediators from mast cells and other white cells such as cytokines, chemokines, interleukins, growth factors, and interferon have helped scientists understand the pathology of allergy at the molecular level. It helps clinically to divide the allergic reaction into immediate reaction (onset within a few minutes after exposure to allergens) and delayed or late-phase reaction (onset hours after exposure to antigens and a reaction that may last for days). The definition of allergy has now expanded from the traditional, immediate allergic reaction to the inclusion of chronic inflammatory processes in the tissues. With a better understanding of how allergies develop, better treatments can be offered to patients who suffer from this disorder.

The eventual goal of the research was to understand the molecular defects that result in allergies and ultimately to find a means to eliminate the problem, rather than simply offer palliative measures. For example, it is now known that interleukin-4 (one of the mediators of T cells) raises IgE production, while interferon (another mediator of T cells) lowers IgE production. By understanding the regulation of IgE production, it may become possible to inhibit IgE production in allergic persons selectively, without affecting the desired functions of the immune response.

—Richard Adler, Ph.D.;
updated by Shih-Wen Huang, M.D.

See also Antihistamines; Asthma; Autoimmune disorders; Bites and stings; Celiac sprue; Decongestants; Dermatitis; Dermatology; Diaper rash; Food poisoning; Gastroenterology; Gastroenterology, pediatric; Gastrointestinal disorders; Gastrointestinal system; Hay fever; Hives; Host-defense mechanisms; Immune system; Immunization and vaccination; Immunology; Lungs; Mold and mildew; Multiple chemical sensitivity syndrome; Poisonous plants; Pulmonary medicine; Pulmonary medicine, pediatric; Rashes; Shock; Skin; Skin disorders; Sneezing.

For Further Information:

Adelman, Daniel C., et al., eds. *Manual of Allergy and Immunology*. 4th ed. Philadelphia: Lippincott Williams & Wilkins, 2002. Examines research developments and the clinical diagnosis and treatment of allergies and immune disorders. Topics include asthma, disorders of the eye, diseases of the lung, anaphylaxism, insect allergies, drug allergies, rheumatic diseases, transplantation immunology, and immunization.

Brostoff, Jonathan, and Linda Gamlin. *Food Allergies and Food Intolerance: The Complete Guide to Their Identification and Treatment*. Rochester, Vt.: Inner Traditions, 2000. Examines the role of food allergies in chronic health conditions such as migraines and persistent fatigue and gives a step-by-step process for identifying and treating food allergies.

Cutler, Ellen W. *Winning the War Against Asthma and*

Allergies. Albany, N.Y.: Delmar, 1998. This clearly written book provides practical information on all aspects of allergies—what they are, their causes, testing, diagnosis, and treatment, including nontraditional therapies. Preventive measures are covered, as are scenarios for various allergy elimination therapies.

Delves, Peter J., et al. *Roitt's Essential Immunology*. 11th ed. Malden, Mass.: Blackwell, 2006. Written by a leading author in the field, the text provides a fine description of immunology. The section on hypersensitivity is clearly presented and profusely illustrated. Though too detailed in places, most of the material can be understood by individuals who have taken high school biology.

Joneja, Janice M. V., and Leonard Bielory. *Understanding Allergy, Sensitivity, and Immunity*. New Brunswick, N.J.: Rutgers University Press, 1990. The authors provide extensive discussion of allergies and the roles played by the immune system. They describe the means by which one can learn to cope with allergies and discuss various testing methods for the identification of allergens.

Kindt, Thomas J., Richard A. Goldsby, and Barbara A. Osborne. *Kuby Immunology*. 6th ed. New York: W. H. Freeman, 2007. The section on hypersensitivity in this immunology textbook is well written and includes a mixture of detail and overview of the subject. Particularly useful are discussions of the various types of hypersensitivity reactions. Some knowledge of biology is useful.

Life, Death, and the Immune System. New York: W. H. Freeman, 1994. This comprehensive collection of articles from *Scientific American* provides basic information and research directions on AIDS, autoimmune disorders, and allergies as well as an excellent discussion of the immune system in general.

Walsh, William. *The Food Allergy Book*. New York: J. Wiley, 2000. In this excellent guide to one highly prevalent form of allergy, the author presents useful background information on food allergies and a pragmatic guide to identifying and eliminating food allergens from one's diet.

Young, Stuart, Bruce Dobozin, and Margaret Miner. *Allergies*. Rev. ed. New York: Plume, 1999. In addition to discussing the diagnosis and treatment of allergies, the authors evaluate the various remedies on the market at the time of publication. Also useful are lists of organizations to contact for further information.

Allied health

Health care system

Definition: A designation used to describe the services and personnel that support the providers of direct patient care within the larger health care system.

Key terms:

anesthetist: a health care specialist who administers an agent (anesthetic) that makes the patient insensitive to sensation or pain

audiologist: a hearing impairment specialist involved in evaluation, measurement, and rehabilitation

chiropractic: a health care strategy which teaches that disease can be caused by the pinching of spinal nerves, the treatment of which involves spinal adjustment

kinesiotherapist: a health care specialist who provides therapy to a patient's muscles through muscular movement and exercise

nuclear medicine: an area of medicine that uses radioactive nucleotides in diagnostic and treatment procedures

optometry: a specialty that deals with problems in the refractive power of the eyes and with the making of corrective lenses

paramedical: related to the science or practice of medicine

perfusionist: a health care specialist who operates extracorporal circulation equipment when it is necessary to support or replace a patient's circulatory or respiratory function

podiatry: the specialty that deals with the diagnosis and treatment of foot problems, including minor surgery

sonographer: a health care specialist who records and displays the results of an ultrasonic scan which produces a sonogram of a specific anatomical area

Boundaries Within Medicine

Allied health refers to a field of health care workers who participate with physicians and/or nurses in a team effort to promote health and prevent disease in the patient. Allied health occupations may be either professional or technical, depending on the extent and caliber of didactic learning and clinical study as well as on the duties associated with the occupation.

Throughout the evolution of the American health care system, the role of the physician has remained relatively stable and of primary importance. The American Medical Association (AMA) successfully developed specialty categories to solidify the role of the physician and to protect the doctorate in medicine.

The designation "allied health" appears to be a creation of the AMA to describe those paramedical occupations that developed within the evolving health care system in response to the advancing technology and expanding health care facilities, such as hospitals, clinics, medical centers, and laboratories. The AMA, through its various societies and committees, guided the formation of a variety of occupations to perform tasks that would not or could not be performed by the medical doctor or nurse. These occupations were carefully husbanded by strict job descriptions, educational guidelines, and evaluation criteria. For the most part, allied health professions are those fields that the Committee on Allied Health Education and Accreditation (CAHEA) of the AMA has scrutinized according to essential criteria that have been adopted by the particular profession. These criteria are primarily the standards that are established by a profession as a means to establish education programs that instruct new professionals, to perform a self-study by each program, and to be evaluated by an outside visiting team. A profession is also characterized by the establishment of a society or association by those practitioners of the occupation for the purpose of supporting the research, teaching, and learning of its members. The society sets standards of job performance and evaluation and also establishes a code of ethics to which its members adhere.

Those professions not accredited by the CAHEA are dentistry, optometry, podiatry, chiropractic, veterinary medicine, physical therapy, and nursing. Whether a profession finds the designation "allied health" complimentary or acceptable appears to depend on the status of the profession with respect to its age, the amount of education and responsibility required, and whether autonomy from the AMA is desired. The more autonomous a profession, the more impressive the identity and social status of its practitioners with respect to salary, power, and influence. For example, although a physical therapist can have a private practice rather than be employed in a hospital or another setting that guarantees a certain number of patients, a therapist is not legally allowed to treat a patient without an order from a physician. In 1998, the average salary for a hospital physical therapy (PT) supervisor was $50,000, while those in private practice earned $55,000 or more. In order to have a private practice, a physical therapist must cultivate a list of local physicians for referrals.

The nursing profession is a good example of a health profession that, to a greater or lesser extent, is not under the allied health umbrella. It is not listed by either the CAHEA or the Association of Schools of Allied Health Professions (ASAHP). Although the U.S. government provided scholarships for nurses in the Allied Health Personnel Training Act of 1966, nursing is excluded from the definition in the Health Professions Education Amendment of 1991. Nursing has been continuously able to maintain its integrity as a profession for a number of reasons: It has always had solidarity provided by the National League of Nursing (NLN), it has continued to develop its education requirements and responsibilities, it requires government licensure, and it has a very visible role in health care delivery—to some extent more than that of the physician.

The nursing profession continues to develop and is reaching into areas that were traditionally considered to be the domain of the physician. Nurse practitioners are able to take medical histories, read X rays, order and read tests, and diagnose conditions. They are able to prescribe medications in thirty-five states and can be reimbursed for some services by Medicare and Medicaid. Nurse anesthetists can work independently of a doctor in a variety of health care delivery settings.

According to the 1991 federal legislation cited above, the term "allied health profession" excludes both the nurse and the physician assistant. It includes all those who have had educational training in a science program relating to health services, earning anything from a certificate to a doctorate. It further defines allied health care personnel as individuals who share in the responsibility of the delivery of health care services or those related to health care. Such services include the identification, evaluation, and prevention of disease and disorders, as well as those related to diet and nutrition, health promotion, rehabilitation, and health systems management.

Those professionals who are excluded from the label of allied health care personnel by the government are doctors of medicine, osteopathy, dentistry, veterinary medicine, optometry, podiatry, pharmacy, chiropractic, and clinical psychology. Also excluded are pharmacists with bachelor's degrees, social workers, and those with graduate degrees in public health and health administration. It is confusing, however, to have physician assistants excluded from allied health by the government and the CAHEA but included in the designation by the ASAHP. Physical therapy is included by the government and the ASAHP but excluded by the CAHEA. The reason for such apparent confusion rests with the various points of view. The government is interested in the service provided by the particular occupation. The ASAHP is interested in promoting allied health education, professional growth, and collaboration between the professions and in influencing public policy as it relates to these factors. The CAHEA has the responsibility of overseeing the allied health education programs that are under the AMA umbrella.

According to the ASAHP, allied health professionals serve in a variety of autonomous and service positions. Therapists and counselors function in private practice and are directly involved with their patients. The medical technologist practices in a laboratory profession at least once removed from patient contact. Allied health care professionals work in every aspect of the health delivery system in a variety of disciplines with a variety of educational experiences. They work throughout the country in a number of physical settings, including hospitals, physicians' office laboratories, clinics, hospices, community programs, schools, and extended care facilities.

Because of the dynamic state of health care, many allied health care occupations eventually become professions. The expansion of knowledge and evolving technology require increased learning and understanding. The aspiring practitioner of a particular occupation is confronted with a body of information that must be mastered. Those involved with the occupation must organize the information, find new applications, and teach what they know to students interested in the occupation. Essentials or standards are adopted, and a new allied health profession is born. The evolution of the medical technologist or clinical laboratory scientist from the help hired by the pathologist provides a good example of how a profession begins and then sustains itself. The first allied health professions to establish essential criteria and have their education programs evaluated by the AMA were occupational therapy, medical technology, and physical therapy.

Science and Profession

Allied health is a designation that can be understood only in the context of direct health care providers and patients. Direct health care providers are those who are licensed to interact directly with the patient in diagnosis and/or treatment. Examples are medical doctors of various specialties, nurses, dentists, optometrists, chiropractors, and podiatrists. Ancillary activities that support direct care would be described as allied health. Those careers that are involved with these activities are allied health careers or professions.

The ancillary activities to primary care have come about for many reasons. Among them are the advances in technology that have resulted in more sophisticated diagnostic testing. Only the direct caregiver such as a medical doctor (and in some cases, a nurse practitioner) can make a diagnosis. This activity may require data, however, that are provided by the medical technologist, audiologist, diagnostic medical sonographer, or radiologic technologist; some data are provided only after time-consuming and specialized laboratory activity provided by the cytotechnologist or the blood bank technology specialist. Health care often involves specialized equipment and someone specifically trained in running it, such as the perfusionist, the radiation therapy technologist, and the cardiovascular technologist; the more mundane but very important task of medical record keeping is performed by an administrator and technicians; highly specialized areas of therapy have resulted in careers that require a very narrow area of medical understanding or a specialized area that complements the medical activity of the doctor, such as art therapist, music therapist, occupational therapist, physical therapist, and respiratory therapist.

Allied health has become an important aspect of the American health care system. Sophisticated technology and equipment, new therapeutic techniques, routine record keeping, complex laboratory tests, and specialized therapies have resulted in careers that complement the duties of the direct caregiver. Clinical care can only be as good as the primary care professionals supported by allied health care professionals. An adequate allied health system depends on the support of allied health educational institutions, professional organizations, and clinical settings that support service delivery, research, and education.

If the designation "allied health" is to be related to those professions whose essential criteria for their education programs are adopted by the CAHEA, then three things must be considered when describing each of the allied health professions: first, the educational background in terms of degree requirements and of didactic and clinical experience; second, the occupational duties to be performed; and third, the association or organization that takes on the responsibility of sponsoring the profession with regard to organizing, developing, teaching, and evaluating.

For a number of allied health occupations, either a bachelor's degree is not required or this requirement varies among programs. Examples of such occupations often use the designation "technician," as in emergency medical technician, histologic technician, medical laboratory technician, medical record technician, and respiratory therapist technician. Others receive very specialized training, such as the diagnostic medical sonographer and the perfusionist. Examples of those allied health professionals in fields whose essential criteria are evaluated and accredited by the CAHEA and that have maintained the bachelor's degree are anesthesiology assistants, athletic trainers, specialists in blood bank technology, cytotechnologists, medical illustrators, medical records administrators, nuclear medicine technologists, occupational therapists, radiation therapy technologists, radiographers, and respiratory therapists.

Even under the aegis of the AMA, however, CAHEA evaluation and accreditation are not enough to be used to define allied health personnel. The ASAHP lists the twenty-eight careers regulated by the AMA (except physician assistant) and thirty-nine others that fall under the definition of allied health professions as outlined by the federal government. Among those careers are art therapist, audiologist, dance therapist, dental assistant, dietitian, educational therapist, genetic counselor, health care administrator, histotechnologist, kinesiotherapist, music therapist, nutritionist, ophthalmic medical technologist, optician, optometric technician, physical therapist, psychiatric technician, recreational therapist, speech/language pathologist, veterinary technician, and vocational rehabilitation counselor. The ASAHP listing of allied health careers demonstrates an allied health view that extends beyond the medical profession into autonomous professional areas such as dentistry, optometry, dietetics, nutrition, physical therapy, and veterinary medicine.

Credentials such as certification, registry, or licensure of an occupation/profession are the final aspect that has an impact on the allied health professions. Certification implies that an individual has met certain ethical criteria and has achieved the minimal standards required to practice a particular occupation. Certification is usually provided by a nongovernment agency. Registry, which is usually provided by a government agency, involves being placed on a government listing. It is usually used with occupations that involve a minimal threat to public safety.

Licensure is an important part of the health care system because it attempts to protect both the public (which must rely on competent care) and the health care personnel (who must protect the profession to which they belong). Public safety is achieved when a government agency is given the responsibility of overseeing the credentials of a person who attempts to practice a particular occupation or use a particular title. The health care worker is protected because licensure prevents unqualified practitioners from entering the occupation or profession. It also appears to increase salary benefits and prestige, as well as to provide the profession with greater visibility with respect to legislative government and the public in general.

Probably one of the most important aspects of licensure is that it legally defines the extent of the activities that may be performed in the profession or occupation. For example, medical technologists and respiratory therapists can monitor arterial blood gases and electrolytes. If licensure to perform the tests were given to only one of the occupations, however, it would be illegal for individuals in the unlicensed profession to perform the tests. Licensure is particularly significant to the allied health professions because duties may overlap, especially in the variety of health care settings that are being developed.

The negative aspects to licensure should also be considered for their impact on allied health and most health care professions. There is a decrease in mobility when each state has its own licensing commission or agency. Some studies indicate that many rural areas do not have adequate care, and it is believed the licensure of professions not already licensed in some states, such as medical technology, could add to this problem by discouraging the movement of health care workers to these areas.

Finally, licensure affects not only individuals but also the facilities in which health care is practiced. Laboratories and direct care facilities such as hospitals are usually regulated by government licensure. The movement of health care treatment from hospitals to the many alternative facilities that now exist may also require that standards be established and evaluated.

Because of the uniformity of the health care system, there is ease of mobility horizontally (from location to location) for those in allied health occupations. There is consistency of facilities, equipment, job opportunity, job description, operating procedures, and regulations. Yet the very reason for the creation of most allied health occupations or professions—the requirement for specialized knowledge, procedures, or technology—makes them narrow in focus. Consequently, many people agree that there is less vertical mobility within some allied health positions.

Nevertheless, the educational requirements for some allied health occupations, particularly a bachelor's degree in liberal arts, provide greater opportunity for advancement. Job advancement opportunities can also increase with advanced degrees. For example, a bachelor's degree in medical technology or a master's degree in business administration provides an individual with professional opportunities in many of the ancillary industries that support the American health care system.

Perspective and Prospects

The health care system in the United States is the product of three major forces: private enterprise, government, and charity. Although each of these forces may have had different objectives, their united goal has been the improved health of the American population. The primary location for the delivery of health care has been the hospital. The health care professions that evolved within this system and that have, in large part, given direction to its evolution are the medical profession and the nursing profession.

With the establishment of hospitals as the site of health care delivery, the nursing profession made itself fundamental to the continued evolution of health care. The hospital became the keystone of the entire health care system, as well as the focal point where each of the three forces would exert its influence.

As a result of health care moving from the private home to the public setting of the hospital, the health care of the patient improved, but at the same time it became more technology-oriented and more costly. Since the 1950's, technological advances have had a direct effect on patient care and therefore on the ever-evolving professions of medicine and nursing. During this same time of technological growth and specialized care, new areas of health care have begun to develop that are outside the accepted areas of medicine and nursing but allied to them because their common goal is the health of the patient.

As many as sixty-seven professions can be described as allied health. They complement the activities of not only the physician and nurse but also a variety of direct caregivers such as dentists, optometrists, and clinical psychologists. Allied health activities take place in hospitals, physicians' office laboratories, private laboratories, clinics, schools, extended care facilities, and the variety of other facilities utilized by direct care providers.

Advanced technology, the professions that constitute the health care team, and the administrative bureaucracy form the $500 billion health care industry in the United States. In 2000, it was estimated that health care spending was 13.2 percent of the gross domestic product of the United States. The health care system also provides one of the most rapidly expanding areas for job opportunities in the American economy.

Allied health occupations and professions are an integral part of the American health care system. Their role is indispensable to those professions responsible for patient diagnosis and treatment. Allied health provides a vast market for scientific products and instrumentation. It is composed of and supported by an array of professional organizations and educational institutions that will provide the impetus for its continued growth and evolution.

—*Patrick J. DeLuca, Ph.D.*

See also American Medical Association (AMA); Anesthesiology; Audiology; Blood banks; Cardiac rehabilitation; Cytopathology; Environmental health; Health maintenance organizations (HMOs); Hospice; Hospitals; Imaging and radiology; Laboratory tests; Nuclear radiology; Occupational health; Paramedics; Physical rehabilitation; Physician assistants; Preventive medicine; Pulmonary medicine; Sports medicine; Surgical technologists.

For Further Information:

American Medical Association. *Health Professions: Education Standards*. Chicago: Author, 1999. This directory is an excellent catalog of those allied health professions that have been developed and regulated by the AMA through the CAHEA. Professions are listed and described with regard to their duties and educational requirements.

Clerc, Jeanne M. *An Introduction to Clinical Laboratory Science*. St. Louis: Mosby Year Book, 1992. This introductory text provides an excellent treatment of the development of the clinical laboratory and the clinical laboratory scientist as they relate to the health care system.

Corder, Brice W., ed. *Medical Professions Admission Guide: Strategy for Success*. Champaign, Ill.: National Association of Advisors for the Health Professions, 1998. An excellent resource for students, health profession advisers, and anyone who is interested in learning about health professions. Careers are described in the context of the health care settings in which they are practiced.

Miller, Benjamin F., Claire Brackman Keane, and Marie T. O'Toole. *Miller-Keane Encyclopedia and Dictionary of Medicine, Nursing, and Allied Health*. Rev. 7th ed. Philadelphia: W. B. Saunders, 2005.

Provides comprehensive definitions, background information, and clinical implications, as well as pronunciation guides; a list of stems, prefixes, and suffixes; and a forty-page insert of full-color illustrations of human anatomy and common disorders.

Mosby's Medical Dictionary. 7th ed. St. Louis: Mosby/Elsevier, 2006. Illustrated definitions of a wide variety of medical terms, especially those pertaining to anatomy, equipment, and pathophysiology.

Alternative medicine

Specialty

Anatomy or system affected: All

Specialties and related fields: Osteopathic medicine, preventive medicine, public health

Definition: A wide variety of medical practices and therapies which fall outside traditional, Western medical practice. The approaches emphasize the individual as a biopsychosocial whole, or, in some cases, as a biopsychosocial-spiritual whole. They deemphasize focusing treatment on specific diseases or symptoms.

Key terms:

physiological: characteristic of or appropriate to an organism's healthy or normal functioning

therapeutic: relating to the treatment of disease or disorders, but mostly pertaining to healing or curing and not merely the absence of disease or symptoms

toxin: a poisonous substance that is a product of the chemical processes of a living organism

Science and Profession

Alternative medicine—known also as natural healing, complementary medicine, integrative medicine, or holistic medicine—focuses on the relationship among the mind, body, and spirit. The underlying philosophy is that people can maintain health by preventing disease in the first place by keeping the body in "balance" and by utilizing the body's "natural" healing processes when people succumb to disease. Alternative medicine approaches contrast with Western medicine's traditional focus on treating symptoms and curing disease and its underemphasis of preventive medicine. Thought radical at one time, complementary medicines and therapies are gaining wide appeal as their anecdotal efficacy and reputation grow.

Alternative medicine practitioners treat everything from diseases such as cancer and acquired immunodeficiency syndrome (AIDS) to chronic pain and fatigue, stress, insomnia, depression, high blood pressure, circulatory and digestive disorders, allergies, arthritis, diabetes mellitus, and drug and alcohol addictions.

The major risks associated with alternative medicine include costly delays in seeking appropriate treatment, misinformation, side effects from self-administered remedies, and psychological distress if patients believe that they are responsible for their own illness or lack of recovery. In addition, many alternative medicine practitioners have little or no formal health training and may discourage traditional medical treatment or oppose proven health measures such as immunization and pasteurization.

Diagnostic and Treatment Techniques

Numerous alternative medicine treatments exist, and they vary widely in the nature of their claims, their acceptability to conventional doctors, and the manner in which they can and cannot be tested. The treatments can be divided into three main types.

The first type consists of those treatments that deal with the mind/body connection or that have recognized benefits and accepted applications and so are often used together with conventional medicine. These approaches include acupuncture and acupressure, biofeedback, chiropractic, hydrotherapy, light therapy, meditation, oxygen therapy, qi gong, sound therapy, Tai Chi Chuan, and yoga. The second type comprises treatments that can be tested by conventional methods and have some accepted applications. These treatments include aromatherapy, cell therapy, colon therapy, detoxification, energy medicine, enzyme therapy, homeopathy, kinesiology, magnetic field therapy, and neural therapy. Treatments of the third type are very difficult to study because they seem to be at odds with Western medicine and cannot readily be tested through standard methods. An example of this type of treatment is herbal medicine.

Acupressure and acupuncture. These treatments are both based on the belief that the body has a vital energy that must be balanced in order to maintain good health. Acupressure uses pressure from the fingertips or knuckles to stimulate specific points on the body, while acupuncture uses needles inserted into the skin to restore the balance of energy. Both acupressure and acupuncture have been shown to stimulate the release of endorphins, the body's natural painkillers. Acupressure is useful for relieving chronic pain and fatigue and increasing blood circulation. Acupuncture has been used successfully for relieving chronic pain and treating drug and alcohol withdrawal symptoms. Although hepatitis, transmission of infectious disease, and internal injuries have been reported in connection with acupuncture, such problems are uncommon.

Biofeedback. This technique involves learning to control automatic physiological responses such as blood pressure, heart rate, circulation, digestion, and perspiration in order to reduce anxiety, pain, and tension. The patient concentrates on consciously controlling the body's automatic responses while a machine monitors the results and displays them for the patient. Biofeedback can be useful in treating asthma, chronic pain, epilepsy, drug addiction, circulatory problems, and stress.

Chiropractic. Chiropractic treatment uses traditional medicine techniques such as X rays, physical examinations, and various tests in order to diagnose a disorder. Muscle spasms or ligament strains are treated by manipulation or adjustment to the spine and joints, thus reducing pressure on the spinal nerves and providing relief from pain. Recent research suggests chiropractic should be considered in treating certain types of lower back pain, as it is often superior to conventional interventions. Practitioners should be state licensed, and caution should be taken with practitioners who often repeat full-spine X rays or who ask patients to sign contracts at any time during treatment. Chiropractic is practiced either "straight," involving only spinal manipulation, or "mixed," involving other biomedical technologies such as electrical stimulation. Chiropractic treatment can be harmful if it is practiced in patients with fractures or undetected tumors or if it is practiced incorrectly.

Hydrotherapy. The use of water for healing or therapeutic purposes is termed hydrotherapy. It is used to treat chronic pain; to relieve stress; to improve circulation, mobility, strength, and flexibility; to reduce swelling; and to treat injuries to the skin. Because the buoyancy of water offsets gravity, more intense exercise can be done when standing in water, while a lower heart rate is maintained and pain is decreased. The risks associated with hydrotherapy are minimal, such as overdoing exercise, or rare, such as slipping or drowning.

Light therapy. Phototherapy, or light therapy, is used to treat health disorders that are related to problems with the body's inner clock, or circadian rhythms. These rhythms govern the timing of sleep, hormone production, body temperature, and other biological functions. People need the full wavelength spectrum of light found in sunlight in order to maintain health. If the full wavelength is not received, the body may not be able to absorb some nutrients fully, resulting in fatigue, tooth decay, depression, hostility, hair loss, skin conditions, sleep disorders, or suppressed immune functions. Treatment involves spending more time outdoors, exercising, and using light boxes that mimic natural sunlight. Phototherapy is commonly used to treat seasonal affective disorder, a recognized subtype of depressive illness.

Meditation. Meditation is used to relax the mind and body, to reduce stress, and to develop a more positive attitude. By focusing on a single thought or repeating a word or phrase, a person can release conscious thoughts and feelings and enter deep relaxation. Meditation can affect the pulse rate and muscle tension and so is effective in treating high blood pressure, migraines, insomnia, and some digestive disorders.

Oxygen therapy. Hyperbaric oxygenation therapy, or oxygen therapy, is used to treat disorders in which the oxygen supply to the body is deficient. This therapy can help with heart disease, circulatory problems, multiple sclerosis, gangrene, and strokes. Oxygen therapy is also used for traumas such as crash injuries, wounds, burns, bedsores, and carbon monoxide poisoning. Treatment consists of exposing the patient to 100 percent pure oxygen under greater-than-normal atmospheric pressure. The body tissues receive more than the usual supply of oxygen and so can compensate for conditions of reduced circulation. The increased oxygen helps keep tissues alive and promotes healing.

Qi gong. Qi gong (pronounced "chee-kung") translates from the Chinese as "breathing exercise." The Chinese believe that exercise balances and amplifies the vital energy force—Ch'i or qi—within the body. Qi gong is used to increase circulation; to reduce stress; to promote health, fitness, and longevity; and to cure illness. The most common exercises involve relaxation, strengthening, and inward training. Because the exercise involves movement done with gentle circular and stretching movements, people with decreased flexibility or disabilities can participate.

Sound therapy. The use of certain sounds can reduce stress, lower blood pressure, relieve pain, improve movement and balance, promote endurance and strength, and overcome learning disabilities. The body has its own rhythm, and illness can arise when the rhythm is disturbed. Tests have shown that particular sounds can slow breathing and a racing heart, create a feeling of well-being, alter skin temperature, influence brain-wave frequencies, and reduce blood pressure and muscle tension.

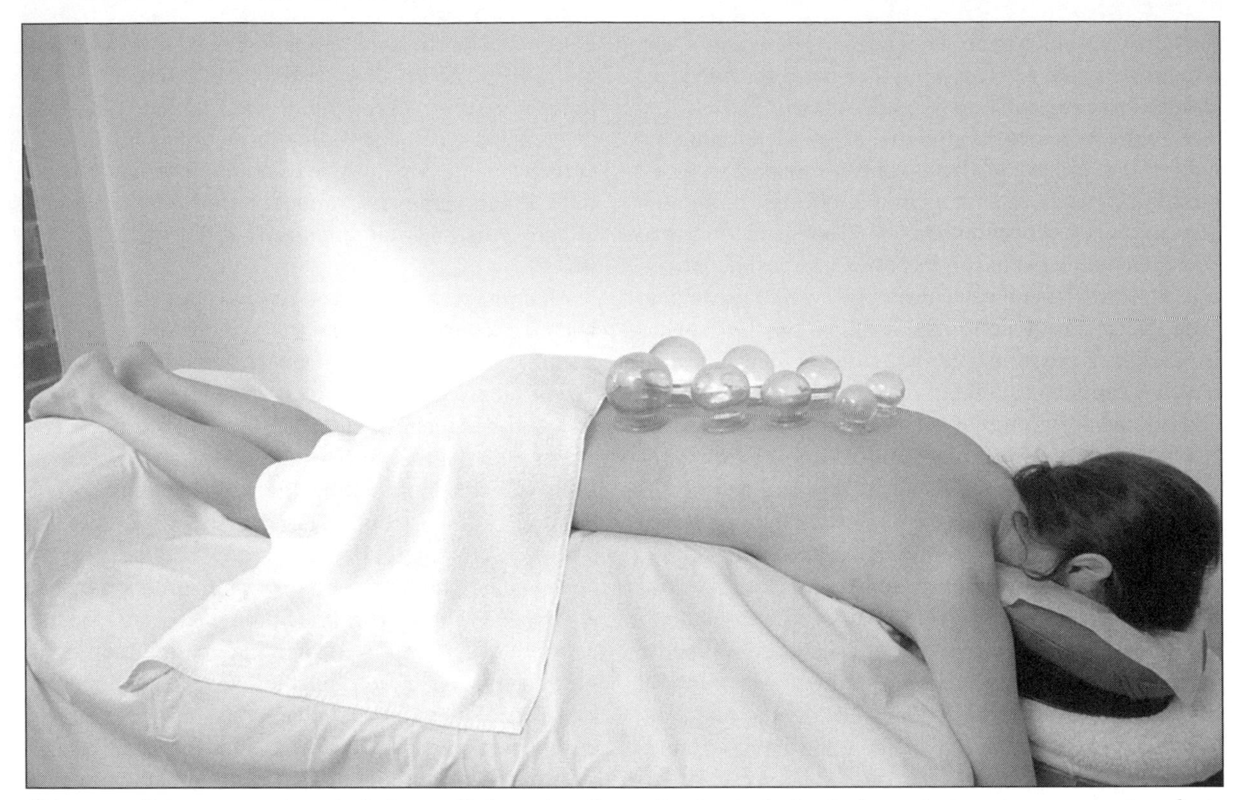

Chinese medicine may employ a technique called cupping, the application to the back of cups that create a vacuum, in order to restore proper circulation. (PhotoDisc)

Tai Chi Chuan. Originally designed as a form of self-defense, Tai Chi Chuan is now practiced as physical exercises based on rhythmic movement, equilibrium of body weight, and effortless breathing. The exercises involve slow and continuous movement without strain. Tai Chi Chuan is beneficial because it demands no physical strength initially. The exercises increase circulation, stimulate the nervous system and glandular activity, and increase joint movement and concentration.

Yoga. The ancient art of yoga seeks to achieve the balance of mind, body, and spirit. Practitioners believe that good health is created through proper breathing, relaxation, meditation, proper diet and nutrition, and exercise. The deep breathing and stretching exercises bring relaxation, release of tension and stress, improved concentration, and oxygenation of the blood. The exercises can also provide muscle toning and aerobic respiration, which are beneficial to the heart.

Aromatherapy. Used extensively in Europe and Japan, aromatherapy involves the use of the essential oils or essence from the flowers, stems, leaves, or roots of plants or trees. These essences can be absorbed through the skin, eaten, or inhaled in vapor form. There is evidence that inhaling some scents may help prevent secondary respiratory infections and reduce stress. Practitioners believe that aromatherapy can benefit people suffering from muscle aches, arthritis, digestive and circulatory problems, and emotional or stress-related problems. Absorption through the skin and inhalation are considered safe, but eating any essence could result in poisoning.

Cell therapy. Although not approved in the United States, cell therapy is widely used worldwide. It involves the injection of cells from the organs, fetuses, or embryos of animals and humans. These cells are used for revitalization purposes; that is, they promote the body's own healing process for damaged or weak organs. Cell therapy seems to stimulate the immune system and is used to treat cancer, immunological problems, diseased or underdeveloped organs, arthritis, and circulatory problems.

Colon therapy. This technique involves the cleaning and detoxification of the colon by flushing with water, using enemas, or ingesting herbs or other substances. A healthy colon will absorb water and nutrients and eliminate wastes and toxins. Most modern diets, however, are low in fiber, a substance which helps clean out the colon. Further, most people are relatively sedentary and eat acidic foods. For adults, most digested food takes fifty to seventy hours after digestion to move through the bowels. (In contrast, evidence indicates that in the early twentieth century, fecal material was released within twelve to twenty hours after ingestion.) A baby's food is defecated within four to ten hours after ingestion. If not completely eliminated, layers of wastes can build up in the colon and toxins can leak into the bloodstream, causing many health problems; in exact, the theory goes that the more time fecal material spends in the body, the more time there is for impacted feces, bacteria, viruses, fungi, parasites, and toxemia to develop. If not completely eliminated, layers of wastes can build up in the colon and toxins can leak into the bloodstream, causing many health problems. Although not a specific cure for any disease, colon therapy removes the source of toxins and allows the body's natural healing processes to function properly. Practitioners claim that symptoms related to colon dysfunction, such as backaches, headaches, bad breath, gas, indigestion and constipation, sinus or lung congestion, skin problems, and fatigue can be relieved when the toxins are removed from the colon.

A person trained in colonic therapy guides a speculum into the rectum and cleanses the area by gently guiding water, herbs, vitamins, or oxygen through the entire five feet of the colon. Enemas cleanse only the lower or sigmoid colon, which is only eight to twelve inches of the bowel.

Detoxification. This therapy focuses on ridding the body of the chemicals and pollutants present in water, food, air, and soil. The body naturally eliminates or neutralizes toxins through the liver, kidneys, urine, and feces, and through the processes of exhalation and perspiration. Detoxification therapy accelerates the body's own natural cleansing process through diet, fasting, colon therapy, and heat therapy. Symptoms of an overtaxed body system include respiratory problems, headaches, joint pain, allergy symptoms, mood changes, insomnia, arthritis, constipation, psoriasis, acne, and ulcers.

Energy medicine. Bioenergetic medicine, or energy medicine, uses an energy field to detect and treat health problems. A screening process to measure electromagnetic frequencies emitted by the body can detect imbalances that may cause illness or warn of possible chemical imbalances. One of several machines is then used to correct energy-level imbalances. Energy medicine claims to relieve conditions such as skin diseases, headaches, migraines, muscle pain, circulation problems, and chronic fatigue.

Enzyme therapy. This treatment uses plant and pancreatic enzymes to improve digestion and the absorption of nutrients. Since enzymes provide the stimuli for all chemical reactions in the body, improper eating habits may cause a lack of certain enzymes, resulting in general health problems.

Homeopathy. Based on the belief that "like cures like," homeopathy is thought to provide relief from most illnesses. During therapy, the patient receives small doses of prepared plants and minerals in order to stimulate the body's own healing processes and defense mechanisms. These substances mimic the symptoms of the illness. While studies on this approach remain inconclusive, homeopathic medicine has wide appeal, possibly because most (but not all) homeopathic practitioners are traditionally trained medical physicians.

Kinesiology. This therapy employs muscle testing and standard diagnosis to evaluate and treat the chemical, structural, and mental aspects of the patient. The principle behind kinesiology is that certain foods can cause biochemical reactions that weaken the muscles. Diet and exercise, as well as muscle and joint manipulation, are part of the treatment. There are risks of injury caused by an unqualified practitioner.

Magnetic field therapy. Also called biomagnetic therapy, magnetic field therapy uses specially designed magnets or magnetic fields applied to the body. Electrically charged particles are naturally present in the bloodstream, and when magnets are placed on the body, the charged particles are attracted to the magnets. As a result, currents and patterns are created that dilate the blood vessels, allowing more blood to reach the affected area. Magnetic field therapy is used to speed healing after surgery, to improve circulation, and to strengthen and mend bones. It is also used to improve the quality of healing in sprains, strains, cuts, and burns, as well as to reduce or reverse chronic conditions such as degenerative joint disease, some forms of arthritis, and diabetic ulcers.

Neural therapy. This therapy is used to treat chronic illness or trauma (injury) caused by changes in the natural electrical conductivity of the nerves and cells. Every cell has its own frequency range of electricity, and tissue remains healthy as long as the energy flow through the body is normal. Neural therapy uses anesthetics injected into the body to deliver energy to cells blocked by disease or injury. Conditions that respond to neural therapy are allergies; arthritis; asthma; kidney, liver, and heart disease; depression; head and back pain; and muscle injuries.

Herbal medicine. This field uses plants and flowers to treat most known symptoms of physical and emotional illnesses. Almost 75 percent of the world's population relies on herbal remedies as their primary source of health care, and much of traditional medicine is derived from plants. Herbal medicine mixtures can be complicated, however, and some, like any medications, are toxic if taken incorrectly.

Perspective and Prospects

Many alternative or complementary therapies, while new to Western society and medicine, are ancient and derive from nontechnologically based understandings of how the human body and the world work. What specifically works for whom, when, and for what conditions remains a complex problem. Anecdote and hearsay, and the limits and failures of Western medicine, guide and motivate interest in these approaches.

Renewed interest in alternative therapies occurred in the 1970's and has grown since. By 1998, an estimated one-third of all Americans had used some form of complementary therapy. In 1992, with Americans spending more than fourteen billion dollars annually on alternative medicine, the U.S. government established the Office of Alternative Medicine as a part of the National Institutes of Health (NIH). This office evaluates complementary treatments on a scientific basis and provides public information. Health insurers maintain a key interest in alternative medicine, and an increasing number are paying for it. Many traditionally trained physicians are prescribing or recommending some form of alternative medicine as a complement to their own.

In 2004, the National Center for Complementary and Alternative Medicine found that 36 percent of adults use some form of complementary or alternative medicine. If one includes megavitamin therapy and prayer that is associated with health concerns, the number rises to 62 percent. The survey found that the main reasons that people use complementary and alternative medicine were beliefs that it would improve their health when combined with conventional medicine, or that it would be interesting to try, or that conventional treatment either would not or did not work. People most likely to use complementary or alternative medicine are women, those with a high level of education, those who have been hospitalized in the last year, and former smokers.

In 2006, the American Holistic Medical Association had approximately eight hundred members. Physicians can become board certified in holistic medicine, meaning that they are committed to treating the whole person, emphasize prevention rather than merely treating symptoms, believe in integrating other modes of treatment and not limiting themselves to only Western medicine, and believe in the importance of the healing relationship and in treating the patient as a unique individual. In 2005, the Association of the American Medical Colleges reported that 95 of 125 medical schools offer complementary and alternative coursework and training.

—Virginia L. Salmon;
Paul Moglia, Ph.D.;
updated by LeAnna DeAngelo, Ph.D.

See also Acupressure; Acupuncture; Allied health; Aromatherapy; Chiropractic; Colon therapy; Enzyme therapy; Herbal medicine; Holistic medicine; Homeopathy; Hydrotherapy; Hypnosis; Kinesiology; Light therapy; Magnetic field therapy; Massage; Meditation; Oxygen therapy; Pain management; Stress reduction; Supplements; Yoga.

For Further Information:

Center for Applied Physiology. http://www.menninger.edu/. The Menninger Clinic is one of the foremost clinical and research centers in self-regulation and biofeedback.

Ditchek, Stuart, Andrew Weil, and Russell H. Greenfield. *Healthy Child, Whole Child: Integrating the Best of Conventional and Alternative Medicine to Keep Your Kids Healthy*. New York: HarperCollins, 2002. Provides recommendations for common childhood ailments and focuses on children's mind-body wellness and their naturally superior healing abilities.

Freeman, Lyn. *Mosby's Complementary and Alternative Medicine: A Research-Based Approach*. 2d ed. St. Louis: Mosby, 2004. Provides comprehensive coverage in a textbook format. Addresses the history, philosophy, and mechanisms of alternative medicine. Includes a review of clinical trials, indications, and contraindications for each type of therapy.

Jacobs, Jennifer, ed. *The Encyclopedia of Alternative Medicine: A Complete Family Guide to Complementary Therapies*. Rev. ed. Boston: Journey Edition,

1997. Discusses current alternative medicine approaches.

Kastner, Mark, and Hugh Burroughs. *Alternative Healing: The Complete A-Z Guide to over 160 Different Alternative Therapies*. New York: Henry Holt, 1996. The encyclopedic, one-page to four-page entries are brief but include sources of additional information. Also offers a useful resource section and bibliography.

Mauskop, Alexander, and Brill Marietta Abrams. *The Headache Alternative: A Neurologist's Guide to Drug-Free Relief.* New York: Dell Paperbacks, 1997. A practical review of how to apply complementary and alternative approaches to treating migraine, sinus, and tension headaches. Contains excellent resources and a bibliography section.

Mills, Simon, and Steven J. Finando. *Alternatives in Healing*. London: Grange Books, 1995. Provides detailed introductory chapters discussing the principles, philosophy, and techniques of diagnosis and treatment with alternative medicine. Includes case studies comparing various treatment methods.

Pelletier, Kenneth. *Best Alternative Medicine*. New York: Simon & Schuster, 2002. Explains mind/body medicine, herbal and homeopathic remedies, spiritual healing, and traditional Chinese systems. Discusses the effectiveness of each therapeutic approach, the ailments each is most appropriate for, and how they can help prevent illness.

Trivieri, Larry, Jr., and John W. Anderson, eds. *Alternative Medicine: The Definitive Guide*. 2d ed. Berkeley, Calif.: Ten Speed Press, 2002. The bible of alternative medicine. Includes the sections "Medicine for the 21st Century," "Alternative Therapies," and "Health Conditions" with a quick reference A-Z section of additional health conditions.

Weil, Andrew. *Healthy Aging: A Lifelong Guide to Your Physical and Spiritual Well-Being*. New York: Knopf, 2005. Provides an excellent overview of the scientific basis for alternative medicine in a manner that is engaging for the reader.

ALTITUDE SICKNESS

DISEASE/DISORDER

ANATOMY OR SYSTEM AFFECTED: Brain, ears, head, lungs, nervous system, respiratory system

SPECIALTIES AND RELATED FIELDS: Emergency medicine, neurology, occupational health

DEFINITION: A condition resulting from altitude-related hypoxia (low oxygen levels).

INFORMATION ON ALTITUDE SICKNESS

CAUSES: Rapid ascent to high altitudes, hypoxia (low oxygen levels)

SYMPTOMS: Headache, decreased appetite, insomnia, fatigue, nausea, death in severe cases

DURATION: A few days

TREATMENTS: Descent to lower altitudes, corticosteroids, oxygen

CAUSES AND SYMPTOMS

There are four types of altitude sickness: acute mountain sickness, high-altitude pulmonary edema (HAPE), high-altitude cerebral edema (HACE), and high-altitude retinopathy (HAR). Though most patients have mild symptoms, death is not uncommon in severe cases. Illness is associated with rapid ascent to mountain areas by tourists, skiers, and mountaineers. Residents of mountainous regions are less susceptible because their bodies have adapted to lower oxygen levels. It is estimated that up to one-quarter of tourists skiing in the mountains of the western United States have experienced some manifestations, although mild ones, of altitude sickness.

Acute mountain sickness is characterized by headache, decreased appetite, insomnia, fatigue, nausea, and onset at altitudes above 1,980 meters (6,500 feet). The risk of becoming affected increases with young age, quick ascent, and a past history of acute mountain sickness. Symptoms usually last for a few days. Between 5 and 10 percent of patients with acute mountain sickness progress to HAPE, which occurs when the small pulmonary blood vessels leak, allowing fluid accumulation in the lungs. Mortality from HAPE ranges from 11 to 44 percent. The related condition HACE occurs when fluid accumulation in the brain causes increased pressure within the skull. Neurologic signs such as confusion and coma may be noted.

TREATMENT AND THERAPY

Prevention is crucial to the reduction of morbidity and mortality from altitude sickness. Ascents should be slow, especially those involving physical exertion. Sedatives and salt should be avoided. Most people adapt to altitude changes within three days. Returning to lower altitudes at night is advised. Premedication with acetazolamide, a prescription drug, will hasten adaptation and reduce symptoms. In serious cases, descent to lower altitudes is vital. Corticosteroids, oxygen, and hyperbaric treatments may be used. Chronically ill persons should check with their doctors before attempting strenuous activity at high altitudes.

—*Louis B. Jacques, M.D.*

See also Asphyxiation; Brain; Brain disorders; Coma; Cyanosis; Edema; Hyperbaric oxygen therapy; Hyperventilation; Lungs; Nervous system; Neurology; Neurology, pediatric; Oxygen therapy; Pulmonary diseases; Pulmonary medicine; Pulmonary medicine, pediatric; Respiration.

For Further Information:

Auerbach, Paul S. *Medicine for the Outdoors*. Rev. ed. Boston: Little, Brown, 1999. This is a revised and updated edition of Auerbach's first-rate guide, providing brief explanations of a wide variety of vacation/exploration medical problems (from diarrhea to Gila monster bites).

Reeves, John T., and Robert F. Grover. *Attitudes on Altitude: Pioneers of Medical Research in Colorado's High Mountains*. Boulder: University of Colorado Press, 2001. Brings together the personal stories and findings of the innovative researchers who examined altitude sickness in the Rocky Mountains.

Rennie, D. "The Great Breathlessness Mountains." *Journal of the American Medical Association* 256 (July 4, 1986): 81-82. Findings on high-altitude cerebral and pulmonary edema (HACE and HAPE) are discussed in an editorial. The history of acute mountain sickness (AMS) is outlined.

Ward, Michael P., John B. West, and James S. Milledge. *High Altitude Medicine and Physiology*. 3d ed. New York: Oxford University Press, 2001. Examines the practice and management of common medical and surgical conditions in the mountains.

Wilkerson, James A., ed. *Medicine for Mountaineering and Other Wilderness Activities*. 5th ed. Seattle: The Mountaineers Books, 2001. This book is a first-aid manual that goes beyond traditional treatment protocols. It was written for those who need information to care for serious injuries when organized medical help is not available.

Alzheimer's disease

Disease/disorder

Anatomy or system affected: Brain, cells, nerves, nervous system, psychic-emotional system

Specialties and related fields: Geriatrics and gerontology, internal medicine, neurology, nursing, psychiatry

Definition: A relentlessly progressive disease resulting in the loss of higher cognitive function; the most common form of dementia.

Key terms:

Alzheimer's beta peptide (Aβ): the principal proteinaceous component of certain brain lesions in Alzheimer's disease

amyloid: extracellular proteinaceous deposits having distinctive tinctorial properties

neurofibrillary tangles: a hallmark lesion of Alzheimer's disease and several other disorders consisting of intracellular aggregates of the structural protein tau

presenilins: proteins linked to several forms of inherited Alzheimer's disease, which are believed to play a role in the production of Aβ

senile plaques: a hallmark lesion of Alzheimer's disease, composed of Aβ amyloid

Causes and Symptoms

In 1906, Alois Alzheimer described the pathological correlates of presenile dementia. Once considered rare, Alzheimer's disease is now recognized as the most common form of dementia, affecting more than 10 percent of people in the sixth decade of life and nearly 50 percent of people in the eighth decade. The cognitive impairments include agnosia, the loss of perceptual ability regarding the interpretation of sensory perceptions; apraxia, the inability to understand the meaning or appropriate use of things; and dysphasia, the failure to arrange words in a meaningful manner. It is a relentlessly progressive neurodegenerative disorder which leads ultimately to death. While neurological and psychiatric examination provide an assessment of impairment, definitive diagnosis is arrived at only through autopsy. On the level of observable behavior level, in persons affected by Alzheimer's dementia the symptoms often develop gradually, usually after the age of sixty. However, the disease has also been known to develop in younger individuals and to have a more rapid onset. As such, when symptoms such as those noted develop at any age, they deserve attention.

On a more neurologic and cellular level, Alzheimer's disease is characterized by a triad of pathological changes in the brain including senile (or neuritic) plaques, which consist of extracellular proteinaceous deposits surrounded by dystrophic neurons; the presence of similar extracellular proteinaceous deposits in the brain vasculature, termed amyloid (or congophilic) angiopathy; and the presence within nerve cells of tangled fibrillary protein aggregates, called neurofibrillary tangles. These pathological hallmarks are accompanied by significant neuronal loss and brain atrophy, particularly in areas of the brain involved in memory and cognition, such as the hippocampus and temporal and prefrontal cortex. Neuronal loss disproportionately affects nerve cells that use the neurotransmitter acetylcholine (cholinergic neurons). It should be noted, however, that the tangles and plaques have also been found postmortem in the brains of individuals who did not have Alzheimer's disease, so the association of these hallmarks is not completely understood in all individuals.

The extracellular protein deposits in the plaques and brain vasculature have distinct optical and staining properties, suggesting that there is significant underlying organization of their constituent molecules. There are many distinct, typically rare, diseases in which proteins are deposited in this organized fashion in various parts of the body. In 1842, these deposits were called waxy degenerations or lardaceous diseases, and in 1854, they were termed amyloid ("starchlike"). The diseases are now termed amyloidoses. Examples of amyloidoses include the familial amyloidotic polyneuropathies and cardiomyopathies, senile systemic amyloidosis, lattice corneal dystrophy, the Dutch and Icelandic variants of hereditary cerebral hemorrhage with amyloid (HCHWA), and the spongiform encephalopathies, such as "mad cow disease" and kuru. In 1922, the most rigorous histological test for amyloid was devised, staining with congo red: amyloid deposits bind congo red (are congophilic) and rotate polarized light rays (are birefringent), resulting in a transition from red stain in bright-field microscopy to an apple green coloration under polarized light microscopy. Large segments of the proteins that form amyloid deposits have a particular molecular configuration called the beta pleated sheet. These proteins precipitate from solution and aggregate to form organized structures called amyloid fibrils. The parallel alignment of the congo red dye with the organized amyloid fibril results in the optical activity recognized as birefringence.

Because the beta pleated sheet was recognized as the principal configuration of the molecules in amyloid deposits, the primary component of the amyloid deposits in Alzheimer's disease was termed beta (for beta pleated sheet) amyloid protein (βAP), or, more recently, Alzheimer's beta peptide (Aβ).

The identity of the primary protein component of Alzheimer's amyloid was deduced in 1987. Aβ is derived from a much larger protein, the β-amyloid precursor protein (APP), by two proteases, β-secretase, and γ-secretase. When added to cultures of neurons, Aβ is toxic, and the degree of toxicity is correlated with the degree to which the Aβ has aggregated. APP is also a substrate for a third secretase, α-secretase, which cleaves in the middle of the Aβ sequence and thereby precludes formation of the neurotoxic Aβ peptide. In contrast to Aβ, the α-secretase-cleaved derivatives of APP are believed to be neurotrophic.

The identification of β- and γ-secretase has been a particularly vexing problem for biologists. A mutation in two amino acids of APP adjacent to the β-secretase site is known to increase β-secretase activity and thus to increase Aβ production. However, it is a matter of debate whether this mutation (lysine and methionine mutated to asparagine and leucine, or, in biochemical annotation, KM to NL) is due to the increased activity of β-secretase or to an unrelated "NLase" enzyme. Furthermore, although most Aβ is forty amino acids long,

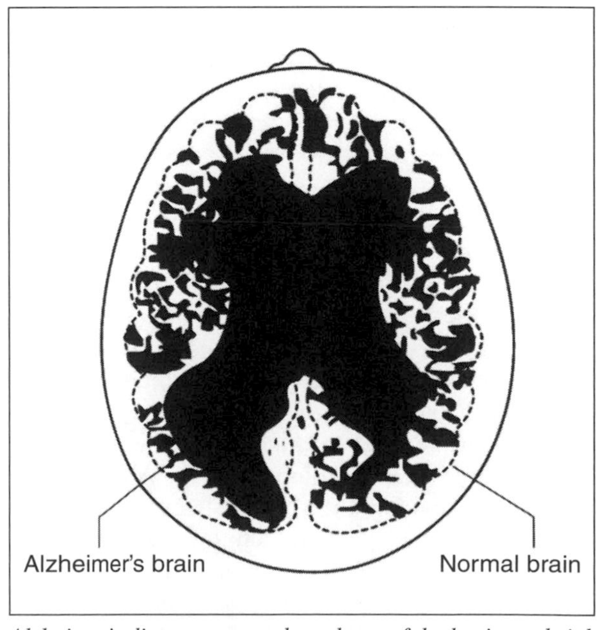

Alzheimer's disease causes the volume of the brain to shrink substantially.

Aβ is heterogeneous in size, ranging from thirty-nine to forty-three amino acids in length, and the forty-two amino acid form appears to be particularly pathogenic. Most of this variation occurs at the γ-secretase site, and because of the variations in observed forms of Aβ, there are different hypotheses regarding the type of activity that would be expected of a γ-secretase. For example, Aβ 40 and 42 might be generated by two distinct secretases. Alternatively, both Aβ 40 and Aβ 42 might be generated from the same enzyme, but the particular cleavage site might be influenced by local factors: prior to γ-secretase cleavage the Aβ domain of APP resides in the membrane, and factors that influence membrane thickness, such as cholesterol content, may lead to preferential cleavage at one of the sites. Still a third possibility is that γ-secretase generates a peptide several amino acids longer than the mature Aβ 40/2 peptide and that a second enzyme chews back on this "pre-Aβ" to yield the mature Aβ 40/2. Here, too, factors such as membrane thickness might influence the relative abundance of the Aβ 40 and Aβ 42 forms.

Nevertheless, β-secretase has recently been identified by several groups as the beta-site APP cleaving enzyme (BACE), and animals whose expression of BACE has been "knocked out" produce virtually no Aβ. Although the identity of γ-secretase has long eluded researchers, γ-secretase activity is now closely associated and sometimes identified with expression of the presenilins (see below). However, since it has never been demonstrated that presenilins have γ-secretase-like catalytic activity, there is still debate regarding whether they are γ-secretase or a requisite component of a secretase complex. γ-secretase has been identified with tumor necrosis factor-alpha converting enzyme (TACE).

APP is a member of a family of proteins, including two amyloid-precursor-like proteins (APLP1 and 2) for which several possible functions have been proposed, including the formation of specific brain structures, neurite outgrowth, and neurobehavioral development. Several mutations have been identified in APP in association with familial Alzheimer's disease, and these mutations are believed to influence the rate of secretase cleavage or to alter the solubility of the Aβ peptide. A further mutation in APP is associated with hereditary cerebral hemorrhage with amyloid-Dutch variant (HCHWA-Dutch), a rare disorder with Alzheimer's-like cerebrovascular pathology. APP has been localized to chromosome 21, and those afflicted with trisomy 21 (Down syndrome) suffer many of the same neurodegenerative hallmarks of Alzheimer's disease, perhaps through a gene dosage effect.

INFORMATION ON ALZHEIMER'S DISEASE

CAUSES: Unknown
SYMPTOMS: Decreased ability to interpret sensory perceptions or to understand the meaning or appropriate use of things, dysphasia
DURATION: Progressive, eventually fatal
TREATMENTS: None for underlying cause; some second-generation drugs slow disease progression

In addition to mutations in APP, mutations in other genes have been identified as causative factors in inherited forms of Alzheimer's disease that appear to affect APP processing. A tremendous amount of interest has recently focused upon presenilin 1, originally designated as S182, a gene associated with chromosome-14-linked Alzheimer's disease. Soon after the discovery of presenilin 1 in 1995, mutations in another gene, originally designated as STM2, were identified as causative in chromosome-1-linked Alzheimer's disease. The amino acid sequences of these proteins are remarkably similar, and STM2 is now called presenilin 2. Mutations in either of these genes result in early-onset Alzheimer's disease, but presenilin 1 mutations result in a far more malignant disease. Presenilin 1 mutations often result in an extraordinarily early onset (third decade of life), and Alzheimer's plaques are abundant in regions of the brain, such as the cerebellum, which are unaffected in the sporadic disease. This results in motor signs, such as myoclonus and seizure, which are absent in the sporadic disease. Mutations in both presenilin 1 and presenilin 2 result in increased production of Aβ, especially of a slightly larger and more pathogenic peptide, Aβ 42. Because these mutations appear to primarily influence the length of Aβ, their activity has primarily been associated with γ-secretase activity.

Initially, the mechanisms by which the presenilin mutations might result in Alzheimer's disease were unclear. By coincidence, researchers in the field of programmed cell death, or apoptosis, found a gene they identified as ALG-3, which they believed rescued cells from programmed cell death. ALG-3 had significant identity with a portion of presenilin 2, and the researchers speculated that mutations in the presenilins might lead nerve cells to an aberrant entry into apoptosis, resulting in the neuronal cell atrophy and death observed in Alzheimer's disease. However, there is considerable debate about whether necrosis, as opposed to apoptosis, is the primary means of cell death in Alzheimer's disease, and the role of the presenilins in apoptosis remains controversial.

The presenilins had no similarity to any known mammalian proteins but had limited identity with two proteins found in the nematode worm *C. elegans*. One protein with very limited identity is spe-4, a protein involved in spermatogenesis in the worm. The other protein with more significant identity (43 percent) is sel-12, a protein involved in the signaling of Notch, a protein involved in many developmental processes. Attempts to knock out the expression of presenilin 1 result in severe defects that are lethal to the late-stage embryo and that closely resemble the defects obtained with knockout of Notch expression. Conversely, expression of the normal human presenilin in worm cells is defective for sel-12 expression and restores Notch signaling, suggesting that both γ-secretase activity and Notch expression converge in the activity of presenilin.

Notch signaling requires the proteolysis of a membrane-bound precursor in a manner that is very similar to the γ-secretase cleavage of APP. While the presenilins do not resemble any known proteases, a certain class of proteases has an obligate amino acid residue which, when mutated in presenilin, eliminates both γ-secretase and Notch cleavage. Also, drugs that are believed to be γ-secretase inhibitors inhibit both γ-secretase cleavage and Notch cleavage. Thus, the presenilins appear to be intimately involved with the proteolysis of APP and Notch. Although Notch activity does not appear to be directly related to Alzheimer's pathology, there is a concern that drugs designed to reduce Aβ production by inhibiting γ-secretase activity might also have an impact on normal Notch signaling, thereby adversely influencing such things as blood cell maturation.

The presenilins are synthesized by all cells in the body, and they appear to be localized within the cell primarily if not exclusively in the endoplasmic reticulum/golgi apparatus. While Aβ was believed to be derived primarily from the cell-membrane-associated APP through a specific pathway (the endosomal/lysosomal pathway), the localization of the presenilins and their association with γ-secretase activity to the endoplasmic reticulum led to a reevaluation of the cellular site of Aβ generation. There is a consensus now that most Aβ, particularly the more pathogenic Aβ 42, is produced within the cells at the endoplasmic reticulum/golgi apparatus. These results are significant because they suggest that, rather than forming from extracellular circulating Aβ proteins, amyloid plaques may begin as aggregates of Aβ within the cell. Those aggregates may, in turn, lead to neuronal injury and death.

Although the presenilins are intimately associated with γ-secretase activity, there has not yet been any definitive proof that the presenilins are involved in proteolytic activity. One would expect, for example, that if the portion of human APP cleaved by γ-secretase and presenilin were coexpressed in a cell that has no endogenous γ-secretase activity (such as a yeast cell), that presenilin would cleave APP, yet this does not occur, and controversy remains over whether enzymatic activity resides with the presenilins or whether the presenilins are an obligate component of multiprotein complexes. Recently, a protein that forms a complex with presenilin and that binds APP was identified. This protein, Nicastrin, named for the Italian village of Nicastro, where key early studies on familial Alzheimer's disease took place, also appears to play an important role in γ-secretase activity and in Notch processing. It is possible that there are other key components to this γ-secretase complex that are yet to be elucidated. A number of additional proteins that interact with presenilin or with APP have been identified; their role in Alzheimer's disease pathogenesis is being investigated. These include calsenilin, Fe65, X11, and BBP-1 (β-amyloid binding protein-1).

Aβ is, therefore, a neurotoxic peptide and a component of two of the predominant features of Alzheimer's disease. Since senile plaques occur within specific regions of the brain, while sparing other regions (especially the cerebellum), investigators originally believed that this distribution of pathology was due to regional differences in the production of APP. However, it soon became apparent that APP was synthesized by virtually all cells and that Aβ is present in abundance throughout the brains and indeed in other tissues of normal nondemented individuals. How, then, does a normal biological molecule become a pathological agent in the aging brain to cause nonfamilial (sporadic) cases of Alzheimer's disease?

It has been proposed that multiple genetic and environmental factors may play a role in this transformation. Some investigators have proposed that one or more of the minor components of amyloid plaques may act as "pathological chaperone" molecules by binding Aβ and altering its solubility. The identification of such components might lead to new drug research strategies and to new insight into the mechanisms of amyloid formation. For example, heparin sulfated proteoglycans (HSPGs) have been identified as components of amyloid deposits, and some investigators have attempted to block amyloid formation by inhibiting the interaction of Aβ with HSPGs. Alpha-synuclein was identified as the nonamyloid component of Alzheimer's disease plaques (NAC peptide); interestingly, mutations in α-synuclein have been identified in familial forms of Parkinson's disease, and this protein is a major constituent of the inclusion bodies found in Parkinson's-disease-associated Lewy body dementia. Aluminum has been identified as a component of the senile plaques found in Alzheimer's disease, and aluminum toxicity results in the formation of neurofibrillary tangles. It has been proposed that aluminum exposure may be a predisposing factor, but this hypothesis is very controversial. Similarly, zinc has been implicated in the formation of Aβ plaques, and a drug that chelates (absorbs) zinc appears to reduce the abundance of plaques in transgenic animal models of Alzheimer's disease.

Soluble Aβ may circulate in the serum and cerebral spinal fluid bound to one of several chaperone proteins, including apolipoprotein e, apolipoprotein J, and transthyretin. Polymorphisms in these proteins might alter the affinity of these proteins for Aβ, thereby leaving more free Aβ available to aggregate into amyloid fibrils. A particular isoform of apolipoprotein E (ApoE4), for example, has an altered affinity for Aβ, and the inheritance of this isoform is associated with increased risk for Alzheimer's disease.

Genes that may play roles in the degradation of proteins may also be involved in the development of Alzheimer's disease pathology. For example, polymorphisms in the cystatin C gene may alter the susceptibility to late-onset Alzheimer's. Cystatin C is a protease inhibitor, and mutant cystatin C is an amyloid component in the Icelandic variant of hereditary cerebral hemorrhage with amyloid (HCHWA-I). Also, the normal process by which cells target proteins for disposal may be altered in Alzheimer's disease. Cells normally target proteins for degradation by conjugating them to the protein ubiquitin, and there are reports that the ubiquitination pathway is altered in the brain afflicted with Alzheimer's disease.

Neuritic plaques and less organized forms of plaques (diffuse plaques) are not unique to Alzheimer's disease but are also found in dementia pugilistica, as a sequelae to severe trauma, are found in Down syndrome, and are coexistent with other diseases, such as Parkinson's disease. Likewise, as already noted, the amyloid (congophilic) angiopathy is also found in other familial amyloidoses. It is the combination of these cardinal findings with the finding of neurofibrillary tangles that forms the triad of primary pathological signs of Alzheimer's disease.

Neurofibrillary tangles are intracellular aggregates of an unusually modified (hyperphosphorylated) form of the structural protein tau (τ). Neurofibrillary tangles are not unique to Alzheimer's disease but occur in several other neurodegenerative diseases, such as amyotrophic lateral sclerosis (ALS)-Parkinson's dementia complex as a consequence of measles infections of the central nervous system (subacute sclerosing panencephalitis), in the rare spongiform encephalopathies (including Creutzfeldt-Jakob disease and kuru) and in frontotemporal dementia. The number of neurofibrillary tangles correlates well with the severity of behavioral impairment.

There has been a long-standing debate regarding the significance of the pathological findings in Alzheimer's disease. The debate has focused on whether Aβ-associated pathology or the tau-protein-associated pathology is the primary lesion in the disease, thus dividing investigators jocularly into βaptist and τaoist camps.

There has been a general consensus that Aβ plays a central causative role in the disease. According to this "amyloid hypothesis," the excessive production, rapid deposition, or aberrant metabolism of Aβ results in the formation of toxic aggregates of Aβ, which in turn result in injury to neurons, neuronal death, and behavioral impairment. The tau pathology manifested as neurofibrillary tangles is a consequence of Aβ effects. Consistent with this view is the fact that all genes that have thus far been associated with familial Alzheimer's disease play a role in Aβ processing or solubility.

However, others would argue that amyloid plaques in Alzheimer's disease are an epiphenomenon, that they are a result of the neurodegenerative process rather than its cause. According to this "tau hypothesis," neurofibrillary tangles are the central pathological finding in the disease, and Aβ plaques are a relatively inert consequence of normal aging or of neurofibrillary tangle-associated neuronal degeneration. Consistent with this viewpoint is the strong correlation between behavioral impairment and neurofibrillary tangle burden. In contrast, amyloid plaques may be found in the brains of normal nondemented individuals, and total plaque burden (the number of plaques found in a given brain section) does not correlate well with behavior. Indeed, it has been difficult to demonstrate significant behavioral impairment in transgenic animal models of Alzheimer's disease (animals that overproduce human APP in the brain), even in the presence of significant amyloid deposits in the brain. It is noteworthy that those animals fail to develop neurofibrillary tangles. However, there have been no direct links between the genetics of Alzheimer's disease and tau protein, although recently a mutation has been identified in tau associated with a non-Alzheimer's dementia (frontotemporal dementia).

Recently there has been a significant convergence of opinion that Aβ is central to Alzheimer's disease pathogenesis. This is due to recent reports that total brain amyloid protein burden (a measure of the total Aβ protein, including protein from plaques) and not plaque number correlates well with severity of dementia.

In the News: Drugs to Slow the Progress of Alzheimer's Disease

Although there is no cure for Alzheimer's disease, certain drugs are shown to improve cognitive functioning. Pharmacological treatment of Alzheimer's disease consists of drugs that prevent the breakdown of acetylcholine in the synapses. Four cholinesterase inhibitors approved for mild to moderate forms of Alzheimer's disease are Cognex, Aricept, Reminyl, and Exelon. These agents inhibit an enzyme called acetylcholinesterase that degrades the neurotransmitter acetylcholine.

One of the most recent drugs to hit the market is called Namenda. It is the first approved medication to treat moderate to severe forms of Alzheimer's disease. Studies have shown that its use results in a slower decline in mental function. Namenda can be taken alone or in combination with donepezil (Aricept).

New drugs in clinical trial investigations include cholinesterase inhibitors such as epastigmine and physostigmine (Synapton)—a sustained release formation—and cholinergic agonist drugs such as milameline, AF 102B, and SB202026 (Memric). Clinical trials provide measurable means of hope for patients with Alzheimer's disease and their families. Two newer drugs in phase 2 of clinical trials include heptylphysostigmine (a cholinesterase inhibitor) and xanomeline (a cholinergic agonist).

In addition to approved Food and Drug Administration (FDA) medications, nonconventional treatment have been shown to improve the cognitive ability of some patients with Alzheimer's disease. Vitamin E, ginkgo biloba, estrogen, coenzyme Q10, nonsteroidal anti-inflammatory drugs (NSAIDs) such as aspirin and ibuprofen, and cholesterol-lowering agents are such treatments. More research is needed, for the effectiveness and safety of these remedies has not been evaluated by the FDA.

—Janet Mahoney, R.N., Ph.D., A.P.R.N.

Treatment and Therapy

There are presently no therapies available for Alzheimer's disease that target the putative underlying mechanisms for the genesis and progression of the disease, although there are extraordinary efforts under way throughout the world to address these mechanisms. Treatment options at present are primarily palliative. This means that they address the symptoms, perhaps providing some temporary relief, but not providing any cure.

Since Alzheimer's disease neurodegeneration appears to affect primarily cholinergic neurons, cholinergic agents such as tacrine (Cognex), and other second-generation drugs that are better tolerated, such as donepezil (Aricept), rivastigmine (Exelon), and galantamine (Reminyl), have shown efficacy in terms of temporarily slowing progression of the disease. These agents all inhibit an enzyme (acetylcholinesterase) which degrades the neurotransmitter acetylcholine. Clinical trials using an agent that mimics the actions of acetylcholine (nicotine) ended abruptly due to side effects that included severe anxiety.

Because the amyloid lesions in Alzheimer's disease may elicit a limited inflammatory response in the brain, which in turn may be a major component of the neurotoxic effects of Aβ, nonsteroidal anti-inflammatory drugs (NSAIDs), such as aspirin and ibuprofin, have been proposed as agents having possible ameliorative effects.

Certain retrospective studies have shown a negative correlation between the use of estrogen replacement therapy (ERT) and both the age of onset and severity of

Alzheimer's disease in postmenopausal women, suggesting that ERT may have a protective function in these subjects.

Cholesterol may influence the production of Aβ by altering the characteristics of cell membranes, and Aβ is transported by lipoproteins. Thus, lipid metabolism may have an impact on the development of Alzheimer's disease. It has recently been shown that the cholesterol-lowering agents lovastatin and pravastatin may significantly reduce the risk of Alzheimer's disease in older patients.

PERSPECTIVE AND PROSPECTS

The pharmaceutical manufacturer Lilly has patented the first orally active β-secretase inhibitor, and it is likely that there are many such drugs currently in development. It is possible that some of these drugs may suffer liabilities due to alterations of Notch signaling. Nevertheless, they will provide key information regarding the validity of the amyloid hypothesis. With the recent cloning of β-secretase, drug discovery efforts surrounding β-secretase will likely be greatly facilitated.

Another potential target for drug intervention in Alzheimer's disease is the inhibition of Aβ aggregation. Although a number of agents have been reported that inhibit aggregation, they are all characteristically large molecular weight peptides that have very limited access across the blood/brain barrier. Thus, although this approach may work in principle, the development of a useful drug from this approach may be severely limited by issues regarding access of the drug to the brain.

Neurofibrillary tangles are an additional feature of Alzheimer's disease that may serve as a target for drug development. Since neurofibrillary tangles are composed of hyperphosphorylated tau protein, inhibitors of tau phosphorylation might be developed as useful therapeutic entities.

It has recently been reported that experimental vaccination of transgenic animals, showing features of Alzheimer's disease such as amyloid plaques with Aβ peptide, results in the reduction of amyloid burden. The exciting implications of these experiments are that Alzheimer's disease might one day be treated or even prevented by vaccination. This approach to the treatment of Alzheimer's disease has entered early clinical trials.

Other approaches to therapeutics for Alzheimer's disease include the development of neurotrophic factors that may enhance neuron survival. Research into stem cells has provided evidence for the presence of neuronal stem cells within the brain. Research into the mechanisms of stem cell migration and development might yield drugs that would enhance the recruitment of such primitive stem cells into dystrophic areas of the brain.

Because early detection of Alzheimer's disease increases the effectiveness of current drugs and treatments and helps keep some of the disease's more devastating symptoms at bay, research is focused on ways to detect the disease definitively. A Canadian study released in 2002 notes possible connections between scores of verbal memory tests and the likelihood of developing the disease. The study examined patients' performance on a variety of psychological tests to gauge the tests' reliability in detecting preclinical Alzheimer's disease. The researchers discovered that verbal memory tests—for example, recalling the categories of words or being able to remember terms for a short period of time—were highly accurate in determining which individuals went on to develop the disease. These findings seem to support what other researchers have found: the evident decline in verbal memory in elderly individuals in the one- to two-year period prior to the development of Alzheimer's disease symptoms.

The search for causes of Alzheimer's dementia remains a topic of interest in the effort to develop prevention strategies. For instance, recent research has demonstrated that isoflurane, a common anesthetic, can lead to the development of amyloid protein in cultured neuronal cells and to cell death. Research following this discovery may lead to recommendations to avoid the use of such anesthetics, in favor of others, as a way of preventing exposure of vulnerable persons to what may be a causative factor in Alzheimer's dementia.

—Robert L. Martone;
updated by Nancy A. Piotrowski, Ph.D.

See also Aging; Aging: Extended care; Amnesia; Brain; Brain disorders; Dementias; Geriatrics and gerontology; Memory loss; Neurology; Pick's disease; Psychiatry, geriatric.

FOR FURTHER INFORMATION:

Alzheimer's Association. http://www.alz.org/. Site of a voluntary organization dedicated to researching the prevention, cures, and treatments of Alzheimer's disease. The Benjamin B. Green-Field Library and Resource Center collects a wide range of materials related to Alzheimer's disease and related disorders and provides service to family members, educators and students, health professionals, social service agencies, and the general public.

Bellenir, Karen, ed. *Alzheimer's Disease Sourcebook: Basic Consumer Health Information About Alzheimer's Disease, Other Dementias, and Related Disorders*. 3d ed. Detroit: Omnigraphics, 2003. Provides comprehensive information for health consumers on symptoms, research, related disorders, and other dementia. Includes a glossary and resource listings.

Brioni, Jorge D., and Michael W. Decker, eds. *Pharmacological Treatment of Alzheimer's Disease: Molecular and Neurobiological Foundations*. New York: Wiley-Liss, 1997. Reviews many current approaches to treatment.

Esiri, Margaret M., Virginia M.-Y. Lee, and John Q. Trojanowski, eds. *The Neuropathology of Dementia*. 2d ed. New York: Cambridge University Press, 2004. A thorough and rigorous presentation of the neuropathology that underlies dementia.

Gauthier, Serge, ed. *Clinical Diagnosis and Management of Alzheimer's Disease*. 3d ed. Abingdon, Oxfordshire, England: Informa Healthcare, 2006. A clinical textbook designed for medical students. Covers the etiology, clinical and laboratory assessment, natural evolution, and medical and nonmedical management of Alzheimer's disease.

Mace, Nancy L., and Peter V. Rabins. *The Thirty-Six-Hour Day: A Family Guide to Caring for Persons with Alzheimer Disease, Related Dementing Illnesses, and Memory Loss in Later Life*. 4th ed. Baltimore: Johns Hopkins University Press, 2006. Provides a wealth of information for families coping with Alzheimer's disease, including topics such as the evaluation of persons with dementia, hospice care, assisted living facilities, financing care, and the latest findings on eating and nutrition.

Rowland, Lewis P., ed. *Merritt's Textbook of Neurology*. 11th ed. Philadelphia: Lippincott Williams & Wilkins, 2005. An essential text for all neurological disorders.

Wasco, W., and R. E. Tanzi, eds. *Molecular Mechanisms of Dementia*. Totowa, N.J.: Humana Press, 1997. A useful survey of research regarding recent research in the field of dementia.

Whitehouse, Peter J., Konrad Maurer, and Jesse F. Ballenger, eds. *Concepts of Alzheimer Disease: Biological, Clinical, and Cultural Perspectives*. Baltimore: Johns Hopkins University Press, 2003. Explores the social and intellectual history of Alzheimer's disease, especially the evolution in the way in which the disease has been viewed and studied.

AMENORRHEA

DISEASE/DISORDER

ANATOMY OR SYSTEM AFFECTED: Endocrine system, reproductive system

SPECIALTIES AND RELATED FIELDS: Endocrinology, family medicine, gynecology

DEFINITION: The absence of menstrual cycles.

KEY TERMS:

anorexia nervosa: a psychiatric disease characterized by a distorted body image in which the individual severely limits food intake because of fear of weight gain

estrogen: a hormone secreted from the ovaries that is crucial for the buildup of the uterine lining, ovulation, and bone density maintenance

premature ovarian failure: cessation of menses prior to the age of forty because of the early loss of ovarian follicles

prolactin: a hormone secreted from the posterior pituitary gland; at high levels (for example, resulting from tumors in the pituitary), prolactin can cause amenorrhea and increase breast secretions, a condition known as galactorrhea

secondary sexual characteristics: in females, the development of breast tissue and pubic hair

CAUSES AND SYMPTOMS

Amenorrhea, or the absence of menses, can be physiologic, such as during pregnancy, or pathologic. Amenorrhea can be primary or secondary in nature. Primary amenorrhea is defined as the absence of menses by age sixteen, even in the presence of normal growth and secondary sexual characteristics. In girls with abnormal growth, primary amenorrhea is defined as the absence of menses by age fourteen. Causes of primary amenorrhea include abnormalities of the reproductive outflow tract which prevent the flow of menstrual blood. Examples include imperforate hymen, transverse vaginal septum, and Asherman's syndrome, whereby scar tissue within the uterus prevents the outflow of menstrual fluid. Girls with these conditions may experience cyclic cramping and discomfort from the buildup of menstrual blood. Other causes of primary amenorrhea include genetic problems such as Turner syndrome, in which the individual has a single X chromosome, or androgen insensitivity syndrome, in which the individual appears female but is genetically male and lacks ovaries and a uterus. Turner syndrome and androgen insensitivity tend to be asymptomatic regarding their amenorrhea. Rare congenital causes of primary amenorrhea

> **Information on Amenorrhea**
>
> **Causes:** Stress, psychological disorders, hormone deficiency, extremely low body fat
> **Symptoms:** Cessation of menstrual periods
> **Duration:** Often chronic
> **Treatments:** Hormone replacement, oral contraceptives, counseling

include Kallman syndrome and empty sella syndrome.

Secondary amenorrhea refers to the absence of menstrual periods after menstrual cycles have occurred previously. It is defined as the absence of menses for the duration of three regular menstrual cycles or six months. Physiological causes of secondary amenorrhea include pregnancy, the postpartum state, and the menopause. Pathologic causes of secondary amenorrhea include disorders of the central nervous system or hypothalamus, such as extreme stress or exercise and anorexia nervosa. Disorders of the pituitary gland, such as tumors, can cause secondary amenorrhea as well. These tumors may be accompanied by galactorrhea, from high levels of prolactin, or by visual impairment. Hormonal disturbances can also lead to secondary amenorrhea. One example is hypothyroidism, which is often accompanied by fatigue and cold intolerance. Polycystic ovary syndrome, an endocrinologic disorder characterized by insulin resistance and hirsutism, may also lead to amenorrhea. Another cause of secondary amenorrhea is premature ovarian failure, which may be attributable to radiation or chemotherapy. These individuals may experience the symptoms of early menopause, such as hot flashes and vaginal dryness.

Treatment and Therapy

The treatment for amenorrhea depends on the cause. If the disorder is the result of anatomic causes, then surgery may cure it. For instance, an imperforate hymen or transverse vaginal septum can be corrected surgically, allowing for normal outflow of menstrual fluid. If the disorder is the result of hormonal imbalances, then medications may be given, such as thyroid hormone for hypothyroidism or bromocriptine for hyperprolactinemia. In individuals with polycystic ovary syndrome, metoformin may be given to regulate the menstrual cycles. By correcting these hormonal imbalances, the resumption of regular menstrual cycles may occur, thus allowing for conception and pregnancy, if the individual so desires.

In cases of amenorrhea caused by extreme stress or exercise and anorexia nervosa, removal from the stressful conditions, a decrease in exercise levels, or an increase in caloric intake to maintain normal ideal body weight often remediates amenorrhea. Individuals who suffer from anorexia nervosa also require psychiatric treatment.

Individuals with genetic causes or premature ovarian failure leading to amenorrhea are unlikely to attain menstruation via medical therapy. For these individuals, therapy is aimed at preventing or treating the sequelae of estrogen deficiency that accompany amenorrhea. For instance, women with premature ovarian failure are at risk for the depletion of bone mineral density and osteoporosis. These individuals may benefit from hormone replacement therapy in the form of estrogen and progesterone.

Perspective and Prospects

The cause for amenorrhea can often be found, since a vast array of diagnostic tests are available. Anatomic abnormalities may be detected on physical examination or via imaging of the reproductive structures such as ultrasound. Hormonal causes of amenorrhea can often be found through blood tests of hormones produced by the hypothalamus, pituitary gland, ovaries, thyroid gland, and adrenal glands. These tests can identify the hormone derangement and which organ is responsible. Genetic tests have allowed physicians to understand the basis of primary amenorrhea on a molecular level. While many cases of amenorrhea can be treated effectively once the cause has been identified, the future holds promise that better therapies with fewer side effects will be found.

—Anne Lynn S. Chang, M.D.

See also Anorexia nervosa; Dysmenorrhea; Eating disorders; Exercise physiology; Gynecology; Hormones; Menstruation; Puberty and adolescence; Reproductive system; Weight loss and gain; Women's health.

For Further Information:

Kasper, Dennis L., et al., eds. *Harrison's Principles of Internal Medicine*. 16th ed. New York: McGraw-Hill, 2005.

Stenchever, Morton A., et al. *Comprehensive Gynecology*. 4th ed. St. Louis: Mosby, 2006.

Tierney, Lawrence M., Stephen J. McPhee, and Maxine A. Papadakis, eds. *Current Medical Diagnosis and Treatment 2007*. New York: McGraw-Hill Medical, 2006.

American Indian health

Overview

Anatomy or system affected: All

Specialties and related fields: All

Definition: Statistics and medical problems of persons descended from the original inhabitants of North America.

Key terms:

alcoholism: a disorder characterized by the excessive consumption of alcohol, leading to dependency

cirrhosis: a chronic disease of the liver in which normal tissue is replaced with fibrous tissue, resulting in the loss of functional liver cells

diabetes mellitus: a disorder of carbohydrate metabolism, resulting in excessive amounts of glucose in the blood and urine

hepatitis: inflammation of the liver characterized by jaundice, liver enlargement, and fever

obesity: a weight more than 20 percent above normal

otitis media: inflammation of the middle ear, characterized by pain, dizziness, and impaired hearing

sudden infant death syndrome: a fatal sudden cessation of breathing in healthy sleeping infants under a year old

syphilis: a chronic infectious disease either transmitted by direct contact (usually in sexual intercourse) or passed from mother to child in utero

tuberculosis: an infectious disease of humans and animals caused by the tubercle bacillus and characterized by the coughing up of mucus and sputum, fever, weight loss, and chest pain

years of potential life lost: a measure of the burden of premature deaths

Population and Statistics

More than three million residents of the United States are of American Indian ancestry. This diverse population consists of more than five hundred tribes speaking more than three hundred different languages. There are three hundred American Indian reservations in the continental United States. In the American Indian population, 33 percent are below the age of fifteen and 6 percent are older than sixty-four. In comparison, in the total U.S. population, 22 percent are younger than fifteen and 13 percent are over the age of sixty-four. Of American Indians, 8.9 percent have at least a college degree (compared to 20.3 percent of the total U.S. population). The unemployment rate among American Indians is 14.8 percent (6.3 percent for the total U.S. population), and 31 percent of American Indians are below poverty level (13.1 percent for the total U.S. population).

The Urban Indian Health Institute analyzed census and vital statistics data from 1990 to 2000 and found health disparities between American Indians and the general U.S. population. The Federal Indian Health Service reported health trends for 2000 to 2001. Average life expectancy of American Indians was 70.6 years, compared to 76.5 for the total U.S. population. The years of potential life lost (YPLL) rate (per 1,000) for American Indians was 88, compared to the total U.S. population of 48.4. The death rate (per 1,000) for all ages was 715.2 for American Indians and 479.1 for the total U.S. population. For American Indians aged five to fourteen, the top two causes of death were unintentional injuries and homicide. For the corresponding U.S. population, the top two were unintentional injuries and malignant neoplasms. American Indians aged fifteen to twenty-four were most likely to die from unintentional injuries or suicide (for the U.S. population, they were unintentional injuries or homicide). For ages twenty-five to forty-four, the top two causes of death in American Indians were unintentional injuries and chronic liver disease, whereas the top causes of death in the U.S. population were unintentional injuries and malignant neoplasms. For the total U.S. population, the top five leading causes of death were heart disease, malignant neoplasms, stroke, chronic lower respiratory disease, and unintentional injuries. The top five leading causes of death for American Indians of all ages were heart disease, malignant neoplasms, unintentional injuries, diabetes mellitus, and chronic liver disease.

Major Health Concerns

Heart disease is the leading cause of death in American Indians. The incidence is twice that of the general U.S. population. Diabetes mellitus plays a large part in heart disease. While mortality rates from heart disease have decreased in general in the United States, American Indians have seen no change in the death rate from heart disease, which is 8 percent higher than the rate for all races.

Malignant neoplasm, or cancer, was unknown to American Indians until the latter part of the twentieth century. Cancer is the third leading cause of death in American Indian women. Furthermore, American Indians have a lower survival rate from all cancers than any other group. The five-year survival rate for American Indian women is 35.2 percent. For Caucasian women, that number is 50.3 percent. Although the rates of breast cancer are lower in American Indians than in Caucasians, breast cancer mortality rates are increasing in American Indians. For breast cancer, the five-year survival rates are 49 percent for American Indians and 76 percent for Caucasian women. In American Indian men, the five major cancer sites that lead to death are the lungs, prostate, colon, stomach, and liver. The overall cancer mortality rate for American Indian men aged fourteen to twenty-four years is 3.7 percent. The rate for U.S. men of all races in the same age range is 3.3 percent. Gallbladder cancer rates are high for both male and female American Indians. This form of cancer is 8.9 times more likely to occur in American Indians than in Caucasians. Death rates from lung cancer have been increasing in American Indian populations. This increase may be due, in part, to the observation that urban American Indians are more likely to be habitual tobacco users than people of other races. For example, in 1998 the Catawba tribe of South Carolina reported that 30.2 percent of their population were current smokers (the rate was 20 percent for African Americans and 25.7 percent for Caucasians). Maternal tobacco use is also a serious risk factor for infant death.

American Indian infant health status is lower compared with most children in the United States. Premature births and infant mortality rates are higher for American Indians than for the general population. Sudden infant death syndrome (SIDS) was the leading cause of American Indian infant mortality between 1995 and 2000 at twice the rate of the general population. One risk factor, maternal alcoholism, is three to four times more common in American Indians than in the total population. In one study, first trimester binge drinking was related to six times the risk for SIDS.

Approximately 75 percent of all American Indian childhood deaths are the result of injuries, twice the rate for the total U.S. population. Although rarely fatal, otitis media is another health concern for American Indian children. Otitis media is seen twice as often in American Indian children than in the general U.S. population. For infants, the rate of otitis media in American Indians was three times higher than in the general population.

While diabetes mellitus was virtually nonexistent in American Indians before 1950, Type II diabetes is now the fourth leading cause of death in this population. The common cold and diabetes are the two most frequent causes of outpatient visits to American Indian health centers. The prevalence of diabetes mellitus is 15 percent in American Indian adults, compared with 7 percent in total U.S. adults. In adult American Indians over age fifty-five, the prevalence doubles to 30 percent, with a higher frequency in women than in men. There is an increasing incidence in American Indians under the age of twenty. Diabetes mellitus is associated with thyroid disease and impaired circulation that occurs with high blood sugar (glucose). Complications of diabetes mellitus include blindness, kidney failure, lower extremity amputation, heart disease, circulation problems, coma, and depression. Of all people with diabetes, American Indians are six times more likely to suffer kidney failure. Amputations related to diabetes mellitus are three to four times higher in American Indians than in others with the disease. American Indians have the highest death rate in the world from diabetes mellitus. American Indians are three times more likely to die from diabetes mellitus than the general U.S. population.

The increase in the prevalence of diabetes mellitus may be explained, in part, by genetics. One theory is that American Indians have a "thrifty genotype." Because they were hunter-gatherers, their bodies had to adapt to fluctuations in weight, from famine to feast. When food was available, body fat was stored quickly in preparation for periods without food. When this lifestyle changed, this genotype became maladaptive. Food is now no longer scarce. Whereas hunter-gatherer diets consisted of wild game, fish, nuts, fruits, and vegetables, U.S. government commodities given to American Indians have high fat and sugar content. This diet promotes fat storage in a body that is already genetically predisposed to store fat rapidly, an adaptation that is no longer necessary for survival. Consequently, obesity, a risk factor in diabetes mellitus, is a major health concern for American Indians.

American Indians exhibit the highest prevalence of obesity among all racial groups. Obesity starts early in the lives of American Indians. In the general U.S. population, 11 percent of six- to eleven-year-olds are overweight. The rate is 28.6 percent in American Indian children of the same age. A survey conducted by the Indian Health Services in 1990 showed that 40 percent of five- to eighteen-year-old American Indians were overweight. From the study of the Catawba, 63.4 percent reported being overweight and 42.8 percent were physically inactive. In American Indian men, 34 percent are overweight. The rate for American Indian women is 40 percent. Diet plays a large part in obesity. One study indicated that American Indians' high consumption of sugary drinks may be a major contributor to obesity. In support of this conclusion, American Indian children have five times the dental decay than the average U.S. child. Dental problems are also associated with alcohol abuse.

Alcohol-related hospitalizations for American Indians are 1.6 times greater than in the general population. A variety of medical problems are associated with alcoholism: kidney and bladder problems, hearing and vision problems, and head injuries. Alcohol abuse has a high rate of co-occurrence with smoking, suggesting a genetic predisposition to both addictions. A genetic basis to alcoholism is also indicated by the reduced ability of some Asians and American Indians to metabolize alcohol. This same genetic predisposition affects vulnerability to alcohol cirrhosis. Alcoholism is related to some of the leading causes of American Indian deaths that occur at rates three to four times the national average: accidents, suicides, homicides, and cirrhosis. Excessive use of alcohol can lead to drug-related hepatitis.

PERSPECTIVE AND PROSPECTS

Research in genetics led to the conclusion that American Indians migrated to the North American continent from east-central Asia. European contact reduced the population of American Indians. Major health concerns of the American Indians were infectious diseases against which they had no immunity, such as typhoid, diphtheria, measles, smallpox, syphilis, and tuberculosis. For example, following the Spanish colonization of California, between 1800 and 1802 there was a diphtheria epidemic among the Chumash. As a result, 15 percent of the tribe's population died.

The Indian Removal Act of 1830 forced American Indians to leave their homelands and travel to designated reservations. The combination of stress and poor nutrition made them susceptible to infectious diseases. For example, the Choctaws were devastated by cholera. Between 1836 and 1840, ten thousand American Indians died from smallpox. Some American Indians dealt with the stress of disease and removal by drinking alcohol. American Indians began dying of alcohol poisoning.

As a result of the move to reservations, inadequate housing and nutrition led to infant deaths from pneumonia, gastrointestinal disorders, tuberculosis, heart disease, and syphilis. Yakama infants died most frequently from pneumonia, which developed from influenza. Bacilli spread through the air and on blankets, dishes, and clothing. Malnutrition, heart disease, tuberculosis, and infection increased the risk of developing pneumonia. Children died from vomiting, diarrhea, and infections resulting from gastrointestinal disorders. Tuberculosis developed quickly as a result of malnutrition and unsanitary housing. A fetus developed congenital heart disease as a result of the mother's poor nutrition, lack of prenatal care, and infection or disease such as rubella. Syphilis in adults caused increased sterility. In the Yakama tribe, 79 percent of people who died of syphilis were children who had contracted the disease from their mothers. In all, a child's life expectancy was 6.4 years.

Acculturation resulting from European contact is associated with the major health concerns of American Indians. Forced cultural changes have resulted in changed lifestyles. For example, between 1936 and 1946, American Indians went from an agricultural to an industrial society. The increased incidence of diabetes mellitus among American Indians is associated with urban, industrialized, and sedentary lifestyles added to an increase of store-bought foods in their diet. More generally, profound cultural changes can result in stress that leads to health problems.

Improvements in American Indian health can be made through research, education, and community-based prevention programs. For example, educational programs emphasize breast cancer awareness and screenings. As another example, to reduce the incidence of diabetes mellitus, interventions promote exercise, a reduced-fat diet, and glucose control. Efforts to change diets must take into account what foods are currently part of the diet and what importance those foods have for a particular American Indian tribe. Educational programs to promote weight loss must pay attention to some tribal beliefs that large bodies indicate wealth, while skinny bodies represent weakness and illness. Breast-feeding programs encourage and support American Indian women to breast-feed their babies for at least two months. Research indicates that breast-fed babies are less likely to develop diabetes. Prevention strategies are aimed at the leading causes of injury-related death, such as car wrecks and suicide. Programs to reduce the incidence of alcoholism show an encouraging reduction in the number of alcohol-related American Indian deaths.

—Elizabeth Marie McGhee Nelson, Ph.D.

See also Accidents; Addiction; African American health; Alcoholism; Asian American health; Cancer; Cirrhosis; Diabetes mellitus; Ear infections and disorders; Gallbladder cancer; Heart disease; Hepatitis; Liver; Liver disorders; Men's health; Obesity; Smoking; Sudden infant death syndrome (SIDS); Suicide; Syphilis; Tobacco; Tuberculosis; Women's health.

For Further Information:

Castor, Mei L., et al. "A Nationwide Population-Based Study Identifying Health Disparities Between American Indians/Alaska Natives and the General Populations Living in Select Urban Counties." *American Journal of Public Health* 96, no. 8 (August, 2006): 1478-1484. This article examines the health status of American Indian populations living in urban areas through an analysis of U.S. census and vital statistics data.

Denny, Clark H., et al. "Disparities in Chronic Disease Risk Factors and Health Status Between American Indian/Alaska Native and White Elders: Finding from a Telephone Survey, 2001 and 2002." *American Journal of Public Health* 95, no. 5 (May, 2005): 825-827. Compares American Indians and Caucasians for prevalence of smoking, physical inactivity, obesity, diagnosed diabetes, and general health status.

Grossman, David C., et al. "Disparities in Infant Health Among American Indians and Alaska Natives in U.S. Metropolitan Areas." *Pediatrics* 109, no. 4 (April, 2002): 627-633. Addresses the health status of American Indian children.

Joe, Jennie R. "Out of Harmony: Health Problems and Young Native American Men." *Journal of American College Health* 49 (March, 2001): 237-242. This article emphasizes the major health problems in American Indian men.

MedlinePlus. *Native-American Health*. http://www.nlm.nih.gov/medlineplus/nativeamericanhealth.html. Provides online health information on American Indian health issues.

Rhodes, Everett R., ed. *American Indian Health: Innovations in Health Care, Promotion, and Policy*. Baltimore: Johns Hopkins University Press, 2000. From a native perspective, this book looks at American Indian health taking into account history and politics. It includes a review of the most important diseases emphasizing cultural and medical perspectives.

Trafzer, Clifford E., and D. Weiner, eds. *Medicine Ways: Disease, Health, and Survival Among Native Americans*. Walnut Creek, Calif.: AltaMira Press, 2001. From the perspective of American Indians, the authors of this collection of essays examine health issues in a historical and socioeconomic context.

American Medical Association (AMA)

Organization

Definition: The largest voluntary association of physicians in the United States, with most of its members engaging directly in the practice of medicine.

Key terms:

Accreditation Council for Continuing Medical Education (ACCME): the organization that promotes and accredits continuing education for physicians, which the AMA sponsors

Accreditation Council for Graduate Medical Education (ACGME): the council that accredits physician residency programs in 1,500 U.S. medical schools; it is sponsored by the AMA and four other organizations

House of Delegates: the representative body that decides official policy and action on behalf of the AMA membership; state medical societies are allocated most of the delegate positions in the house, since 90 percent of all physicians affiliate with them, while medical specialty societies, military and other federal service groups, and five special sections also are given representation

Liaison Committee on Medical Education (LCME): an organization formed by the AMA and the Association of American Medical Colleges to set standards and accredit all U.S. and Canadian medical schools offering M.D. degrees

Role in the United States

Since its inception, the American Medical Association (AMA) has worked to improve the credibility of medicine as a profession in the United States. The AMA helped to shape and develop the physician licensing system used now in every state. Through the auspices of various accreditation bodies that it sponsors, such as the LCME, ACGME, and ACCME, the AMA monitors medical education programs to ensure that they continue to meet high standards. The AMA established a professional code of ethics for physicians and revises it periodically to guide physicians through the ever-changing health care environment. The AMA Council on Ethical and Judicial Affairs regularly issues interpretations of the principles of medical ethics; the council can censure, suspend, or expel a physician who violates the code of ethics. The *Journal of the American Medical Association* (or *JAMA*) was first published in July, 1883, and is now the world's most widely circulated medical journal. The AMA also publishes ten medical specialty journals and the weekly *American Medical News*. In addition, the AMA produces and distributes press releases, video news releases, and radio and television news programs.

The AMA advocates a "patient's bill of rights," which supports patient autonomy, dignity, confidentiality, and ongoing access to needed medical care. The AMA believes that the practice of medicine should be based on sound scientific principles, which are promulgated in *JAMA* and in the many specialty journals that it sponsors and publishes. The AMA also houses one of the nation's largest medical libraries, subscribes to more than 150 computer databases, and maintains comprehensive computer files on all physicians and medical students in the United States.

GUIDELINES FOR HEALTH

The AMA acknowledged early in its development the role that it should play in promoting the improvement of public health. Among the public health initiatives that the AMA has sponsored are the clear labeling of poison containers, early childhood screening for hearing and vision problems, the inspection of milk to ensure its quality, the installation of seat belts in automobiles, low tolerance in state laws regarding drunk driving, and the banning of tobacco product advertisement. More recently, the AMA was among the first professional associations to advocate significant reform of the American health care delivery system, especially to respond to the needs of uninsured and underinsured people. The communications arm of the AMA produces services and products designed to increase public knowledge regarding significant health care issues and medical care advances.

PERSPECTIVE AND PROSPECTS

Nathan Smith Davis, a medical doctor and a delegate of the New York State Medical Society, introduced resolutions that led to the holding of the first national medical convention in May, 1846. Davis's tireless leadership during the first convention enabled the establishment of the American Medical Association in May, 1847. Davis also served as an AMA president and the first editor-in-chief of the *Journal of the American Medical Association*.

The original AMA constitution set out several enduring principles for the organization. The AMA would be governed by representatives elected from the membership, and officers would serve only one year. The purposes of the AMA would be to advance medical knowledge, to work to improve medical education, to establish high ethical and practice standards, to encourage the formation and maintenance of state and local medical societies, and to work against medical quackery.

In order to ensure that the association speaks with a unified voice, the AMA has used, since its founding, the principle of representative democracy. State medical societies are entitled to a voting delegate and an alternate for each one thousand members; this represents the overwhelming majority of voting delegates. Other organizations, such as the Veterans Administration and medical schools sections, are also given one delegate and one alternate. The delegates form the AMA House of Delegates, which meets twice a year to evaluate and decide on policy issues. In order to prepare properly for a meeting of the House of Delegates, reference committees consider and hold open hearings on important medical issues, such as testing for acquired immunodeficiency syndrome (AIDS). The reference committees then make recommendations to the House of Delegates, which often decides hundreds of policies during each session.

The AMA is a powerful lobbyist in Washington, D.C., where it seeks to influence national legislation affecting the delivery of medical care. It also represents the interests of its members in important cases brought before various courts.

—Russell Williams, M.S.W.

See also Animal rights vs. research; Centers for Disease Control and Prevention (CDC); Education, medical; Ethics; Hippocratic oath; Law and medicine; National Institutes of Health (NIH).

FOR FURTHER INFORMATION:

American Medical Association. *Caring for the Country: A History and Celebration of the First 150 Years of the American Medical Association*. Chicago: Author, 1997. Written as a lively, thoughtful narrative, this book examines the role a great institution and its physician members have played in creating the world's finest system of medical care.

Baker, Robert B., ed. *The American Medical Ethics Revolution: How the AMA's Code of Ethics Has Transformed Physicians' Relationships to Patients, Professionals, and Society*. Baltimore: Johns Hopkins University Press, 1999. Twenty essays offer a detailed analysis of the political and philosophical maneuvering behind the preparation of the 1847 Code of Ethics and explore the resulting impact on modern health care.

Campion, Frank. *The AMA and U.S. Health Policy Since 1940*. Chicago: Chicago Review Press, 1984. A thorough study of the American Medical Association's medical policy since 1940. Includes bibliographical references and an index.

Fishbein, Morris. *A History of the American Medical Association, 1847 to 1947*. Philadelphia: W. B. Saunders, 1947. A historical look at the American Medical Association, including biographies of the organization's presidents and the histories of publications, councils, bureaus, and other official bodies.

Amnesia

Disease/disorder

Anatomy or system affected: Brain, nervous system, psychic-emotional system

Specialties and related fields: Neurology, psychiatry, psychology

Definition: The loss of memory due to physical and/ or psychological conditions.

Key terms:

anterograde: referring to amnesia in which events following a biological or psychological trauma are forgotten; new learning is impaired

episodic memory: the remembrance of personal information in one's life, such as the events of the previous day

procedural memory: the ability to reproduce learned skills, particularly perceptual-motor activities such as riding a bike

retrograde: referring to amnesia in which events preceding a biological or psychological trauma are forgotten; retrieving previously formed memories is impaired

semantic memory: the storage of factual information, such as the meaning of words

Information on Amnesia

Causes: Head trauma, various diseases, psychological or emotional trauma

Symptoms: Loss of memory for a specific time period

Duration: Episodic, sometimes long term

Treatments: Psychological intervention, drugs affecting neurotransmitter levels

Causes and Symptoms

The primary attribute of amnesia is a loss of memory for a specific time period. The extent, duration, and type of that memory loss can vary greatly. In anterograde amnesia, the formation of new memories is impaired, while in retrograde amnesia, the retrieval of previously formed memories is impaired. In rare cases, anterograde amnesia is continuous, in which there is great impairment of memory formation for the remainder of a person's life. Retrograde amnesia in rare cases may be generalized, in which the totality of an individual's personal memory preceding the onset of amnesia is lost. More commonly, both anterograde and retrograde amnesias are localized, in which the memory of a period of time ranging from seconds to minutes (although occasionally days or longer) is lost. The memory loss may be selective, with only some aspects of a particular time period being absent. In all these forms of amnesia, the most common type of information lost is episodic; rarely are procedural memories destroyed.

Amnesia is typically caused by either psychological circumstances, in which case it is termed psychogenic, or by biological processes, where it is referred to as biogenic or organic. Sometimes, however, the cause involves both psychological and biological factors. Psychogenic amnesias are usually caused by some sort of emotional trauma. Emotional trauma is the common thread that runs through the amnesia associated with the following disorders: dissociative amnesia (the inability to recall significant personal information), fugue (memory loss accompanied by sudden, unexpected travel from home), dissociative identity disorder (the presence of two or more distinct personalities, with inability to recall extensive time periods), and post-traumatic stress disorder (significant distress and memory disturbances following an extreme traumatic event). Emotional trauma is typically absent in posthypnotic amnesia, which is induced by hypnotic suggestion, and childhood amnesia, in which adult memories of early childhood experiences before the age of five are typically vague and fragmentary. Psychogenic memories, while principally involving episodic information, may extend to semantic information, which is rarely seen in biogenic amnesia.

Biogenic amnesia is usually the result of trauma to the brain or disease processes. Anterograde and retrograde amnesia are common following a concussion or brain surgery, particularly involving the temporal lobe. Electroconvulsive treatments induced by a current passed through electrodes on the forehead (sometimes used to treat depression) tend to have a more anterograde effect. A diversity of toxic and infectious brain illnesses can lead to Korsakoff's syndrome, first described in chronic alcoholics. The primary feature is anterograde disturbance, with the ability to store new information limited to a few seconds. Dementia typically begins with the loss of recent memories and gradually spreads retrograde into the person's more distant past as the condition progresses. Hardening of the brain arteries, Alzheimer's disease, and numerous infectious agents can lead to dementia. Transient global amnesia is an abrupt anterograde and retrograde loss leaving some degree of permanent memory loss; it is thought to be caused by temporary reductions in the blood supply to specific brain regions.

Treatment and Therapy

As time passes from the emotional and physiological traumas that precipitate amnesia, there is usually some degree of memory recovery. The less severe the trauma, the better the prognosis. Psychological interventions involving the use of careful interrogation, the use of emotionally significant stimuli, or hypnosis can help the amnesic fill in the gaps of memory deficits. Drugs that affect levels of neurotransmitters such as acetylcholine, aspartate, glutamate, norepinephrine, and serotonin can also have an impact on memory recovery. For example, John Krystal reported in 1993 that Vietnam War veterans given yohimbine, a drug that activates norepinephrine, experienced vivid flashbacks of combat trauma.

Some amnesias can be either prevented—using electrodes on only one side of the head in electroconvulsive treatment lessens the likelihood of amnesia—or significantly ameliorated by psychological and/or biological intervention. Severe amnesias, however, such as in dementia, have no effective treatment. Major memory loss in the elderly has a particularly poor prognosis for recovery and is often indicative of imminent death. Where memory recovery is poor, optimizing the use of the remaining mental abilities and available environmental resources can help those with amnesia better adapt to their living environments.

Perspective and Prospects

The first scientific explanations of amnesia came in the late nineteenth century. Théodule-Armand Ribot (1839-1916) proposed a "law of regression," in which memory loss was thought to progress from the least stable to the most stable memories. Sergey Korsakoff (1853-1900) was one of the first to demonstrate that amnesia need not be associated with the loss of reasoning abilities found in dementia. While Ribot and Korsakoff focused on organic causes of amnesia, Pierre Janet (1859-1947) described amnesics who apparently had no underlying biological disease. He explained these cases in terms of mental fragmentation that he called dissociation.

Prevention, rather than treatment, of amnesia became the focus of attention as the twentieth century drew to a close. Two promising research areas are drugs to limit the effects of brain damage and the beneficial impact of a stimulating environment in staving off the effects of aging on the brain.

—Paul J. Chara, Jr., Ph.D., and Kathleen A. Chara, M.S.

See also Aging; Aging: Extended care; Alcoholism; Alzheimer's disease; Brain; Brain disorders; Delusions; Dementias; Geriatrics and gerontology; Hypnosis; Memory loss; Post-traumatic stress disorder; Psychiatric disorders; Psychiatry; Psychiatry, child and adolescent; Psychiatry, geriatric; Shock therapy; Stress.

For Further Information:

Baddeley, Alan, et al., eds. *Episodic Memory: New Directions in Research.* New York: Oxford University Press, 2002. Provides fifteen contributions on the subject of memory from leading researchers in cognitive psychology, neuropsychology, and neuroscience.

Berrios, German E., and John R. Hodges, eds. *Memory Disorders in Psychiatric Practice.* New York: Cambridge University Press, 2000. Explores the psychiatric approach to memory disorders and covers such topics as historical aspects of memory and its disorders, mood and memory, memory impairments seen in the dementias, amnesic syndrome, transient epileptic amnesia, confabulation, and the Ganser syndrome.

Damasio, Antonio R. *Descartes' Error: Emotion, Reason, and the Human Brain.* New York: G. P. Putnam's Sons, 1994. Damasio brings some fascinating cases to bear on one of the oldest problems in philosophy and psychology. The book is a good read on an important subject, an excellent contribution to scholarship on the effects of emotion on rationality.

Herman, Judith L. *Trauma and Recovery: The Aftermath of Violence from Domestic Abuse to Political Terror.* New York: Basic Books, 1992. This book addresses parallels between private and public traumas, including the experiences of rape survivors, combat veterans, battered women, physically abused children, and concentration camp victims.

Schacter, Daniel L. *Searching for Memory: The Brain, the Mind, and the Past*. New York: Basic Books, 1996. Schacter describes what memory is and how it works, discussing such subjects as the hippocampus and other pertinent areas of the brain and how they function.

Squire, Larry R., and Daniel L. Schacter, eds. *Neuropsychology of Memory*. 3d ed. New York: Guilford Press, 2002. Examines the physiology of memory and memory disorders.

Amniocentesis

Procedure

Anatomy or system affected: Abdomen, reproductive system, uterus

Specialties and related fields: Embryology, genetics, obstetrics, perinatology

Definition: The removal of amniotic fluid from a pregnant woman for analysis; this fluid provides biochemical and genetic information about the fetus, enabling physicians to identify congenital problems in the second trimester as well as to determine the presence of fetal or intraamniotic disease in the third trimester.

Key terms:

amniotic sac: a thin, tough, membranous sac that contains amniotic fluid and that encloses the embryo or fetus

chorionic villi: the fingerlike projections of the placenta that function in oxygen, nutrient, and waste transportation between a fetus and its mother

chromosomal defect: an abnormality in the chromosomes, the threadlike, darkly staining bodies found in all cells that carry genetic information in the form of deoxyribonucleic acid (DNA)

Down syndrome: a common genetic disorder characterized by mental retardation and a number of other abnormal findings, including heart malformations

gestational age: the age of a fetus, as determined from the first day of the last menstrual period, which is approximately two weeks before the date of conception; when the date of the last menstrual period is not known, the gestational age can be estimated via ultrasound

karyotype: the chromosomal makeup of an individual; also refers to the arrangement of chromosomes in standard paired fashion on a photomicrograph, which can facilitate analysis of the chromosomes

respiratory distress syndrome: a disease of lung immaturity that can be fatal and is found in children who are born prematurely

Rh isoimmunization: a condition in which a woman who is lacking a substance on red blood cells called Rh factor carries a fetus with the Rh factor on its red blood cells; in these cases, the woman may produce antibodies that attack the red blood cells of the fetus, leading to fetal anemia

trimester: any of the three consecutive three-month periods during pregnancy; the first trimester generally refers to weeks zero to twelve of gestation, the second trimester refers to weeks thirteen to twenty-four of gestation, and the third trimester refers to weeks twenty-five to forty-two of gestation

trisomy 18: a condition caused by extra pieces of chromosome 18 in the cells of the fetus; characterized by mental retardation and a number of other abnormalities, often including severe heart malformations

ultrasonography: the use of sound waves, directed at the body, to create visual images of the tissues being examined

Indications and Procedures

Human pregnancy begins after an egg cell and a sperm cell unite to become a fertilized egg. This process, called conception, occurs in one of the Fallopian tubes, and about a week later the fertilized egg enters the uterus. Cell division during the time period between fertilization and its entry into the uterus converts the fertilized egg into an organized cell cluster that attaches to the lining of the uterus. Following this attachment, the cluster penetrates the lining and becomes intimately commingled with uterine tissues, developing three parts: the placenta, the embryo, and an amniotic sac (filled with the fluid within which the embryo is suspended). Two months after conception, the embryo—then an inch-long fetus—possesses all the anatomic features that will be present when it is born. During the remainder of the pregnancy, the fetus will grow much larger, and all its internal and external anatomic details will be elaborated.

Amniocentesis is used to provide diagnostic information before a fetus is born. It can be carried out anytime after fourteen weeks gestational age. At this point, the amniotic fluid pockets are large enough to sample safely with minimal risk to the fetus, and an adequate volume of amniotic fluid may be obtained for genetic and biochemical analysis. In general, amniocentesis or other forms of prenatal diagnosis in early pregnancy

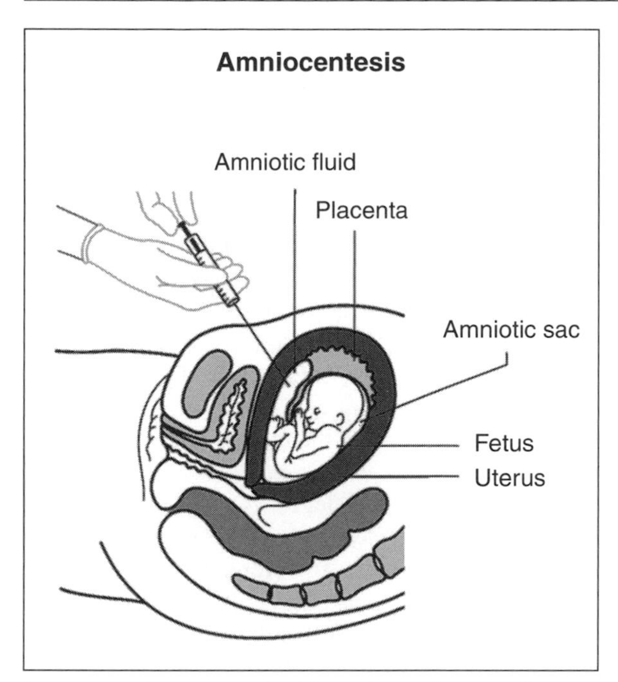

Removal and analysis of fluid from the amniotic sac that surrounds a fetus during gestation can be used to rule out or confirm the presence of serious birth defects or genetic diseases.

(that is, before twenty-four weeks gestational age) are indicated when the risk that the fetus is abnormal is as least as great as the risk of miscarriage from the procedure.

Amniocentesis is indicated in cases where a fetal anomaly is suspected or found on ultrasound, and additional information can be gained through the amniotic fluid regarding the nature of the defect. It is also indicated in women over the age of thirty-five, as the risk for chromosomal defects increases with maternal age. At the age of thirty-five, the risk of Down syndrome outweighs the risk of performing amniocentesis, thereby making the procedure a reasonable one to perform routinely. Other indications for an amniocentesis include women with a previous pregnancy complicated by chromosomal abnormalities and in cases where either parent is a carrier for a chromosomal abnormality.

Another indication for amniocentesis is in the setting of a known family history of a genetic defect. The types of disorders that can be ruled out via amniocentesis tend to be single-gene defects, and either parents have usually been diagnosed as having the disease or are known carriers of the disease. Examples of these diseases include cystic fibrosis, Duchenne or Becker muscular dystrophy, fragile X syndrome, hemophilia, Huntington's disease, neurofibromatosis type 1, sickle cell disease, Tay-Sachs disease, phenylketonuria (PKU), and thalassemias.

In the third trimester, amniocentesis is indicated if fetal developmental maturity and well-being need to be assessed. These factors help guide decision making in treating a patient and her fetus. Commonly, amniocentesis is used to determine fetal lung maturity. This piece of information will help the obstetrician better weigh the risks of early delivery versus prolonging a pregnancy in cases where the pregnancy is complicated by conditions that put the infant and/or mother at risk. Another indication for amniocentesis in the third trimester is to assess the level of fetal anemia, such as in cases of Rh isoimmunization. Amniocentesis can provide samples of amniotic fluid that can be analyzed to determine the degree of fetal red blood cell destruction and anemia. Futhermore, these samples also can be analyzed for fetal lung maturity. If the fetal lungs are mature and the fetal anemia is profound, then the obstetrician may opt for early delivery of the infant in order to minimize the risks posed to the fetus by remaining in utero.

Another indication for performing amniocentesis in the third trimester is to rule out an infection. When an intra-amniotic infection is suspected, an analysis of amniotic fluid via amniocentesis can determine the presence or absence of an infection and help the obstetrician determine a treatment plan, such as antibiotics or delivery of the infant.

Amniocentesis in the third trimester may also be indicated for therapeutic purposes. For instance, it may be performed in cases in which the amount of amniotic fluid is excessive, which is termed polyhydramnios. In this situation, the removal of amniotic fluid may relieve maternal symptoms of extreme discomfort and pressure. Another example of a therapeutic use for amniocentesis is in cases of twin gestation in which unequal sharing of the placenta is present. This can lead to a condition in which the amniotic sac of one twin contains dramatically more fluid than that of the other twin. In such cases, amniotic fluid may be aspirated from the twin with the excess amniotic fluid in order to relieve the uneven distribution of fluid between the two fetuses.

Amniocentesis can be an office procedure. The woman is usually supine or lying on her side. Ultrasound is performed to determine the location of the fetus, the location of the placenta, and the location of the largest and most accessible pockets of amniotic fluid. The optimal location for needle insertion is then determined, and the site of needle puncture on the abdomen is cleaned to prevent infection. Local anesthetic may be injected at the puncture site to minimize discomfort. Under ultrasound guidance, a needle attached to a syringe is inserted through the skin, subcutaneous fat, and uterine wall and finally into a pocket of amniotic fluid. Correct placement of the needle is confirmed by the aspiration of amniotic fluid. A sample of the fluid is then aspirated into the syringe. The syringe is disconnected from the needle, and the needle is removed. Obstetricians will almost always monitor the well-being of the fetus through fetal heart tones before and after the procedure in order to ensure that the fetus tolerated the procedure well.

Uses and Complications

In the second trimester, amniocentesis can be very helpful in identifying chromosomal abnormalities, particularly in women over the age of thirty-five. The amniotic fluid obtained from amniocentesis contains fetal cells that can be grown in tissue culture and examined for abnormalities in the chromosomes. Chromosomal problems can lead to a fetus with syndromes such as Down syndrome or trisomy 18. After a woman tests positive for a chromosomal abnormality, she should receive genetic counseling regarding the nature of the abnormality and known consequences of fetuses carrying it. Knowledge of the chromosomal abnormality can help the pregnant woman plan for the future and can help the obstetrician and pediatrician plan for the safest delivery possible for the baby. Some women who discover that they are carrying a fetus with a chromosomal abnormality may opt for termination of the pregnancy; others may wish to continue it. In cases in which the amniocentesis results are normal, the woman's anxiety and fears regarding having an abnormal baby may be greatly reduced.

Other uses of amniocentesis include analysis of the fetal cells to determine the presence of hereditary diseases such as cystic fibrosis. Amniocentesis can also identify the sex of the fetus. The amniotic fluid from amniocentesis may also be used to identify levels of biochemical markers such as acetyl cholinesterase, which may be indicative of structural abnormalities in the fetus.

In the third trimester, the most common use of amniocentesis is to determine fetal lung maturity in cases where the obstetrician anticipates an early delivery of the baby. The amniotic fluid can be analyzed for levels of substances secreted by the developing fetal lung (such as the ratio of lecithin and sphingomyelin). Because the respiratory system is one of the last organs to mature in the fetus, the level of these chemical markers which indicate fetal lung maturity enables physicians to assess whether the lungs are mature. Immature fetal lungs can lead to a serious condition called respiratory distress syndrome after the baby is born. In cases in which amniocentesis indicates that the fetal lungs are not yet mature, steroid injections may be given to the mother to induce fetal lung maturity prior to the delivery of the infant.

Another use of amniocentesis in the third trimester is to follow the severity of fetal anemia in Rh isoimmunization. In these cases, the mother produces an antibody, a type of protein, which attacks the fetus's red blood cells, leading to anemia. As the pregnancy progresses, fetal anemia can become very severe and can even lead to fetal death. Therefore, the ability to track the progression of fetal anemia is extremely important. This is possible through serial amniocenteses. The amniotic fluid obtained from amniocentesis is analyzed for its optical density. The result helps guide the physician in determining whether it is safer for the fetus to continue in the uterus or whether it should be delivered. In cases in which the fetus is very premature and early delivery is undesirable, drastic measures such as an intrauterine transfusion of blood to the fetus via the umbilical cord may be performed.

For most patients, amniocentesis is relatively painless and involves only an initial pinprick and/or a sensation of pressure. Amniocentesis is very safe for both mother and fetus, and it may be repeated more than once during a pregnancy if necessary. The chances of a complication from an amniocentesis are on average less than 0.5 percent. The risk is even lower in the hands of experienced practitioners. Potential complications include fetal loss when the amniocentesis is performed in early pregnancy. When performed in the third trimester of pregnancy, complications include precipitation of labor, placental trauma leading to bleeding, and injury to the fetus, for example if the needle punctures delicate parts of the fetus. As with any invasive procedure, there is always a risk of bleeding or infection (in this case, to both the mother and the fetus). However, these risks are small when the proper procedures are followed.

Perspective and Prospects

The ability for physicians to diagnose fetal abnormalities essentially began with the development of amniocentesis in the 1950's. Its first application was in the diagnosis of Rh isoimmunization. In 1966, M. W. Steele and W. R. Breg, Jr., demonstrated that the fetal cells from the amniotic fluid could be cultured and the chromosomal makeup of the fetus could be analyzed. This led to the development of the field of prenatal diagnosis.

Besides amniocentesis, a common technique used for prenatal diagnosis is chorionic villus sampling. In this procedure, placental tissue and amniotic fluid are sampled and sent for analysis. A catheter is inserted into the uterus through the vaginal opening and then guided by ultrasonography until its tip reaches the many chorionic villi that edge the placenta at its connection to the uterus. Gentle suction is applied, and a few of the villi are sucked out, first into the catheter and then into a sampling device. The cells that are obtained are tested in the same manner as with cells obtained through amniocentesis.

Chorionic villus sampling arose from the demonstration of the clear value of the information derived from fetal cells obtained from amniotic fluid. This useful procedure was devised to shorten the time period after amniocentesis, often several weeks long, that is needed to grow enough fetal cells in tissue culture to provide the amount of tissue required for successful karyotyping or DNA sequencing work. Another advantage of the chorionic villus sampling procedure is that it can be carried out with younger fetuses, as young as twelve weeks old, although the risk to such a fetus (fetal loss) is somewhat higher than that which is seen after amniocentesis. However, earlier diagnosis of a fetal abnormality allows for more time to obtain counseling and for decision making. If termination of the pregnancy is desired, then the earlier it is performed, the safer it is for the mother.

Prenatal diagnosis has multiple purposes beyond the diagnosis of fetal abnormalities in utero. Traditionally, many couples have been discouraged from obtaining prenatal diagnosis if termination of the pregnancy is not an option for them. Nevertheless, prenatal diagnosis can be invaluable in helping parents make informed choices when their fetus is at risk for an abnormality. Often, couples find it difficult to make decisions regarding the pregnancy, and the more information available to them, the more likely the best decisions will be made in keeping with the couple's values. Another purpose of prenatal diagnosis is that normal results from prenatal testing can go a long way in reassuring women and their partners who are at high risk for an abnormal fetus. Finally, a third purpose of prenatal diagnosis is to allow couples who are afraid to have children because of a known familial or personal history of abnormalities to proceed with pregnancy, with the knowledge that abnormalities can be detected early in utero.

Unfortunately, most fetal abnormalities that are found are not easily repairable, reversible, or curable prior to birth. In recent years, a small number of research-oriented medical centers in the United States have started pioneering programs for fetal surgery. Fetal surgery involves surgical correction of anomalies while the fetus is in utero, with the hope that early correction will result in better results and fewer morbidities than waiting until after the baby is born. In fetal surgery, both the mother and the fetus must undergo surgery. The uterus is accessed through incisions on the mother's abdomen. The fetus may be temporarily removed from the uterus while the defect is being repaired. The fetus is then replaced in the uterus, and the woman's uterus and the abdominal incision are closed. Neural tube defects and congenital diaphragmatic hernias (in which a defect in the fetal diaphragm enables the fetal bowel to enter the thoracic cavity and prevent the fetal lungs from developing) are examples of fetal defects that can be repaired through fetal surgery. Fetal surgery carries considerable risks to the mother and fetus. There are the usual risks of major surgery to the mother, such as bleeding, infection, and risk of internal injury. The fetus is at increased risk of premature delivery and of persistent loss of amniotic fluid from leaks in the amniotic sac. Hence, fetal surgery is still considered experimental, and results from these procedures have been mixed at best.

Finally, amniocentesis has enabled physicians to minimize morbidity and mortality of infants in many situations in which an effective intervention exists, once the diagnosis of a disease state is established. This is especially true for maternal or fetal problems in the third trimester. Hence, the utility of amniocentesis not only involves potentially decreased stays in neonatal intensive care units but in many cases may be cost effective in the long run as well. However, the complexity of determining which specific parameters should be used to determine cost effectiveness (for example, relevant clinical options, variables, outcomes, and placement of values on the outcomes) makes this analysis extremely difficult.

—Sanford S. Singer, Ph.D.;
updated by Anne Lynn S. Chang, M.D.

See also Abortion; Birth defects; Chorionic villus sampling; Cystic fibrosis; Down syndrome; Embryology; Fetal surgery; Genetic counseling; Genetic diseases; Genetics and inheritance; Gynecology; Karyotyping; Laboratory tests; Mental retardation; Obstetrics; Placenta; Pregnancy and gestation; Rh factor; Screening; Sickle cell disease; Spina bifida; Ultrasonography; Women's health.

FOR FURTHER INFORMATION:

Filkins, Karen, and Joseph F. Russo, eds. *Human Prenatal Diagnosis*. 2d ed. New York: Marcel Dekker, 1990. This book attempts to "clarify and rationalize aspects of diagnosis, genetic counseling, and intervention." It is meant as a guide for health professionals and is also useful to general readers.

Gabbe, Steven G., Jennifer R. Niebyl, and Joe Leigh Simpson, eds. *Obstetrics: Normal and Problem Pregnancies*. New York: Churchill Livingstone, 2002. An excellent comprehensive resource that provides the indications, uses, and procedures related to amniocentesis.

Heyman, Bob, and Mette Henriksen. *Risk, Age, and Pregnancy: A Case Study of Prenatal Genetic Screening and Testing*. New York: Palgrave, 2001. Examines prenatal testing in the context of a British hospital, exploring the perspectives of pregnant women, hospital doctors, and midwives and the way in which the decision to undertake prenatal testing is made.

Nussbaum, Robert L., Roderick R. McInnes, and Willard F. Huntington. *Thompson and Thompson Genetics in Medicine*. Rev. 6th ed. Philadelphia: W. B. Saunders, 2004. A clear and concise summary of the science behind prenatal diagnosis and the basics of genetic analysis in the medical setting.

Rapp, Rayna. *Testing Women, Testing the Fetus: The Social Impact of Amniocentesis in America*. New York: Routledge, 1999. Rapp, an anthropologist, combines personal experience and professional expertise. She interviewed women of many different racial, cultural, religious, educational, and financial backgrounds for this study.

Sherwood, Lauralee. *Human Physiology: From Cells to Systems*. 6th ed. Belmont, Calif.: Thomson/Brooks/Cole, 2007. This college textbook contains useful biological information about pregnancy and genetic defects, as well as facts useful to understanding amniocentesis and its advantages and disadvantages. Provides many valuable definitions and diagrams.

Turnpenny, Peter, and Sian Ellard. *Emery's Elements of Medical Genetics*. 12th ed. New York: Elsevier Churchill Livingstone, 2005. Contains good chapters on prenatal diagnosis (includes amniocentesis) and recent developments in medical science.

AMPUTATION

PROCEDURE

ANATOMY OR SYSTEM AFFECTED: Arms, bones, hands, joints, knees, legs, muscles, musculoskeletal system, nervous system, skin

SPECIALTIES AND RELATED FIELDS: Critical care, emergency medicine, general surgery, oncology, orthopedics, physical therapy, plastic surgery, vascular medicine

DEFINITION: The removal of a limb or other body part in order to prevent more serious harm to the patient.

KEY TERMS:

disarticulation: the amputation of a limb through a joint, without cutting the bone

edema: the accumulation of an excessive amount of fluid in cells or tissues

fascia: a sheet of fibrous tissue which envelops the body beneath the skin and also encloses the muscles or groups of muscles, separating their many layers or groups

gangrene: necrosis (tissue death) caused by obstruction of the blood supply; it may be localized to a small area or involve an entire extremity

ischemia: a local anemia or area of diminished or insufficient blood supply caused by mechanical obstruction (commonly narrowing of an artery) of the blood supply

periosteum: the thick, fibrous membrane that covers the entire surface of a bone except for the cartilage within a joint

peripheral: referring to a part of the body away from the center

prosthesis: a fabricated, artificial substitute for a missing part of the body, such as a limb

prosthetist: an individual skilled in constructing and fitting prostheses

vascular: relating to or containing blood vessels

INDICATIONS AND PROCEDURES

Amputations are performed in order to preserve life or to avoid more extensive damage or destruction to an individual or a portion of the body. They are performed in response to pathological processes (bacterial or viral infections, ischemia, or cancer, for example) that do not respond to treatment or to address the aftereffects of violent trauma (accidents, crushing injuries, or bullet wounds) in which tissues have been injured so extensively that they cannot be repaired, restored, or otherwise salvaged or saved.

Extremities are the most common sites for amputations, and there are four reasons for removing all or part of an extremity. The first is trauma which is so severe that surgical or other repair is not possible. The second reason is the presence of a tumor in the bones, soft tissues, muscles, blood vessels, or nerves of the extremity. A third cause is extensive infection that does not respond to usual or conservative treatment or that may lead to septicemia, a generalized infection which spreads throughout the entire body. The final indication for performing an amputation is the presence of peripheral vascular disease, a group of conditions that compromise or reduce the blood supply in an extremity.

Most amputations of the leg are performed because of impaired circulation, or ischemia. Several conditions may lead to ischemia, the most common of which is inadequately controlled diabetes mellitus. Others include atherosclerosis (a buildup of plaque in a blood vessel which restricts circulation), cellulitis, and vascular diseases. Bacterial infection can also lead to impaired circulation. When circulation continues to be inadequate, gangrene develops; infection can also contribute to or accelerate existing gangrene.

There are three general classes of amputation: provisional or open, conventional or standard, and osteomyoplastic. The techniques for each are briefly described.

The technique for a provisional amputation is often referred to as guillotine. In the past, this approach was commonly used in battle situations where speed was important to minimize both blood loss and subsequent infection. Currently, the technique is used mainly to remove a victim from a dangerous situation, typically one causing a crushing injury in which the alternative to amputation is death. All tissues are cut circularly. Skin is retained to the greatest degree possible, muscle and fascia are cut shorter, and the bone is cut shorter still. The hope is that the soft tissues (skin and muscles) will ultimately cover the bone, but the results are generally unsatisfactory. Large scars are common, and muscle frequently adheres to the bone. Long periods are required for healing, infections are common, and prostheses do not fit well. Another, more definitive amputation is usually required at a later date.

In a conventional amputation, skin, underlying tissues, muscle, and fascia are all cut in curved flaps that originate at the end of the remaining, unamputated bone. The muscles, fascia, bone, and major blood vessels are divided at the base of the remaining bone; nerves are cut at a slightly higher level, approximately 2.5 centimeters (1 inch) above the end of the bone. The nerves will retract somewhat into the muscle, minimizing postoperative pain. Muscles are tapered so that large masses of tissue are not present over the end of the stump; this will enhance the fit of a later prosthesis. At the cut end of the bone, the outer layer of bone is removed in order to reduce the possibility of bone spurs forming at some time in the future. The skin over the amputation site is closed loosely to avoid stretching as it heals.

The purpose of an osteomyoplastic amputation is to improve function after a prosthesis is fitted. The preparation of skin and fascia is the same as for a conventional amputation. Nerves and blood vessels are also divided. Muscles are separated for about 5 centimeters (2 inches) past the point where the bone will be cut. A portion of the outer surface (periosteum) from the bone to be amputated is sutured to the divided muscle. The bone is then cut. The prepared flap of periosteum and muscle is sutured to the periosteum of the stump. This procedure covers the marrow cavity of the stump, helps to preserve the remaining bone, and reduces postopera-

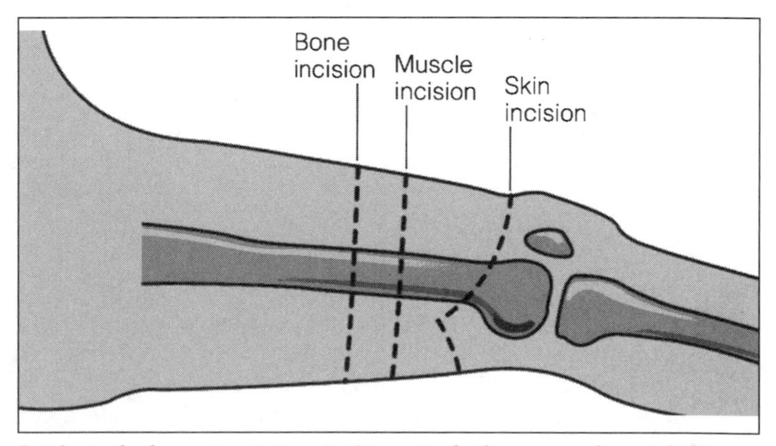

In above-the-knee amputation, incisions in the bone, muscles, and skin are made in such a way that the muscles and skin can be folded over the remaining bone, thus creating a stump to which a prosthesis may later be molded and attached.

tive infections. The remaining muscles are then sutured across the end of the stump. The skin is closed as in a conventional amputation. In an alternative procedure, holes are drilled in the bone of the stump. Muscles are inserted in the holes and sutured in place. The net effect of these osteomyoplastic procedures is to strengthen the musculature of the stump and to improve mobility for a prosthesis.

There are several common sites or levels for amputations of the leg. Syme's amputation is performed when most of the foot has been destroyed by trauma or compromised by poor circulation. In this type of amputation, the bones of the foot are removed, and the end of the tibia becomes the weight-bearing surface for the prosthesis.

A below-the-knee (BK) amputation is used to provide additional mobility for a prosthesis. It also leads to more complete rehabilitation because the knee is still available for movement. It is also associated with a reduction in phantom limb pain.

An above-the-knee (AK) amputation is frequently selected when gangrene extends into the muscles or skin of the calf. When the muscles of the leg are contracted, a prosthesis is not likely to be fitted or used; thus there is no advantage to a BK amputation in this situation. The AK amputation is associated with the highest healing rate for amputations among patients with peripheral vascular disease. The rate of a repeat amputation performed at a higher level on the leg is also low. Prostheses that permit walking, however, are less efficient with amputations at this level.

Both amputations have about the same rate of healing, but a higher percentage of individuals with BK amputations walk on prostheses than do those with AK amputations. The choice between BK and AK amputation is determined by the general health of the patient and the potential for rehabilitation. The most important determinant of level of amputation, however, is the vascular status of the patient.

The leg can also be amputated at either the knee or the hip; such a procedure is a disarticulation, an amputation through a joint. A knee disarticulation is most commonly used with children to preserve the growing portion (epiphysis) of the remaining thigh bone. A hip disarticulation is used with tumors or extensive soft tissue injuries in the thigh. Special prostheses that permit walking after such procedures are available, but they are relatively uncommon.

Portions of the upper extremity are usually amputated after extensive trauma. Malignant disease of the bone or muscle is a less common reason for amputation at these sites. The considerations described for the lower extremity are applicable for the upper extremity, namely, preserving as much tissue as possible for later rehabilitation and recovery of function. The sites for amputation are also analogous. Individual fingers can be amputated, or the entire hand can be amputated at the wrist (a location similar to the Syme's amputation of the foot). Similarly, the forearm can be amputated either below the elbow or above the elbow. Portions of the arm can be disarticulated at the elbow or at the shoulder. Restoration of function is far more difficult, however, in an upper extremity amputation than for a lower extremity amputation. It is easier to restore the ability to walk than it is to restore hand function.

USES AND COMPLICATIONS

The level or site of an amputation is critical to recovery and rehabilitation. When an amputation is performed because of cancer or some other malignant disease, the principal concern is a wide excision of any apparent tumor. When amputation is performed after the patient has sustained significant trauma or to treat peripheral vascular disease, the major factor determining the best site is usually the extent of healthy tissue. Other important factors include preserving sufficient length in the remaining bone or stump so that a prosthesis may be used. Furthermore, the prosthesis must be functional, must have adequate space for attachment, and must be cosmetically acceptable. The scar must be placed so that it will not break down from mechanical traction or interfere with the fit of the prosthesis.

In general, the more bone that can be left in place, the more functional a prosthetic limb will be; patients will also have better control of their prostheses. Frequently, special procedures will have to be used to save skin or to graft skin to the site of an amputation so as to preserve the length of the bone. The issue of bone length is especially critical in amputations of the upper extremities, as arms, hands, and fingers are so important in daily functions. The prospects for rehabilitation are also considered when an amputation is contemplated. For example, there is less need to preserve bone for a prosthesis if an individual is not inclined—because of temperament, age, or physical condition—to rehabilitate a lost body part.

There are different regional considerations for patients requiring an amputation for peripheral vascular disease. The ability of the skin and other tissues to heal is directly dependent on an adequate supply of blood.

Injections of dye into local small arteries, a procedure called arteriography, are used to determine if the vessels can deliver sufficient blood to a proposed amputation site or around joints such as the knee.

Amputations for extensive trauma should be performed soon after the injury is sustained in order to reduce the chances for contamination or infection. This practice will also assist in subsequent psychological adjustment to the loss of the body part.

Bedridden patients frequently suffer from ulcers of the skin, or bedsores, lesions that do not heal well if at all. In combination with impaired circulation (ischemia), these ulcers can lead to the need for amputations. This group of patients must be carefully prepared for surgery by conditioning muscles that will remain after the amputation. Before an amputation is attempted, extensive efforts must be made to heal all skin ulcers. Physical therapy is frequently used before the surgery to strengthen and improve the tone of muscles. Antibiotics, moist heat, and frequently changed dressings are employed to fight infection. Patients should be moved frequently to avoid the formation of new skin ulcers. Special beds are often used to avoid concentrating pressure on body parts; this can be accomplished with pillows and lambskin mats. In some cases, ice packs are used in the days immediately prior to amputation to limit the spread of infection and to reduce pain.

Conventional postoperative care for amputation focuses on providing optimal tissue care: movement and specific exercises to prevent contractures (the loss of use for muscles), the compression of tissue to prevent edema, and the initiation of physical therapy to regain or retain the optimum use of the remaining body part. The ultimate goal is to provide a prosthesis wherever possible and appropriate in order to improve the patient's quality of life and vocational opportunities.

Edema is minimized by applying tight dressings to the amputation site. After sutures are removed, elastic bandages are used for the next several weeks. Exercises and movement of the stump will prevent contractures. These exercises should be started as soon as possible after the amputation. When a portion of an arm or leg has been removed, it is important to move and stretch the entire limb.

One problem associated with amputations is called phantom limb pain: the perception of pain in a body part that is no longer attached to the body. Typically, a patient who has lost a limb will experience pain or other sensation as if the limb were still intact. This phenomenon occurs because of stimulation in the nerve endings of the remaining stump. Such sensations are amplified in the posterior horn, a portion of the spinal cord. The nervous impulses are processed by the brain and interpreted as pain; it is this subjective feeling that the patient experiences. Phantom limb pain can usually be prevented by surgical techniques employed at the time of amputation.

Traumatically amputated body parts can sometimes be reattached. Portions of fingers, hands, and entire upper extremities have been successfully reattached; lower extremity reattachments are less common. The regeneration of nerves, however, is not uniformly accomplished. The myelin sheaths of nerves—the cells that surround many nerves to provide insulation and to increase the velocity of nerve impulse conduction—must be approximated for successful regeneration. The lack of nerve regeneration can affect either motor or sensory aspects of the body part. Lack of motor nerve regeneration leads to disuse atrophy and loss of functional use of the body part. Cosmetically, the body usually appears normal. Loss of sensory innervation requires adaptation, but the ability to move the body part is not affected. If the sensory loss is from skin only, the deficit is usually not significant. Sensory loss in fingers and toes is more serious; other senses such as sight and position receptors in joints must be relied upon to compensate for the lack of direct input from fingers or toes. These deficits can be overcome with rehabilitation.

Amputations performed by surgeons skilled in techniques appropriate for ischemic or necrotic tissue have the lowest incidence of postoperative complications and the highest degree of success for subsequent rehabilitation. The death rate for amputations required for isolated trauma, infection, or tumors is less than 3 percent. In contrast, amputations related to vascular diseases result in death for approximately one patient in four. Mortality rates rise with the removal of increasing amounts of a body part: The removal of a toe or foot is less likely to end in death than the removal of an entire leg.

PERSPECTIVE AND PROSPECTS

Historically, techniques for amputation evolved on the battlefield. Amputation was the only treatment available for battle casualties; the alternative was death. Military surgeons were known for speed. In the early part of the twentieth century, antibiotics were discovered. Improved instrumentation and operative techniques were first developed in the 1950's. Microscopic procedures have been perfected more recently. The net effect of these developments has been to reduce the need for amputation following trauma. These same techniques have enabled the reattachment or reimplantation of fingers or other extremities.

When amputation is necessary, however, the surgeon must weigh the desires of the patient against his or her best interests. It is natural for patients to want to retain as much original tissue as possible, but surgeons prefer to perform an amputation only once. Impaired circulation compromises tissues. When individuals with conditions such as diabetes require amputation and insufficient tissue is removed, the result is frequently another amputation. Individuals with poorly controlled diabetes may lose their entire legs in a series of amputations.

After an amputation, physical therapy begins the rehabilitation process. As soon as the patient can tolerate movement, exercises are undertaken. The goal of these activities is to return the person to as normal a level of function as possible. The services of an occupational therapist are used to regain old motor skills or to learn new ones. An artificial body part is fitted by a prosthetist. The sooner a prosthesis is fitted, the greater is the probability that the patient will adapt successfully to it. Temporary prostheses initially fitted within the first twenty-four hours following surgery have had high degrees of acceptance.

Prostheses typically are of two varieties: functional and cosmetically appealing. Prostheses with wires attached to movable hooks allow limited motor function of hands. Muscles of the forearm are retrained to provide movement of the hook. Lower limb prostheses are usually more anatomically correct and cosmetically appealing. They allow walking and other movements but do not usually allow fine motor control of toes. This does not preclude the adaptation and eventual recovery of fairly complex motor skills, including those required for participation in sports activities.

One predictor of eventual success with the prosthesis is the age at which it is fitted. Young children adapt rapidly, but the older the patient is, the more difficult adaptation to a prosthesis becomes. Older persons often merely tolerate an artificial limb while younger persons accept the prosthesis and continue with the activities of their lives. Much of the rehabilitation after an amputation is psychological. With appropriate support and therapy, the potential for a nearly normal life exists for most persons experiencing an amputation.

—*L. Fleming Fallon, Jr., M.D., Ph.D., M.P.H.*

See also Arteriosclerosis; Bacterial infections; Bone cancer; Bone disorders; Bone grafting; Bones and the skeleton; Cancer; Circulation; Critical care; Critical care, pediatric; Diabetes mellitus; Emergency medicine; Fracture and dislocation; Fracture repair; Frostbite; Gangrene; Grafts and grafting; Ischemia; Lower extremities; Muscles; Oncology; Orthopedic surgery; Orthopedics; Orthopedics, pediatric; Osteonecrosis; Physical rehabilitation; Plastic surgery; Prostheses; Skin; Tumor removal; Tumors; Upper extremities; Vascular medicine; Vascular system; Wounds.

For Further Information:

Barnes, Robert W. *Amputations: An Illustrated Manual.* Philadelphia: Hanley & Belfus, 2000. Examines methods and results of amputation surgeries.

Brunicardi, F. Charles, et al., eds. *Schwartz's Principles of Surgery.* 8th ed. New York: McGraw-Hill, 2005. A standard textbook of surgery. Its intended audience is practicing surgeons, and thus technical language is used. The serious reader can find greater detail in this work.

May, Bella J. *Amputations and Prosthetics: A Case Study Approach.* 2d ed. Philadelphia: F. A. Davis, 2002. Details advances in bioengineering research that have affected prosthetic components and examines topics such as postsurgical management, lower and upper limb amputations, psychosocial issues, and working with children with amputations.

Smith, Douglas G. "General Principles of Amputation Surgery." In *Atlas of Amputations and Limb Deficiencies: Surgical, Prosthetic, and Rehabilitation Principles*, edited by Smith, John W. Michael, and John H. Bowker. Rosemont, Ill.: American Academy of Orthopaedic Surgeons, 2004. A fairly technical account of surgical techniques of amputation. General readers are advised to approach this work with a medical dictionary for assistance.

Townsend, Courtney M., Jr., et al., eds. *Sabiston Textbook of Surgery.* 17th ed. Philadelphia: Elsevier Saunders, 2005. A standard textbook of surgery intended for practicing professionals but can be generally understood by the layperson.

Amyotrophic lateral sclerosis

Disease/Disorder

Also known as: Lou Gehrig's disease

Anatomy or system affected: Musculoskeletal system, nervous system, respiratory system

Specialties and related fields: Alternative medicine, biochemistry, family medicine, gastroenterology, internal medicine, neurology, physical therapy, psychiatry, psychology, pulmonary medicine, speech pathology

DEFINITION: A progressive, degenerative neurological disorder that affects the cells in the brain and spinal cord.

KEY TERMS:

electromyography (EMG): a technique used to diagnose various nerve and muscle disorders, entailing continuous recording of the electrical activity in a muscle through the use of electrodes

fasciculation: a brief, spontaneous contraction of muscle fibers associated with disorders of the lower motor neurons

lower motor neuron: one type of nerve with a cell body in the spinal cord and an axon that extends into the brain

motor neuron: one of several units that make up the nerve pathway between the brain and the particular organ connected to it

spasticity: a rigidity or resistance to passive limb movement, usually occuring in limbs that are weak, respond in an impaired way to voluntary control, and whose weakness is thought to be due to observed lesions in the upper motor neurons

upper motor neuron: one type of nerve with a cell body in the brain and an axon that extends into the spinal column

INFORMATION ON AMYOTROPHIC LATERAL SCLEROSIS

CAUSES: Unknown

SYMPTOMS: Slurred speech, weakening grip, clumsiness and unsteadiness, weakened limbs

DURATION: Progressive and fatal

TREATMENTS: None; symptomatic relief and comfort measures

CAUSES AND SYMPTOMS

Amyotrophic lateral sclerosis (ALS) plagues twenty thousand Americans, with five thousand cases newly diagnosed each year. In spite of extensive epidemiological, controlled, and clinical research, the cause or causes of ALS are unknown. In most cases, it does not run in families, there are no known risk factors, and it does not seem to develop following exposure to toxins, radiation, or any particular environmental sources. Diet appears to have no effect. It appears to occur at random, while tending to strike individuals between the ages of forty to sixty, and it is more common in men than women.

However, 5 to 10 percent of all ALS cases are inherited in what is referred to as "the familial form." Of these familial cases, 20 percent may have a mutation in the gene responsible for the production of superoxide dismutase 1 (SOD1). Nonetheless, this finding does not explain most other cases.

ALS researchers have also noted the presence of increased glutamate in the spinal cord and serum in some familial and nonfamilial cases. They theorize that its existence may play a key role in the mechanism of nerve damage. Other theories about what causes ALS assign important roles to the body's own immune system, suggesting that ALS may essentially be an autoimmune disease, similar in mechanism (if not effect) to lupus.

The signs and symptoms of ALS are almost always gradual and subtle in its early stages. People may begin occasionally to slur speech, spill food, or experience weakening grip. Oddly, but not particularly troublingly, their feet may miss stairs and their fingers may miss the correct keys when typing. They tend to report that they are becoming clumsy and unsteady, their penmanship is worsening, and their limbs are weakening. Frequently, people put up with these early signs believing they will go away spontaneously, or that they are the result of fatigue, an undiagnosed infection, or the side effects of medication. Further along this early stage, however, fasciculation and spasticity commonly become clinically evident due to both upper and lower motor neuron damage.

For the neurological specialist, the key to diagnosing and differentiating ALS from other motor neuron disorders is the presence of simultaneous upper and lower motor neuron damage. The diagnosis of ALS is made because other, more common, motor neuron diseases have been excluded. This exclusion is important because several of these diseases mimic ALS but are far more treatable.

There are several diagnostic procedures helpful in determining the patient's diagnosis. Electromyography (EMG) is a diagnostic technique that detects electrical activity in the muscles. Specific EMG patterns and findings can be diagnostic of ALS, though not all patterns are clear, distinct, and unambiguous. Nerve conduction studies are also used to help differentiate ALS from peripheral neuropathy or myopathies. Magnetic resonance imaging (MRI), a procedure commonly used for helping to diagnose many conditions, provides visual images of the brain and spinal cord. While MRI readings are usually unremarkable in ALS patients, an MRI is often ordered to help the physician decide that the troubling symptoms are not from another disorder, evident in an abnormal or significant MRI reading.

The progression of the disease varies widely from individual to individual; however, the course or stages of deterioration remain fairly universal. As the disease progresses and attacks voluntary motor functions, patients develop increasing difficulty with walking, swallowing, talking, and dressing themselves. Further along, patients may need more aggressive support with feeding tubes and mechanical ventilators.

Perhaps the most insidious aspect of ALS is that while voluntary muscles deteriorate, thinking and emotions remain completely unaffected. Individuals are aware of the entire disease process, loss of independence, and decreasing ability to express themselves. Perhaps even more important than the medical management of the disease is the attention to the existential, psychological, and family challenges that ensue.

Treatment and Therapy

There is no specific treatment or cure for ALS. The mainstays of therapy rely on supportive assistance with mobility and communication, symptomatic relief, and comfort measures. Medications such as riluzole (Rilutek) can decrease the release of glutamate, and a few studies have shown that riluzole may prolong survival and slow the rate of deterioration. Unfortunately, it does not halt or reverse neuron damage.

Not much pain accompanies ALS. More problematic are feelings of stiffness, soreness, and discomfort. Both pharmacologic and nonpharmacologic treatments can bring symptomatic relief of spasticity, fatigue, and fasciculations, significantly improving patients' comfort and quality of life.

Allied health care providers such as physical, occupational, and speech therapists play a large role in helping keep patients, and often their families, functional, maintaining independence and mobility as much as possible. As muscle weakness progresses, assistive devices such as communication and sign boards, leg splints, and wheelchairs may be needed. Mental and behavioral health specialists, as well as hospice programs, provide much needed support and relief for both patients and family members, who are typically the caregivers of the ALS patient.

Perspective and Prospects

Scientists are searching for a biological marker for ALS. Such a discovery may yield a method of early detection and possible prevention. An interesting case study presented a scenario that ALS may be associated with a virus. A patient with acquired immunodeficiency syndrome (AIDS) was simultaneously diagnosed with ALS. Treatment with antiviral AIDS therapy combated the signs and symptoms of ALS as well. This critical observation may link ALS to a viral cause and possible cure. However, far more research needs to be done.

In conclusion, ALS is a varyingly progressive degenerative neurologic disorder. At this time, there is no cure or treatment. Comfort measures and supportive care are the mainstay of treatment for patients and their families. Providing both physical and emotional support is crucial to both. National and local support agencies offer multiple services to assist them.

—Paul Moglia, Ph.D., and Debra Ellen Margolis, D.O.

See also Aphasia and dysphasia; Motor neuron diseases; Muscle sprains, spasms, and disorders; Muscles; Nervous system; Neuralgia, neuritis, and neuropathy; Neurology; Palsy; Paralysis; Spinal cord disorders; Spine, vertebrae, and disks.

For Further Information:

ALS Association. http://www.alsa.org/. A group that works toward a cure for ALS and helps to improve the lives of those suffering from the disease.

Feigenbaum, David, ed. *Journeys with ALS*. Virginia Beach, Va.: DLRC Press, 1998. A collection of personal stories about coping with the disease, from ALS sufferers and their caregivers.

Kimura, Jun, and Ryuji Kaji, eds. *Physiology of ALS and Related Diseases*. New York: Elsevier Science, 1997. A collection of reports on clinical aspects and treatment approaches to ALS and related diseases, aimed at professionals in the treatment field but also of use to those interested in theoretical and practical aspects of ALS research and patient care.

McFarlane, Rodger, and Philip Bashe. *The Complete Bedside Companion: No-Nonsense Advice on Caring for the Seriously Ill*. New York: Simon & Schuster, 1998. A comprehensive and practical guide to caregiving for patients with serious illnesses. The first section deals with the general needs of caring for the sick, while the second section covers specific illnesses in depth. Includes bibliographies and lists of support organizations.

Mitsumoto, Hiroshi, and Theodore L. Munsat, eds. *Amyotrophic Lateral Sclerosis: A Guide for Patients and Families*. 2d ed. New York: Oxford University Press, 2001. Comprehensive, clinically focused coverage of current knowledge of ALS. Topics include history, terminology and classification, epidemiology, clinical features, course and prognosis, familial ALS, the immune hypothesis, hypotheses for viral and other transmissible agents, and treatment and management, including unconventional or unorthodox treatments, drug development, physical rehabilitation, and speech and communication management.

Oliver, David, Gian Domenico Borasio, and Declan Walsh, eds. *Palliative Care in Amyotrophic Lateral Sclerosis*. New York: Oxford University Press, 2001. Provides an evidence based guide to the care of people with ALS, including the control of symptoms, the psychosocial care of patients and their families, and care in bereavement. Aimed at all those involved in the care of ALS patients.

Parker, James N., and Philip M. Parker, eds. *Official Patient's Sourcebook on Amyotrophic Lateral Sclerosis*. San Diego, Calif.: Icon Health, 2003. Provides comprehensive information drawn from public, academic, government, and peer-reviewed research, and gives myriad sources for basic and advanced information on the disease.

ANATOMY

ANATOMY OR SYSTEM AFFECTED: All

SPECIALTIES AND RELATED FIELDS: All

DEFINITION: The structure of the human body—its parts, systems, and organs.

KEY TERMS:

abdomen: the rib-free part of the trunk, below the diaphragm

head: the part of the body containing the major sense organs (such as the eyes and ears) and the brain

lower extremities: the thigh, lower leg, and foot

thorax: the part of the trunk above the diaphragm, containing the ribs; the chest

trunk: the central part of the body, to which the extremities are attached

upper extremities: the arm, forearm, and hand

STRUCTURE AND FUNCTIONS

The body's parts can be categorized either regionally or functionally. Regionally, the body consists of a trunk to which are attached two upper extremities, two lower extremities, and a head, attached by means of a neck. Functionally, the body consists of a digestive system, a circulatory system, an excretory system, a respiratory system, a reproductive system, a nervous system, an endocrine system, an integument (skin), a skeleton, and a series of muscles.

Regionally, the body consists of a central portion called the trunk, to which other parts are attached. The trunk itself may be divided into an upper portion called the chest (or thorax), containing ribs, and a lower, rib-free portion called the abdomen. Internally, the thorax and abdomen are separated by a muscular sheet called the diaphragm. Attached to the trunk are two upper extremities, two lower extremities, and a head. The upper extremities include the arms, forearms, and hands; the lower extremities include the thighs, lower legs, and feet. The head includes the brain and the major sense organs such as the eyes and ears; the neck is the narrower, flexible part that connects the head to the trunk. The ventral (front) surface of the abdomen is often divided around the umbilicus into upper-left, upper-right, lower-left, and lower-right quadrants.

Functionally, the body consists of a number of organ systems: a digestive system, a circulatory system, an excretory system, a respiratory system, a reproductive system, a nervous system, an endocrine system, an integument (skin), a skeleton, and a series of muscles. The digestive system breaks down foods into simpler substances and absorbs them. The circulatory system transports oxygen and other materials around the body. The excretory system rids the body of many waste products, while the respiratory system rids the body of carbon dioxide and adds oxygen to the blood. The reproductive system produces sex cells and, in females, provides an environment for the development of an embryo. The nervous system sends signals in the form of nerve impulses from one part of the body to another, and the endocrine organs send chemical messengers (hormones) through the bloodstream. The integument, or skin, protects the outer surface of the body from infection, from injury, and from drying out (desiccation); it also maintains the body's internal temperature by providing insulation and preventing the body from overheating during exercise through sweating. The skeleton serves as the body's framework and consists of 206 separate bones; these bones support the body's other organs and also protect the heart, the lungs, and especially the central nervous system (including the brain and the spinal cord). The muscles produce movements by their contractions.

Each major organ system is constructed of several major organs. The major organs contained within the thorax are the heart, lungs, and thymus body. The major organs contained within the abdomen include the stomach, spleen, liver, pancreas, small intestine (consisting of the duodenum, ileum, and jejunum), large intestine (consisting of the cecum, colon, and rectum, with the colon further divided into an ascending colon, transverse colon, descending colon, and sigmoid colon), and bladder. The kidneys and urinary ducts lie along the dorsal body wall of the abdomen. Also contained within the lower abdomen are the uterus, ovaries, and Fallopian tubes in the female and the vas deferens and prostate gland in the male. In males, two downward extensions of the abdominal cavity form the scrotal sacs that surround the testes.

The thoracic and abdominal cavities (and the scrotal cavities in males) are all considered part of the general body cavity, or coelom. Each part of the coelom is lined on all sides with a thin, single layer of flat (squamous) cells known as the peritoneum. The peritoneum forming the outer wall of these cavities is called the parietal peritoneum; the peritoneum on the outer surface of the internal organs, or viscera, is called the visceral peritoneum.

Each type of organ is made of a number of different tissues. The four major types of tissues are epithelium, connective tissue, muscle tissue, and nervous tissue. Epithelial tissues (or epithelium) include those tissues that originate in broad, flat surfaces; their functions include protection, absorption, and secretion. Epithelia can be one-layered (simple) or many-layered (stratified). Their cells can be flat (squamous), tall and skinny (columnar), or equal in height and width (cuboidal). Some simple epithelia have nuclei at two different levels, giving the false appearance of different layers; these tissues are called pseudostratified. Some simple squamous epithelia have special names: The inner lining of most blood vessels is called the endothelium, while the lining of the body cavities (including all parts of the coelom) is called the mesothelium. Kidney tubules and most small ducts are also lined with simple squamous epithelia. The pigmented layer of the retina and the front surface of the lens are examples of simple cuboidal epithelia. Simple columnar epithelia form the inner lining of most digestive organs and the linings of the small bronchi and the gallbladder. The epithelia lining the Fallopian tubes, nasal cavities, and bronchi are ciliated, meaning that the cells have small, hairlike extensions called cilia.

The outer layer of skin is a stratified squamous epithelium; other stratified squamous epithelia line the inside of the mouth, esophagus, and vagina. Sweat glands and other glands in the skin are lined with stratified cuboidal epithelia. Most of the urinary tract is lined with a special kind of stratified cuboidal epithelium, called a transitional epithelium, that allows a large amount of stretching. Parts of the pharynx, the larynx, the urethra, and the ducts of the mammary glands are lined with stratified columnar epithelium.

Glands are composed of epithelial tissues that are highly modified for secretion. They may be either exocrine glands (in which the secretions exit by ducts to targets nearby) or endocrine glands (in which the secretions are carried by the bloodstream to targets some distance away). The salivary glands in the mouth, the glandular lining of the stomach, and the sebaceous glands of the skin are examples of exocrine glands. The thyroid gland, adrenal gland, and pituitary gland are examples of endocrine glands. The pancreas has both exocrine and endocrine portions: The exocrine parts secrete digestive enzymes, while the endocrine parts, called the islets of Langerhans, secrete the hormones insulin and glucagon.

Connective tissues are tissues containing large amounts of material called extracellular matrix, located outside the cells. The matrix may be a liquid (such as blood plasma), a solid containing fibers of collagen and related proteins, or an inorganic solid containing calcium salts (as in bone). Blood and lymph are connective tissues with a liquid matrix (plasma) that can solidify when the blood clots. In addition to plasma, blood contains red cells (erythrocytes), white cells (leukocytes), and the tiny platelets that help form clots. The many kinds of leukocytes include granular types (basophils, neutrophils, and eosinophils, all named according to the staining properties of their granules), the monocytes, and the several types of lymphocytes. Lymph contains lymphocytes and plasma only.

Most connective tissues have a solid matrix, which includes fibrous proteins such as collagen and elastic fibers in some cases. If all the fibers are arranged in the same direction, as in ligaments and tendons, the tissue is called regular connective tissue. The dermis of the skin is an example of an irregular connective tissue in which the fibers are arranged in all directions. Loose connective tissue and adipose (fat) tissue both have very few fibers. The simplest type of loose connective tissue, with the fewest fibers, is sometimes called areolar connective tissue. Adipose tissue is a connective tissue in which the cells are filled with fat deposits.

Hemopoietic (blood-forming) tissue occurs in bone marrow and in the thymus, and it contains the immature cell types that develop into most connective tissue cells, including blood cells. Cartilage tissue matrix contains a shock-resistant complex of protein and sugarlike (polysaccharide) molecules. Cartilage cells usually become trapped in this matrix and eventually die, except for those closest to the surface. Bone tissue gains its supporting ability and strength from a matrix containing calcium salts. Its typical cells, called osteocytes, contain many long strands by which these cells exchange nutrients and waste products with other osteocytes, and ultimately with the bloodstream. Bone also contains osteoclasts, large cells responsible for bone resorption and the release of calcium into the bloodstream.

Mesenchyme is an embryonic connective tissue made of wandering, amoeba-like cells. During embryological development, the mesenchyme cells develop into many different cell types, including hemocytoblasts, which give rise to most blood cells, and fibroblasts, which secrete protein fibers and then usually differentiate into other cell types.

Muscle tissues are specially modified for contraction. When a nerve impulse is received, overlapping fibers of the proteins actin and myosin slide against one another to produce the contraction. The three types of muscle tissue are smooth muscle, cardiac muscle, and skeletal muscle. The term "striated muscle" is sometimes used to refer to cardiac and skeletal muscle, both of which have cylindrical fibers marked by cross-bands, also called cross-striations. The striations are caused by the lining up of the contractile proteins actin and myosin. Smooth muscle contains cells with tapering ends and centrally located nuclei. Muscular contractions are smooth, rhythmic, and involuntary, usually not subject to fatigue. The cells are not cross-banded. Smooth muscle occurs in many digestive organs, reproductive organs, and skin, as well as in many other organs. Cardiac muscle occurs only in the heart. Its cross-striated fibers branch and come together repeatedly. Contractions of these fibers are involuntary, rhythmic, and without fatigue. Nuclei are located in the center of each cell; cell boundaries are marked by dark-staining structures called intercalated disks. Skeletal muscle occurs in the voluntary muscles of the body. Their cylindrical, cross-striated fibers contain many nuclei but no internal cell boundaries; a multinucleated fiber of this type is called a syncytium. Skeletal muscle is capable of rapid, forceful contractions, but it fatigues easily. Skeletal muscle tissue always attaches to connective tissue structures.

Nervous tissues contain specialized nerve cells (neurons) that respond rapidly to stimulation by conducting nerve impulses. All neurons contain RNA-rich granules, called Nissl granules, in the cytoplasm. Neurons with a single long extension of the cell body are called unipolar. Those with two long extensions are called bipolar, and neurons with more than two long extensions are called multipolar. There are two types of extensions: Dendrites conduct impulses toward the cell body, while axons generally conduct impulses away from the cell body. Many axons are surrounded by a multilayered fatty substance called the myelin sheath, which is composed of many layers of cell membrane wrapped around the axon.

Nervous tissues also contain several types of neuroglia, cells that hold nervous tissue together. Many neuroglia cells have projections that wrap around the neurons and help nourish them. The many types of

DIRECTIONAL TERMS FOR THE BODY

Superior: upward; toward the top of the head
Inferior: downward; toward the ground or the feet
Cranial: toward the head; the same as superior in humans
Caudal: toward the tail
Dorsal: toward the back
Ventral: toward the belly surface
Medial: toward the midline
Lateral: away from the midline
Radial: on the medial side (or thumb side) of the arm, forearm, and hand
Ulnar: on the lateral side (or little finger side) of the arm, forearm, and hand; the same side that contains the ulna
Anterior: forward, in the customary direction of motion; equivalent to ventral in humans, but the same as cranial in other animals
Posterior: toward the rear, opposite to the customary direction of motion; equivalent to dorsal in humans, but the same as caudal in other animals

neuroglia include the tiny microglia and the larger protoplasmic astrocytes, fibrous astrocytes, and oligodendroglia.

Two major tissue types make up most of the brain and spinal cord, or central nervous system. The first type, gray matter, contains the cell bodies of many neurons, along with smaller amounts of axons, dendrites, and neuroglia cells. The second type, white matter, contains mostly the axons, and sometimes also the dendrites, of neurons whose cell bodies lie elsewhere, along with the myelin sheaths that surround many of the axons. Clumps of cell bodies are called nuclei when they are found within the brain and ganglia when they occur elsewhere. Bundles of axons are called tracts within the central nervous system and nerves when they appear peripherally.

The body can be described by the use of directional terms, which are defined in a relative manner according to the location of a given body part or segment. Some important directional terms are "superior," "inferior," "cranial," "caudal," "dorsal," "ventral," "medial," "lateral," "radial," "ulnar," "anterior," and "posterior."

Disorders and Diseases

Diseases or disorders that affect the entire body are called systemic or multisystem diseases. For example, fevers or febrile diseases raise the body's temperature. Many fevers are caused by infectious diseases such as influenza (actually a series of different viral infections). Influenzas cause fever, sore throat, muscle aches, coughs, headache, fatigue, and a general feeling of malaise.

Edema, or tissue swelling, is marked by an increase in the amount of extracellular fluid in several parts of the body at once. In the case of pulmonary edema, the fluid stains pink and fills the usually empty lung spaces (alveoli).

Most cancers are recognized by abnormalities of the cells in which they occur. The most dangerous cancers are marked by large tumors with ill-defined, irregular margins. If the cancer tumor is well defined, is small, and has a smooth, circular margin, then it is much less of a threat. Cancers are especially dangerous when they undergo metastasis, a process by which they produce wandering cells that spread throughout the body.

Juvenile diabetes mellitus (also called diabetes mellitus, Type I, and insulin-dependent diabetes mellitus, or IDDM), like most endocrine disorders, has systemic consequences throughout the body, including damage to nearly all the blood vessels. The primary defect in this disorder is a lack of insulin, which impairs the body's ability to use glucose. Another endocrine disorder with systemic consequences is Addison's disease, which is caused by a deficiency of the hormone adrenocorticotropic hormone (ACTH) that normally stimulates the cortex of the adrenal gland. Symptoms include weakness, loss of appetite, fatigue, weight loss, and reduced tolerance to cold. These symptoms result from imbalances in the levels of glucose and mineral salts throughout the body.

Systemic lupus erythematosus, a connective tissue disease, often produces red skin lesions marked by degeneration and flattening of the lower layers of the epidermis, drying and flaking of the outermost layer, dilation of the blood vessels under the skin, and the leakage of red blood cells out of these vessels, adding to the red color. (The word "erythematosus" means "red.")

Muscular dystrophy has several forms; the most common is marked in its advanced stages by enlarged muscles in which the muscle tissue is replaced by a fatty substance. Another muscular disease, myasthenia gravis, is often marked by overall enlargement of the thymus and an increase in the number of thymus cells. Myocardial infarction, a form of heart disease marked by damage to the heart muscle, is noticed in histological section by dead, fibrous scar tissue replacing the muscle tissue in the heart wall. In patients with arteriosclerosis, the usually elastic walls of the arteries become thicker and more fibrous and rigid; many of the same patients also suffer from atherosclerosis, a buildup of deposits on the inside of the blood vessel, partially or completely blocking blood flow.

In nervous tissue, damage to peripheral nerves often results in a process called chromatolysis in the cell bodies of the neurons from which these axons arise. The nuclei of these cells enlarge and become displaced to one side, while the Nissl granules disperse and the cell body as a whole undergoes swelling. Increased deposits of fibrous tissue characterize multiple sclerosis and certain other disorders of the nervous system. Some of these diseases are also marked by a degeneration of the myelin sheath around nerve fibers. In the case of a cerebrovascular stroke, impaired blood supply to the brain causes degeneration of the neuroglia, followed by general tissue death and the replacement of the neuroglia by fibrous tissue. Cranial hematoma (abnormal bleeding) results in the presence of blood clots (complete with blood cells and connective tissue fibers) in abnormal locations. Alzheimer's disease is marked by granules of a proteinlike substance called amyloid, often containing aluminum, surrounded by additional concentric layers of similar composition.

PERSPECTIVE AND PROSPECTS

The Latin names that are used today for most body parts are derived in large measure from the writings of Galen, or Caius Galenus, the physician to the Roman army in the second century. The study of anatomy was furthered in the Renaissance by artists such as Leonardo da Vinci (1452-1519) and Michelangelo (1475-1564), both of whom dissected human corpses illegally in order to gain further knowledge of the anatomical structures visible on the body's surface. Such studies were followed by the well-illustrated anatomical texts of Andreas Vesalius (1514-1564), who corrected many of Galen's errors regarding the structure of the human body.

A medical understanding of the circulatory system began with the studies of the Renaissance physician William Harvey (1578-1657), who examined the veins in the arms of many patients. It was Harvey who first described the presence of valves in the veins and who proved that the blood circulates outward from the heart, throughout the body, and then back again to the heart.

Microscopes were first developed around 1700 by Antoni van Leeuwenhoek (1632-1723) and others. Electron microscopes first became commercially available in the 1950's. Microscopy using instruments of these two types was widely used for distinguishing between healthy and diseased tissue, in tissue taken either from bodies at autopsy or from biopsies of living patients. Modern diagnostic radiology began with the discovery of X rays by Wilhelm Conrad Röntgen (1845-1923). Computed tomography (CT) scanning, which was developed in the 1960's and 1970's, allows for the creation of a three-dimensional X-ray picture.

—Eli C. Minkoff, Ph.D.

See also Genomics; Physiology; Systems and organs; *specific parts or systems.*

FOR FURTHER INFORMATION:

Abrahams, Peter H., Sandy C. Marks, Jr., and Ralph Hutchings. *McMinn's Color Atlas of Human Anatomy.* 5th ed. New York: Mosby, 2003. A useful set of color illustrations covering all parts of the body.

Agur, Anne M. R., and Arthur F. Dalley. *Grant's Atlas of Anatomy.* 11th ed. Philadelphia: Lippincott Williams & Wilkins, 2005. Offers many excellent, detailed illustrations of the human body.

Crouch, James E. *Functional Human Anatomy.* 4th ed. Philadelphia: Lea & Febiger, 1985. An easy-to-read book which offers helpful explanations. A good reference source for the beginning anatomy student or nonscientist.

Marieb, Elaine N. *Essentials of Human Anatomy and Physiology.* 8th ed. San Francisco: Pearson/Benjamin Cummings, 2006. This introductory anatomy and physiology textbook, easily accessible to those with little science background, is richly illustrated with diagrams and photographs, which help to illuminate body systems and processes.

Moore, Keith L., and Anne M. R. Agur. *Essential Clinical Anatomy.* 3d ed. Philadelphia: Lippincott Williams & Wilkins, 2007. A basic text that examines the importance and function of anatomy.

Netter, Frank H. *The CIBA Collection of Medical Illustrations.* 8 vols. West Caldwell, N.J.: CIBA Pharmaceutical, 1983. A large-format set of excellent medical illustrations for college students.

Rohen, Johannes W., Chihiro Yokochi, and Elke Lütjen-Drecoll. *Color Atlas of Anatomy: A Photographic Study of the Human Body.* 6th ed. Philadelphia: Lippincott Williams & Wilkins, 2006. An excellent compendium of color photographs of various anatomical structures.

Rosse, Cornelius, and Penelope Gaddum-Rosse. *Hollinshead's Textbook of Anatomy.* 5th ed. Philadelphia: Lippincott-Raven, 1997. Good descriptions and illustrations are highlights of this thorough, modern, and detailed reference work.

Standring, Susan, et al., eds. *Gray's Anatomy.* 39th ed. New York: Elsevier Churchill Livingstone, 2005. The classic anatomy text. Thorough descriptions and excellent, detailed color illustrations are provided.

ANEMIA

DISEASE/DISORDER

ANATOMY OR SYSTEM AFFECTED: Blood, heart, kidneys

SPECIALTIES AND RELATED FIELDS: Cardiology, family medicine, hematology, internal medicine, nephrology, oncology, preventive medicine

DEFINITION: Anemia is defined as a decrease in the oxygen-carrying capacity of blood with a reduction in the red blood cell count and/or hemoglobin.

KEY TERMS:

erythrocytes: red blood cells of the circulatory system that contain hemoglobin and are responsible for delivering oxygen to the tissues

erythropoietin: the hormone protein that is produced in the kidneys and acts on the bone marrow helping in red blood cell synthesis
hematopoiesis: the process of production of red blood cells by bone marrow
hemoglobin: the pigmented protein that imparts red color to the blood and carries oxygen from the lungs to the rest of the body
hemolytic anemia: anemia attributable to increased destruction of red blood cells
macrocytic anemia: anemia with red blood cells of increased size
microcytic anemia: anemia with red blood cells of decreased size
normocytic anemia: anemia with red blood cells of normal size

Information on Anemia

Causes: A deficiency in the oxygen-carrying material of the blood and/or vitamin B_{12}
Symptoms: Pallor, shortness of breath, heart palpitations, lethargy and fatigue, low blood pressure
Duration: Acute or chronic
Treatments: Replacement of deficient iron, vitamin B_{12}, or folate; blood transfusions

Causes and Symptoms

Red blood cells or erythrocytes are continuously produced in the bone marrow by a process known as hematopoiesis. This complex process requires adequate amounts of iron, vitamins such as B_{12} and folic acid, and hormones such as erythropoietin. Iron is required to form hemoglobin, which is the oxygen-carrying protein contained in red blood cells. Deficiency of any of the above can cause a decrease in hemoglobin or red blood cell counts, resulting clinically in anemia. Certain medications, environmental toxins, and cancers that affect the bone marrow can also cause anemia. As erythropoietin is produced in the kidneys, anemia is seen with chronic kidney disease as well.

The normal life span of a red blood cell, from its production in the bone marrow to its destruction in the liver and spleen, is about 120 days. If the life span is decreased in any way, either by increased destruction due to various reasons or through blood loss (during trauma, vaginal bleeding, gastrointestinal bleeding, or surgery), anemia can result. Increased destruction can also occur if the red blood cells are abnormal or the liver or spleen are enlarged. Anemia is recognized by laboratory tests when the hemoglobin falls below the normal values expected for the age and sex of the patient. The normal range of hemoglobin is 13.5 to 17.5 milligrams per deciliter in males and 12 to 16 milligrams per deciliter in females.

Anemia is generally classified into three broad categories: microcytic, macrocytic, and normocytic, based on red blood cell size measured as the mean corpuscular volume (MCV) of red blood cells in blood tests. Microcytic anemia refers to decreased red blood cell size, usually with decreased hemoglobin as well. The most common cause of microcytic anemia is iron deficiency. Other causes include lead poisoning, thalassemia, sideroblastic anemia, and anemia of chronic disease.

Iron-deficiency anemia is a type of microcytic anemia with low serum iron caused by decreased intake, malabsorption, or increased loss of iron. The most common cause of iron deficiency in the United States is chronic blood loss, usually seen in women of reproductive age (menstrual loss) and the elderly (gastrointestinal blood loss due to tumors or cancers). Pregnant women may have iron deficiency as a result of inadequate intake that does not meet the requirements of the growing fetus; they require iron supplementation. Iron is absorbed in the small intestine, and any disease or procedure that causes problems with absorption, such as celiac sprue, inflammatory bowel disease (IBD), or intestinal surgery, can lead to iron-deficiency anemia. Iron-deficiency anemia is also prevalent in developing nations due to parasitic infestations such as hookworm. Iron deficiency is usually diagnosed by blood tests, but occasionally a bone marrow biopsy may be required in which absent iron stores are noted.

Chronic lead poisoning can also cause anemia by a direct toxic effect on the bone marrow. Lead is found in old house paints, pipes, bullets, batteries, and other items. Children living or playing in old houses are usually affected and may develop learning and behavioral problems in addition to anemia. The characteristic feature of lead poisoning in anemia is basophilic stippling of red blood cells.

Thalassemias are inherited disorders of the hemoglobin involving alpha or beta chains. These defective hemoglobin chains result in very small red blood cells that are fragile and destroyed in the spleen, causing hemolytic anemia. Patients with thalassemia may be revealed to suffer from anemia early in their childhood.

Hydrops fetalis is a very severe form of thalassemia that results in fetal death. Thalassemia is most commonly seen in people of Mediterranean and Southeast Asian origin. Cooley's anemia or beta thalassemia major occurs early in childhood and causes growth retardation.

Sideroblastic anemia is also caused by defective hemoglobin in red blood cells, resulting in hemolytic anemia. Certain toxins such as lead, alcohol, drugs such as chloramphenicol, and hypothermia can cause acquired sideroblastic anemia. Occasionally, sideroblastic anemia may be normocytic. A diagnosis is made when blood tests reveal an excess of iron and a characteristic bone marrow study shows ringed sideroblasts.

Macrocytic anemia is characterized by an increase in red blood cell size. Common causes of macrocytic anemia are vitamin B_{12} and folic acid deficiencies, alcoholism, hypothyroidism, myelodysplastic syndromes (MDS), and hemolytic anemias.

Vitamin B_{12} and folate deficiency cause megaloblastic or macrocytic anemia. Vitamin B_{12} or cobalamin is essential for DNA synthesis. Cobalamin that is ingested in food is bound to the intrinsic factor that is essential for absorption of the vitamin in the small intestine. Most cobalamin deficiency is the result of chronic dietary deficiency or pernicious anemia, which is a deficiency in the intrinsic factor. Folate (folic acid) is present in green leafy vegetables and fruits such as bananas. Folate deficiency is generally attributable to dietary deficiency, increased need as in pregnancy, or decreased absorption in the small intestine. Dietary deficiency is especially common in alcoholics. Pregnant women and patients on certain medications such as methotrexate have increased folic acid needs and require folic acid supplements.

Hemolytic anemias are characterized by increased fragility of the red blood cells and hence their increased destruction in the spleen and liver. The types of hemolytic anemias are sickle cell anemia, hereditary spherocytosis, thalassemia, and autoimmune hemolytic anemias.

Sickle cell anemia is common in those with African ancestry. It is characterized by an abnormal "sickle" shape to the red blood cell that occurs when it is ex-

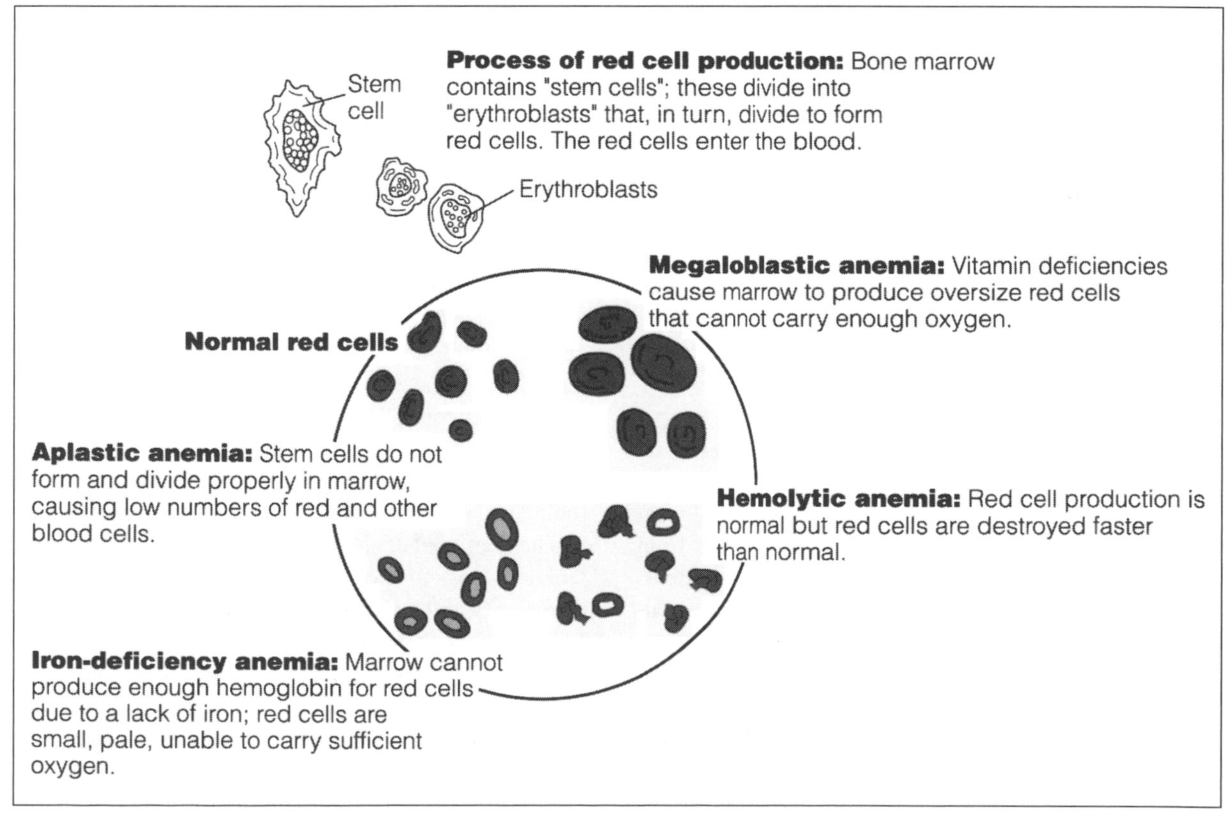

Anemia may take several different forms.

posed to certain triggers. These abnormal red blood cells are unable to carry adequate oxygen to the tissues. As these fragile cells pass through the capillaries of the spleen, they rupture easily, resulting in anemia. In hereditary spherocytosis, red blood cells are spherical and rigid instead of being biconcave flexible discs. These cells are trapped in the spleen and are destroyed before completing their normal life span of 120 days. In autoimmune hemolytic anemia, antibodies are produced against the red blood cells, which enable them to be targets of destruction by the white blood cells of the immune system. This type of anemia is seen with unmatched blood transfusion or with the ingestion of certain drugs.

Normocytic anemia is characterized by a normal red blood cell size and is seen in anemia of chronic disease, acute blood loss, and anemia of chronic kidney disease.

Chronic inflammatory diseases such as rheumatoid arthritis or osteomyelitis result in the production of certain toxins that act directly on the bone marrow and decrease red blood cell production. Normocytic anemia ensues, in which there is simply an overall decrease in red blood cell production without a maturation defect. The anemia usually improves when the chronic inflammation subsides. In chronic kidney disease, a decrease in erythropoietin production results in decreased red blood cell production. Aplastic anemia is another condition characterized by a marked decrease in red blood cell production because of the effect of toxins, medications, or infections such as parvovirus B19 (fifth disease). Other blood cell types may also be affected in aplastic anemia, resulting in severe infections and bleeding problems.

The symptoms of anemia are generally the same irrespective of the cause. Patients are generally pale and fatigued easily and can experience palpitations or rapid heartbeat. Most of the symptoms are attributable to compensatory mechanisms of the body trying to overcome decreased oxygenation. These compensatory mechanisms result in an increased circulating fluid volume that can eventually cause heart failure. Patients may have symptoms of heart failure such as foot swelling, shortness of breath, palpitations, chest pain, lightheadedness, or episodes of passing out. Patients whose anemia is caused by blood loss may have these symptoms if the loss is chronic and the body has adequate time to compensate. In cases of acute blood loss or when hemoglobin falls below 5 milligram per deciliter, however, patients may experience shock, low blood pressure, heart attack, stroke, and confusion, sometimes leading to death. On the other hand, chronic mild anemia may be asymptomatic and is detected as an incidental finding on a routine laboratory test.

Other symptoms may be specific to the cause of the anemia. Iron deficiency may sometimes manifest itself as pica (a craving for materials such as clay or ice) and flattened or spoon-shaped nails. Severe thalassemia in children is usually displayed in multiple fractures, a characteristic chipmunk face, an enlarged liver and spleen, heart failure, and gallstones. Patients with anemia caused by vitamin B_{12} deficiency may have neurological and psychiatric problems. There may be an associated thick red tongue and cracking at the angles of the mouth due to other associated vitamin deficiencies. Patients with hemolytic anemia can suffer from jaundice, dark urine, and gallstones because of the bilirubin released from the hemolysed red blood cells and enlarged spleen. Patients with sickle cell anemia may have acute pain crises and multiple infections. As a result of decreased oxygenation in peripheral tissues, stroke, angina, or lung clots may be the primary presentation in sickle cell disease. Patients with anemia of chronic disease usually have an obvious source of inflammation. Patients with bone marrow failure may also display symptoms of infection and bleeding.

Treatment and Therapy

The most important step in the management of anemia is an evaluation of the patient's condition and the cause of anemia by a physician. A detailed history is usually elicited and should include dietary habits, occupation, associated symptoms, family history, medication history, and other medical problems. A complete physical examination is performed looking specifically for jaundice, pallor, signs of heart failure, and enlarged liver and spleen. The most helpful tool in the diagnosis of anemia is the blood test. The physician may order further tests when the diagnosis is difficult, which may include invasive tests such as a bone marrow biopsy.

The treatment of anemia is directed toward the cause and acuteness of the problem. Acute blood loss is an emergency and requires close monitoring in a hospital. It is treated with blood transfusions and fluid resuscitation. Some patients displaying signs of shock may need to be monitored in an intensive care setting. Patients with chronic anemia may be managed on an outpatient basis.

Iron deficiency is usually treated with oral iron sulfate tablets. Antacids interfere with iron absorption and hence should not be taken simultaneously. Patients who cannot tolerate oral iron may be given iron intravenously. Lead poisoning is treated with chelating agents to remove the lead from the body. Thalassemia requires multiple blood transfusions and, if severe enough, bone marrow transplantation. Iron overload may become a problem with multiple blood transfusions, and chelating treatment with desferrioxamine may be needed to remove the excess iron. Hereditary spherocytosis may be treated with pyridoxine, and acquired spherocytosis caused by alcohol and medications is treated with discontinuation of the offending agent. Megaloblastic anemia due to vitamin B_{12} and folic acid deficiency is treated with oral supplements of these vitamins. Vitamin B_{12} may also be given intramuscularly. The neurological abnormalities are reversible if treated early. Autoimmune hemolytic anemias are treated by removal of the offending agent and with steroids. Some patients may require splenectomy (surgical removal of the spleen). Sickle cell crises are treated in the hospital with intravenous fluids, oxygen, and blood transfusion. Supportive care is generally required, and patients may need antibiotics for infections and high doses of painkillers. The number of attacks may be reduced by oral hydroxyurea therapy as an outpatient.

The treatment of anemia caused by chronic kidney disease due to low erythropoietin will require supplementation with weekly subcutaneous erythropoietin and iron. In patients undergoing dialysis, hemoglobin must be maintained above 11 milligrams per deciliter. Patients with aplastic anemia will require multiple blood transfusions and immunosuppressive therapy and may benefit from bone marrow transplantation.

PERSPECTIVE AND PROSPECTS

The earliest mention of iron therapy is in Greek mythology in the story of Iphiclus being cured of impotence by drinking a tea made from the rust of an iron blade. The use of iron for the treatment of anemia, however, occurred much later, after the discovery of blood and blood transfusion.

Jan Swammerdam first described red blood cells in 1658, and the first blood transfusion was dog-to-dog in 1665 by Oxford physician Richard Lower. The first human-to-human blood transfusion was performed successfully in 1818 by British obstetrician James Blundell for the treatment of postpartum hemorrhage. Death from hemolytic anemias caused by mismatched blood transfusions, however, was a problem until Karl Landsteiner identified the ABO blood groups in 1901, for which he received the Nobel Prize in Medicine in 1930. He subsequently discovered Rh groups in blood that further reduced the incidence of hemolytic anemias resulting from blood transfusions. The first case of sickle cell anemia was described by James Herrick in 1910, but it was Linus Pauling who postulated that the disease was the result of the presence of mutant hemoglobin HbS.

The mortality rate of anemia has improved significantly over the past century thanks to advances in blood transfusion and bone marrow transplantation. Current research is focusing on the therapeutic potential of anemia correction in cancer, rheumatoid arthritis, human immunodeficiency virus (HIV) infection, heart failure, and kidney disease. It is being shown that the correction of anemia improves quality of life significantly. Synthetic blood may become the treatment of anemia in the future.

—Venkat Raghavan Tirumala, M.D., M.H.A.

See also Blood and blood disorders; Blood testing; Hematology; Hematology, pediatric; Phlebotomy; Serology; Sickle cell disease; Thalassemia; Vitamins and minerals.

FOR FURTHER INFORMATION:

Anemia.com. http://www.anemia.com/. A good source for anemia education. The site describes in detail, in simple terms, how anemia affects the body, its symptoms and signs, and its treatment. Also provides information about anemia in chemotherapy and chronic kidney disease.

Bloodbook.com. http://www.bloodbook.com/. This Web site describes the history of blood transfusion medicine.

Greer, John, et al., eds. *Wintrobe's Clinical Hematology*. 11th ed. Philadelphia: Lippincott Williams & Wilkins, 2004. A thorough textbook on blood and hematological diseases. Anemia is described in great detail.

Kasper, Dennis L., et al., eds. *Harrison's Principles of Internal Medicine*. 16th ed. New York: McGraw-Hill, 2005. A very comprehensive medical textbook with detailed descriptions of the pathophysiology, diagnosis, and treatment of various types of anemia.

National Anemia Action Council. http://www.anemia.org/. This Web site by the National Anemia Action Council provides information for medical professionals as well as patients and the public.

Anesthesia

Procedure

Anatomy or system affected: Brain, muscles, musculoskeletal system, nerves, nervous system, psychic-emotional system, skin, spine

Specialties and related fields: Anesthesiology, critical care, dentistry, emergency medicine, general surgery, neurology, ophthalmology

Definition: The administration of drugs to block the transmission of nerve impulses and thus to prevent pain, especially during surgery or childbirth; anesthesia may be general (causing total unconsciousness) or regional and local (deadening sensation and decreasing awareness, without causing loss of consciousness).

Key terms:

epidural anesthesia: anesthesia produced by injecting a local anesthetic between the vertebral spines and beneath the ligamentum flavum into the extradural space; also known as extradural anesthesia

local anesthesia: anesthesia produced by injecting a local anesthetic solution directly into the tissues; also known as local block

local anesthetics: drugs that produce a reversible blockade of nerve impulse conduction

regional anesthesia: insensibility caused by the interruption of nerve conduction in a region of the body

spinal anesthesia: anesthesia produced by injecting a local anesthetic around the spinal cord; also known as subarachnoid block

Indications and Procedures

Anesthetics are given primarily to prevent the pain of surgery during operations. They also are given to reduce fear, relax tissues, and prevent a sympathetic nervous system response to surgery. Some believe, erroneously, that being "put to sleep" with a general anesthetic is the only way an operation can be performed pain-free.

General anesthesia is a type of anesthesia that produces total unconsciousness and affects the entire body. Regional anesthesia, another type of anesthesia, does not produce unconsciousness but allows surgery to be performed without pain by producing loss of sensation in a region of the body—by interrupting the transmission of nerve impulses from the area to be incised.

With general anesthesia, patients receive drugs that are delivered both intravenously and by inhalation. With regional anesthesia, the anesthetic agents are deposited either on the surface of the area to be anesthetized or near a particular nerve or pathway that lies between the area and receptors for painful stimuli that are part of the central nervous system. As a result, transmission of noxious stimuli to the brain is effectively "blocked," allowing a surgical procedure to be performed without the patient feeling pain. Regional anesthesia is frequently referred to as regional nerve blockade.

Local anesthetics operate in several ways. Those injected near the nerves diffuse into the nerves and bind to receptors on their membranes. Once in the nerve sheath, local anesthetic agents prevent sodium from moving into the nerve interior by physically occluding sodium channels. Impulses traveling from the surgical area to the central nervous system are blocked such that nerves transmitting touch, temperature, and pain sensation are temporarily interrupted. Nerve impulses traveling from the central nervous system to the surgical area are also blocked, leading to an interruption of motor power to the surgical area.

The number of nerves blocked depends on where the local anesthetic is deposited—that is, on the type of regional anesthetic technique utilized. The duration of the nerve blockade depends on the type and dosage of local anesthetic injected as well as on the technique utilized. Diffusion of the local anesthetic out of the nerve and its absorption into the vascular bed causes the effect of the local anesthetic to be terminated. The blood flowing around the nerve removes the drug from the area. Decreasing the flow of blood to the area by adding vasoconstricting agents, such as epinephrine, to the local anesthetic to be injected is a method commonly utilized to prolong the duration of the nerve block.

Local anesthetics are weak bases whose structure consists of an aromatic moiety connected to a substituted amine through an ester or amide linkage. The two major families of local anesthetics are the amino amides and the amino esters. The clinical differences between the ester and amide local anesthetics involve their potential for producing adverse side effects and the mechanisms by which they are metabolized.

Local anesthetics are also classified on the basis of their potency and duration of action: a short duration of action (thirty to forty-five minutes), an intermediate duration of action (one to two hours), or a long duration of action (four to eight hours). The range in duration of nerve blockade is attributable primarily to two factors: the concentration of the drug used and the addition of vasoconstricting agents, such as epinephrine.

Local and regional anesthesia are excellent ways of supplying surgical anesthesia and postoperative analgesia (pain control). Local anesthetics are now being given in combination with narcotic analgesics (painkillers). Narcotics injected in combination with local anesthetics work through a different mechanism of action; they bind to narcotic receptors in the area and provide analgesia without interrupting nerve transmission. The combination of local anesthetic agents with narcotics is gaining popularity in postoperative and labor pain control; longer durations of pain relief can be obtained while avoiding the systemic side effects of intravenously administered narcotics.

There are six categories of regional anesthesia: topical anesthesia, local block and field block, nerve block, intravenous (IV) neural blockade, subarachnoid block (spinal anesthesia), and epidural anesthesia, including caudal block. The major differences are the size of the region that is anesthetized and the duration of the neural blockade.

Topical anesthesia. In this technique, also known as surface anesthesia, an anesthetic drug is sprayed or dropped onto an area to be desensitized. This short-acting form of anesthesia blocks nerve endings in the skin as well as mucous membranes, such as those of the nasopharynx (nose and throat), mouth, rectum, and vagina. Topical anesthesia is employed in minor procedures such as eye or rectal examinations. The advantages of topical anesthesia include quick onset of action, ease of administration, and general nontoxicity. Disadvantages include lack of deeper-tissue anesthesia and lack of tissue relaxation. A frequently used topical anesthetic is the drug benzocaine, often utilized for traumatic tissue pain secondary to sunburn.

Local blocks and field blocks. In local blocks, the local anesthetic is injected with a needle and syringe into the skin and tissues of an area to be incised. As a result, the nerves in the area of the incision are blocked. Local blocks are used in short minor operations and prior to the insertion of intravenous or spinal needles. A field block is another type of local block. In a field block, the area surrounding the incision is also injected with local anesthetics, preventing impulses transmitted from a larger area from reaching the central nervous system.

Nerve blocks. Nerve blocks interrupt the transmission of nerve impulses by nerves or by bundles of nerves that are further removed from the surgical site. Nerve blocks may be used to anesthetize a single finger or toe (digital nerve block), a foot (ankle block) or hand, or an entire arm (axillary, supraclavicular, and interscalene blocks) or leg (leg block). In each type of neural blockade, the physician or nurse anesthetist injects local anesthetic agents around the major nerves that supply the area to be incised. The number of injections depends on the location of the nerves to be blocked. For example, in performing a leg block, four nerves—the femoral, sciatic, lateral femoral cutaneous, and obturator nerves—because of their separate locations, may be blocked individually. An arm block can be accomplished by a single injection of a larger volume of local anesthetic into the axillary sheath or between the middle and anterior scalene muscles in the neck. Upper extremity blocks can be performed with a single injection because the brachial plexus (the nerves innervating the arm) is collectively encased in a sheath. Distal to the axillary area, the nerves innervating the arm are no longer encased in a sheath. Consequently, separate injections of the radial, median, and ulnar nerves are required to block the arm at the elbow or wrist.

Intercostal nerve blocks. Intercostal nerves innervate the outer and inner surfaces of the abdominal wall. Intercostal nerve blockade is utilized for postoperative pain control following thoracic or upper abdominal surgeries. A sterile needle is inserted into the skin over the lower margin of the rib along the posterior axillary line. The needle is then directed toward the intercostal groove located inferior to the rib. A local anesthetic is injected into the intercostal space containing the intercostal nerve, vein, and artery. The anesthetic lasts from six to twelve hours and may be prolonged by the addition of epinephrine to the solution.

Intravenous neural blockade. Intravenous (IV) neural blockade was discovered by August Bier in 1908; he was also the first to utilize spinal anesthesia routinely. Today, IV regional neural blockade is also referred to as Bier blockade. With Bier blockade, the local anesthetic agent is injected into a vein, lying distal to a tourniquet, in an upper or lower extremity (instead of around a nerve). Inflation of the tourniquet prevents the local anesthetic from being released into the general circulation. The local anesthetic, thus contained in the extremity, travels to the major nerves in the limb and blocks neural transmission. The duration of the neural blockade is governed by the length of time that the tourniquet is inflated. Once the tourniquet is deflated, the local anesthetic enters the systemic circulation, the neural blockade recedes, and normal sensation and power to the extremity are rapidly returned. Intravenous regional blockade of the extremities has many advantages: ease of performance, rapid onset, controllable duration of action, and rapid recovery. The disadvantages include possible tourniquet discomfort, possible reaction to the local anesthetic when it is released into the general circulation, and rapid return of sensation, including pain.

Spinal anesthesia. Spinal anesthesia, also called subarachnoid block, is a commonly utilized form of anesthesia. Spinal anesthesia can be used for almost any type of surgical procedure below the umbilicus, such as surgical procedures performed on the legs and hips, hysterectomies, appendectomies, and cesarean sections.

A lumbar puncture (spinal tap) is performed in the lower back, usually between the second and third lumbar vertebrae, the third and fourth lumbar vertebrae, or the fifth lumbar and first sacral vertebrae. The patient is placed on his or her side in a flexed position (or sometimes in a sitting position). The physician or nurse anesthetist, wearing sterile gloves, prepares the skin in the area to be punctured with a skin antiseptic, such as betadine, and then drapes the area with a sterile towel. The anesthetist then infiltrates the area of the puncture with lidocaine, producing a local block. Once the skin is anesthetized, the lumbar puncture is performed; a needle is inserted through the intraspinous space into the subarachnoid space. The needle passes through the supraspinous ligament, intraspinous ligament, and ligamentum flavum. Proper placement of the needle is identified through an observation of freely flowing spinal fluid. A local anesthetic agent is then injected into the spinal fluid. Cerebrospinal fluid (CSF) is a clear, colorless ultrafiltrate of the blood that fills the subarachnoid space. The total volume of CSF is 100 to 150 milliliters; the volume contained in the subarachnoid space is 25 to 35 milliliters.

Once injected into the subarachnoid CSF, the local anesthetic agent spreads in both a cephalad (toward the head and anterior) and a caudad (toward the feet and posterior) direction. Factors influencing this spread include the dose and volume of the agent used, patient position, and the specific gravity (weight) of the anesthetic solution relative to the CSF. One of three types of solutions—isobaric, hypobaric, or hyperbaric—can be used. Hyperbaric solutions are heavier than CSF; thus, placing the patient in Trendelenburg's position (with the head tilted downward) will increase the cephalad spread of the anesthetic. With the patient in Trendelenburg's position, hypobaric solutions (with a specific gravity less than that of CSF) of local anesthetic agents spread caudally. Spread of the local anesthetic in the subarachnoid space usually stops (fixation) within five to thirty-five minutes after injection. After fixation has occurred, patient position changes will not influence the spread of local anesthetic or the subsequent level of anesthesia.

Within minutes after a subarachnoid injection of a local anesthetic, patients experience a warm sensation in their lower extremities, followed by a loss of sensation and inability to move the legs. The duration of the neural blockade is dependent on the type of local anesthetic utilized, as well as the addition of any vasoconstrictor.

Epidural anesthesia and caudal block. Like spinal anesthesia, epidural blockade can be used for the prevention of pain during surgery. It can also be used to relieve pain after surgery, chronic pain, and the pain in labor; to supplement a light general anesthetic; and to diagnose and treat autonomic nervous system dysfunction. The technique is excellent for the operations performed on the lower abdomen, pelvis, and perineum; for laminectomies; and in obstetrics for the relief of labor pains and the facilitation of delivery.

As with spinal anesthesia, the patient is placed on his or her side in a flexed position (or sometimes in a sitting position). The physician or nurse anesthetist, wearing sterile gloves, prepares the skin in the area of the puncture with an antiseptic such as betadine and drapes the area with a sterile towel. The anesthetist infiltrates the area of the puncture with lidocaine, producing a local block. Once the skin is anesthetized, an epidural needle is inserted between the appropriate lumbar vertebrae (occasionally between thoracic vertebrae). With epidural blockade, however, the needle is not advanced into the subarachnoid space; needle advancement is terminated when the needle tip is in the epidural space. Thus, the dura is not penetrated as in spinal anesthesia. (As a result, postdural puncture headache does not occur with a properly placed epidural needle.) Once the epidural space has been identified, local anesthetic agents (in larger volumes than utilized with subarachnoid anesthesia) are injected through the needle or through a small catheter threaded through the needle. Placement of a catheter through the needle allows reinjection to take place without subsequent needle punctures; this is particularly desirable for long surgeries, postoperative pain control, and the control of labor pains. Local anesthetic agents injected through a catheter for postoperative or labor pain control are usually given at lesser concentrations so that nerve motor fibers are not interrupted.

Caudal block is another type of epidural anesthesia. In this case, the needle (with or without a catheter) is placed through the sacroccygeal ligament just superior to the coccyx. The technique is gaining popularity as an adjunct to general anesthesia in children, for the purpose of postoperative pain control.

USES AND COMPLICATIONS

Regional anesthesia has several advantages over general anesthesia. The first is ease of administration: The agents used are injectable, the equipment required is minimal, and the costs are reasonable. Second is relative safety: A localized area of the body can be operated upon while avoiding most of the undesirable and potentially harmful side effects of general anesthesia, such as loss of consciousness and the depression of the cardiovascular and respiratory systems. In addition, advantages include excellent muscle relaxation, which is often required in order to facilitate surgical procedures; improved peripheral blood flow; an antithrombitic effect; a decreased loss of blood in some cases; and postoperative pain relief, a benefit most patients find highly desirable. Regional anesthesia is also utilized in combination with general anesthesia in an effort to increase the benefits of both while decreasing the adverse side effects of each.

Yet regional anesthesia has some disadvantages. First, some operations cannot be performed under regional anesthesia (for example, major surgical procedures involving the brain, heart, and lungs). Second, some patients may be allergic to the local anesthetics. Local anesthetics of the amino ester type may result in allergic reactions because of the metabolite p-aminobenzoic acid. Local anesthetics of the amino amide class are essentially devoid of allergic potential. Many anesthetic solutions, however, contain methylparaben as a preservative, and this compound can produce an allergic reaction in persons sensitive to p-aminobenzoic acid. Third, some patients desire to be unaware of the operation and may be anxious at the thought of being "awake." They erroneously believe that the total unconsciousness produced by general anesthesia is the only method to produce unawareness. In the majority of cases, patients who receive a regional anesthetic also receive intravenous sedation to decrease their level of awareness. Subsequently, many patients report having no recollection whatsoever of the surgical procedure.

In addition, the advantages of spinal anesthesia, one of the most popular types of regional anesthesia, far outweigh the disadvantages, which include hypotension, a high level of anesthesia, and postdural puncture headache. Hypotension is treated with intravenous fluids and, if necessary, the administration of vasoconstricting drugs. Postdural puncture headache (spinal headache) is thought to be caused from a loss of spinal fluid (which cushions the brain) through the dural hole produced by the spinal needle. Recent advances in the technique of spinal anesthesia administration, including the use of very small needles introduced in a manner that separates the dural fibers, have significantly decreased the incidence of postdural puncture headache. Should this complication arise, however, it is treated with analgesics, intravenous fluids, and, if necessary, an injection of saline (or a sample of the patient's own blood) around the site of the dural puncture, effectively "patching" the dural hole created by the spinal needle.

The first successful demonstration of anesthesia (diethyl ether) by William T. G. Morton occurred in 1846 at the Massachusetts General Hospital. The discovery of anesthesia occurred prior to the discovery of germ theory and aseptic techniques: Although anesthesia made surgery painless in the early nineteenth century, there was still a high rate of surgical morbidity and mortality as a result of infection. In the late 1860's, germ theory had evolved from the work of Robert Koch and Louis Pasteur, and Joseph Lister's subsequent work on principles of asepsis contributed significantly to a decline in surgical mortality from infection by the late 1880's. There remained, however, a high surgical mortality rate caused by anesthesia. At that time, general anesthetic agents were commonly utilized, and few, if any, practitioners specialized in the administration of anesthesia.

Regional anesthesia was first utilized in 1884 when a German physician named Carl Koller performed an operation to correct glaucoma using a local anesthetic. In this case, cocaine, an alkaloid obtained from the coca plant, was instilled into the eye. This successful operation brought significant acceptance to the principle of local anesthesia. The great advantage of local anesthesia was that it anesthetized only the part of the body on which the operation was to be performed: Patients could be spared the depressive effects of general anesthesia, especially those on the cardiovascular and respiratory systems.

By the 1930's, various regional anesthesia techniques had been developed, including subarachnoid block (spinal anesthesia), lumbar epidural, caudal epidural, intravenous, and brachial plexus anesthesia.

The occurrence of these regional anesthetic techniques, along with the evolution of local anesthetic agents, allowed anesthetists to tailor the type and duration of regional anesthesia to the requirements of each patient. As a result, regional anesthesia has become a popular choice among surgeons, anesthetists, and patients.

—*Maura S. McAuliffe*

See also Acupuncture; Anesthesiology; Catheterization; Hypnosis; Lumbar puncture; Narcotics; Nervous system; Neurology; Neurology, pediatric; Pain; Pain management; Pharmacology; Surgery, general; Surgical procedures.

For Further Information:

Cousins, Michael J., and P. O. Bridenbaugh, eds. *Neural Blockade in Clinical Anesthesia and Management of Pain*. 3d ed. Philadelphia: J. B. Lippincott, 1998. This bible of regional anesthesia principles and techniques contains chapters written by experts in the field.

Katz, Jordan. *Atlas of Regional Anesthesia*. 2d ed. Norwalk, Conn.: Appleton & Lange, 1999. An atlas of nerve block techniques explained in a simple and straightforward manner. The exquisite drawings and meticulous details of the illustrations make this an exceptional text.

Palmer, C. M., M. Paech, and R. D'Angelo, eds. *Handbook of Obstetric Anesthesia*. 6th ed. Oxford, England: Bios Scientific, 2002. An accessible text that outlines a variety of uses of anesthesia during normal and high-risk pregnancies. Topics include maternal physiology and pain pathways, procedures for cesarean sections, and common clinical scenarios such as preeclampsia, obesity, multiple gestation, and coexisting disease.

Sweeney, Frank. *The Anesthesia Fact Book: Everything You Need to Know Before Surgery*. Cambridge, Mass.: Perseus, 2003. Designed to help the health consumer become more informed and confident prior to surgery. Covers topics such as how general anesthesia works and how it differs from twilight, spinal, or epidural anesthesia; the credentials one should look for in an anesthesiologist; and questions that are important to ask prior to surgical procedures.

Winnie, A. P. *Plexus Anesthesia: Perivascular Techniques of Brachial Plexus Block*. Reprint. Philadelphia: W. B. Saunders, 1993. This book, written by the leading expert in regional anesthesia for the upper extremities, is one of the best of its kind. A well-organized, comprehensive text.

Anesthesiology

Specialty

Anatomy or system affected: Brain, muscles, musculoskeletal system, nerves, nervous system, psychic-emotional system, skin, spine

Specialties and related fields: Anesthesiology, critical care, dentistry, emergency medicine, general surgery, neurology, ophthalmology

Definition: The science of administering anesthesia during a surgical procedure.

Key terms:

anesthesia: a new word coined in the 1840's, derived from a Greek word meaning "not feeling"

electric anesthesia: the use of pulses of electricity to deaden nerve cells or cause unconsciousness

endotracheal tube: a flexible tube inserted through the mouth or nose into the trachea (windpipe) to carry anesthetic gas and oxygen directly to the lungs

ether: a volatile liquid that causes unconsciousness when inhaled; first demonstrated during surgery in 1846

nitrous oxide: called "laughing gas" because people appeared to become intoxicated from inhaling it; first used in 1844 to pull a tooth painlessly

novocaine: a local anesthetic, commonly used in dentistry, whose chemical structure is similar to that of cocaine

sodium pentothal: a fast-acting anesthetic that is injected into the vein; first developed for military hospitals during World War II

spinal anesthesia: the injection of an anesthetic at the base of the spine to produce loss of feeling in the lower part of the body and legs

The History of Anesthesiology

In a modern hospital, the surgical operating room normally is a very quiet place. The anesthesiologist, surgeon, assisting doctors, and nurses perform their duties with little conversation while the patient sleeps. Family members sit quietly in a nearby waiting room until the operation is over. Before the advent of anesthesiology in the 1840's, however, surgery had been a thoroughly gruesome experience. Patients might drink some whiskey to numb their senses, and several strong men were recruited to hold them down. Surgeons cut the flesh with a sharp knife and sawed quickly through the bone while patients screamed in agony. The operating room in the hospital was located as far as possible from other patients awaiting surgery so that they would not hear the cries so plainly.

Many kinds of operations were performed before anesthetics were discovered. Among these were the removal of tumors, the opening of abscesses, amputations, the treatment of head wounds, the removal of kidney stones, and cesarean sections and other surgeries during childbirth. The frightful ordeal of "going under the knife," however, often caused patients to delay surgery until it was almost too late. Also, for the surgeon it was nerve-racking to work without anesthetics, trying to operate while the patient screamed and struggled.

Sir Humphry Davy (1778-1829) was a distinguished British chemist who studied the intoxicating effect of a gas called nitrous oxide. While suffering from the pain of an erupting wisdom tooth, he sought relief by inhaling some of the gas. In 1800, he published a paper suggesting the use of nitrous oxide to relieve pain during surgery. There was no follow-up on his idea, however, and it was forgotten until after anesthesia had been discovered independently in America.

The next episode in the history of anesthesiology was the work of Crawford W. Long (1815-1878), a small-town doctor in Georgia. In the early 1800's, "ether frolics" had become popular, in which young people at a party would inhale ether vapor to give them a "high" such as from drinking alcohol. One young man was to have surgery on his neck for a tumor. Long was the town druggist as well as the doctor, so he knew that this fellow had purchased ether and enjoyed its effects. Long suggested that he inhale some ether to ready himself for surgery. On March 30, 1842, the tumor was removed with little pain for the patient. It was the first successful surgery under anesthesia.

Unfortunately, Long did not recognize the great significance of what he had done. He did not report the etherization experiment to his colleagues, and it remained relatively unknown. He used ether a few more times in his own surgical practice, one time while amputating the toe of a young slave. Long finally wrote an article for a medical journal in 1849 telling about his pioneering work, three years after anesthesia had been publicly demonstrated and widely adopted by others.

The story of anesthesiology then moved to Hartford, Connecticut, where a young dentist named Horace Wells (1815-1848) played a major role. P. T. Barnum, of show business and circus fame, was advertising an entertaining "GRAND EXHIBITION of the effects produced by inhaling NITROUS OXIDE or LAUGHING GAS!" Wells decided to attend. He was one of the volunteers from the audience and "made a spectacle of himself," according to his wife.

Another volunteer who had inhaled the gas began to shout and stagger around; finally he ran into a bench, banging his shins against it. The audience laughed, but the observant Wells noticed that the man showed no pain, even though his leg was bleeding. This demonstration gave Wells a sudden insight that a person might have a tooth pulled or even a leg amputated and feel no pain while under the influence of the gas.

Wells became so excited by the idea of eliminating pain that he arranged to have some nitrous oxide gas brought to his office on the next day. Then he had a long talk with a young dentist colleague, John Riggs, about the potential risks of trying it out on a patient. Finally, Wells decided to make himself the first test case, if Riggs would be willing to extract one of his wisdom teeth.

On the morning of December 11, 1844, a bag of nitrous oxide gas was delivered by the man who had been in charge of the previous evening's exhibition. Wells sat in the dental chair and breathed deeply from the gas bag until he seemed to be asleep. Riggs went to work with his long-handled forceps to loosen and finally pull out the tooth, with no outcry from the patient. After a short time, Wells regained consciousness, spit out some blood, and said that he had felt "no more pain than the prick of a pin."

After this success, Wells immediately set to work on further experiments. He acquired the apparatus and chemicals to make his own nitrous oxide. Within the next month, he used the gas on more than a dozen patients. Other dentists in Hartford heard about the procedure and started using it. By the middle of January, 1845, Wells was confident enough to propose a demonstration to a wider audience.

Wells was able to arrange for a demonstration at Massachusetts General Hospital in Boston. While the audience watched, he anesthetized a volunteer patient with gas and extracted his tooth. Unfortunately, the patient groaned at that moment, causing laughter and scornful comments from the onlookers. Wells was viewed as another quack making grandiose claims without evidence. His demonstration had failed, and he returned to Hartford in discouragement. He later commented that he had probably removed the gas bag too soon, before the patient was fully asleep.

It was another dentist, William T. G. Morton (1819-1868), who finally provided a convincing demonstration of anesthesia. Morton tried to obtain some nitrous oxide from a druggist, who did not have any on hand and suggested that ether fumes could be substituted. Morton then used ether on several dental patients, with

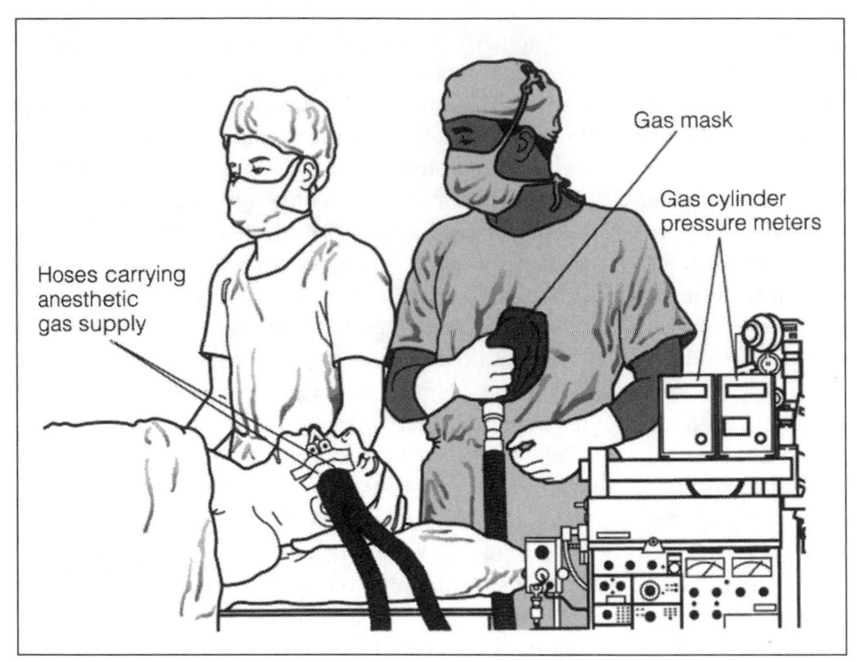

The anesthesiologist, as a crucial team member in every major surgery, must constantly monitor the vital signs and level of consciousness of the anesthetized patient.

excellent results. In 1846, he obtained permission for a demonstration at the same hospital where Wells had failed two years earlier. Famous Boston surgeon John Warren and a skeptical audience watched as Morton instructed a patient to breathe the ether. When the patient was fully asleep, Warren removed a tumor from his neck. To everyone's amazement, there was no outcry of pain during the surgery. After the patient awoke, he said that he felt only a slight scratch on his neck. Warren's words have been recorded for posterity: "Gentlemen, this is no humbug!" Another doctor said, "What we have seen here today will go around the world."

The result of this dramatic demonstration of October 16, 1846, spread quickly to other hospitals in America and Europe. Several hundred surgeries under anesthesia were done in the next year. In England, John Snow experimented with a different anesthetic, chloroform, and began to use it for women in childbirth. In 1853, Queen Victoria took chloroform from Snow during the delivery of her eighth child. Acceptance of anesthesia, and the science of anesthesiology, by the medical profession and the general public grew rapidly.

Science and Profession

Nitrous oxide, ether, and chloroform were the big three anesthetics for general surgery and dentistry for nearly a hundred years after their discovery. All three were administered by inhalation, but there were differences in safety, reliability, and side effects for the patient.

Wells, the dentist who had unsuccessfully tried to demonstrate nitrous oxide anesthesia in 1844, came to a tragic end in 1848 because of chloroform. He was testing the gas on himself to find out what an appropriate dosage should be. Unfortunately, he became addicted to the feeling of intoxication that it gave him. While under the influence of a chloroform binge, he accosted a woman on the street and was arrested. He committed suicide while in prison.

Nitrous oxide is a nearly odorless gas that must be mixed with oxygen to prevent asphyxiation. Storing the gases in large, leakproof bags was awkward. By comparison, ether and chloroform were much more convenient to use because they are liquids that can be stored in small bottles. The liquid was dripped onto a cloth and held over the patient's nose. Ether is hazardous, however, because it is flammable, and it also has a disagreeable odor. Chloroform is not flammable but is more difficult to administer because of the danger of heart stoppage.

Anesthesiology was practiced primarily by dentists, eye doctors, chemists, and all types of surgeons for many years. The Mayo Clinic in Rochester, Minnesota, was one of the first hospitals to recognize the need for specialists to administer anesthesia. In 1904, a nurse from Mayo named Miss Magaw gave a talk on what she had learned from eleven thousand procedures performed under anesthesia. Her concluding comment was that "ether kills slowly, giving plenty of warning, but with chloroform there is not even time to say goodby." Ether takes more time to induce anesthesia, but Miss Magaw asserted that the patient's life was in less danger than from chloroform.

A Scottish physician, James Y. Simpson, was one of the early advocates of using chloroform for partial anesthesia during childbirth. The woman could breathe the vapor intermittently for several hours as needed without the disagreeable odor of ether. She would remain conscious, but the anesthetic apparently produced a kind of amnesia so that the pain was not fully remembered. Simpson received much public acclaim for his help to women in labor, including a title of nobility. (One humorist of the day suggested a coat-of-arms for Sir Simpson, showing a newborn baby with the inscription, "Does your mother know you're out?")

In the 1920's, several new anesthetic gases were created by chemists working closely with medical doctors. The advantages and drawbacks of each new synthesized compound were tested first on animals, then on human volunteers, and finally during surgery. One of the most successful ones was cyclopropane: It was quick-acting and nontoxic and could be mixed with oxygen for prolonged operations. Like other organic gases, however, it was explosive under certain conditions and had to be used with appropriate caution.

A major development in 1928 was the invention of the endotracheal tube by Arthur Guedel. A rubber tube was inserted into the mouth and down the trachea (windpipe) to carry the anesthetic gas and oxygen mixture directly to the lungs. The space around the rubber tube had to be sealed in some way in order to prevent blood or other fluid from going down the windpipe. Guedel's ingenious idea was to surround the tube with a small balloon. When inflated, it effectively closed off the gap between the tube and the trachea wall. He gave a memorable demonstration at a medical meeting using an anesthetized dog with a breathing tube in its throat. After inflating the seal, the dog was submerged under water for several hours and then revived, showing that no water had entered its lungs.

The first local anesthetic was discovered in 1884 by Carl Koller, a young eye doctor in Vienna. He was a colleague of the famous psychoanalyst Sigmund Freud, and together they had investigated the psychic effects of cocaine. Koller noticed that his tongue became numb from the drug. He had the sudden insight that a drop of cocaine solution might be usable as an anesthetic for eye surgery. He tried it on a frog's eye, with much success. Following the tradition of other medical pioneers, he then tried it on himself. The cocaine made his eye numb. Koller published a short article, and the news spread quickly. Within three months, other doctors reported successful local anesthesia, using cocaine for dentistry, obstetrics, and many kinds of general surgery.

Chemists investigated the molecular structure of cocaine and were able to develop synthetic substitutes such as novocaine, which was faster-acting and less toxic. Another improvement was to inject local anesthetic under the skin with a hypodermic needle. With this technique, it was possible to block off pain from a whole region of the body by deadening the nerve fibers. A spinal or epidural block is often used to relieve the pain of childbirth or for various abdominal surgeries.

There is another class of anesthetic drugs called barbiturates which were originally developed for sleeping pills. Any medication that induces sleep automatically becomes a candidate for use as an anesthetic. The most successful barbiturate anesthetic has been sodium pentothal. It is normally administered by injection into a vein in the arm and puts the patient to sleep in a matter of seconds. When the surgery is over, the needle is withdrawn and consciousness returns, with few aftereffects for most people. The anesthesiologist may use sodium pentothal in combination with an inhaled anesthetic if the surgery is expected to be lengthy.

DIAGNOSTIC AND TREATMENT TECHNIQUES

Suppose that a man is scheduled to have some kind of abdominal surgery, such as the repair of a hernia or hemorrhoids or the removal of the appendix, an intestinal blockage, or a cancerous growth. The anesthesiologist would select a sequence of anesthetics that depends primarily on the expected length of the operation and the physical condition of the patient.

About an hour before surgery, the patient receives a shot of morphine to produce relaxation and drowsiness. After he is wheeled into the operating room, the anesthesiologist inserts a needle into a vein in the patient's arm and injects a barbiturate such as sodium pentothal. This drug puts him to sleep very quickly because it is rapidly distributed through the body, but it is not suitable for maintaining anesthesia.

A muscle-paralyzing agent such as curare is now injected, which allows the anesthesiologist to insert an endotracheal tube into the lungs. The tube delivers a mixture of nitrous oxide and oxygen, supplemented with a small amount of other organic additives or of a more potent gas such as ether. The seal around the tube must be inflated to prevent fluids from entering the windpipe. The patient is now in a state of surgical anesthesia.

For a difficult surgery, additional curare may be injected to paralyze the abdominal muscles completely. In this case, the breathing muscles would also become paralyzed, which means that a mechanical respirator would be needed to inflate and deflate the lungs.

The anesthesiologist monitors the patient's condition with various instruments, such as a stethoscope, blood pressure and temperature sensors, and an electrocardiograph (EKG or ECG) with a continuous display. A catheter may be inserted into a vein to inject drugs or to give a blood transfusion if necessary. When the surgery is completed, the anesthesiologist is responsible for overseeing procedures undertaken in the recovery room as the patient slowly regains consciousness.

PERSPECTIVE AND PROSPECTS

Many modern surgeries would be impossible without anesthesia. Kidney or other organ transplants, skin grafts for a burn victim, or microsurgery for a severed finger all require that the patient remain still for an extended period of time. Anesthesiologists choose from a variety of local and general anesthetics as the individual situations require.

In the emergency room of a hospital, patients are brought in with injuries from industrial, farm, or car accidents. Gunshot and knife wounds, the ingestion of toxic chemicals, or sports injuries often require immediate action to reduce pain and preserve life. Soldiers who are wounded or burned in battle can be given relief from pain because of the available anesthetics. Beyond operating room patients, another category of people who benefit greatly from anesthesia are those who suffer from chronic pain, including that from arthritis, back pain, asthma, brain damage, cancer, and other serious ailments.

A more recent innovation is electric anesthesia, which employs an electric current. It is widely used for animals and is gaining acceptance for humans. A marine biologist can submerge two electrodes into water and cause nearby fish to become rigid and unable to swim. After being netted and tagged, the fish are released with no harmful aftereffects. Veterinarians can use a commercially available device with two electrodes that attach to the nose and tail of a farm animal. Pulses of electricity are applied, causing the animal to remain immobilized until surgery is completed.

The most common human application of electric anesthesia is in dentistry. The metal drill itself can act as an electrode, sending pulses of electric current into the nerve to deaden the sensation of pain. The discomfort of novocaine injections and the possible aftereffects of the drug are avoided. Another application is to provide relief for people with chronic back pain, using a small, battery-powered unit attached to the person's waist.

Experiments have been done using electricity for total anesthesia, both on animals and on human volunteers. Electrodes are strapped to the front and back of the head. When an appropriate voltage is applied, the subject falls into deep sleep in a short time. When the electricity is turned off, consciousness is regained almost immediately. In one experiment, two dogs underwent "electrosleep" for thirty days with no apparent ill effects. Long-term studies with more subjects are needed to establish this new technology.

People who have misgivings about becoming a subject for electric anesthesia today perhaps can appreciate the feelings of anxiety that the early volunteers for inhalation anesthesia experienced in the 1840's. Moreover, the contribution of anesthesiology to modern medicine, in all of its forms, has been spectacular when one recalls the suffering of preanesthesia patients.

—Hans G. Graetzer, Ph.D.

See also Acupuncture; Anesthesia; Hypnosis; Narcotics; Neurology; Neurology, pediatric; Nursing; Pain management; Pharmacology; Physician assistants; Surgery, general; Surgical procedures.

FOR FURTHER INFORMATION:

Gregory, George A., ed. *Pediatric Anesthesia.* 4th ed. New York: Churchill Livingstone, 2002. A good text overview of anesthesia for children, accompanied by black-and-white photographs, figures, and diagrams.

Gross, Amy, and Dee Ito. "All About Anesthesia: What Are the Choices When It Comes to Childbirth and Surgery?" *Parents Magazine* 65 (April, 1990): 213-221. A question-and-answer format is used to clarify the differences between spinal, epidural, and general anesthesia during childbirth. Several questions deal with potential recovery problems for mother and baby.

Longnecker, David E., and Frank L. Murphy. *Dripps, Eckenhoff, Vandam Introduction to Anesthesia.* 9th ed. Philadelphia: W. B. Saunders, 1997. This classic text is intended for medical students, anesthesia residents, nurse anesthetists, and nonanesthesia personnel. Each chapter includes a brief list of important references.

Miller, Ronald D., ed. *Miller's Anesthesia.* 6th ed. Philadelphia: Elsevier/Churchill Livingstone, 2005. A mainstay text that examines all aspects of the practice and effects of anesthesia.

Palmer, C. M., M. Paech, and R. D'Angelo, eds. *Handbook of Obstetric Anesthesia.* 6th ed. Oxford, England: Bios Scientific, 2002. An accessible text that outlines a variety of uses of anesthesia during normal and high-risk pregnancies. Topics include maternal physiology and pain pathways, procedures for cesarean sections, and common clinical scenarios such as preeclampsia, obesity, multiple gestation, and coexisting disease.

Postotnik, Pauline. "Anesthesia: A Long Way from Biting Bullets." *FDA Consumer*, June, 1984, pp. 24-27. A brief history of the development of anesthesia. Provides a good overview of sedatives, barbiturates, narcotics, muscle relaxants, and gaseous anesthetics. The monitoring equipment used during surgery is also described.

Rushman, G. B., N. J. H. Davies, and R. S. Atkinson. *A Short History of Anaesthesia*. Oxford, England: Butterworth-Heinemann, 1996. A historical text that examines the first 150 years of the practice of anesthesia. Includes a bibliography and an index.

Sweeney, Frank. *The Anesthesia Fact Book: Everything You Need to Know Before Surgery*. Cambridge, Mass.: Perseus, 2003. Designed to help the health consumer become more informed and confident prior to surgery. Covers topics such as how general anesthesia works and how it differs from twilight, spinal, or epidural anesthesia; the credentials one should look for in an anesthesiologist; and questions that are important to ask prior to surgical procedures.

Wolfe, Richard J. *Tarnished Idol: William Thomas Green Morton and the Introduction of Surgical Anesthesia—A Chronicle of the Ether Controversy*. San Francisco: Norman, 2000. Wolfe provides the first scholarly biography of Morton, the man credited with the first successful public demonstration of anesthesia. This exhaustive work includes much new material.

Aneurysmectomy

Procedure

Anatomy or system affected: Abdomen, brain, chest, heart

Specialties and related fields: Anesthesiology, critical care, emergency medicine, preventive medicine

Definition: A surgical procedure to repair an aneurysm, which occurs when an arterial or venous wall balloons.

Indications and Procedures

An aneurysm occurs when an artery or vein swells as pressure builds within it. Although aneurysms can occur wherever there are arteries or veins, typical occurrences are cranial (called cerebral aneurysms), thoracic, or abdominal. A major cause of aneurysms is a narrowing or blockage of clogged arteries or veins.

People who experience acute aneurysms are sometimes mistaken for stroke victims. Typical indications are a cessation of eye movement accompanied by a drooping of the eyelids and dilation of the pupil, rigidity in the neck, intense headache, and loss of consciousness.

Many aneurysms are repaired through bypass surgery, in which the affected area is clamped shut and excised. The area is then replaced by a section of artery or vein from the patient's leg, which is sutured into place. Controlling blood loss during such surgery is essential. If an aneurysm has ruptured, then numerous blood transfusions are likely to be required during the surgery, and preoperative blood typing is indicated. Patients are anesthetized when the surgeon is ready to make the first incision. A sterile surgical field is of the utmost importance for this procedure. As they are exposed, blood vessels are sealed immediately with hemostats (forceps) to control bleeding.

Uses and Complications

Aneurysmectomies are used to remove weakened tissue in arteries and veins at the site where ballooning has occurred or is imminent. The immediate danger posed by aneurysms is rupture, which can lead quickly to fatal blood loss. It is, therefore, imperative that medical assistance be rendered immediately. Treatment usually involves surgery to remove the aneurysm. In cases requiring emergency surgery, the prognosis is poor.

Aneurysms are sometimes diagnosed through X rays and angiograms before they become symptomatic. Cerebral aneurysms are best detected through computed tomography (CT) scans or magnetic resonance imaging (MRI). When an early diagnosis is made, surgery can be performed under more controlled conditions than those that accompany emergency surgery. For aortic aneurysms, surgery before a rupture occurs usually has a recovery rate of 80 to 90 percent, whereas the recovery rate for surgery performed after an aneurysm has ruptured is less than 5 percent.

An aneurysm that occurs in the aorta is particularly dangerous because it creates a buildup in pressure around the heart so intense that it can cause the heart to stop beating. Although blood loss presents the greatest immediate risk in aneurysmectomy, seizures, cerebral edema, hydrocephalus, and infection may also present significant risks for patients.

—R. Baird Shuman, Ph.D.

See also Aneurysms; Angiography; Brain; Brain disorders; Cardiology; Circulation; Computed tomography (CT) scanning; Craniotomy; Heart; Neurosurgery; Vascular medicine; Vascular system.

For Further Information:

Melander, Sheila Drake, ed. *Case Studies in Critical Care Nursing: A Guide for Application and Review*. 3d ed. Philadelphia: W. B. Saunders, 2004.

Phillips, Nancymarie Fortunato. *Berry and Kohn's Operating Room Technique*. 10th ed. St. Louis: Mosby, 2004.

Phippen, Mark L., and Maryanne Papanier Wells. *Patient Care During Operative and Invasive Procedures*. Philadelphia: W. B. Saunders, 2000.

Aneurysms

Disease/disorder

Anatomy or system affected: Blood vessels, brain, circulatory system, head, heart, nervous system

Specialties and related fields: Cardiology, emergency medicine, general surgery, neurology, vascular medicine

Definition: A localized dilatation of a blood vessel, particularly an artery, that results from a focal weakness and distension of the arterial wall.

Causes and Symptoms

The arterial distension associated with aneurysms will take one of several forms. For example, fusiform aneurysms create a uniform bulge around an artery, while those of the saccular variety distend on one side of the blood vessel. Some saccular aneurysms found in the brain are called berry aneurysms for their protruding shapes.

Hypertension and arteriosclerosis commonly produce dilatation of the thoracic aorta. Very large aneurysms

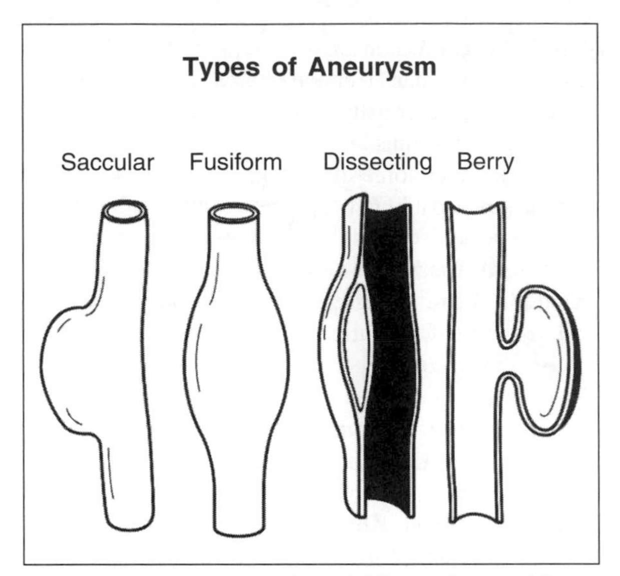

Aneurysms may cause a variety of different shapes of distension of the affected blood vessel.

of the abdominal aorta (possibly the most common type) are usually caused by advanced atherosclerosis. The pathologic processes associated with the production of aortic aneurysms are varied, but certain factors are common to all. The media (middle arterial layer) of the normal aorta must remain intact in order for the aorta to withstand the systolic blood pressure. When the media is damaged, there is progressive dilation of the weakened area and an aneurysm develops. An aortic aneurysm is a serious disease with poor prognosis. Many such aneurysms rupture and cause death before surgical intervention can take place.

There are several types of aneurysms. Dissecting aneurysms are actually hematomas. Blood enters the wall of the aorta and splits the media of the vessel. The dissection of the media usually begins as a transverse tear in the region above the aortic valve. Some believe that hypertension promotes the tear by increasing the tension on the aorta. Traumatic aneurysm is usually caused by penetrating wounds or by blunt trauma; the most common cause of such injuries is automobile accidents. Mycotic aneurysms of the aorta may be associated with bacterial endocarditis and sometimes with organisms such as salmonella. Aneurysms of the sinuses of Valsalva may be attributable to syphilitic aortitis, bacterial endocarditis, or congenital defect.

Information on Aneurysms

Causes: Dilatation of a blood vessel (particularly an artery) from hypertension, arteriosclerosis, blunt trauma, bacterial endocarditis

Symptoms: Often none; sometimes sudden and severe pain, lump, or pulsing sensation near blood vessels

Duration: Acute

Treatments: Surgery

Treatment and Therapy

Surgical therapy for thoracic aortic aneurysms varies with the type and location of the lesion. Aneurysms involving the aortic arch are often surgically corrected by employing a bypass technique. One method sutures a large prosthetic graft between the ascending and descending aortas, thus bypassing the diseased area. Surgical techniques sometimes offer the only hope for the survival of a patient with aneurysm.

—*Jane A. Slezak, Ph.D.*

See also Aneurysmectomy; Arteriosclerosis; Brain; Brain disorders; Bypass surgery; Cardiology; Cardiology, pediatric; Circulation; Heart; Hypertension; Neurology; Neurology, pediatric; Neurosurgery.

For Further Information:

Goldman, Lee, and Dennis Ausiello, eds. *Cecil Textbook of Medicine*. 22d ed. Philadelphia: W. B. Saunders, 2004. A comprehensive text which provides a valuable reference for all diseases, disorders of the nervous and neuromuscular systems, and environmental and physical factors in disease.

Keen, Richard R., and Philip B. Dobrin, eds. *Development of Aneurysms*. Georgetown, Tex.: Landes Bioscience, 2000. A compilation of thirteen papers that explore the pathology, etiology, and epidemiology of aneurysm.

Parker, James N., and Philip M. Parker, eds. *The Official Patient's Sourcebook on Cerebral Aneurysm*. San Diego, Calif.: Icon Health, 2002. Designed for the health consumer and drawn from public, academic, government, and peer-reviewed research, provides a guide for obtaining information covering virtually all topics related to cerebral aneurysm.

Yao, James S. T., and William H. Pearce, eds. *Aneurysms: New Findings and Treatments*. Norwalk, Conn.: Appleton & Lange, 1994. Discusses the diagnosis of aneurysms and therapies to treat them. Includes bibliographic references and an index.

Angina

Disease/disorder

Anatomy or system affected: Circulatory system, heart

Specialties and related fields: Cardiology, family medicine, internal medicine

Definition: Chest pain ranging from mild indigestion to a severe crushing, squeezing, or choking sensation.

Information on Angina

Causes: Arteriosclerosis, coronary artery spasms, low blood pressure, low blood volume, vasoconstriction, anemia, chronic lung disease

Symptoms: Severe crushing, squeezing, or choking sensation in chest

Duration: Often chronic, with three- to five-minute episodes

Treatments: Nitrates, beta-blockers, calcium-channel blockers

Causes and Symptoms

Usually located below the sternum, angina may radiate down the left arm and/or left jaw, or down both arms and jaws. It is ischemic in nature, meaning that the pain is produced by a variety of conditions that result in insufficient supply of oxygen-rich blood to the heart. Some examples include arteriosclerosis (hardening of the arteries), atherosclerosis (arteries clogged with deposits of fat, cholesterol, and other substances), coronary artery spasms, low blood pressure, low blood volume, vasoconstriction (a narrowing of the arteries), anemia, and chronic lung disease.

Precipitating factors for angina include physical exertion, strong emotions, consumption of a heavy meal, temperature extremes, cigarette smoking, and sexual activity. These factors can cause angina because they may increase heart rate, cause vasoconstriction, or divert blood from the heart to other areas, such as the gastrointestinal system. Angina usually lasts from three to five minutes and commonly subsides when the precipitating factors are relieved. Typically, it should not last more than twenty minutes after rest or treatment.

Diagnosis consists of a physical examination which includes a chest X ray to determine any cardiac abnormalities; blood tests to screen risk factors such as lipids or to detect enzymes that can indicate if a heart attack has occurred; electrocardiography (ECG or EKG); nuclear studies such as thallium stress tests, which measure myocardial perfusion; coronary angiography to evaluate the anatomy of the coronary arteries and to note the location and nature of artery narrowing or constriction; cardiac catheterization to measure cardiac output; and Holter monitor studies to evaluate chest pain during the performance of daily activities for a twenty-four-hour period.

Treatment depends on the specific cause of the angina. Three types of drugs are the most common form of treatment: nitrates, to increase the supply of oxygen to the heart by dilating the coronary arteries; beta-blockers, to lower oxygen demand during exercise and improve oxygen supply and demand; and calcium blockers, to decrease the work of the heart by decreasing cardiac contractility.

—*John A. Bavaro, Ed.D., R.N.*

See also Arteriosclerosis; Cardiology; Cardiology, pediatric; Chest; Echocardiography; Heart; Heart attack; Heart disease; Hyperlipidemia; Hypertension; Ischemia; Pain; Thrombosis and thrombus.

For Further Information:

Dranov, Paula. *Random House Personal Medical Handbook: For People with Heart Disease*. New York: Random House, 1991.

McGoon, M. *The Mayo Clinic Heart Book*. 2d ed. New York: William Morrow, 2000.

Pantano, James. *Living with Angina: A Practical Guide to Dealing with Coronary Artery Disease and Your Doctor*. New York: First Books, 2000.

Parker, James M., and Philip M. Parker, eds. *The 2002 Official Patient's Sourcebook on Angina*. San Diego, Calif.: Icon Health, 2002.

Zaret, Barry L., Marvin Moser, and Lawrence S. Cohen, eds. *Yale University School of Medicine Heart Book*. New York: William Morrow, 1992.

Angiography

Procedure

Anatomy or system affected: Blood, blood vessels, brain, circulatory system, head, heart

Specialties and related fields: Cardiology, emergency medicine, radiology, vascular medicine

Definition: The X-ray analysis of the cardiovascular system following the injection of a radiopaque contrast dye into an artery.

Indications and Procedures

Angiography (also called arteriography) is a procedure utilized for the detection of abnormalities in arteries of the heart, brain, or other organs. The procedure is carried out when symptoms suggest the narrowing or blockage of an artery, most frequently in the heart or brain. Such symptoms include chest pain or similarly associated discomfort in the region of the stomach or left side of the body. Even if pain is absent, shortness of breath may indicate a cardiac or pulmonary problem. Slurred speech or vision may likewise suggest narrowing of an artery in the brain. Angiography can therefore indicate the likelihood of a heart attack or stroke, as well as other problems which may produce similar symptoms, such as blood clots or cancer.

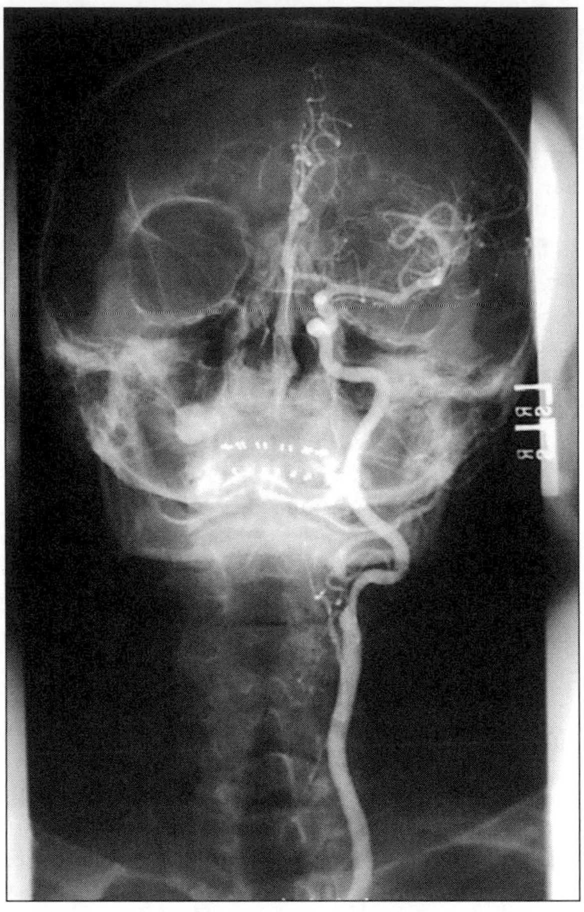

An angiogram showing the path of the carotid artery through the head and neck. (Digital Stock)

The patient must avoid food or drink for approximately eight hours prior to the procedure. A catheter is inserted through the skin, usually in the groin area, and placed into the artery to be examined. A sedative is not necessary, although it may be given to the patient to aid in relaxation.

Once the catheter is in place, a radiopaque dye is injected, and X-ray photographs of the area in question are taken. The procedure generally takes about three hours.

Uses and Complications

Since any blockage or narrowing of an artery will result in accumulation of the radiopaque dye, the radiologist can pinpoint the site of the block. Based on the symptoms, the physician can discuss the diagnosis and recommend further procedures.

The most common complication associated with angiography is the mild discomfort resulting from insertion of the catheter. The dye itself may cause a slight burning sensation, and on rare occasions it may trigger an allergic response. In 1 to 2 percent of cases, more serious complications develop. If the blockage results from an atherosclerotic plaque or from a blood clot, in rare circumstances a piece of this material may break off and lodge elsewhere in the arterial system. The result can be a stroke or heart attack.

—*Richard Adler, Ph.D.*

See also Angioplasty; Arteriosclerosis; Bypass surgery; Cardiology; Catheterization; Circulation; Echocardiography; Heart; Heart attack; Imaging and radiology; Radiopharmaceuticals; Strokes; Vascular medicine; Vascular system.

For Further Information:

Dranov, Paula. *Heart Disease*. New York: Random House, 1990.

Higgins, Charles B., and Albert de Roos. *Cardiovascular MRI and MRA*. Philadelphia: Lippincott Williams & Wilkins, 2002.

Karch, Amy Morrison. *Cardiac Care: A Guide for Patient Education*. New York: Appleton-Century-Crofts, 1981.

Ludinghausen, Michael. *Clinical Anatomy of Coronary Arteries*. New York: Springer, 2003.

Prince, Martin R., et al. *3-D Contrast MR Angiography*. New York: Springer-Verlag, 2003.

Rutherford, Robert B., ed. *Vascular Surgery*. 5th ed. Philadelphia: W. B. Saunders, 2000.

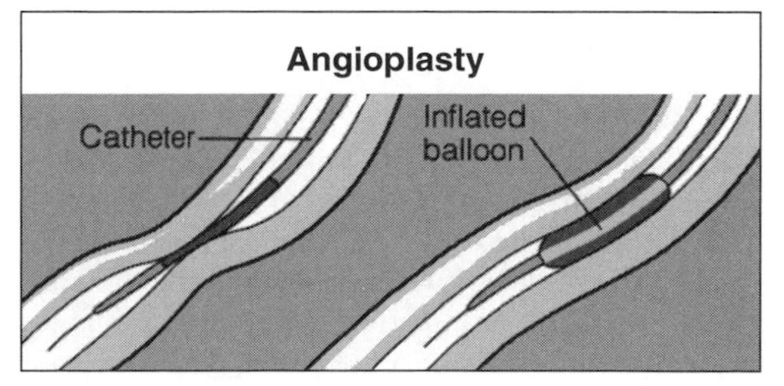

Balloon angioplasty involves the insertion of a catheter into an artery that has narrowed and the inflation of a small balloon in order to expand the vessel; this procedure is usually performed to counteract the effects of atherosclerotic disease, in which plaque deposits accumulate in the arteries.

Angioplasty

Procedure

Anatomy or system affected: Blood vessels, circulatory system, heart

Specialties and related fields: Cardiology, vascular medicine

Definition: The insertion of a long, flexible tube into a narrowed or blocked blood vessel in order to repair it; in balloon angioplasty, a small balloon at the end of the tube is inflated to compress a fatty blockage in the blood vessel and thus increase blood flow.

Indications and Procedures

Angioplasty, particularly balloon angioplasty, may be performed on any blocked or narrowed blood vessel, such as in the legs, but it is most commonly used to open heart valves blocked by coronary artery disease.

More than six million people in the United States have a history of heart disease, a condition often signaled by chest pain known as angina pectoris. Other symptoms include shortness of breath, heart palpitations, or an actual heart attack. Probable causes of heart disease can be diagnosed by stress tests and angiography. If the cause is blockage of the coronary arteries, the cardiologist may order angioplasty to open the blocked vessels and restore a better blood flow to the heart muscle.

The patient cannot eat or drink anything after midnight the day before the procedure is to be performed. A mild sedative may be given. The site for insertion of the catheter, often the inside of the elbow or the groin, is shaved and is cleaned with an antiseptic solution. A local anesthetic is injected at the insertion site, but the patient remains awake during the procedure. The surgeon makes a small opening in the skin at the insertion site, inserts the catheter into an artery, watches the progress of the catheter on an X-ray monitor, and guides the tip into the blocked arteries.

In balloon angioplasty, the most common type, the tube is equipped with a balloon. Once the tip is in place in the blocked area, the balloon is inflated and deflated several times in order to compress the fatty material (plaque) and increase blood flow through the artery. The catheter then is slowly withdrawn.

If the arm site was used, the small incision is stitched closed. If the groin site was used, the puncture opening is closed with pressure. A dressing is applied to the insertion site. Barring any complications, the usual hospital stay is four to seven days.

Uses and Complications

The cardiac catheters used in angioplasty can also remove plaque with special cutting or laser tips. The balloon tip may be used to place a stent, a metal device, permanently in the coronary artery to keep it open.

About 80 percent of the angioplasty treatments are successful, with the patient being able to resume a reasonably normal lifestyle and enjoy a good quality of life. Complications of coronary artery angioplasty seldom occur, but they may include bleeding or clotting, an abnormal heartbeat, perforation of the heart muscle or artery, and, rarely, a heart attack, stroke, or even death.

—*Albert C. Jensen, M.S.*

See also Angina; Angiography; Arteriosclerosis; Bypass surgery; Cardiology; Catheterization; Heart; Heart attack; Heart disease; Heart valve replacement; Palpitations; Stents; Thrombolytic therapy and TPA; Vascular medicine; Vascular system.

For Further Information:

American Heart Association. *AHA Focus Series: Arteriosclerosis*. Washington, D.C.: Author, 1988.

Editors of the University of California, Berkeley, Wellness Letter. *The New Wellness Encyclopedia*. Boston: Houghton Mifflin, 1995.

McGoon, M. *The Mayo Clinic Heart Book*. 2d ed. New York: William Morrow, 2000.

Ohman, Magnus, Gail Folger Cox, and Victoria K. Folger. *So You're Having a Heart Cath and Angioplasty*. New York: Wiley, 2003.

Rutherford, Robert B., ed. *Vascular Surgery*. 5th ed. Philadelphia: W. B. Saunders, 2000.

Tcheng, James E. *Primary Angioplasty in Acute Myocardial Infarction*. Totowa, N.J.: Humana Press, 2002.

Animal rights vs. research

Ethics

Definition: The debate concerning medical research techniques using animals as test specimens in order to obtain information regarding procedures, drugs, or products to be used on human beings.

Key terms:

amyloidosis: a condition characterized by the deposit of waxy substances in animal organs

biomedical research: investigation or experimentation relating to biological, medical, and physical science

biomedicine: the branch of medical science concerned with the capacity of human beings to survive and function in abnormally stressful environments and with the protective modification of such environments

cardiomyopathy: a typically chronic disorder of heart muscle that may involve obstructive damage to the heart

commissurectomy: the removal of a connecting band of tissue in the brain or spinal cord

endocarditis: inflammation of the lining of the heart and its valves

hemophilia: a hereditary blood defect (occurring almost exclusively in males) characterized by delayed clotting of the blood and consequent difficulty in controlling hemorrhage after even minor injuries

neuritis: an inflammatory or degenerative lesion of a nerve, marked by pain and the loss of normal reflexes

toxoplasmosis: an infection caused by parasitic microorganisms that invade tissues and that may cause damage to the central nervous system, especially in infants

uveitis: inflammation of the uvea of the eye

Controversy Surrounding Animal Experimentation

The practice of utilizing animals as test subjects in research has resulted in the informal formation of two basic factions: those who support its role as providing information regarding the contagion and transmission of diseases, their treatment, and their potential cure; and those who deplore the use of animals, citing miserable living conditions for captive animals, which are subjected to painful and debilitating experiments that sometimes result in disfigurement, permanent injury, or death. Those in the first party include doctors, medical researchers, and the patients and their families who have benefited from the information gained. They believe that the performance of experiments on animals has been invaluable, leading to the discovery of many medical treatments and cures for humans afflicted with disease, as well as information related to the risks and benefits of drugs or other products. The second party, often referred to as animal rights activists, is made up of people dedicated to halting the testing and killing of animals in experiments. Groups such as People for the Ethical Treatment of Animals (PETA) and the Animal Liberation Front (ALF) have picketed laboratories, incensed critics, and, in extreme cases, destroyed testing facilities and released the animals kept in them in order to prevent or impede further testing. These groups believe that animals have a right to live in their normal habitats without human intervention.

Since second century Rome, doctors and scientists have conducted experiments on animals, including dissections. The discoveries have yielded untold amounts of information which can be assimilated to human medical conditions. Animal experiments have become so commonplace, however, that animals are sometimes regarded as mere tools in the laboratory. "To me, a monkey was as expendable as a screwdriver or a pair of pliers," indicates Donald Barnes, a former experimental psychologist who has become an animal activist.

Animal rights activists seek an end to animal experimentation, claiming that much of it is unnecessary. According to PETA, the major infectious diseases, such as poliomyelitis, tuberculosis, cholera, and typhoid fever, are dying out in developing countries mostly because of improved living conditions and sanitation, rather than because of vaccines. Furthermore, the ALF reminds scientists that insulin, a treatment for diabetes mellitus that was created using animal research, is not a cure for the disease. Some test procedures, such as scalding or electrocution, are pointless, as the outcome of the experiment is already known. Barnes explains why he was fired from a research position: "One day I refused to carry out a particular military experiment on four perfectly healthy primates, but only because we already knew the answer to the question. It was an invalid experiment, and as the principal investigator I knew that its only purpose was to ensure further funding for the lab."

Animal rights activists can take two different approaches to the issue. The more conventional and more peaceful method is the pursuit of stricter regulations for animal research. In announcements and letters to researchers, activists may state that they are seeking the enactment of laws and regulations that ban all research using animals. Bills to prevent or limit animal research have been introduced in several American states. Other efforts include an attempt to win legal standing to act on behalf of animals and endeavors to divert federal funds earmarked for biomedical research into the development of alternatives for experimentation.

Other activists have taken extreme measures to display their disgust through demonstrations, break-ins, and vandalism to research laboratories across the United States. Such acts cost research firms more than $17 million annually. Damage to the laboratories and equipment and the releasing or stealing of animals impede the research process and call attention to the activists' concerns. The efforts of some of these activists have become increasingly violent, including the use of bombs and other explosives at or near testing facilities. PETA, an organization of more than 325,000 members, says that it disavows violence, but the ALF has actually claimed credit for some of the attacks.

In direct contrast to the activists' perceptions of animal research are doctors, scientists, beneficiaries, and others who argue in favor of animal biomedical testing. According to David Chernof, the former president of the Los Angeles County Medical Association, "Animal research has been the basis for every medical advance which has benefitted humanity in the past 100 years—from insulin to heart surgery to polio and a cure for childhood leukemia." The American Medical Association (AMA) and other medical organizations support the use of animal testing for its importance in advancing the treatment and cure of human diseases. Animals are considered indispensable in biomedical research because of structural similarities between animals and humans, who often react to illnesses in the same way and suffer from many of the same diseases. The AMA actively opposes all laws, regulations, and social protesting that seek to limit such research. The medical field believes that it is only through continued support of the research process, including funding and experimentation, that the United States can continue to be a leader in medical discoveries.

Consumers of a variety of health, hygiene, and beauty products also benefit from animal testing. Such testing has protected consumers from pain, discomfort, and allergic reactions to such products as shampoo, lipstick, and dyes. While testing that does not involve the use of animals often can achieve these goals, sometimes animal testing is the only way to establish the safety of a product for use by humans.

Scientists point out that the information gained from the research often benefits the animals as well. For example, research has shown that feeding monkeys a low-cholesterol diet helps to relieve arteriosclerosis in that particular animal. Other experiments have resulted in the discovery of vaccines to treat infected cattle, poultry, horses, cats, and dogs. In addition, the researchers indicate that the federal government's rules and regulations regarding the housing conditions and care of test animals are so strict that the medical centers probably provide better care for these animals than that received by human patients.

Another group that supports animal biomedical research are the patients who have survived an illness or catastrophe because research had allowed the development of proper treatments, or patients currently receiving treatment. The Incurably Ill for Animal Research (IIFAR), a U.S. organization made up of people suffering from chronic diseases (and their families), supports the humane use of animals for research. In 1990, the group presented the U.S. Congress with a petition signed by 70,000 members requesting that such research be allowed to continue. While the members of IIFAR express regret that animals have been sacrificed, they argue that the technology and information gained have helped many of them cope with illness and receive treatment and have sometimes cured diseases that otherwise would have proven fatal to humans.

Caught in the middle of the controversy are veterinarians, who by trade seek to alleviate pain and illness of animals. Veterinarians are the caretakers of research animals and at the same time are the targets of the campaigns of animal rights activists. The American Veterinary Medical Association basically agrees with the AMA on this issue, but it has not taken such a high-profile role in proclaiming this position. Some veterinarians believe that they are fighting a war of facts versus emotions and that education is the only answer, that the public should be informed that animal welfare is not necessarily equated with animal rights.

A go-between group needs to be established, one that could assuage the fears of animal rights activists while still promoting humane methods of experimentation with animals. One organization, the Physicians for Responsible Medicine, could perhaps lead the way for more answerable research practices.

The Benefits of Animal Research

Whether the use of animals in experiments is ethical is a matter of debate. Not all animal experimentation is equal. The goals of animal experimentation for product safety, such as for cosmetics versus a drug for heart disease, may need to be weighed separately. The merit and the pros and cons may differ substantially in the eyes of both animal testing advocates and animal rights advocates.

Nevertheless, such research has had many successes. Breakthroughs using animal research have resulted in the development of a vaccine for polio, treatments for cancer, safer heart surgery, and even the artificial heart. Some other medical discoveries made through animal research, listed in the *Journal of the American Medical Association*, are in aging, anesthesia, behavioral studies, cardiovascular medicine, the study of hearing (audiology), ophthalmology, organ transplantation, pulmonary medicine, radiology, reproductive biology, virology, and the treatment and study of AIDS, cancer, hemophilia, hepatitis, malaria, rabies, and toxoplasmosis.

Aging. Direct relationships between infections and immunologic disease have made dogs an excellent example to study in cases of amyloidosis. Dogs also serve as models for the study of Alzheimer's disease because of similar pathological changes—an increase in neuritic plaques—seen with Alzheimer's disease in humans. Primates also exhibit this abundance of neuritic plaques. Mice have been used in aging studies because their functional ability declines with age in a fashion similar to that of humans. Rats have been studied extensively for their age-related characteristics and behavior.

Anesthesia. The development of equipment and use of positive-pressure ventilation in performing chest surgery on dogs led to an adapted use for humans. A classic success story in the development of anesthetic techniques was when the first lung cancer patient to have a lung removed survived another forty years.

Behavioral studies. Research involving dogs, rats, and mice provides feedback on environmental adaptation, hereditary characteristics, and learned behaviors. Relationships between behaviors such as fear and stress and between physiological changes such as cardiac rate changes and anorexia nervosa can provide assimilations for humans. Research on depression in primates provides information about sleep disturbances, which can resemble depression and disordered physiology in humans. The study of the communicative abilities of primates helps in the development of teaching practices for mentally retarded children. Animals who suffered from intractable epilepsy have undergone commissurectomy, which has led to the understanding of left-right brain hemisphere cognitive differences in humans. Experiments with rats have shown that obesity shortens the life span. Finally, mice have been utilized as principal research subjects because of the availability of inbred strains and mutants with differing neuroanatomy and biochemistry. Furthermore, the generally short life span of a mouse allows researchers to observe the animal and its changes in its normal lifetime, yielding information within a short time frame.

Cardiovascular medicine. Endocarditis develops naturally in dogs—no inducement or intervention is necessary—and provides scientists with information on bacterial endocarditis in humans. Many inherited cardiovascular problems occur in dogs, and the surgical techniques to correct such defects have also proven effective in humans. Rats develop hypertension spontaneously, increasing with age and occurring more frequently in male rats. Tests of blood pressure controls and the use of antihypertensive agents work on both rats and humans. Cats are used as models to evaluate therapeutic approaches to cardiomyopathy, as well as the role of the liver and how the gastrointestinal tract functions.

Audiology. Hearing loss patterns in mice closely resemble those in humans. The mouse has become an excellent source of information about age-induced hearing loss as well as about the effects of noise exposure.

Ophthalmology. Common retinal diseases such as glaucoma, cataracts, and uveitis occur in dogs; these animals have been used to find effective strategies for alleviating these eye conditions in humans. Cat research involving cataracts has provided information on postsurgical corneal healing. Primates have also been used in the study of vision disorders and visual maturation in children.

Organ transplantation. The first successful kidney transplants were performed on dogs in the late 1950's, which led to correct procedures for human organ transplantation. Studies of tissue rejection in rats can be assimilated to the same affliction in humans.

Pulmonary medicine. Rats have proven valuable in the study of decompression sickness as well as of the effects of air emboli in the lungs. Dogs have been used to study emphysema, pulmonary edema, and thermal burns of the lung associated with fire or the ingestion of chemicals. Lung surgery on dogs led to the development of the pulmonary pump oxygenator.

Radiology. Research in radiology shows that some animals are more sensitive to radiation than others and that survival is dependent on the age when the first dosages of radiation were received.

Reproductive biology. Primates, rats, and mice are excellent subjects for reproductive research, including studies on endocrinology and menstruation. This research has led to advances in fertility control methods for humans. Pregnancy, fetal development, and birth are studied in primates because of their similarities to the human condition of pregnancy. The identification of the Rh factor was an immunological breakthrough resulting from tests on primates.

Virology. Understanding of viral transmissions and diseases has been furnished by research done on mice; these findings have led to the formulation of vaccines for influenza, polio, encephalomyelitis, and rabies.

Acquired immunodeficiency syndrome (AIDS). Simians provide an excellent study population for AIDS because their immunodeficiency symptoms, syndromes, and viruses are almost identical to those of humans. In addition, the AIDS virus itself was isolated in captive rhesus monkeys.

Cancer. One of the first studies of chemotherapy was performed on dogs, which resulted in the knowledge that some cancers may be caused by infectious agents. Cats are used as subjects in breast cancer studies because of similarities in structure to humans. In addition, rats and mice are used extensively in cancer research, especially in the study of tumors and in the screening of carcinogenic (cancer-causing) compounds.

Hemophilia. Hemophilia in dogs is nearly identical to that in humans, so the dog has served as a model for this research. The first successful bone marrow transplant occurred in laboratory mice and served as the example for such transplants in humans.

Hepatitis. The dog is used as a research subject because viral hepatitis occurs naturally in dogs. The dog also is used for comparative studies of cirrhosis of the liver. Research involving chimpanzees led to the discovery of the hepatitis B vaccine.

Malaria. Potential therapies for malaria, which affects 200 million people worldwide, can be discovered through tests on primates.

Rabies. The original vaccine produced for the treatment of rabies resulted from experimentation on rabbits.

Toxoplasmosis. The study of cats infected with toxoplasmosis has led to treatments for the 4,500 human babies born annually in the United States with this infection.

PERSPECTIVE AND PROSPECTS

Through the use of animals as test subjects, benefits have been gained for both humans and animals. Many therapies and cures have been discovered through careful experimentation with animals in which a particular animal is found to be suited to a particular test. Animal research has been performed for centuries, and the information gleaned from the procedures has provided modern medicine with many vaccines and treatments that probably would not have been possible without such research.

Animal rights activists have struck a nerve in the field of research and have increased awareness among animal researchers about ensuring the use of humane methods of experimentation. Continued dialogue between these groups will be necessary to avoid the halting of important medical research and to discourage the unnecessary use of animals when other methods are available.

—*Carol A. Holloway;*
updated by Nancy A. Piotrowski, Ph.D.

See also American Medical Association (AMA); Ethics; Laboratory tests; National Institutes of Health; Veterinary medicine.

For Further Information:

Breo, Dennis L. "Animal Rights vs. Research? A Question of the Nation's Scientific Literacy." *The Journal of the American Medical Association* 264 (November 21, 1990): 2564. An excellent source of information regarding all aspects of animal biomedical research.

Cohen, Carl, and Tom Regan. *The Animal Rights Debate*. Lanham, Md.: Rowman and Littlefield, 2001. An exploration of the philosophical debate with the authors representing the opposite poles.

Cooke, Patrick. "A Rat Is a Pig Is a Dog Is a Boy: The Debate over Animal Rights Is Full of Equations That Don't Add Up." *Health* 5 (July/August, 1991): 58-64. An excellent article examining the highly emotional issue of animal experimentation in medical research.

Fox, James G., et al., eds. *Laboratory Animal Medicine*. 2d ed. New York: Elsevier, 2002. A text that covers the biological and disease aspects of laboratory animal medicine. Also explores the biohazards associated with the use of animal experimentation and factors complicating the bioethics of animal research.

Groves, Julian McAllister. *Hearts and Minds: The Controversy over Laboratory Animals*. Philadelphia: Temple University Press, 1997. This book describes the controversies involved in the use of laboratory animals for different types of testing.

Jackson, Christine. "Dissection: Science or Violence?" *Mothering*, no. 9 (Spring, 1991): 91. A list of sources for further information is provided at the end of the article, as well as a directory of sources offering alternatives to the dissection of animals.

Kistler, John M., and Marc Bekoff. *Animal Rights: A Subject Guide, Bibliography, and Internet Companion*. Westport, Conn.: Greenwood Press, 2000. A comprehensive bibliography of 916 annotated entries that cover a range of topics surrounding animal rights, from vegetarianism to vivisection to feminist perspectives. Topic discussions are balanced and accompanied by Web page information that lists reviews, related articles, and books available online.

Rudacille, Deborah. *The Scalpel and the Butterfly: The War Between Animal Research and Animal Protection*. New York: Farrar, Straus & Giroux, 2000. In this useful survey, Rudacille takes a middle ground between biomedical researchers who defend animal experimentation and animal rights activists who would abolish such research.

Sterna, James P. *Earth Ethics: Introductory Readings on Animal Rights, and Environmental Ethics*. 2d ed. Upper Saddle River, N.J.: Prentice Hall, 2000. An anthology of writings that explore the opposing debates of a range of ethical issues, including the use of animals for scientific research.

Wise, Stephen M. *Drawing the Line: Science and the Case for Animal Rights*. Cambridge, Mass.: Perseus, 2002. The former president of the Animal Legal Defense Fund explores the intelligence and abilities of myriad animals in an effort to demonstrate how animals often meet the criteria for legal personhood.

Anorexia nervosa

Disease/disorder

Anatomy or system affected: Brain, endocrine system, gastrointestinal system, hair, heart, immune system, kidneys, musculoskeletal system, nails, nervous system, psychic-emotional system, reproductive system, skin

Specialties and related fields: Family medicine, neurology, nutrition, psychiatry, psychology

Definition: Self-induced malnutrition resulting in a body weight 15 percent or more below normal for age and height, and, in women, characterized by the absence of three or more consecutive menstrual periods.

Key terms:

eating disorder: weight gain or loss resulting from compulsive overeating, anorexia nervosa, or bulimia

obsessive-compulsive: having a preoccupation with a specific idea (such as body image) and showing uncontrollable related behavior (such as dieting)

refeeding: the reintroduction of nutritional substances into the diet of a patient suffering from malnutrition

Causes and Symptoms

Anorexia nervosa is an obsessive-compulsive disorder characterized by a body weight at or below 85 percent of normal and an intense fear of weight gain. Anorexia nervosa is typically a physical manifestation of under-

Information on Anorexia Nervosa

Causes: Emotional and psychological disorders pertaining to body image
Symptoms: Extreme weight loss, amenorrhea, malnutrition, forgetfulness, attention deficits, confusion, fatigue, apathy, irritability, brittle nails, hair loss, dry skin, cold hands and feet
Duration: Chronic
Treatments: Medical refeeding, individual and/or family counseling, antidepressants

lying emotional conflicts such as guilt, anger, and poor self-image. Eating disorders such as anorexia nervosa are the third most common chronic condition among girls ages fifteen to nineteen. Approximately 90 percent of people with anorexia are female.

Anorexia nervosa often occurs following a successful dieting experience, and frequent dieting may contribute to the development of the disorder. Dieters may experience positive feedback regarding weight loss and feel compelled to continue losing weight.

Although the term "anorexia" means "loss of appetite," most anorexics continue to experience hunger but ignore the body's normal craving for food. Anorexics frequently identify specific areas of the body that they believe are "fat," despite their emaciated condition. Secrecy and ritual eating habits may be signs of anorexia nervosa. Sufferers often lie to family and friends to avoid eating meals and may eat only a set diet at a specific time of day.

Many people with anorexia are high achievers, exhibiting perfectionist or "people-pleasing" personalities. In addition, a strong correlation exists between anorexia nervosa and athletic activities that emphasize the physique, such as track, tennis, gymnastics, cheerleading, and dance. People with anorexia may demonstrate additional obsessive-compulsive behaviors such as weighing themselves and/or examining themselves in the mirror several times per day, being overly concerned with calorie or fat content, exercising compulsively, maintaining unusually consistent eating patterns, and kleptomania (compulsive stealing).

Anorexia nervosa is frequently a symptom of depression, and the accompanying weight loss can be seen as a cry for help. Eating disorders tend to run in families, particularly those that equate thinness with success and happiness. The condition may also occur as a result of a traumatic situation such as death, divorce, pregnancy, or sexual abuse.

Symptoms and resulting physical conditions include amenorrhea, the abnormal interruption or absence of menstrual discharge, which can occur when body fat drops below 23 percent. Anorexia nervosa may also be characterized by a distended abdomen as a result of a buildup of abdominal fluids and the slowing of the digestive system.

Resulting malnutrition can impair the immune system and cause anemia or decreased white blood cell counts. Brain and central nervous system functions may also be affected, resulting in forgetfulness, attention deficits, and confusion. Anorexics frequently experience fatigue, apathy, irritability, and extreme emotions.

Additional symptoms can include thyroid abnormalities, fainting spells, irregular heartbeat, brittle nails, hair loss, dry skin, cold hands and feet, hypotension (low blood pressure), infertility, broken blood vessels in the face, and the growth of downy body hair called lanugo as the body attempts to insulate itself because of the loss of natural fat.

The occurrence of eating disorders in adolescents is especially dangerous because the condition can retard growth and delay or interrupt puberty. Anorexia nervosa can also result in the erosion of heart muscle, which lowers the heart's capacity and can lead to congestive heart failure. Anorexics may experience musculoskeletal problems such as muscle spasms, atrophy, and osteoporosis as a result of potassium and calcium deficiencies. In extreme cases, patients may also experience kidney failure.

Treatment and Therapy

Treatment of anorexia nervosa generally consists of medical treatment, including electrolyte balance, and diagnosing and addressing any related health problems, such as heart problems, depression, and osteoporosis; psychotherapy, either group, family, individual, or some combination; and nutrition counseling, as most people with anorexia need to focus away from weight loss and toward nutritional gain.

Research indicates that eating disorders are one of the psychological problems least likely to be treated, and anorexia nervosa has the highest mortality rate of all psychosocial problems. The National Institute of Mental Health estimates that one in ten anorexia cases ends in death from starvation, suicide, or medical complications such as heart attacks or kidney failure.

Psychologists play a vital role in the successful treatment of eating disorders and are integral members of the multidisciplinary team that may be required to provide patient care. As part of this treatment, a physician may be called on to rule out medical illnesses and determine that the patient is not in immediate physical danger. A nutritionist may be asked to help assess and improve nutritional intake.

It is frequently necessary first to treat the acute physical symptoms associated with anorexia nervosa. Most patients—especially those with severe cases—benefit from treatment in a controlled environment that allows medically supervised "refeeding" to achieve a target rate of weight gain. Less severe cases may be treated on an outpatient basis.

During the initial phase of refeeding, the patient may receive a low-calorie diet to avoid overwhelming low-functioning organs. Patients who do not comply with the recommended diet may receive caloric supplements and, in serious cases, intravenous feeding.

Successful treatment also involves resolution of underlying emotional conflicts through individual and/or family counseling and may also include use of antidepressants such as fluoxetine (Prozac).

Anorexia nervosa is extremely difficult to treat, with a fatality rate of 5 percent to 10 percent within ten years. Nearly half of all sufferers never recover fully from the condition.

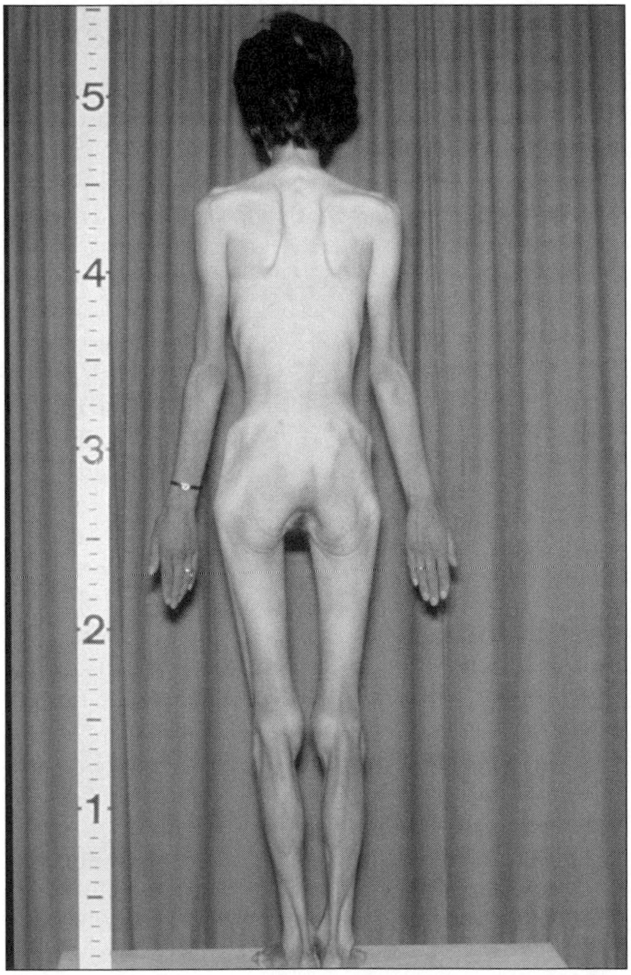

A woman suffering from severe anorexia nervosa. (Custom Medical Stock Photo)

Perspective and Prospects

Anorexia is a multifaceted problem that has physical, emotional, and cultural components. More than three-quarters of adolescent girls in the United States report being unhappy with their bodies and, on average, 25 percent of women are on a diet at any given time.

Most eating disorders were not recognized as illnesses until the late nineteenth century. Conditions such as anorexia nervosa gained the attention of medical professionals during the 1960's and beyond as a result of the media's obsession with thinness.

The media are prime contributors to this trend. Television and magazines send confusing messages to young consumers, such as depicting painfully thin models promoting high-fat snacks. Most models weigh about 23 percent less than the average American woman, and up to 60 percent of models suffer from eating disorders. In addition, the media frequently portray overweight people as having a lower socioeconomic status than people who are thin. Obese people are generally portrayed as comical, while thin people are often depicted as more intelligent, sophisticated, and successful, and as happier with their lives.

It appears likely that the incidence of eating disorders will continue to escalate as the media persist in depicting an idealized female body image significantly below normal body weight.

—*Cheryl Pawlowski, Ph.D.;*
updated by LeAnna DeAngelo, Ph.D.

See also Addiction; Amenorrhea; Anxiety; Appetite loss; Bulimia; Depression; Eating disorders; Hyperadiposis; Malnutrition; Menstruation; Nutrition; Obesity; Obesity, childhood; Obsessive-compulsive disorder; Psychiatric disorders; Psychiatry, child and adolescent; Puberty and adolescence; Sports medicine; Stress; Vitamins and minerals; Weight loss and gain; Weight loss medications; Women's health.

For Further Information:

Broccolo-Philbin, Anne. "An Obsession with Being Painfully Thin." *Current Health 2* 22, no. 5 (January, 1996): 23. Bulimia and anorexia nervosa are two eating disorders that affect young people. Depression can be a major factor in determining whether a person develops an eating disorder, as can a poor self-image.

Brumburg, Joan Jacobs. *Fasting Girls: The History of Anorexia Nervosa*. Rev. ed. New York: Vintage Books, 2000. An award-winning exploration of the history of women's ambiguous relationship with food, tracing the problem back to the sixteenth century and examining the modern medical and social aspects of the problem.

Costin, Carolyn. *The Eating Disorder Sourcebook*. 3d ed. New York: McGraw-Hill, 2006. Costin is the director of an eating disorders clinic, and a recovered anorexic person. The book offers unique information about risk factors, prevention, medications, and various treatment for eating disorders.

Gordon, Richard A. *Eating Disorders: Anatomy of a Social Epidemic*. 2d ed. Malden, Mass.: Blackwell Scientific, 2000. Explores the roles that biological factors, sexual abuse, and the fashion industry play in eating disorders; new findings about males with eating disorders; and how eating disorders are shaped in children.

Lucas, Alexander R. *Demystifying Anorexia Nervosa: An Optimistic Guide to Understanding Healing*. New York: Oxford, 2004. Offers comprehensive guidance on the most effective treatments for anorexia nervosa.

National Association of Anorexia Nervosa and Associated Disorders. http://www.anad.org/site/anadweb/. A site that provides hotline counseling, a national network of free support groups, referrals to health care professionals, and education and prevention programs to promote self-acceptance and healthy lifestyles.

Parker, James N., and Philip M. Parker, eds. *The 2002 Official Patient's Sourcebook on Binge Eating Disorder*. San Diego, Calif.: Icon Health, 2002. Draws from public, academic, government, and peer-reviewed research to provide a wide-ranging handbook for patients with eating disorders.

Anthrax

Disease/disorder

Also known as: Woolsorter's disease

Anatomy or system affected: Gastrointestinal system, immune system, nervous system, respiratory system, skin

Specialties and related fields: Bacteriology, critical care, dermatology, emergency medicine, internal medicine, microbiology, pathology

Definition: A bacterial infection of humans and other animals, especially herbivores, which occurs following entrance into the body of *Bacillus anthracis* spores through abrasions in the skin or by ingestion or inhalation.

Key terms:

eschar: a thick, crusty, blackish skin lesion that follows a burn, other injury, or some unusual types of infection; derived from the Greek *eschara*, meaning "fireplace"

spores: highly resistant structures produced by certain gram-positive bacteria under environmental pressure to allow survival until more favorable conditions exist

virulence: the degree of pathogenicity, or ability to cause disease; derived from the Latin *virulentus*, meaning "full of poison"

Causes and Symptoms

The bacterium that causes anthrax is a large, encapsulated, gram-positive rod which produces exotoxins and spores. The capsule and exotoxins are important virulence factors, and both are necessary for disease to occur. Spores are ellipsoidal or oval and are located within the bacilli. The endospores have no reproductive significance, as only one spore is formed by each bacillus and a germinated spore yields a single bacillus. Spores form in soil or dead tissue and with no measurable metabolism may remain dormant for years. They are resistant to drying, heat, and many disinfectants.

Anthrax is primarily a disease of herbivorous animals that has spread to humans through association with domesticated animals and their products. Herbivorous animals grazing in pastures with soil contaminated with endospores become infected when the spores gain entry through abrasions around the mouth and germinate in the surrounding tissues. Omnivores and carnivores can become infected by ingesting contaminated meat. Human infection is often a result of a close association with herbivores, particularly goats, sheep, or cattle (including their products of hair, wool, and hides). Anthrax has been an uncommon infection in the United States, and only 233 human cases were reported from 1955 to 1987.

The most common clinical illness in humans is skin infection acquired when spores penetrate through cuts or abrasions. After an incubation period of three to five days, a papule develops and evolves into a vesicle, which ruptures to leave an ulcer that dries to form a characteristic black eschar. Inhaled spores reach the alveoli of the lung, where they are engulfed by macrophages and germinate into bacilli. Bacilli are carried to lymph nodes, where release and multiplication are followed by bloodstream invasion and spread to other parts of the body, including the brain, causing meningitis. The illness begins with flulike symptoms a few days after the inhalation of anthrax spores and may be associated with substernal (under the breastbone) discomfort. Cough, fever, chills, and respiratory distress with dyspnea (abnormal or uncomfortable breathing) and stridor (noisy breathing) ensue. The least common type of infection is that of the gastrointestinal tract.

The laboratory criteria for the diagnosis of anthrax are cultural growth of *Bacillus anthracis* from a clinical specimen collected from an affected tissue or site or other supportive laboratory data, such as polymerase chain reaction (PCR), immunohistochemical staining, or serology that shows evidence of anthrax infection.

Treatment and Therapy

Antibiotic treatment of cutaneous anthrax does not change the course of the evolving skin lesion, but it reduces edema (swelling) and systemic symptoms such as fever, headache, and malaise which may be part of the illness. Antibiotic therapy is also initiated to prevent complications from spreading infection and, most important, bloodstream invasion. The mortality rate of cutaneous infection with appropriate antibiotic treatment is less than 1 percent. Virtually all patients with

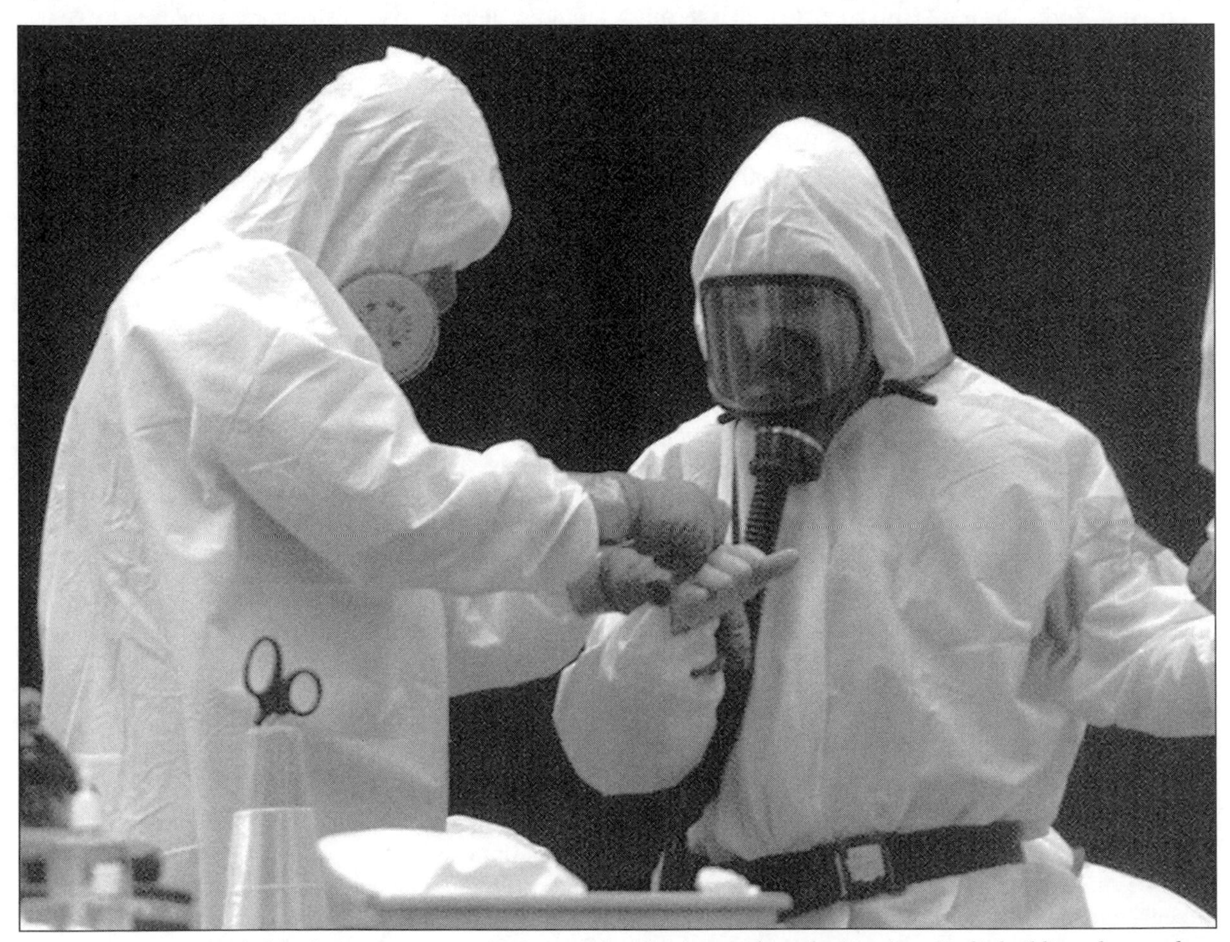

In October, 2001, a firefighter decontaminates an FBI agent after they emerge from the American Media building where anthrax sent through the mail caused the death of a photo editor. (AP/Wide World Photos)

inhalation anthrax will die if untreated. Antibiotic therapy, especially if administered during the early part of this biphasic illness, combined with other intensive supportive measures, may save up to 50 percent of patients, although long-term effects may be noted. The paucity of gastrointestinal anthrax cases has resulted in limited mortality data, but mortality has been estimated to be as high as 50 percent, with disease limited to the mouth and throat having a better prognosis. If recovery ensues, the disease subsides within two weeks. Antibiotic therapy is indicated for all cases.

Initial antibiotic therapy is with either ciprofloxacin or doxycline, plus one or two additional antibiotics for more severe cases until the patient is stable. Prolonged antibiotic therapy (one hundred days) is indicated for more serious illness. Antibiotics may also be used to prevent illness in the case of possible exposure, and an anthrax vaccine is available for persons at high risk of exposure.

PERSPECTIVE AND PROSPECTS

A disease killing cattle in 1491 B.C.E., likely to have been anthrax, is recounted in the Book of Genesis. In Exodus 9, the Lord instructs Moses to take "handfuls of ashes of the furnace" and "sprinkle it toward the heaven in the sight of the Pharaoh." Moses performed the deed, and "it became a boil breaking forth with blains upon man and upon beast." This may represent the first use of anthrax as a biological agent. Greek peasants tending goats suffered from anthrax. *Anthrax* in Greek means "coal," which refers to the coal-black center of the skin lesion.

Anthrax was the first pathogenic bacillus to be seen microscopically when it was described in infected animal tissue by Aloys-Antoine Pollender in 1849. Studies by Robert Koch in 1876 resulted in the four postulates which form the basis for the study of infectious disease causation. In 1881, Louis Pasteur demonstrated the protective efficacy of a vaccine for sheep made with his attenuated vaccine strain.

Anthrax spores can be easily packaged to act as aerosolized agents of war, and the genome may be bioengineered to alter the virulence of anthrax or the ability of current vaccines to protect against it. In 1979, anthrax spores were accidentally released from a Soviet biowarfare facility in the city of Sverdlovsk, resulting in at least seventy-seven human cases, with sixty-six deaths. In the United States, a bioterrorism attack with anthrax spores placed in letters and sent through the mail caused twenty-two cases, with five deaths, in 2001.

INFORMATION ON ANTHRAX

CAUSES: Infection with bacterial spores through skin or by ingestion or inhalation

SYMPTOMS: After skin exposure, vesicle that ruptures to leave an ulcer; after inhalation, flulike symptoms a few days later (cough, fever, chills, respiratory distress); systemic spread causes fever, headache, malaise, and sometimes meningitis

DURATION: Two weeks, with long-term effects; inhalation type often fatal

TREATMENTS: Prolonged antibiotic therapy and intensive supportive measures

In the future, more rapid molecular based diagnostic methods promise to identify cases earlier so that appropriate antibiotic therapy can be initiated, ensuring a maximum opportunity for recovery. A need also exists for safer and more effective vaccines that would offer protection even against bioengineered strains.

—*H. Bradford Hawley, M.D.*

See also Bacterial infections; Bacteriology; Biological and chemical weapons; Epidemiology; Immunization and vaccination; Microbiology; Toxicology; Zoonoses.

FOR FURTHER INFORMATION:

Bartlett, John G., Thomas V. Inglesby, Jr., and Luciana Borio. "Management of Anthrax." *Clinical Infectious Diseases* 35 (October 1, 2002): 851-858.

Centers for Disease Control and Prevention. "Bioterrorism-Related Anthrax." *Emerging Infectious Diseases* 8 (October, 2002): 1013-1183.

Dixon, Terry C., et al. "Anthrax." *New England Journal of Medicine* 341 (September 9, 1999): 815-826.

ANTIBIOTICS

TREATMENT

ANATOMY OR SYSTEM AFFECTED: All

SPECIALTIES AND RELATED FIELDS: Bacteriology, immunology, microbiology, pharmacology

DEFINITION: The use of drugs that are selectively toxic to microorganisms.

KEY TERMS:

chemotherapeutic index: for antibiotics, the ratio of the maximum dose that can be administered without causing serious damage to a person to the minimum dose that will cause serious damage to the infecting microorganism; a measure of selective toxicity

minimal inhibitory concentration: the amount of an antibiotic needed to inhibit the growth of a microorganism in the laboratory; may be correlated to the dose of the antibiotic needed to control an infection

normal microbiota: the collection of microorganisms that inhabit tissues of healthy persons and that to some degree establish environments hostile to pathogens (the causative agents of disease)

resistance determinants: genes found in some bacteria that permit them to resist the action of particular antibiotics; these genes can be transferred between cells, allowing rapid spread of antibiotic resistance among bacteria

semisynthetic: used to refer to natural products, such as antibiotics, that have been chemically modified to be more useful for a particular application

spectrum of activity: the range of microbial species that can be inhibited by an antibiotic; broad-spectrum antibiotics can control more than one kind of infection, but narrow-spectrum antibiotics avoid unintentional damage to the normal microbiota

superinfection: an infection caused by destruction of the normal microbiota by antibiotic therapy, which allows for proliferation of a pathogen other than the one targeted by the antibiotic

Indications and Procedures

Humans live in the midst of a microbial world of bacteria, fungi, and protozoa. Microorganisms were the first inhabitants of the earth. When multicellular animals arose, some microbes adapted to use them as a source of nutrients. Most of these microorganisms did no harm to their hosts. In fact, humans carry around bacteria numbering in the trillions. Some were not as harmless and possessed the means to penetrate tissues and invade internal organs. As a result, animals evolved a variety of defensive strategies, referred to as immune responses, to resist such invasion. Infections develop when these responses fail to repel the invaders. To combat such infections, humans can turn to antibiotics for help.

Antibiotics are drugs that kill, or inhibit the reproduction of, microorganisms. In the strict use of the term as defined by Selman Waksman, the discoverer of streptomycin, an antibiotic is "a chemical substance produced by microorganisms which has the capacity to inhibit the growth of bacteria and even destroy bacteria and other microorganisms in dilute solution." In everyday communication, however, use of the term has been expanded to include a variety of synthetic and semisynthetic chemicals exhibiting antimicrobial activity.

The effectiveness of antibiotics arises from their selective toxicity, which relies on differences between the fundamental biology of pathogenic microorganisms and that of an infected person. The sulfonamides, or sulfa drugs, the first class of antimicrobial compounds to achieve widespread use, are chemically similar to molecules used by bacteria for the synthesis of folic acid, an essential vitamin. When sulfonamides are present, they interfere with folic acid synthesis, preventing growth of the bacteria. Because humans lack the ability to synthesize folic acid (which is obtained from food), their cells are unaffected by sulfonamides. The beta-lactams, a class of antimicrobial chemicals that includes the penicillins and cephalosporins, interfere with the synthesis of peptidoglycan, an essential component of bacterial cell walls that is totally lacking in human cells. Other antibiotics target unique aspects of microbial protein synthesis and nucleic acid metabolism. Antibiotics are sometimes used in combination; for example, beta-lactams may be used to weaken bacterial cell walls, promoting access of a second antibiotic directed against an internal target.

The clinical microbiology laboratory can assist physicians in determining appropriate antibiotic therapy by identifying infectious agents and determining the susceptibility or resistance of the agent to a range of potential antibiotics. An increased need for such services has accompanied the evolution of pathogenic microorganisms in response to the use of antibiotics. In the early days of antimicrobial chemotherapy, it was often sufficient to diagnose an infection from its symptoms, from which one could infer the type of microorganism causing the infection (for example, gram-positive or gram-negative bacteria) and prescribe one of a limited number of broad-spectrum agents with confidence that it would be effective. Today, while immediate application of broad-spectrum antibiotics may be called for to contain a serious infection, concern over creating resistant pathogens leads more physicians to request the identification and testing of microorganisms. Furthermore, the extensive resistance encountered among pathogens suggests that a broad-spectrum agent may be ineffective.

Advances in clinical microbiology are directed toward increasing the speed and accuracy of the identification of infectious agents, with a primary goal of providing information useful in prescribing antimicrobial

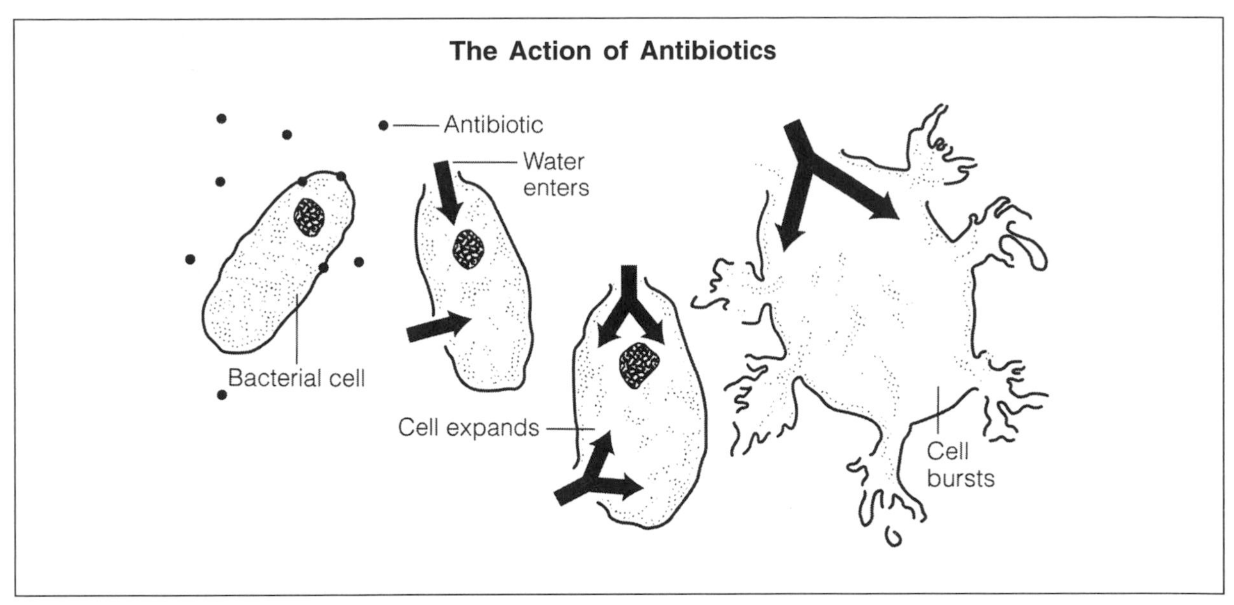

An antibiotic destroys a bacterium by causing its cell walls to deteriorate; water will then enter the bacterium unchecked until it bursts.

chemotherapy. Clinical samples (infected fluids, biopsy samples, or tissue swabs) are used to inoculate selective and differential media that favor the growth of a suspected pathogen. Material from isolated colonies is then subjected to a variety of tests designed to characterize aspects of the microorganism's physiology and metabolic biochemistry, which provide criteria for the taxonomic identification of the organism. While some smaller laboratories rely on the manual inoculation of test media and reference to printed diagnostic tables for identification, the trend is toward greater automation to allow more rapid processing of multiple samples. Panels of test media prepared in multiwell plates can be simultaneously inoculated, and because many of the tests are evaluated by color changes, test results can be read with spectrophotometers designed to scan the individual tests. Test data are entered into computer programs that match the test results with probability matrices to provide a probable identification of the organism used to inoculate the tests. In the largest laboratories, efficiency can be enhanced by using robotics to conduct many of the steps, from inoculation to the reporting of test results and probable identification.

While automation can help to speed up the rate at which test information is obtained, classic identification tests are limited by the need for the incubation and growth of the test organism; this limitation can be particularly burdensome in the case of microorganisms that are especially slow-growing, among which are the mycobacteria that cause tuberculosis. In response, laboratories increasingly rely on identification methods that allow direct examination of the microorganism. Serological tests, which use antibodies directed against antigens specific to a particular microbe, and DNA probes, targeted to species-specific genes, are being applied to an increasing range of pathogenic microorganisms. Some of these tests have advanced to the point that infectious agents can be identified directly in clinical samples, circumventing the need for isolation in the laboratory.

In evaluating the susceptibility of a microorganism to an antibiotic, microbiologists seek to determine the minimal inhibitory concentration (MIC) at which an antibiotic will inhibit the growth of the microbe in a standard growth medium; the MIC can be correlated with an effective dose of the antibiotic. In broth dilution tests, a defined number of microbial cells is inoculated into a series of broth tubes containing different concentrations of an antibiotic; the MIC is reported as the lowest concentration of the antibiotic that prevents growth of the organism in the broth. The same technologies used to automate identification can be used to allow a large number of broth dilution tests to be carried out in multiwell plates, so that susceptibility to a range of antibiotics can be determined simultaneously.

Where automation is unavailable, broth dilution testing is impractical because of the labor involved, and laboratories may rely on an indirect method called a disk diffusion test, or Kirby-Bauer assay. In this method, disks of filter paper impregnated with a defined amount of antibiotic are placed on a plate of solid growth medium that has been seeded with cells of the microorganism being tested. During incubation, the antibiotic diffuses from the disk, leading to a gradient of antibiotic concentration extending in all directions from the disk. If the microbe is susceptible to the antibiotic, its growth will be inhibited in a circular zone surrounding the disk; the diameter of the zone of inhibition varies directly with the MIC for that antibiotic. As with traditional identification methods, tests for antibiotic susceptibility are limited by the requirement that the test organism be allowed time to grow in the laboratory. It is likely that commercial DNA probes will be developed to allow the direct detection of genes that encode resistance to individual antibiotics.

USES AND COMPLICATIONS

Given the importance of differences between the biology of infectious microorganisms and the biology of the infected host to the effectiveness of antibiotics, it is not surprising that antibiotics have been used most successfully to control infections caused by bacteria, whose molecular and cellular biology differs vastly from that of humans. Consequently, most antibiotics directed against bacteria show a favorable chemotherapeutic index, which is the ratio of the maximum dose that can be administered without causing serious harm to the recipient of the drug to the minimum dose that will be effective in controlling the infection.

Infections caused by eukaryotic fungi and protozoa are particularly difficult to treat because of the similarities between the cell structure and function of these organisms and those of human cells. While the topical application of antifungal agents such as miconazole is very effective in the treatment of fungal skin infections and vaginal candidiasis, the treatment of systemic fungal infections (usually with amphotericin B) is much more difficult to perform and is more likely to cause serious side effects. Similar complications accompany efforts to treat protozoal infections with antimicrobial agents; this situation is especially frustrating, since parasitic infections such as malaria and schistosomiasis pose a major worldwide health problem. The number of methods available for the chemical treatment of viral infections is extremely limited, in view of the fact that viruses rely on the molecular machinery of the infected host for their reproduction. One antiviral strategy that has met with limited success is to design nucleotide analogues that interfere with viral nucleic acid synthesis; both acyclovir, used for infections caused by the herpes simplex virus, and azidothymidine, the first agent shown to affect the course of human immunodeficiency virus (HIV) infection, belong to this class of drugs.

In addition to potential toxicity, other factors need to be considered when choosing an antibiotic for treatment of a particular infection. Attention must be given to the fate of an antibiotic once it is administered, so that a sufficient concentration is maintained at the site of infection. If an antibiotic is administered orally, then it must be able to survive the environment of the gastrointestinal tract in order to reach the targeted tissues. Only certain antibiotics are able to cross the blood-brain barrier for effective treatment of infections of the central nervous system. Although the rapid clearance of an antibiotic may be detrimental in the treatment of many infections, it can be advantageous in the treatment of urinary tract infections, in which effectiveness requires the accumulation of the antibiotic in the bladder.

Antibiotics can be classified according to their spectrum of activity (the range of pathogenic organisms that they effectively kill or inhibit); broad-spectrum antibiotics are effective against many species, while narrow-spectrum antibiotics target a specific group. A broad-spectrum antibiotic can be prescribed upon diagnosis of an infection, without identification of the particular pathogen responsible; this trait can be important when immediate containment of the infection is essential to the health of the patient. Yet the indiscriminate use of broad-spectrum antibiotics can harm microorganisms other than those causing an infection. External surfaces, including the skin, gastrointestinal tract, upper respiratory tract, and vagina, are inhabited by large numbers of microorganisms, collectively referred to as the normal microbiota. While this relationship is hardly a symbiotic one, such organisms do help to maintain environments that inhibit the growth of pathogenic microbes. Administration of broad-spectrum antibiotics can cause the depletion of normal microbiota organisms, leading to conditions favoring superinfection by a pathogen other than the one targeted by the antibiotic. For example, vaginal candidiasis (often called a yeast infection) can develop with the administration of antibacterial drugs. The bacteria that normally inhabit the vagina maintain an acidic environment that inhibits the growth of the pathogenic fungus *Candida albicans*, which may nevertheless persist in low numbers. If these bacteria are adversely affected by antibiotic treatment, then the vagina may become less acidic, allowing *C. albicans* to grow and cause tissue damage. Other superinfections can lead to serious damage to the gastrointestinal tract. There is also concern that the use of broad-spectrum antibiotics may encourage the growth of antibiotic-resistant strains among the microorganisms that constitute the normal microbiota. Because antibiotic resistance can be transferred from one bacterial species to another, conditions that favor the growth of any antibiotic-resistant microbes can contribute to the development of antibiotic-resistant pathogens.

Specific resistance to the action of antibiotics is a matter of great concern to medical personnel who deal with infectious diseases. In the early 1940's, when the first antibiotics came into widespread use, virtually all strains of *Staphylococcus aureus* (a bacterium that causes a variety of infections) were susceptible to penicillin G, a beta-lactam that can be administered orally. By the 1990's, it was rare to isolate a strain of *S. aureus* from an infection that was not resistant to multiple beta-lactams. Similar situations prevail with other pathogenic microorganisms, seriously impairing the ability to control many infections. Antibiotic resistance usually develops when a pathogen possesses specific genes encoding proteins that allow the organism to avoid the action of the antibiotic. Such proteins may inactivate the antibiotic molecule, interfere with the uptake of the antibiotic, or modify the target of the antibiotic so that it is no longer affected by the antibiotic. In bacteria, the genes encoding antibiotic resistance (called resistance determinants, or R-factors) are usually found on plasmids, small circular deoxyribonucleic acid (DNA) molecules that are separate from the bacterial chromosome. A single plasmid may contain genes for resistance to several antibiotics. Many plasmids also contain genes that allow them to be transferred from one cell to another, even if the cells are of different species. These genes can cause antibiotic resistance to spread rapidly among microorganisms.

Because the presence of an antibiotic in an animal's tissues favors the survival of bacteria carrying resistance determinants for that antibiotic, continued application of an antibiotic tends to increase the incidence of resistance to that antibiotic. Overcoming this dilemma is difficult. Narrow-spectrum antibiotics should be used whenever practical, since they limit the range of species subject to selection for antibiotic resistance. Some microbiologists have urged that the nontherapeutic application of antibiotics, such as the use of tetracycline as a growth-promoting factor in animal feeds, be discontinued because it can contribute to the spread of resistance determinants. The identification of new natural and synthetic compounds for which resistance has not yet been encountered can help to defeat pathogens that have developed resistance to the current repertoire of antibiotics, but experience teaches one to expect that such victories will be temporary; the implementation of each new antibiotic will lead to the discovery of new resistance determinants. Humans must accumulate knowledge of the biology of their adversaries in order to design narrow-spectrum drugs that are precisely targeted to the metabolism of a pathogen.

PERSPECTIVE AND PROSPECTS

The latter decades of the nineteenth century are often referred to as the golden age of microbiology, because it was during this time that microbiologists identified many of the pathogenic microorganisms responsible for infectious diseases. Although such knowledge was very useful in helping to control the transmission of infectious diseases in populations through public health measures and vaccination programs, it did little to alleviate the suffering of the individual already infected with the now-identifiable pathogen. Actual treatment of infections required the identification of chemical compounds that would be selectively toxic to the microorganisms, and such compounds were unknown at that time. Nevertheless, the potential value of such compounds motivated many scientists to devote their research to the search for chemicals that would destroy microorganisms without damaging an infected person.

The few compounds used at this time (mostly heavy metal salts) tended to exhibit a very low chemotherapeutic index, and some scientists despaired of finding poisons that were poisonous for only some forms of life. Then, in 1910, Paul Ehrlich demonstrated that Salvarsan (arsphenamine), an arsenical compound, was selectively toxic to the bacterial agent of syphilis. Although Salvarsan was useless for other infections, it provided evidence that selective toxicity was possible and encouraged the medical community to find other selective toxins. Extensive chemical screening programs led, in 1935, to the commercial production of the sulfanilamides, which are active against multiple species of bacteria.

The greatest conceptual advance in the development of antimicrobial drugs was made by those bacteriologists who concentrated on the phenomenon of antagonism, whereby certain microorganisms produce compounds that inhibit others. Study of these compounds eventually led to the practical application of gramicidin (described by René Dubos in 1939), penicillin (described by Alexander Fleming in 1928), and streptomycin (described by Selman Waksman in 1943). Penicillin receives special attention in the history of antibiotics because the industrial processes developed to allow production of massive quantities of the drug proved valuable in the commercial exploitation of other antibiotics. With the goal of increasing the yield of penicillin, motivated in part by a desire to have an alternative to the sulfonamides for the treatment of infections attending World War II, industrial microbiologists optimized the composition and aeration of the growth media and selected mutant strains of the penicillin-producing fungus that secreted the drug in amounts far greater than those seen by Fleming. In doing so, they established some of the engineering principles that allowed for the growth of biotechnology.

Eventually, major pharmaceutical companies committed themselves to extensive screening programs to identify additional natural antibiotics. Microorganisms isolated from soil were tested for their ability to inhibit the growth of pathogens. Eventually it was realized that, although a diverse range of organic molecules possess antibiotic properties, such compounds are produced by a limited range of microorganisms. More than half of the natural antibiotics currently in use are produced by mycelial bacteria called actinomycetes. One approach that has complemented the identification of new natural antibiotics is the chemical modification of such drugs through the addition or removal of groups of atoms. Compared to natural antibiotics, such semisynthetic derivatives may have properties that promote accumulation at high levels in the target tissue or prevent recognition of the antibiotic molecule by products of resistance determinants. All the beta-lactams in common use today are semisynthetic molecules.

While microbiologists have been discovering further natural antibiotics and synthesizing others, they have also been learning more about the molecular biology of infectious pathogens. Research is also progressing on ways to decrease the unnecessary use of antibiotics. Rapid flu tests can now be used by doctors to determine whether patients need antibiotics at all. New uses for antibiotics are also being discovered every day. For instance, researchers have begun to explore ways to attach powerful implants to medical devices in order to decrease infection postoperatively. Together, all these types of knowledge will allow antibiotic development to become increasingly useful and important to helping humans attempt to stay ahead of the evolution of their ancient adversaries.

—Kenneth A. Pidcock, Ph.D.;
updated by Nancy A. Piotrowski, Ph.D.

See also Bacterial infections; Bacteriology; Candidiasis; Chemotherapy; Cytology; Cytopathology; Drug resistance; Fungal infections; Genetic engineering; Gram staining; Herbal medicine; Immune system; Immunology; Immunopathology; Infection; Laboratory tests; Microbiology; Parasitic diseases; Pharmacology; Pharmacy; Protozoan diseases; Viral infections.

For Further Information:

Black, Jacquelyn G. *Microbiology: Principles and Explorations*. 6th ed. Hoboken, N.J.: John Wiley & Sons, 2004. One of numerous microbiology textbooks in print, each of them having strengths and weaknesses in the presentation of different topics.

Brock, Thomas, ed. *Milestones in Microbiology*. Englewood Cliffs, N.J.: Prentice Hall, 1961. A collection of classic papers in microbiology published before World War II. Includes papers by Paul Ehrlich, Alexander Fleming, and Gerhard Domagk describing the first classes of antimicrobial compounds.

Conte, John E. *Manual of Antibiotics and Infectious Diseases: Treatment and Prevention*. 9th ed. Philadelphia: Lippincott Williams & Wilkins, 2002. Chapter topics include antibiotic pharmacology, prophylaxis and clinical usage, common infectious diseases, HIV infection, immunobiologic agents and vaccines, and hospital epidemiology. Provides useful tables of dosages and recommendations for empiric, prophylactic, and antibiotic therapies.

Gale, E. F., et al. *The Molecular Basis of Antibiotic Action*. London: John Wiley & Sons, 1981. The definitive scientific reference work on antibiotics. The text is organized by target of antimicrobial effect, with extensive citation of original papers that provide the current models of antibiotic action.

Levy, Stuart B. *The Antibiotic Paradox: How the Misuse of Antibiotics Destroys Their Curative Powers*. Cambridge, Mass.: Perseus, 2001. A leading researcher in molecular biology explores a modern-day massive evolutionary change in bacteria due to misuse of antibiotics. He argues that a build-up of new antibiotic-resistant bacteria in individuals and in the environment is leading medicine into a dangerous territory where "miracle" drugs may be obsolete.

Moberg, Carol L., and Zanvil A. Cohn, eds. *Launching the Antibiotic Era*. New York: Rockefeller Press, 1990. A collection of papers from a 1989 symposium at Rockefeller University honoring René Dubos, whose discovery of gramicidin provided evidence that microbial antagonism could be exploited for chemotherapy.

Neu, H. C. "The Crisis in Antibiotic Resistance." *Science* 249 (August 21, 1992): 1064-1073. One of a series of articles in this issue of *Science* that deal with "emerging pathogens," microorganisms that have been found to be unexpectedly difficult. Contains somewhat technical but clear descriptions of the molecular mechanisms used by bacteria to defeat antibiotic action.

Walsh, Christopher. *Antibiotics: Actions, Origins, Resistance*. Washington, D.C.: ASM Press, 2003. Examines such topics as how antibiotics block specific proteins, how the molecular structure of drugs enables such activity, the development of bacterial resistance, and the molecular logic of antibiotic biosynthesis.

Antidepressants

Treatment

Anatomy or system affected: Brain, nervous system, psychic-emotional system

Specialties and related fields: Biochemistry, family medicine, neurology, psychiatry, psychology

Definition: A group of drugs used for the treatment of clinical depression.

Key terms:

bipolar disorders: mood disorders characterized by significant swings in mood from depression to persistent feelings of elation; also known as manic-depressive illness

depression: a mood disorder characterized by loss of energy, depressed mood, diminished interest in pleasurable activities, feelings of worthlessness, and difficulty in concentrating

fluoxetine: the generic name for the antidepressant commonly called Prozac

monoamine oxidase inhibitors (MAOIs): a class of drugs that relieve the symptoms of depression by inhibiting the enzyme that deactivates the brain chemical monoamine oxidase

neurotransmitters: chemicals produced by the brain that allow for cells to transmit electrical signals

obsessive-compulsive disorder: a psychiatric disorder that causes a person to ruminate on a particular thought and then act out a ritualistic behavior

selective serotonin reuptake inhibitors (SSRIs): a class of antidepressant drugs, first introduced in 1987, that work by inhibiting the reuptake of the neurotransmitter serotonin, thus making more of it available to brain cells

tricyclics: antidepressant drugs that interfere with several neurotransmitters, making more of them available to the brain

Indications and Procedures

Antidepressants are prescribed most often to individuals suffering from symptoms of clinical depression, a severe form of depression that interferes with the person's ability to function (for example, to hold down a job or to handle the responsibilities of being a student). The symptoms of depression should be present for at least several months before a diagnosis is made and medication is recommended.

Fortunately, several classes of antidepressants can be considered as treatment options. Each class of drugs acts on the nervous system in its own unique way, and each class produces different kinds of side effects. Monoamine oxidase inhibitors (MAOIs) and tricyclic antidepressants are regarded as two different classes of first-generation drugs. These two classes and the new-generation selective serotonin reuptake inhibitors (SSRIs), including fluoxetine (Prozac), all affect the nervous system by increasing the availability of neurotransmitters such as norepinephrine or serotonin.

Although physicians have several classes of drugs at their disposal to combat the effects of depression, no single drug or class of drugs has been found to be significantly more effective in treating symptoms. In fact, no reliable test exists to discover which antidepressant will be most effective for a particular patient. However, it is clearly the case that most patients will respond favorably to one class of drugs over the others. The effectiveness of antidepressants can be evaluated on two fronts: the degree to which symptoms of clinical depression are reduced, and the pervasiveness of any adverse side effects that may result from a particular medication.

Uses and Complications

For a single episode of depression, antidepressants will be prescribed for six to twelve months in order to minimize the possibility of a relapse. In instances of chronic depression, it is not unusual for someone to remain on antidepressants for several years. Since all antidepressant medications cause some adverse side effects, periodically physicians will attempt to adjust the amount of drug that a patient takes in order to find the minimum clinically effective dose. MAOIs may produce a serious adverse side effect known as a hypertensive crisis, which results in a rapid elevation of blood pressure. This condition can be caused by an interaction of the drug with foods containing tyramine, such as aged cheeses, aged meats, and red wines; thus, these foods must be avoided. Less serious side effects produced by MAOIs include constipation, diarrhea, or difficulty falling asleep.

Tricyclic antidepressants may produce dry mouth, blurred vision, or weight gain. However, the most serious aspect of tricyclics is the danger if an overdose is taken. Given that patients suffering from depression may be predisposed to thoughts of suicide, the amount of prescription given at one time must be carefully monitored and should be limited. SSRIs have fewer and more easily tolerated side effects than the first-generation antidepressants, although some patients will experience weight gain and sexual dysfunction resulting in the loss of the sexual drive.

Abruptly stopping an antidepressant prescription will lead to a range of withdrawal symptoms, from feeling more depressed to becoming irritable to developing flulike symptoms. Although the withdrawal symptoms are not dangerous, it is recommended that antidepressants be reduced in dosage over a period of several days.

Perspective and Prospects

Since the introduction of Prozac in 1987, those suffering from depression have had access to a medication that has been every bit as effective as other classes of antidepressants without producing many of the adverse side effects. Investigators are also learning that antidepressants can help patients with other psychological conditions, such as bipolar disorders, anxiety disorders, panic attacks, and obsessive-compulsive disorder.

Despite the successes that have come with the availability of several classes of antidepressants, there still remains a group of patients suffering from depression who do not benefit from them. Investigators are continuing to look for more effective drugs, particularly ones that can alleviate the symptoms of depression more quickly.

—*Bryan C. Auday, Ph.D.*

See also Anxiety; Bipolar disorders; Depression; Emotions: Biomedical causes and effects; Grief and guilt; Neurology; Neurology, pediatric; Obsessive-compulsive disorder; Panic attacks; Pharmacology; Postpartum depression; Psychiatric disorders; Psychiatry; Psychiatry, child and adolescent; Psychiatry, geriatric; Stress; Stress reduction; Suicide.

For Further Information:

American Psychiatric Association. *Diagnostic and Statistical Manual of Mental Disorders: DSM-IV-TR*. Rev. 4th ed. Washington, D.C.: Author, 2000.

Diamond, Ronald J. *Instant Psychopharmacology: Up-to-Date Information About the Most Commonly Prescribed Drugs for Emotional Health*. 2d ed. New York: W. W. Norton, 2002.

Feldman, Robert S., Jerrold S. Meyer, and Linda F. Quenzer. *Principles of Neuropsychopharmacology*. Sunderland, Mass.: Sinauer Associates, 1997.

Lickey, Marvin E., and Barbara Gordon. *Medicine and Mental Illness: The Use of Drugs in Psychiatry*. New York: W. H. Freeman, 1991.

Ray, Oakley, and Charles Ksir. *Drugs, Society, and Human Behavior*. 9th ed. New York: McGraw-Hill, 2002.

Antihistamines

Treatment

Anatomy or system affected: Chest, circulatory system, ears, eyes, head, immune system, lungs, nose, psychic-emotional system, respiratory system, throat

Specialties and related fields: Family medicine, immunology, otorhinolaryngology, pharmacology, preventive medicine, pulmonary medicine

Definition: Over-the-counter and prescription-type drugs that are commonly prescribed for allergy symptoms in order to reduce the effects of histamines.

Key terms:

addictive drugs: drugs that are controlled in terms of their administration, dispensation, sales, and use because of their reinforcing nature and relationships with conditions such as substance use disorders

allergic rhinitis: an uncomfortable condition of the nose resulting from the sensitivity of the nasal passageway to pollen or other substances

arrhythmias: problems with the rhythm of the heart, such as irregular heartbeat

decongestants: drugs that are taken in order to break up

congested mucus, fluids commonly found in the sinuses during allergic reactions and colds, in order to reduce swelling in the sinuses

drug synergy: a process by which drugs taken in combination with each other interact and can have a greater effect than the drugs taken separately

histamines: proteins released by the immune system as part of allergic reactions

mucous membranes: the lining covering the parts of the body in the major air passageways and in the alimentary tract

Indications and Procedures

Antihistamines serve the purpose of providing a rapid form of treatment for controlling histamine-based physical reactions, including cold and allergy symptoms, rashes and hives, and insect bites and stings. They are also especially helpful for the allergic condition known as hay fever, which is related to seasonal allergies, and allergic rhinitis. Antihistamines serve largely to decrease the discomfort and symptoms caused by histamine reactions. Symptoms of histamine reactions may include sneezing, itchy skin, rashes, a swollen throat, watery or itchy eyes, and a runny nose. In reducing these effects, antihistamines may also be useful in helping to decrease the risk of additional infections caused by the swelling of sensitive mucous membranes in the body, particularly in the sinuses, nose, and throat. Typically if such membranes remain swollen, the passageways of the body, such as the sinuses, can become congested, making it easier for infections to develop.

Antihistamines are typically administered orally, in pill form, one or more times per day, but they are also available in the form of eye drops, nose sprays, and liquids. They are also combined frequently with other drugs such as decongestants in order to ameliorate further any uncomfortable cold symptoms and to prevent consequent problems such as sinus infections. Antihistamines alone are generally considered to be ineffective at reducing nasal congestion.

Uses and Complications

In addition to reducing histamine reactions, antihistamines also have a number of helpful side effects, including mild reductions in nausea and motion sickness, a general effect of drying secretions, and an ability to induce drowsiness, which can help individuals initiate and maintain sleep. This ability to induce drowsiness can be helpful, particularly for both adults and children needing a mild, nonaddictive sleep medication. It should be noted, however, that mild tolerance to the sedating effects of antihistamines has been observed and so use for such a purpose should be time limited.

Furthermore, any drug, including antihistamines, can be abused if used in larger quantities than prescribed or recommended. For instance, some individuals may use high quantities of antihistamines in order to experience a more pronounced sedating effect or other psychoactive effects. This is dangerous, as use of any substance outside of its recommended use, particularly in situations requiring safety (for instance, driving, operating machinery, being around strangers, being in strange places) may lead to unexpected negative consequences.

Of the side effects mentioned, drowsiness persists in being the most problematic, as people needing to take the drugs more than once a day may have their daytime activities interrupted by feeling sleepy. Additionally, if antihistamines are combined with other substances, both prescription drugs or others such as alcohol, then drug synergies can occur. With sedating drugs such as alcohol, for instance, the onset of drowsiness can hasten and its strength can be greater than might be expected with either the antihistamine or the alcohol alone. As such, the use of antihistamines, particularly in combination with other sedating drugs (opioids, barbiturates, anesthetics, benzodiazepines, sedating pain medications), or even sedating alternative medicines, is not advised in situations requiring attention and alertness, such as driving or operating machinery.

In response to these problems, newer antihistamines have been developed in order to cause less drowsiness. These newer drugs have sometimes had other side effects, however, such as arrhythmia. Therefore, the ideal antihistamine does not yet exist.

Because of issues such as drug interactions and how the drug may affect the body, antihistamines should be taken cautiously. They also should not be used without the supervision of a physician by women who are trying to become pregnant, by individuals using antibiotics, or by individuals who are undergoing surgery because the effects of the drugs may interfere with these conditions. Other contraindications may exist as well. The advice of a physician or pharmacist is best followed when taking any drug.

Perspective and Prospects

New antihistamines are being developed at a rapid pace. Part of this activity is driven by a desire to make them more effective. For instance, antihistamines have been paired with substances such as decongestants so that they may relieve more symptoms. The development of antihistamines has also been spurred by the desire to decrease the general sedating effects of earlier versions. In the past, however, some additions have come with both advantages and disadvantages. The addition of pseudoephedrine to antihistamine medications, for example, increased their ability to address symptoms and decreased some of the drowsiness. Pseudoephedrine, however, has stimulating properties that have been identified as problematic and has had to be removed from many types of medications.

Antihistamine development is also driven by a desire to make them more specific. For instance, one person may need an antihistamine to reduce nasal irritation while another may need one to alleviate itchy eyes. As such, it is expected that antihistamines will be developed to have much more specific effects on the body and to have little to no sedating or other side effects while still being effective at reducing allergy and cold symptoms. Nevertheless, some of the familiar antihistamines known today are likely to remain available, as they are generally useful. Also, mildly sedating medicines, such as antihistamines taken at a normally recommended dose, may continue to have a place in medicine, as they serve as a good substitute for individuals needing nonaddictive sleep medication and who are unlikely to abuse these substances.

—Nancy A. Piotrowski, Ph.D.

See also Allergies; Anti-inflammatory drugs; Bites and stings; Common cold; Decongestants; Hay fever; Hives; Host-defense mechanisms; Immune system; Immunology; Itching; Multiple chemical sensitivity syndrome; Nasopharyngeal disorders; Over-the-counter medications; Otorhinolaryngology; Pharmacology; Pharmacy; Rashes; Sinusitis; Skin; Skin disorders; Sleep disorders; Smell; Sneezing.

For Further Information:

American Psychiatric Association. *Diagnostic and Statistical Manual of Mental Disorders: DSM-IV-TR*. Rev. 4th ed. Washington, D.C.: Author, 2000.

Julien, Robert M. *A Primer of Drug Action*. 10th ed. New York: Worth, 2004.

Siegfried, D. R. *Anatomy and Physiology for Dummies*. New York: John Wiley & Sons, 2002.

Anti-inflammatory drugs

Treatment

Anatomy or system affected: All

Specialties and related fields: Dermatology, endocrinology, family medicine, internal medicine, ophthalmology, otorhinolaryngology, rheumatology, vascular medicine

Definition: Medicines used to relieve inflammation, pain, redness, and swelling; generally grouped into two categories: nonsteroidal anti-inflammatory drugs (NSAIDs) and corticosteroids (steroid hormones that have an anti-inflammatory effect).

Key terms:

arthritis: a painful condition that involves inflammation of one or more joints

bursitis: inflammation of the tissue around a joint

hormone: a substance that is produced in one part of the body and travels through the bloodstream to another part of the body, where it has its effect

inhalant: medication that is inhaled into the lungs

salicylates: a group of drugs that includes aspirin and related compounds used to relieve pain, reduce inflammation, and lower fever

steroids: any of various compounds that contain hormones

tendinitis: inflammation of a tendon or a tough band of tissue that connects muscle to the bone

Indications and Procedures

Nonsteroidal anti-inflammatory drugs (NSAIDs) relieve painful conditions such as arthritis, bursitis, gout, menstrual cramps, tendinitis, sprains, and strains. While some drugs are sold only with a doctor's prescription, other drugs are sold over the counter. Some common NSAIDs, with the brand name in parentheses, are diclofenac (Voltaren), etodolac (Lodine), flurbiprofen (Ansaid), ibuprofen (Motrin, Advil, Rufen, Nuprin), nabumetone (Relafen), naproxen (Naprosyn or Aleve), and oxaprozin (Daypro). These drugs are sold as capsules, caplets, tablets, liquids, and suppositories.

Corticosteroids make up the second group of anti-inflammatory drugs that relieve inflammation and allergic reactions (and the itching, swelling and redness that are associated with them, as well as with various skin conditions). They are similar to the natural hormone cortisone used in the treatment of arthritis. Corticosteroids are available in numerous forms, including inhalants, creams and ointments, and oral (systemic) medications. Common corticosteroids are beclomethasone (Beconase, Vancensase, Vanceril), betamethosone (Diprolene, Lotrisone), hydrocortisone, mometasone (Elocon), prednisone (Deltasone, Orasone), and triamcinolone (Azmacort, Nasacort).

Aspirins and NSAIDs are commonly used in the treatment of arthritis. Because high doses of aspirins are required to control joint inflammation, NSAIDs are effective for arthritis treatment and are useful for people who cannot tolerate the required dosage of aspirin. Individual responses to NSAIDs vary, and only through careful and controlled trial and evaluation can effective dosages be determined. These drugs tend to lose their effectiveness after prolonged use, and others may need to be substituted.

Uses and Complications

NSAIDs can cause some serious side effects, especially if they are taken for a long period of time or in large doses or if several NSAIDs are taken together. Older persons who take NSAIDs are likely to develop stomach problems. NSAIDs can also increase the possibility of bleeding after surgery or sensitivity to sunlight. The following persons should consult their physicians before taking NSAIDs: individuals who are taking other medications, women who are pregnant or who plan to become pregnant, women who are breast-feeding, and individuals with stomach or intestinal problems, liver disease, heart disease, high blood pressure, bleeding difficulties, diabetes, Parkinson's disease, or epilepsy.

For most individuals who are prescribed these drugs, however, common side effects are mild and may include stomach pain or cramps, nausea, vomiting, indigestion, headache, and dizziness. It is also important to note that research has been used to identify new anti-inflammatory painkillers that produce fewer of these kinds of effects. One recent example is licofelone, an NSAID that is reported to be gentler on the stomach.

For most individuals using these substances, serious side effects are rare. For some, however, they can be life-threatening. In fact, research has shown that some NSAIDs can increase the risk of strokes and heart attacks. These types of NSAIDs are COX-2 inhibitors. Such risks underscore the need for medical consultation when using these drugs. Any feelings of tightness in the chest, irregular heartbeat, swelling, and fainting are reasons to discontinue taking NSAIDs and consult a physician.

Corticosteroid therapy produces dramatic, immediate relief from pain, swelling, and inflammation due to arthritis. However, the beneficial effects tend to be temporary. Long-term use causes harmful reactions to corticosteroids, which may be reduced if the drugs are taken on alternate days. Also, small amounts of steroid may be injected into the inflamed joint.

Corticosteroids are a common treatment for persons suffering from more serious asthmatic conditions or when treatment with bronchodilators is not effective. Corticosteroids, which are not bronchodilators and do

In the News: Dangers of COX-2 Inhibitors

In a 2001 issue of the *Journal of the American Medical Association*, Debabrata Mukherjee and coauthors summarized the results of two major randomized trails of COX-2 inhibitors: the Vioxx Gastrointestinal Outcomes Research Study (VIGOR), with 8,076 patients, and the Celecoxib Longterm Arthritis Safety Study (CLASS), with 8,059 patients, as well as several smaller trials of these drugs. The VIGOR study found that treatment with rofecoxib (trade name Vioxx) increased the risk of developing a thrombotic cardiovascular event (myocardial infarction, unstable angina, cardiac thrombus, resuscitated cardiac arrest, sudden or unexplained death, ischemic stroke, and transient ischemic attacks) by twofold over naproxen treatment. Myocardial infarction rates for COX-2 inhibitors were found to be significantly higher than the placebo group in both large studies. Other smaller-scale studies are consistent with the findings from the VIGOR and CLASS trials.

Some of these adverse effects of Vioxx could be mitigated by simultaneous treatment with aspirin; however, such an approach significantly detracts from the utility of nonsteroidal anti-inflammatory drugs (NSAIDs) such as Vioxx, since one would experience the same degree of stomach irritation from the aspirin that NSAIDs are prescribed to avoid. In September, 2004, the pharmaceutical company Merck pulled Vioxx, which had been a popular pain reliever for arthritis, off the market because of the preponderance of evidence suggesting that it poses serious risks of heart attack and stroke. It has been estimated that as many as 30,000 to 100,000 patients have had heart attacks or strokes as a result of taking Vioxx.

—Michael R. King, Ph.D.

not open the airways, work to reduce inflammation and allow the lungs to function properly. They should be taken regularly and over a long term to achieve full benefits. While oral corticosteroids are used largely in the prevention of asthma attacks, inhaled corticosteroids may be sprayed into the nose for relief of stuffy nose, irritation, hay fever, or other allergies.

Ophthalmic anti-inflammatory medicines can be used to reduce problems that occur during or following eye surgery and soothe some eye inflammations; they can be obtained only with a doctor's prescription. Corticosteroids also relieve inflammation of the temporal arteries, or blood vessels that run along the temples. Inflammation here disrupts the blood supply and can result in blindness, loss of vision, strokes, and heart attacks.

Long-term use of corticosteroids causes a large number of serious side effects, including puffiness, weight gain, facial hair, reduced resistance to infection, gastrointestinal ulcers and bleeding, and diabetes. It may increase the risk of high blood pressure and osteoporosis, which is more likely to develop in older women. Corticosteroids can slow or stop growth in children and teenagers.

Individuals who have medical conditions such as allergies, diabetes, pregnancy, osteoporosis, glaucoma, infections, thyroid problems, liver disease, kidney disease, heart disease, or high blood pressure should discuss these conditions with their physician before taking corticosteroids.

If corticosteroids are used for a short time, serious side effects are rare. However, breathing problems or tightness in the chest, pains, rash, swelling, extreme tiredness, irregular heartbeat, or wounds that will not heal should be reported to the patient's physician.

PERSPECTIVE AND PROSPECTS

The bark of the willow tree, which contains salicylates, was known in eighteenth century England to reduce fever and aches, and in 1876 the first successful treatment of acute arthritis with sodium salicylate (aspirin) was reported. In the 1970's, John Vane amassed evidence of the effectiveness of NSAIDs.

The earliest demonstration of the importance of corticosteroids as anti-inflammatory agents occurred in the 1940's in regard to rheumatoid arthritis. The challenge of corticosteroid therapy lies in achieving the desired results with a minimum of side effects.

—Mary Hurd;
updated by Nancy A. Piotrowski, Ph.D.

See also Allergies; Antihistamines; Arthritis; Asthma; Back pain; Bursitis; Dermatitis; Dermatology; Dermatology, pediatric; Eye surgery; Fever; Gout; Hay fever; Inflammation; Itching; Narcotics; Over-the-counter medications; Pain; Pain management; Pharmacology; Poisonous plants; Rashes; Rheumatoid arthritis; Rheumatology; Skin disorders; Steroids; Tendinitis; Tendon disorders.

FOR FURTHER INFORMATION:

American Medical Association. *American Medical Association Family Medical Guide*. 4th ed. Hoboken, N.J.: John Wiley & Sons, 2004.

Liska, Ken. *Drugs and the Human Body with Implications for Society*. Englewood Cliffs, N.J.: Prentice Hall, 2003.

Subak-Sharpe, Genell J., and Thomas O. Morris, eds. "Drug Therapy." In *The Columbia University College of Physicians and Surgeons Complete Home Medical Guide*. 3d ed. New York: Crown, 1995.

Wood, Paul L. *Neuroinflammation: Mechanisms and Management*. 2d ed. Totowa, N.J.: Humana Press, 2003.

ANTIOXIDANTS

TREATMENT

ANATOMY OR SYSTEM AFFECTED: All

SPECIALTIES AND RELATED FIELDS: Alternative medicine, family medicine, internal medicine, nutrition, oncology

DEFINITION: A group of vitamins, minerals, and enzymes that help protect the body from damage-causing free radicals.

FREE RADICALS AND CELL DAMAGE

The role of antioxidants in preventing aging has received considerable interest in recent years. Antioxidants are substances that neutralize the harmful effects of free radicals in the body. Free radicals are highly reactive chemicals that form in normal metabolism or are produced by radiation and environmental stress. These volatile chemicals react with cell components, causing mutations in deoxyribonucleic acid (DNA) and destroying cell proteins and lipids. The aging process and various degenerative diseases of aging are believed to be caused in part by the lifetime accumulation of cell damage caused by free radicals. Both antioxidants and free radicals are produced naturally by the body to help the body stay in a balanced state of health. The disruption of the balance, by things such as aging, stress, and pollution, damages DNA in the cells. Antioxidants may provide protection and reduce the risk of stroke, heart disease, cancer, and other health problems associated with aging.

Antioxidant defenses occur naturally in the body to inactivate free radicals and repair damaged tissues. The body's natural supply of antioxidants is limited, however, and a small amount of destruction occurs to cells daily. Dietary antioxidants—in the form of fruits and vegetables or vitamin supplements—are believed to improve health and to prevent aging by boosting the body's natural supply of antioxidants.

Extensive research, including many large-scale studies, has demonstrated the beneficial role of dietary antioxidants in preventing such age-related disorders as cardiovascular disease, cancer, immune dysfunction, brain and neurological disorders, and cataracts. Fruits and vegetables, long recognized for their protective and healthful effects, are particularly rich sources of antioxidants, which may be the basis for their antiaging and anticarcinogenic properties.

IMPORTANT ANTIOXIDANTS

Vitamin E, vitamin C, and beta carotene are the main dietary antioxidants. Vitamin E (tocopherol) is a fat-soluble antioxidant found in oil, nuts, seeds, and whole grains. This antioxidant appears to protect arteries against damage. Two recent studies have shown that taking vitamin E supplements appears to reduce the risk of heart disease dramatically. In addition, studies in mice suggest that vitamin E supplements slow the decline of brain and immune system function caused by aging. Vitamin C (ascorbate) works in the water-soluble part of tissues. Citrus fruits, strawberries, sweet peppers, and broccoli are good sources of vitamin C. This antioxidant boosts the immune system, strengthens blood vessel walls, and increases levels of a natural antioxidant, glutathione. Vitamin C also helps restore levels of active vitamin E in the body. Beta carotene, a precursor of vitamin A, is found in carrot juice, sweet potatoes, and apricots. Many studies have demonstrated the anticancer and antiaging effects of beta carotene.

Other antioxidants include coenzyme Q_{10}, gingko, lipoic acid, grapeseed, and various substances found in green and black teas. The micronutrients zinc and selenium also have antioxidant properties; they aid the immune system and boost the levels of natural antioxidant enzymes in the body. Antioxidants appear to work together, as a combination of antioxidants is more potent than each substance alone.

PERSPECTIVE AND PROSPECTS

Evidence for the beneficial role of antioxidants in human health is growing. Clinical studies have not definitively confirmed, however, whether consuming large amounts of antioxidants offers increased protection against aging. It is not clear what the optimal levels of antioxidants are to prevent the damaging effects of aging. Adequate levels of vitamins may vary greatly for each person, depending on levels of environmental stress, smoking, how well supplements are absorbed, and other factors. In addition, it is unclear whether vitamin supplements are superior to fruits and vegetables, since other factors in these foods (fiber, micronutrients) may be responsible for their healthful effects.

In general, people who eat five to eight servings of fruits and vegetables per day are thought to be getting an adequate amount of antioxidants. Taking antioxidant supplements is controversial, as some researchers believe that they may interfere with the body's natural production of antioxidants.

—Linda Hart, M.S., M.A.;
updated by LeAnna DeAngelo, Ph.D.

See also Aging; Alternative medicine; Cancer; Food biochemistry; Herbal medicine; Immune system; Melatonin; Nutrition; Phytochemicals; Self-medication; Supplements; Vitamins and minerals.

FOR FURTHER INFORMATION:

Balch, James F., and Phyllis A. Balch. *Prescription for Nutritional Healing: A Practical A-to-Z Reference to Drug-Free Remedies Using Vitamins, Minerals, Herbs, and Food Supplements*. 3d ed. Garden City Park, N.Y.: Avery, 2000.

Bourassa, Martial G., and Jean-Claude Tardif, eds. *Antioxidants and Cardiovascular Disease*. New York: Springer, 2006.

Busch, Felicia. *The New Nutrition: From Antioxidants to Zucchini*. New York: Wiley, 2000.

Cadenas, Enrique, and Lester Packer, eds. *Handbook of Antioxidants*. 2d ed. New York: Marcel Decker, 2002.

Knight, Joseph A. *Free Radicals, Antioxidants, Aging and Disease*. Washington, D.C.: AACC Press, 1999.

Morello, Michael J., et al., eds. *Free Radicals in Food: Chemistry, Nutrition, and Health Effects*. Washington, D.C.: American Chemical Society, 2002.

Weil, Andrew, M.D. *Healthy Aging: A Lifelong Guide to Your Physical and Spiritual Wellbeing*. New York: Knopf, 2005.

Anxiety

Disease/disorder

Anatomy or system affected: Heart, nervous system, psychic-emotional system, skin

Specialties and related fields: Cardiology, internal medicine, psychiatry, psychology

Definition: Heightened fear or tension that causes psychological and physical distress; the American Psychiatric Association recognizes six types of anxiety disorders, which can be treated with medications or through counseling.

Key terms:

anxiety: abnormal fear or tension, which may occur without any obvious trigger

brain imaging: any of several techniques used to visualize anatomic regions of the brain, including X rays, magnetic resonance imaging, and positron emission tomography

compulsion: a repetitive, stereotyped behavior performed to ward off anxious feelings

GABA/benzodiazepine receptor: an area on a nerve cell to which gamma aminobutyric acid (GABA) attaches and that causes inhibition (quieting) of the nerve; benzodiazepine drugs enhance the attachment of GABA to the receptor

obsession: a recurrent, unwelcome, and intrusive thought

panic: a sudden episode of intense fearfulness

Causes and Symptoms

Anxiety is a subjective state of fear, apprehension, or tension. In the face of a naturally fearful situation, anxiety is a normal and understandable condition. When anxiety occurs without obvious provocation or is excessive, however, anxiety may be said to be abnormal or pathological (existing in a disease state). Normal anxiety is useful because it provides an alerting signal and improves physical and mental performance. Excessive anxiety results in a deterioration in performance and in emotional and physical discomfort.

There are several forms of pathological anxiety, known collectively as the anxiety disorders. As a group, they constitute the fifth most common medical or psychiatric disorder. In the United States, 14.6 percent of the population will experience anxiety at some point in their lives. More women suffer from anxiety disorders than do men, by a 2:1 ratio.

The anxiety disorders are distinguished from one another by characteristic clusters of symptoms. These disorders include generalized anxiety disorder, panic disorder, obsessive-compulsive disorder, phobias, adjustment disorder with anxious mood, and post-traumatic stress disorder. The first three disorders are characterized by anxious feelings that may occur without any obvious precipitant, while the latter three are closely associated with anxiety-producing events in a person's life.

Generalized anxiety disorder is thought to be a biological form of anxiety disorder in which the individual inherits a habitually high level of tension or anxiety that may occur even when no threatening circumstances are present. Generally, these periods of anxiety occur in cycles which may last weeks to years. The prevalence is unknown, but this disorder is not uncommon. The male-to-female ratio is nearly equal.

Evidence suggests that generalized anxiety disorder is related to an abnormality in a common neurotransmitter receptor complex found in many brain neurons. These complexes, the GABA/benzodiazepine receptors, decrease the likelihood that a neuron will transmit an electrochemical signal, resulting in a calming effect on the portion of the brain in which they are found. These receptors exist in large numbers in the cerebral cortex (the outer layer of the brain), the hippocampus (a structure inside the temporal lobe shaped like a sea horse), and the amygdala (the almond-shaped gray matter inside the temporal lobe). The hippocampus and amygdala are important parts of the limbic system, which is significantly involved in emotions. Benzodiazepine drugs enhance the efficiency of these receptors and have a calming effect. In contrast, if these receptors are inhibited, feelings of impending doom result.

Panic disorder is found in 1.5 percent of the United States population, and the female-to-male ratio is 2:1. This disorder usually begins during the young adult years. Panic disorder is characterized by recurrent and unexpected attacks of intense fear or panic. Each discrete episode lasts about five to twenty minutes. These episodes are intensely frightening to the individual, who is usually convinced he or she is dying. Because people who suffer from panic attacks are often anxious about having another one (so-called secondary anxiety), they may avoid situations in which they fear an attack may occur, in which help would be unavailable, or in which they would be embarrassed if an attack occurred. This avoidance behavior may cause restricted activity and can lead to agoraphobia, the fear of leaving a safe zone in or around the home. Thus, agoraphobia (literally, "fear of the marketplace") is often secondary to panic disorder.

Panic disorder appears to have a biological basis. In those people with panic disorder, panic attacks can often be induced by sodium lactate infusions, hyperventilation, exercise, or hypocalcemia (low blood calcium). Highly sophisticated scans show abnormal metabolic activity in the right parahippocampal region of the brain of individuals with panic disorder. The parahippocampal region, the area surrounding the hippocampus, is involved in emotions and is connected by fiber tracts to the locus ceruleus, a blue spot in the pons portion of the brain stem that is involved in arousal.

In addition to known biological triggers for panic attacks, emotional or psychological events may also cause an attack. To be diagnosed as having panic disorder, however, a person must experience attacks that arise without any apparent cause. The secondary anxiety and avoidance behavior often seen in these individuals result in difficulties in normal functioning. There is an increased incidence of suicide attempts in people with panic disorder; up to one in five have reported a suicide attempt at some time. The childhoods of people with panic disorder are characterized by an increased incidence of pathological separation anxiety and/or school phobia.

Obsessive-compulsive disorder (OCD) is an uncommon anxiety disorder with an equal male-to-female ratio. It is characterized by obsessions (intrusive, unwelcome thoughts) and compulsions (repetitive, often stereotyped behaviors that are performed to ward off anxiety). The obsessions in OCD are often horrifying to the afflicted person. Common themes concern sex, food, aggression, suicide, bathroom functions, and religion. Compulsive behavior may include checking (such as repeatedly checking to see if the stove is off or the door is locked), cleaning (such as repetitive handwashing or the wearing of gloves to turn a doorknob), or stereotyped behavior (such as dressing by using an exact series of steps that cannot be altered). Frequently, the compulsive behaviors must be repeated many times. Sometimes, there is an exact, almost magical number of times the behavior must be done in order to ward off anxiety. Although people with OCD have some conscious control over their compulsions, they are driven to perform them because intense anxiety results if they fail to do so.

The most common psychological theory for OCD was proposed by Sigmund Freud, who believed that OCD symptoms were a defense against unacceptable unconscious wishes. Genetic and brain imaging studies, however, suggest a biological basis for this disorder. Special brain scans have shown increased metabolism in the front portion of the brain in these patients, and it has been theorized that OCD results from an abnormality in a circuit within the brain (the cortical-striatal-thalamic-cortical circuit). Moreover, OCD is associated with a variety of known neurological diseases, including epilepsy, brain trauma, and certain movement disorders.

Phobias are the most common anxiety disorders. A phobia is an abnormal fear of a particular object or situation. Simple phobias are fears of specific, identifiable triggers such as heights, snakes, flying in an airplane, elevators, or the number thirteen. Social phobia is an exaggerated fear of being in social settings where the phobic person fears he or she will be open to scrutiny by others. This fear may result in phobic avoidance of eating in public, attending church, joining a social club, or participating in other social events. Phobias are more common in men than in women, and they often begin in late childhood or early adolescence.

In classic psychoanalytic theory, phobias were thought to be fears displaced from one object or situation to another. For example, fear of snakes may be a displaced fear of sex because the snake is a phallic symbol. It was thought that this process of displacement took place unconsciously. Many psychologists now believe that phobias are either exaggerations of normal fears or that they develop accidentally, without any symbolic meaning. For example, fear of elephants may arise if a young boy at a zoo is accidentally separated from his parents. At the same time that he realizes he is alone, he notices the elephants. He may then associate elephants with separation from his parents and fear elephants thereafter.

INFORMATION ON ANXIETY

CAUSES: Abnormality in common neurotransmitter receptor complex, genetics, emotional or psychological events

SYMPTOMS: Motor tension (muscle tension, trembling, fatigue) and autonomic hyperactivity (shortness of breath, palpitations, cold hands, dizziness, gastrointestinal upset, chills, frequent urination)

DURATION: Often chronic, with discrete episodes lasting five to twenty minutes

TREATMENTS: Sedatives, psychotherapy

Adjustment disorder with anxious mood is an excessive or maladaptive response to a life event in which the individual experiences anxiety. For example, an individual may become so anxious after losing a job that he or she is unable to eat, sleep, or function and begins to entertain the prospect of suicide. While anxiety is to be expected, this person has excessive anxiety (the inability to eat, sleep, or function) and a maladaptive response (the thought of suicide). The exaggerated response may be attributable to the personality traits of the individual. In this example, a dependent person will be more likely to experience an adjustment disorder than a less dependent person.

Adjustment disorders are very common. In addition to adjustment disorders with anxious mood, people may experience adjustment disorders with depressed mood, mixed emotional features, disturbance of conduct, physical complaints, withdrawal, or inhibition in school or at work. These disorders are considered to be primarily psychological.

Post-traumatic stress disorder (PTSD) is similar to adjustment disorder because it represents a psychological reaction to a significant life event. PTSD only occurs, however, when the precipitating event would be seriously emotionally traumatic to a normal person, such as war, rape, natural disasters such as major earthquakes, or airplane crashes. In PTSD, the individual suffers from flashbacks to the precipitating event and "relives" the experience. These episodes are not simply vivid remembrances of what happened but a transient sensation of actually being in that circumstance. For example, a Vietnam War veteran may literally jump behind bushes when a car backfires.

People who suffer from PTSD usually are anxious and startle easily. They may be depressed and have disturbed sleeping and eating patterns. They often lose normal interest in sex, and nightmares are common. These individuals usually try to avoid situations that remind them of their trauma. Relationships with others are often strained, and the patient is generally pessimistic about the future.

In addition to the anxiety disorders described, abnormal anxiety may be caused by a variety of drugs and medical illnesses. Common drug offenders include caffeine, alcohol, stimulants in cold preparations, nicotine, and many illicit drugs, including cocaine and amphetamines. Medical illnesses that may cause anxiety include thyroid disease, heart failure, cardiac arrhythmias, and schizophrenia.

Treatment and Therapy

When an individual has difficulty with anxiety and seeks professional help, the cause of the anxiety must be determined. Before the etiology can be determined, however, the professional must first realize that the patient has an anxiety disorder. People with anxiety disorders often complain primarily of physical symptoms that result from the anxiety. These symptoms may include motor tension (muscle tension, trembling, and fatigue) and autonomic hyperactivity (shortness of breath, palpitations, cold hands, dizziness, gastrointestinal upset, chills, and frequent urination).

When an anxiety disorder is suspected, effective treatment often depends on an accurate diagnosis of the type of anxiety disorder present. A variety of medications can be prescribed for the anxiety disorder. In addition, several types of psychotherapy can be used. For example, patients with panic disorder can be educated about the nature of their illness, reassured that they will not die from it, and taught to ride out a panic attack. This process avoids the development of secondary anxiety, which complicates the panic attack. Phobic patients can be treated with systematic desensitization, in which they are taught relaxation techniques and are given graded exposure to the feared situation so that their fear lessens or disappears.

The origin, diagnosis, and treatment of anxiety disorders can best be portrayed through case examples. Three fictional cases are described below to illustrate typical anxiety disorder patients.

Ms. Smith is a twenty-four-year-old married mother of two young children. She works part-time as a bookkeeper for a construction company. Her health had been good until a month ago, when she began to experience spells of intense fearfulness, a racing heart, tremors of her hands, a dry mouth, and dizziness. The spells would come on suddenly and would last between ten and fifteen minutes. She was convinced that heart disease was causing these episodes and was worried about having a heart attack. As a result, she consulted her family physician.

Physical examination, electrocardiogram, and laboratory studies were all normal. Her physician had initially considered cardiac arrhythmia (abnormal rhythm of the heartbeat) as a cause but diagnosed panic disorder on the basis of Ms. Smith's history and the outcome of the tests. Treatment consisted of medication and comforting explanations of the nonfatal nature of the disorder. Within three weeks, the panic attacks stopped altogether.

This case illustrates many common features of panic disorder. The patient is a young adult female with classic panic attacks striking "out of the blue." Most patients fear that they are having a heart attack or a stroke or that they are going insane. Typically, they present their symptoms to general medical physicians rather than to psychiatrists. Treatment with medication and simple counseling techniques is usually successful.

Mr. Jones is a thirty-five-year-old single man who works as an accountant. He has always been shy and has adopted leisure activities that he can do alone, such as reading, gardening, and coin collecting. As a child, he was bright but withdrawn. His mother described him as "high-strung," "a worrier," and "easily moved to tears." Recently, he has been bothered by muscle achiness, frequent urination, and diarrhea alternating with constipation. He thinks constantly about his health and worries that he has cancer.

Mr. Jones makes frequent visits to his doctor, but no illness is found. His doctor tells him that he worries too much. The patient admits to himself that he is a worrier and has been his whole life. He ruminates about the details of his job, his health, his lack of friends, the state of the economy, and a host of other concerns. His worries make it hard for him to fall asleep at night. Once asleep, however, he sleeps soundly. Finally, Mr. Jones is given a tranquilizer by his physician. He finds that he feels calm, no longer broods over everything, falls asleep easily, and has relief from his physical symptoms. To improve his social functioning, he sees a psychiatrist, who diagnoses a generalized anxiety disorder and an avoidant (shy) personality disorder.

This case illustrates many features of patients with generalized anxiety disorder. These individuals have near-continuous anxiety for weeks or months that is not clearly related to a single life event. In this case, some of the physical manifestations of anxiety are prominent (muscle tension, frequent urination, and diarrhea). Difficulty falling asleep is also common with anxiety. In contrast, patients who are depressed will often have early morning wakening. In this case example, the patient also has a concomitant shy personality that aggravates his condition. Such a patient usually benefits from treatment. Medication may be required for many years, although it may be needed only during active cycles of anxiety. Because some patients attempt to medicate themselves with alcohol, secondary alcoholism is a potential complication.

Ms. Johnson is a forty-two-year-old married homemaker and mother of four children. She works part-time in a fabric store as a salesclerk. She is friendly and outgoing. She has also been very close with her family, especially her mother. Ms. Johnson comes to her family physician because her mother has just had a stroke. Because her mother lives on the other side of the country, Ms. Johnson needs to take an airplane if she is to get to her mother's bedside quickly. Unfortunately, Ms. Johnson has a long-standing fear of flying; even the thought of getting into an airplane terrifies her. She has not personally had a bad experience with flying but remembers reading about a plane crash when she was a teenager. She denies any other unusual fears and otherwise functions well.

Her family physician refers her to a psychologist for systematic desensitization to relieve her phobia for future situations. As a stopgap measure for the present, however, she is taught a deep-muscle relaxation technique, is shown videotapes designed to reduce fear of flying, and is prescribed a tranquilizer and another drug to reduce the physical manifestations of anxiety (a beta-blocker). This combination of treatments allows her to visit her mother immediately and, eventually, to be able to fly without needing medication.

This case illustrates a typical patient with an isolated phobia. Phobias are probably the most common anxiety disorders. Treatments such as those described above are usually quite helpful.

PERSPECTIVE AND PROSPECTS

Anxiety has been recognized since antiquity and was often attributed to magical or spiritual causes, such as demoniac possession. Ancient myths provided explanations for fearful events in people's lives. Pan, a mythological god of mischief, was thought to cause frightening noises in forests, especially at night; the term "panic" is derived from his name. An understanding of the causes of panic and other anxiety disorders has evolved over the years.

Sigmund Freud (1856-1939) distinguished anxiety from fear. He considered fear to be an expected response to a specific, identifiable trigger, whereas anxiety was a similar emotional state without an identifiable trigger. He postulated that anxiety resulted from unconscious, forbidden wishes that conflicted with what the person believed was acceptable. The anxiety that resulted from this mental conflict was called an "anxiety neurosis" and was thought to result in a variety of psychological and physical symptoms. Psychoanalysis was developed to uncover these hidden conflicts and to allow the anxiety to be released.

Freud's theories about anxiety are no longer universally accepted. Many psychiatrists now believe that several anxiety disorders have a biological cause and that they are more neurological diseases than psychological ones. This is primarily true of generalized anxiety disorder, panic disorder, and obsessive-compulsive disorder. It is recognized that anxiety can also be triggered by drugs (legal and illicit) and a variety of medical illnesses.

Psychological causes of anxiety are also recognized. Adjustment disorder with anxious mood, phobias, and post-traumatic stress disorder are all thought to be primarily psychological disorders. Unlike with Freud's conflict theory of anxiety, most modern psychiatrists consider personality factors, life experiences, and views of the world to be the relevant psychological factors in such anxiety disorders. Nonpharmacological therapies are no longer designed to uncover hidden mental conflicts; they provide instead support. Specific therapies include flooding (massive exposure to the feared situation), systematic desensitization (graded exposure), and relaxation techniques.

—Peter M. Hartmann, M.D.

See also Antidepressants; Appetite loss; Arrhythmias; Bipolar disorders; Death and dying; Depression; Emotions: Biomedical causes and effects; Grief and guilt; Gulf War syndrome; Hyperhidrosis; Hyperventilation; Hypochondriasis; Midlife crisis; Neurosis; Obsessive-compulsive disorder; Palpitations; Panic attacks; Paranoia; Phobias; Postpartum depression; Post-traumatic stress disorder; Psychiatric disorders; Psychiatry; Psychiatry, child and adolescent; Psychiatry, geriatric; Psychoanalysis; Psychosomatic disorders; Sexual dysfunction; Stress; Stress reduction; Suicide; Sweating.

For Further Information:

American Psychiatric Association. *Diagnostic and Statistical Manual of Mental Disorders: DSM-IV-TR*. 4th rev. ed. Washington, D.C.: Author, 2000. This textbook contains the official diagnostic criteria and classification for all the anxiety disorders. Provides useful descriptions, definitions, and prevalence data.

Barlow, David H. *Anxiety and Its Disorders*. 2d ed. New York: Guilford Press, 2002. Examines the subject in the context of recent developments in emotion theory, cognitive science, and neuroscience. Reviews the implications for treatment and integrates them into newly developed treatment protocols for the various anxiety disorders.

Bourne, Edmond J. *The Anxiety and Phobia Workbook*. Oakland, Calif.: New Harbinger, 1995. This is an excellent self-help book for problems related to anxiety. It may also be helpful for family members seeking to understand anxiety better or to support those affected by anxiety.

Davidson, Jonathan, and Henry Dreher. *The Anxiety Book*. New York: Penguin, 2003. The director of the Anxiety and Traumatic Stress Program at Duke University Medical Center provides an informed overview of each category of chronic anxiety, including its symptoms and manifestations. Self-assessment tests are included to help readers identify which type of anxiety is troubling them.

Kleinknecht, Ronald A. *Mastering Anxiety: The Nature and Treatment of Anxious Conditions*. New York: Plenum Press, 1991. This book provides a good overview, with statistics and good explanations of the different types of anxiety disorder.

Leaman, Thomas L. *Healing the Anxiety Diseases*. New York: Plenum Press, 1992. A helpful text written by a family physician with an interest in anxiety disorders. Provides a good overview of the subject in nontechnical terms and contains practical advice on dealing with anxiety.

Saul, Helen. *Phobias: Fighting the Fear*. New York: Arcade, 2001. Traces the historical and cultural roots of phobias, examining case studies and literature in the process.

Sheehan, David V. *The Anxiety Disease*. New York: Bantam Books, 1983. A classic book written for the layperson that explains the nature of anxiety, the different types of anxiety disorder, and treatment approaches.

Apgar score

Procedure

Anatomy or system affected: Circulatory system, heart, lungs, muscles, nervous system, respiratory system

Specialties and related fields: Critical care, neonatology, obstetrics

Definition: Dr. Virginia Apgar, an obstetrical anesthesiologist, developed the Apgar score in 1952 to assess the clinical status of newborns and the effectiveness of resuscitation.

Indications and Procedures

The five categories evaluated by the Apgar score—heart rate, respiratory effort, muscle tone, response to

The Apgar Score

Sign	Score 0	Score 1	Score 2
Heart rate (beats per minute)	Absent	Below 100	Above 100
Respiratory effort	Absent	Slow, irregular	Good crying
Muscle tone	Limp	Some	Active motion
Response to nasal catheter	None	Grimace	Cough, sneeze
Color	Blue or pale	Body pink, extremities blue	Pink

stimulus, and color—reflect functions necessary to sustain life. The accompanying table lists the components in descending order of importance. The Apgar score is the sum of scoring each of the five parameters.

The first Apgar score is traditionally assigned at one minute after birth. It reflects the baby's condition in the womb and indicates the degree of resuscitation that may be required. A low one-minute score is not predictive of adverse neurologic outcome.

A second Apgar score is assigned at five minutes after birth. A score of 7 to 10 is considered normal, while a score of 4 to 6 is considered borderline. A five-minute Apgar score of 3 or less has been associated with cerebral palsy in full-term infants; however, only approximately 4 to 5 percent of infants with low five-minute Apgar scores have long-term neurologic abnormalities. A stronger relationship exists between low Apgar scores and future neurologic disability when the assessment is taken at times greater than ten minutes after birth.

Perspective and Prospects

In the United States, approximately 1 percent of all babies are born with Apgar scores of less than 6. The highest proportions of infants with low Apgar scores at five minutes are among infants born to mothers under sixteen years of age or over forty years of age and to those who did not receive prenatal care.

Current research using the Apgar score focuses increasingly on the neonatal heart rate and respiratory effort, looking for long-term subtle behavioral disabilities that may be associated with low and borderline Apgar scores.

—*David A. Clark, M.D.*

See also Blue baby syndrome; Cardiovascular system; Childbirth; Childbirth complications; Jaundice; Multiple births; Neonatology; Physical examination; Pregnancy and gestation; Premature birth; Reflexes, primitive; Respiration; Respiratory distress syndrome; Screening; Well-baby examinations.

For Further Information:

Apgar, Virginia, and Joan Beck. *Is My Baby All Right?* New York: Trident Press, 1972.

Barness, Lewis A. *Manual of Pediatric Physical Diagnosis*. 6th ed. St. Louis: Mosby Medical, 1991.

Schwartz, M. William, ed. *Clinical Handbook of Pediatrics*. 2d ed. Baltimore: Williams & Wilkins, 1999.

Zitelli, Basil J., and Holly W. Davis, eds. *Atlas of Pediatric Physical Diagnosis*. 4th ed. St. Louis: Mosby-Wolfe, 2002.

Aphasia and dysphasia

Disease/disorder

Anatomy or system affected: Brain, nervous system

Specialties and related fields: Neurology, speech pathology

Definition: Aphasia is loss of the comprehension or production of language, while dysphasia is impairment of comprehension or production of language.

Key terms:

angiography: a series of X-ray films taken in a fixed sequence using contrast dye so that pictures of the arteries, smaller vessels, and veins can be obtained

ataxia: lack of coordination and irregularity of voluntary, purposeful movements

computed tomography (CT) scan: a noninvasive diagnostic study consisting of a series of X-ray films scanning different levels of the brain and resulting in pictures that show hemorrhages, tumors, cysts, edema, infarction, atrophy, and hydrocephalus
electroencephalography (EEG): recording of the electrical activity of the brain by using eight to sixteen electrodes placed on specific areas of the scalp; used to evaluate cerebral disease, as well as metabolic and systemic disorders, and to diagnose brain death
hemiparesis: weakness on one side of the body
myoclonus: a series of shocklike contractions that cause throwing movements of a limb
nystagmus: involuntary oscillations of one or both eyes
paresthesia: numbness and tingling sensations in the extremities
ptosis: sagging or drooping; often refers to ptosis of the eyelids, usually as a result of muscle weakness

Information on Aphasia and Dysphasia

Causes: Dysfunction in the left cerebral hemisphere, primarily from stroke but also from various vascular, neoplastic, traumatic, degenerative, metabolic, or infectious diseases or injuries
Symptoms: Various language dysfunctions (fluency, volume, or quantity of speech)
Duration: Acute, chronic, or progressive, depending on cause
Treatments: Speech therapy, treatment of underlying cause

Causes and Symptoms

Dysphasias are usually associated with cerebrovascular accident (CVA), or stroke, involving the middle cerebral artery or one of its many branches. Language disorders may arise, however, from a variety of injuries and diseases: vascular, neoplastic, traumatic, degenerative, metabolic, or infectious.

Dysphasia results from dysfunction in the left cerebral hemisphere, most commonly in the frontotemporal region of the brain and particularly around the insula. Most language disorders are attributable to acute processes that either resolve or cause a chronic residual deficit, while others result from degenerative disorders that cause the dysfunction to be progressive.

Dysphasias have been classified both anatomically and functionally. Other classifications are linguistic and describe the fluency, volume, or quantity of speech. Pure forms of any language dysfunction, however, are very rare. Expressive dysphasias are primarily characterized by expressive deficits, but a verbal comprehension deficit may be present. Receptive dysphasias have expressive deficits. Transcortical dysphasias involve the ability to repeat and to recite. Speech is fluent but with striking paraphrases. The individual is unable to read and write, and comprehension is impaired.

Transcortical dysphasias are caused by hypoxia (oxygen deficiency) from prolonged hypotension (low blood pressure), carbon monoxide poisoning, or other mechanisms that destroy the border zone between the anterior, middle, and posterior cerebral arteries. Blood supply is marginal in this region. Hypoxia in this area may occasionally isolate the posterior speech areas or all the speech areas from the remainder of the cortex, although both areas remain intact. The sensory and motor speech areas are, therefore, functional, but connections with other sensory or motor areas are impaired. Information from the remaining areas of the cortex cannot be transmitted to be transformed into language.

Aphasias can be classified into Broca's, Wernicke's, anomic, or global aphasias. Aphasia reflects damage to one or more of the brain's primary language centers, which, in most persons, are located in the left hemisphere. Broca's area lies next to the region of the motor cortex that controls the muscles necessary for speech, and presumably coordinates their movement. Wernicke's area, which helps control the content of speech and affects its auditory and visual comprehension, lies between Heschl's gyrus, the primary receiver of auditory stimuli, and the angular gyrus, a "way station" between the auditory and visual regions. Connecting Wernicke's and Broca's areas is a large nerve bundle, the arcuate fasciculus, which also helps control the content of speech and enables repetition.

The left hemisphere is dominant for language in all right-handed people and in the majority of left-handed people. When a stroke occurs in the dominant hemisphere, the patient may experience dysphasia or aphasia. Language disorders involve the expression and comprehension of written or spoken words. When the lesion involves Wernicke's area of the brain, the patient experiences receptive aphasia; neither the sounds of speech nor its meaning can be distinguished, and comprehension of both written and spoken language is impaired. The lesion causing expressive aphasia affects Broca's area, the motor area for speech. The patient has difficulty speaking and writing. Aphasias may be classified as either nonfluent or fluent. In nonfluent aphasia, the patient speaks very little and produces speech slowly and with obvious effort. In fluent aphasia, the patient may speak, but the phrases have little meaning because of impaired comprehension. Conduction aphasia is a type of fluent aphasia in which the lesion is in the pathway between Broca's and Wernicke's areas. Most aphasias are mixed, with some impairment of both expression and understanding. A massive lesion may result in global aphasia, in which virtually all language function is lost.

Stroke is the most common cause of aphasia. Associated findings usually include decreased level of consciousness, right-sided hemiparesis, and paresthesia. Another communication problem experienced by many stroke patients is dysarthria, or slurred speech. Dysarthria results from a disturbance in muscular control and produces impairment of pronunciation, articulation, and phonation. Dysarthria does not result in any disturbance of language function itself. However, an occasional stroke patient may be unfortunate enough to have both aphasia and dysarthria.

A transient ischemic attack (TIA) can produce any type of aphasia. Usually, the aphasia occurs suddenly and resolves within twenty-four hours of the TIA. Brain abscess may result in any type of aphasia. Usually, the aphasia develops insidiously and may be accompanied by hemiparesis, ataxia, facial weakness, and signs of increased intracranial pressure. A brain tumor may cause anomic aphasia, which may be an early sign of the condition. Encephalitis (brain inflammation) usually produces transient aphasia. Its earlier signs include fever, headache, and vomiting. Accompanying the aphasia may be convulsions, confusion, stupor or coma, hemiparesis, asymmetrical deep tendon reflexes, positive Babinski's reflex, ataxia, myoclonus, nystagmus, ocular palsies, and facial weakness. Head trauma may cause any type of aphasia. Typically, aphasia resulting from severe trauma occurs suddenly and may be transient or permanent, depending on the extent of brain damage. Anomic aphasia may begin insidiously and then progress; associated signs include behavioral changes, memory loss, poor judgment, restlessness, myoclonus, and muscle rigidity. Alzheimer's disease, a degenerative dementia, may also cause aphasia. Drug abuse, particularly heroin overdose, can cause any type of aphasia.

Depending on its severity, aphasia may impede communication slightly or may make it impossible. Anomic aphasia eventually resolves in more than 50 percent of patients, but global aphasia is irreversible.

In the pediatric population, aphasia is sometimes mistakenly attributed to children who fail to develop normal language skills but who are not considered mentally retarded or developmentally delayed. Aphasia refers solely to loss of previously developed communication skills, however, and should not be used in this context. Brain damage associated with aphasia in children most commonly follows anoxia (oxygen deprivation), the result of near-drowning or airway obstruction.

Treatment and Therapy

If a person suddenly develops aphasia, a physician should be notified immediately. The patient is assessed quickly for signs of increased intracranial pressure, such as papillary changes, decreased level of consciousness, vomiting, seizures, bradycardia (slow heart rate), widening pulse pressure, and irregular respirations. If signs are detected related to increased intracranial pressure, appropriate medications are administered to decrease cerebral edema. Emergency resuscitation equipment may be used to support respiratory and cardiac function, if necessary. Emergency surgery may be indicated.

If the patient does not display signs of increased intracranial pressure, or if the aphasia has developed gradually, then a thorough neurologic assessment is performed, starting with the patient history. Information may be obtained from the patient's family or companion because of the patient's impairment. The staff member assigned to the patient's care will ask about a history of headaches, hypertension, or seizure disorders, as well as about any drug use. The patient's ability to communicate and to perform routine activities before the aphasia began is assessed. The patient is checked for obvious signs of neurologic deficit, such as ptosis or fluid leakage from the nose and ears. The patient's vital signs are taken and level of consciousness assessed. Assessing the level of consciousness is often difficult, however, because the patient's verbal responses may be unreliable. In addition, dysarthria or speech apraxia (the inability to control voluntarily the muscles of speech) may accompany aphasia. The patient should be allowed ample time to respond and should be spoken to slowly. Assessment of pupil response, eye movements, and motor function, especially mouth and tongue movement and swallowing, is conducted. To best assess motor function, the care provider will first demonstrate and then have the patient imitate responses, rather than merely providing verbal directions.

Immediately after aphasia develops, the patient may become confused or disoriented. The care provider can help restore a sense of reality by frequently telling the patient what has happened, where he or she is and why, and the date. The patient needs careful explanation of diagnostic tests, such as computed tomography (CT) scans, angiography, and electroencephalography (EEG). Later, periods of depression are expected as the patient recognizes the handicap. The patient can be aided in attempts at communication through a relaxed, accepting environment with a minimum of distracting stimuli. When speaking to the patient, the staff assigned to care cannot assume that he or she understands. The patient may simply be interpreting subtle clues to meaning, such as social context, facial expressions, and gestures. To help avoid misunderstanding, care providers should speak in simple phrases and use demonstration to clarify verbal directions. Because aphasia is a language disorder, not an emotional or auditory one, a normal tone of voice should be used when speaking to the patient. Necessary aids, such as eyeglasses or dentures, should be provided to facilitate communication. Referrals to speech pathologists early in the development of the problem will help the patient cope with aphasia.

—Jane C. Norman, R.N., Ph.D.

See also Brain; Brain disorders; Neurology; Neurology, pediatric; Speech disorders; Strokes; Transient ischemic attacks (TIAs).

FOR FURTHER INFORMATION:

Greenberg, David A., Michael J. Aminoff, and Roger P. Simon. *Clinical Neurology*. 5th ed. New York: McGraw-Hill, 2002.

Rowland, Lewis P., ed. *Merritt's Textbook of Neurology*. 11th ed. Philadelphia: Lippincott Williams & Wilkins, 2005.

Samuels, Martin A., ed. *Manual of Neurologic Therapeutics*. 6th ed. New York: Lippincott Williams & Wilkins, 1999.

Victor, Maurice, and Allan H. Ropper. *Adams and Victor's Principles of Neurology*. 7th ed. New York: McGraw-Hill, 2002.

APHRODISIACS

TREATMENT

ALSO KNOWN AS: Love potions

ANATOMY OR SYSTEM AFFECTED: Genitals (theoretically), psychic-emotional system

SPECIALTIES AND RELATED FIELDS: Alternative medicine

DEFINITION: A substance capable of inducing sexual desire or lust or enhancing sexual performance.

INDICATIONS AND PROCEDURES

The word "aphrodisiac," derived from Aphrodite, the mythical Greek goddess of love, describes a number of animal and plant products reputedly capable of promoting sexual desire. All aphrodisiacs are hoped to function in one of three ways: promote a desire for sexual stimulation or sexual appetite, increase the ability to indulge in sexual activity, or increase the capability and prolong the ability to maintain successful sexual activity. In theory, aphrodisiacs are an exciter of lust, but in practice an aphrodisiac may be anything, of any means, that increases the appetite and capacity for sexual pleasure. Only those cultures treating sex as a pleasurable activity, rather than as an act strictly to ensure a new generation, seem to have sought out drugs, potions, elixirs, charms, and spells as a means to increase sexual activity.

The concept of natural substances being used to promote sexual activity has been a feature of art and literature throughout history, but modern medical and scientific opinions have been dismissive, concluding that no such substances that can be quantitatively measured exist in natural products. Despite this knowledge, the market for aphrodisiacs flourishes, in many cases to the detriment of rare or endangered plants and animals whose natural characteristics are falsely considered to harbor the means of enhancing sexual pleasure.

At the same time, a number of modern drugs are being manufactured, prescribed, and used in Western clinical medicine to restore the sexual capability of patients who suffer either physical or pathological disorders resulting in organic impotence (lack of the physical capability for sexual performance). Modern pharmaceutical manufacturers aggressively market numerous proprietary hormone and testosterone replacement therapies and priapitic drugs. A clinical drug prescribed for penile dysfunction, such as Viagra (sildenafil), by strict definition could be considered an aphrodisiac.

Uses and Complications

Traditionally, women use aphrodisiacs as a means to stimulate feelings of sexual desire in a partner or to increase their own personal sexual enjoyment. Male aphrodisiac usage is often more complicated. Sexual potency is a major component of the male ego, and anxiety associated with lack of sexual prowess is a phenomenon that crosses cultural, economic, educational, and class boundaries.

One major motive for the use of aphrodisiacs is a feeling of sexual inadequacy. For individuals who consider themselves sexually adequate yet still use aphrodisiacs, mere physical performance and sexual stamina are less important. These people tend to use aphrodisiacs in the hope of increasing their sexual pleasure. From a biological perspective, a successful sexual encounter is one in which the male achieves penetration and ejaculation. Socially, however, both partners want sexual pleasure and satisfaction: male orgasm and ejaculation in concert with female orgasm or climax. This requires timing and experience, usually with a familiar partner. Thus, increasing the sensitivity of the female clitoris to encourage female orgasm or delaying the male orgasm by decreasing the sensitivity of the penis has become the focused use of some aphrodisiacs.

—Randall L. Milstein, Ph.D.

See also Hormones; Masturbation; Reproductive system; Sexual dysfunction; Sexuality.

For Further Information:

Stanley, Autumn. *Mothers and Daughters of Invention*. Metuchen, N.J.: Scarecrow Press, 1993.

Stark, Raymond. *The Book of Aphrodisiacs*. New York: Stein and Day, 1981.

Taberner, P. V. *Aphrodisiacs: The Science and the Myth*. Philadelphia: University of Pennsylvania Press, 1985.

Apnea

Disease/disorder

Anatomy or system affected: Brain, lungs, nervous system, respiratory system

Specialties and related fields: Internal medicine, neonatology, neurology, pulmonary medicine

Definition: Cessation of breathing, from the Greek meaning "without wind."

Information on Apnea

Causes: Inspiratory muscle inactivity, airway obstruction

Symptoms: Choking, snoring, gasping, stridor, bradycardia, cyanosis, depression, irritability, learning difficulty, daytime sleepiness

Duration: Chronic, with multiple episodes during sleep

Treatments: Medication (xanthines), mechanical treatment (continuous positive airway pressure mask), surgery

Causes and Symptoms

People normally experience brief pauses in breathing. When these pauses last more than twenty seconds or are accompanied by bradycardia (slow heart rate) or cyanosis (bluish skin from poor blood oxygenation), however, it can be life-threatening. This condition is referred to as apnea.

Apnea can be categorized into three types based on whether inspiratory muscle activity is present. In central apnea, which has a neurological cause, there is no activity of inspiratory muscles following expiration. Central apnea is uncommon except in apnea of prematurity in infants. Obstructive apnea, the most common type, occurs when the person is making an effort to breathe, so inspiratory muscles are moving. As a result of a blockage, however, air cannot flow into or out of the person's nose or mouth. This condition typically occurs while the patient is asleep and is characterized by snoring, gasping for air, or stridor (noisy breathing). It is seen in people who have a physical obstruction in the airway, who experience gastroesophageal reflux, or who are overweight. The third type of apnea is mixed apnea, which is a combination of central and obstructive apnea. It is usually seen in young children and can occur while asleep or awake.

Individuals with apnea will often show decreases in heart rate, oxygen saturation, peripheral blood flow, and muscle tone. Adults suffering from sleep apnea may exhibit depression, irritability, learning difficulty, and sleepiness during the day. With sleep apnea, there can be up to sixty apneic episodes per hour, with snoring and/or choking in between.

All forms of apnea can be diagnosed by electrophysiological testing. Pneumograms are often done on premature babies to record their pattern of breathing over a twelve-hour period. Polysomnography is used for older children and adults to record electrical activity of the brain, muscle activity, heart rate, airflow, oxygen levels in the body, and eye movement.

Treatment and Therapy

The treatment of apnea can be based on medication, mechanical treatment, or surgery. The category of drugs used to treat apnea are xanthines. Mechanical treatment involves the use of continuous positive airway pressure (CPAP), a mask worn over the nose during sleep that forces air through the nasal passages. Surgery may be performed to remove an obstruction or to increase the size of the airway.

Perspective and Prospects

Studies have indicated that people with obstructive sleep apnea have less gray matter in their brains. Research is being done to determine if the lack of gray matter leads to the apnea or the lack of oxygen with apnea causes deterioration in the brain.

—*Robin Kamienny Montvilo, Ph.D.*

See also Asphyxiation; Cyanosis; Lungs; Pulmonary diseases; Pulmonary medicine; Pulmonary medicine, pediatric; Respiration; Resuscitation; Sleep; Sleep apnea; Sleep disorders; Wheezing.

For Further Information:

George, Ronald B. *Current Pulmonology and Critical Care Medicine*. Vol. 17. Philadelphia: C. V. Mosby, 1996.

Klaus, Marshall H., and Avroy A. Fanaroff, eds. *Care of the High-Risk Neonate*. 5th ed. Philadelphia: W. B. Saunders, 2001.

Pack, Allan, ed. *Sleep Apnea: Pathogenesis, Diagnosis, and Treatment*. New York: Marcel Dekker, 2002.

Appendectomy

Procedure

Anatomy or system affected: Abdomen, gastrointestinal system, intestines

Specialties and related fields: Emergency medicine, general surgery

Definition: Corrective surgery to remove the appendix, which is required when acute appendicitis produces severe abdominal pain and the probability of peritonitis or health complications, which may be fatal if untreated.

Key terms:

cecum: a pouchlike portion of the large intestine

fecalith: a hardened piece of fecal matter which often begins events leading to appendectomy by blocking the appendix

peritonitis: infection of the abdominal (peritoneal) cavity in which the visceral organs are found

septic pyelophlebitis: inflammation of the veins which carry blood away from the kidneys; it results from neglecting symptoms of acute appendicitis and can be fatal

Indications and Procedures

The appendix, more correctly named the vermiform appendix, is a hollow tube of muscle attached to the pouchlike beginning of the large intestine (the cecum) and closed at the end farthest from this point of attachment. It does not serve a known purpose and is thought to be a disappearing vestige of an organ that once had a purpose. Hence the appendix is called a vestigial organ.

A vermiform appendix exists only in humans and other primates. In humans, it is approximately 7.6 to 10.2 centimeters (3 to 4 inches) long and 1.3 centimeters (0.5 inch) in diameter. The cavity of the appendix (its lumen) is narrowest at the point of attachment to the cecum, and the muscular walls of the organ normally contract periodically to expel into the cecum both mucus made by the appendix and intestinal contents which may have accidentally entered the lumen.

When the narrow opening of the appendix into the cecum is blocked so as to prevent expulsion of mucus or fecal material, the organ becomes infected, a condition called appendicitis. The most frequent obstructions found in appendix openings are fecaliths. These objects are hardened pieces of fecal matter that entered the appendix from the large intestine. Swelling of the inner walls of the appendix as a result of other causes (such as bacterial infection) can also begin such a blockage.

Following blockage, the events leading to appendicitis usually occur in the following order. First, fluids and mucus secreted by the cells lining the walls of the appendix collect in the blocked organ. This makes the appendix swell, causing the blood vessels that feed the organ's tissues gradually to close off. In the absence of an adequate blood supply, the tissue begins to die. At the same time, bacteria originating in the cecum grow vigorously in the affected appendix, increasing the inflammation and swelling of the dying organ.

Quick and appropriate treatment by surgical removal of the infected appendix—appendectomy—is often required at this time. Otherwise, the walls of such an appendix, one weakened by tissue death and subjected to increasing pressure by both bacterial growth and the buildup of mucus, may burst. When this happens, the contents spill into the abdominal cavity and infect the membranes which line it. Such infection, peritonitis, can be very painful. In most cases, however, the use of antibiotics will keep peritonitis from becoming fatal.

Where appendectomy is required, the patient is usually given a general anesthetic. A 5- to 7.6-centimeter (2- to 3-inch) incision is made directly over the site of the appendix, and the surgeon ties off and cuts the blood vessels that feed the organ. The appendix is then tied off near its connection to the cecum and carefully cut free without allowing its contents to enter the abdominal cavity. The operation usually takes under an hour and produces minor postoperative discomfort for a few days. The surgical risks of this procedure are very slight.

USES AND COMPLICATIONS

Acute infection of the appendix, requiring its surgical removal, is the most frequent cause for abdominal surgery. It is most likely to occur between the ages of eight and thirty, but no age group is exempt. Acute appendicitis is often symptomized by initial generalized abdominal pain which rapidly becomes localized. The pain, which can be quite severe and which is felt whenever the patient moves or coughs, frequently occurs in the lower-right quadrant of the abdomen (an area between the navel and the front edge of the right hipbone). This location is common because many appendixes are located in the underlying abdominal cavity. The appendix may be found, however, in any of several other positions. Hence, the pain can occur elsewhere in the abdomen, and acute appendicitis may be mistaken for other abdominal disorders.

Other symptoms useful in diagnosing acute appendicitis are nausea and vomiting, increased pulse rate, and mild fever. In addition, the patient's white blood count will often increase from the normal range of 7,000 to 10,000 per cubic millimeter to 25,000. Doctors can also use CT (computed tomography) scanning for diagnostic purposes. When symptoms of acute appendicitis occur, medications should not be given unless quick access to surgical facilities is available. For example, cathartics are a poor treatment choice because they stimulate intestinal contractions that may accelerate intestinal rupture. Similarly, the use of hot water bottles to relieve pain is inappropriate because it may also speed rupture. In cases of acute pain, the patient should be taken to a hospital emergency room as quickly as possible.

The dangers associated with appendicitis arise from its neglect. Peritonitis is rarely fatal because of the use of antibiotics. Much more serious are localized abscesses of the abdominal wall and the inflammation of the veins that carry blood away from the kidneys (septic pyelophlebitis). Both of these problems can be fatal, even when extensive and aggressive antibiotic therapy is carried out.

If a clear diagnosis of acute appendicitis cannot be made, it has become customary, in recent years, to wait and observe the patient's symptoms for up to twenty-four hours before surgery. This waiting period allows the physician an exact diagnosis without unduly subjecting the patient to the risk of peritonitis. In some cases, abdominal X rays are useful diagnostic tools. During such waiting periods, patients are under careful surveillance, and a surgical facility is kept ready for quick use, if needed.

—*Sanford S. Singer, Ph.D.*

The Removal of the Appendix

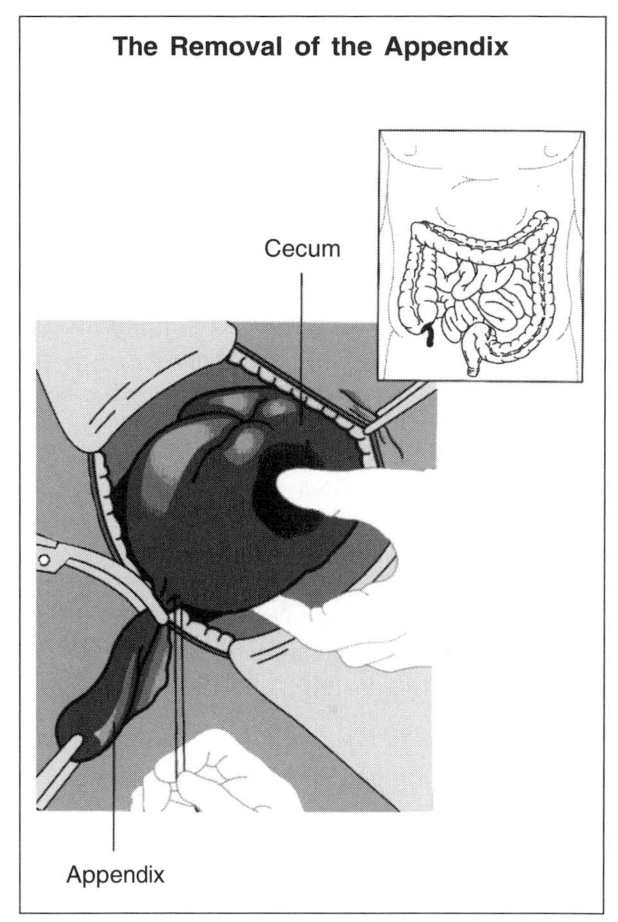

Inflammation of the appendix, a vestigial organ attached to the colon, usually requires an emergency appendectomy to avoid rupture and more extensive, life-threatening infection; the inset shows the location of the appendix.

See also Abdomen; Abdominal disorders; Appendicitis; Emergency medicine; Gastroenterology; Gastroenterology, pediatric; Gastrointestinal system; Infection; Inflammation; Intestinal disorders; Intestines; Laparoscopy; Pediatrics; Peritonitis.

For Further Information:

Beers, Mark H., et al. *The Merck Manual of Diagnosis and Therapy*. 18th ed. Whitehouse Station, N.J.: Merck Research Laboratories, 2006. This is a reference work for physicians, and the nomenclature can be daunting. It is best consulted after more general introductory reading.

Krahenbuhl, L. *Acute Appendicitis: Standard Treatment or Laparoscopic Surgery?* New York: Karger, 1998. Examines methods for diagnosing and treating appendicitis.

Tierney, Lawrence M., Jr., et al., eds. *Current Medical Diagnosis and Treatment 2004*. 43d ed. New York: McGraw-Hill, 2003. This text, updated yearly, is the point of reference for physicians and other health care practitioners. It incorporates each year's biomedical research discoveries.

Zinner, Michael J., et al., eds. *Maingot's Abdominal Operations*. 10th ed. Stamford, Conn.: Appleton & Lange, 1997. This textbook has long been considered the classic work on all surgical disciplines.

Appendicitis

Disease/disorder

Anatomy or system affected: Abdomen, gastrointestinal system, intestines

Specialties and related fields: Emergency medicine, gastroenterology, pediatrics

Definition: Inflammation of the human vermiform appendix.

Causes and Symptoms

Appendicitis may be acute or chronic. The inflammation characteristic of the condition may be associated

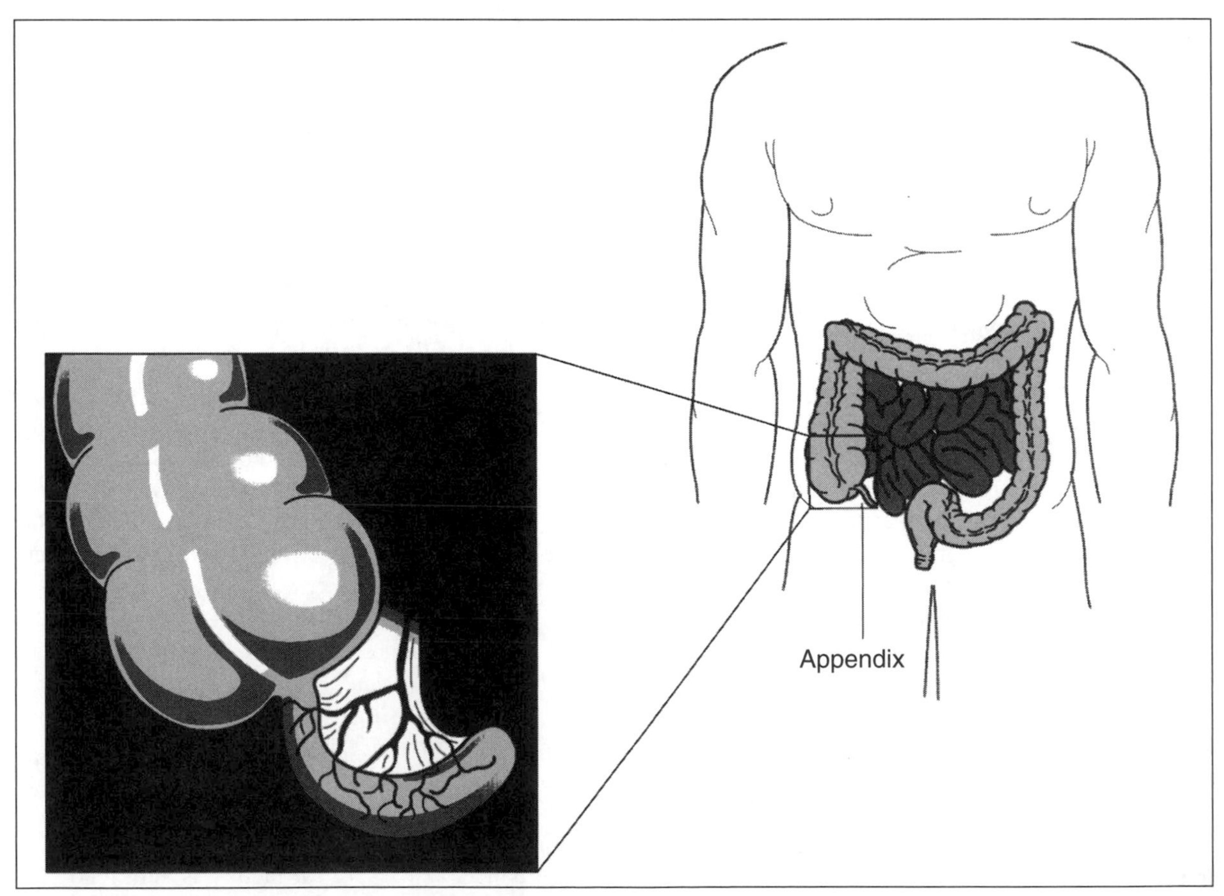

The vermiform appendix, located in the lower-right abdomen at one end of the large colon, may become inflamed as a result of obstruction; surgery is nearly always required to avoid bursting and the release of deadly toxins into the body.

Information on Appendicitis

Causes: Infection or unknown
Symptoms: Abdominal pain, nausea, fever, elevated white blood cell count
Duration: Acute or chronic
Treatments: Surgical removal of appendix

with infection or the causes may be various or even unknown.

In the human digestive system, the small intestine empties into the large intestine, or colon, in the lower right abdomen. Movement of waste from that point is generally upward through the ascending colon, but the colon begins with a downward-projecting blind end called the cecum, to which is attached the vermiform ("wormlike") appendix. The appendix has no known function. Occasionally, its opening into the cecum becomes obstructed, and inflammation, swelling, and pain follow. Sometimes the cause of the obstruction is identifiable, such as pinworms or other parasites, or hardened fecal material; more often, it is not. Symptoms, including pain that is general at the outset but localizes in the lower right abdomen, can include nausea, fever, and an elevated white blood cell count. If the swollen appendix bursts, peritonitis—infection and poisoning of the abdominal cavity—can result. Peritonitis is usually signaled to the patient by an abrupt cessation of pain, when the swelling is relieved, but is followed by serious and life-threatening complications.

Treatment and Therapy

The treatment of choice is almost invariably surgical removal of the inflamed appendix, an operation that is no longer considered major surgery. The patient is usually out of bed in a day or two and fully recovered in a few weeks. Peritonitis, however, calls for emergency surgery to remove the toxic material released by the ruptured appendix, as well as the appendix itself. Because a greater or lesser portion of the abdominal cavity must be cleansed with saline solution and treated with antibiotics, this surgery can become a major procedure.

—Robert M. Hawthorne, Jr., Ph.D.

See also Abdomen; Abdominal disorders; Appendectomy; Gastroenterology; Gastroenterology, pediatric; Gastrointestinal disorders; Gastrointestinal system; Infection; Intestinal disorders; Intestines; Obstruction; Pediatrics; Peritonitis.

For Further Information:

Clayman, Charles B., ed. *The American Medical Association Encyclopedia of Medicine*. New York: Random House, 1994. A concise presentation of numerous medical terms and illnesses. A good general reference.

Krahenbuhl, L. *Acute Appendicitis: Standard Treatment or Laparoscopic Surgery?* New York: Karger, 1998. Examines methods for diagnosing and treating appendicitis.

Litin, Scott C., ed. *Mayo Clinic Family Health Book*. 3d ed. New York: HarperResource, 2003. Perhaps the best general medical text for the layperson, this book covers the entire medical field. While the information is derived from a wide variety of highly technical sources, the articles are written to be easily understood by a general audience.

Wagman, Richard J., ed. *The New Complete Medical and Health Encyclopedia*. 4 vols. Chicago: J. G. Ferguson, 2002. Thorough and clear, with good illustrations.

Appetite loss

Disease/disorder

Also known as: Anorexia

Anatomy or system affected: Gastrointestinal system, heart, immune system, liver, nervous system, psychic-emotional system

Specialties and related fields: Alternative medicine, cardiology, internal medicine, nutrition, psychiatry, psychology

Definition: Loss of interest in food, which may be physical or psychological in origin.

Key terms:

anorexia: loss of appetite

anorexia nervosa: a pathological condition in which victims intentionally starve themselves

nausea: an unpleasant sensation followed by stomach and intestinal discomfort, which may lead to vomiting

Causes and Symptoms

Loss of appetite is an almost universal condition that occasionally affects nearly everyone. It becomes a significant health problem only when it persists. Its causes can be psychological or emotional. For example, often when someone dies, those most affected by the death may stop eating, but they will likely return to normal eating patterns with the passage of time. Chronic depression, however, may result in sustained appetite

> **Information on Appetite Loss**
>
> **Causes:** Psychological or emotional factors (grief, depression); physical factors (infections, intestinal obstructions, cancer, leukemia, pancreatitis, autoimmune diseases, chemotherapy, other medications, dementia)
> **Symptoms:** Lack of interest in eating
> **Duration:** Temporary or sustained
> **Treatments:** Depends on cause; may include psychotherapy, treatment of underlying disease or disorder, cessation of medication

loss. Loss of appetite may also be triggered by such physical causes as infections, intestinal obstructions, cancer (particularly of the colon and stomach), leukemia, pancreatitis (inflammation of the pancreas), autoimmune diseases such as rheumatoid arthritis or scleroderma, chemotherapy and various other medications, and dementia, especially Alzheimer's disease. In many such cases, the cause can be eliminated or controlled in such a way that the appetite returns.

Anorexia nervosa is self-starvation that can have dangerous health consequences. The condition is more prevalent in young women than in older women or in men. Anorexics have a pathological fear of gaining weight, even when their condition results in becoming perilously thin. Although the term "anorexia" means "loss of appetite," most anorexics continue to experience hunger but ignore the body's craving for food.

Treatment and Therapy

Because persistent loss of appetite can result in dangerous weight loss and malnutrition, immediate professional treatment is indicated. Where the causes are physical, internists, oncologists, nutritionists, and other health professionals attempt to remove or limit the cause, although this may not always be possible. They must initially determine when the loss of appetite began and whether its onset was gradual or sudden. They need to know whether their patients frequently feel nauseated and whether they can keep down the food that they ingest.

It is also important to determine whether the appetite loss is constant or intermittent. Some patients' loss of appetite does not include all foods but is limited to some particular foods. In many cases, patients' moods influence their appetites. In all cases, the starting point for treatment is an extensive physical examination that includes broad-spectrum blood tests and urinalysis. Such tests may detect diabetes, kidney infections, and, in women, pregnancy, all of which may affect appetite and eating habits. When loss of appetite is triggered by such factors as a high and/or persistent fever, controlling the fever by attacking the infection that causes it should control the problem.

More difficult to treat are situations in which loss of appetite is attributable to psychological factors such as depression. Patients in such situations are usually referred to psychiatrists or psychologists. Sometimes they become involved in group therapy that can provide them with support while they cope with their problems. If their anorexia is not controlled, it can prove fatal: Patients can lose muscle tone to such as an extent that the heart cannot continue to pump blood through the body, and death from heart failure may occur.

Perspective and Prospects

When the causes of appetite loss are physical, they can usually be treated aggressively and effectively. With medical advances that include such sophisticated diagnostic equipment as ultrasound, magnetic resonance imaging (MRI), or computed tomography (CT) scans, physical abnormalities can be detected while they are still in their early developmental stages. Also, advanced techniques of assessing the information provided by blood tests and urinalysis have opened important windows into the area of physical diagnosis.

—R. Baird Shuman, Ph.D.

See also Aging; Alzheimer's disease; Anorexia nervosa; Antidepressants; Anxiety; Autoimmune disorders; Bariatric surgery; Cancer; Chemotherapy; Death and dying; Dementias; Depression; Eating disorders; Gastrointestinal disorders; Grief and guilt; Leukemia; Malnutrition; Nutrition; Obstruction; Pancreatitis; Psychiatric disorders; Psychiatry; Psychiatry, child and adolescent; Psychiatry, geriatric; Rheumatoid arthritis; Scleroderma; Weight loss and gain; Weight loss medications.

For Further Information:

Clarke, Julie M., and Ann Kirby-Payne. *Understanding Weight and Depression*. New York: Rosen, 2000.

Dockray, Graham J., and Gerard P. Smith, comps. and eds. *Appetite: Papers of a Theme Issue*. London: Royal Society, 2006.

Shuchter, Stephen R., Nancy Downs, and Sidney Zisook. *Biologically Informed Psychotherapy for Depression*. New York: Guilford Press, 2006.

Whitney, Ellie, and Sharon Rady Rolfes. *Understanding Nutrition*. 10th ed. Belmont, Calif.: Thomson/Wadsworth, 2005.

Aromatherapy

Treatment

Anatomy or system affected: Brain, nervous system, nose, psychic-emotional system

Specialties and related fields: Alternative medicine, otorhinolaryngology, preventive medicine, psychology

Definition: The use of scents to facilitate physical, mental, and emotional well-being.

Indications and Procedures

Aromatherapy is best thought of as a complement to other procedures or treatments. Essential oils and aromatic plants are used to stimulate memories, bring about feelings of calm, aid meditation, and enhance visualization exercises. Aromatherapy helps create conditions requiring the enhanced ability to concentrate, mental or physical relaxation, or the discussion of personal information or memories. As such, aromatherapy may be an appropriate adjunctive treatment for stress-related disorders or disorders treated with psychotherapies. Some practitioners suggest that specific scents have extraordinary properties (such as memory enhancers or aphrodisiacs), but little scientific evidence exists for such claims.

Methods of aromatherapy are varied but chiefly involve scent inhalation alone or in combination with massage. With massage, essential oils (oils from aromatic plants) are applied directly to the body and massaged into the skin. Otherwise, essential oils are inhaled briefly, as one might use "smelling salts," or in a more diffuse manner, as with incense or perfume. Oils may be dabbed on pulse points, disbursed by fragrance diffusers, simmered in potpourri vessels, added to boiling water to be diffused by steam, or added to baths.

Uses and Complications

Allergic reactions to the aromatic oils are the greatest complication of aromatherapy. The substances typically used are highly concentrated and not safe for internal use. In the hands of an unskilled user, the oils may create unpleasant odors or medically dangerous allergic reactions. Aromatherapy is probably not advisable for adults or children without the consultation of an allergist. In addition, the long-term effects of such inhalants on lung functioning are not well documented; caution must be advised.

Perspective and Prospects

Historically, perfumes were sacrificed to the gods among Greeks, were essential for burial rites among Egyptians, and attracted good spirits among American Indians. Today, scents are used widely by therapists and individuals alike to facilitate well-being. Future work will likely include greater research on aromatherapy's safety and the role of olfaction on memory functioning.

—*Nancy A. Piotrowski, Ph.D.*

See also Allergies; Alternative medicine; Anxiety; Herbal medicine; Stress; Stress reduction.

For Further Information:

Lawless, Julia. *The Complete Illustrated Guide to Aromatherapy: A Practical Approach to the Use of Essential Oils for Health and Well-Being*. New York: HarperCollins, 2002. An accessible guide to use of aromatherapy.

Ryman, Daniele. *Aromatherapy: The Complete Guide to Plant and Flower Essences for Health and Beauty*. New York: Bantam, 1993. From a leading international authority, the definitive guide to the enriching therapeutic practices of aromatherapy—perfect for anyone interested in natural health and beauty.

Arrhythmias

Disease/disorder

Also known as: Dysrhythmias, conduction disturbances

Anatomy or system affected: Heart

Specialties and related fields: Cardiology

Definition: A disturbance of electrical conduction activity in the heart. Potential causes range from medications to diseases or conditions that delay or block an impulse in the conduction system.

Key terms:

atria: the two upper chambers of the heart, which receive blood from the body and lungs and send it to the ventricles; the sinoatrial node is located in the upper right atrium

conduction pathway: a system of nodes and tracts through the heart that conduct electrical impulses to its muscle cells, creating coordinated contraction

electrocardiogram (ECG or EKG): a recording of the electrical activity of the heart

sinoatrial (S-A) node: the pacemaker of the heart; also called the sinus node

ventricles: the two lower chambers of the heart, which receive blood from the atria and send it to the body and lungs

Causes and Symptoms

The heart is a unique muscle with characteristics of each of the other two types of muscle, skeletal and smooth. Like skeletal muscle cells, myocardial cells are striated and contract following the all-or-none principle, but individual cells can contract independently. Like smooth muscle, the heart is controlled by the autonomic nervous system but able to contract independently because it has its own unique conduction system, composed of the sinoatrial (S-A) node; the interatrial and internodal conduction tracts; the atrioventricular (A-V) junction, including the A-V node and bundle of His; the right and left bundle branches; and the Purkinje fibers.

The heart delivers blood to all tissues needing nutrients and oxygen. The ability to contract effectively twenty-four hours a day, seven days a week for years requires a system with good internal control and many backup systems. Blood flow through the heart needs to move progressively through the right atrium and ventricle to the lungs in order to oxygenate the blood and through the left atrium and ventricle and out to the body to deliver the nutrients and oxygen. Control of heart rate and rhythm by the autonomic nervous system and conduction tissues creates effective pumping.

When something goes awry with this pumping, the condition is called an arrhythmia and is defined by where the problem originates. Arrhythmias range from benign to life-threatening, depending on which portion of the heart is involved. The description of arrhythmias follows the conduction system, from S-A node or sinus arrhythmias to independent ventricular myocardial cells producing ectopic (extra) beats, called premature ventricular contractions (PVCs). The determination of what type of arrhythmia is present is made by interpreting the electrocardiogram (ECG or EKG).

Two types of arrhythmias may occur: impulse propagation, in which an area of the heart or conduction tissue blocks the passage of an impulse, or impulse initiation, in which an area of the heart or conduction tissue becomes excited and creates one or more extra beats. They may occur because of something acute and reversible, such as inadequate oxygenation (myocardial infarction, or heart attack), or a chronic condition, possibly from damage to the myocardial tissue or the conduction system.

Information on Arrhythmias

Causes: Inadequate oxygenation (as from heart attack), medications, various conditions
Symptoms: Often none; blood clots possible
Duration: Acute or chronic
Treatments: None, medications, or surgery (pacemaker implantation, heart transplantation), depending on severity

Treatment and Therapy

Depending on the diagnosis, treatments range from nothing to hospitalization. An example of a benign arrhythmia is sinus bradycardia, a normal rhythm but a very slow rate, less than sixty beats per minute. Athletes often have well-conditioned cardiovascular systems which pump more blood each beat than do those of nonathletes; thus, their heart rates are slower when the same amount of blood needs to be delivered.

The other extreme, ventricular fibrillation, is characterized by ventricular cells contracting wildly. Blood flow is totally disrupted, and if the arrhythmia is not controlled by defibrillation (the application of electricity), then sudden death will occur. In between these extremes would be someone who reacts to caffeine. Premature atrial contractions (PACs), isolated early beats coming from irritated cells in the atrium, may occur when a person is under stress or has taken stimulants. The obvious treatment is to remove the stress or the stimulant in order to return the heart to normal.

The treatment of arrhythmia may depend on whether it has an impact on blood flow. It is important to keep blood moving smoothly and progressively through the heart. When blood flow is turbulent, the cells suspended in the blood bump into one another, and some are damaged. When this happens, blood clots can form. If an abnormal number of clots occur, a greater chance exists that they could also block a blood vessel either in the heart or the lungs, which can be life-threatening.

The decision to treat the arrhythmia or to treat only the symptoms (blood clots) is a question for patients and physicians. Medications can be used to reduce clotting, but this requires long-term treatment with possible side effects. Surgery may be able to correct the arrhythmia. Knowing the risks and benefits of each treatment helps the patient decide.

If damaged myocardium is the cause of the arrhythmia, then the physician will determine the extent of the damage and offer treatment options, ranging from medications to surgery. The medication may interrupt or keep the arrhythmia from occurring, or it may help the weakened muscle pump blood, which will increase the flow of oxygen and help reduce the chance for further arrhythmias.

If the conduction system is not functioning, then a pacemaker may be inserted and attached to the heart to create a regular rhythm. At the extreme, a heart transplant has the ability to correct an arrhythmia, but this is not usually the reason that a transplant occurs. A transplanted heart has its internal conduction system intact and so should be able to beat on its own.

Perspective and Prospects

The longer one lives, the greater the chance that the heart muscle or conduction system will be damaged. Therefore, it is essential that pharmaceutical companies continue to search for effective drugs and that surgeons continue to refine the techniques required to best treat arrhythmias. Pacemakers have advanced dramatically since the early 1980's, from bulky instruments with nonrechargeable batteries to sophisticated, miniature combination machines which can adjust the heart rate depending on need and, in the extreme, defibrillate with a shock to convert a problem arrhythmia. A concerted effort by emergency medical personnel and technicians has created automatic external defibrillators (AEDs) that anyone can use to allow those people suffering from fibrillation to be saved. Such devices are necessary because cardiopulmonary resuscitation (CPR) is effective in only about 20 percent of cases, often because fibrillation persists during CPR and continues to interrupt blood flow.

—*Wendy E. S. Repovich, Ph.D.*

See also Arteriosclerosis; Cardiology; Cardiology, pediatric; Cardiopulmonary resuscitation (CPR); Echocardiography; Heart; Heart attack; Heart disease; Hypertension; Ischemia; Mitral valve prolapse; Pacemaker implantation; Palpitations; Panic attacks.

For Further Information:

Angelopoulos, Theodore J. "Electrocardiography." In *ACSM's Clinical Certification Review*, edited by Michael S. Wegner, Jeanne E. Ruff, and Walter R. Thompson. Philadelphia: Lippincott Williams & Wilkins, 2001.

Berne, Robert M., and Matthew N. Levy. *Cardiovascular Physiology*. 8th ed. St. Louis: C. V. Mosby, 2001.

Boyer, Mary Jo. *Lippincott's Need-to-Know ECG Facts*. Philadelphia: Lippincott Williams & Wilkins, 1997.

Arteriosclerosis

Disease/disorder

Anatomy or system affected: Blood vessels, circulatory system, heart

Specialties and related fields: Cardiology, internal medicine, vascular medicine

Definition: Also called atherosclerotic disease or "hardening of the arteries," a generalized disease that causes narrowing of the arteries because of deposits on the arterial walls and leads to a multitude of serious medical conditions, notably stroke and heart attack.

Key terms:

angina: chest, jaw, or shoulder pain with exercise or stress—a symptom of atherosclerotic heart disease

embolus: a small piece of atherosclerotic plaque, thrombus, or other debris that breaks off and lodges in a blood vessel

infarct: tissue death resulting from lack of blood flow

intermittent claudication: a symptom of lower extremity arteriosclerosis manifested by pain or cramping in the leg while walking, relieved by rest; from the Latin word *claudicatio*, "to limp"

ischemia: lack of blood in a particular tissue

rest pain: pain noted in the most distal portion of the extremity at rest, relieved by analgesics

revascularization: procedures to reestablish the circulation to a diseased portion of the body

thrombosis: aggregation of platelets and other blood cells to form a clot

Causes and Symptoms

The human body's arterial system is designed to carry oxygen, hormones, various types of blood cells (such as red and white blood cells), and other nutrients in the blood from the heart to the periphery and all organ structures of the body. The arteries are composed of three separate layers: adventia (the outer layer), media (the middle layer), and intima (the inner layer). Atherosclerosis or arteriosclerosis, derived from the Greek words that mean "hardening of the arteries," refers to the different diseases that compromise one or more of the layers of the large or medium-sized arteries or smaller arterioles. Most commonly, fat, cholesterol,

Information on Arteriosclerosis

Causes: Increased levels of fat, cholesterol, and/or calcium deposits that form plaques in arteries
Symptoms: Angina, cramping in extremities, pallor, parathesias
Duration: Chronic
Treatments: Drugs, bypass surgery, lifestyle changes

and calcium deposits are laid down along the intima and inner portion of the media. These components build up, forming plaques, which then may produce stenosis (narrowing) or occlusion (closure) of the arterial lumen. Accumulation of platelets and other blood cells can form a thrombus along with plaque buildup, which also obstructs the arteries. Pieces of plaque or thrombotic material can break off, causing emboli to lodge in the vessels acutely. Atherosclerosis begins with some form of damage to the delicate lining of the intima (the endothelium), by infections, inflammation, hypertension, or even natural toxins. That damage induces platelet adherence and other repair mechanisms, creating an opportunity for the accumulation of fat and calcium deposits in plaques.

Depending on the arterial segment in the body that is affected, various diseases and symptoms may occur. As the blood vessels become diseased with plaque buildup, the body will try to compensate by the development of collaterals, small vessels that bypass the diseased artery. Collateral vessels are smaller than the native arteries and cannot accommodate the same amount of blood. Normally, during exercise, there is an increased demand for additional blood flow to the muscles; flow will increase and the arteries will dilate. With atherosclerosis, since the arteries are blocked and collaterals cannot accommodate the additional blood volume, waste products in the muscles build up, causing pain. In the heart, this process affects the flow in the coronary arteries, and angina (chest pain) may occur. In lower extremity arteriosclerosis, stenosis or occlusions of the aorta, iliac, femoral, popliteal, or tibial arteries may occur, producing intermittent claudication.

As the disease progresses, more blood vessels become stenosed or occluded and collateral formation will maximize, but the circulation is severely limited and ischemia may result. In atherosclerotic heart disease, significant ischemia may then result in a myocardial infarct, or heart attack. In the lower extremities, patients may develop rest pain. The most severe symptoms of lower extremity arteriosclerosis are the development of nonhealing ulcers and gangrene (tissue death) in the lower portion of the foot, similar to a heart attack. When the disease process has become this severe, there are multisegmental areas of arterial occlusions and no further compensatory mechanisms.

Acute arterial ischemia is a sudden onset of ischemia as opposed to the more common chronic processes described above. The usual cause of acute arterial ischemia is an embolus (portion of a clot) that lodges in the arteries. The most common source of embolization is the heart; embolization from the heart occurs in patients who have recently had a heart attack, who have mitral valvular disease, or who have atrial fibrillation (irregular heartbeats). Another cause of acute arterial ischemia is thrombosis of, or embolization from, an aneurysm. In such cases, since no significant collaterals have developed in the area of the acute blockage, immediate revascularization is mandatory to prevent significant tissue death.

Aneurysms—another disease entity that may be associated with the atherosclerotic disease process—produce a weakening of the adventia and a "ballooning" of the arteries with a thrombus (clot). Rupture or thrombosis (clotting off) may be a consequence of aneurysmal disease.

In cerebrovascular disease, atherosclerosis affects the arteries supplying the circulation to the brain (the carotid and vertebral-basilar system). The most common symptoms noted are transient ischemic attacks (TIAs), also referred to as ministrokes. TIAs usually last less than twenty-four hours. Most TIAs are produced by embolization, in which pieces of plaque in the major arteries break off and temporarily block the blood flow to certain areas of the brain. Once the symptoms last more than twenty-four hours, a cerebrovascular accident (CVA), cerebral infarct, or stroke has occurred. Atherosclerosis in the cerebrovascular system will behave in a manner similar to that previously described, with increasing stenosis and eventual occlusion. Collateral development seems to be especially prominent in the cerebrovascular system, since the brain is a greedy organ needing blood at all times. The majority of CVAs are caused by occlusion or thrombosis of a major vessel, producing significant ischemia in a portion of the brain.

Other sources of CVAs are hemorrhaging (bleeding) from ruptured cerebral aneurysms or from uncontrolled hypertension. This significant bleeding can cause spasm of the arteries in the brain and eventual ischemia. Monckeberg's sclerosis, not usually thought of as a true form of atherosclerosis, refers to the disease in which calcification of the tibial arteries is noted, often in diabetic patients.

Contributing or significant risk factors in the development of atherosclerosis include hypertension (high blood pressure), hyperlipidemia (high amounts of fats or lipids in the blood), smoking, diabetes mellitus, and family history. Inflammation, especially from infections, is a newly discovered and significant risk factor as well. Also, depending on the significance and the location of atherosclerosis, a variety of symptoms and conditions can result. In atherosclerotic heart disease, the first symptom is angina. As in intermittent claudication, chest, shoulder, or upper back pain may occur during exercise or stress as a result of the decreased blood supply to the tissues of the end organ, the myocardium (heart muscle). As the disease progresses, the angina will become more unstable and patients will become progressively limited in minor activities. Symptoms of a heart attack may include severe, crushing chest pain, shortness of breath, pain in the left arm, and tingling of the fingers. Cessation of breathing and cardiac arrest indicate a significant heart attack. Immediate medical attention during the severe symptomatic phase or with cardiac arrest will aid in reducing further damage to the heart muscle and may prevent death. Many heart attacks are "silent" in that, although portions of the cardiac muscle are "dead," symptoms will have been negligible or minor, because of sufficient collateralization.

In lower extremity atherosclerosis, patients with intermittent claudication will complain of pain or cramping in their calves, thighs, or buttocks while walking or exercising; symptoms will be relieved by rest. Claudication is usually described by distances, such as "one block" claudication or "half a mile" claudication. Rest pain occurs mostly at night at the most distal portion of the extremity, usually the toes and forefoot. Often patients will sleep in chairs or with their legs hanging off the bed to relieve the pain. On physical examination, the foot is usually cool to the touch, with a slightly bluish discoloration. There is hardening of the nails, dryness of the skin, and loss of hair in the lower portion of the leg. Pulses are absent or diminished. Often, when the leg is in a dependent position, dependent rubor, a purplish discoloration of the leg, is seen, produced by dilation of the small blood vessels in the skin to provide the maximum amount of blood. Elevating the leg will produce a cadaverous white pallor. Because of the limited blood supply, ulcers will not heal and gangrene can develop. Patients with symptoms of severe claudication, rest pain, or neuropathic diabetes should be evaluated prior to undergoing any podiatry procedures because their compromised circulation will result in poor healing. Patients with acute arterial ischemia of the lower extremity will complain of the "five P's": pain, pallor, pulselessness, parathesia (decrease of feeling), and paralysis. As previously described, emergent revascularization of the acutely ischemic limb is necessary to prevent limb loss or amputation.

Although aneurysmal disease is a separate entity, it may be associated with atherosclerotic disease in certain cases. Most aneurysms produce no symptoms. Detection of aneurysms is usually incidental; during a physical examination, for example, a physician may note a pulsatile mass in the abdomen (aorta, iliac), in the groin (femoral), or behind the knee (popliteal). Incidental diagnosis of aneurysms may also occur during routine chest X rays; the X ray may reveal a calcium rim around the body of the aneurysm. As aneurysms increase in size, the probability of rupture increases; therefore, elective surgery is usually recommended

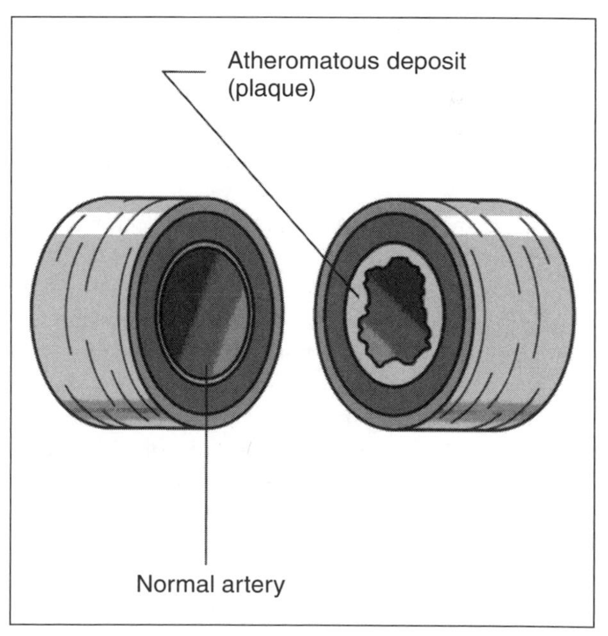

Arteriosclerosis leads to the buildup of fatty plaques on the walls of arteries, which inhibits blood flow and may lead to obstructions resulting in stroke, heart attack, and other life-threatening events.

once certain sizes are achieved: more than 6 centimeters for an abdominal aneurysm and more than 2 centimeters for femoral and popliteal aneurysms. Symptoms of a rupturing abdominal aneurysm include severe lower back pain and a decrease in blood pressure, whereas thrombosis of a popliteal or femoral aneurysm will cause an acutely ischemic leg. Symptomatic aneurysms are considered medical emergencies, since ruptures may result in death and thrombosis in limb loss.

Symptoms of TIAs in the carotid arteries, which supply the front of the brain, include hemiparesis (numbness) or hemiplegia (weakness) of an arm and/or leg, affecting the carotid artery on the side opposite the symptom; aphasia (speech disorder), usually affecting the left carotid artery; or amaurosis fugax (blindness in one eye, similar to the sensation of a shade over the eye), which is from the carotid artery on the same side as the blindness. Other symptoms include dizziness, vertigo, imbalance, and other visual disturbances. These more generalized symptoms are referable to the vertebral-basilar circulation, which supplies the back portions of the brain, or are a result of multisegmental cerebrovascular disease in which a low-flow state can affect multiple areas of the brain and produce diverse symptoms. A stroke is an event whose symptoms will last more than twenty-four hours. Often these are permanent deficits, affecting the patient for the rest of his or her life.

Many patients will be asymptomatic (have no symptoms) and not develop TIAs but will have a stroke, which may result from eventual occlusion or thrombosis of the cerebral vessels and infarcts in a particular section of the brain. Asymptomatic cerebrovascular disease is often detected by the presence of a bruit (French for "noise"). Stenosis in arteries resembles rapids in a river: Flow will go very fast through the blockage and then be turbulent. The turbulence will produce a bruit which can be detected with a stethoscope. Turbulence from stenoses ranging from 20 to 80 percent can cause a bruit. The absence of a bruit does not mean that the arteries are disease-free. Once the stenosis reaches critical proportions, the flow is diminished and turbulence may be negligible. An occluded artery will also have no bruit, since there is no flow. Once the narrowing has reached 60 to 80 percent, many doctors will recommend elective surgery to reestablish flow and prevent eventual occlusion and possible stroke. About 75 percent of strokes are ischemic, resulting from this process. Bruits may be appreciable in other parts of the body and can also indicate the presence of atherosclerosis in those areas.

Atherosclerosis of the renal arteries, which supply the kidneys, may cause a condition known as renovascular hypertension. This type of high blood pressure is often difficult to control with medication, and continued high blood pressure will contribute to progression of the atherosclerotic process elsewhere in the body.

Another condition that results from atherosclerosis is chronic mesenteric ischemia. Here the blood vessels supplying the intestines, the stomach, and many of the organs associated with the digestive process are affected. Patients may experience pain with eating and significant weight loss. This condition is often missed until an extensive workup for cancer or other chronic diseases yields negative results. In acute mesenteric ischemia, by contrast, thrombosis of the superior mesenteric artery occurs. As with other acute arterial conditions, emergent revascularization is necessary to prevent gangrene of the intestines.

TREATMENT AND THERAPY

A complete history and physical examination are usually the first methods of diagnosing atherosclerosis. Eliciting symptoms, noting significant risk factors and physical findings, will aid the physician in determining areas at risk.

In lower extremity atherosclerosis, a common noninvasive method utilizes Doppler ultrasound. A series of blood pressure cuffs are attached to the extremity, and segmental blood pressure and plethysmographic waveforms are measured. A drop of more than 20 millimeters of mercury (mm Hg) of pressure between segments or extremities is indicative of a significant stenosis at that level. Exercise testing will demonstrate whether there are significant drops in pressure, confirming the diagnosis and severity of claudication. A similar method, ocular pneumoplethysmography (OPG), developed by William Gee, utilizes eye cups placed in the eye to measure the ocular pressure. A vacuum is applied to the eyes, effectively occluding the ophthalmic arteries, the first major branch of the internal carotid artery. As the vacuum is released, the blood flow is reestablished and the appearance of arterial pulsations is noted on a strip chart, denoting the systolic ophthalmic pressures. A difference of 5 mm Hg is consistent with significant (greater than 50 to 70 percent) carotid disease.

Duplex ultrasound machines utilize B-mode (brightness-mode) ultrasound to visualize the vessels and type of plaque, while Doppler ultrasound can audibly evaluate the blood flow in the vessels. Using real-time spectrum analyzers, the Doppler signals are then analyzed in terms of velocities and waveform characteristics. The greater the velocities, the greater the amount of stenosis. Absence of blood flow will denote occlusions. The use of color duplex ultrasound, in which the Doppler signals are color-coded in terms of flow direction and speed to denote the various flow patterns in normal and diseased vessels, has enhanced the diagnostic accuracies in the examinations. The use of color Doppler in many of the ultrasound machines is aiding in more rapid detection of arterial lesions in the heart, cerebrovascular, and lower extremity arterial circulation.

Arteriography or angiography is an invasive procedure. The delineation of the blockages and collateral pathways detected through this method—in which the patient is hospitalized and a catheter is used to inject dye containing iodine into the arteries—is then used to plan a revascularization procedure.

Ultrasound is the primary diagnostic tool for detecting and measuring the size of aneurysms. Computed tomography (CT) scanning is an alternative radiological modality to visualize aneurysms.

The majority of patients with mild to moderate intermittent claudication can be treated conservatively. Cessation of smoking, alterations to diet, and a carefully controlled exercise plan will alleviate or decrease the progression of symptoms. Less than 5 percent of patients with intermittent claudication will develop gangrene sufficient to warrant a major amputation within a five-year period.

Some medications available work by decreasing the stickiness of the platelets in the blood; these are often prescribed for patients with claudication. Aspirin is often prescribed to alleviate symptoms of TIAs and to protect patients from strokes or heart attacks. Although it is a powerful drug in decreasing the incidence of embolization, a national study has demonstrated that patients with TIAs and severe stenosis of the carotid arteries should undergo surgical revascularization to protect against major strokes. It has become clear that aspirin may also be helpful because of its anti-inflammatory properties, particularly now that the role of damage to the endothelium from inflammation and infections is understood.

Severe disabling claudication, rest pain, ulceration or gangrene of the lower extremity, and unstable angina and heart attacks require some sort of surgical intervention. Usually bypass surgery is planned to revascularize the ischemic portion of the extremity or myocardial tissue to prevent limb loss or further cardiac events. The arteriogram will illustrate the areas of blockage, and, depending on the results of this test, various types of bypasses can be performed. Inflow procedures refer to bypasses performed above the groin. Aorto-iliac or aorto-femoral are the most common types performed, usually utilizing a prosthetic (plastic) material. Outflow procedures are those performed below the groin; these include femoral-popliteal or femoral-tibial bypasses. Prosthetics are sometimes used, but the best bypass material in terms of durability is the patient's own vein, either removed and reversed, or in situ (in place). Depending on the type of bypass procedure performed, the five-year patency rates (number of bypasses open at five years) exceed 85 percent for aorto-iliac/aorto-femoral bypasses and 75 percent for lower extremity reconstructions. Coronary artery bypass grafts (CABGs) typically employ the saphenous veins of the legs or the mammary artery of the chest wall to bypass the diseased segments in the heart vessels.

Endarterectomy, a surgical technique in which the intima and part of the media are excised, effectively "scrapes out" atherosclerotic plaques. Although used in other arterial segments, endarterectomy is the most common surgical procedure used to revascularize the carotid arteries.

Other interventional modalities have been developed. Percutaneous balloon angioplasty involves placing a balloon catheter in the diseased segment during an angiogram and opening up the area of stenosis or small segmental occlusion. This method has been employed in the coronary arteries as well as in the vessels of the aorta, iliacs, and lower extremities.

New lytic drugs, which "dissolve" clots, are sometimes employed alone, or in combination with balloon angioplasties or surgery, especially in the more acute cases of lower extremity arterial ischemia and myocardial infarctions.

Perspective and Prospects

Atherosclerosis of the coronary and cerebrovascular system is a major cause of death. Heart attacks are the primary cause of death in the United States, with approximately 650,000 people dying annually. Half of those deaths are sudden, with no prior significant symptoms. Stroke is the third leading cause of death in the United States, with approximately 155,000 deaths annually. There are 400,000 strokes annually, and about one-fourth of all nursing home patients are permanently impaired from strokes. These statistics have a great impact on the amounts of health care monies spent annually to care for victims of heart disease and strokes.

Since the 1960's, the rates of death from both heart attacks and strokes in the United States have decreased significantly. Control of blood pressure and diet, the development of new drugs and diagnostic techniques, and the advent of cardiovascular surgery in the early 1950's have aided in this decrement. Unfortunately, atherosclerotic diseases are still prevalent. Autopsies of Korean War and Vietnam War American soldiers demonstrated that atherosclerotic plaque was evident even at an early age. This was attributed to the high-fat diet of most Americans. It is recognized that this disease is more prevalent in young males and that females are more protected until the onset of menopause; then the death rates tend to equalize. High-salt diets, which may increase the incidence of hypertension, also contribute to the development and progression of atherosclerosis. Since the 1960's, extensive education of the American public regarding dietary control has had a favorable impact. More recently, the benefits of exercise have helped to stem the atherosclerotic process.

The 1950's saw the development of cardiovascular surgery. The first bypass (arterial autograft) probably occurred during the Korean War. Coronary artery bypass surgery and carotid endarterectomies are among the most common surgical procedures performed today. Recognition of and prompt treatment of cardiac and cerebrovascular symptoms remain the key to better survival rates. With development of newer bypass materials for lower extremity bypass surgery in the 1970's, as well as better surgical techniques for utilization of the saphenous veins, the amputation rate has significantly decreased. Research into graft materials that better mimic the native arteries and veins continues.

Since the 1950's, a number of noninvasive and invasive procedures have been developed to diagnose atherosclerotic disease. The development of ultrasound devices in the 1950's initiated the research into using these noninvasive devices to diagnose atherosclerotic disease. The duplex devices, introduced commercially in the late 1970's and early 1980's, opened a new diagnostic field for detection of atherosclerotic disease. These devices allow for visualization of plaque morphology (composition of the plaque such as thrombus, calcium, and hemorrhage) and the blood-flow characteristics for a better understanding of the atherosclerotic process. Future developments in the field of ultrasound include holographic imaging for three-dimensional visualization of plaques. These noninvasive technologies will also allow physicians to monitor the effects of new drugs and techniques in the treatment of atherosclerosis. Advances in digital subtraction and computer enhancement of angiographic techniques, along with new contrast media, are making arteriograms safer and more accurate.

Technologies being developed for future diagnostic use include magnetic resonance imaging (MRI), a nonradiological modality for visualizing structures in the brain and other portions of the body. MRI is being expanded with the aid of computerization to do MR angiography. Magnetic resonance is also being utilized to measure, noninvasively, actual flow in individual arterial segments of the body in terms of cubic centimeters per minute. Positron emission tomography (PET) scanning, a non-X-ray method, gives brilliant, color-enhanced visualization of blood flow to tissues.

—Silvia M. Berry, M.Sc., R.V.T.;
updated by Connie Rizzo, M.D., Ph.D.

See also Angina; Angiography; Angioplasty; Bypass surgery; Cardiac arrest; Cardiology; Cholesterol; Circulation; Claudication; Edema; Embolism; Endarterectomy; Echocardiography; Heart; Heart attack; Heart disease; Heart failure; Hypercholesterolemia; Hyperlipidemia; Hypertension; Ischemia; Metabolic syndrome; Phlebitis; Stents; Strokes; Thrombolytic therapy and TPA; Thrombosis and thrombus; Transient ischemic attacks (TIAs); Vascular medicine; Vascular system; Venous insufficiency.

For Further Information:

Crawford, Michael, ed. *Diagnosis and Treatment in Cardiology*. New York: McGraw-Hill, 2002. Discusses advances in cardiac diagnostics, treatments, and prognostic indicators and includes extensive information on prevention techniques.

Eagle, Kim A., and Ragavendra R. Baliga. *Practical Cardiology: Evaluation and Treatment of Common Cardiovascular Disorders*. Philadelphia: Lippincott Williams & Wilkins, 2003. Details advances in cardiac medicine.

Goldman, Lee, and Dennis Ausiello, eds. *Cecil Textbook of Medicine*. 22d ed. Philadelphia: W. B. Saunders, 2004. This is a standard textbook of medicine. Although it is somewhat difficult, it is complete, beginning with normal conditions and progressing through disease process, diagnosis, and treatment.

Hoffman, Gary S., and Cornelia M. Weyand. *Inflammatory Disease of Blood Vessels*. New York: M. Decker, 2002. International contributors examine a range of topics pertinent to vascular inflammation in health and disease, including neutrophils in vasculitis, oxygen metabolites and vascular damage, T cells in vascular disease, and primary and secondary vasculitides such as Kawasaki disease, Takayasu's arteritis, relapsing polychondritis, and dyslipidemia in rheumatic disorders.

The New Good Housekeeping Family Health and Medical Guide. New York: Hearst Books, 1989. A popular and useful health care reference book emphasizing the prevention of illness. Includes a color atlas of the body and an encyclopedia of medicine. The encyclopedia section of the book provides a good source for understanding basic health and medical terms.

Rutherford, Robert B., ed. *Vascular Surgery*. 6th ed. Philadelphia: W. B. Saunders, 2005. The definitive textbook for the understanding, diagnosis, and treatment of vascular disorders.

Tierney, Lawrence M., Stephen J. McPhee, and Maxine A. Papadakis, eds. *Current Medical Diagnosis and Treatment 2007*. New York: McGraw-Hill Medical, 2006. This text is the point of reference for physicians and other health care practitioners. It incorporates each year's biomedical research discoveries that have immediate, relevant, and applicable use for the patient.

Arthritis

Disease/disorder

Anatomy or system affected: Bones, hands, hips, immune system, joints, knees, legs, musculoskeletal system

Specialties and related fields: Internal medicine, orthopedics, physical therapy, rheumatology

Definition: A group of more than one hundred inflammatory diseases that damage joints and their surrounding structures, resulting in symptomatic pain, disability, and systemwide inflammation.

Key terms:

anti-inflammatory drugs: drugs to counter the effects of inflammation locally or throughout the body; these drugs can be applied locally or introduced by electric currents (in a process called ionthophoresis), by injections into the joint or into the muscles, or by mouth; the three classes of these drugs are steroidal, immunosuppressant, and nonsteroidal

cartilage: material covering the ends of bones; it does not have a blood supply or nerve supply but may swell or break down

inflammation: the body's defensive and protective responses to trauma or foreign substances by dilution, cellular efforts at destruction, and the walling-off of irritants; characterized by pain, heat, redness, swelling, and loss of function mediated through a chemical breakdown

physical modalities: the physical means of addressing a disease, which include heat, cold, electricity, exercises, braces, assistive devices, and biofeedback

rehabilitation: a physician-led program to evaluate, treat, and educate patients and their families about the sequelae of birth defects, trauma, disease, and degenerative conditions, with the goals of alleviating pain, preventing complications, correcting deformities, improving function, and reintegrating individuals into the family and society

synovium: the cellular lining of a joint, having a blood supply and a nerve supply; the synovium secretes fluid for lubrication and protects against injury and injurious agents

Causes and Symptoms

Approximately one in six people (more than 15 percent) suffers from one of approximately one hundred varieties of arthritis, and 2.6 percent of the population suffer from arthritis that limits their activities. Although many people over seventy-five years of age experience arthritis, the disease can occur in the young as a result of infections, rheumatic conditions, or birth defects. Young and middle-aged adults experience the disease as a result of trauma, infections, and rheumatic or immune reactions. Arthritis may be located in joints, joint capsules, the surrounding muscles, or diffusely throughout the body. Inflammation of the joint lining (synovium) can similarly afflict the linings of other organs: the skin, colon, eyes, heart, and urinary passage. Those suffering from the disease may therefore suffer from psoriasis and rashes, spastic colitis and diarrhea, dryness of the eyes, inflammations of the conjunctiva or iris, frequent urination, discharge and burning upon urination, and other symptoms.

The collagen-type arthritic diseases involve the binding materials in the body or connective tissues and may be rheumatologic, generally more diffuse and in the distal joints (as in juvenile rheumatoid arthritis and rheumatic fever), or located in the skin and muscles (dermatomyositis). Psoriatic arthritis causes severe punched-out defects in the joints. Reiter's and Sjögren's syndromes involve the eyes and the joints. Genetic conditions, such as Gaucher's disease, frequently run in families. Metabolic disturbances, such as gout, can leave uric acid deposits in the skin and in the joints. Gout sufferers experience very painful, hot, tender, and swollen joints—often in the large toe. Immunologically mediated arthritides may be associated with infections, liver diseases, bowel disturbances, and immune deficiencies. Localized infections may be bacterial, viral, or fungal. "Miscellaneous disorders," a basket category, include conditions that do not fit into any of the aforementioned categories: Psychogenic disorders and arthritis associated with cystic disorders are examples. Arthritis may also be associated with tumors that grow from cartilage cells, blood vessels, synovial tissue, and nerve tissue. Blood abnormalities may give rise to hemorrhages into joints (a side effect of sickle cell disease and hemophilia) and can be disabling and very painful, sometimes requiring surgery. Traumatic and mechanical derangements—sports and occupational injuries, leg-length disparity, and obesity—may elicit acute synovial inflammation with subsequent degenerative arthritis. Finally, wear-and-tear degeneration can occur in joints after years of trauma, repetitive use, and (especially in the obese) weight-bearing. The most common arthritic entities are rheumatoid arthritis (also called atrophic or proliferative arthritis), osteoarthritis, hypertrophic arthritis, and degenerative arthritis.

The inflammatory reactions in response to injury or disease consist of fluid changes—the dilation of blood vessels accompanied by an increase in the permeability of the blood vessel walls and consequent outflow of fluids and proteins. Injurious substances are immobilized with immune reactions and removed by the cellular responses of phagocytosis and digestion of foreign materials, resulting in the proliferation of fibrous cells to wall off the injurious substances and in turn leading to scar formation and deformities. The chemical reactions to injury commence with a degradation of phospholipids when enzymes are released by injured tissue. Phospholipids—fatty material that is normally present—break down into arachidonic acid, which is further broken down by other enzymes, lipoxygenase and cycloxygenase, resulting in prostaglandins and eicosanoid acids. Most anti-inflammatory medications attempt to interfere with the enzymatic degradation process of phospholipids and could be damaging to the liver and kidneys and to the body's blood-clotting ability.

The physician bases the diagnosis of arthritic disease on the patient's medical history and a physical examination. Specific procedures such as joint aspiration, laboratory studies, and X-ray or magnetic resonance imaging (MRI) may help to establish the diagnosis and the treatment. The history will elicit the onset of pain and its relation to time of day and difficulties performing the activities of daily living. A functional classification has evolved that is similar to the cardiac functional classification: Class 1 patients perform all usual activities without a handicap; class 2 patients perform normal activities adequately with occasional symptoms and signs in one or more joints but still do not need to limit their activities; class 3 patients find that they must limit some activities and may require assistive devices; and class 4 patients are unable to perform activities, are largely or wholly incapacitated, and are bedridden or confined to a wheelchair, requiring assistance in self-care.

A person's medical history or surgical conditions and the medications that he or she is taking can influence the physician's diagnosis and prescription for treatment. Patients may present a gross picture of the body to the physician showing the joints involved in their symmetry (whether distal or proximal, and whether weight-bearing or post-traumatic in distribution). Physicians may ask (verbally or by questionnaire) for a history of other system complaints, which can then be checked more thoroughly. During a physical examination, the physician will check the joints, skin, eyes, abdomen, heart, and urinary tract. The neuromuscular evaluation may reveal localized tenderness of the joints or muscles, swelling, wasting, weakness, and abnormal motions. Joints may have weak-

INFORMATION ON ARTHRITIS

CAUSES: Infection, rheumatic conditions, birth defects, trauma, immune reactions, wear-and-tear degeneration

SYMPTOMS: Joint pain, psoriasis and rashes, spastic colitis and diarrhea, dryness of the eyes, frequent urination

DURATION: Chronic

TREATMENTS: Anti-inflammatory drugs; application of heat, cold, or electricity; exercise; biofeedback; assistive devices

ened ligamentous, muscle, and tendon supports that could give rise to instability or grinding of joints, with subsequent roughening of cartilage surfaces. The arthritides are frequently associated with muscular pains, called fibrositis and myofascial pain syndromes.

Fibrositis is a diffuse muscular pain syndrome with tenderness in the muscles, no muscle spasm, and no limitations in motion; all laboratory tests are within normal limits. It is frequent in postmenopausal women who have a history of migraines, cold extremities, spastic colitis, softening of the bone matrix accompanied by loss of minerals, and irritability. Myofascial trigger points can be found in both men and women, at all ages, with acutely tender nodules or cords felt in muscles. The pain of these trigger points is referred to more distal areas of the muscles that may not be tender to touch. Physicians may frequently miss the acutely tender trigger points. Tests will show whether pain is elicited when muscles are contracted with motion, when muscles are contracted without motion, or when motion is carried out passively by the examiner without muscular effort by the patient.

Joint pathology is generally associated with some limitation in the range of motion. Sensation testing, muscle strength, and reflex changes may also indicate nerve tissue damage. Nerves occasionally pass close to joints and may be pinched when the joint swelling encroaches upon the passage opening. This condition may result in carpal tunnel syndrome, in which the median nerve at the wrist becomes pinched, causing pain, numbness, and weakness in the hand. Pinched nerves may also be associated with tarsal tunnel syndrome, in which the nerve at the inner side of the ankle joint may be compressed and cause similar complaints in the feet. Other nerves may be constricted in exiting from the spine and when passing through muscles in spasm.

The medications used to treat arthritis can involve the nervous system. An evaluation and estimation of the severity of the disease can be obtained by electrical testing, as in electroneuromyography. The nerves are stimulated, and their rate of transmitting the stimulus is measured. The normal transmission rate for nerves is 45 meters per second. Delays at areas of impingement can be determined by measuring the transmission rate of a stimulus from different points along the nerve paths. Abnormal or damaged muscles will cause muscle fibers to contract spontaneously, or "fibrillate." Chest expansion during inspiration and after expiration may be limited because of arthritis at the spine or because of lung pathology. Involvement of the spine can also be measured by the posture, the ability to move the neck, and the ability to move the lower back.

Arthritis of the spine leads to progressive loss in motion. The amount lost can be measured by comparing the normal motion with the restricted motion of the patient. The neck may be limited in all directions, rotation of the head to the sides can restrict the driving view, and the head may gradually tilt forward. The lower back may also exhibit restriction in all directions; for example, it may be limited in forward bending because of spasms in the muscles in the back. Tilting backward of the trunk may be limited and painful when the vertebral body overgrowth of osteoarthritis or degenerative arthritis restricts the space for the spinal cord. The nerves pinched in their passage from the vertebrae may thus cause radiculitis, irritation of the nerves as they exit from the spine that leads to pain and muscle involvement. Circumferential measurements of the involved joints and the structures above and below can confirm swelling, atrophy from disuse or inaction, or atrophy from a damaged nerve supply. When measurements are repeated, they can indicate improvement or deterioration. One type of arthritis that most often affects the spine, ankylosing spondylitis, occurs predominantly in males in their late teenage and early adult years.

Testing of blood for cells, chemicals, or enzymes is helpful. The simplest test—the sedimentation (or "sed") test—measures the rate at which blood cells settle out of the plasma. Normally, women have a more rapid rate of sedimentation than men. When this rate exceeds the normal range, active inflammation in the body is indicated. Comparisons of sed tests performed at different stages can reveal the disease's rate of progression or improvement. The chemicals tested may include uric acid for gout and sugar for diabetes. Blood tests for immune substances and antibodies are also possible. The joint fluid can be aspirated and analyzed, particularly for appearance, density, number of blood cells, and levels of sugar. Cloudy fluid, the tendency to form clots, a high cell count, and lower-than-normal levels of sugar in the joint fluid (compared to the overall blood sugar level) indicate abnormalities. With inflammatory arthritides, the X rays will show the results of synovial fluid and cellular overabundance. Clumps of pannus break off and may destroy the cartilage and bone. Bones about these joints, because of increased vascularity and blood flow, have less minerals and will appear less dense, a condition known as osteoporosis.

Deformities in inflammatory arthritis may be the result of unequal muscle pulls or the destruction or scarring of tissues; such deformities can occasionally be prevented by the use of resting splints, which is most important for the hands.

Degenerative and post-traumatic arthritis show joint narrowing, thinning of the cartilage layer, hardening of the underlying bone (called eburnation), and marginal overgrowth of the underlying bone (called osteophytes), resulting in osteoarthritis. Osteophytes, or marginal lipping in the back, may enhance symptoms of lower back pain. The cushions between the vertebrae, called discs, are more than 80 percent water, a figure which diminishes with aging, bringing the joints in the back (the facets) closer together and compressing the facet joints between the vertebrae. Irritation and arthritis of these joints are the result. Other organ structures may be involved as well.

A diagnosis of rheumatoid arthritis should include two to four of the following criteria: morning stiffness, three or more joints involved symmetrically (especially the hands), six weeks or longer in duration, rheumatoid nodules that can be felt under the skin, blood tests showing a serum rheumatoid factor, and the radiographic evidence described above.

Treatment and Therapy

Treatment of arthritis may vary from home treatment to outpatient treatment to hospitalization for acute, surgical, and/or rehabilitative care. Educating patients as to their condition, the prognosis, the treatment goals, and the methods of treatment is necessary. Patients must be made aware of warning signs of progression, drug effects, local and systemic side effects of drug therapy, and diet associated with relieving pain, stiffness, and inflammation. If surgery is contemplated for joint replacement or other reasons, patients should be fully informed as to expectations and rate of functional activities. Postoperative restrictions in the range of motion must be given; in hip replacement, for example, hip bending should not exceed 90 degrees. The rotation and overlapping of legs must be limited initially after surgery.

Some physicians provide a questionnaire that outlines the activities of daily living and recommends how a patient should perform such activities and how much time should be spent at rest. The goals generally are to maintain function, to alleviate pain, to limit the progression of deformities, to prevent complications, and to treat associated and secondary disease states. In patients with degenerative arthritis—most often the elderly, who are at risk for other organ failures—arthritides associated with systemic diseases and other organ involvements may require care. Patients with rheumatoid arthritis, for example, frequently are anemic. Anti-inflammatory drugs, normally used to treat the arthritis, may cause blood loss through the gastrointestinal tract and even ulcerations. The physician may therefore prescribe alternative therapies.

Other therapies can include assistive devices, counseling patients and their families regarding home management, medicinal regimen and compliance, behavior modification, sexual advice, and biofeedback. The aim is to reduce the need for and frequency of medical care, through a balance between rest and activity and between effective drug dose, toxicity, and physical modalities. To protect joints and allow function, various braces and assistive devices may be needed. Scarring of a wrist joint can be alleviated by avoiding positions that inhibit function. Shoulders should not be left with arms close to the body, since frozen shoulders aggravate neck and arm problems.

Physicians may offer physical therapy, occupational therapy, assistive devices for self-care, ambulation, or home and automobile modifications. Assistive devices may include reachers, an elongated shoehorn handle, thickened handles for utensils, walkers, canes, crutches, and wheelchairs. Homes may require ramps for easier access, widened doors to allow wheelchair passage, grab bars in bathtubs, or raised toilet seats for easier transference from a wheelchair.

Heat therapy may reduce the pain, loosening and liquefying tightened tissues. Somewhat like gelatin, tissue liquefies when heated and solidifies when cooled. Patients frequently will be stiffer after protracted rest periods (for example, on waking) and feel better after some activity and exercise. Heated pools offer an excellent heating and exercise modality. The type of heat modality used will depend upon the depth of heating desired. Hot packs and infrared lamps will heat predominantly the skin surface areas and some underlying muscles. Diathermy units heat the muscular layers, and ultrasound treatments heat the deepest bony layers. Ultrasound (but not diathermy) can even be used in patients who have metallic implants such as joint replacements.

Transcutaneous electrical nerve stimulation can be used to alleviate pain. The units can regulate the frequency of electrical impulses. The usual starting rate is 100 cycles, which can alleviate pain in a few minutes; this rate is later changed to 4 cycles, which will give hours of relief even when discontinued. The intensity

In the News: Glucosamine and Chondroitin

Medical, surgical, and rehabilitative techniques have been used in the treatment of arthritis. Recently more people have turned to complementary and alternative medicine for treatment of medical disorders, including arthritis. Two nutritional supplements that have been widely used to treat osteoarthritis are glucosamine (a substance involved in cartilage formation and repair) and chondroitin sulfate (which provides cartilage with elasticity). While these substances are produced naturally by the human body, when marketed as dietary supplements glucosamine is usually derived from shellfish, while chondroitin either comes from cow or shark cartilage. Since dietary supplements are not regulated by any federal agency, one must be sure to deal with a reputable manufacturer to assure product quality.

A large-scale study of glucosamine and chondroitin in treating osteoarthritis of the knee was undertaken at sixteen rheumatology centers in the United States with funding from the National Institutes of Health. This Glucosamine/Chondroitin Arthritis Intervention Trial (GAIT) compared five groups taking 1,500 milligrams of glucosamine, 1,200 milligrams of chondroitin sulfate, 1,500 milligrams of glucosamine with 1,200 milligrams chondroitin sulfate, 200 milligrams of a COX-2 inhibitor (a nonsteroidal anti-inflammatory drug, or NSAID, available by prescription to treat osteoarthritis), and a placebo. All substances used in this study were assessed to ensure their purity and quality. For patients who suffered moderate to severe pain (but not those suffering mild pain), the combination of glucosamine and chondroitin sulfate provided greater pain relief than did the placebo or the COX-2 inhibitor. Based on this study, the Arthritis Foundation has concluded that the combination of these two substances could serve as an important component of an overall treatment plan for moderate to severe osteoarthritis of the knee. They suggest that these nutritional supplements should be used in conjunction with prescription medications, exercise, weight control, and possibly surgery.

Individuals considering glucosamine/chondroitin therapy should be aware that glucosamine is contraindicated for people with shellfish allergies and may affect blood sugar levels in diabetics. Chondroitin may affect blood-clotting ability in individuals taking anticoagulants. Research into the usefulness of glucosamine and chondroitin sulfate continues.

—Robin Kamienny Montvilo, Ph.D.

can also be varied. The sensation desired is a slight tingle. The effect described induces an increase in the release of beta endorphin, a substance naturally produced by the body with effects similar to those of morphine. Endorphin is produced by other physical therapy procedures as well: hypnosis, acupuncture, suggestion, and stress, among others.

Patients in chronic pain may show a reduced level of the beta endorphin and an increase in a substance P, and they may find no relief of pain with physical therapy. The P chemical increases the nerves' sensitivity to stimuli, producing greater pain. Patients with chronic pain may show depression, hysteria, and hypochondriasis on the Minnesota Multiphasic Personality Inventory and may require antidepressants. Exercise programs can help to increase endorphin levels. These exercises may range from simple movements performed by a therapist (the patient remaining passive) to active exertion against loads for strength. Stretching or gentle, intermittent traction may gradually decrease contractures, but neck traction should not be used in patients with rheumatoid arthritis of the neck.

Surgery may occasionally be necessary to alleviate pain, to replace joints, or to alleviate contractures. Isometric or static exercises can mobilize muscles without joint movement and maintain muscle viability during joint pain. Individuals can, however, be trained to perform activities more efficiently and effectively, thus saving energy. Posture training may alleviate postural muscle fatigue. In acute stages of inflammation, the treatment choices are rest, ice, compression, and proper positioning and medicinals for pain and inflammation. The stepped-up medicinal approach utilizes nonsteroidal anti-inflammatory drugs (NSAIDS)—such as aspirin, indomethacin, ibuprofen, naproxen, piroxicam, and nabumetone—and adds other drugs as necessary, including antimalarials and gold, immune suppressants, and systemic corticosteroids. Irradiation of lymphoid tissues may also be used at the acute stages. Heat modalities should not be used in acute cases, since the speed of chemical reactions increases on heating; the chemical enzyme activity of collagenase that destroys cartilage could increase the rate and extent of damage. The simplest way to prepare cold applications is to fill a plastic container with water and refrigerate it. Physicians may also use fluoromethane or other refrigerant sprays. The hot packs sold in pharmacies can similarly be soaked in water and placed in the refrigerator to create an ice pack.

In 2002, researchers announced a new type of anti-inflammatory painkiller that showed promise in initial studies on people with arthritis in their knees. Licofelone works just as well as NSAIDs but seems to be gentler on the stomach. Medical experts believe that it will prove a better alternative to arthritis drugs such as Vioxx, Bextra, and Celebrex. Vioxx was removed from the market in September, 2004, and Bextra in April, 2005. All three are COX-2 selective inhibitors, the newest of the NSAIDS. These drugs selectively block the enzyme COX-2, the enzyme controlling the production of prostaglandins, natural chemicals that contribute to body inflammation and cause the pain and swelling of arthritis. They do not affect COX-1, however, so the selective aspect offers the benefit of diminishing inflammation without accelerating the risk of stomach ulceration and bleeding.

Perspective and Prospects

Historically, arthritis was treated with electric eels (as the source of electric shocks) and warm baths or sands. Some experimental treatments presently being tried include electric current to joints to bring about reductions in intra-articular pressures and in the fluid and cellular content in joints. Acupuncture has been shown to bring an increase in the beta endorphin levels and consequent relief of pain. Topical use of capsaicin, an extract from peppers, is reported to counteract substance P. One group is attempting the experimental procedure of washing out inflamed joints with a saline-type solution. Exercises continue to maintain and improve strength, dexterity, the range of motion, and endurance. Good health habits—including adequate rest, good nutrition, and nutritional supplements—can be beneficial.

—Eugene J. Rogers, M.D.;
updated by Victoria Price, Ph.D.

See also Bone disorders; Bones and the skeleton; Bursitis; Fracture and dislocation; Gout; Hip fracture repair; Hip replacement; Inflammation; Juvenile rheumatoid arthritis; Massage; Muscle sprains, spasms, and disorders; Orthopedic surgery; Orthopedics; Orthopedics, pediatric; Osteoarthritis; Over-the-counter medications; Pain management; Physical rehabilitation; Reiter's syndrome; Rheumatoid arthritis; Rheumatology; Spinal cord disorders; Spine, vertebrae, and disks; Tendon disorders; Tendon repair.

For Further Information:

Aesoph, Lauri M. *How to Eat Away Arthritis*. Englewood Cliffs, N. J.: Prentice-Hall, 1996. Focuses on dietary therapy as an important mode of treatment for various types of arthritis, including gout.

Arthritis Foundation. *The Arthritis Foundation's Guide to Good Living with Fibromyalgia*. Atlanta: Author, 2001. A guide to self-managing aspects of the disease, offering advice on such topics as exercise, nutrition, and stress management.

Flynn, John A., and Lora Brown Wilder, eds. *Recipes for Arthritis Health*. New York: Rebus, 2003. The writers collaborate by combining their respective expertise in medicinal aspects and nutritional aspects of treating arthritis.

Fries, James F. *Arthritis: A Take-Care-of-Yourself Guide to Understanding Your Arthritis*. 5th ed. Reading, Mass.: Addison-Wesley, 1999. This book is recommended by the Arthritis Foundation. Discusses the major categories of arthritis, as well as pathology, quackery, surgery, employment, prevention, home treatment, and the effects of medications.

Hunder, Gene G. *Mayo Clinic on Arthritis*. Rev. ed. Rochester, Minn.: Mayo Clinic, 2002. Accessible handbook about living with the most common forms of arthritis, osteoarthritis and rheumatoid arthritis.

Lahita, Robert G. *Rheumatoid Arthritis: Everything You Need to Know*. New York: Avery, 2001. Addresses such topics as the occurrence, symptoms, diagnosis, treatment, medications, and alternative and complementary therapy for rheumatoid arthritis.

Lane, Nancy E., and Daniel J. Wallace. *All About Osteoarthritis: The Definitive Resource for Arthritis Patients and Their Families*. New York: Oxford University Press, 2001. Two leading doctors discuss a range of relevant topics, including how diagnosis is made, how the body is affected, methods to alleviate pain, good exercise regimens, and how to find the best resources to cope with the disorder.

Lorig, Kate, and James F. Fries, eds. *The Arthritis Helpbook: A Tested Self-Management Program for Coping with Arthritis and Fibromyalgia*. 6th ed. Cambridge, Mass.: Da Capo Press, 2006. This book states that it is recommended by the Arthritis Foundation. The contributors, who include allied health professionals from the fields of physical therapy, occupational therapy, and public health, address pain management principles, body mechanics, and exercises.

Nelson, Miriam E., et al. *Strong Women and Men Beat Arthritis*. New York: G. P. Putnam's Sons, 2003. Discusses strategies for dealing with arthritis, including nutrition and exercise, medication, surgery, and complementary approaches.

Sands, Judith K., and Judith H. Matthews. "Medications: Arthritis Drugs Hit Their Mark." *Harvard Health Letter* 24, no. 4 (February, 1999): 4-5. Evaluates new arthritis drugs.

Shlotzhauer, Tammi L., and James L. McGuire. *Living with Rheumatoid Arthritis*. 2d ed. Baltimore: Johns Hopkins University Press, 2003. Offers straightforward advice on coping with the disorder, exploring topics such as the emotional challenges of arthritis; why medication, joint protection, physical activity, and good nutrition are essential components of care; and effective exercises to cope with pain, stiffness, and fatigue.

Weinblatt, Michael E. *The Arthritis Action Program: An Integrated Plan of Traditional and Complementary Therapies*. New York: Simon & Schuster, 2000. Focuses on individual responsibility for taking charge of treatment for various kinds of arthritis. Discusses complementary therapies such as yoga, aromatherapy, biofeedback, and acupuncture. Warns against possible adverse effects of complementary therapies that could interact adversely with other medications being taken.

Arthroplasty

Procedure

Anatomy or system affected: Arms, bones, hands, hips, joints, knees

Specialties and related fields: Anesthesiology, general surgery, geriatrics and gerontology, orthopedics, rheumatology, sports medicine

Definition: The replacement of joints—hips, fingers, knees, shoulders, or elbows—by metal or plastic prostheses.

Key terms:

acetabulum: the portion of the pelvic bone joining the femoral head to create the hip joint

cartilage: flexible, connective tissue between bones

epidural: the injection of an anesthetic into the fluid around the spine or into the epidural space in the back

femur: the leg bone extending from the knee to the hip

orthopedics: a medical specialty emphasizing the prevention and correction of skeletal deformities

patella: the flat, triangular bone in the front of the knee; also called the kneecap

tibia: the shin bone

Indications and Procedures

Joints become painful when the cartilage keeping bone from pressing on bone deteriorates, a process called osteoarthritis. They can become sufficiently painful, particularly among the elderly, to indicate more than the analgesic treatment resorted to initially by most people suffering from painful joints.

Arthroplasty, surgery undertaken to replace deteriorating joints, may be performed on the fingers, shoulders, and elbows. The most common sites of such surgery, however, are the hips and knees. Most patients requiring hip or knee replacements are over age fifty, but arthroplasty may be indicated for younger people who have suffered trauma. Specialists in sports medicine frequently prescribe arthroplasty, which is typically performed by orthopedic surgeons.

The hip is a ball-and-socket joint. When people walk, the top of the femur slides into the acetabulum. Cartilage normally covers both bones where they meet, permitting smooth, painless contact between them. When this cartilage deteriorates, bones rub against each other, causing pain and restriction in movement that is best relieved by hip replacement surgery.

A similar situation can afflict the knee. Using an arthroscope or endoscope, an orthopedist makes a small incision in the knee and inserts a narrow illuminated tube with a camera attached into the affected site in order to examine it. If this examination reveals worn bone and cartilage, then a knee replacement, in which the knee joint is replaced with metal and plastic substitutes, is indicated.

Typically, hip and knee replacements are performed on patients under general anesthetic, although a local anesthetic, either spinal or epidural, is sometimes used. In most cases, general anesthetic is preferred because patients must remain completely still during this surgery and general anesthetic causes temporary paralysis.

In hip surgery, an incision, varying in length from 2 to 12 inches, is made over the back of the hip. Tissue and muscles are cut or pushed aside to expose the hip joint. The femur and acetabulum are separated. A declivity made in the acetabulum accommodates the replacement cup and allows for the insertion of a plastic-lined metal shell. The ball atop the femur is removed and replaced with a metal ball attached to a metal stem, usually made of titanium, that is inserted into the femoral canal. The two parts are then cemented into place, making them adhere to the bone. Damaged muscles and tendons are repaired before the incision is closed with staples or sutures.

In knee surgery, a long incision is made in the front of the knee and the patella is removed to make the joint accessible. Holes are drilled into the lower femur to affix the metal replacement. Holes are also drilled in the upper tibia to anchor a plastic plate. The back part of the patella is excised to create a flat surface into which holes are drilled to receive a plastic button. The prosthesis is then secured with cement, and the incision closed, usually with sutures or staples.

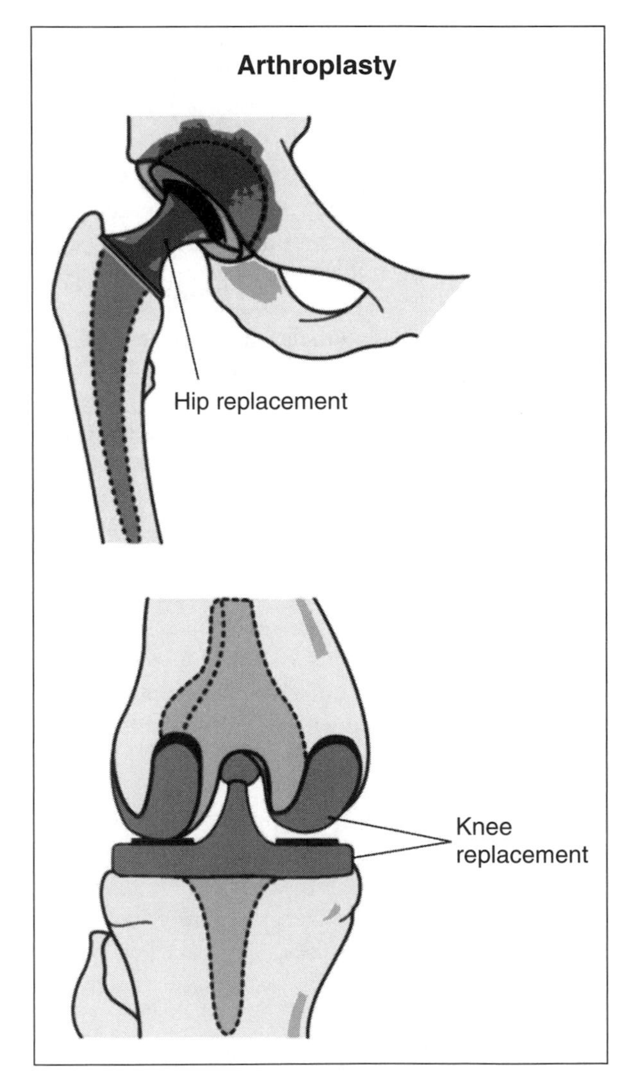

The hip and knee joints can be replaced by metal or plastic ball-and-socket prostheses when disease or injury is too extensive to repair the existing joints.

Uses and Complications

Arthroplasty is used to relieve pain and restore mobility in patients who are reasonable surgical risks. Many have been disabled by their conditions. Because many such patients are elderly, extensive preoperative evaluation is necessary. Conditions such as diabetes mellitus, hypertension, heart or lung disease, and anemia increase the surgical risk. Open lesions increase the risk of infection.

Nerve damage can result from cutting muscles and tendons during surgery. Blood clots can form in the lungs or legs of patients undergoing arthroplasty, and this risk may continue for two months following surgery. Blood thinners are usually administered postoperatively.

Physical therapy, essential following arthroplasty, usually begins two or three days following the surgery and continues for eight weeks. Most patients are completely ambulatory within six weeks postoperatively.

Perspective and Prospects

As the population of the United States ages and its life expectancy increases, incidence of joint problems is increasing exponentially. In the early twentieth century, many people who lived beyond their sixties were immobilized by chronic arthritis, osteoporosis, and painful joints. When an elderly person suffered a broken hip, it often marked the beginning of a physical decline with a fatal outcome.

Medical advances made during World War II had a profound effect on treating many physical problems that, although experienced in combat by relatively young people, required treatment that was soon used in dealing with the joint problems of the elderly. Hip and knee surgery were once more disabling than they currently are. Hip surgery now requires incisions as small as one inch long, although four-inch incisions are more common and ten-inch incisions are used by some surgeons.

Although arthroplasty usually involves a hospital stay of two to four days, it is likely that soon such surgery will become an outpatient procedure. The use of titanium in prostheses has extended the effectiveness of such surgery, with these devices currently expected to last for about two decades.

—R. Baird Shuman, Ph.D.

See also Arthritis; Arthroscopy; Bones and the skeleton; Fracture and dislocation; Fracture repair; Hip fracture repair; Kneecap removal; Orthopedic surgery; Orthopedics; Osteoarthritis; Rheumatoid arthritis; Rheumatology; Rotator cuff surgery; Sports medicine.

For Further Information:

An, Yuehuei H., ed. *Orthopaedic Issues in Osteoporosis*. Boca Raton, Fla.: CRC Press, 2003.

Doherty, Gerard M., and Lawrence W. Way, eds. *Current Surgical Diagnosis and Treatment*. 12th ed. New York: Lange Medical Books/McGraw-Hill, 2006.

Morris, Peter J., and William C. Wood. *Oxford Textbook of Surgery*. 2d ed. New York: Oxford University Press, 2000.

Rose, Eric A. *The Columbia Presbyterian Guide to Surgery*. New York: St. Martin's Griffin, 2000.

Rothrock, Jane C., ed. *Alexander's Care of the Patient in Surgery*. 13th ed. St. Louis: Mosby, 2006.

Arthroscopy

Procedure

Anatomy or system affected: Hips, joints, knees, legs

Specialties and related fields: Orthopedics, rheumatology

Definition: A technique for examining joints through a thin scope inserted into the joint; it may be used to visualize and perform surgical procedures.

Indications and Procedures

The arthroscope is a rigid tube enclosing a series of lenses around which are wrapped glass fibers for transmitting light. The arthroscope is placed inside a larger metal sheath, which allows fluid to flow between the components. After disinfecting the skin, the surgeon inserts a cannula (tube) into the desired cavity using an obturator, a prosthetic device which is removed and replaced by the arthroscope.

Instruments passed through the cannula include probes, forceps, knives, scissors, and a variety of clamps. Cutting may be done manually or with a motor-driven tool. The surgeon uses a small light and lens on the instrument to see the operative field. The eyepiece of an arthroscope may be replaced by a video camera to allow viewing on a television monitor.

After the skin is prepared and the instruments are inserted, diagnostic or operative procedures are begun.

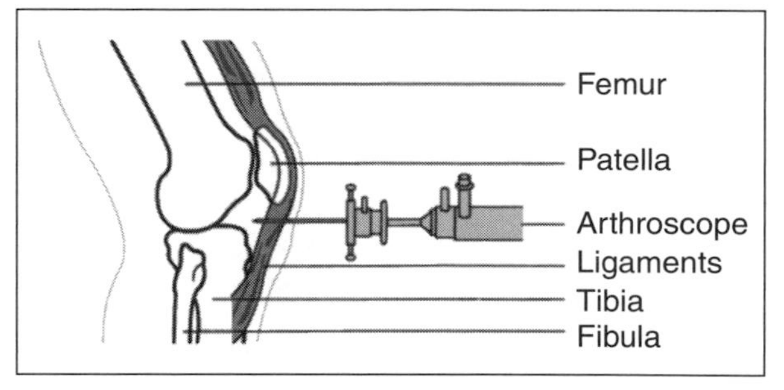

Arthroscopy is a diagnostic procedure in which a fiber-optic instrument is inserted into a joint for direct examination without the complications that accompany a larger incision; sometimes surgical instruments are also passed through the arthroscope.

The joint or tissue is thoroughly explored before any further steps are taken. An assistant positions the body part, freeing the surgeon to operate. The most common site for an arthroscopic procedure is the knee; other sites include the elbow, shoulder, and ankle.

After the procedure is completed, the joint is flushed to remove all debris. The instruments are withdrawn, and the skin punctures are closed with a single suture or bandage closure. The patient returns in a week for a postarthroscopic examination and removal of sutures. Rehabilitation is important; it should begin on the day following arthroscopy and can require up to several months, depending on the site and procedure.

Uses and Complications

Arthroscopy is a technique originally developed for diagnosis in joints; it is now used for surgical procedures as well. Typically, arthroscopy is used for knee and shoulder joint injuries, but it can also be used in the ankle, hip, or elbow. The technique has also been applied in innovative ways by podiatric foot and ankle surgeons to relieve different ankle problems, including ligament damage, bone chips, and recurrent pain from end-stage arthritis.

Many simple procedures can be done using local anesthesia, although regional or general anesthesia is preferred. Arthroscopy can be carried out in either a fluid or a gas environment within the joint. A saline solution is often used; it disperses light more evenly but requires a system to pump the fluid in and out. A gas environment is more useful for visualizing surface irregularities of cartilage.

Such techniques have significantly changed orthopedic surgery. The use of arthroscopy for diagnosis and treatment reduces postoperative infections, the time needed for rehabilitation, and costs. Most arthroscopic procedures are now done on an outpatient basis.

—*L. Fleming Fallon, Jr., M.D., Ph.D., M.P.H.*

See also Arthritis; Arthroplasty; Bones and the skeleton; Endoscopy; Fracture and dislocation; Fracture repair; Hip fracture repair; Kneecap removal; Laparoscopy; Orthopedic surgery; Orthopedics; Osteoarthritis; Rheumatoid arthritis; Rheumatology; Sports medicine.

For Further Information:

Chow, James C. Y., ed. *Advanced Arthroscopy*. New York: Springer, 2001.

Clark, Glenn T., Bruce Sanders, and Charles N. Bertolami, eds. *Advances in Diagnostic and Surgical Arthroscopy of the Temporomandibular Joint*. Philadelphia: W. B. Saunders, 1993.

Miller, Mark D., Daniel E. Cooper, and Jon J. P. Warner. *Review of Sports Medicine and Arthroscopy*. 2d ed. Philadelphia: W. B. Saunders, 2002.

Sherman, Orrin Howard, and Jeffrey Minkoff, eds. *Arthroscopic Surgery*. Baltimore: Williams & Wilkins, 1990.

Tibone, James E., Felix H. Savoie III, and Benjamin S. Shaffer, eds. *Shoulder Arthroscopy*. New York: Springer-Verlag, 2003.

Zarins, Bertram, and Richard A. Marder, eds. *Revision of Failed Arthroscopic and Ligament Surgery*. Malden, Mass.: Blackwell Science, 1998.

Asbestos exposure

Disease/disorder

Anatomy or system affected: Gastrointestinal system, lungs, respiratory system

Specialties and related fields: Environmental health, occupational health, oncology

Definition: Asbestos is a naturally occurring fire-resistant mineral fiber historically used in a variety of applications ranging from lamp wicks to roofing shingles. Asbestos fibers consist of silica compounds that can irritate human tissue, resulting in disorders such as asbestosis as well as cancers of the lung, larynx, and gastrointestinal system.

Key terms:

asbestos: a naturally occurring mineral fiber composed of silica compounds

mesothelioma: a specific type of cancer occurring when asbestos fibers irritate the pleural lining of the lungs

metastasis: the migration of cancer from its original location in the body to other organs

pleura: the thin membrane that lines the interior of the chest walls and covers the lungs

silicon dioxide: a compound formed when silica is exposed to air

Information on Asbestos Exposure

Causes: Irritation of tissue of skin or lungs by silica fibers

Symptoms: For skin, calluslike growths; for lungs, scarring resulting in asbestosis and mesothelioma (cancer)

Duration: Chronic and progressive

Treatments: None; support for symptoms

Causes and Symptoms

Asbestos is a naturally occurring mineral fiber whose fire-resistant properties have been known since antiquity. Although there are a variety of forms of asbestos, with some being more associated with occupational illness and disease than others, all asbestos shares a common characteristic: Because asbestos consists of silica crystals, the fibers are inherently irritating to human tissue. On the surface of the skin, they can become embedded and lead to the formation of calluslike growths, termed "asbestos warts," as the body attempts to encapsulate the irritating fibers.

Inhaled or ingested asbestos fibers are a more serious matter. Asbestos exposure has been associated with cancers of the stomach, liver, and other organs, but asbestosis and mesothelioma are the two most common asbestos-related health disorders.

Asbestosis, a lung disorder caused by the fibers causing scarring of lung tissue, was one of the first disorders recognized as being associated with asbestos exposure. It is now known that the fibers do not scar the lungs directly, but rather trigger the production of acid by the lung tissue as the body attempts to break down the silica crystals. Asbestosis is similar to disorders such as silicosis, "black lung," and "brown lung" in that lung capacity is reduced as cumulative damage reduces victims' ability to breathe.

Mesothelioma, a particularly invidious cancer, is also associated with asbestos exposure. With this form of cancer, the cells between the walls of the pleura (the outer covering of the lungs that separates the lungs from the chest wall) or the peritoneum (the sac containing the abdominal organs) form malignant growths.

Both asbestosis and mesothelioma may take many years to develop, with some victims not developing mesothelioma until as many as forty years had passed since the initial exposure. On the other hand, there have been cases of adolescents developing mesothelioma within only a few months of initial asbestos exposure.

Treatment and Therapy

Localized "asbestos warts" on the skin may be unattractive, but they are generally benign. The lung diseases associated with asbestos exposure, however, are progressive and ultimately fatal. In asbestosis, the scarred lung tissue becomes increasingly stiff, and the person becomes unable to take in sufficient oxygen. In its terminal stage, the sufferer literally feels as though he or she is suffocating.

Mesothelioma has a high mortality rate, as it is rarely detected in its early stages. Symptoms such as shortness of breath are attributed to more common diseases such as asthma. As the cancer spreads, lung capacity is diminished, and the victim eventually dies from the inability to take in sufficient oxygen, if he or she has not already succumbed to other organs failing after the cancer metastasizes.

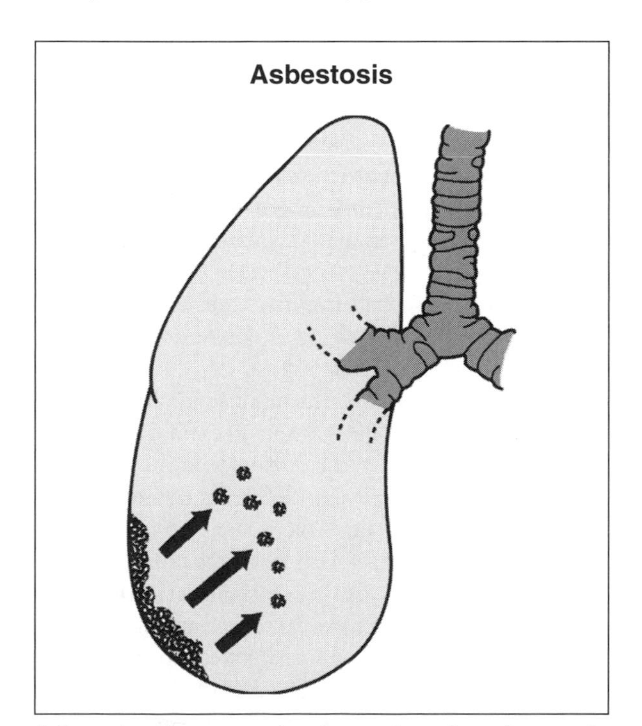

Asbestosis—the progressive destruction of respiratory tissues via inhalation of dust-sized asbestos fibers that attach to the walls of the lung and then spread outward—is often the result of prolonged exposure to asbestos-containing materials (in shipyards, office buildings, manufacturing plants); it is one of a wide variety of environmental diseases.

Perspective and Prospects

The ancient Romans mined asbestos for use in manufacturing fireproof mats and garments, as did various other cultures throughout recorded history. During the nineteenth century, asbestos became a popular material for lamp wicks, as it could convey the lamp oil without being consumed by the flame itself. As industrialization progressed, asbestos became widely used in such applications as brake shoes for automobiles, oven linings in electric stoves, and building materials. Asbestos was impregnated into siding and shingles for exterior walls and roofs, insulation for attics and walls, and ceiling and floor tiles. By the mid-twentieth century, asbestos had become ubiquitous in society, from the materials on which people walked to the roofs over their heads. The Romans recognized that mining asbestos was effectively a death sentence, as slaves working in asbestos production quickly developed coughs and wasted away from lung diseases. Mining being a generally dusty and dangerous occupation, however, the special risks that asbestos presented were not well recognized. For centuries, many physicians assumed that all miners' lung ailments were forms of consumption (tuberculosis), when in fact tuberculosis was an opportunistic infection that followed after a miner became weakened by disorders such as silicosis and asbestosis.

By the 1930's, researchers had established that asbestos presented especially high risks of causing lung diseases in miners, shipyard workers, and others who either manufactured or worked with with materials incorporating asbestos, such as insulation. By the mid-twentieth century, it had become evident that extremely small amounts of asbestos exposure could lead to asbestos-related disorders. Miners' spouses developed mesothelioma after being exposed to asbestos through doing laundry, for example, while children became victims through exposure to their parents' work clothes in the home.

The widespread use of asbestos fibers in multiple applications means that exposure remains a concern in the twenty-first century. Although asbestos is no longer as widely used in industry, reducing the prevalence of workplace exposures, people can still risk asbestos exposure when engaging in home improvement projects as they rip out old flooring or replace ceiling tile.

—Nancy Farm Mannikko, Ph.D.

See also Cancer; Chronic obstructive pulmonary disease (COPD); Environmental diseases; Environmental health; Interstitial pulmonary fibrosis (IPF); Lung cancer; Lungs; Occupational health; Pulmonary diseases; Pulmonary medicine; Pulmonary medicine, pediatric; Skin disorders.

For Further Information:

Bowker, Michael, *Fatal Deception: The Terrifying True Story of How Asbestos Is Killing America*. New York: Touchstone, 2003. Includes a description of the thousands of applications of asbestos in modern society. May ensure that a home remodeler puts on a dust mask before tearing out the old ceiling tiles. Readily understandable by a general audience.

Frank, A. L. "Global Problems from Exposure to Asbestos," *Environmental Health Perspectives Supplements* 101, no. 3 (1993): 165-168. A summary of asbestos-related problems worldwide.

Roggli, Victor L., and others, *Pathology of Asbestos-Associated Diseases*. 2d ed. New York: Springer, 2004. A comprehensive overview of diseases linked to asbestos exposure. Includes a mineralogical explanation of asbestos as well as thorough explication of both the pathology and the history of the diseases.

Asian American health

Overview

Anatomy or system affected: All

Specialties and related fields: All

Definition: Statistics, health profiles, and health concerns of Asian Americans, who are extremely diverse with representations of nearly fifty countries and ethnic groups.

Key terms:

alternative medicine: therapeutic practices that are not currently considered an integral part of conventional medical practice

health: a state of complete physical, mental, and social well-being, and not merely the absence of disease or infirmity

minority: a sociological group that does not constitute a politically dominant plurality of the total population of a given society

Population and Statistics

Asian Americans are U.S residents who have origins in the Far East, Southeast Asia, or the Indian subcontinent. Asian Americans represent nearly fifty countries and ethnic groups, each with distinct cultures, traditions, and histories. According to the 2000 U.S. Census, the largest Asian American subgroup was Chinese, followed by Filipinos and then Asian Indians. Other main Asian American subgroups include Japanese, Korean, Vietnamese, Cambodians, Indonesians, Laotians, Malaysians, Pakistanis, Sri Lankans, and Thais. Pacific Islanders, such as Native Hawaiians, are often grouped with Asian Americans. The majority of Asian Americans are only Asian, while about 14 percent of Asian Americans are combinations of Asian and some other race, with the most common combination being Asian and white.

The Asian American population is a rapidly growing minority group in the United States. According to the 2004 Census Bureau population estimate, there are 13.9 million Asian Americans living in the United States, accounting for 5 percent of the nation's population. This number represents an increase of 63 percent from the 1990 census, a rate that was faster than that in the total U.S population. The Census Bureau projects that the Asian American population will grow to 37.6 million individuals by the year 2050, constituting 9.3 percent of the U.S. population. Asian Americans are generally concentrated in the Western states, the Northeast, and parts of the South. The states with the greatest concentration of Asian Americans are Hawaii, California, Washington, New Jersey, and New York.

More than one hundred languages and dialects are used by Asian Americans. About 67 percent of Asian Americans speak a language other than English at home. The percentage of persons aged five years or older who do not speak English varies among Asian American groups: 61 percent of Vietnamese, 51 percent of Chinese, 24 percent of Filipinos, and 24 percent of Asian Indians are not fluent in English.

According to the 2000 U.S. Census, about 80 percent of Asian Americans aged twenty-five or older had at least a high school diploma. This high school graduation rate among the Asian American youth is similar to that of all people in the United States. However, 44 percent of Asian Americans, in comparison to 20 percent of the total U.S. population, had earned at least a bachelor's degree. Among Asian subgroups, Asian Indians had the highest percentage of bachelor's degree attainment, at 64 percent. Regarding employment, about 45 percent of Asian Americans were employed in management, professional, and other related occupations, compared to 34 percent of the total population in the United States.

The median family income of Asian American families is $9,000 higher than the median for all other ethnic groups in the United States, as shown by the U.S. Census data. A total of 9.4 percent of Asian Americans, compared to 11.5 percent of Caucasians, live in poverty, while 2.2 percent of Asian Americans compared to 1.3 percent of Caucasians live on public assistance. Health insurance coverage among Asian Americans is comparable to the total U.S. population but varies among Asian American subgroups, according to some studies. Private insurance coverage rates are 75.8 percent for Vietnamese, 81.5 percent for Filipino, 84.2 percent for Chinese, and 81.3 percent for other Asian groups. Public insurance coverage rates are 11.2 percent for Vietnamese, 4.9 percent for Filipino, 3.8 percent for Chinese, and 5.5 percent for other Asian groups. Uninsured rates are 13.0 percent for Vietnamese, 13.6 percent for Filipino, 12.0 percent for Chinese, and 13.2 percent for other Asian groups.

Asian Americans represent both extremes of socioeconomic and health indexes. While more than a million Asian Americans live at or below the federal poverty level, it is significant to note that Asian American women have the highest life expectancy (85.8 years) of any ethnic group in the United States, although life expectancy varies among Asian American subgroups: Filipino women (81.5 years), Japanese women (84.5 years), and Chinese women (86.1 years). Furthermore, Asian American babies have the lowest infant mortality rate of any ethnic group. Asian American men are 40 percent less likely to have prostate cancer than non-Hispanic white men. Asian American women are 30 percent less likely to have breast cancer than non-Hispanic white women. Although strokes are more common in some Asian countries, Asian American adults are less likely than Caucasian adults to suffer from a stroke, and they are also less likely to die from a stroke. Asian Americans are 20 percent less likely than non-Hispanic whites to die from diabetes. In general, Asian Americans have lower rates of being overweight or obese, and they are also less likely to be current cigarette smokers, as compared to other ethnic groups.

As a result of poverty, lack of health insurance, and language and cultural barriers among some Asian Americans, however, they suffer disproportionately from certain health problems. Asian Americans account for over half of chronic hepatitis B cases and half of the deaths resulting from the hepatitis B infection in the United States. Asian Americans also account for more than 20 percent of all tuberculosis cases in the United States. Compared to other ethnic groups, Asian American women have the lowest cancer screening rates and are usually diagnosed at the later stages of cancer. Asian American women are 1.5 times more likely to have cervical cancer, compared to non-Hispanic white women. Asian American adults have a higher chance of developing stomach cancer and liver cancer, as well as a higher death rate from these two cancers. While Asian Americans have a lower human immunodeficiency virus (HIV) infection rate than their non-Hispanic white counterparts, they are more likely to be diagnosed at an advanced stage of acquired immunodeficiency syndrome (AIDS) and to suffer from opportunistic infections at the time of diagnosis. Although Asian Americans are less likely to have heart disease and to die from that condition compared to non-Hispanic whites, Native Hawaiians have an unusually high rate of cardiovascular disease.

Because of language and cultural barriers, Asian American elders are less likely to receive social services and medical care and to benefit from social interaction. Asian American adults aged sixty-five years and older are 50 percent less likely to have ever received a pneumonia vaccine, compared to non-Hispanic white adults of the same age group. Many Asian cultures stigmatize mental health problems, and many Asian Americans have difficulty accessing culturally appropriate mental health care. Additionally, several states have reported alarming trends in domestic violence within Asian American communities. Research studies showed increased trends in substance abuse among Asian American adults and increased smoking rates in seventh through twelfth grades of Asian American youths as well.

Major Health Concerns

The ten leading causes of death for Asian Americans in the United States in 2002 were cancer, heart disease, stroke, unintentional injuries, diabetes, influenza and pneumonia, chronic lower respiratory disease, suicide, nephritis, and septicemia. Although they share the similar leading causes of death and suffer from the same health problems as the population at large in the United States, Asian Americans have disproportionately high prevalence of certain illnesses.

Cancer is the number one cause of death for both Asian American men and women, and certain types of cancer are extremely common in Asian American communities. The incidence rate of liver cancer for Asian Americans is 13.8 per 100,000, which is more than double of the rate for other minority groups and more than triple of the rate for whites. The incidence rate of stomach cancer among Asian Americans is 18.5 per 100,000, which is also substantially higher than any other ethnic groups. Lung cancer is the most common cancer among Vietnamese (70.9 per 100,000), Korean (53.2 per 100,000), and Chinese (52.1 per 100,000) men. Lung cancer is also the most common cause of death resulting from cancer among men of these Asian American subgroups.

Asian American women have the third highest incidence rate of breast cancer (93.4 per 100,000), following whites and African Americans. Breast cancer is the most common cancer among Japanese women (82.3 per 100,000), Filipino women (73.1 per 100,000), Chinese women (55.0 per 100,000), and Korean women (28.5 per 100,000). A study found that Asian American females born in the West have a breast cancer rate that is 60 percent higher than those born in the country of origin, and this risk doubles after a decade of residence in the West. Less than half of the Asian American women aged fifty and older reported having a mammography or clinical breast examination in the past two years, the lowest rate for breast cancer screening among all ethnic groups.

Cervical cancer is the most common cancer among Vietnamese women (43.0 per 100,000), a rate that is five times higher than that for Caucasian women. As a result of lack of health-related knowledge, a large number of Vietnamese women cannot correctly explain the purpose of the Pap tests that are used for the early diagnosis of cervical cancer. Compared to other ethnic groups, Southeast Asian women tend to have more severe cases of cervical cancer because of late diagnosis.

Heart disease is the second leading cause of death for most Asian Americans. Cardiovascular disease accounts for over one-third of all deaths for Asian American men and women. Native Hawaiians disproportionately suffer from the burden of heart disease, compared to other ethnic groups in Hawaii. Research shows that the death rate resulting from heart disease for full-Hawaiians is 4.7 times greater than that for all races and 2.5 times greater than that for part-Hawaiians; the death rate for part-Hawaiians was 1.9 times higher than that for all races. Although far less is known about the prevalence of heart disease among other Pacific Islanders and other Asian Americans, anecdotal evidence suggests that cardiovascular risks vary greatly among Asian American subpopulations. Asian Americans from Southeast Asian present more cardiovascular risk factors, such as high blood cholesterol level and high blood pressure (hypertension). Some study found that mean cholesterol levels were highest among Japanese men and women compared to other Asian Americans populations. However, the prevalence of hypertension for Japanese aged fifty and older was less than half of any other ethnic groups in the same age range. Filipinos aged fifty and older had hypertension prevalence rates of more than 60 percent, compared to 47 percent of people in the same age group in the U.S. general populations. One important risk factor for cardiovascular disease is lack of physical activity, and limited research showed that Asian Americans typically are less likely than the general U.S. population to engage in physical activities.

Hepatitis B is a chronic viral infection of the liver. Compared to the U.S. average, hepatitis B is twenty-five to seventy-five times more common among immigrants from Cambodia, Laos, Vietnam, and China. Although a vaccine is available for preventing hepatitis B, Asian American individuals and families with limited access to preventive services may not be vaccinated against the virus. Furthermore, because of language barriers and lack of knowledge, Asian American populations generally are not aware of the benefits of the hepatitis B vaccine for helping prevent disease and liver cancer, which is usually caused by long-term exposure to hepatitis B virus. Thus, liver cancer is one of the common causes for cancer-related death among Asian Americans. In addition to hepatitis B, the hepatitis C infection is also more prevalent in Asian immigrants.

Asian American communities are at high risk for tuberculosis, a bacterial infection of the lung and other body organs. In San Francisco, the infection rate of tuberculosis was reported as 60 per 100,000 for Asian Americans, the highest rate among all ethnic groups in the city. In New York City, Asian Americans also have a higher rate of tuberculosis than any other ethnic group, accounting for more than 24 percent of all tuberculosis cases in New York City. In some Asian American communities, the rate of tuberculosis is increasing. Tuberculosis is especially common among certain Asian American subgroups, such as Cambodians, Chinese, Laotians, Koreans, Asian Indians, Vietnamese, and Filipinos.

Many Asian American cultures believe in and widely use alternative medicines, such as herbal therapy, acupuncture, and massage. With the increase in the number of Asian Americans in the United States, the use of alternative medicine is also increasing. Some types of alternative medicines, such as acupuncture, have gained a level of acceptance in Western medicine; however, governmental health programs such as Medicare and Medicaid do not cover the cost of alternative therapies. A lack of such coverage limits Asian Americans, especially the elderly, in their access to alternative medicine.

On the other hand, concerns have also arisen over the use of alternative medicines. Many products used by alternative healers are unmonitored, and there is a deficiency in regulation. Also, little research has been conducted to evaluate the effectiveness of these alternative medicines. One common form of alternative medicine is dietary supplements, but some of these products may be contaminated. Some Asian cultures view illness as an imbalance of the body, physically and mentally. This concept sometimes interferes with many Asian Americans in seeking proper health care, which results in delayed diagnosis and treatment.

Perspective and Prospects

Asian Americans have historically been overlooked due to the myth of the "model minority"—the erroneous notion that Asian Americans are passive, compliant, and without problems or needs. Some refer to Asian Americans as a "model minority" because the Asian American culture contains a strong work ethic, respect for elders, close family bonds, and successful lives. These perceptions can lead to inadequate attention from American society toward the needs of Asian Americans, especially in health and medicine. Health promotion and disease prevention messages are rarely targeted to Asian American populations in linguistically and culturally appropriate ways. Asian American communities usually lack sufficient health care providers trained to understand Asian cultures. Overall, there is general lack of research on health issues specifically for Asian American populations.

With the rapid increase of Asian American populations in the United States, it is necessary to make their health a public health priority in the nation. As suggested by some experts and organizations, certain approaches can be taken to improve the health of Asian Americans, including establishing a federal government agency that acts as a national resource center on Asian American health, increasing access to health care for Asian American populations by improving access to public-sector health insurance programs, improving cultural competency in health care settings and among health care providers, and supporting new research, health education, and public awareness efforts among Asian Americans.

—Kimberly Y. Z. Forrest, Ph.D.

See also African American health; Alternative medicine; American Indian health; Breast cancer; Cancer; Cervical, ovarian, and uterine cancer; Heart disease; Hepatitis; Hypertension; Men's health; Tuberculosis; Women's health.

For Further Information:

Barnes, Jesse S., and Claudette E. Bennett. *The Asian Population, 2000*. Washington, D.C.: U.S. Department of Commerce, Economics, and Statistics Administration, U.S. Census Bureau, 2002. This report provides demographic statistics specifically for Asian Americans from the 2000 U.S. Census data.

MedlinePlus. *Asian-American Health*. http://www.nlm.nih.gov/medlineplus/asianamericanhealth.html. This Web site provide information related to issues affecting the health and well-being of Asian Americans in the United States.

President's Advisory Commission on Asian Americans and Pacific Islanders. *Asian Americans and Pacific Islanders Addressing Health Disparities: Opportunities for Building A Healthier America*. http://www.aapi.gov/Commission_Final_Health_Report.pdf. This report, published in 2003, describes the health status of Asian Americans and identifies strategies for improving the health of this population. It provides detailed health statistics for Asian Americans.

Asperger's syndrome

Disease/Disorder

Anatomy or system affected: Psychic-emotional system

Specialties and related fields: Psychiatry, psychology

Definition: A pervasive developmental disorder involving clinically significant impairment in social interactions and repetitive or stereotyped patterns of behavior, but no particular problem with cognitive functioning.

Key terms:

autism: a disorder characterized by disturbed language development, a lack of interpersonal responsiveness, odd and repetitive behaviors, and resistance to changes in the environment

pervasive developmental disorders: disorders characterized by delayed and severely impaired social interaction or communication skills, or stereotyped behavior, interests, and activities

Causes and Symptoms

Asperger's syndrome has social and behavioral components. Socially, the person is significantly impaired in the ability to engage in meaningful interaction. Behaviorally, the person has restricted, repetitive patterns of behaviors, interests, and activities. Unlike autism, however, Asperger's syndrome does not involve severe delays in language or other cognitive skills, although subtle aspects of social communication, such as give-and-take conversation, may be impaired. Also, during the first three years, the child has no clinically significant delays in cognitive development. Rather, the child expresses normal curiosity and age-appropriate learning skills and adaptive behavior. This is why clinicians prefer not to refer to Asperger's syndrome as high-functioning autism; they are truly different disorders, despite the fact that they share some commonalities.

The impairment in social interaction is gross and sustained. The child may be unable to maintain normal eye-to-eye contact or may show unusual facial expressions, body posture, or gestures. The child may fail to develop age-appropriate peer relationships. A younger child may show little or no interest in establishing friendships. An older individual may have an interest in friendship but lack understanding of the conventions of social interaction. The individual may lack a spontaneous seeking to share enjoyment, interests, or achievements. The individual may lack social or emotional reciprocity, preferring solitary activities, involving others in activities only as tools or mechanical aids, or not participating actively in simple social play or games. The social impairment typically is manifested as an eccentric and one-sided approach to others, such as pursuing a conversational topic regardless of others' reactions, rather than as social and emotional indifference.

The behavioral impairment takes the form of stereotypical behavior. Persons with Asperger's syndrome may have encompassing preoccupations about a specific topic, such as a professional baseball team, about which they can amass a great deal of information and pursue with great intensity, often to the exclusion of other activities. In contrast to autism, however, language development is normal, with the exception that these individuals are preoccupied with talking about their own arcane interests. They can be verbose, and they fail to self-monitor. In addition, they often exhibit clumsiness and poor coordination.

Because language development is normal, parents or caregivers are not usually concerned about the child's development until the child begins to attend a preschool or is exposed to peers. At this point, the child's social difficulties typically become apparent.

The course of Asperger's syndrome is continuous and lifelong. The patient's verbal abilities may, to some extent, mask the severity of the social dysfunction and may prove misleading for parents and teachers, who are blinded by the child's vocabulary. Despite these problems, however, follow-up studies suggest that, as adults, many individuals with Asperger's syndrome are capable of gainful employment and personal self-sufficiency.

Some diagnosticians are relatively unfamiliar with Asperger's syndrome, and some experts believe that many individuals go undiagnosed. Asperger's syndrome is one of the pervasive developmental disorders and so is similar to autism, Rett's syndrome, and disintegrative disorder. Controversies exist, however, concerning the precise definitions of these autistic spectrum disorders and the boundaries between the milder manifestations of these disorders and nonautistic conditions. As such, the causes and estimates of these disorders are still a topic of debate.

In 2000, Fred R. Volkmar and Ami Klin estimated that the prevalence of Asperger's syndrome varied between 1 and 36 out of 10,000; in 1991, Volkmar and Donald J. Cohen found that more boys than girls are affected. Taking into account the entire spectrum of autistic disorders, a 1992 study by Peter Szatmari indicated that as many as one child in one hundred shows autistic traits. In 2001, a study by Jacquelyn Bertrand and colleagues indicated a prevalence of approximately 6.7 per 1,000 for autism spectrum disorders.

Information on Asperger's Syndrome

Causes: Unknown, possibly genetic
Symptoms: Gross and sustained social impairment; restricted and repetitive patterns of behaviors, interests, and activities
Duration: Lifelong
Treatments: Psychotherapy to enhance communication skills and reduce problem behaviors

Some of the differences demonstrated may be the result of sampling or diagnostic practice.

Little is known about the causes of Asperger's syndrome, although experts Susan E. Folstein and Susan L. Santangelo suspect a genetic contribution because it appears to run in some families. Recent research has not identified any one gene as being responsible for the disorder. Two genes, however, GABRB3 (GABA receptor B3) and Engrailed-2, have been shown to have a relationship with some of the behavioral traits Asperger's syndrome shares with autism. Other research has started to examine whether any abnormalities may have occurred during fetal development, thus affecting how the brain grows.

Treatment and Therapy

As with the other pervasive developmental disorders, no completely effective treatment exists for Asperger's syndrome. Most treatment efforts focus on enhancing communication skills and reducing problem behaviors. In the mid-1960's, Ivar Lovaas and colleagues developed treatment for autism that involved the basic behavioral procedures of shaping and discrimination training. This therapy is also used with persons with Asperger's syndrome. Therapists reward social behaviors, such as playing with peers, by giving food or praise.

Medication typically focuses on specific behaviors or symptoms. Little research support exists for the benefits from vitamins or dietary changes. To the extent that improper habits can generally be disruptive to any person, however, such an approach may be worthy of consideration in the management of pervasive developmental disorders, such as taking care to eat nutritious foods and to avoid foods that are linked to hyperactivity or otherwise are unhealthy.

For children with Asperger's syndrome, most therapy consists of school education combined with special psychological supports for communication and socialization problems. Parents also need support because of the great demands and stress involved in living with and caring for such children.

Occasionally, persons with Asperger's syndrome may be quite successful as adults, especially in professions in which their attention to routine, concentration on detail, and relative indifference to sentiment are an asset. A 1991 study by Christopher Gillberg of individuals with Asperger traits included a dentist, a financial lawyer, a military historian, and a university professor.

Perspective and Prospects

In the 1940's, while working as a pediatrician, Hans Asperger identified what is now known as Asperger's syndrome. In the mid-1960's, psychologists Lovaas and Charles Ferster developed a behavioral approach for treating autism and related disorders. Though refined since that time, the basic tenet, that people with autistic spectrum disorders can learn and be taught some of the skills that they lack, remains the treatment of choice.

—Lillian M. Range, Ph.D.;
updated by Nancy A. Piotrowski, Ph.D.

See also Autism; Bonding; Cognitive development; Developmental stages; Learning disabilities; Psychiatric disorders; Psychiatry; Psychiatry, child and adolescent.

For Further Information:

American Psychiatric Association. *Diagnostic and Statistical Manual of Mental Disorders: DSM-IV-TR*. Rev. 4th ed. Washington, D.C.: Author, 2000.

Ariel, Cindy N., and Robert A. Naseef, eds. *Voices from the Spectrum: Parents, Grandparents, Siblings, People with Autism, and Professionals Share Their Wisdom*. Philadelphia: Jessica Kingsley, 2006.

Bertrand, Jacquelyn, et al. "Prevalence of Autism in a United States Population: The Brick Township, New Jersey, Investigation." *Pediatrics* 108 (2001): 1155-1161.

Folstein, Susan E., and Susan L. Santangelo. "Does Asperger Syndrome Aggregate in Families?" In *Asperger Syndrome*, edited by Ami Klin, Fred R. Volkmar, and Sara S. Sparrow. New York: Guilford Press, 2000.

Gillberg, Christopher. "Clinical and Neurobiological Aspects of Asperger Syndrome in Six Family Studies." In *Autism and Asperger Syndromes*, edited by Uta Frith. Cambridge, England: Cambridge University Press, 1991.

Szatmari, Peter. "The Validity of Autistic Spectrum Disorders: A Literature Review." *Journal of Autism and Developmental Disorders* 22 (1992): 583-600.

Volkmar, Fred R., and Ami Klin. "Diagnostic Issues in Asperger Syndrome." In *Asperger Syndrome*, edited by Klin, Volkmar, and Sara S. Sparrow. New York: Guilford, 2000.

Aspergillosis

Disease/disorder

Anatomy or system affected: Blood, bones, brain, ears, eyes, heart, kidneys, liver, lungs, spleen

Specialties and related fields: Cardiology, family medicine, immunology, internal medicine, microbiology, nephrology, ophthalmology, otorhinolaryngology, pulmonary medicine, radiology

Definition: Infection with fungi from the genus *Aspergillus*, which initially produce pulmonary hypersensitivity reactions or colonize the lung and then either grow within a pulmonary cavity or disseminate through the blood to other organs.

Causes and Symptoms

Members of the fungal genus *Aspergillus* are widely distributed in soil and decaying plant material. Inhalation of fungal spores can cause allergic reactions in people with asthma, a condition called allergic bronchopulmonary aspergillosis. In someone with a preexisting lung cavity caused by tuberculosis or cystic fibrosis, the fungus can grow within this cavity and form a fungus ball (aspergilloma) that moves within the cavity but does not invade the cavity wall. However, if the immune system works poorly because of chronic steroid treatment, alcoholism, or underlying lung disease, then the fungus ball can invade the surrounding lung tissue, a condition called chronic necrotizing pulmonary aspergillosis. If the immune system is profoundly weakened because of a recent organ transplant, advanced acquired immunodeficiency syndrome (AIDS), or genetic diseases that cripple the immune system, then initial colonization of the lung with *Aspergillus* leads to dissemination of the organism through the bloodstream to other organs (invasive aspergillosis). This results in a rapidly progressing and often fatal systemic infection.

Allergic reactions to *Aspergillus* or fungus balls usually cause fever, coughing that sometimes produces blood or brownish mucus, wheezing, recurrent epi-

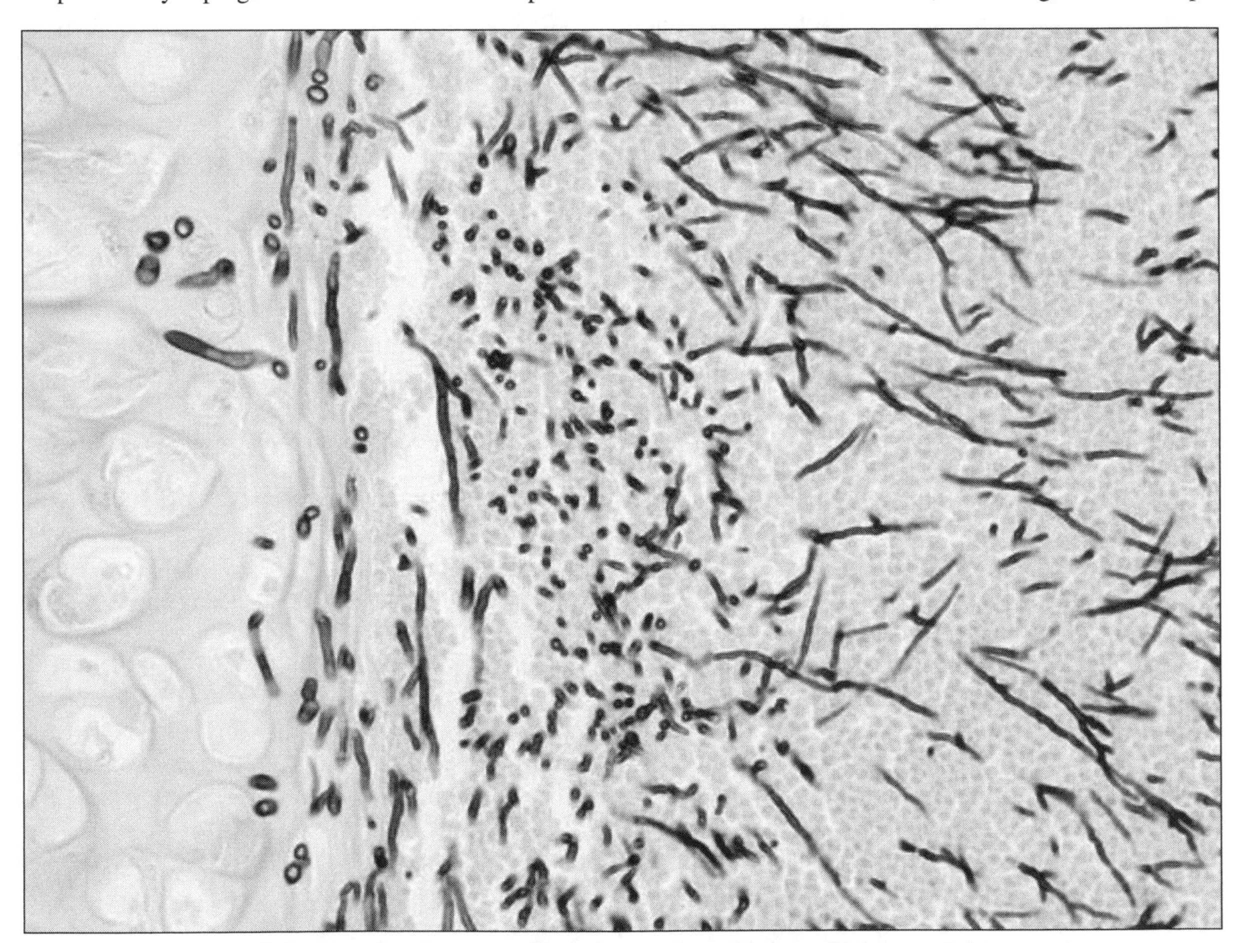

Pulmonary invasive aspergillosis in a patient with interstitial pneumonia.

Information on Aspergillosis

Causes: Infection with *Aspergillus* fungal spores
Symptoms: Fever, coughing, wheezing, lung obstruction, sinus infections; sometimes also chills, headaches, shortness of breath, chest pain, bone pain, blood in the urine, decreased urine output
Duration: Acute
Treatments: Oral corticosteroids, antifungal agents, surgical resection if needed

sodes of lung obstruction, and sometimes sinus infections. The symptoms of invasive aspergillosis may additionally include chills, headaches, shortness of breath, chest pain, coughs that produce blood-filled material, bone pain, blood in the urine, decreased urine output, and symptoms involving specific organs, such as meningitis (brain), blindness or visual impairment (eye), sinusitis, and endocarditis (heart).

Treatment and Therapy

For allergies to *Aspergillus*, oral corticosteroids are used, since inhaled steroids are typically ineffective. Addition of the antifungal drug itraconazole to steroids might be necessary for patients whose allergies fail to resolve. Fungus balls are usually not treated unless they cause symptoms. Surgical resection of the affected part of the lung can cure fungus balls permanently, but only in people who have enough lung capacity to survive such a procedure. Invasive aspergillosis requires immediate therapy, and voriconazole is the usual first treatment choice. Amphotericin B is also a viable option, but its toxicity makes voriconazole the better choice. Caspofungin or posaconazole are also effective in those patients who do not tolerate or respond to other drugs. Fungus balls that invade the lung require prolonged treatment with voriconazole, itraconazole, or amphotericin B formulations to cure the patient completely, but surgical resection of the affected portion of the lung might be necessary.

—Michael A. Buratovich, Ph.D.

See also Acquired immunodeficiency syndrome (AIDS); Alcoholism; Allergies; Asthma; Corticosteroids; Cystic fibrosis; Fungal infections; Immune system; Immunodeficiency disorders; Immunology; Lungs; Pulmonary diseases; Pulmonary medicine; Respiration; Steroids; Transplantation; Tuberculosis.

For Further Information:

Kauffman, Carol A., and Sara Hedderwick. "Opportunistic Fungal Infections: Filamentous Fungi and Cryptococcosis." *Geriatrics* 52 (October, 1997): 40-42.

Parker, James M., and Philip M. Parker, eds. *The Official Patient's Sourcebook on Aspergillosis: A Revised and Updated Directory for the Internet Age*. San Diego, Calif.: Icon Health, 2002.

Richardson, Malcolm D., and Elizabeth M. Johnson. *The Pocket Guide to Fungal Infection*. 2d ed. Malden, Mass: Blackwell, 2006.

Asphyxiation

Disease/disorder

Anatomy or system affected: Lungs, respiratory system

Specialties and related fields: Emergency medicine, occupational health

Definition: The state of unconsciousness or death resulting from oxygen deprivation.

The phenomenon whereby the body experiences a decrease in oxygen below normal levels is called hypoxia; extreme cases lead to anoxia, a complete lack of oxygen. The difference between anoxia and asphyxia is that in asphyxia an accumulation of excess carbon dioxide takes place, as the normal exchange of oxygen and carbon dioxide in the lungs is obstructed.

Respiration is regulated in the medulla, while chemoreceptors present in the aortic arch and the carotid sinus respond to levels of oxygen, carbon dioxide, and the pH in blood and the cerebrospinal fluid. The concentration of carbon dioxide pressure in the plasma is proportional to the oxygen pressure. Generally, oxygen deprivation may be the consequence of one or more of several conditions. In all cases, damage results that leads first to hypoxia and eventually to death.

Types of oxygen deprivation. In the first condition, respiration may be slowed or stopped by injury or foreign material blocking the air passage. The most common example of this case is asphyxia that results from the inhalation of water by exhausted swimmers or persons who cannot swim. Large quantities of water fill the lungs and cut off the oxygen supply. Other examples include the entrapment of food or liquid in the respiratory tract, strangulation, and residence in high altitude. In these cases, the carbon dioxide pressure is drastically increased. Artificial respiration may save the victim's life; it should be performed as soon as possible and after the

Information on Asphyxiation

Causes: Injury, airway obstruction, strangulation, high altitude, poor ventilation, anemia, trauma, hemorrhage, circulatory disease
Symptoms: Increased heart and pulse rate, vision and hearing impairment
Duration: A few minutes
Treatments: Resuscitation with oxygen

removal of the inhaled foreign substance via vomiting. Strangulation provides the more serious problem of capillary rupturing and internal bleeding.

A second condition, hypoxic anoxia, is caused by an inadequate concentration of oxygen in the atmosphere, which occurs in poorly ventilated enclosed spaces such as in mine tunnels, sewers, or industrial areas. Odorless gases such as methane (which is produced in decomposing sewage) or nitrogen may be dangerous because they generally go undetected. A former way of detecting such gases involved taking along a bird in a cage and monitoring its well-being during the exploration of unknown caves or ancient tombs.

In anemic anoxia, respiration may not be effective because of the reduced capacity of the blood to become oxygenated; as a result, less oxygen is transferred to the tissues. Carbon monoxide behaves differently from methane or nitrogen, since it binds much more strongly to hemoglobin than oxygen does. Thus the hemoglobin, which is the oxygen-carrying component of blood, does not transfer oxygen to the tissues, which are starved of it. The passage of oxygen from the lung alveoli to the adjacent blood capillaries may also be affected, such as with chronic lung disease, infections, or developmental effects.

A fourth category is stagnant anoxia, whereby a reduced flow of blood through the blood tissues takes place. This may be a generalized condition, attributable to heart disease, or localized, which may take place in a pilot during aerial maneuvers. A blackout of an aviator is a result of the heart's inability to pump enough blood to these regions against the high centrifugal force. In some cases, the carbon dioxide pressure cannot be removed in the usual manner by the lung. Any lung disease will decrease the effective removal of carbon dioxide and therefore result in elevated levels of it in the blood. Thus in emphysema, a disease in which the alveoli increase in size and which leads to a reduction of the surface area available for gas exchange, carbon dioxide will be retained in the blood. In bronchopneumonia, the alveoli contain secretions, white cells, bacteria, and fibrin, which prevent an efficient gas exchange.

In histotoxic anoxia, the failure of cellular respiration is observed. The body's cells are unable to utilize oxygen as a result of poisoning, as from cyanide. The supply of oxygen is normal, but the cells are unable to metabolize the oxygen that is delivered to them.

Symptoms. All cases of anoxia may lead to oxygen deprivation in the brain, which may be fatal if it lasts more than a few minutes. Nerve cell degeneration may start and continue, despite the fact that the original cause of anoxia is removed and normal breathing is resumed. Many health conditions may interfere with the blood transport of oxygen, which is accomplished via the red blood cells. Such diseases include cases of anemia, trauma, hemorrhage, and circulatory disease.

The body responds to oxygen deprivation with an increase in the rate or depth of breathing. The normal, sea-level oxygen pressure of the air is approximately 160 millimeters (6.2 inches) of mercury. When the oxygen pressure is reduced to 110 millimeters (4.2 inches) of mercury at an altitude of about 3,000 meters (10,000 feet), the pulse rate increases and the volume of blood pumped from the heart also increases. Although prolonged exposure to low oxygen pressure may bring the pulse rate back to normal, the output of the heart remains elevated. Despite the lack of oxygen, both the heart and the brain function because of the dilation of their blood cells and the increased oxygen extraction from the blood. Anoxia leads to vision problems first, while hearing is generally the last sense to go. It is not unusual for a person who is suffering from anoxia to be incapable of moving but able to hear.

—*Soraya Ghayourmanesh, Ph.D.*

See also Altitude sickness; Amyotrophic lateral sclerosis; Apnea; Asthma; Choking; Cyanosis; Drowning; Emphysema; Heimlich maneuver; Hyperbaric oxygen therapy; Hyperventilation; Lungs; Pulmonary medicine; Pulmonary medicine, pediatric; Respiration; Resuscitation; Unconsciousness.

For Further Information:

Heartsaver Manual: A Student Handbook for Cardiopulmonary Resuscitation and First Aid for Choking. Dallas: American Heart Association, 1987.

Kittredge, Mary. *The Respiratory System*. Edited by Dale C. Garell. Philadelphia: Chelsea House, 1989.

Krementz, Jill. *How It Feels to Fight for Your Life*. Boston: Little, Brown, 1989.

Lutz, Peter L., and Goran E. Nilsson. *The Brain Without Oxygen: Causes of Failure—Physiological and Molecular Mechanisms for Survival*. 3d ed. Boston: Kluwer Academic, 2003.

West, John B. *Pulmonary Pathophysiology: The Essentials*. 6th ed. Baltimore: Lippincott Williams & Wilkins, 2003.

Assisted reproductive technologies

Procedure

Anatomy or system affected: Endocrine system, genitals, glands, reproductive system, uterus

Specialties and related fields: Biotechnology, embryology, endocrinology, ethics, genetics, gynecology, obstetrics, perinatology

Definition: A range of medical procedures that are used to assist couples in conception and prenatal care, with special focus on infertility and its cure. Assisted reproductive technologies currently include techniques such as in vitro fertilization, artificial insemination, and surgical procedures to repair or diagnose reproductive problems and in the future may include cloning or gene therapy.

Key terms:

endometrium: the lining of the uterus, which thickens around the time of ovulation in preparation for an embryo to implant, should conception occur

endometriosis: excessive growth of the endometrium, which can result in large clumps of tissue called fibroids that can interfere with ovulation and menses and in some cases can fill the uterus

ovulation: release of an egg from an ovary into a Fallopian tube

tubal ligation: a surgical procedure to prevent the possibility of pregnancy permanently by blocking the Fallopian tubes, thus preventing eggs from passing into the uterus

vasectomy: a surgical procedure for preventing sperm from being released during ejaculation; involves the removal of a portion of the vas deferens in the penis

Indications and Procedures

Although most couples experience little or no difficulty conceiving and carrying a child to term, about 15 percent experience infertility. Infertility is defined as an inability to conceive after a year of having regular, unprotected intercourse. Not all couples can be helped, but an increasing number of reproductive technologies are available, from in vitro fertilization (IVF) and artificial insemination to drug therapies and surgical repair.

Typically, the first step is to determine whether the man's sperm is fertile by performing a simple sperm count. If sperm counts are low or the sperm are abnormal, then the primary treatment is artificial insemination, also called intrauterine insemination (IUI). Cryopreserved sperm are obtained from a sperm bank, which collects ejaculate from healthy, fertile men. The donors of the sperm remain anonymous, and the samples are usually a mixture of sperm from two or more men. This method maintains even greater anonymity and increases the amount of sperm available, thus increasing the chances of conception.

To assure the highest probability of success, IUI should be performed when the woman is ovulating and is most fertile. Most women experience a slight rise in their basal body temperature when they ovulate, and monitoring daily body temperature upon waking can be used in some cases. A more reliable method is detection of a surge in luteinizing hormone (LH) in the urine. LH usually stimulates ovulation within thirty-six to forty hours after the surge. A home urine LH analysis kit can be used, and when the LH surge is detected, insemination can be scheduled for the following day. Self-observation of cervical mucous changes can also be used to detect ovulation. Insemination is a simple office procedure in which the physician uses a special catheter to transfer the semen sample into the uterus.

If adequate numbers of sperm are present, and they appear normal and active, then the diagnostic focus shifts to the woman. Because the female reproductive system is primarily internal, diagnosis is often more complicated and expensive and in some cases can pose risks to the woman. The primary cause of infertility in women is inability to ovulate. Factors that may prevent ovulation can include lifestyle factors (drug abuse, obesity, weight loss, prolonged acute stress), hormone imbalance, ovarian tumors or cysts, previous infection, an unusually short menstrual cycle, previous surgery, or birth defects. Sorting out the specific cause or causes can be a daunting task, and the causes remain unknown in some cases.

The initial diagnosis involves extensive consultation on health status and lifestyle, a complete physical examination, urine and blood tests to check for infection or hormone imbalance, and often tests on samples of cervical mucous and a portion of the endometrium (lining of the uterus). The primary goal of these initial tests is to determine whether ovulation is occurring. If ovulation is occurring, the problem likely involves an abnormal uterine condition or an endocrine imbalance that is interfering with implantation. Other problems might include some fault with the eggs that are released or with the ability of sperm to penetrate or fuse with the nucleus of the egg.

If the ova (eggs) are abnormal, then donor ova can be collected from another woman, followed by IVF with the male partner's sperm. Often the fault with abnormal ova is with the cytoplasm, so another possible treatment is to remove the nucleus from an abnormal ovum and place it into a donor ovum from which the nucleus has been removed. The resulting ovum would then have a nucleus derived from the mother and a cytoplasm derived from the donor. Currently, although this approach is technically feasible, it has ignited ethical concerns similar to those raised about cloning.

If ovulation is not occurring, which is true in the majority of cases, then additional tests are required. Continued monitoring of hormone levels may identify an imbalance or timing problem that can be corrected with hormone treatments. Sometimes hormone treatments alone are able to normalize ovulation and restore fertility. In other cases, the problem involves a blockage or abnormal shape of the Fallopian tubes or uterus. Diagnostic procedures at this stage typically involve some form of imaging technology so that the condition of the reproductive organs can be assessed.

Hysteroscopy is a procedure for viewing the interior of the uterus; it can be done either in a doctor's office or in an outpatient setting at a hospital. In preparation for the procedure, the woman is usually given a mild analgesic such as acetaminophen or ibuprofen, as some minor cramping is common. The doctor then washes the vagina and cervix. A local anesthetic is administered to the cervix. The cervix is carefully dilated, and the hysteroscope is inserted through the cervix into the uterus. The hysteroscope contains a small light for illuminating the interior of the uterus and a small camera for viewing. Some conditions that can be detected using hysteroscopy include a septum that divides the uterus, fibroid growths or polyps, and cancerous or precancerous lesions. Often, the location where the Fallopian tubes enter the uterus can also be viewed. Many of these conditions can be asymptomatic. Surgical removal of a septum or other growths may restore fertility. If a woman is able to produce an egg to fertilize but is unable to carry the child herself, another option is surrogacy, which then involves legal procedures to establish parentage.

Hysterosalpingography can be used to view both the uterus and the Fallopian tubes. This X-ray procedure uses a contrast dye to visualize internal structures. Placing the dye into the uterus involves insertion of a special flexible catheter through the cervix. A balloon at the end of the catheter is inflated to hold the catheter in place as the contrast dye is pumped into the uterus. X rays are taken every few seconds as the dye travels through the uterus. Eventually, the dye travels the length of the Fallopian tubes. The images obtained can be used to identify many of the anomalies also detectable using hysteroscopy and can also identify problems with the Fallopian tubes. If the Fallopian tubes are blocked, then the dye will not travel their length, which will be visible in the X-ray photographs.

In some cases, none of these minimally invasive diagnostic procedures identifies a problem. In such cases, diagnostic laparoscopy can be used. Using a laparoscope, a flexible tube with a light and special lens at the end, a doctor can view internal organs directly. After administering regional or general anesthesia, an incision is made near the region of the peritoneal cavity to be imaged. Carbon dioxide is used to fill the peritoneal cavity to improve viewing conditions. The laparoscope is then inserted through the incision. If an abnormality is detected, then the doctor may insert another instrument to collect tissue for a biopsy. After laparoscopic examination is completed, the incision is closed. Laparoscopy is usually done in a hospital as an outpatient procedure, and the patient can go home the same day. Even after diagnostic laparoscopy, the cause of infertility may remain unknown.

Uses and Complications

Assisted reproductive technologies are best suited to couples in which one or the other is infertile but otherwise in good health. Age may also be an important factor for the woman, as fertility, implantation, and normal development of the fetus are all affected as a woman ages, especially beyond thirty-five. Although these technologies can be successful in older women, the risks involved need to be assessed carefully with a doctor. They can also be more costly in older women, because more attempts using IUI and IVF are often required.

Hysteroscopy and hysterosalpingography are the most commonly used procedures for diagnosing infertility, once the more obvious causes have been ruled out. Although both can cause mild to moderate discomfort, they have very few associated risks and can be performed in most obstetrics/gynecology (OB/GYN) offices. If a clear diagnosis is obtained, then a number of problems may require surgery. Blockage, abnormalities of the Fallopian tubes or other reproductive organs, ectopic pregnancies, and abnormal growths (cysts or tumors) can be treated or repaired surgically. In most cases, laparoscopic surgery is used, as it is less invasive than traditional abdominal surgery. Laparoscopic surgery is performed in the same way as diagnostic laparoscopy and may be done at the same time if a problem is discovered in the process.

Diagnostic laparoscopy is typically the method of last resort, as some potentially life-threatening risks are involved, such as damage to abdominal organs, inflammation or infection of the peritoneum or other organs, hemorrhaging, and formation of embolisms that may block an important artery. The procedure can also be more painful in cases where anesthesia is only partially effective. Current research suggests that the benefits may outweigh the risks, but some women choose not to have diagnostic laparoscopy, and not all doctors consider the risks appropriate.

When surgical intervention is unable to restore fertility, the most common option is in vitro fertilization (IVF). As long as the woman's uterus is anatomically and physiologically normal, IVF can be an effective, although expensive, option. It is the method of choice for women who have blocked Fallopian tubes or an abnormal pelvic anatomy or who have had tubal ligation and are considering reversal. It also tends to increase the chances of pregnancy in older women and women with endometriosis. Low sperm count or vasectomy reversal in the male partner may also require IVF, as the sperm may require concentration for effective fertilization. IVF can also be an effective solution for women who cannot ovulate or who have very few or faulty eggs, in which case donated eggs can be used. Gamete intrafallopian transfer (GIFT) collects multiple eggs and places them into a catheter along with sperm. Ovum and sperm are then together injected surgically into the Fallopian tubes, where conception may take place. In zygote intrafallopian transfer (ZIFT), ovum are mixed with sperm in the laboratory, and the resulting zygotes are surgically placed into the Fallopian tubes.

IVF is not without its risks and potential failings. Carefully designed hormone injection protocols are used to stimulate multiple follicle formation and to prevent premature ovulation. Progress is typically monitored using ultrasound. If the number of follicles is too small, then the cycle may be cancelled, as the cost of retrieval, given the number of eggs that could be available, is too high. Overstimulation can also occur, which can lead to abnormal levels of estrogen that may pose a health threat. If an appropriate number of follicles are produced, then eggs are retrieved using a needle inserted through the top of the vagina. The placement of the needle is guided using ultrasound, and once the ovaries are reached, the eggs are aspirated into it.

A final concern with IVF is the increased incidence of multiple pregnancies. To increase the chance of a pregnancy, multiple fertilized eggs are placed in the uterus. When only a single embryo is transferred, live births occur less than 10 percent of the time. In recent years, as IVF procedures have steadily improved, the incidence of multiple pregnancies has increased. A study published in 2003 showed that when two embryos were transferred and a live birth resulted, approximately 16 percent of the time twins resulted. This percentage rose to almost 30 percent when three embryos were transferred. When more than three embryos were transferred, triplets and higher numbers occurred with increasing frequency as well. Due to the number of premature births resulting from in vitro fertilization, most reproductive endocrinologists limit the number of embryos transferred in order to limit the number of multiple births.

IVF is only a solution when sperm quantity is adequate or donor sperm is acceptable to the couple. In some cases the sperm count for the male may be so low that even concentrating the sperm would be insufficient to achieve fertilization. Sperm can still be obtained from the male in some cases. If no sperm are found in the ejaculate, there may be an obstruction, and sperm may still be obtained by using a needle inserted near the obstruction. In some cases, the male's sperm may lack the ability to penetrate the egg. If a couple insists that they do not want to use donor sperm, then the last option available is typically intracytoplasmic sperm injection (ICSI), in which a single sperm is injected directly into the cytoplasm of an egg. This technique has been so successful that even males with only a few sperm have been able to father a child. If sperm count is low or motility is poor, sperm from the male may be mixed with donor sperm, so that if pregnancy occurs, the identity of the father can remain uncertain if so desired by the parents.

Perspective and Prospects

Assisted reproductive technologies arose during the latter half of the twentieth century. Prior to this period, infertility was poorly understood and treatments were essentially nonexistent. The first attempt at treating infertility involved artificial insemination in 1785 by the Scottish surgeon John Hunter. A child was born that same year, apparently as a result of his attempts. The next documented attempt at IUI was by Robert Dickinson in 1890. His attempts were highly secretive because the Anglican Church condemned such procedures. The first comprehensive guidelines for determining male infertility based on sperm count and quality were published in 1934.

In 1945, a report of early IUI experiments was published in the *British Medical Journal*. As a result, in 1948 the archbishop of Canterbury proposed making IUI a criminal offense. Although the British government did not follow his advice, it did discourage the use of IUI. During the 1950's, the public demand for solutions to infertility far exceeded medical solutions. By 1955, there had been four successful pregnancies using frozen donor sperm. In spite of these successes, IUI was not to become an acceptable and widely used procedure until the 1970's.

The first fertility drug was developed in 1949, but it took until 1962 for this discovery to be applied successfully, resulting in ovulation and a successful birth. Throughout the 1960's and beyond, the use of fertility hormones was further refined, allowing more infertile women to ovulate and bear children. Use of fertility hormones has become a key part of IVF as well, allowing the harvesting of viable eggs.

The first step toward IVF occurred in 1944, when the first in vitro fertilization took place. It took another thirty-one years for the first IVF pregnancy, and unfortunately it was an ectopic pregnancy. Three years later, in 1978, Louise Brown became the first "test tube" baby born as a result of IVF. In 1981, Elizabeth Jordan Carr became the first IVF baby in the United States. Use of IVF is now routine, and success rates continue to rise.

The 1980's and 1990's saw even greater improvements. Surgical procedures using laparoscopy continued to improve, and diagnostic procedures became ever more sensitive. In the 1980's, donor eggs became widely available. One of the difficulties in using donor eggs had always been preserving them until use, because they seemed much more sensitive than sperm. The first baby derived from a frozen egg occurred in 1983, and methods of preservation are now even better. In 1986, the first baby derived from a frozen donor egg was born in Australia.

In 1992, researchers in Belgium reported the first pregnancies resulting from ICSI, and a year later the first successful birth from ICSI was reported in the United States. IVF was so routine by this time that in 1994 a sixty-two-year-old woman gave birth, and a year later a sixty-three-year-old woman who lied to her doctor about her age also gave birth.

To work around the use of defective eggs, in 1997 the first cytoplasmic transfer birth occurred and ignited controversy over the continued use of the technique. Some ethicists saw it as being too much like human cloning and germline genetic manipulation and advocated banning the technique. In the United States, the Food and Drug Administration (FDA) quickly stepped in and claimed jurisdiction over use of the technique. It remains an experimental technique, and its implications are still being addressed.

The cloning of the first mammal from adult cells, Dolly the sheep, brought the possibility of reproductive cloning in humans to the forefront. In response to the many concerns about the potential for cloning humans, President Bill Clinton issued a moratorium on funding to those performing research on human cloning. Human cloning remains a very controversial issue and has been banned by most countries.

The future of assisted reproductive technologies will probably include ever more improved techniques and may also include germline gene modification. Embryos can currently be screened for a number of genetic defects, so that parents can be given the opportunity to use only healthy embryos. The potential for screening for a variety of genetic defects or traits means that parents in the future could choose embryos that meet certain criteria such as sex, intelligence, or personality. It may even be possible to engineer improvements in embryos. The ethics of using these kinds of techniques are still being debated and are considered questionable by many. Regardless of the outcome of these discussions, the future certainly will hold the prospect for almost all couples to have a baby derived from their own genetic material, a dream that was once unattainable for many infertile couples.

—Bryan Ness, Ph.D.;
updated by Robin Kamienny Montvilo, Ph.D.

See also Cloning; Conception; Embryology; Ethics; Gamete intrafallopian transfer (GIFT); Genetic engineering; Gynecology; In vitro fertilization; Infertility, female; Infertility, male; Multiple births; Obstetrics; Pregnancy and gestation; Reproductive system.

FOR FURTHER INFORMATION:

American Society for Reproductive Medicine. *Guidelines on Number of Embryos Transferred: A Practice Committee Report—A Committee Opinion.* Birmingham, Ala.: Author, 1999. Recommendations for in vitro fertilization to prevent problems of prematurity due to multiple births.

Blackley, Michelle. "'EGGS FOR SALE': The Latest Controversy in Reproductive Technology." *USA Today* 132, no. 2698 (July, 2003): 56-58. Discusses one of the ethical dilemmas facing application of the new technologies.

De Jonge, Christopher J., and Christopher L. R. Barratt, eds. *Assisted Reproductive Technology: Current Accomplishments and New Horizons.* Cambridge, England: Cambridge University Press, 2002. An in-depth overview of the current technologies, written by professionals from medical and biological disciplines.

Henig, Robin Marantz. "Pandora's Baby." *Scientific American* 288, no. 6 (June, 2003): 62-67. A comparison between the controversy surrounding IVF when it was first introduced and the more recent controversy over human cloning.

Khamsi, F., et al. "Recent Advances in Assisted Reproductive Technologies." *Endocrine* 9, no. 1 (August, 1998): 15-25. An overview of the many new technologies that have arisen and a call for more careful assessment of the causes of infertility and the application of the procedures.

Powledge, Tabitha M. "Looking at ART." *Scientific American* 286, no. 4 (April, 2002): 20-21. Discusses the current outlook for assisted reproductive technologies, the government's involvement in regulating them, and criticisms of the techniques.

Schultz, Richard M., and Carmen J. Williams. "The Science of ART." *Science* 296, no. 5576 (June, 2002): 2188-2190. Overviews the scientific underpinnings of assisted reproductive technologies and expresses concern that their use may be outpacing science.

Shanley, Mary Lyndon. *Making Babies, Making Families.* Boston: Beacon Press, 2001. A wide-ranging overview of the many issues involved in using the latest technologies, including the ethical and legal aspects.

Tan, Seang Lin, and Togas Tulandi, eds. *Reproductive Endocrinology and Infertility: Current Trends and Developments.* Basel, Switzerland: Marcel Dekker, 2003. A comprehensive text covering recent technology used in the treatment of infertility.

Wilcox, Melynda Dovel, and Josephine Rossi. "What Price a Miracle?" *Kiplinger's Personal Finance* 56, no. 9 (September, 2002): 116-119. Discusses the economic issues involved in IVF, including whether health insurance will cover it.

Yoshida, T. M. "Infertility Update: Use of Assisted Reproductive Technology." *Journal of the American Pharmaceutical Association* 39, no. 1 (January/February, 1999): 65-72. A review of the recent clinical literature on assisted reproductive technologies, with an emphasis on how complete the information is.

ASTHMA

DISEASE/DISORDER

ANATOMY OR SYSTEM AFFECTED: Chest, immune system, lungs, respiratory system

SPECIALTIES AND RELATED FIELDS: Environmental health, immunology, pulmonary medicine

DEFINITION: A chronic inflammatory obstructive pulmonary disease that obstructs the airways to the lungs and makes it difficult or, in severe attacks, nearly impossible to breathe.

KEY TERMS:

allergen: any substance that causes an overreaction of the immune system; also called an antigen

allergic reaction: the presence of adverse symptoms that are part of the body's overreaction to an antigen

allergy: an overreaction of the immune system to a substance that does not affect the general population; the tendency to be allergic is inherited

beta-agonists: chemicals that attach to the beta-receptors on cells; often used in inhalers, they cause the bronchioles to dilate, or open

bronchioles: small air tubes leading to the air sacs of the lungs; the functional units of the airway that are involved in asthma

mast cells: cells in connective tissue capable of releasing chemicals that cause allergic reactions

trigger: the substance or event that sets off an asthma attack; triggers may be allergens or some other type of stimulus

CAUSES AND SYMPTOMS

Asthma is a Greek word meaning "gasping" or "panting." It is a chronic obstructive pulmonary (lung) disease that involves repeated attacks in which the airways in the lungs are suddenly blocked. The disease is not completely understood, but asthma attacks cause the person to experience tightening of the chest, sudden breathlessness, wheezing, and coughing. Death by asphyxiation is rare but possible. Fortunately, the effects can be reversed with proper medication. The severity of symptoms and attacks varies greatly among individuals, and sufferers can be located on a continuum running from mild to severe. Mild asthmatics have fewer than six minimal attacks per year, with no symptoms between attacks, and they require no hospitalizations and little or no medication between attacks. Severe asthmatics have more than six serious attacks each year, have symptoms between attacks, lose more than ten school days or workdays, and require two or more hospitalizations per year. Attacks are typically spaced with symptom-free intervals but may also occur continuously. Rather than focusing only on the specific attacks, one should view and treat asthma as a chronic disease, a nagging, continuing condition that persists over a long period of time.

Information on Asthma

Causes: Environmental factors, allergens, viral infections, stress, exercise
Symptoms: Tightening of the chest, sudden breathlessness, wheezing, coughing
Duration: Chronic, with acute episodes
Treatments: Medications (bronchodilators, anti-inflammatory drugs, trigger-sensitivity reducers); lifestyle modification to avoid triggers

A review of the path of air into the body during normal breathing helps in understanding asthma. During inhalation, air travels into the nose and mouth and then into the trachea (windpipe); it then divides into the two tubes called bronchi and enters the lungs. Inside each lung, the tubes become smaller and continue to divide. The air finally moves into the smallest tubes, called bronchioles, and then flows into the millions of small, thin-walled sacs called alveoli. Vital gas exchange occurs in the alveoli.

This gas exchange involves two gases in particular, oxygen and carbon dioxide. Oxygen must cross the membrane of the alveoli into the blood and then travel to all the cells of the body. Within the cells, it is used in chemical reactions that produce energy. These same reactions produce carbon dioxide as a by-product that is returned by the blood to the alveoli. This gas is removed from the body through the same pathway that brought oxygen into the lungs.

The parts of this airway that are involved in asthma are the bronchioles. These tubes are wrapped with smooth, involuntary muscles that adjust the amount of air that enters. The lining of the bronchioles also contains many cells that secrete a substance called mucus. Mucus is a thick, clear, slimy fluid produced in many parts of the body. Normal production of mucus in the lungs catches foreign material and lubricates the pathway to allow smooth airflow. People suffering from asthma have very sensitive bronchioles.

Three pathological processes in the bronchioles contribute to an asthma attack. One is an abnormal sensitivity and constriction of the involuntary muscles surrounding the airways, which narrows the diameter of the airway. Another is an inflammation and swelling of the tissues that make up the bronchioles themselves. The third is an increased production of mucus, which then blocks the airways. These three mechanisms may work in combination and are largely caused by the activation of mast cells in the airways. The result can be extreme difficulty in taking air into the lungs until the attack subsides. The characteristic "wheeze" of asthma is caused by efforts to exhale, which is more difficult than inhaling. In the most serious attacks, the airways may close down to the point of suffocating the patient if medical help is not given.

Attacks can vary in severity at different times because of variations in tension within the bronchiole muscles. Although there is still debate about the general function of these muscles, they probably help to distribute the air entering the alveoli evenly. Control of the tension in these smooth muscles is involuntary and follows a circadian (twenty-four-hour) rhythm influenced by neurohormonal control. Accordingly, for most people this cycle causes maximum constriction to occur at about 6:00 A.M. and maximum relaxation to occur at about 6:00 P.M. Hence, asthma attacks tend to be more severe in the late night and early morning.

Following a given asthma attack, patients are sometimes susceptible to additional, more severe attacks. This period of high risk, called a late-phase response, occurs five or six hours after the initial symptoms pass and may last as long as several days. Some researchers believe that the increase in deaths from asthma in the United States may be tied to this danger, which often goes unrecognized.

The initial cause and mechanism of an asthma attack can vary from person to person. Accordingly, asthma is usually divided into two types. One type is extrinsic, that is, caused by external triggers that bring about an allergic response. Allergic reactions involve the immune system. Normal functioning of the immune system guards the body against harmful substances. With an allergy, the body incorrectly identifies a harmless substance as harmful and reacts against it. This substance is then called an allergen. If the symptoms of this reaction occur in the lungs, the person has extrinsic or allergic asthma.

Researchers have discovered that many people with asthma have elevated levels of immunoglobulin E (IgE), a substance that indicates an allergic reaction within the body. Allergic triggers for asthma include dust, pollens, animal dander, cockroaches, and other substances. Infants may have an IgE response to respiratory syncytial virus. Improved asthma treatments may lie in substances that interfere with interleukin-4 (IL-4), which promotes IgE production in the body.

When allergens enter the body, the white blood cells make specific IgE antibodies that can bond with the invaders. Next, the IgE antibodies attach to the surfaces of mast cells; these cells are found all over the body and are numerous in the lungs. The allergens attach to the IgE antibodies located on the mast cells, and the mast cells are stimulated to produce and release chemicals called mediators, such as histamine, prostaglandin D_2, and leukotrienes. These mediators cause sneezing, tighten the muscles in the bronchioles, swell the surrounding tissues, and increase mucus production.

The second type of asthma is intrinsic and does not involve allergies. People who suffer from intrinsic asthma have hyperactive or twitchy airways that overreact to irritating factors. The mechanism for this form is not always understood, but no IgE antibodies for the irritant are placed on the mast cells. Examples of such nonallergic stimuli are cigarette smoke, house dust, artificial coloring, aspirin, ozone, or cold air. Odors from insecticides, cleaning fluids, cooking foods, and perfume can also trigger attacks. Also included in this category are attacks that are caused by viral infections (including colds and flu), stress, and exercise. Asthma can be triggered by many different substances and events in different people. While the symptoms are the same whether the asthma is intrinsic or extrinsic, asthmatics need to identify what substances or events trigger their attacks in order to gain control of the disease.

Why people develop asthma is not well understood. Asthma can begin at any age, but it is more likely to arise in childhood. While it is known that heredity predisposes an individual to asthma, the pattern of inheritance is not a simple one. Most geneticists now regard allergies as polygenic, which means that more than one pair of genes is involved. Height, skin color, and intelligence are other examples of polygenic traits. Exposure to particular external conditions may also be important. The children who develop asthma are more likely to be boys, while girls are more likely to show signs of the disease at puberty (about age twelve). Childhood asthma is also most likely to disappear or to be "outgrown" at puberty; about half of the cases of childhood asthma eventually disappear.

Early exposures to some triggers may be a key in the development of asthma. Increasingly, studies indicate that air pollution is an important risk factor for developing asthma, especially in children. Smoking by mothers can cause children who have a genetic disposition to develop asthma, as early exposure to secondhand smoke can cause an allergy to develop. Early studies in this area were confusing until the data were sorted by level of education. Lung specialist Fernando Martinez of the University of Arizona believes that less-educated women who smoke are more likely to cause this effect because their homes tend to be smaller and therefore

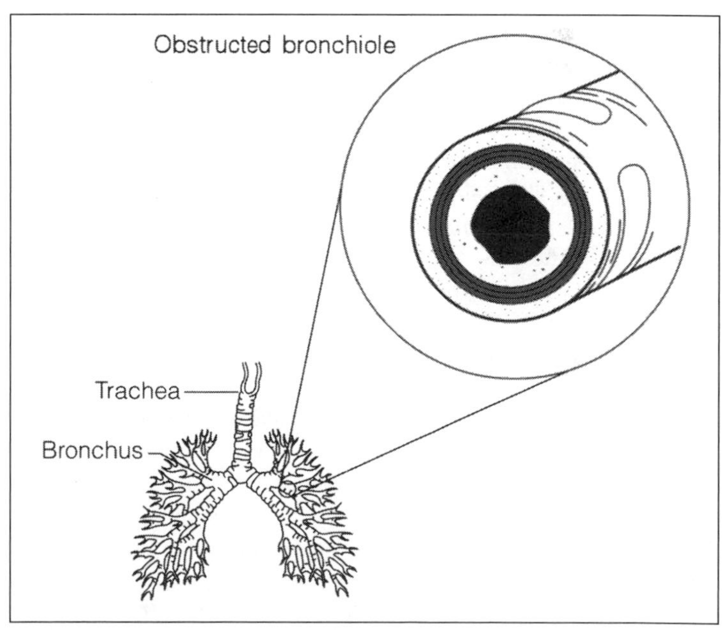

During an asthma attack, obstructed bronchioles limit or halt airflow, resulting in severely restricted breathing.

expose the children to more concentrated levels of smoke. Another study, this one in Great Britain, indicated that more frequent and thorough housecleaning might keep children from developing asthma. Early exposure by genetically susceptible children to dust and the mites that thrive in dust may also cause some to develop asthma.

Asthma is a major health problem in the United States. As many as 20 million Americans may have the disease, and the number has been mysteriously increasing since 1970. The disease affects people of all races, but African Americans are more likely than Caucasians to be hospitalized for and die from asthma attacks.

While attacks can cause complications, there is no permanent damage to the lungs themselves, as there is in emphysema. Complications include possible lung collapse, infections, chronic dilation, rib fracture, a permanently enlarged chest cavity, and respiratory failure. However, millions of days of work and school are lost as victims recuperate; asthma is the leading cause of missed school days. Even though attacks can be controlled by medication, occasionally fatalities do occur. The total number of deaths from asthma in the United States was 4,487 in 2000.

TREATMENT AND THERAPY

The key to gaining control of asthma is discovering the particular factors that act as triggers for an attack in a given individual. These factors vary and at times can be surprising; for example, one person found that a mint flavoring in a particular toothpaste was a trigger for his asthma. A 2007 study from the American College of Chest Physicians indicates that an obscure and toxic ecological phenomenon known as the Florida Red Tide, occurring along shorelines and caused by blooms of the aquatic organism *Karenia brevis*, can trigger asthma in coastal residents in the American Southeast and around the Gulf of Mexico. Nevertheless, most common triggers fall in the following groups: allergies; irritants, including dust, fumes, odors, and vapors; air pollution, temperature, and dryness; colds and flu; and stress. Even types of food may be important. Diets low in vitamin C, fish, or a zinc-to-copper ratio, as well as diets with a high sodium-to-potassium ratio, seem to increase the risk of asthma attacks and bronchitis. There have also been correlations between low niacin levels in the diet and tight airways and wheezing.

Some doctors have improved their diagnosis of asthma with a tool called the peak flow meter. The meter can also be used by patients at home to predict im-

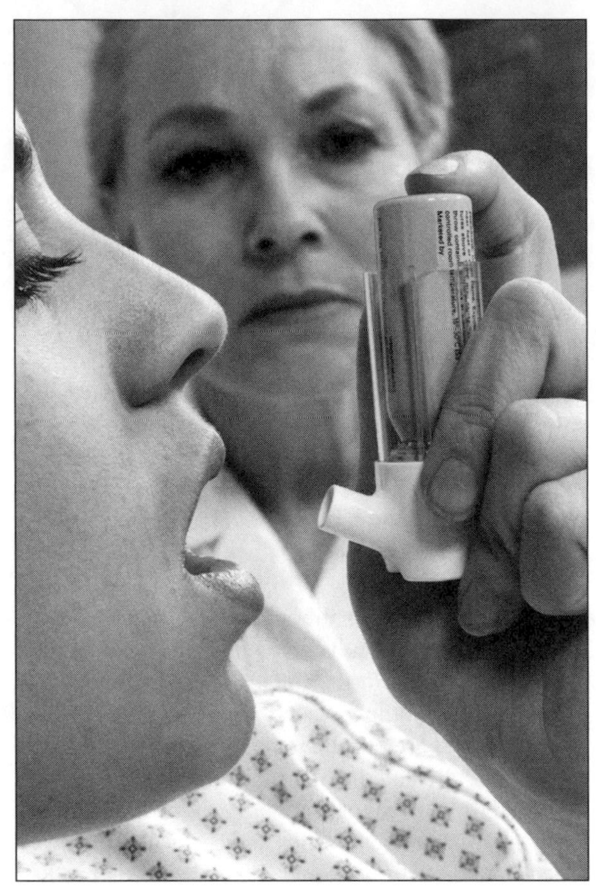

Many asthma medications are delivered using an inhaler. (PhotoDisc)

pending attacks. This inexpensive device measures how fast air can be moved out of the lungs. Therefore, it can be discovered that airways are beginning to tighten before other symptoms occur. The early warning allows time to adjust medications to head off attacks. This tool can help asthmatics take charge of their disease.

Various medications are available to keep the airways open and to lower their sensitivity. In an emergency, drugs may be injected, but medications are usually either inhaled or taken orally as pills. Because inhaling transports the medication directly to the lungs, lower doses can be used. Many asthmatics carry inhalers, which allow them to breathe in the medication during an attack. Because this action requires a person to coordinate inhaling with the release of the spray, young children are sometimes better off with a device that requires them to wear a mask. The choice and dosage of medicine vary with the patient, and physicians need to determine what is safest and most effective for each individual. Self-treatment with nonprescription drugs should be avoided.

Some of the most commonly prescribed drugs are bronchodilators, inflammation reducers, and trigger-sensitivity reducers. The bronchodilators include albuterol, metaproterenol, and terbutaline. They are beta-agonists that mimic the way in which the body's nervous system relaxes or dilates the airways. (Any drug that functions as a beta-blocker should be avoided by asthmatics because of its opposite effects.) Another bronchodilator is adrenaline (or epinephrine), but it is a less specific drug that also affects the heart and increases the pulse rate. Theophylline, a stimulant chemically related to caffeine, relaxes the airways and also helps clear mucus. Cromolyn sodium decreases sensitivity to triggers and is sometimes inhaled on a daily basis as a long-term treatment to prevent attacks.

The use of inflammation reducers known as corticosteroids play an important role in the treatment of asthma. Whether administered via the mouth or an inhaler, these powerful medications can both prevent and treat the airway inflammation that leads to asthma attacks. Their anti-inflammatory effects mean fewer symptoms and attacks, better airflow, and airways that are less likely to react to triggers in an exaggerated or hyperresponsive manner. Inhaled steroids are preferred for long-term treatment of asthma. Inhalation delivers the medication directly to the site of inflammation and is associated with fewer side effects, which can include osteoporosis, thinning and easily bruised skin, cataracts, and suppression of the adrenal glands. However, oral steroids play an important role in the treatment of asthma, especially during periods of sudden, life-threatening symptoms or for patients with severe and ongoing disease. To minimize possible side effects, oral steroids are given every other day or in decreasing dosage over a limited period of time. Initially, corticosteroids were used if other drugs were ineffective, but in 1991 they were strongly

IN THE NEWS: INCREASED ASTHMA RATES IN THE UNITED STATES

Asthma rates in the United States are increasing, especially in children, but the cause has yet to be determined. The American Lung Association reported a rise in prevalence of the disease from 34 cases per 1,000 people in 1982 to 56 cases per 1,000 in 1994. The Environmental Protection Agency reported that in the last two decades of the twentieth century, cases of childhood asthma more than doubled.

A study covered in the August, 2002, issue of *Pediatrics* reported that the prevalence of asthma increased on average 4.3 percent per year between 1980 and 1996. From 1997 to 2000, however, asthma attacks leveled off and may have reached a plateau. Nevertheless, office visits for children with asthma increased 3.8 percent from 1980 to 1999. Hospitalization of children with asthma grew 1.4 percent each year during this period, and child deaths from asthma increased 3.4 percent per year from 1980 to 1998. Statistics also show that children four years of age and younger had the greatest increase in prevalence and use of health care, but the highest mortality was in adolescents. There was a highly disproportionate number of cases in African American children.

Causes for the increase are unknown, but theories include factors in the environment, such as increasing air pollutants and allergens. The "hygiene hypothesis" suggests that more sterile living environments, the use of antibiotics and antibacterial products, and vaccinations may be contributing factors. Another possibility, according to Dr. Lara J. Akinbami of the Centers for Disease Control and Prevention's National Center for Health Statistics, is diagnostic transfer, which refers to a change in the labeling of other respiratory diagnoses of children to asthma. Diagnostic transfer may be the result of greater awareness of the disease but alone would not account for the rise in rates. Adding to the complexity of this issue is that, in 1997, the National Health Interview Survey was redesigned and began using a different childhood asthma measure.

Public health efforts may have contributed to the recent plateau by providing greater access to care for children through the State Children's Health Insurance Program. Other public health interventions have promoted prevention and a decline in mortality from the disease. Although it is not completely clear that rates have reached a true plateau, or what the exact causes of increased rates may be, most researchers and physicians agree that more research and data are needed.

—Martha Oehmke Loustaunau, Ph.D.

recommended for long-term preventive use. Calcium and vitamin D supplements are used to prevent bone loss in these patients.

Concerns about safety with these medications increase when asthmatics use high doses (more than two hundred inhalations monthly) of beta-agonist inhalers or take combined beta-agonist/anti-inflammant drugs for a long period of time. A higher risk of fatal or near-fatal attacks has been found with a high usage of fenoterol, a beta-agonist that is not used in the United States. A study published in the *Annals of Internal Medicine* in 2006 found similar risks with inhalers containing another beta-agonist, salmeterol. The popular asthma inhaler Advair, the fourth best-selling drug in the world, is an example of an inhaler containing this beta-agonist. The study surveyed published trials and found that patients taking either salmeterol or fenoterol combined with an anti-inflammatory drug for extended periods were 2.5 times more likely to be hospitalized and 3.5 times more likely to die than were patients taking the anti-inflammatory drug alone. This study followed a Food and Drug Administration (FDA) advisory released in 2005 warning the public that beta-agonists can cause a worsening of symptoms, and the *Annals of Internal Medicine* study recommended that inhalers containing this combination be taken off the market.

Paul Scanlon, a chest physician at the Mayo Clinic, warns that individuals should not exceed their prescribed dosage when using an inhaler. An individual who feels the need to use an inhaler more often to obtain adequate relief should see a doctor. The increased need is a sign of worsening asthma, and a doctor needs to investigate and perhaps change the treatment.

Over-the-counter drugs are often used by asthmatics to treat their symptoms. These drugs often use ephedrine, metaraminol, phenylephrine, methoxamine, or similar chemicals. All these drugs are structurally related to amphetamine or adrenaline. Unfortunately, some people may be getting relief without discovering the cause of their asthma. The National Asthma Education Panel (NAEP) maintains that self-treatment without a doctor's guidance is risky.

That asthmatics should generally avoid exercise is a myth. With a doctor's approval, regular sports and exercise may be pursued. Furthermore, exercise may be helpful in reducing the frequency and severity of attacks. Many athletes compete at high levels in spite of their asthma. An outstanding example is Olympic gold medalist Jackie Joyner-Kersee, who is asthmatic and who was named the best all-around female athlete in the world in 1988. Another is Jeanette Bolden, who had been especially affected as a child but sprinted to an Olympic gold medal in 1984. Sports that do not require continuous activity or exposure to cold, dry air are preferred. Swimming is considered ideal. Doctors can help the athlete with a pre-exercise medication plan and a backup plan if symptoms occur during or after the exercise.

Another damaging belief about asthma needs comment. Early Freudian psychology held that asthma could be caused by a mother who failed to answer her baby's crying. Accordingly, the onset of asthma, with its gasping for air, was seen as a continuation of that crying. This sad hypothesis is false: Asthma is not connected to any abnormal relationships between mother and child, and it is not caused by early or deep psychological problems.

Researchers continue to search for new ways to reduce the frequency and the effects of asthmatic attacks. The National Heart, Lung, and Blood Institute in Bethesda, Maryland, found that caffeine in coffee seems to help. The study showed that asthmatics who are regular coffee drinkers suffer one-third fewer symptoms (particularly, less wheezing) than those who do not drink coffee. The most promise, however, seems to be in developing a new line of drugs that will prevent the mast cells from releasing their chemicals. Such a medication could stop inflammation before it takes hold, either by curbing the production of leukotrienes or by preventing these chemicals from acting on the airways.

New drugs that interfere with the chemical moderators such as leukotriene have been approved for treatment. Zileuton, approved for use in 1997 and sold as Zyflo, interferes with leukotriene production in the mast cells. In 1998, montelukast sodium, sold as Singular, received FDA approval in the United States and Canada. Singular blocks the actions of leukotrienes as they attach to receptors on the outside of airway cells and turn on the cellular responses that lead to the asthma reaction: contraction of the airway muscles, swelling of the airway lining, and flooding of the remaining airway space with sticky mucus.

Perspective and Prospects

Asthma was recognized in ancient times in both the East and the West. The Chinese people have a rich collection of traditional remedies going back more than two thousand years that includes the use of *ma huang*, an Asiatic species of the genus *Ephedra*, for asthma and other lung conditions. *Ma huang* is a shrubby, almost leafless gymnosperm. In 1887, the alkaloid ephedrine was isolated from *Ephedra* as the active ingredient in the plant; the drug is similar in effect to adrenaline. Alkaloids are bitter in taste and often affect the nervous system. Scientists used the ending *-ine* to identify alkaloids, many of which have strong physiological effects on humans (such as caffeine, morphine, nicotine, and cocaine). *Ma huang* was used in both ancient China and India.

Pliny the Elder (23-79 C.E.) believed that everything had been created for the sake of humans and therefore that nature was a complete storehouse of natural remedies. His encyclopedia *Historia Naturalis* recommended ephedron, a source of ephedrine, for asthma, coughing, and hemorrhages. Some believe that Pliny may have suffered from asthma. He died from the fumes of Mount Vesuvius while investigating the volcano and trying to help refugees.

In the eighteenth century, the discovery of oxygen, nitrous oxide, and other gases led to serious efforts to determine medical uses for these gases. Inhalation allowed a gaseous medication to be removed as soon as the effect was achieved; precise dosage did not have to be calculated. There were legitimate efforts to find painkillers for surgery and dentistry. Soon charlatans falsely claimed, however, to be able to use the new gases to cure asthma and other diseases. Anesthetics such as ether, nitrous oxide, and chloroform were used by doctors in the 1850's to treat asthma and other conditions.

As early as 1190, Maimonides, the physician to the court of Saladin, the sultan of Egypt, noted that asthma tended to run in families. Unfortunately, Maimonides' thoughts about heredity were forgotten until much later. Early in the twentieth century, researchers did find that 48 percent of the asthmatics surveyed had an immediate family history of allergies.

In 1991, the NAEP, a federal panel of experts brought together by the National Heart, Lung, and Blood Institute, issued the first national guidelines for the diagnosis and treatment of asthma. These guidelines recommended that doctors should not approach asthma as treatment for the attacks alone. Rather, NAEP experts urged a focus on long-term prevention, increasing the use of inhaled steroids, especially with severe and moderate asthmatics. The report also urged increased use of the peak flow meter to predict attacks.

—Paul R. Boehlke, Ph.D.;
Shih-Wen Huang, M.D.;
updated by Caroline M. Small

See also Allergies; Asphyxiation; Environmental diseases; Lungs; Multiple chemical sensitivity syndrome; Pulmonary diseases; Pulmonary medicine; Pulmonary medicine, pediatric; Respiration; Wheezing.

FOR FURTHER INFORMATION:

Adams, Francis V. *The Asthma Sourcebook*. 3d ed. New York: McGraw Hill, 2006. The revised edition of this valuable guide by pulmonary specialist and respected New York City physician Adams contains up-to-date information on medications and treatment, as well as on childhood asthma and myths about asthma.

American Lung Association. http://www.lungusa.org/. Includes in-depth information and recent research findings, a guide to local events and programs, and a section to share personal stories, among other features.

American Medical Association. *Essential Guide to Asthma*. New York: Pocket Books, 1998. Although sparsely illustrated, this handy book presents the essential details on asthma from diagnosis to treatment and prevention, as well as a chapter covering alternative therapies, a glossary, and a resources list.

Barnes, Peter J., and Simon Godfrey. *Asthma*. 2d ed. London: Martin Dunitz, 2000. A pocket-sized guide that describes clinical features, treatment, and management guidelines.

Berger, William E. *Asthma for Dummies*. New York: John Wiley & Sons, 2004. The well-known Dummies series covers the mechanisms of the disease and its treatment and management in easy-to-understand language. The author is a former president of the American College of Allergy, Asthma, and Immunology.

Clark, T. J. H., et al., eds. *Asthma*. 4th ed. New York: Oxford University Press, 2001. A clinical text with eighteen chapters covering a range of topics including molecular biology of asthma to education of patients and healthcare providers.

Haas, François, and Sheila Sperber Haas. "Living with Asthma." In *The World Book Medical Encyclopedia*. Chicago: World Book, 1988. This special report carefully explains the disease and encourages asthmatics to take control of their lives. A chart details how a house can be asthma-proofed. Side effects and drawbacks of various drugs are charted.

Krementz, Jill. *How It Feels to Fight for Your Life*. Boston: Little, Brown, 1989. A collection of fourteen case studies of children who have serious chronic diseases. In one chapter, Anton Broekman, a ten-year-old, describes what living with asthma is like.

Ostrow, William, and Vivian Ostrow. *All About Asthma*. Morton Grove, Ill.: Albert Whitmany, 1989. A children's book written to inform and encourage. The writers, a boy and his mother, tell about his experience with asthma. He explains causes, symptoms, and ways to lead a normal life. A must for children with asthma.

Parker, James M., and Philip M. Parker, eds. *The 2002 Official Patient's Sourcebook on Asthma*. San Diego, Calif.: Icon Health, 2002. Draws from public, academic, government, and peer-reviewed research to provide a wide-ranging handbook for patients with asthma.

Welch, Michael J., and the American Academy of Pediatrics. *American Academy of Pediatrics Guide to Your Child's Asthma and Allergies: Breathing Easy and Bringing up Healthy, Active Children*. New York: Random House, 2000. A user-friendly guide to living with and managing childhood asthma, including discussions of identifying allergies and asthma, preventing attacks, understanding and choosing medications, and explaining the disorder to young children.

Astigmatism

Disease/disorder

Anatomy or system affected: Eyes

Specialties and related fields: Ophthalmology, optometry

Definition: A slight deformation of the eyeball that makes it impossible for a person to form a sharp image of two perpendicular lines simultaneously.

Causes and Symptoms

The problem of astigmatism is caused by a difference in the focal length of the eye for two perpendicular directions, which can occur if the eyeball becomes slightly deformed, like a grape being squeezed between two fingers. The curvature of the cornea would be flattened in one plane but remain more rounded in the other one. A deformed eye lens can also cause astigmatism.

During an eye examination, the optometrist tests for astigmatism by showing the patient a diagram of straight lines radiating outward from the center of the picture. A person with normal eyes will see all the lines in focus, but someone with astigmatism will see only one line sharply focused while the other ones are fuzzy.

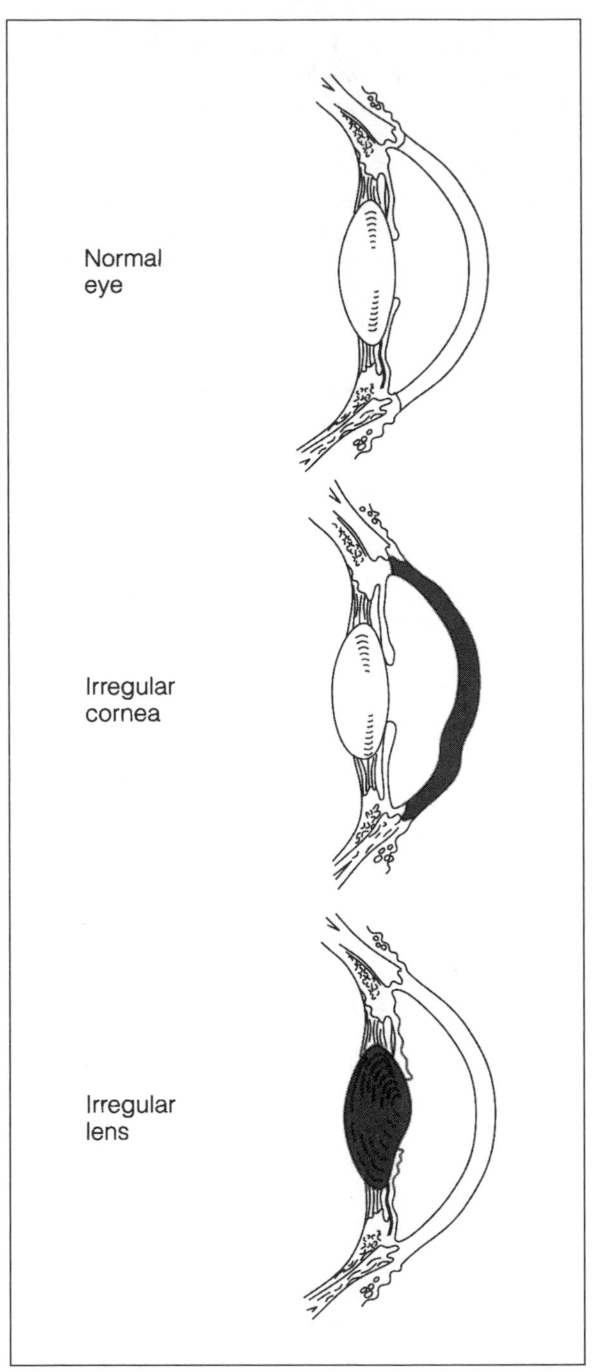

Astigmatism results when either the cornea or the lens is irregular, distorting the image that reaches the retina.

For example, if the horizontal line is perceived to be in focus, then the vertical line will be blurred while the lines in between will be partially out of focus. Each eye must be tested individually because the amount of astigmatism can differ.

Information on Astigmatism

Causes: A slight deformation of the eyeball or lens
Symptoms: Inability to form a sharp image of two perpendicular lines simultaneously
Duration: Chronic
Treatments: Eyeglasses, hard contact lenses, laser surgery

Treatment and Therapy

To correct for astigmatism, the optometrist can add a cylindrical correction to the eyeglass prescription, which changes the focal length of the eye in only one plane. A cylindrical lens can be pictured to be thick in the middle and thin at the edges, like a slice cut off from the outside edge of a cylindrical object.

A typical prescription for a person who is farsighted and also has astigmatism might be "+2.0D + 0.5 cyl axis 90." The "+2.0D" is the strength of a typical converging lens for a farsighted person, expressed in diopters. Diopters are equal to the inverse of the focal length, so 2.0 diopters equals a focal length of 0.5 meter, or 50 centimeters. The correction for astigmatism here specifies a cylindrical lens of +0.5 diopters situated at an angle of 90 degrees to the horizontal axis.

Astigmatism can be corrected with hard contact lenses because the lens makes contact with the cornea over a layer of tears. The tears fill the space between the lens and the misshapen eyeball, providing the extra focusing that is required.

Laser surgery has become a highly successful procedure to correct for vision problems, including astigmatism. The surgeon first cuts through a paper-thin layer of the outer eye surface (called the cornea) and lifts it like a flap. A computer-controlled laser beam is then used to remove layers of the inner cornea, reshaping it to restore horizontal and vertical symmetry for the eyeball. When the flap is replaced, it molds itself to the reshaped inner cornea.

—Hans G. Graetzer, Ph.D.

See also Blurred vision; Eye infections and disorders; Eye surgery; Eyes; Laser use in surgery; Myopia; Ophthalmology; Optometry; Refractive eye surgery; Sense organs; Vision disorders.

For Further Information:

American Medical Association. *American Medical Association Family Medical Guide*. 4th rev. ed. Hoboken, N.J.: John Wiley & Sons, 2004.
Cameron, John R., James G. Skofronick, and Roderick M. Grant. *Medical Physics: Physics of the Body*. Madison, Wis.: Medical Physics, 1992.
Slade, Stephen G., Richard Baker, and Dorothy Brockman. *The Complete Book of Laser Eye Surgery*. Naperville, Ill.: Sourcebooks, 2000.

Ataxia

Disease/disorder

Anatomy or system affected: Brain, musculoskeletal system, nervous system
Specialties and related fields: Exercise physiology, family medicine, geriatrics and gerontology, internal medicine, neurology, nursing, occupational health, orthopedics, pediatrics, physical therapy, speech pathology
Definition: A lack of coordination while performing voluntary movements that may appear as clumsiness, inaccuracy, or instability.

Causes and Symptoms

Ataxia most often results from disorders of the cerebellum (a large structure at the lower back of the brain, just above where the spinal cord enters the skull at the bottom) or its connections. Disorders resembling ataxia can also be seen following parietal or frontal lobe lesions of the brain. Ataxia is a symptom, not a diagnosis. Ataxia may affect any part of the body.

Some medical conditions can cause ataxia to appear suddenly, such as head trauma, stroke, brain hemorrhage, brain tumor, congenital abnormality, postviral infections, exposure to certain drugs or toxins (for example, alcohol or seizure medications), and cardiac or respiratory arrest. Other conditions may cause ataxia to appear gradually, such as hypothyroidism, some vitamin deficiencies (vitamins E or B_{12}), exposure to certain drugs or toxins (heavy metals, chronic alcohol use, and some cancer drugs), certain kinds of cancer (ovarian and lung cancer), congenital abnormality, heredity disorders, multiple sclerosis, syphilis, and unknown causes of cerebellar degeneration disorders.

Treatment and Therapy

A careful neurologic and general physical examination, including blood tests and X rays, can determine whether other parts of the nervous system are impaired and whether a medical illness may be causing ataxia. No medicine specifically treats the symptom of ataxia. If ataxia is the result of a stroke, a low vitamin level, or

Information on Ataxia

Causes: Head trauma, stroke, brain hemorrhage, brain tumor, congenital abnormality, postviral infections, exposure to certain drugs or toxins, cardiac or respiratory arrest, hypothyroidism, some vitamin deficiencies, certain cancers, multiple sclerosis, syphilis

Symptoms: Lack of coordination while performing voluntary movements (clumsiness, inaccuracy, instability)

Duration: Acute, chronic, or progressive, depending on cause

Treatments: Medications or surgery, depending on underlying condition; physical and occupational therapy

exposure to a toxic drug or chemical, then treatment would involve minimizing the effects of the current stroke and preventing further ones, instituting vitamin therapy, or avoiding the toxic drug or chemical, respectively. In some cases, the metabolic disorders that cause ataxia may be treated with controlled diet and medication. If ataxia is the result of a tumor, then surgery may be necessary. Many people with hereditary or idiopathic forms of ataxia have additional symptoms. Medications or other therapies might be appropriate for some of these symptoms, such as tremor, stiffness, spasticity, depression, and sleep disorders.

The mainstay of treatment for ataxia is the provision of physical and occupational therapy directed at maintaining function for as long as possible. Gait training and assistive devices such as canes, crutches, or a walker are useful to prevent falls and enhance mobility. Other adapted utensils and tools may be helpful to assist with writing, feeding, and self-care if hand or arm coordination is impaired, as can speech therapy and communication devices for those with impaired speech.

Extremity ataxia that interferes with activities of daily living, such as feeding or dressing, may be treated with proximal splinting. Distal weights may dampen intention tremor. If the ataxia is exacerbated by weakness, strengthening exercises can be beneficial. Specific coordinated exercises are often helpful in treating static causes of ataxia (stroke or head injury) but not as useful in treating progressive disorders such as hereditary ataxias. Ataxia of eye movements rarely requires treatment, but it may be disabling if the patient has difficulty reading.

—Linda L. Pierce, Ph.D., R.N.

See also Alcoholism; Brain; Brain damage; Brain disorders; Brain tumors; Head and neck disorders; Multiple sclerosis; Muscle sprains, spasms, and disorders; Muscles; Nervous system; Neuroimaging; Neurology; Occupational health; Speech disorders; Strokes; Vitamins and minerals.

For Further Information:

Braddom, Randall L., ed. *Physical Medicine and Rehabilitation*. 3d ed. Philadelphia: Saunders Elsevier, 2007.

Gillen, G. "Improving Activities of Daily Living Performance in an Adult with Ataxia." *American Journal of Occupational Therapy* 54, no. 1 (January/February, 2000): 89-96.

_______. "Improving Mobility and Community Access in an Adult with Ataxia." *American Journal of Occupational Therapy* 56, no. 4 (July/August, 2002): 462-466.

Athlete's foot

Disease/disorder

Also known as: Tinea pedis

Anatomy or system affected: Feet, nails, skin

Specialties and related fields: Dermatology, podiatry

Definition: A microscopic fungal infection that lives on the outer layers of skin, nails, or hair on the feet.

Causes and Symptoms

Several different dermatophytes (microscopic fungi) can cause tinea pedis through contact with the skin on the bottom of the foot. Once contact is made, the dermatophytes grow if the environmental conditions are right. These fungi thrive in warm, moist surroundings such as wet shoes and socks or the floors of pool decks, showers, and locker rooms. Since sweat is a common source of moisture for fungal growth, this disorder is often associated with athletes—thus the term "athlete's foot." It is commonly believed that athlete's foot is highly contagious. However, the presence of the fungus on the healthy foot does not necessarily result in the disorder; a warm, moist environment is also required.

The most common symptom of athlete's foot is constant itching or burning of the skin between the toes, particularly the outside, smaller toes. The skin turns white and begins to peel. A scaly, dry rash develops and

Information on Athlete's Foot

Causes: Presence of fungi and warm, moist surroundings
Symptoms: Constant itching or burning between toes; peeling skin; dry, scaly rash; skin cracks or fissures
Duration: Acute or chronic
Treatments: Good hygiene; removal of moist, warm environment; antifungal drugs (creams, powders, sprays, liquids)

frequently progresses to cracks or fissures. A clear fluid may be released. If untreated, the infection may spread to the toenails and other areas of the foot. Also, the person becomes more susceptible to secondary bacterial infections.

Another form of athlete's foot results in a red, scaly rash that spreads across the bottom and sides of the foot. Because the rash pattern resembles a moccasin, this form is often called "moccasin foot."

Treatment and Therapy

With good hygiene and the removal of moist, warm environmental conditions, the fungus may die off on its own. If these conditions are not treated, however, the fungus can persevere for years. The best results occur with the use of antifungal drugs. Many types are available over the counter in creams, powders, sprays, or liquids. Imidazole drugs attack the cell walls of the fungus and keep the cells from growing and reproducing. Eventually, the infection will die off. More severe infections are treated with allylamine drugs. These drugs, which must be obtained with a prescription, cause a buildup of toxins that kill the fungi.

The best treatment for athlete's foot is to prevent it by using good foot hygiene. Feet should be washed daily with soap and water. Wet feet should always be dried thoroughly, especially between the toes. Shoes and socks should be kept dry by regular changing and the use of foot powder to absorb moisture, if needed. Wearing light, airy shoes to reduce perspiration of the feet is also beneficial.

—*Bradley R. A. Wilson, Ph.D.*

See also Dermatology; Feet; Foot disorders; Fungal infections; Itching; Lower extremities; Over-the-counter medications; Podiatry; Rashes; Skin; Skin disorders.

For Further Information:

Alexander, Ivy L., ed. *Podiatry Sourcebook.* 2d rev. ed. Detroit: Omnigraphics, 2007.

Donowitz, Leigh G., ed. *Infection Control in the Child Care Center and Preschool.* 4th ed. Philadelphia: Lippincott Williams & Wilkins, 1999.

Richardson, Malcolm D., and Elizabeth M. Johnson. *The Pocket Guide to Fungal Infection.* Malden, Mass.: Blackwell Science, 2000.

Attention-deficit disorder (ADD)

Disease/disorder

Also known as: Attention-deficit hyperactivity disorder (ADHD)

Anatomy or system affected: Brain, nervous system, psychic-emotional system

Specialties and related fields: Family medicine, genetics, neurology, pediatrics, psychiatry, psychology

Definition: A condition characterized by an inability to focus attention or to inhibit impulsive, hyperactive behavior; it is associated with poor academic performance and behavioral problems in children but also may be diagnosed in adults under certain conditions.

Key terms:

antianxiety medication: a medication that acts in the brain to decrease negative reactions to stress and anxiety and to decrease avoidance behavior

antidepressant: a medication that acts in the brain to decrease a sad or depressed mood and other behaviors associated with depression

nervous system: the system in the body, including the brain, that receives and interprets stimuli and transmits impulses to other organs; the brain is the center of thinking and behavior

neurotransmitter: a chemical in the brain that sends a signal from one brain cell to another

Causes and Symptoms

Most experts think that 2 to 5 percent of children may have attention-deficit disorder (ADD), which is more formally known as attention-deficit hyperactivity disorder (ADHD). The cause of ADD is unknown, although the fact that it often occurs in families suggests some degree of genetic inheritance. The condition is more common in boys, but it does occur in girls. ADD is usually diagnosed when a child enters school, but it may be discovered earlier. Adolescents and even adults who were not diagnosed earlier in life may be diagnosed later in life when their symptoms cause particularly severe problems. Some causes of ADD that have been suggested, but never proved, include low blood sugar, food additives, the sweetener aspartame, allergies, and vitamin deficiencies. Other causes being explored include head injury, exposure to emotionally traumatic situations such as abuse or violence, and exposure to environmental contaminants such as lead or substances of abuse such as nicotine in utero.

Children who do not have ADD may, at times, have some of the symptoms of this disorder, but children who can be diagnosed with ADD must have most of the symptoms most of the time—in school, at home, or during other activities. The symptoms are usually grouped into three main categories: inattention, hyperactivity, and impulsiveness.

Children who have symptoms of inattention often make careless mistakes at school or do not pay close attention to details in play or work. They may have problems sustaining attention over time and frequently do not seem to listen when spoken to, especially in groups. Children with ADD have difficulty following instructions and often fail to finish chores or schoolwork. They do not organize well and may have messy rooms and desks at school. They also frequently lose things necessary for play or school. Because they have trouble sustaining attention, children with ADD dislike tasks that require this skill and will try to avoid them. One of the key symptoms is distractibility, which means that children with ADD are often paying attention to extraneous sights, sounds, smells, and thoughts rather than focusing on the task that they should be doing. Particularly frustrating to parents is the symptom of forgetfulness in daily activities, in spite of numerous reminders from parents about such common, everyday activities as dressing, hygiene, manners, and other behaviors. Children with ADD have a poor sense of time; they are frequently late or think that they have more time to do a task than they really do.

Not all children with ADD have symptoms of hyperactivity, but many have problems with fidgeting, or squirming. It is common for these children to be constant talkers, often interrupting others. Other symptoms of hyperactivity include leaving their seat in school, church, or similar settings and running around excessively in situations where they should be still. Children with ADD have difficulty playing quietly, although they may watch television or play video games for long periods of time. Some of these children seem to be driven by a motor, or are continuously on the go.

Information on Attention-Deficit Disorder (ADD)

Causes: Unknown, possibly genetic
Symptoms: Inattention, hyperactivity, impulsiveness
Duration: Chronic
Treatments: Medication, counseling

All children with ADD will have some symptoms of impulsiveness, such as blurting out answers before questions are completed. Another example of impulsiveness would be or intruding upon others in conversation or in some activity. They may also have difficulty standing in lines or waiting for their turn in games.

It is important to recognize that children with ADD are not bad children who are hyperactive, impulsive, and inattentive on purpose. Rather, they are usually bright children who would like to behave better and to be more successful in school, in social life with peers, and in family affairs, but they simply cannot. One way to think about ADD is to consider it a disorder of the ability to inhibit impulsive, off-task, or undesirable attention. Consequently, the child with ADD cannot separate important from unimportant stimuli and cannot sort appropriate from inappropriate responses to those stimuli. It is easy to understand how someone whose brain is trying to respond to a multitude of stimuli, rather than sorting stimuli into priorities for response, will have difficulty focusing and maintaining attention to the main task.

It is also important to remember that it is not only the presence of symptoms that categorizes a child as having ADD but also the intensity and prevalence of the symptoms in more than one setting. For example, a child may not seem to pay attention in school and often may be disruptive in class but be a normal child at home, playing Little League baseball, and in church school. This child may have a learning disability without ADD or a specific conflict with the teacher.

Children most likely to be diagnosed correctly with ADD will have many of the following characteristics. They will have a short attention span, particularly for activities that are not fun or entertaining. They will be unable to concentrate because they will be distracted by peripheral stimuli. They will have poor impulse control so that they seem to act on the spur of the moment. They will be hyperactive and usually rather clumsy, resulting in their being labeled "accident-prone." They will certainly have school problems, especially when classwork requires more thinking and planning—often seen about third grade and beyond. They may display attention-demanding behavior and/or show resistant or overpowering social behaviors. Last, children with ADD often act as if they were younger, and "immaturity" is a frequent label. Along with this trait, they have wide mood swings and are seen as very emotional.

Many experts think that ADD is a developmental problem, caused by the failure of the brain and nervous system to grow and mature normally. Thus, while some behavior might be acceptable at earlier ages, when it persists into later ages, it may signal a developmental problem. For an average, normal two-year-old child, a short attention span, impulsivity, distractibility, clumsiness, recklessness, and less-than-perfect planning abilities would not be unexpected or very troublesome. All these characteristics are acceptable for the toddler. When those symptoms persist into and beyond kindergarten, however, they are of greater concern and may signal a need for further evaluation. For some, this slowed development may improve during childhood. For others, however, it may persist into adolescence and create additional problems.

Adolescents who have ADD are usually not hyperactive, although they may have problems with impulsive talking and behavior. They have considerable difficulty complying with rules and following directions. They may be poorly organized, causing problems both with starting projects and with completing them. Their inability to monitor their own behavior leads to problems making and keeping friends and causes them to have conflicts with parents and teachers beyond those normally seen in teenagers. Adolescents with ADD usually have problems in school in spite of average or above-average potential. They may have poor self-esteem and a low frustration tolerance. Because of these and other factors related to ADD, they may also be at greater risk of developing substance use problems and other mental health problems.

Several other neurologic or psychiatric disorders have symptoms that can overlap with ADD, so diagnosis is often difficult. When a child is suspected of having ADD, he or she should have a thorough medical interview with, and physical examination by, a physician familiar with child development, ADD, and related conditions. A psychological evaluation to determine intelligence quotient (IQ) and areas of learning and performance strengths and weaknesses should be obtained. School records need to be reviewed, and teachers may be asked to submit rating forms or similar instruments to document school performance. A thorough family history and a discussion of family problems such as divorce, violence, alcoholism, or drug abuse should be part of the evaluation. Other conditions that might be found to exist along with ADD, or to be the underlying cause of symptoms thought to be ADD, include oppositional defiant disorder, conduct disorder (usually seen in older children), depression, or anxiety disorder. Many physicians, teachers, psychologists, and parents do not believe that ADD is a "real" condition, but this disorder is widely accepted in the United States as a credible diagnosis for a child who demonstrates many of the above symptoms at home, at play, and at school. In 1998, the National Institutes of Health (NIH) held a Consensus Development Conference on the Diagnosis and Treatment of Attention Deficit Hyperactivity Disorder. While most experts support the ADD diagnosis, the final report noted a need for further research into the validity of the diagnosis.

TREATMENT AND THERAPY

Treatment and therapy for ADD will usually begin with the diagnostic process and involves the family of the child affected. Generally, treatment will consist of some combination of psychotherapy, medication, and education. In some cases, therapy for the child and/or the family may be indicated. This therapy may be help the family learn about ADD. It also may be recommended when things happening in the family are seen as related to the type or severity of symptoms that the child may be experiencing. For instance, if the family is undergoing a stressful event, such as a divorce, serious loss, or death, or other problems such as economic stress, then the symptoms of ADD may worsen. Therefore, treatment may focus on trying to minimize the impact of such stressors on the child.

The medical treatment of ADD is one of the most controversial issues in education and in medicine. Although scientific studies clearly show the value of certain medications, and scores of parents and teachers have noticed remarkable improvement with treatment, some people take issue with using medications to change a child's behavior. Clearly, medications alone are not the answer for ADD. Families and children need guidance and support in the form of counseling, as well as considerable information about the condition. Special accommodations can be arranged with most schools and are mandated by federal law. Once educational adjustments have been made and counseling is in place, however, medications can play an important role.

The most frequently prescribed medications are stimulants; they include dexedrine, methylphenidate (Ritalin), and a combination of dexedrine salts (Adderall). A similar medication, pemoline (Cylert), has been related to side effects, which may limit its usefulness. The stimulant medications may function by influencing chemicals in the brain called neurotransmitters, which help transmit messages among brain and nerve cells. In ADD, it is thought that the medications improve the function of cells that direct the brain to focus attention, resist distraction, control behavior, and perceive time correctly. These medications are generally thought to be safe and effective, although they can have such adverse effects as headache, stomachache, mood changes, heart rate changes, appetite suppression, and interference with going to sleep. All children receiving medication must be monitored at regular intervals by a physician.

Other medications that may be used for ADD include antidepressants and antianxiety medications. Some children are treated with combinations of two medications; in unusual circumstances, there may be even more than two. Some of these medications are Imipramine and Desipramine, antidepressants that act mainly to control impulsiveness and hyperactivity; Bupropion, an antidepressant, and Buspar, an antianxiety medicine, both of which have been used largely in older children and adolescents; and clonidine and guanfacine, which work on brain nerve message transmitters and are sometimes helpful in calming aggressive behavior. Behavior modification and several forms of psychotherapy or counseling are also held to be effective, whether concurrently with or as a replacement for medication. Critics of medication have expressed concerns not only with side effects but also with the potential for contributing to drug abuse, and a belief in the greater long-term effectiveness of psychotherapy alone. The latter view suggests that medication may interfere with promoting true self-control. The 1998 NIH Consensus report emphasized the continuing controversies and the need for outcomes research pertaining to these issues.

Costs and risks for adverse effects should be discussed with the physician who has made the diagnosis of ADD before implementing any treatment, to ensure safety and a reasonable expectation of efficacy.

Perspective and Prospects

Attention-deficit disorder remains controversial, largely because of the subjective nature of its symptoms. For about 5 percent of all children and adolescents, however, ADD is a real issue that can cause great harm if not recognized and managed correctly. Diagnosis should be based on documentation of the child's and family's history, careful examination, and educational and psychological assessment. Treatment should always include educational accommodations and counseling for the child and the family. When symptoms create problems at home and at school, properly prescribed and managed medications have been shown to offer great relief in most cases.

Children and parents in the United States can share experiences and resources through organizations that assist families dealing with attention-deficit disorder. The national organization Children and Adults with Attention Deficit/Hyperactivity Disorder (CHADD) has state and local chapters helping families cope with the condition. CHADD chapters often have libraries and provide resources on ADD. Learning Disabilities Association of America (LDA) has state and local chapters helping schools and families cope with a wide range of learning disabilities, including ADD.

—Robert W. Block, M.D.;
Nancy E. Macdonald, Ph.D.;
updated by Nancy A. Piotrowski, Ph.D.

See also Anxiety; Brain; Brain disorders; Emotions: Biomedical causes and effects; Learning disabilities; Pediatrics; Psychiatry, child and adolescent; Puberty and adolescence; Stress.

For Further Information:

Accardo, Pasquale J., ed. *Attention Deficits and Hyperactivity in Children and Adults: Diagnosis, Treatment, Management*. 2d ed. New York: Marcel Dekker, 2000. A medically oriented text covering a range of multidisciplinary topics including the physiological substrate, an overview of clinical diagnosis, associated deficits, therapy, legal issues, and adolescent transitions and ADHD.

Barkley, Russell A. *Taking Charge of ADHD*. Rev. ed. New York: Guilford Press, 2000. A comprehensive guide for parents that discusses how to understand ADD, how to be a successful parent, how to cope with the child at home and at school, and how to evaluate medications.

Breggin, Peter R. *Talking Back to Ritalin*. Monroe, Maine: Common Courage Press, 1998. This book details the major concerns of critics of stimulant treatment for ADD. Also discusses alternative approaches and resources for concerned parents and educators.

Children and Adults with Attention Deficit/Hyperactivity Disorder. http://www.chadd.org/. Site describes this parent-based organization formed to improve the lives of individuals with attention-deficit disorders and their families.

Phelan, Thomas W. *All About Attention Deficit Disorder: Symptoms, Diagnosis and Treatment—Children and Adults*. 2d rev. ed. Glen Ellyn, Ill.: Child Management, 2000. A very accessible handbook that covers all the important facets of the disorder: what to look for, how to diagnose, and how to treat attention deficit disorder, as well as tools for research and emotional support.

Quinn, Patricia O. *ADD and the College Student: A Guide for High School and College Students with Attention Deficit Disorder*. Rev. ed. American Psychological Association, 2001. Answers important questions from young ADD patients preparing for or attending college about such topics as physiology, ADD-friendly colleges, and legal rights.

Rief, Sandra F. *The ADHD Book of Lists: A Practical Guide for Helping Children and Teens with Attention Deficit Disorders*. New York: Wiley, 2003. Designed for school personnel and parents, this resource book details recent research and strategies, supports, and interventions that help minimize the problems and optimize the success of children and teens with ADHD.

Wender, Paul H. *The Hyperactive Child, Adolescent, and Adult*. New York: Oxford University Press, 1987. This book offers concise information about ADD in children, adolescents, and adults. Clearly defines the characteristics of individuals with symptoms of ADD and discusses the reasons for using medications.

Zeigler Dendy, Chris A. *Teenagers with ADD: A Parents' Guide*. Bethesda, Md.: Woodbine House, 1995. This resource is a workbook for parents and teachers of adolescents who have ADD. Includes useful lists of problem behaviors at home and at school, with practical solutions to these problems.

AUDIOLOGY

SPECIALTY

ANATOMY OR SYSTEM AFFECTED: Ears

SPECIALTIES AND RELATED FIELDS: Neurology, otorhinolaryngology, speech pathology

DEFINITION: The study of the auditory system and its measurement, including the assessment of the medical, surgical, or rehabilitation implications arising from a number of disorders affecting hearing.

KEY TERMS:

audiologist: one who is specifically trained at an approved institution of learning to provide diagnostic testing and rehabilitative training to those with hearing disorders

audiometer: a calibrated electronic device for the purpose of measuring human hearing to determine the magnitude of loss and the probable rehabilitative course

auditory system: the human hearing mechanism, including the pinna, the external ear canal, the middle ear structures, the cochlea, and the ascending neural pathway that terminates in the auditory cortex of the brain

auditory system disorder: any condition or state that interferes with or alters the normal function of acoustic information transfer from the outer ear to the brain

aural rehabilitation: a program for hearing-impaired individuals that may include auditory prostheses, auditory training, and speech-reading training

communicative skills: those skills required to express thoughts, desires, and feelings effectively through verbal communication

habilitative: referring to the process of creating or teaching a function involving human behavior, thought, and reason

mixed hearing loss: the combined effects of the loss of sensory or neural integrity and the presence of a barrier to the normal transmission of sound (such as wax in the ear, a hole in the eardrum, or some congenital anomaly affecting the transmission pathway of the auditory system)

rehabilitative: referring to the process of re-creating or teaching a function that has been impaired as a result of injury, disease, or aging

retrocochlear hearing loss: any disruption of neural information processing beyond the cochlea

sensorineural hearing loss: the loss of sensory or neural tissue of the auditory system as a result of disease, age, and acquired or congenital factors

SCIENCE AND PROFESSION

The field of audiology has become an indispensable adjunct in the objective diagnosis of hearing loss and auditory disorders. The scope of audiology practice is rather extensive and includes broad categorical services. According to the U.S. Department of Labor, the audiologist "specializes in diagnostic evaluation of hearing, prevention, habilitative and rehabilitative services for auditory problems and research related to hearing and attendant disorders." Among other functions, the audiologist

> determines range, nature, and degree of hearing function . . . using electroacoustic instrumentation; . . . coordinates audiometric results with other diagnostic data, such as educational, medical, social, and behavioral information; . . . differentiates between organic and nonorganic hearing disabilities through evaluation of total response pattern and use of acoustic tests; . . . [and] plans, directs, conducts, or participates in conservation, habilitative and rehabilitative programs, including hearing aid selection and orientation, counseling guidance, auditory training, speech reading, language rehabilitation, and speech conservation.

Audiologists may have primary affiliations in private practice, clinics and hospitals, military installations, universities and colleges, or in public and private school systems.

Because of the significant advances that have been made in providing differential diagnosis of impaired auditory behavior, the number of institutions providing audiology programs increased dramatically in the latter half of the twentieth century. Although the highest degree offered in audiology is the Ph.D., there is a strong movement supporting the introduction of a professional doctorate of audiology, which would stress clinical diagnosis, auditory prosthetic evaluation, and rehabilitative practice.

The membership of the American Speech-Language-Hearing Association (ASHA) consists of speech pathologists and audiologists, with the former having significantly greater numbers. ASHA provides two major, bimonthly sources of information: the *Journal of Speech and Hearing Research* and the *Journal of Speech and Hearing Disorders*. In 1988, James Jerger and other prominent audiologists in the United States formed the American Academy of Audiology. Its members consist exclusively of audiologists holding a master's or Ph.D. degree in that field. A quarterly publication of the Academy is the *Journal of the American Academy of Audiology*. Its content reflects the increase in knowledge of the human auditory system, its measurement and rehabilitative care.

DIAGNOSTIC AND TREATMENT TECHNIQUES

One of the most common services associated with the practice of audiology is the basic assessment of the auditory system relative to pure-tone air conduction thresholds. This is a procedure in which the patient's ability to just detect the presence of a tone delivered through earphones or a speaker is determined. Additionally, speech threshold detection is determined by assessing the patient's ability to identify correctly 50 percent of a list of two-syllable words. Measurements of the acoustic reflex provide information about hearing loss, as do reflex-eliciting auditory tests. The acoustic reflex is the contraction of the stapedial muscle produced by a strong acoustic signal. The strength of the response and the level at which it is elicited are important diagnostic indicators of system malfunction, as is the absence of a reflex response. The degree to which the reflex response deviates in morphology and amplitude from normal is diagnostically significant. Communication handicap inventories also are an essential part of the basic assessment procedure. Such inventories provide useful information as to the degree of social handicap as a concomitant part of hearing impairment. Serial communication inventories serve as indicators of the effectiveness of habilitative or rehabilitative programs designed to enhance communicative skills. The term "basic" is applied to indicate a routine assessment of auditory function. Basic assessment does not provide the preponderance of clinical evidence needed to determine the site of injury or disease or to suggest its medical or surgical management.

Another service associated with audiology is an extended evaluation of the auditory system, which is composed of all anatomical structures that contribute to human hearing. Such an evaluation may include the determination of air conduction, bone conduction, and speech thresholds, as well as the administration of word and sentence recognition tests. Air conduction tests are performed by placing calibrated headphones over the patient's ears and presenting a broad range of discrete frequencies. In practice, that frequency range extends from 250 to 8,000 hertz. Even though the normal human ear is capable of perceiving a much broader frequency range (from 20 hertz to 20,000 hertz), the range between 250 hertz and 8,000 hertz contains all the essential frequencies needed to understand speech.

Bone conduction thresholds are determined by placing a vibrator, or bone oscillator, at the mastoid bone and presenting the same frequency range. Often, differences in the patient's response to air-conducted and bone-conducted signals provide essential diagnostic information and suggest the site of injury or disease.

Speech threshold and word or sentence evaluations provide the clinician with performance scores that indicate the degree to which speech understanding has been compromised by the hearing disorder. Such measurements also indicate the probability of understanding connected discourse in communicative situations. There are a number of speech tests that provide information about the status of the auditory system. The most commonly used speech stimuli are two-syllable words to determine an individual's speech reception threshold and one-syllable words to assess the auditory system's discrimination function.

Another standard audiological practice is a comprehensive behavioral evaluation to determine the sensorineural site of lesion, that is, the place in the auditory system from which the hearing disorder originates. For most hearing disorders affecting auditory performance, it is critical that this site be located. It may be found in the peripheral system (the cochlea), which contains specialized sensory tissue that responds to sound pressure changes. The problem could also lie in the ascending auditory pathway, including its terminal projection in the auditory cortex of the brain. To arrive at an accurate diagnosis, the audiologist employs a number of advanced tests, such as sophisticated acoustic reflex tests, tests of frequency discrimination (the ability to detect differences between two or more signals), tests of intensity discrimination, and tests of auditory adaptation. The latter is a clinical procedure in which one determines whether a continuous sound decays over time to the point of inaudibility; such abnormal decay of the test signal indicates possible malfunction of the neural pathway of the auditory system. The results of these several tests increase significantly the probability that the site of lesion can be found.

One of the most promising clinical advances in audiology has been the development of evoked response audiometry (ERA). ERA is best defined as the mea-

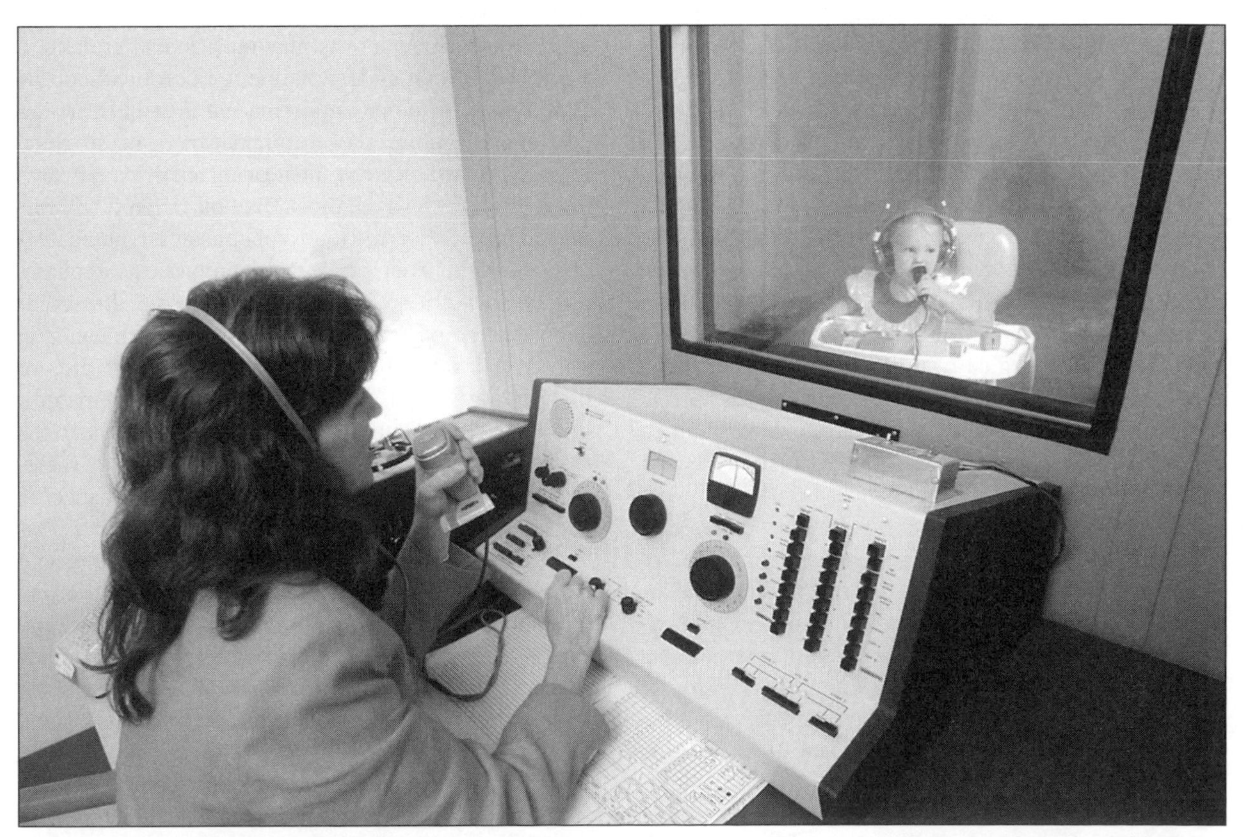

An audiologist administers a hearing test to a child. Routine screening is often used to detect problems in children. (Digital Stock)

surement of neuroelectrical activity generated in the brain stem or of higher orders of brain function elicited by an acoustic signal. Acoustic signals, clicks, and tone pips are submitted to the external auditory ear. If the signals are detected by the auditory system, there is a change in neuroelectrical activity for each signal presented. A computer stores these minute changes in activity. When a sufficient number of acoustic signals have been processed, the computer prints out a response pattern consistent with the transmission of the electrical response from cochlear and subsequent responses as the signal travels to the brain. Response patterns have been classified as first (from the cochlea, 0 to 2 milliseconds), fast (from the acoustic nerve and auditory brain stem, 2 to 10 milliseconds), slow (from the primary and secondary areas of the cerebral cortex, 50 to 300 milliseconds), and late (from the primary and associated areas of the cerebral cortex, more than 300 milliseconds). More recent terminology of these time-related events refers to them as early, middle, and late responses.

Evoked potential measurement is significant because it offers a method of auditory assessment for those patients unwilling or unable to give reliable voluntary responses to acoustic stimuli. For example, evoked response audiometry provides a means of detecting hearing impairment in the neonate and very young. It also provides a clinical method of determining normal or abnormal hearing function for those who are mentally retarded. Evoked responses to acoustic stimuli aid in the diagnosis of various types of tumors or neuromas that affect the transmission of auditory signals to the brain. If such lesion sites are detected early, it may be possible to remove them surgically and save the patient's hearing. Certainly, early detection of retrocochlear pathology increases the probability that surgical intervention will preserve auditory system performance.

In 1978, D. T. Kemp published a germinal paper identifying the presence of otoacoustic emissions. Spontaneous emissions are generated within the cochlea and can be measured by a probe microphone assembly inserted into the external ear canal. Not all individuals have spontaneous otoacoustic emissions that can be measured by current probe microphone systems. Evoked otoacoustic emissions can be measured, however, in individuals having normal hearing or hearing loss of no more than 40 to 45 decibels. Such emissions are evoked by presenting a series of clicks or other compatible acoustic stimuli to the patient's auditory system. The cochleomechanical activity induced by these acoustic signals is "picked up" by a probe microphone and processed by a computer. The graphic information obtained has proven to be of significant benefit in the screening of neonates and the very young. The literature would seem to suggest that otoacoustic emission measurement is fast, reliable, and repeatable. Research is under way to assess the range of losses that can be measured and the most appropriate stimuli to be employed in order to gain specific bits of information about cochlear behavior.

Auditory prosthetic evaluations have become common practice in audiology. When tests for hearing function determine that a hearing impairment exists, medical referral is mandatory for appropriate clinical management. For a sizable number of hearing-impaired individuals, however, medical or surgical intervention will not alter the hearing loss. For cases in which hearing impairment is a permanent sensorineural condition, a hearing aid or assistive listening device (or both) is often the preferred treatment modality in the rehabilitative process. To determine the appropriate electroacoustic characteristics of the hearing aid device to compensate best for the hearing deficit, special tests are conducted. Such tests may measure differences in word and speech understanding with and without the hearing aid. Another important test measures the degree of comfort or discomfort resulting from the sound level that is produced by the hearing aid device; if such a test is not performed, the patient may reject the hearing aid because it is too loud and unpleasant. Other tests designed to help determine the appropriate level of amplified sound involve narrow-band noise thresholds and various environmental sounds to which the patient may be periodically exposed during the activities of daily living. The use of environmental sound recordings provides the audiologist with objective indications of the electroacoustic responses that will yield maximum speech discrimination in the presence of specific background noises.

Audiology has helped many children and adults with hearing impairment through the use of hearing aids and the practice of aural rehabilitation. The selection and fitting of hearing aid devices have become important parts of the professional responsibilities of the clinical audiologist. With the many advances in hearing aid technology that have occurred, the audiologist has been given a much broader array of electroacoustic devices from which to select the one that offers the best correspondence with a patient's needs. For example, some commercial hearing aid systems can be digitally programmed to meet the specific acoustic requirements of the hearing-impaired individual. In some cases, programmable hearing aids provide more than one acoustic response at the immediate command of the user. Should the device fail to meet the acoustic requirements of the patient, it can be reprogrammed in a short period of time to achieve a better correlation with the patient's need for amplification.

Auditory (aural) rehabilitation is also of clinical concern to the audiologist, and a major branch of audiological practice is in this field. In this context, rehabilitation refers to the development and conduct of special programs to assist the hearing impaired in utilizing and understanding more efficiently verbal language (speech). For example, for those children born with a severe auditory deficit, the early introduction of aural rehabilitation programs is of paramount importance to the development of verbal language. Consistent with the development of rehabilitation programs is the early detection of hearing impairment that cannot be ameliorated by surgical or medical intervention. From a rehabilitative point of view, early introduction of hearing aid amplification and supportive auditory and speech-reading training programs have been of inestimable value in speech and language development for the hearing-impaired child. In some of the major school systems throughout the United States, there is an "educational audiologist" whose task it is to develop and maintain special programs intended to assist hearing-impaired children.

Equally as important are auditory rehabilitation programs for the hearing-impaired adult. Hearing impairment is a rather insidious phenomenon, gradually worsening over time. Consequently, adult patients are somewhat unaware of hearing loss until they fail to recognize enough of speech sounds to understand intended messages. When speech understanding has been degraded by hearing impairment, rehabilitative programs stress the use of hearing aid amplification and the value of speech reading. Training programs may assist the adult in learning speech-reading skills or in adapting to a hearing aid device. It is important that the audiologist be aware of attitudes or behaviors that may restrict or limit a patient's acceptance of and participation in programs designed to assist the hearing impaired.

Perspective and Prospects

Audiology, as a recognized academic discipline, originated during World War II. At that time, thousands of military personnel needed diagnostic and rehabilitative services for ear injuries incurred during active service. It was essential that an organized program be developed to meet the demand. Several military hospitals and selected universities and colleges undertook the task of developing programs to accomplish these diagnostic and rehabilitative tasks. One of the first textbooks dealing exclusively with audiological practice was authored by Dr. Hayes Newby in 1958 while he was teaching at Stanford University. Since that memorable introduction, hundreds of special texts have been published relative to various aspects of audiological practice.

Since the early pioneering days during World War II, the field of audiology and the clinical skills of audiologists have expanded appreciably. Significant advances in auditory disorder diagnosis and in prosthetic and rehabilitative care have been made. Although audiology is a relatively new academic and professional discipline, its contributions to the understanding and treatment of auditory system disorders have greatly advanced the understanding of its role in human communication.

—Robert Sandlin, Ph.D.

See also Aging; Aging: Extended care; Biophysics; Deafness; Dyslexia; Ear infections and disorders; Ear surgery; Ears; Hearing loss; Hearing tests; Ménière's disease; Motion sickness; Neurology; Neurology, pediatric; Otorhinolaryngology; Sense organs; Speech disorders.

For Further Information:

Alpiner, Jerome G., and Patricia A. McCarthy, eds. *Rehabilitative Audiology: Children and Adults*. 3d ed. Philadelphia: Lippincott Williams & Wilkins, 2000. Designed for both student and practitioner, offers information for assessing and treating hearing impaired individuals and includes the special needs of children, early identification of hearing loss, assessment and intervention with preschool and school-age children, rehabilitative assessment for the aging population, and hearing aid selection.

Gelfand, Stanley A. *Essentials of Audiology*. 2d ed. New York: Thieme, 2001. Undergraduate text covering a wide range of relevant topics, including acoustics, anatomy and physiology, sound perception, auditory disorders, and the nature of hearing impairment.

Jerger, James, ed. *Pediatric Audiology*. San Diego, Calif.: College-Hill Press, 1984. This text is devoted exclusively to explaining the various clinical tests conducted to determine the extent of hearing disorders in children. Brings together a number of distinguished authors dealing with specific aspects of pediatric audiology.

Katz, Jack, ed. *Handbook of Clinical Audiology*. 5th ed. Philadelphia: Lippincott Williams & Wilkins, 2002. Text that examines advances in the scientific, clinical, and philosophical understanding of audiology. Sections of the book cover behavioral tests, physiologic tests, special populations, and the management of hearing disorders.

Lubinski, Rosemary, and Carol M. Frattali, eds. *Professional Issues in Speech-Language Pathology and Audiology*. San Diego, Calif.: Singular/Thomson Learning, 2001. For those interested in entering the field of audiology. Covers the practicalities of a career path, ethical-legal considerations, professional organizations, and ongoing issues in health care, among other topics.

Mendel, Lisa Lucks, Jeffrey L. Danhauer, and Sadanand Singh. *Singular's Illustrated Dictionary of Audiology*. San Diego, Calif.: Singular, 1999. A comprehensive reference guide to the field that includes numerous photographs, charts, and diagrams. Appendices cover acronyms, illustrations, topic categories, and physical quantities.

Newby, Hayes, and Gerald Popelka. *Audiology*. 6th ed. Englewood Cliffs, N.J.: Prentice Hall, 1992. A well-organized introductory text on the practice of audiology. Each chapter reviews a specific aspect of audiological practice from the bases of hearing to the various audiological tests designed to yield clinical information about the normal and abnormal behavior of the human auditory system.

Auras

Disease/disorder

Anatomy or system affected: Arms, brain, ears, eyes, legs, mouth, nervous system, nose, psychic-emotional system, skin, throat

Specialties and related fields: Internal medicine, neurology, psychiatry, psychology

Definition: Warning sensations of varying kinds received by the patient prior to a seizure, migraine, or psychotic episode.

Causes and Symptoms

Causes of auras include seizures (epilepsy), drug side effects, delirium, dementia, migraines, cerebral palsy, brain cancers, convulsions, hallucinations, and the aging process. General symptoms include skin sensations and motor, vegetative, and psychological phenomena. More specific symptoms include epigastric discomfort, dizziness, faintness, and basic elementary phenomena, such as seeing brilliant dots and lines, hearing sounds, and experiencing strange and disagreeable odors. Symptoms occasionally include a "pins-and-needles" feeling on one side of the face or body, followed by numbness, or numbness without tingling. Other symptoms include speech problems, confusion, weakness on one side, mood swings, mental fuzziness, and fluid retention.

> **Information on Auras**
>
> **Causes:** Seizures, migraines, drug side effects, delirium, dementia, cerebral palsy, brain cancers, convulsions, hallucinations, aging process
>
> **Symptoms:** Skin sensations, dizziness, faintness, seeing brilliant dots and lines, hearing sounds, experiencing disagreeable odors, tingling and/or numbness, speech problems, confusion, weakness on one side, mood swings
>
> **Duration:** Temporary
>
> **Treatments:** Surgery, medications

Treatment and Therapy

Auras (seizures) are of diagnostic importance because they suggest a cerebral localization. For these sufferers, surgery of the affected brain area may bring some relief, as might the use of appropriate medication.

Migraine aura sufferers benefit from the use of several antimigraine drugs, including Inderal (propranolol) and Sansert (methysergide), as well as analgesics and ergotamines. All of the above are effective drugs in stopping a migraine attack once it has begun. The sufferers of auras related to psychosis will also benefit from the use of appropriate psychotropic medications.

Perspective and Prospects

"Aura" derives from a Greek word for breeze. The term was introduced by Galen, a Greek physician and writer of the second century B.C.E., to designate a momentary gasping sensation experienced by some patients before an epileptic attack.

Current U.S. laws permit epilepsy patients with controlled seizures to drive. Factors that significantly decrease the odds of patients with epilepsy having motor vehicle crashes due to seizures are long seizure-free intervals, reliable auras, few prior nonseizure-related accidents, and having had their antiepileptic drugs (AEDs) reduced or switched. Patients who have rare seizures without definite auras should not drive alone.

The majority of current research related to auras is in the area of seizures (epilepsy). Advances have been made in the treatment of auras through surgery and medications. Research and medical advances in the twenty-first century will help health care professionals understand better the causes of auras, refine existing treatment methods, and develop new medications and treatments.

—Carol A. Heintzelman, D.S.W.

See also Aging; Brain; Brain disorders; Cerebral palsy; Dementias; Dizziness and fainting; Epilepsy; Hallucinations; Headaches; Migraine headaches; Numbness and tingling; Psychiatric disorders; Psychosis; Seizures; Sense organs; Speech disorders.

FOR FURTHER INFORMATION:

Collin, P. H., ed. *Dictionary of Medicine*. 2d ed. Chicago: Fitzroy Dearborn, 1998.

Farley, D. "Migraine, Cluster, and Tension: Headache Misery May Yield to Proper Treatment." *FDA Consumer* 26 (September, 1992): 26-32.

Krauss, G. L., et al. "Risk Factors of Seizure-Related Motor Vehicle Crashes in Patients with Epilepsy." *Neurology* 52 (April 22, 1999): 1321-1329.

Lindgren, C. E. *Capturing the Aura: Integrating Science, Technology, and Metaphysics*. Nevada City, Calif.: Blue Dolphin, 2001.

Redlich, F. C., and D. X. Freedman. *The Theory and Practice of Psychiatry*. New York: Basic Books, 1966.

AUTISM

DISEASE/DISORDER

ALSO KNOWN AS: Autistic disorder, autism spectrum disorder, Asperger's syndrome, pervasive developmental disorder

ANATOMY OR SYSTEM AFFECTED: Brain, psychic-emotional system

SPECIALTIES AND RELATED FIELDS: Family medicine, genetics, pediatrics, pharmacology, psychiatry, speech pathology

DEFINITION: A neurodevelopmental disorder characterized by impairment in emotional expression and recognition, difficulty with social relationships, delayed and/or abnormal language and communication, and preoccupation with repetitive, stereotyped behaviors or interests.

KEY TERMS:

behavior modification: a type of psychotherapy designed to change specific problematic behaviors through punishment and reward

echolalia: verbal repetitions of the words of others, sometimes modified with each repetition

functional magnetic resonance imaging (fMRI): the use of magnetic radiology to generate fairly detailed images of brain activity during specific functional activities (such as speech or visual imagery)

mental retardation: defined as a score of 70 or less (100 is average) on standardized intelligence quotient (IQ) tests, together with significant difficulties in some or all aspects of daily adaptive functioning (such as self care, travel, and monetary exchanges)

mirror neuron system: a network of neurons in the brain that are activated equally when producing an action and when observing the production of that same action by another person; thought to comprise at least part of the neural substrate for empathy and interpersonal understanding

occupational therapy: a form of therapy that focuses on teaching basic life skills

pica: the ingestion of nonfood substances

positron emission tomography (PET): a technique that uses radioactive tracers to produce images of the brain based on metabolism and blood flow

stereotypies: ritualistic, rhythmic, repeated movements of the hands, body, or head

CAUSES AND SYMPTOMS

Autism is a lifelong neurodevelopmental disorder that is almost always diagnosed in early childhood, though mild presentations may not be diagnosed until middle childhood. According to the handbook of mental health, the American Psychiatric Association's *Diagnostic and Statistical Manual of Mental Disorders: DSM-IV-TR* (4th rev. ed., 2000), autism is diagnosed if there is evidence of qualitative impairment in both social interaction and communication, together with a marked participation or interest in restricted and repetitive behaviors or activities. Autism also typically involves delays or abnormal functioning in imaginative and symbolic play in childhood. At least one of these symptoms must have been observed prior to age three for a diagnosis of autism to be made.

In the DSM-IV-TR, autistic disorder is grouped under the general classification of pervasive developmental disorder, together with Asperger's syndrome, childhood disintegrative disorder, Rett's disorder, and "pervasive developmental disorder (not otherwise specified)." These disorders have similar symptom profiles; however, children with these diagnoses tend to demonstrate a wide range of behavioral, psychological, and physical symptoms. For this reason, practitioners often refer to "autistic spectrum disorder" in order to capture the breadth of symptom profiles and varying severity levels that are characteristic of children with autism and related disorders.

In the early twenty-first century, studies suggest that as many as 1 in 166 children are diagnosed with autism. Some researchers have argued that autism became increasingly prevalent over the course of the twentieth century, citing studies from the 1950's and 1960's that listed the incidence of autism at 4 to 5 per 10,000. However, it has also been suggested that the apparent rise in the incidence of autism simply reflects a rise in awareness of the disorder and an increase in the accuracy of the diagnostic criteria. Autism is more common in males than in females, with a ratio of approximately 4:1.

The social interactions of individuals with autism are strikingly abnormal, ranging from self-imposed social isolation to somewhat engaged but inappropriate social behavior. Typically, those with autism avoid eye contact. They also demonstrate little if any facial expressiveness, and they generally do not produce social gesturing or body language. Individuals with autism generally lack empathy; they do not smile in response to other people's expressions of happiness, nor do they attempt to comfort others in distress. While the majority of children with autism develop attachments to their parents and/or other caregivers, there is a marked aloofness and lack of social reciprocity in their interactions even with close others. In adults with autism, close friendships and romantic attachments are not common. It is often said that individuals with autism do not relate to other people as people, but rather treat people more like objects. A classic example of this is a child with autism leading an adult by the hand and then placing the adult's hand on a door, rather than verbally or gesturally requesting that the door be opened.

Language development in children with autism is almost always delayed, and between 25 and 30 percent never acquire spoken language, despite having normal hearing abilities. Those individuals with autism who do develop language often show evidence of low-level linguistic disorders such as echolalia, persistent use of neologisms, pronoun reversals, and other grammatical anomalies. The subset of individuals with autism who develop fluent speech typically demonstrate poor conversational skills, related to the general lack of social reciprocity seen in autism. Their speech is often delivered in a monotone, is repetitive, and focuses mainly on their own concerns. Autistic speakers typically show little awareness of the perspectives or interests of their listeners. Individuals with autism also show deficits in receptive communication; there is reduced attention to human voices in general, poor understanding of nonverbal language, including gesture and vocal intonation, and difficulties with nonliteral language such as metaphor and irony.

Individuals with autism demonstrate a preoccupation with restricted and repetitive behaviors, interests, and activities. This focus on repetition can take a range of forms, from performance of stereotypies to compulsive insistence on daily routines to an intense focus upon specific, narrow topics of interest. Common stereotypies seen in autistic individuals are hand flapping, head banging, or more complex whole-body movements. Autistic children sometimes engage in self-injurious behavior patterns, such as self-biting or head banging, and/or self-soothing behaviors, such as rocking or self-stroking. Some children with autism also develop pica, eating such things as paper, paperclips, or dirt. More complex ritualistic behavior patterns might include compulsive hand washing, counting, or arrangement of possessions. This aspect of autism can also include intense preoccupation with highly restricted topics, such as weather patterns, buttons, or television schedules.

Another defining characteristic included in the diagnostic criteria for autism is a lack of imaginative or pre-

Information on Autism

Causes: Unknown

Symptoms: Difficulty with social relationships, language, and communication; preoccupation with repetitive or stereotyped behaviors and interests; general resistance to changes in routine

Duration: Chronic

Treatments: Behavior modification, social skills training, speech/language therapy, occupational therapy, music therapy

tend play in childhood. This symptom may be related to the general literalness seen in autistic communication. The play of children with autism tends to be solitary and to involve the repetitive manipulation of objects. The one-sidedness of autistic children's play and their generally impaired social interactions typically result in failure to develop peer relationships appropriate to their developmental level. Children with autism are therefore often cut off from their peer groups, which can cause feelings of loneliness and depression, especially as they approach adolescence.

Up to three-quarters of children with autism are also mentally retarded, with an intelligence quotient (IQ) below 70. The mental profiles of autistic children can be uneven, however, with particularly low verbal IQ scores but normal or near-normal scores on measures of mathematical and spatial IQ.

As of the early twenty-first century, there is no known cause of autism. Risk factors include genetic relatedness, difficult birth, and comorbid disorders such as attention deficit hyperactivity disorder (ADHD) and obsessive-complusive disorder (OCD). In the 1990's, scientists investigated the claim, initially made by parents and bolstered by apparently rising rates of autism, that the measles, mumps, and rubella (MMR) vaccine, typically given around age eighteen months, caused autism in some cases. A number of thorough epidemiological studies found no evidence for a link between the MMR vaccine and autism, although some researchers suggested that the vaccine could exacerbate already-present autistic symptoms in toddlers.

Treatment and Therapy

There is no cure for autism, nor is there one single treatment. Because children with autism can display such a wide range of symptoms, the range of available treatments is also wide. Physicians, psychologists, and other health professionals focus on alleviating the symptoms that are the most disruptive to a particular individual with autism. Available treatments include behavior modification, social skills training, speech/language therapy, occupational therapy, play therapy, music therapy, dietary interventions, and medication, among others. Often a combination of these types of treatments will be used to address the therapeutic needs of an autistic individual.

One of the most successful treatments for autism has been intensive behavior modification therapy. In his book *The Autistic Child: Language Development Through Behavior Modification* (1977), Dr. O. I. Lovaas described a program of intensive one-on-one behavior modification therapy that can be highly effective in alleviating disturbing symptoms and in engendering positive social behaviors in autistic children. Lovaas's technique is controversial because it involves both rewards for appropriate behaviors, such as making eye contact or maintaining conversation, as well as punishments for inappropriate behaviors, such as self-damaging acts, stereotypies, or pica. In a well-publicized legal case in the 1990's, Massachusetts banned the use of punishment in a school for autistic children. As a result, the children's levels of self-injurious behavior increased, to the extent that the parents petitioned for punishment to be reinstated in the school's behavior modification program. While the utility of punishment is generally acknowledged, many behavior modification therapists now suggest that the positive reinforcement of rewarding appropriate behavior is effective enough that punishment for inappropriate behavior is not necessary. Despite variations in philosophy and technique, behavior modification aimed at increasing social responsiveness and decreasing inappropriate behaviors is generally an essential component of therapy for autistic children.

Social skills training is used to encourage individuals with autism to adhere to the implicit rules of conversation and social interaction (for example, looking at people's faces when speaking to them). Occupational therapy focuses on teaching skills that allow individuals with autism to participate in daily life: crossing a street, preparing simple meals, making purchases, and answering the telephone. Play therapy involves entering the world of the autistic individual—in the case of children, spending "floor time" with them to break through their aloofness. Music therapy has been used to draw emotional responses from children with autism, with varied levels of success. Dietary interventions have also been found to alleviate some of the symptoms of autism in certain cases.

No drug is specifically prescribed for autism; however, various medications are sometimes used to treat the symptoms of autism. Stimulant drugs may be used to treat the inattentiveness of autistic children who are particularly isolated and unresponsive. Tranquilizing drugs may be prescribed to manage obsessive-compulsive behaviors that are disruptive to normal functioning. Antidepressant drugs are also sometimes prescribed for autistic children to heighten emotional responsiveness and/or to stabilize mood. As many as one-third of children with autism develop seizures, often in adolescence, that are similar to epileptic seizures. These seizures are usually treated with medication.

Outcomes for individuals with autism depend on the severity of their symptoms. Autistic individuals with mild impairments can live at home, participate in family and social life, go to mainstream schools, and eventually take on appropriate paid work. In fact, some highly repetitive occupations, such as shelving books in a library or entering computer data, may fit extremely well with the desires and talents of individuals with autism. Those with more profound autistic symptoms or significant mental retardation may go to special schools, participate in remedial programs, or live in special residential facilities. Whatever the setting, individuals with autism respond most positively to a highly structured environment in which the other people are understanding and tolerant of their social and communicative abnormalities.

Parents, siblings, and friends of individuals with autism may also benefit from therapy. Life with an autistic person can be rewarding, especially when progress is made, but it can also be frustrating and depressing. Often the parents, siblings, and friends of children with autism, as well as professionals working with such children, feel rejected by the autistic tendency to avoid close social contact. Most professionals suggest that anyone who spends extended periods of time with an individual with autism will benefit from some form of training and/or emotional support.

Perspective and Prospects

Though it is likely to be an old syndrome, autism was first described in the 1940's. Dr. Leo Kanner in the United States and Dr. Hans Asperger in Austria independently published papers describing children with severe social and communicative impairments. Both Kanner and Asperger used the term "autism" (meaning "alone") to describe the syndromes they had identified. Kanner described children who had impoverished social relationships from early in life, employed deviant language, and were subject to behavioral stereotypies. Asperger's description identified children with normal IQ's and normal language development who suffered from social and some types of communicative impairments. As of the early twenty-first century, there is ongoing controversy as to whether autism and Asperger's syndrome represent two ends of a single spectrum disorder or whether individuals with Asperger's syndrome constitute a distinct clinical group.

In his original report, Kanner observed that the parent-child relationships in cases of children with autism appeared to be somewhat unusual. This suggestion fit with the tenor of the times, in which psychology and psychiatry were dominated by Freudian theories. Thus early explanations of autism, now discredited, suggested that children developed the syndrome as a result of cold, abusive, or confusing home environments (references were made to "refrigerator mothers"), and early treatments of autism focused on improving parent-child relationships or removing children with autism from their home environments.

In the early twenty-first century, work on autism has focused on the physiological and cognitive aspects of the disorder. Brain studies utilizing functional magnetic resonance imaging (fMRI) and positron emission tomography (PET) scanning have uncovered several abnormalities in the brains of individuals with autism, including larger than normal brains, and abnormal functioning in the areas thought to be responsible for social interactions. In particular, the structure and functioning of the mirror neuron system, hypothesized to be the structural substrate for empathy, have been shown to be abnormal in individuals with autism. Cognitive studies into autism have suggested that the perceptual and reasoning proclivities of individuals with autism are abnormal. One hypothesis is that autistic individuals' minds are characterized "weak central coherence," such that they prefer to focus on details and parts rather than on global wholes, leading to the tendency to focus on concrete minutia while avoiding complex and dynamic human interaction. Another hypothesis is that individuals with autism lack a "theory of mind," which results in an inability to consider others' emotions, perspectives, desires, and thoughts.

—*Virginia Slaughter, Ph.D.*

See also Anxiety; Asperger's syndrome; Bonding; Cognitive development; Developmental stages; Learning disabilities; Mental retardation; Neuroimaging; Psychiatric disorders; Psychiatry; Psychiatry, child and adolescent; Speech disorders.

For Further Information:

Autism Society of America. http://www.autism-society.org/. A leading source of information and referral on autism, focusing on access and opportunity for all individuals within the autism spectrum, education, advocacy at state and federal levels, active public awareness, and the promotion of research.

Frith, Uta. *Autism: Explaining the Enigma*. 2d ed. New York: Blackwell Science, 2003. This book, by one of the world's leading researchers into autism, provides an overview of current knowledge and scientific research on the behavioral, cognitive, and brain characteristics of individuals with autism.

Greenspan, Stanley and Serena Wieder. *Engaging Autism: Using the Floortime Approach to Help Children Relate, Communicate, and Think.* Cambridge, Mass.: Da Capo Press, 2006. This book highlights the positive, potentially productive side of autism and outlines a program for engaging individuals with autism in social interactions.

Happe, Francesca. *Autism: An Introduction to Psychological Theory.* London: UCL Press, 1994. This readable book gives an historical overview of autism and presents various theories that have been proposed to explain the disorder, including the "weak central coherence" and "theory of mind" hypotheses.

Park, Clara. *The Siege: The First Eight Years of An Autistic Child, With an Epilogue, Fifteen Years Later, Vol. 1.* New York: Little, Brown, 1991. A compelling and poetic personal story of a parent's experience with autism.

Autoimmune disorders

Disease/disorder

Anatomy or system affected: All

Specialties and related fields: All

Definition: Damage to the tissues or organs of the body caused by failure of the immune system to distinguish between "self" and "nonself," producing autoantibodies or autoreactive T lymphocytes (T cells).

Key terms:

allele: a specific variation of a gene in deoxyribonucleic acid (DNA); many genes have only two alleles (usually referred to as dominant and recessive), while other genes may have one hundred or more alleles

antibody: a molecule of the immune system, produced by B cells and targeted toward eliminating a specific antigen

antigen: a protein or related molecule that is seen as foreign and therefore induces antibody formation in an individual

autoantibody: an antibody which binds to a protein that is a normal part of the human body from which it originates (as opposed to part of a bacteria, virus, or another human being)

B cells: also known as B lymphocytes; the antibody-producing cells of the immune system

multigenic: referring to a trait or characteristic that requires the product of more than one gene in order to be activated

selection: the process by which developing immune system cells are either allowed to continue to maturation or destroyed before they can enter the circulation

T cells: also known as T lymphocytes; the immune system cells involved in cellular immunity and regulation of the immune response

tolerance: the ability of the immune system to remain unresponsive to self antigens

Information on Autoimmune Disorders

Causes: Unknown, possibly hereditary, environmental, or viral

Symptoms: Varies widely; may include pain, fatigue, joint and muscle inflammation, muscle weakness, sleep disturbances, headaches, numbness and tingling, central nervous system disturbances

Duration: Often chronic

Treatments: Alleviation of symptoms, strengthening the immune system

Causes and Symptoms

Autoimmunity refers to a group of widely varying diseases or disorders that include familiar examples (Type I diabetes mellitus, myasthenia gravis, multiple sclerosis, rheumatoid arthritis) and many that are not as familiar (idiopathic thrombocytopenic purpura, Graves' disease, Felty's disease, Hashimoto's thyroiditis). The list is long (see figure 1, p. 237) and growing as researchers continue to ferret out the root causes of many disorders that have been known for one hundred years or more. In many cases, environmental triggers or environmentally controlled flare-ups are common (see figure 2, p. 238). All have one thing in common: the failure of the human immune system to distinguish between self (own) and nonself antigens, thus leading the body to attack itself and destroy tissues or organs.

Autoimmunity is not a rare event; it occurs in all people, and it does not necessarily give rise to disease. For instance, aged or damaged cells of the body are normally destroyed by autoantibodies (antibodies directed against self). However, other autoantibodies, which arise by chance combinations of genes, are normally suppressed during development in the thymus gland. This is referred to as selection. If the thymus fails to do its job, then these autoantibodies may be released into the lymph nodes and into the bloodstream, seeking out tissue or antigens to attack and destroy.

Autoimmune disorders can be classified in several ways. Some diseases affect only one organ system (organ-specific), and some affect multiple systems. Examples of organ-specific disorders are Addison's disease and Graves' disease; non-organ-specific disorders include systemic lupus erythematosus and scleroderma. Alternatively, one can classify autoimmune disorders by the type of immune system cells involved in their onset. Some diseases are caused by the antibody-secreting B cells; they include myasthenia gravis, multiple sclerosis, rheumatic fever, systemic lupus erythematosis, and Graves' disease. Other disorders are the result of the action of the systemic T cells; they include Addison's disease and Hashimoto's thyroiditis.

The onset of an autoimmune disorder hinges on many factors, some of which are still being identified. It is well established, however, that autoimmunity is multifactorial and multigenic. In other words, many environmental factors and many genes are involved in determining susceptibility to autoimmune disorders. In addition, many environmental factors are thought to be involved in controlling remission and flare-ups of autoimmune disorders. Most autoimmune disorders are probably the result of the release of T or B cells that, because they did not properly distinguish between self and nonself, should have been suppressed by the body's immune system but were not. Some autoimmune responses are a result of damage to, or tumors of, the immune system tissues (lymphatic system).

A variety of studies in recent years have established genetic links in autoimmune diseases, but because most are multigenic, there is no simple Mendelian inheritance pattern seen. Nonetheless, there seems to be a clear correlation between certain human leukocyte antigen (HLA) genes and certain autoimmune disorders. For instance, those who have HLA allele B27 have a ninetyfold greater risk than the normal population for developing ankylosing spondylitis. Those with allele DR3 have a twelvefold greater risk of celiac disease and a tenfold greater risk of Sjögren's disease. In the case of insulin-dependent diabetes, the relative risk factor is fivefold if one has the DR3 allele or the DR4 allele, but if both are present then the risk jumps to twentyfold. If the DR3 and DQw8 alleles are present, then the risk factor is one hundredfold. Yet, these alleles themselves do not automatically cause autoimmune disease, as evidenced by several studies on identical twins, where the rate of disease in the twin of an affected person ranges from 25 to 50 percent. Clearly environmental factors can change susceptibility to autoimmune disease into actual manifestation.

Autoimmune disorders are much more common in women than in men. In addition, they are usually more severe in women. This is likely due to the effects of estrogen, which has a role in enhancing the expression of HLA genes and activating macrophages, thus leading to higher tissue destruction. Some autoimmune responses are noted to flare and subside throughout the menstrual cycle, in conjunction with the rise and fall of estrogen levels. Stress has also been shown to be a contributing factor that can cause an autoimmune disorder to flare. This response is likely mediated through the hypothalamus and pituitary glands, which release hormones that directly stimulate the immune system.

It has been known for many years that expression of some autoimmune diseases is preceded by infection by a virulent organism. Infections may contribute to autoimmunity in several ways. Some microbes produce antigens that are very close in structure to human antigens. When antibodies are produced against the invading organism, the antibodies also attack self-antigens because of the chemical similarity. Examples of this response are poststreptococcal glomerulonephritis and rheumatic fever. Other invaders may damage human cells and release proteins that are not normally seen by the immune system (sequestered proteins). These proteins are seen as foreign, and an immune response is set up against these self-antigens (a similar response may be seen when normally sequestered proteins are released through trauma or injury). An example is sympathetic ophthalmia, in which eye lens proteins that are normally not seen in the circulation are released, triggering antibodies that may then attack the opposite (uninjured) eye as well.

The symptoms of autoimmune disorders are as varied as the disorders themselves. No one set of symptoms fits all disorders. Symptoms may be systemic or localized, progressive or stable. Symptoms may also be life-threatening or simply annoying.

Multiple sclerosis (MS) is an autoimmune disorder involving the central nervous system. Nerve axons of the white matter of the brain are normally surrounded by myelin protein sheaths that protect the nerves and speed the process of transmission. In individuals with MS, these myelin sheath proteins are gradually attacked and destroyed, slowing transmission so that patients develop a loss of control of motor function and vision. This disease often progresses irregularly and unpredictably and is irreversible. It appears to be the result of both B cells (producing antibodies against oligodendroglia, the cells that make myelin protein) and T cells (acting against a peptide product from the myelin protein). Although what triggers the initial response is unclear, it has been suggested that onset may follow infection with either Epstein-Barr or hepatitis B virus. More than 2.5 million people worldwide are affected by MS, mostly women diagnosed between age twenty and fifty.

Systemic lupus erythematosus (SLE), known simply as lupus, is a generalized disorder that occurs predominantly in women. It is clearly linked to B cells and the production of antibodies against parts of the DNA molecule. These DNA antibodies cause tissue damage by combining with free DNA (from cells that have been damaged through disease or the normal aging process), and they may form immune complexes that are deposited in the kidneys and arterioles, leading to tissue destruction and fibrosis, and in the joints, leading to arthritis. Autoantibodies against red blood cells or platelets may also be found in SLE. Antibodies against muscles may be present and contribute to muscle inflammation, while the presence of antibodies to heart muscle may lead to myocarditis and endocarditis. Antibodies against skin components lead to a characteristic "butterfly rash" on the bridge of the nose and the area around the eyes seen in many patients with SLE; this rash worsens in the presence of sunlight.

Rheumatoid arthritis is a common, crippling disease. It is controlled by B cells in the joints that are activated to produce several antibodies, including rheumatoid factor. The result is the formation and deposition of im-

FIGURE 1. PARTIAL LIST OF AUTOIMMUNE DISEASES

Disease	*Organ/Target*
Addison's disease	Adrenal glands
Ankylosing spondylitis	Spine
Antiphospholipid antibody syndrome	Blood clotting
Celiac disease	Small intestine
Crohn's disease	Gastrointestinal tract
Diabetes mellitus Type I (some forms)	Pancreas islet cells
Felty's disease	Joints and spleen
Goodpasture's syndrome	Kidneys and lungs
Graves' disease	Thyroid gland
Guillain-Barré syndrome	Peripheral nervous system
Hashimoto's thyroiditis	Thyroid gland
Hemolytic anemia	Red blood cells, platelets
Multiple sclerosis	Brain and spinal cord
Myasthenia gravis	Junctions between nerves and muscles
Pemphigus vulgaris	Skin and mucus membranes
Pernicious anemia	Stomach parietal cells
Polymyositis	Skeletal muscle
Poststreptococcal glomerulonephritis	Kidneys
Psoriasis	Skin
Rheumatic fever	Heart
Rheumatoid arthritis	Connective tissue and joints
Scleroderma	Heart, lungs, kidney, gastrointestinal tract
Sjőgren's syndrome	Saliva and tear glands
Systemic lupus erythematosus	DNA, platelets, all organs
Thrombocytopenic purpura	Platelets
Wegener's granulomatosis	Lungs and kidneys

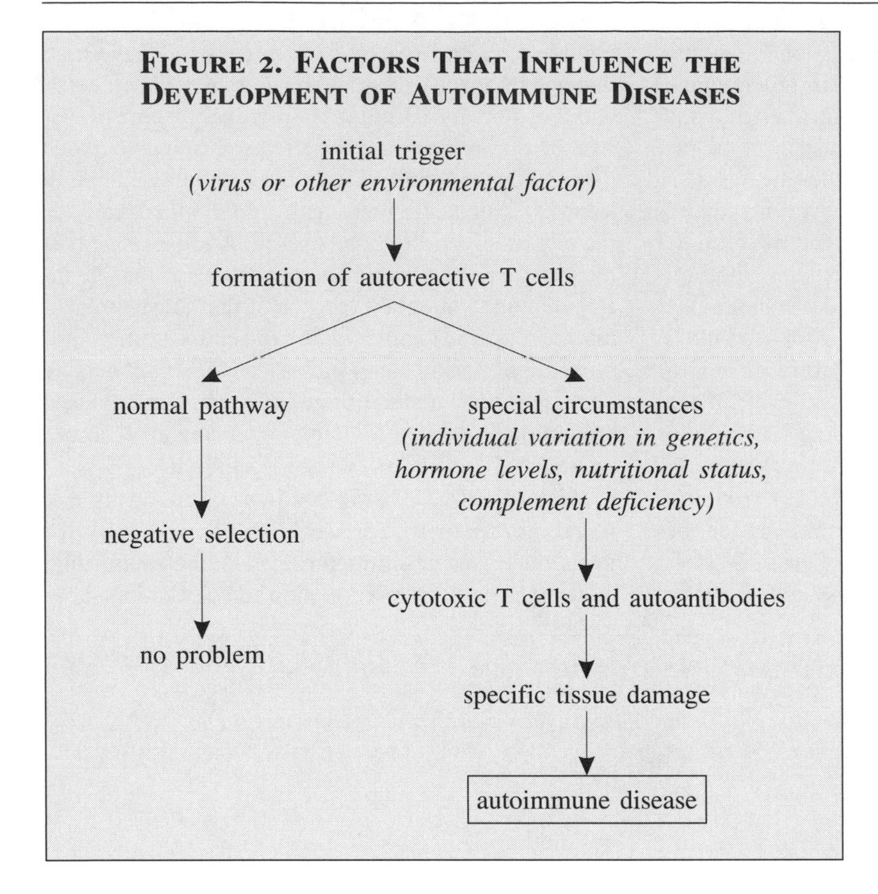

FIGURE 2. FACTORS THAT INFLUENCE THE DEVELOPMENT OF AUTOIMMUNE DISEASES

mune complexes in the joint cartilage. Antibodies directed against cartilage may also be seen. The resulting destruction activates chemicals that stimulate T cells to come to the area, and they in turn release destructive enzymes, just as they would if bacteria were invading the joints. All these responses lead to joint damage, inflammation, and pain. As the disease progresses, the synovia swell and extend into the joints, causing further pain and discomfort along with disfigurement of the joints. The cause of antibody activation is unknown and may be quite variable.

Both Hashimoto's thyroiditis and Graves' disease are forms of autoimmune thyroiditis. In Hashimoto's disease, antibodies are formed against a protein within the thyroid cells, leading to attack of the cells and destruction of much of the thyroid tissue. In Graves' disease, antibodies are formed that bind to the receptors for thyroid-stimulating hormone (TSH), the pituitary hormone that stimulates the thyroid gland to produce thyroid hormone. The receptors in turn are stimulated. Thus, the thyroid gland is hyperstimulated, and excess thyroid hormone is turned out, a condition known as thyrotoxicosis.

An individual with myasthenia gravis experiences muscle fatigue and extreme weakness with only mild exercise (such as walking short distances). It is caused by autoantibodies that are directed against the acetylcholine (ACh) receptor molecule. In normal neural cells that control large muscles, ACh is stimulated to be released from the neuron and bind to receptors on the muscle fiber end plate. If that receptor is blocked or destroyed by an antibody, the ACh cannot bind, and therefore the muscle is not stimulated to respond (contract). If a few receptors are blocked, then the muscle may still respond weakly. If enough antibody is present to block a large number of receptors, however, then the threshold limit for muscle response will not be achieved and the muscle will not respond even in the presence of repeated stimulation from the neuron.

Scleroderma, also known as progressive systemic sclerosis, predominantly affects middle-aged women and is caused by collagen deposition in a variety of tissues of the body. Antibodies may be found against the centromere portion of the DNA. Symptoms include calcium deposition in the skin, sensitivity to cold, and decreased esophageal motility. The lungs often experience fibrosis, as do the kidneys, leading to death from kidney failure in nearly half of all patients.

TREATMENT AND THERAPY

Most autoimmune disorders cannot be cured; they develop into chronic conditions that require a lifetime of care and monitoring. Treatment is quite varied and depends on the underlying cause and etiology of the disease. Overall, the goals of treatment are to reduce the symptoms and to control the disease or disorder while at the same time allowing the immune system to continue fighting the viruses and bacteria affecting the body on a daily basis. The most generalized treatment is the administration of immunosuppressive drugs. The most commonly used drugs are azathioprine and cyclophosphamide; corticosteroids are also used to reduce the inflammatory responses seen in many autoimmune disorders. Drugs such as methotrexate have gained wide acceptance in the treatment of rheumatoid arthritis and other autoimmune disorders, but they have systemic side effects that in some cases may be worse than the autoimmune disorder itself (such as suppression of the basic immune responses involved in fighting off everyday viruses and bacteria). While the doses used to fight autoimmunity are much lower than those used to suppress organ graft rejection, these general effects may still be seen, especially in older individuals whose immune systems are declining as a result of age. Thus, a significant amount of effort has been put into finding drugs that will be able to suppress only the self-reactive antibodies and not the entire immune system.

Hormones, proteins, or other substances normally produced or secreted by the cells or organs damaged in autoimmune disease (such as thyroid hormone or insulin) can usually be supplemented to the point that they are within the proper physiologic range. Sometimes this works well. For instance, Graves' disease can be effectively controlled by removing the overactive thyroid gland and then supplementing thyroid hormone in the patient. Treating Type I diabetes in children by supplementing insulin, however, is a much trickier proposition, as the finely controlled release of insulin from the beta cells of the pancreas cannot be duplicated by a single injection.

Many investigators have worked on vaccinations to autoimmune disorders, using animal models of varying types. Some results have been promising, even if the mechanism of action is still mostly unexplained. Vaccinations against autoimmune thyroiditis, encephalitis, and arthritis have been successful in some animal models.

Another approach that has been tried experimentally is the use of oral tolerance therapy. Large quantities of the offending autoantigen are given to the patient in the hope that tolerance to the particular protein will develop. This approach is similar to the way in which desensitization is used with allergy sufferers. Oral doses of myelin, for instance, have shown some success as a treatment for patients with multiple sclerosis.

Perspective and Prospects

The history of human understanding of autoimmune disorders is quite short. Paul Ehrlich, early in the twentieth century, described a condition of "horror autotoxicus," the attack of the human immune system against self tissues. His studies set the stage for fairly rapid advancement in understanding of the human immune system. Understanding of the genetic and molecular basis for autoimmunity, however, along with the realization that autoimmunity is a normal part of immune system development, began in the 1980's mainly as a result of the development of genetic and biochemical tools that allowed new insights into the cause of symptoms that were established long ago. Even where the cause was well established (such as with insulin-dependent diabetes, established in the 1920's), no significant changes in treatment were made until new genetic tools became available. Indeed, the entire field of immunology, which until the 1970's was in its infancy as a medical field, has grown exponentially as new molecular tools have enabled researchers to elucidate the pathways by which autoimmunity exacts its toll.

There is still plenty to do, both in terms of determining pathways and in developing new therapies aimed at specific targeting of these pathways. With completion of the Human Genome Project, an incredible amount of new knowledge is available that will help researchers produce treatments that are much more targeted and specific than those used in the past. As more is learned about the immune system and pathways of inflammation, new therapies may be designed that will prevent the development of most autoimmune diseases.

—Kerry L. Cheesman, Ph.D.

See also Amyotrophic lateral sclerosis; Anemia; Arthritis; Asthma; Chronic fatigue syndrome; Diabetes mellitus; Immune system; Immunodeficiency disorders; Immunology; Multiple chemical sensitivity syndrome; Multiple sclerosis; Myasthenia gravis; Reiter's syndrome; Rheumatic fever; Rheumatoid arthritis; Scleroderma; Sjögren's syndrome; Systemic lupus erythematosus (SLE); Thyroid disorders.

For Further Information:

Abbas, Abul K., and Andrew K. Lichtman. *Basic Immunology: Functions and Disorders of the Immune System*. 2d ed. Philadelphia: Elsevier Saunders, 2006. An easy-to-read introduction to the human immune system. Includes excellent figures and a thorough glossary.

American Autoimmune Related Diseases Association (AARDA). http://www.aarda.org/. A site that provides information on a range of autoimmune disorders, a section on women and autoimmunity, a newsletter, and links to resources, among other features.

Feldmann, Marc, Fionula M. Brennan, and Ravinder N. Maini. "Rheumatoid Arthritis." *Cell* 85, no. 3

(May 3, 1996): 307-310. A well-written but technical look at this particular autoimmune disease.

Janeway, Charles A., Jr., et al. *Immunobiology: The Immune System in Health and Disease*. 6th ed. New York: Garland Science, 2005. A classic undergraduate text on immunology, containing a well-written and thorough chapter on autoimmunity and transplantation.

Life, Death, and the Immune System. New York: W. H. Freeman, 1994. An easy-to-read special issue of *Scientific American*. Includes a helpful chapter on autoimmune disease.

National Institute of Allergy and Infectious Diseases (NIAID). National Institutes of Health. http://www.niaid.nih.gov/publications/autoimmune.htm. This Web site contains free, easy-to-read pamphlets on autoimmune disorders for those needing basic information.

Pines, Maya, ed. *Arousing the Fury of the Immune System: New Ways to Boost the Body's Defenses*. Chevy Chase, Md.: Howard Hughes Medical Institute, 1998. A free report that outlines new developments in the fight to understand and control the human immune system.

Steinman, Lawrence. "Multiple Sclerosis: A Coordinated Immunological Attack Against Myelin in the Central Nervous System." *Cell* 85, no. 3 (May 3, 1996): 299-302. A well-written but technical look at this particular autoimmune disease.

Walport, M. J., et al. "Complement Deficiency and Autoimmunity." *Annals of the New York Academy of Sciences* 815 (April, 1997): 267-281. A review of knowledge related to the role of the complement system in autoimmunity. Fairly technical.

AUTOPSY

PROCEDURE

ANATOMY OR SYSTEM AFFECTED: All

SPECIALTIES AND RELATED FIELDS: Biochemistry, forensic medicine, histology, microbiology, pathology

DEFINITION: The postmortem (after-death) examination of a body in order to determine the cause of death; it involves both a systematic, orderly inspection of the external and internal structures of the body systems and a chemical and microbiological analysis of visceral contents.

KEY TERMS:

anatomic pathologist: a doctor who is especially concerned with the study of the structural and functional changes in tissues and organs that cause or are caused by disease; this doctor performs autopsies

coroner: an officer, often a layperson, who holds inquests in regard to violent, sudden, or unexplained deaths

diener: a person who assists the pathologist in the morgue and at the autopsy

forensic autopsy: a systematic investigation to determine the cause of death, providing the pathologist with information to state an informed opinion about the manner and mechanism of death in cases that are of public interest

gross pathology: that which is visible to the naked eye, or "macroscopic," during inspection

histopathology: the histologic or microscopic description of abnormal pathologic tissue changes; these changes can be seen under the microscope

morgue: a place, usually cooled, where dead bodies are temporarily kept, pending proper identification, autopsy, or burial

THE FUNDAMENTALS OF PATHOLOGY

Translated literally, pathology is the study (*logos*) of suffering (*pathos*). As a science, pathology focuses on the study of the structural and functional consequences of injury on cells, tissues, and organs and ultimately the consequences on the entire organism (that is, the patient). Oftentimes, cells and fragments of tissues are obtained surgically from living patients; this procedure, called biopsy, is for the purpose of evaluating the nature and extent of injury. The results of a biopsy help direct the treatment. Autopsy, by contrast, is performed to examine the dead body and the internal organs systematically, in order to determine why the patient died.

Four aspects of a disease process form the core of pathology and are searched for diligently during autopsy studies. These are etiology, or cause; pathogenesis, the mechanism of development of disease; morphologic changes, the structural alterations induced in cells, tissues, and organs of the body; and clinical significance, the functional consequences of these morphologic changes.

There are two major classes of etiologic causation factors: genetic and acquired. Examples of acquired factors are infections, physical trauma, chemical injury and poisoning, nutritional factors, and radiation and solar injury (sunburn). When an autopsy is performed, this etiology is sought, but it has been acknowledged that the classic concept of one cause leading to one disease—developed largely from the discovery of specific infectious agents as the causes of specific diseases—is no longer sufficient. More often than not, multiple factors are acting at once. Genetic factors also affect environmentally induced diseases: For example, not all alcoholic patients develop significant liver disease (cirrhosis). Conversely, environment may have a profound influence on genetically induced disease: For example, not all individuals with the chemical and genetic markers for gout will develop that disease. During autopsies, systematic samplings of blood, body fluids, and tissues are taken in order to test for microbial causes and often chemical causes.

Pathogenesis refers to the sequence of events in the cells and organs that results from injury, from the initial responses to the ultimate expression of disease. It has become clear, for example, that many events at the subcellular and molecular levels are interacting and taking shape long before a disease becomes clinically observable. For example, the virus that causes acquired immunodeficiency syndrome (AIDS) destroys lymphocytes (special white blood cells) and causes a gradual loss of immunity in the body long before AIDS becomes clinically observable as a disease.

Morphologic changes are the structural and associated functional alterations in cells, tissues, and organs that are characteristic of a disease process. They are directly observed at the autopsy table by "gross" or "macroscopic" inspection of the body and organs and later by "microscopic" or histologic study of tissue samples removed from these organs. These morphologic studies can be carried out in extreme detail using the electron microscope (ultrastructural studies) and immunologic or even genetic and molecular analysis. In forensic medicine, deoxyribonucleic acid (DNA) evidence is at times used as a definitive "thumbprint" of specific genetic makeup and can be obtained from even a few hairs.

The nature of these morphologic changes and their distribution in different organs influence normal function and determine the observed clinical features—the signs and symptoms of disease, such as fever and pain—and the disease's course and outcome. Thus, the clinical significance of these alterations can be used to assess the cause of death.

PROCEDURES AND TECHNIQUES

Autopsies are performed for several generally recognized purposes, which are closely related. Medical autopsies are performed to improve the diagnosis of disease and to help the practicing or treating physician avoid repeating errors in diagnosis and therapy; it has been repeatedly shown that autopsies contribute to improvements in medical care. The College of American Pathologists (CAP) has stressed the importance and necessity of the autopsy as a service to both the medical community and the public, recognizing it as a useful medical procedure performed by a qualified physician to assess the quality of patient care and evaluate clinical diagnostic accuracy. The autopsy is also a valuable tool for determining the effectiveness and impact of treatment modalities, discovering and defining new and/or changing diseases (as in AIDS), increasing the understanding of biological processes of disease (pathogenesis), and augmenting clinical and basic research. Information gathered from autopsies is used to provide accurate public health and vital statistical information and education as it relates to disease. Finally, the autopsy is used for obtaining legal, factual information.

In the United States, permission to perform an autopsy must be granted. A legal action can arise when the autopsy consent has not been obtained or when it has not been obtained from the proper person. The statutes of individual states usually establish who can consent to the autopsy. In general, a surviving spouse has first priority for authorizing an autopsy, and in the absence of the spouse, the next of kin has legal custody of the body and the right to authorize an autopsy. Some statutes indicate that whoever assumes custody of the body for burial may give permission for autopsy.

At large medical centers, there usually is an autopsy service, the director of which is a qualified anatomic pathologist. At times, there is also a perinatal pathologist, an anatomic pathologist specializing in the pathology of newly born babies. House officers who are medical doctors-in-training often assist in performing the autopsies. The autopsy suite is a well-equipped theater usually in close proximity to the morgue and is served by a diener.

Thus the usual autopsy is performed by professional pathologists. After carefully examining the body as a whole and recording its various attributes, the pathologist makes a surgical incision to allow for the detailed inspection of the body cavities and the organ systems, looking for gross abnormalities. Every organ is thus examined, measured, and weighed and its description recorded. Sampled sections of the organs are then taken for histologic studies, and samples of blood and other body contents may be taken for microbiologic and chemical studies.

The objectives of the autopsy will vary among institutions and even among cases within an institution. For example, an academic institution with a training program in pathology, a private hospital without a training program, and a medical examiner's office might be expected to approach a specific autopsy with very different objectives. Nevertheless, a minimum basic and standard level of examination, description, and tissue sampling is usually done. Photography is also used to document the gross findings.

Histologic study of the tissue samples is completed, and the results of microbiologic and chemical analysis are obtained. After the patient's record is carefully reviewed and all the findings are correlated, often in consultation with the decedent's treating physician, a final document, the autopsy report, is produced.

In many autopsies, the basic gross, histologic, chemical, and microscopic examination will be inadequate to resolve fully all questions raised by the circumstances of the patient's clinical course and death. The ability to carry out additional studies may then become critical to resolving these questions. Ancillary studies to which pathologists may resort include injections of substances into blood vessels to observe blockages (angiography), chromosomal studies, toxicology, X-ray defractions, and histochemical procedures. The results of these studies are also recorded in the final autopsy report.

Two standard techniques are generally used to perform autopsies. They differ from each other in the order in which the organs are removed and in whether single organs or intact organ systems are removed from the body. In Virchow's technique, organs are removed one by one. Originally, the first step was to expose the cranial cavity, the spinal cord, and the thoracic, cervical, and abdominal organs, in that order. This technique, with some modifications, is still widely used. In Rokitansky's technique, the dissection is initially carried out in situ (before the removal) and then combined with en bloc removal. This technique is often modified when used in medical centers, where the en bloc removal of the cervical, thoracic, and abdominal organs is done. Dissection of the various organ systems is performed after removal.

Another technique, Potter's technique, is often used in pediatric autopsies. The external examination, particularly of fetuses and newborns, concentrates on the search for congenital malformations; the face, ears, or hands may reveal characteristic symptoms of a disorder, such as with Down syndrome. The placenta and umbilical cord must be studied in all autopsies for fetuses and newborns.

Few autopsies offer more difficulties than postoperative cases, in which death has occurred during or shortly after a surgical operation. The pathologist must evaluate his or her findings in the light of their medicolegal implications, such as complications from surgical intervention, anesthesia, or drug administration. At times, obtaining permission to conduct an autopsy may require certain restrictions in its performance. In such restricted autopsies, access can be confined to only the chest or abdomen, or to the reopening of surgical wounds.

Medicolegal autopsies are best carried out by forensic pathologists, who must first ascertain that death has, in fact, occurred. (Failure to do so has, on occasion, led to embarrassment and serious repercussions.) Not all medicolegal autopsies deal with violent or unnatural deaths. Generally, more than half of all cases investigated by the office of the chief medical examiner in New York are deaths from natural causes that occur suddenly, unexpectedly, or in an unusual manner. Coronary heart disease (heart attacks) and respiratory infections (pneumonias) are the most common causes of death in such cases, and the greatest incidence is in persons forty-five to fifty-five years of age. Strenuous physical or emotional activity may bring about a heart attack in a patient with undetected but severe narrowing of the coronary vessels.

When a crime is suspected, evaluation of the circumstances of death and investigation of the scene where the body was found may be crucial. The position of the body, the distribution of the blood lost by the victim or the assailant, or objects found in the vicinity may offer important clues. Identification of the body can be a complex issue, especially with mutilated or decomposed bodies, and may involve X-ray and dental studies, as well as detailed studies of body contents and hair samples.

Estimation of the time of death is another concern of the forensic pathologist; at times, this can be determined very simply by the circumstantial evidence. For example, when, after a rainy night, the ground under the body is found to be dry, death probably occurred before the onset of rain. More often, however, the time of death is estimated from physical or chemical measurements of values whose rate of postmortem change has been found to be rather constant, such as body temperature or the chemical analysis of certain body and blood constituents. These methods can be useful for short postmortem intervals. For longer intervals, a determination of the level of potassium in the vitreous humor (a gelatinous fluid in the eyeball) is fairly reliable.

Special procedures are used by the forensic pathologist to investigate questions related to criminal abortion, vehicular and aircraft accidents, air embolism, decompression sickness, drowning, exposure to elements, gunshot wounds, rape, and infanticide (in which the main objective is to decide whether the infant was born alive or was a stillbirth).

Toxicologic autopsies, in which poisoning is suspected, are also the responsibility of the forensic pathologist. The sampling of tissues, especially from the brain, liver, lung, kidneys, fat, hair, fingernails, and stomach contents, is done, and samples are also collected from urine, blood, bile, and the vitreous humor of the eyeball. The list of possible poisons and drugs that can be abused is endless, and the investigation of which poison may be the cause of death is both an art and a science.

PERSPECTIVE AND PROSPECTS

The field of pathology is, next to therapeutics (the study of medicinal substances), the oldest division of the healing arts because it is the study of disease itself. Its historical development can be broadly sketched in five different periods, each one highlighted by a fundamental change in the concept of the "seat of disease." An examination of the steps by which pathology has reached its present state provides a useful perspective on the subject.

At the dawn of history, primitive humans believed that there was only a single disease, one that could produce disturbances as varied as headaches, blood vomit, epilepsy, or the death of mother and child during labor. While, in some of those cases, there were apparent causes of death, the real causes were thought to be hidden and supernatural. Thus, the concept of disease was not localized to any specific organ or even to a war wound or broken bone.

The idea of "humors" soon took over. It began in ancient Egypt, was well articulated by the Greeks, and came to dominate medical thought in the Western world up to the Renaissance. The humoral theory of disease proposes that illness is the result of disturbance in the equilibrium between four qualities (hot, cold, wet, and dry) and four elements (air, water, fire, and earth) to affect four body constituents (blood, yellow bile, black bile, and phlegm). This theory was championed by such intellectual giants as Aristotle, Pythagoras, and even Hippocrates and was fine-tuned by Galen in the second century.

The theory of the "equilibrium of humors" implies that disease affects not the entire organism but only such fluids, or humors, indicated by the specific disease. Thus a man has jaundice because of an imbalance of his humors caused by an excess of yellow bile, an excess resulting from the winds blowing in the wrong direction. One disease had become many diseases, with specific seats within the body, but these seats were not subject to anatomic evaluation.

The study of anatomy and gross pathology (that is, autopsy) became generalized in the sixteenth century, and it sounded the death knell for humoral pathology. Antonio Benivieni (1443-1502) is rightfully considered the founder of gross pathology. He is the first physician who performed autopsies, and his medical text appears to be the first to deal with anatomic and gross changes in different organs in relation to clinical symptoms. He worked in the same hospital in Florence, Italy, where the great anatomist Leonardo da Vinci conducted his anatomic dissections. His book contains the protocols for fifteen autopsies performed to ascertain the cause of death, or the seat of disease. Also of great significance in this period is the work of Jean-François Fernel (1497-1558), from Paris, whose book *Medicina* (1554) was divided into three parts: physiology, pathology, and therapeutics. The section on pathology contains 120 chapters and separates diseases into special groups, with brief autopsy presentations for clinical correlation.

The seventeenth century saw the emergence of a small group of physicians who collected the accounts of all available experiences and published them in enormous volumes. Théophile Bonet (1620-1689) is the most important of these reviewers, and his book, *Corps de medecine et de chirurgie* (1679), appearing about two hundred years after Benivieni's, contains summaries of more than three thousand autopsy protocols, including those of Benivieni himself and other masters such as Andreas Vesalius. This book was the stimulus for the monumental contribution of Giovanni Battista Morgagni (1682-1771), whose work marks the official inauguration of anatomic pathology and autopsy as a science. His classic text, *De sedibus et causis morborum per anatomen indagatis* (1761), contains the clinical histories and autopsy protocols of more than seven hundred cases, correlating the morphologic and clinical findings. More important, he committed his autopsy studies to the revelation of the cause of disease, thus establishing the general principle that "seats of disease" are internal body organs, not humors, and thatlocalization in different organs explains different symptoms. This concept served as the basis for the fundamental work of anatomic pathologists-clinicians such as René-Théophile-Hyacinthe Laënnec and Richard Bright.

The next great step in the development of pathology, and establishing the premiership of autopsy as its medium of study, was the French pathologist Marie-François-Xavier Bichat (1771-1802), who established in *Recherches physiologiques sur la vie et la mort* (1800) that organs are formed of elements called tissues. The work of Rudolf Virchow (1821-1902) raised pathology to the premier medical science; he placed the concept of the microscopic cell as the unit of life at the center of medicine and his theory of cellular pathology, thus making cells the unit and "seat" of disease.

Impressive strides in subcellular and molecular pathology have established many morphologic lesions within subcellular structures, even within genes. Such studies can be performed on minute samples of tissues obtained through fine probes. These biopsy techniques and the great technological advances in nuclear and radiologic investigative techniques have allowed the physician to study the cause and extent of disease during the patient's lifetime and with a high level of sophistication. Thus, the role of the autopsy has declined somewhat as an educational tool, but the practice continues to be used in clinical research, medical statistics, public health, and population genetics and to procure organs for tissue transplantation. In fact, many of the functions of autopsy will be extended and improved. For example, the demand for transplantable tissues and organs, procured from cadavers, is likely to increase. Also, recognition of new diseases will occur, aided by postmortem examinations and the application of new technologies and ancillary studies. The autopsy still has much to contribute to education and research, as it constitutes a priceless, continuing, and intimate contact with the natural history of disease.

—Victor H. Nassar, M.D.

See also Anatomy; Biopsy; Blood testing; Death and dying; Disease; Forensic pathology; Law and medicine; Malpractice; Pathology; Wounds.

For Further Information:

Burton, Julian L., and Guy N. Rutty, eds. *The Hospital Autopsy*. 2d ed. New York: Oxford University Press, 2002. A comprehensive exploration of the history and techniques of autopsy practice. Includes topics such as external examination, evisceration, dissection of internal organs, the production of the autopsy report, and microbiological, biochemical, toxological and immunological analysis.

Camenson, Blythe, and Anita Hufft. *Opportunities in Forensic Science Careers*. New York: McGraw-Hill, 2001. Provides those seeking a career in forensics with information on training, education requirements, and salary statistics. Lists professional and Internet resources.

Dix, Jay, and Robert Calaluce. *Guide to Forensic Pathology*. Boca Raton, Fla.: CRC Press, 1998. Provides a concise overview of forensic pathology. Discusses how to determine the time and manner of death, the roles of experts in death investigation, how effective testimony is presented in court, and the importance of forensic DNA testing.

Hutchins, Grover M., ed. *Autopsy: Performance and Reporting*. Northfield, Ill.: College of American Pathologists, 1990. A multiauthored, detailed manual that is concisely written and illustrated. The chapters examine techniques, various medicolegal and ethical questions, contemporary issues related to the decline in autopsy rates in the 1980's, autopsy utilization, quality assurance, and reimbursement.

Ludwig, Jurden. *Handbook of Autopsy Practice*. 3d ed. Totowa, N.J.: Humana Press, 2002. A revised text designed for residents and practicing pathologists to guide them through the autopsy and to find the essential information relevant for the interpretation of the autopsy data.

Perez-Tamayo, Ruy. *Mechanisms of Disease: An Introduction to Pathology*. 2d ed. Chicago: Year Book Medical, 1985. A fascinating review of the study of disease as life under abnormal conditions. Considers the history and future of pathology, with up-to-date information on new technologies. A textbook for medical students.

Sheaff, Michael T., and Deborah J. Hopster. *Post Mortem Technique Handbook*. 2d ed. London: Springer, 2005. Illustrated text that provides a guide to performing the modern postmortem and covers a range of evisceration and dissection techniques.

Avian influenza

Disease/disorder

Also known as: Bird flu, avian flu

Anatomy or system affected: Blood, blood vessels, circulatory system, gastrointestinal system, heart, intestines, kidneys, lungs, muscles, musculoskeletal system, nerves, nervous system, nose, reproductive system, respiratory system, stomach, throat, urinary system

Specialties and related fields: Biochemistry, epidemiology, immunology, pathology, virology

Definition: Avian influenza is caused by several virus strains that attack birds; occasionally, a strain develops the ability to attack humans, sometimes triggering an epidemic. There is concern that the H5N1 strain could mutate into a form that is highly contagious among humans and result in a pandemic.

Key terms:

antibody: a specific protein made by an organism in response to one kind of antigen; the antibody attaches to that antigen and deactivates the cell, virus, or chemical to which the antigen is attached, thus protecting the organism

antigen: foreign material that stimulates the host organism to produce antibodies specific to that material

epidemic: the spread of a disease through a population or region

epidemiology: the study of the mechanisms by which diseases spread within and among populations and regions

mutation: a change in the instructions, either deoxyribonucleic acid (DNA) or ribonucleic acid (RNA), of a cell or virus that sometimes changes the characteristics of the cell or virus

pandemic: a disease that spreads around the world

pathogenic: causing disease

reassortment: one means of recombination among viruses; it occurs when two strains are present in the same host, where they may exchange genes to form viruses with new capabilities

RNA virus: a virus that uses RNA as its genetic material, or ultimate instructions for its characteristics

vaccine: an antigen from a virus or other disease-causing entity that is artificially prepared in a structure not capable of causing disease but which will stimulate the production of antibodies, thus bringing about immunity to the original disease

Causes and Symptoms

A group of RNA viruses causes influenza in birds. Most such viruses do not attack humans, although human influenza viruses were probably derived from bird influenza viruses. On the rare occasion that a bird flu strain achieves the ability to enter and reproduce in human cells, the human is unlikely to have effective defenses and the viral attack is likely to be severe. If the virus strain combines its ability to reproduce in humans and its highly pathogenic nature with the ability to transfer from human host to human host, then it is particularly dangerous. The most deadly human influenza pandemics in history probably began this way. At the turn of the twenty-first century, public health officials were concerned that the avian influenza virus strain H5N1 might undergo such a transformation and initiate such a pandemic.

Influenza virus strains are named for two of their surface proteins, hemagglutinin (with fifteen or sixteen known types) and neuraminidase (with nine known types). Each different protein is assigned a number, so that H5 in H5N1 refers to the hemagglutinin which was assigned the number five. Similarly, N1 refers to the neuraminidase assigned the number one. Hemagglutinins are responsible for attachment of the virus to host cells and entry into those cells. After production of new viruses in the cell, neuraminidases are used by the new viruses to break out of the cell.

Influenza viruses are notorious for their ability to change their surface antigens and thereby escape host defenses, which are dependent on recognition of those antigens. The H5 and N1, surface proteins that characterize the virus, are also the antigens targeted by host defenses. Both are displayed on the surface of the membranelike coat that surrounds the virus. The hemagglutinin (H5) is the primary target for cell defenses. If an organism has been exposed to a given hemagglutinin, then it will quickly produce antibodies that attach to that hemagglutinin, blocking the site that is normally used to attach to the organism's cells. The virus is rendered harmless if it cannot attach to and enter a cell. If this is the organism's first exposure to the specific hemagglutinin, however, then the response will not be as rapid. The host's immune system will begin making antibodies against the new antigen, but they are made too slowly during this first exposure, and illness results. Most humans have had no exposure to H5 antigens and so are unprotected against H5N1.

Symptoms of avian influenza in humans include the familiar set generally caused by flu viruses. Those

Information on Avian Influenza

Causes: Virus passed among birds and sometimes to humans
Symptoms: Initially fever, appetite loss, clogged sinuses, runny nose, and muscle aches, progressing to the circulatory, nervous, reproductive, and urinary systems
Duration: From one to five days, often fatal
Treatments: Antiviral drugs

symptoms—fever, loss of appetite, clogged sinuses, runny nose, muscle aches, and so forth—pass in three to five days with most influenza strains, and the victim recovers. With H5N1, however, other host systems—such as the circulatory, nervous, reproductive, and gastrointestinal systems—often become involved. In more than 50 percent of human cases reported, death occurs, sometimes within a day of the onset of symptoms.

Treatment and Therapy

The major medical solutions to avian flu infection are medications and vaccination. Antiviral medications were difficult to develop, and few effective drugs are available. Many of the drugs prescribed for viral infections are actually used to combat secondary infections by bacteria attempting to take advantage of the host's weakened condition. Vaccine development against influenza viruses is also problematic. The vaccines target antigens on the surface of the viruses, and the viruses mutate and change their surface antigens so frequently that new vaccines must be developed almost every year to defend against the new strains of influenza. Given these difficulties and the fact that most influenza victims recover in three to five days without treatment, drugs and vaccines against influenza have not been a high priority compared to those against more deadly diseases such as smallpox. Periodically, however, a particularly pathogenic influenza strain has developed, and effective treatment would have saved many lives. Because the H5N1 strain is feared for its potential to be one of those strains, scientists have sought to develop both drugs and vaccines against this virus.

Four medications that act against flu viruses are available, but the virus has quickly developed resistance to the older pair, amantadine and rimantadine. The H5N1 virus populations in Vietnam and other Southeast Asian countries are already resistant to these drugs. In those countries, the virus has been present in poultry, and occasionally in humans, a bit longer than elsewhere. Two newer drugs, oseltamivir (Tamiflu) and zanamivir (Relenza), are expected to be effective, but they have not yet been tested sufficiently against the H5N1 virus strain.

Progress in vaccine development has been encouraging, but no proven vaccine is available. Even when a vaccine becomes ready for use, production of enough to meet the needs of a pandemic would be challenging. Stockpiling a vaccine in anticipation of a pandemic is possible, but the exact antigen against which it must be directed cannot be known until the virus is in the process of initiating the pandemic. Each year, experts predict the most likely antigens for an approaching flu season, and vaccines are produced in advance against those antigens. Should an influenza virus employ an antigen not anticipated by the experts, then the stockpiled vaccines would be worthless.

Vaccine production technology is also improving, but the improvements have not been fully implemented. In the standard technique, the antigenic virus to be used in the vaccine is grown in fertilized eggs—an expensive, slow, and inefficient method. Tissue culture techniques, in which the antigenic virus is grown in cells in artificial media, promise dramatic improvement in vaccine preparation once they are fully integrated into the production system.

Perspective and Prospects

The history of influenza can be traced much further back in time than the understanding of its cause. Reports describing epidemics and pandemics in which the victims showed symptoms of influenza go back to the early 1500's at least, but the first isolation of an influenza virus did not occur until 1933. The worst flu pandemic occurred in 1918-1919 (the Spanish flu), when twenty million to one hundred million people died of influenza. It was one of the deadliest diseases in history. Two more recent flu pandemics, the Asian flu (1957) and the Hong Kong flu (1968), were seriously disruptive, but not as deadly. All these pandemics were caused by influenza type A viruses, the type to which strain H5N1 and the other avian influenza viruses belong.

The concern over avian influenza type A H5N1 began in 1997 in Hong Kong, where poultry and humans came under attack. Three events associated with these infections captured the attention of epidemiologists, because together they suggested H5N1's potential as the agent of an influenza pandemic. First, transmission occurred from poultry to humans. Second, H5N1 proved to be highly pathogenic, as six of the eighteen infected humans died. Third, there was some indication of human-to-human transfer of the virus. If the virus maintained its pathogenic nature and its ability to move from poultry to humans, and if it added the ability to transfer efficiently from one human to another, it would almost certainly initiate another deadly pandemic.

Between 1997 and 2006, a number of human cases of avian influenza type A were documented in a number of countries. Not all were the result of the feared H5N1 strain, but the other strains bear watching as well. Between 2004 and 2006, there were two hundred confirmed cases of human infection with H5N1, most in Southeast Asia (Vietnam, Cambodia, Indonesia, Thailand) but also in Egypt, Iraq, Azerbaijan, and Turkey. No H5N1 infections were documented in North America, but avian influenza virus type A H7N2 caused illness in New York, and H7N3 attacked poultry workers in Canada. No North American infection resulted in a human fatality. None of these infections involved extensive or sustained human-to-human transmission, though a few restricted transfers between humans may have occurred. Most of the human infections were transferred from infected domestic poultry. Some may have been contracted from wild waterfowl (ducks and geese).

Human health is not the only concern regarding the H5N1 strain; there are agricultural and economic concerns as well. Poultry flocks can be destroyed by the virus. There were several poultry outbreaks around the world before 2006, in which an estimated 150 million barnyard birds either died as victims of the virus or were culled to remove the infection focus and prevent further spread of the virus. Although the governments involved frequently compensated individuals for their

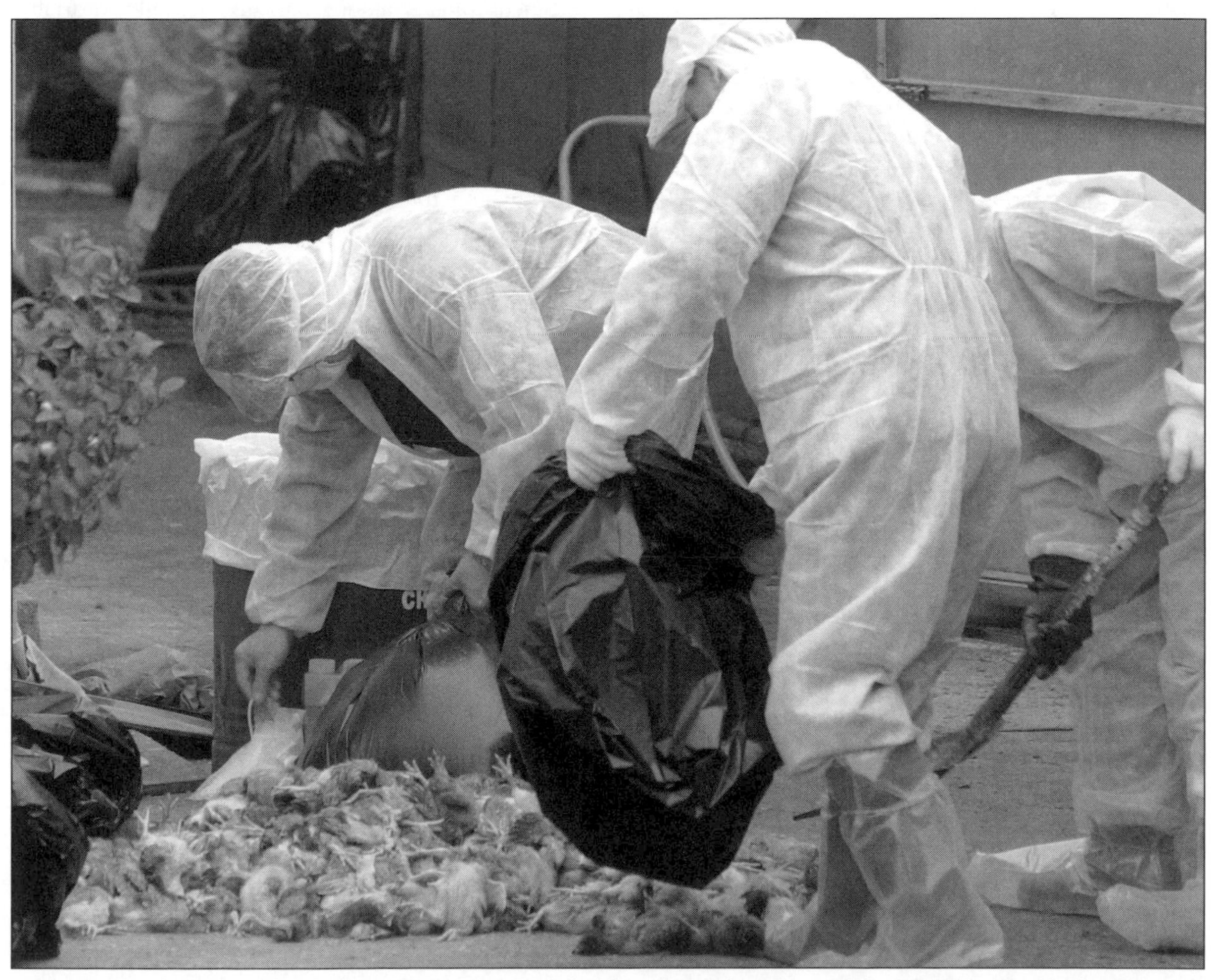

Health officials in Hong Kong collect chickens killed by avian influenza in 2002. (AP/Wide World Photos)

culled animals, the compensation was usually well below market value. This practice encourages farmers to hide infections that occur in their flocks, which slows discovery of potential outbreaks and gives the virus a headstart that it does not need. In addition, several governments were suspected of hiding avian flu outbreaks until they were impossible to conceal, in an attempt to protect their countries' economic interests.

The role played by wild birds is an important piece of this puzzle as well. Wild birds, especially waterfowl, act as the reservoir for H5N1. The birds maintain the virus between epidemics. Waterfowl are known to carry the virus, release virus in their feces and oral secretions, and are usually not sickened by the virus infection. These characteristics of the reservoir indicate how easily a pandemic could start from a mutant virus in the reservoir. In Hong Kong in 2002-2003 and again in China in 2005, large numbers of wild birds were killed by the virus, emphasizing the virus's tendency to mutate. Experts believe that it may take only a few mutations for the virus to gain the ability to transfer between humans. If they are right, then the waterfowl reservoir is always just a step away from creating a pandemic virus strain.

Given their mobility, especially during migration, wild birds also appear to be good candidates for spreading the virus among countries and continents. However, investigations suggest that, while wild bird migration might play a role in viral geographic expansion, it is probably secondary to the role played by commercial poultry exchanges.

Avian influenza virus type A H5N1 has demonstrated its ability to transfer from wild birds to domestic poultry (and perhaps to humans), to decimate domestic poultry flocks, to be transferred from poultry to humans, and to be highly pathogenic for humans. It has not demonstrated the ability to pass freely from one human to another. If it were to add this last ability to its arsenal, it would be a candidate to initiate a pandemic as deadly as the influenza pandemics of the past. The change required to introduce this ability to the H5N1 virus is not thought to be elaborate. A few simple mutations in the viral RNA might suffice.

Epidemiologists have one special concern, the potential for the virus to use pigs for reassortment of its genes. In developing countries, pigs often share living space with chickens and other poultry. Humans often live adjacent to the animals or even share their living space. These associations are troubling because pigs host both human and bird flu viruses, and the intimate association of the three species presents the two viral strains with the opportunity to invade the same pig. Together in the same host, they would be expected to exchange RNA strands. Some reassortments might produce a virus with the capability to transfer from human to human. There was no evidence that such a transformation has occurred. However, the possibility is real and the defenses (antiviral drugs and vaccination) are not in place and fully functional, so the concern is understandable.

Some investigators suggest, however, that the concern has been overblown. They point out that no H5 influenza strain has ever caused a pandemic and that successful pandemic-causing influenza strains attach to receptors in the upper parts of the human respiratory tract, while the receptors to which H5N1 viruses attach are in the lower reaches. Some skeptics also argue that if H5N1 went through the changes necessary to achieve efficient transfer among humans, it would invariably lose pathogenic potency in the process, thus minimizing its pandemic potential.

Governments and public health officials are between the proverbial rock and hard place. They would be criticized if they prepared for a threat that did not materialize, but more tragic results would occur if they failed to prepare and a pandemic broke out. Criticism for a perceived lack of preparation is already widespread. While another pandemic is probably inevitable, no one can know when it will materialize or what specific disease organism will be the cause, so there is no easy answer to their conundrum. For the long-term struggle against avian influenza, however, disease patterns in animal populations might be very helpful in predicting which threats have the potential to cause human pandemics and in otherwise understanding the viruses. This possibility calls for close coordination among students of wildlife, veterinary, and human disease. That coordination will not solve all the mysteries of influenza outbreaks but should aid in understanding them, and the influenza viruses will not be controlled until they are more thoroughly understood.

—Carl W. Hoagstrom, Ph.D.

See also Epidemiology; Immunization and vaccination; Influenza; Viral infections; Zoonoses.

For Further Information:

Clark, Larry, and Jeffrey Hall. "Avian Influenza in Wild Birds: Status as Reservoirs, and Risks to Humans and Agriculture." In *Current Topics in Avian Disease Research: Understanding Endemic and*

Invasive Diseases, edited by Rosemary K. Barraclough. Washington, D.C.: American Ornithologists' Union, 2006. A nice outline of the problem. Also considers human health, agricultural concerns, and the potential effect on wild bird populations.

Davis, Mike. *The Monster at Our Door: The Global Threat of Avian Flu*. New York: The New Press, 2005. A good discussion of the problem from the "sky-is-falling-and-nobody-is-doing-anything" perspective.

Green, Jeffrey. *The Bird Flu Pandemic*. New York: Thomas Dunne Books, 2006. A balanced presentation of the potential for such an event with suggestions for appropriate individual responses.

Sfakianos, Jeffrey N. *Avian Flu*. New York: Chelsea House, 2006. A good discussion of the biology of flu viruses. A balanced presentation of the bird flu problem.

Siegel, Marc. *Bird Flu: Everything You Need to Know About the Next Pandemic*. Hoboken, N.J.: John Wiley & Sons, 2006. A good discussion of the problem from the perspective that "the sky-is-falling" theorists are overreacting.

Wehrwein, Peter, ed. "Bird Flu: Don't Fly into a Panic." *Harvard Health Letter* 31, 8 (June, 2006): 1-3. A concise, balanced description of the problem and protective steps that an individual can take.

Back disorders. *See* Back pain; Spinal cord disorders.

Back pain

Disease/disorder

Also known as: Backache

Anatomy or system affected: Abdomen, back, bones, hips, joints, legs, ligaments, muscles, musculoskeletal system, nerves, nervous system, spine

Specialties and related fields: Alternative medicine, anesthesiology, emergency medicine, exercise physiology, family medicine, general surgery, geriatrics and gerontology, neurology, nursing, obstetrics, occupational health, orthopedics, osteopathic medicine, physical therapy, preventive medicine, radiology, rheumatology, sports medicine

Definition: Acute or chronic and usually severe pain centered along the spine, usually in the lower back but also common in the neck and upper back.

Key terms:

annular bulge: protrusion of a disk beyond its normal circumference, unusally because of compression caused by gravity, strain on the spine, or aging

cervical spine: the highest of three parts of the spine, consisting of seven vertebrae, named C1 (top of the neck) to C7, in a natural lordosis

herniated disk: prolapse of the nucleus through a rupture or weakness in the annulus

intervertebral disk: the flexible, cylindrical pad between each two vertebrae, consisting of the nucleus pulposis (gelatinous center) and the annulus fibrosis (concentric rings of cartilage); the flexibility, moistness, and thickness of the disk decreases naturally with age

kyphosis: backward curvature of the spine or a section of the spine

lordosis: forward curvature of the spine or a section of the spine

lumbar spine: the lowest of three parts of the spine, consisting of five vertebrae, named L1 to L5 (just above the sacrum), in a natural lordosis

radiculopathy: also called nerve root entrapment or pinched nerve; irritation or compression of the root of a spinal nerve between vertebrae, caused by annular bulge, herniated disk, or spinal injury

referred pain: any pain whose origin is elsewhere in the body from where it is felt; with radiculopathy in the lumbar spine, the pain is typically in the leg

sciatica: intense pain in one buttock and down the back of that leg, caused by inflammation of the sciatic nerve, the largest nerve in the body; in some cases this inflammation is referred pain from radiculopathy where the sciatic nerve originates between L4 and the sacrum

scoliosis: sideways curvature of the spine or a section of the spine

thoracic spine: the middle of three parts of the spine, consisting of twelve vertebrae, named T1 (top of the chest) to T12, in a natural kyphosis

Causes and Symptoms

Most back pain is caused by disk problems, but the disk problems themselves have a wide variety of causes and manifestations. Annular bulge, disk herniation, muscular spasms, and strain from overexertion are just a few of these causes. Among these manifestations are sudden and persistent attacks of sharp, debilitating pain that exaggerate spinal kyphosis, may create scoliosis, and make standing up or bending over without assistance either impossible or very difficult.

The more the lumbar spine approaches either kyphosis or scoliosis, the more out of alignment the natural curvature of the whole spine becomes and the more pain results. Scoliosis or uncontrollable listing to one side is a frequent symptom of disk damage, usually either annular bulge or herniation.

Referred pain may appear from any lumbar radiculopathy, but the two most common presentations are in the thigh, from pinching the femoral nerve between L2 and L4 vertebrae, and as sciatica, from pinching the sciatic nerve between L4 and the sacrum. Shooting pains elsewhere in the leg, genital dysfunction, or incontinence and other urinary or bowel complications may result from radiculopathy of any of several other lum-

Information on Back Pain

Causes: Usually disk disorders (herniation, muscular spasms, strain from overexertion or poor posture)

Symptoms: Sudden and persistent attacks of sharp, debilitating pain

Duration: Acute or chronic

Treatments: Good posture and habits, painkillers, muscle relaxants, physical therapy; surgery in extreme cases

bar, sacral, or lower thoracic nerves. In very severe cases, partial paralysis or constant, intolerable pain may occur.

Treatment and Therapy

Many ways of treating back pain exist, and the program of treatment must be adapted to the particular situation of each patient. Good posture is always essential. Learning to sit up straight, perhaps with a lumbar support roll, or a change of habits, such as learning to lift with the legs rather than the back, may be advised. Sometimes drug therapy with painkillers or muscle relaxants, or physical therapy with manipulation and exercises, is the only additional treatment required. As a last resort and in extreme cases, including emergency cases of incontinence or paralysis, surgery to repair a disk may be indicated.

Treatment options come not only from regular medicine but also from alternative, complementary, or allied systems of health care. The McKenzie method of bending the spine backward, thus emphasizing lumbar lordosis, has proved successful. Techniques drawn from chiropractic, osteopathy, yoga, acupuncture, and other styles of therapy have sometimes provided either temporary or permanent relief.

Perspective and Prospects

Low back pain seems to be equally prevalent in all eras and in all countries. Despite socioeconomic improvements in the lives of physical laborers, and despite the fact that a decreasing proportion of people worldwide make their living from physical labor, no concomitant decrease in new low back pain cases has been observed. If anything, there may be a slight increase in the percentage of low back pain cases in industrialized nations since the mid-twentieth century. People with desk-bound occupations and sedentary habits are at great risk for developing low back pain, especially if they slouch in their chairs or fail to protect the natural lordosis of the lumbar spine.

Physicians no longer consider typical low back pain either an injury or a disease. Since the late twentieth century they have understood it as a natural degenerative condition that can usually be delayed by good posture habits and managed by physical therapy, painkilling drugs, and lifestyle changes.

—*Eric v. d. Luft, Ph.D., M.L.S.*

See also Aging; Alternative medicine; Bone disorders; Bones and the skeleton; Chiropractic; Disk removal; Kyphosis; Nervous system; Neuralgia, neuritis, and neuropathy; Pain; Pain management; Physical rehabilitation; Sciatica; Scoliosis; Slipped disk; Spinal cord disorders; Spine, vertebrae, and disks; Yoga.

For Further Information:

Borenstein, David G., Sam W. Wiesel, and Scott D. Boden. *Low Back and Neck Pain: Comprehensive Diagnosis and Management*. 3d ed. Philadelphia: Saunders, 2004.

Burn, Loic. *Back and Neck Pain: The Facts*. New York: Oxford University Press, 2006.

Cailliet, Rene. *Low Back Pain Syndrome: A Medical Enigma*. Philadelphia: Lippincott Williams & Wilkins, 2003.

Fishman, Loren, and Carol Ardman. *Back Talk: How to Diagnose and Cure Low Back Pain and Sciatica*. New York: Norton, 1997.

Hutson, Michael A. *Back Pain: Recognition and Management*. Boston: Butterworth-Heinemann, 1993.

McGill, Stuart. *Low Back Disorders: Evidence-Based Prevention and Rehabilitation*. Champaign, Ill.: Human Kinetics, 2002.

McKenzie, Robin, and Craig Kubey. *Seven Steps to a Pain-Free Life: How to Rapidly Relieve Back and Neck Pain Using the McKenzie Method*. New York: Dutton, 2000.

Twomey, Lance T., and James R. Taylor, eds. *Physical Therapy of the Low Back*. New York: Churchill Livingstone, 2000.

Waddell, Gordon. *The Back Pain Revolution*. 2d ed. New York: Churchill Livingstone, 2004.

Bacterial infections

Disease/disorder

Anatomy or system affected: Gastrointestinal system, immune system, intestines, lungs, lymphatic system, respiratory system

Specialties and related fields: Bacteriology, epidemiology, immunology, internal medicine, microbiology

Definition: Infectious diseases caused by bacteria, of which hundreds exist.

Key terms:

antibiotic: a substance that kills microorganisms, including bacteria; antibiotics are used as a primary therapy in combating bacterial diseases

bacteria: small, single-celled organisms with a very simple structure; they live virtually everywhere and most varieties are harmless, although some types are capable of causing disease

cell: the smallest unit of a living thing; a bacterium consists of one cell, whereas humans are made of billions

immune system: the natural defenses of the body, which kill invading organisms such as harmful bacteria

immunity: resistance to infection by a particular disease-causing microorganism, often acquired by vaccination

infectious disease: diseases that can be passed from person to person through direct or indirect contact; many bacterial diseases are infectious

inflammation: signs and symptoms of the body's immune response to some bacterial infections; may include redness, swelling, heat, pain, and the production of pus

metabolism: the chemical reactions in an organism that sustain life and lead to growth and reproduction

microorganism: any small organism, including bacteria, protozoans, mold, fungi, and viruses; in this context, refers to those which cause disease

vaccination: the process of injecting into an individual a substance that provides immunity to a particular disease

Information on Bacterial Infections

Causes: Exposure to bacteria

Symptoms: Localized pain, fever, inflammation, production of pus

Duration: Ranging from one to several days or weeks

Treatments: Antibiotics, vaccinations for prevention

Causes and Symptoms

Bacteria are very small, one-celled organisms (the cell being the smallest unit of a living organism) with an average size of thousandths of a millimeter. Based on their relatively simple structure, they are classified as prokaryotic cells. Prokaryotic cells have a rigid outer cell wall, very simply organized hereditary material (deoxyribonucleic acid, or DNA) floating free within the cell, and only a few other structures necessary for their survival, growth, and reproduction. Eukaryotic cells, such as those found in humans, plants, and other animals, have highly organized DNA and many more internal structures. Despite the fact that bacteria are relatively "simple," they are still very complex living organisms.

The many types of bacteria can be divided into three categories based on their shape: coccus (round), bacillus (rod-shaped), or spirillum (spiral). Another major distinction between types of bacteria is based on the sugar and lipid (fat) composition of their cell walls. This difference can be identified through Gram staining, the result of the stain determining whether the organism is gram-positive or gram-negative. Various types of bacteria may have additional structures that are useful in their identification. Capsules and slime layers are water-rich sugary materials secreted by the bacteria which cling to their surfaces and form halolike structures. Flagella are long, thin, whiplike structures found in one location on the bacterium or occasionally covering its entire surface. These structures are used to enhance the motility, or movement, of the bacteria.

Some bacteria are normal, harmless inhabitants of human bodies, such as those on the surface of the skin. Others, such as those that live in the human intestinal tract, aid in digestion and are essential for good health. The warm, moist, nutrient-rich human body also provides an excellent breeding ground for numerous harmful bacterial invaders. For bacteria to cause infectious disease, several stages must occur. The bacteria must enter the person, they must survive and multiply on or in the person, they must resist the natural defenses of the human body, and they must damage the infected person. Most bacterial diseases are infectious because of the ease with which they can be transmitted from individual to individual by physical contact with the person, a contaminated object, or bacteria expelled into the air, such as by coughing or sneezing. A few bacterial diseases, such as food poisoning, are not classified as infectious.

Bacterial infections cause disease by a variety of mechanisms. Many of them produce chemical compounds that are toxic to human beings. For example, *Salmonella* and *Staphylococcus aureus* are two types of bacteria that are capable of causing food poisoning. *Clostridium botulinum* produces the deadly botulism toxin. In each case, ingestion of the toxin in contaminated food can lead to serious illness. *Clostridium tetanii* can enter the body through puncture wounds and will multiply rapidly deep in tissue where there is little exposure to the air. The toxin that it produces acts on the central nervous system and causes severe muscle spasms, which can lead to death from respiratory failure. Water that has been contaminated with raw sewage is a potent source of disease-causing bacteria. *Vibrio cholera* produces a potent toxin that causes severe diarrhea leading to death if it is not vigorously treated. Certain varieties of *Escherichia coli* and *Shigella* found in contaminated water can also cause severe intestinal disorders. Toxic shock syndrome is associated with the production of toxins by *Staphylococcus aureus*.

Another common cause of disease from bacterial infections is the result of the physical destruction of tissue by the invading organisms. Leprosy (also called Hansen's disease), caused by *Mycobacterium leprae*, if left untreated, can lead to severe deterioration and disfiguration of large areas of a person's body. If a wound interrupts the blood supply to an area of the body such as a hand or foot, the tissues begin to decay, thereby providing nutrients for many bacteria, especially *Clostridium perfringens*. These bacteria can greatly accelerate the destruction of the tissue, which causes the condition known as gas gangrene.

In many cases, disease results when the infecting bacteria are recognized by the body's natural defense system (the immune system) as "nonself," that is, as invaders. Certain cells within the body are designed to attack intruders and eliminate them. During this process, disease symptoms that are consequences of the immune system's response may be evident: inflammation (redness and swelling), the production of pus, and fever, among other symptoms. In some cases, certain components of the bacteria, such as capsules and slime layers, may protect them from being eliminated by the immune system. The bacteria may also multiply exceedingly rapidly, producing increasing amounts of toxins that overwhelm the capacity of the immune system to eliminate them. In these cases, continued and increasingly elevated disease symptoms such as fever can cause severe, even fatal, damage unless an alternate method for eliminating the infection is found. Failure to eliminate the bacterial invaders can also lead to a long-term, chronic infection that damages body tissues.

Many respiratory diseases are associated with the body's immune response to bacterial invasion. *Streptococcus pyogenes* is the causative agent of strep throat, whose features include severe redness, inflammation, pain, and the production of pus in throat tissue. In a small percentage of cases, strep throat can also lead to an infection of and potential permanent damage to the heart valves in a disease called rheumatic fever. In tuberculosis, *Mycobacterium tuberculosis* enters the lungs through inhalation. The body's defense system walls off the intruders and forms a nodule called a tubercle deep in the lung tissue. Nevertheless, the bacteria continue to multiply in the nodule and can travel to new sites in the lung. Tubercle formation occurs at these new sites. Eventually, this repeated cycle of infection and nodule formation becomes a chronic disease and leads to the destruction of lung tissue. Bacterial pneumonia can be caused by several different organisms, including *Klebsiella pneumoniae* and *Mycobacterium pneumoniae*. A pneumonia-like disease, Legionnaires' disease, was first identified in 1976 after twenty-nine delegates to an American Legion convention died from a mysterious respiratory disorder. The lengthy process of identifying a causative agent led to the discovery of a type of bacteria not previously known, *Legionella pneumophila*.

The human urinary and genital tracts are also potential havens for invading bacteria. Cystitis (bladder infections) are caused by many different types of bacteria. Kidney infections can be acquired as corollaries of urinary tract infections. Sexually transmitted diseases (STDs) are contracted through sexual contact with an infected partner, and two common STDs have a bacterial origin. Gonorrhea is caused by *Neisseria gonorrhoeae* and leads to a severe inflammatory response and rapid spread of the organisms throughout the body. If not treated, it can lead to sterility as well as to diseases of the joints, heart, nerve coverings, eyes, and throat. Syphilis, caused by *Treponema pallidum*, can also have serious consequences if left untreated, including dementia and death. In addition, it can be passed to a fetus developing inside an infected mother in a condition known as congenital syphilis.

Treatment and Therapy

The medical management of the many bacterial infections and the diseases they cause begins with diagnosis. Diagnosis relies on a variety of biochemical tests that are analyzed in conjunction with the signs and symptoms exhibited by the infected individual. Treatment is then designed so that it not only eliminates the disease symptoms but also eradicates all invading bacterial organisms, thereby minimizing the chance of a recurrence of the disease. Prevention involves steps that the individual takes to avoid potential contact with infectious diseases, as well as the use of medical procedures that protect against specific bacterial diseases.

In order to treat a bacterial disease properly, the invading organism must be identified correctly. In some cases, symptomology can be specific enough to identify the offending bacterium, but since there are literally thousands of different types of disease-causing organisms, a systematic approach using a variety of tests is undertaken to make a definitive diagnosis. First, a specimen from the infected person is collected. This may be a blood or urine sample; a swab of the infected area, such as the throat or another skin surface; or a secretion, such as sputum, mucus, or pus. Since human bodies are normally inhabited by a variety of harmless bacteria, the individual types of bacteria are isolated in pure cultures, in which each bacterium present is of the same type. The pure cultures are then tested to deter-

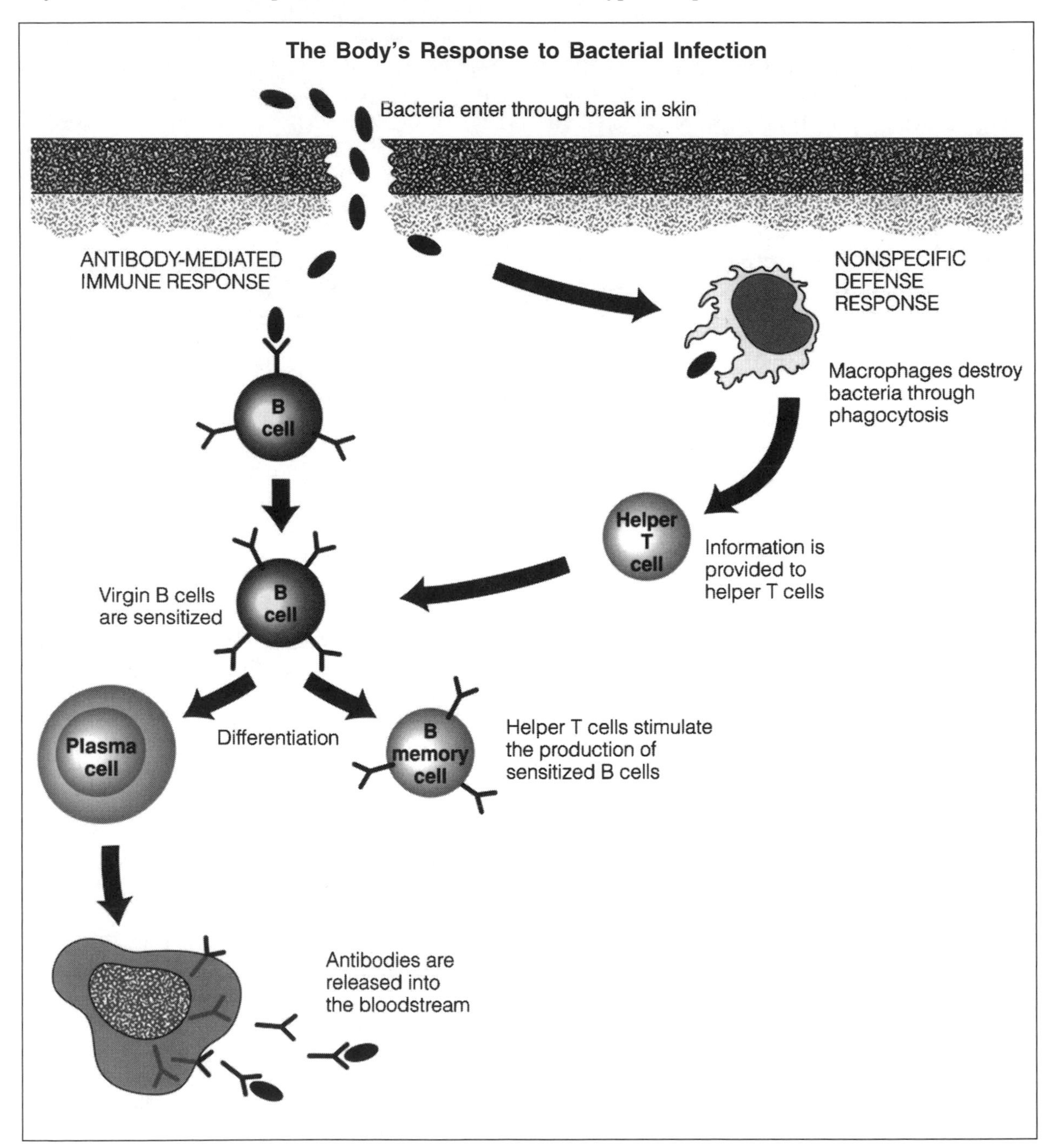

Bacterial infections cause the body to respond with either antibody production or phagocytosis leading to antibody production.

mine the identity of the organisms. Staining procedures, such as Gram's stain, and microscopic examination of the stained bacteria to determine the Gram reaction and the shape of the bacteria can narrow down the identity of the organisms considerably.

Based on these results, a standard series of tests is performed, continually narrowing down the possible identities until only one remains. One test measures the organisms' growth requirements. Many identifications are aided by analyzing the types of sugars and proteins that the organisms can use as food sources. The byproducts of their metabolism (chemical reactions occurring inside the bacteria), such as acids and gas, are identified. Oxygen requirements, motility, and the presence of a capsule are three other common characteristics that are examined. For cases in which the identification of a particular variety of one type of bacteria is necessary, more complex tests may be undertaken, such as an analysis of the particular sugars and proteins on the surface of the organism or tests for the production of specific toxins. Once the bacterium's identity is confirmed, treatment may begin.

The most common type of treatment for bacterial infection is antibiotic therapy. Antibiotics are chemical compounds that kill bacteria. Originally discovered as antibacterial compounds produced by bacteria, molds, and fungi (such as penicillin from bread mold), many more are synthetically produced. Antibiotics work in a variety of fashions. Some, such as penicillin and the cephalosporins, interfere with the synthesis of cell walls by bacteria, thus preventing the organisms from multiplying. Other commonly used antibiotics prevent the bacteria from synthesizing the proteins that they need to survive and multiply. These includes the tetracyclines (a class of antibiotics which act against a large range of bacteria), erythromycin, and streptomycin. A host of other antibiotics target a variety of bacterial functions, including specific chemical reactions and the propagation of genetic material, and the structural components of the bacteria. Each class of antibiotics works best on certain types of bacteria. For example, penicillin is most efficient in killing cocci (such as *Streptococcus* and *Staphylococcus*) and gram-positive bacilli.

Frequently, the symptoms of a bacterial disease may disappear rapidly after the beginning of antibiotic therapy. This reaction is attributable to the inhibition of bacterial multiplication and the destruction of most of the microorganisms. A small number of the bacteria may not be killed during this initial exposure to antibiotics, however, and if antibiotic therapy is ended before all are killed, a recurrence of the disease is likely. A full prescription of antibiotics should be taken to avoid this situation. For example, effective treatment and eradication of all bacteria in tuberculosis may take six months to a year or more of antibiotic treatment, despite the fact that the symptoms are alleviated in a few weeks.

Upon repeated exposure to a type of antibiotic, some bacteria develop the capacity to degrade or inactivate the antibiotic, thus rendering that drug ineffective against the resistant microorganism. In these cases, other antibiotics and newly developed ones are tested for their effectiveness against the bacteria. Such situations have arisen in the bacteria that cause gonorrhea and tuberculosis.

While antibiotics exist to combat infections of most types of bacteria, in some cases the human immune system is capable of clearing the infection without additional intervention. In these instances, the symptoms of the infection are treated until the body heals itself. This is the common treatment path in mild cases of food poisoning, such as those caused by some *Salmonella* and Staphylococcus varieties. Diarrhea and vomiting are treated by replacing water and salts, by drinking large volumes of fluids, and perhaps by using over-the-counter remedies to ease some of the symptoms.

Many bacterial diseases can be easily prevented through good hygiene. Foods, such as eggs and meats, that are not thoroughly cooked may become quickly contaminated by the rapid growth of food-poisoning organisms present on their surfaces. Proper cooking kills these organisms. Similarly, foods that are not properly stored but left out in warm places can also provide a potent breeding ground for toxin-producing bacteria. Picnic food not properly refrigerated is a common source of food poisoning. Similarly, questionable water sources should never be used for drinking or cooking water without proper treatment. Filtering with an ultrafine filter specifically designed to remove bacteria is one safeguard, as is boiling for the required time period based on altitude. Food that may have been washed with contaminated water sources should always be cooked or peeled before consumption.

Many diseases can be prevented with vaccinations. A bacterial vaccine is a mixture of a particular bacterium, its parts, or its inactivated toxins. When this solution is injected into an individual, it provides immunity (resistance to infection) to the particular organism contained in the vaccine. Some vaccines provide lifetime immunity when enhanced with an occasional booster shot, while some are relatively short-acting. Many types of vaccines that are directed against specific diseases are part of standard preventive care given to children. For example, the DPT vaccine confers immunity to diphtheria, pertussis (whooping cough), and tetanus. Some vaccines are useful for individuals who are living, working, or traveling in areas where certain diseases are endemic, or for those who regularly come into contact with infected individuals. Examples of these sorts of vaccines include those for plague (*Yersinia pestis*), typhoid fever (*Salmonella typhi*), cholera, and tuberculosis.

Perspective and Prospects

Bacteria were first described as "animalcules" by the Dutch scientist Antoni van Leeuwenhoek in 1673 after he observed them in water-based mixtures with a crudely designed microscope. In 1860, Louis Pasteur recognized that bacteria could cause the spoiling of wine and beer because of the by-products of their metabolism. Pasteur's solution to this problem was heating the beverages enough to kill the bacteria, but not change the taste of the drink—a process known as pasteurization, which is used today on milk and alcoholic beverages. In addition, Pasteur settled a long-standing debate on the origin of living things that seemed to arise spontaneously in fluids exposed to the air. He demonstrated that these life-forms were seeded by contaminating bacteria and other microorganisms found in the air, in fluids, and on solid surfaces. Pasteur's work led to standard practices in laboratories and food processing plants to prevent unwanted bacterial contamination; these practices are referred to as aseptic techniques.

Prior to the late 1800's, deaths from wounds and simple surgeries were quite common, but the reason for these high mortality rates was unknown. In the 1860's, Joseph Lister, an English surgeon, began soaking surgical dressings in solutions that killed bacteria, and the rate of survival in surgical and wound patients was greatly improved. In 1876, Robert Koch, a German physician, discovered rod-shaped bacteria in the blood of cattle that died from anthrax, a disease which was devastating the sheep and cattle population of Europe. When he injected healthy animals with these bacteria, they contracted anthrax, and samples of their blood showed large numbers of the same bacteria. By these and other experiments, Koch, Lister, and others proved the "germ theory of disease"—that microorganisms cause disease—and appropriate measures were instituted to protect against the transmission of bacteria to humans through medical procedures and food.

A milestone in the prevention of infectious diseases was the development of vaccinations. The first vaccine was developed in 1798, long before the germ theory of disease was proven. The British physician Edward Jenner first used vaccination as a preventive step against the contraction of deadly smallpox, a viral disease. How vaccinations work and their use as a protection against bacterial diseases were discovered around 1880 by Pasteur.

The first antibiotic, penicillin, was discovered by Alexander Fleming in 1928. Since then, scores of others, produced both naturally and synthetically, have been analyzed and used in the treatment of bacterial diseases. All these discoveries have made bacterial disease a much less deadly category of illness than it was in the late 1800's. Yet bacterial diseases are by no means conquered. Overuse of antibiotics in medical practice and in cattle feed results in the appearance of new varieties of bacteria that are resistant to standard antibiotic therapy. Research will continue to develop new means of controlling and destroying such infective organisms. Bacteria also play an important role in synthesizing new antibiotics and other pharmaceuticals in the laboratory through recombinant DNA technology. These organisms will continue to provide challenges and opportunities for human health in the years to come.

—Karen E. Kalumuck, Ph.D.;
updated by Matthew Berria, Ph.D.

See also Anthrax; Antibiotics; Bacteriology; Botulism; Childhood infectious diseases; Cholecystitis; Cholera; Cystitis; Diphtheria; Drug resistance; *E. coli* infection; Endocarditis; Enterocolitis; Epiglottitis; Gangrene; Gonorrhea; Gram staining; Hemolytic uremic syndrome; Impetigo; Infection; Laboratory tests; Legionnaires' disease; Leprosy; Lyme disease; Mastitis; Microbiology; Microscopy; Necrotizing fasciitis; Osteomyelitis; Pelvic inflammatory disease (PID); Plague; Pneumonia; Pyelonephritis; Quinsy; Salmonella infection; Scarlet fever; Serology; Shigellosis; Staphylococcal infections; Strep throat; Streptococcal infections; Styes; Syphilis; Tetanus; Tonsillitis; Toxic shock syndrome; Tropical medicine; Tuberculosis; Tularemia; Typhoid fever; Typhus; Whooping cough.

For Further Information:

Biddle, Wayne. *A Field Guide to Germs*. 2d ed. New York: Anchor Books, 2002. This comprehensive book is easily accessible to the nonspecialist and includes a discussion of nearly every virus, bacterium, and fungus known to cause human and nonhuman animal disease. The history of the microbe and the treatment of diseases are included.

Forbes, Betty A. Daniel F. Sahm, and Alice S. Weissfeld. *Bailey and Scott's Diagnostic Microbiology.* 11th ed. St. Louis: Mosby, 2002. A well-organized text that is accessible to the general reader. Describes in detail methods for the isolation and identification of microorganisms, in particular diagnostic procedures for the identification of bacterial infectious diseases.

Frank, Steven A. *Immunology and Evolution of Infectious Disease.* Princeton, N.J.: Princeton University Press, 2002. Blends research from molecular biology, immunology, pathogen biology, and population dynamics to discuss how and why parasites vary to escape recognition by the immune system, vaccine design, and the control of epidemics.

Joklik, Wolfgang K., et al. *Zinsser Microbiology.* 20th ed. East Norwalk, Conn.: Appleton and Lange, 1992. This is the bible of microbiology, with a heavy emphasis on medical microbiology. Features a detailed analysis of the biochemistry of bacteria and other microorganisms.

Pelczar, Michael J., Jr., E. C. S. Chan, and Noel R. Krieg. *Microbiology: Concepts and Applications.* New York: McGraw-Hill, 1993. This textbook is accessible to the general reader and is a good source of information on bacterial physiology and genetics, diagnostic testing, the prevention and cure of bacterial diseases, and environmental microbiology.

Schlegel, Hans G. *General Microbiology.* 7th ed. Cambridge, England: Cambridge University Press, 1993. This compact version of a classic German textbook provides a concise yet broad account of bacteriology and microbiology for readers with all levels of interest. Topics include cell structure, biochemistry, microbes in the environment, the practical applications of microbes, and the cause, prevention, and cure of diseases.

Shaw, Michael, ed. *Everything You Need to Know About Diseases.* Springhouse, Pa.: Springhouse Press, 1996. This well-illustrated consumer reference, compiled by more than one hundred doctors and medical experts, describes five hundred illnesses and conditions, their causes, symptoms, diagnosis, treatment, and prevention.

Wilson, Michael, Brian Henderson, and Rod McNab. *Bacterial Virulence Mechanisms.* New York: Cambridge University Press, 2002. Basing their discussion on research advances in microbiology, molecular biology, and cell biology, the authors describe the interactions that exist between bacteria and human cells both in health and during infection.

Bacteriology

Specialty

Anatomy or system affected: Cells, immune system

Specialties and related fields: Biochemistry, epidemiology, microbiology, pathology, pharmacology, public health

Definition: The study of bacteria.

Key terms:

anaerobic: free of oxygen

fermentation: a chemical reaction that splits complex organic compounds into relatively simple substances

infection: the invasion of healthy tissue by a pathogenic microorganism, resulting in the production of toxins and subsequent injury of tissue

Science and Profession

Bacteriology is the study of bacteria, unique life-forms that maintain the basic physiological and genetic processes of all other types of cellular life but that have the unusual characteristic of chemicophysiological diversity. Many bacteria live in totally anaerobic environments, converting carbohydrates to acids and alcohol by fermentation, nitrate to nitrogen gas, sulfate to hydrogen sulfide, and hydrogen and carbon dioxide to methane gas. Some bacteria live by photosynthetic processes similar to those of plants, while others survive by using energy obtained through the oxidation of sulfur, hydrogen, ammonia, or ferric minerals.

The history of life on Earth is closely linked to the presence of bacteria. Geologic evidence suggests the early increase in the earth's atmospheric oxygen more than two billion years ago was the direct result of bacteriological activity. Throughout time, bacteria have continued to play a crucial role in recycling materials necessary for the survival of plants and animals. In the biosphere, bacteria are responsible for degrading and converting complex substances into useful products. Bacteria break down carbohydrates, proteins, and lipids to form carbon dioxide, and they convert ammonia to nitrate and nitrogen gas to amino acids, all of which are essential to the life cycle of plants. Bacteria

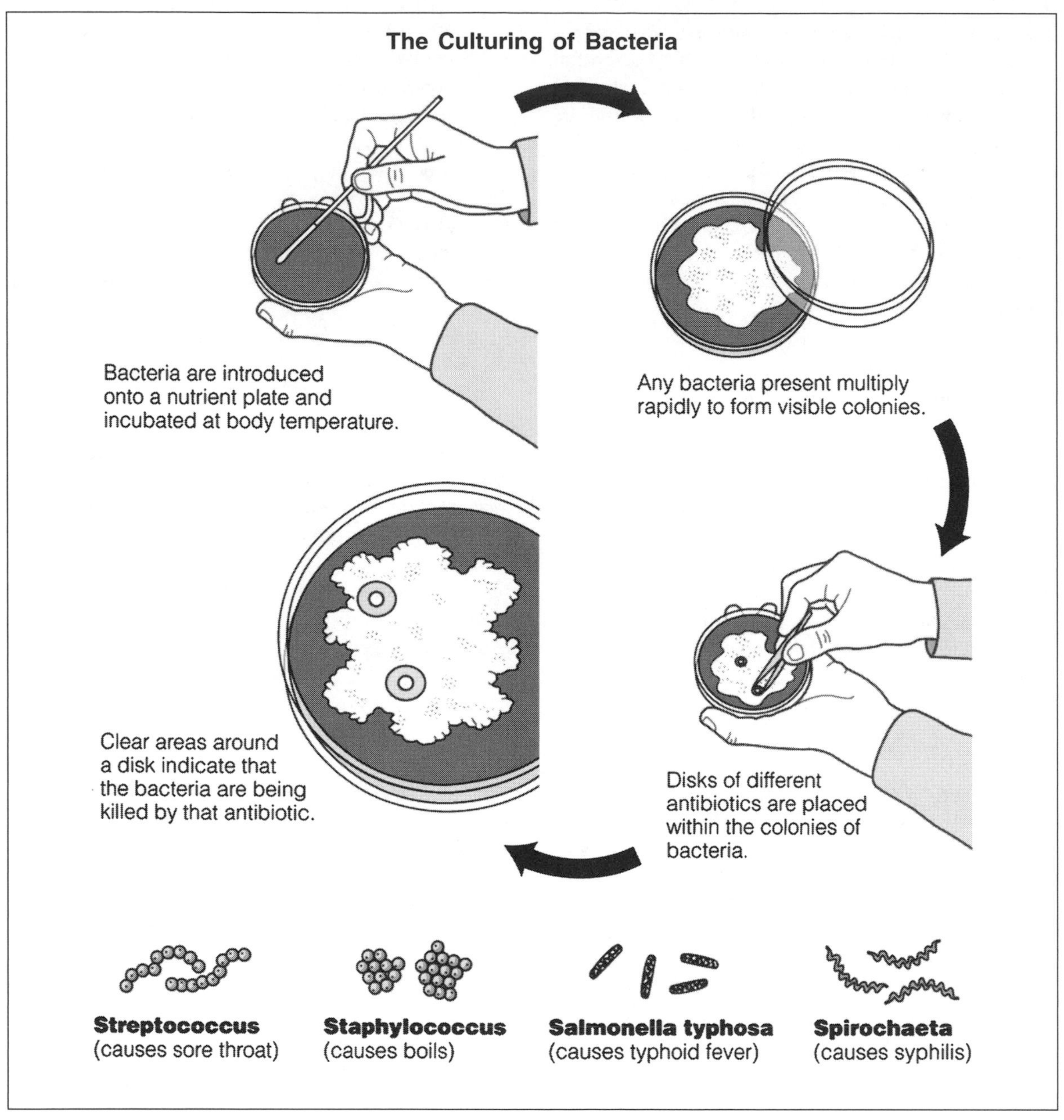

Bacteriologists use culturing techniques to identify types of bacteria and to develop and test antibiotics to destroy them; some bacteria are either harmless or helpful to humans, but harmful bacteria can cause a number of diseases, such as syphilis, typhoid fever, streptococcal infections, and staphylococcal infections.

are the basis of many industrial processes. Bacteria colonies are involved in producing cheeses and fermented foods such as pickles, sausage, and sauerkraut. Bacteria thriving in sewage and landfills produce methane gas, which is used as an alternative energy source by humans. The exploitation of bacteria as a detoxifying agent of environmental pollutants is becoming widespread. Almost all medically important antibiotics are produced by bacteria cultures.

Many types of bacteria live in association with animals. Most bacteria associated with humans live on the surface of the skin, in the mouth, or in the intestinal tract; the majority are harmless, and many are quite beneficial. Some bacteria, known as pathogens, are opportunistic and able to establish themselves in the body of a host, multiply, and produce local or systemic infections. Many pathogens are the causes of severe diseases in humans; most notable are anthrax, tuberculosis, bubonic plague, typhoid fever, pneumonia, gonorrhea, syphilis, gangrene, meningitis, botulism, diphtheria, scarlet fever, tetanus, streptococcal infections, and pertussis (whooping cough).

Medical bacteriology involves the study of infectious diseases produced by bacteria. Medical bacteriologists isolate bacteria suspected of being infectious, relate their role to the disease in question, study the life cycle of the bacteria colony, and seek means to provide therapy to infected victims and prevent further spread of the infectious pathogen.

Bacteriologists are highly skilled scientists having undergone advanced studies in the fields of biology, microbiology, and chemistry; many have additional training in medical specialties such as pathology, epidemiology, and serology.

Diagnostic and Treatment Techniques

The way in which bacterial infections develop usually follows a consistent pattern. Transmission may occur by one of four pathways: direct contact, such as sneezing or sexual intimacy; inhalation; common source contacts, such as food, water, or blood; and vector-borne spreading by insects or parasites. Bacteria first invade the body through some opening, such as a wound or the skin, nose, throat, lung, intestine, urethra, or bloodstream. The bacteria then target specific cells and begin to reproduce, establishing a primary infection. If the infection remains unchecked, it may spread to the lymphatic system or bloodstream, and multiple sites of infection may develop. The resulting infection destroys local tissue by producing toxins that damage cells or by producing compounds that interfere with body metabolism.

The control of bacterial infections is accomplished by breaking the links in the chain of transmission. This can be done by altering the behavior of potential hosts through education programs, quarantine, health inspections of common source contacts, and pest eradication programs. Other efforts to control infections involve altering the defensive capability of the host. The most effective means has been through vaccination. Vaccination immunizes individuals so that they are no longer susceptible to the targeted infection. Additionally, many bacterial infections can be treated with injections or topical and oral applications of antibiotics.

Perspective and Prospects

During the mid-nineteenth century, studies by Louis Pasteur into undesirable fermentation of beers and wines led him to the conclusion that infections in animals might be the result of some type of fermentation process. Pasteur experimented with the microbiological cause of infections by studying the characteristics of anthrax and cholera bacilli. Pasteur noted that the introduction of dead bacterial pathogens into a healthy host did not result in disease. Furthermore, if the host was injected with a virulent supply of the subject bacteria, the host did not contract the disease. The result of this work was the discovery of a method for acquired immunity to disease.

Working during the same period, German physician Robert Koch provided proof that anthrax and tuberculosis are caused by bacteria. Earlier in his career, Koch developed methods for isolating pure cultures of bacteria, then identifying, staining, and cataloging bacilli. The result of this work was that Koch and other investigators were able to view infected blood samples, then quickly isolate and cross-reference noted bacilli with previously identified pathogens.

The work of these two pioneering bacteriologists quickly led to the development of bacterial toxins for diphtheria and tetanus. The groundwork that they provided helped to establish the role that microorganisms play in the development of infectious disease and ushered in a golden age of discovery into the cause of infectious diseases and their control by immunization.

—Randall L. Milstein, Ph.D.

See also Antibiotics; Bacterial infections; Cells; Cholecystitis; Cystitis; Cytology; Cytopathology; Drug resistance; *E. coli* infection; Gangrene; Gram staining; Immunology; Immunopathology; Infection; Laboratory tests; Mastitis; Microbiology; Microscopy; Pathology; Pharmacology; Staphylococcal infections; Strep throat; Streptococcal infections; Tropical medicine.

For Further Information:

Alcamo, I. Edward. *Microbes and Society: An Introduction to Microbiology*. Sudbury, Mass.: Jones and Bartlett, 2002. A nonscientific text for the liberal arts student that explores the importance of microbes to human life and their role in food production and agriculture, in biotechnology and industry, in ecology and the environment, and in disease and bioterrorism.

Shnayerson, Michael. *The Killers Within: The Deadly Rise of Drug Resistant Bacteria*. New York: Little,

Brown, 2002. Traces the evolution of drug-resistant bacteria and how physicians are trying to combat them.

Snyder, Larry, and Wendy Champness. *Molecular Genetics of Bacteria*. 2d ed. Washington, D.C.: ASM Press, 2002. A text that introduces the field of bacterial molecular genetics and describes the mechanisms of mutations and gene exchange in bacteria and phages. Concentrates specifically on the bacterium *E. coli* while using examples from other bacteria as appropriate.

Topley, W. W. C. *Topley and Wilson's Microbiology and Microbial Infections*. Edited by Leslie Collier, Albert Ballows, and Max Sussman. 9th ed. 6 vols. New York: Oxford University Press, 1998. This work contains contributions from more than 320 highly respected medical professionals. All of the contributors deal essentially with diseases of human beings, but animal diseases are mentioned where animal models of infection are relevant.

Volk, Wesley A. *Essentials of Medical Microbiology*. 5th ed. Philadelphia: Lippincott-Raven, 1996. This comprehensive, illustrated text has been expanded to include immunopathology of infectious diseases, gene therapy in immunodeficiency disorders, virulence factors of bacteria, viral pathogenesis, diagnostic virology, and chemotherapeutic agents in virology.

Wilson, Michael, Brian Henderson, and Rod McNab. *Bacterial Virulence Mechanisms*. New York: Cambridge University Press, 2002. Basing their discussion on research advances in microbiology, molecular biology, and cell biology, the authors describe the interactions that exist between bacteria and human cells both in health and during infection.

Balance disorders

Disease/disorder

Anatomy or system affected: Nervous system

Specialties and related fields: Neurology

Definition: Problems with balance that may be described by sufferers as dizziness or vertigo and usually are associated with the inner ear; balance disorders may result in falls and other accidents.

Information on Balance Disorders

Causes: Age-related changes, viral infection in inner ear, motion sickness

Symptoms: Light-headedness, unsteadiness, imbalance in walking, vertigo, nausea, tinnitus

Duration: Temporary or chronic

Treatments: Antibiotics, neurological assessment

Causes and Symptoms

Being able to stand upright and walk with a steady gait is the result of a complex of body systems. For example, sight and hearing provide information about an individual's location and movement, and proprioceptors in muscles and joints help evaluate the individual's position in the environment. Age affects many of these systems, and age-related changes often impair the sense of balance.

Balance disorders include light-headedness, unsteadiness, or imbalance in walking. Such disorders also include vertigo, the feeling that a person's surroundings are moving or spinning around or that the person is spinning. Vertigo is sometimes accompanied by nausea. Because the ears often are involved, dizziness or vertigo may also be accompanied by tinnitus, a hissing, buzzing, or ringing sound in one or both ears.

Balance disorders often involve the labyrinth, a membrane-lined inner-ear chamber filled with fluid. The labyrinth consists of three canals, each at right angles to the other two. Any head movement—shaking, nodding, or tilting—is sensed by the canals, and the information is transmitted to the brain. Sometimes the labyrinth becomes inflamed, often from a viral infection, thus interfering with the signals relating to movement. Interference also occurs in motion sickness, in which the eyes see one kind of movement while the body, via the labyrinth, senses another kind of movement. The result is a confusion of signals and, often, the familiar sensations of dizziness, nausea, and vomiting.

Other causes of balance problems include neural dysfunctions and restrictions on the supply of blood to the brain. Light-headedness, for example, may be the result of changes in the flow of blood to the brain; if the flow is diminished, the result often is a "graying out," or darkening of vision. In extreme cases, the sufferer faints.

A balance disorder such as unsteadiness in walking may be the result of a dysfunction in the cerebellum, the back part of the brain. If the condition persists or worsens, it may be a symptom of a serious neurological disorder. Also, as part of the aging process, fine hairs in the inner ear may be reduced in number or size and thus function imperfectly. This frequently results in balance dysfunctions. Ear pain, nasal congestion, or discharge from the ears may result from middle-ear disorders and accompanying balance problems. Other causes include some medications, poor sleep habits, and vision problems.

Treatment and Therapy

Balance disorders may be symptomatic of serious physical problems and are best dealt with by a physician. If a balance problem is occasional and of short duration, relief may be gained simply by lying down for a brief while in a darkened room.

—*Albert C. Jensen, M.S.*

See also Batten's disease; Brain; Brain disorders; Dizziness and fainting; Eye infections and disorders; Hypotension; Ménière's disease; Vision disorders.

For Further Information:

American Medical Association. *American Medical Association Family Medical Guide*. 4th rev. ed. Hoboken, N.J.: John Wiley & Sons, 2004.

Aminoff, Michael J., David A. Greenberg, and Roger P. Simon. *Clinical Neurology*. 6th ed. New York: McGraw-Hill Medical, 2005.

Bannister, Roger. *Brain and Bannister's Clinical Neurology*. 7th ed. Oxford, England: Oxford University Press, 1992.

Brandt, Thomas. *Vertigo: Its Multisensory Syndromes*. New York: Springer-Verlag, 1999.

Parsons, Malcolm, and Michael Johnson. *Diagnosis in Color: Neurology*. New York: Mosby, 2001.

Baldness. *See* Hair loss and baldness.

Bariatric surgery

Procedure

Also known as: Gastric bypass, stomach stapling, weight loss surgery

Anatomy or system affected: Abdomen, endocrine system, gallbladder, gastrointestinal system, intestines, psychic-emotional system, skin, stomach

Specialties and related fields: Gastroenterology, general surgery, endocrinology, internal medicine, nutrition, orthopedics, plastic surgery, psychiatry, psychology

Definition: Any surgical procedure changing the structure of the digestive system in order to achieve weight reduction.

Key terms:

bariatrics: the medical management of obesity and related conditions

body mass index (BMI): a calculation using an individual's weight in kilograms divided by height in meters squared; a BMI of 30 or more is considered obese

duodenum: the first segment of the small intestine, attached to the stomach

gallstones: solid deposits of cholesterol or calcium salts found in the gallbladder or bile ducts

ileum: the last and usually longest segment of the small intestine

jejunum: the middle segment of the small intestine

laparoscopic surgery: surgery performed with a laparoscope, a slender, tubular instrument with a tiny video camera attached; enables smaller incisions

malabsorption: the abnormal utilization of nutrients from food

sleep apnea: breathing irregularities during sleep

Indications and Procedures

Candidates for bariatric surgery are the severely obese, with a body mass index (BMI) of 40 or more, or a BMI of 35 to 39 with serious medical conditions, such as diabetes mellitus, heart disease, hypertension, and sleep apnea. Typically, to qualify for surgery patients must first have tried other methods of weight loss (dietary modification, exercise, and/or drug therapy) and must be seriously impaired in their ability to perform routine activities. In addition, patients should undergo extensive psychiatric evaluation to ensure that they understand the risks of the procedure and are motivated enough to cope with its dramatic effects and permanent lifestyle changes.

There are two types of procedures. Restrictive surgery—including vertical banded gastroplasty, gastric banding, or laparoscopic gastric banding (lap band)—uses bands or staples near the top of the stomach to create a small pouch that restricts food intake to no more than one-half to one cup. The stoma, a tiny gap in the pouch that opens into the lower stomach, slows the emptying of the pouch to prolong fullness, thus reducing hunger.

Malabsorptive surgery involves surgical rearrangement of the digestive system to bypass parts of the stomach and small intestine, where most nutrients are absorbed. Roux-en-Y gastric bypass is the most commonly performed operation, derived from a procedure developed in 1966 by Dr. Edward E. Mason and named after the Y-shaped connection it creates. Roux-en-Y combines restriction with malabsorption, bypassing the lower stomach and the duodenum to connect the stomach pouch directly to the jejunum, or (less frequently) the iliem. In biliopancreatic diversion, sometimes performed on patients with a BMI of 50 or more, a portion of the stomach is actually removed, with the remaining section attached directly to the ileum, thus shortening the small intestine drastically to produce greater weight loss.

Uses and Complications

To lose weight and keep it off, surgery alone is not enough; strict diet and exercise regimens must be maintained. On average, bypass patients lose 66 percent of their excess weight after two years but gain some back as a result of stretching of the pouch over time. At five years, the loss of excess weight typically stabilizes at 33 to 50 percent. Restrictive procedures tend to result in comparatively less weight loss because there is no malabsorption. Diabetes, hypertension, and high cholesterol may improve significantly after surgery, often before marked weight loss occurs. Arthritis, sleep apnea, and other obesity-related conditions may gradually improve as weight is lost. In addition, patients often experience improved mobility and stamina and may report enhanced self-esteem and social acceptance.

Patients with very severe obesity, heart disease, diabetes, or sleep apnea and those who have inexperienced surgeons are at greater risk of developing complications. Gastric bypass patients face a 0.5 to 1.0 percent fatality rate; restrictive surgery patients fare better at 0.1 percent. Follow-up operations are required in 10 to 20 percent of patients. Most lap band patients experience at least one side effect, including abdominal pain, heartburn, nausea, vomiting, and band slippage to the extent that up to 25 percent may have the bands removed. If staples are used, then the risk of developing a leak or rupture is around 1.5 percent, leading to serious infection and often requiring further surgeries; laparoscopic patients appear to be at higher risk. Because 30 percent of patients develop gallstones after surgery as a result of rapid weight loss, the gallbladder is often removed as well. In 2 percent of cases, the spleen may be injured, necessitating its removal.

Other complications include blood clots, gaseous distention, infection, bowel or esophageal perforation, bowel strangulation, hernias, strictures, ulcers, late staple breakdown, menstrual irregularities, and hair loss. Patients undergoing malabsorptive procedures by definition will suffer from nutritional deficiencies, including anemia and metabolic bone disease resulting in osteoporosis, unless supplements are taken daily; regular vitamin B_{12} shots are necessary for some patients. Many patients will require further cosmetic surgery to remove large, sagging folds of skin.

All patients may experience vomiting from eating too much or too quickly. Pain behind the breastbone can result from insufficient chewing, causing large food particles to lodge in the stoma. About 70 percent of gastric bypass patients will develop dumping syndrome, a condition caused by eating too much fat or sugar, which can result in severe dizziness or weakness, abdominal cramps, nausea, vomiting, and diarrhea. Biliopancreatic bypass is further associated with chronic diarrhea and other long-term complications such as liver disease.

Perspective and Prospects

Surgical treatment for obesity began in the early 1950's with dangerous intestinal bypass procedures. As techniques have improved, the number of surgeries performed has mushroomed. The American Society for Bariatric Surgery reports that its member surgeons performed 28,800 operations in 1999 and 63,100 in 2002. During the same period, however, many more of the lucrative surgeries were performed by nonmembers. As of 2007, no regulatory body oversaw bariatric surgical practices, and board certification was voluntary. Evolving surgical practices and long-term outcomes remain difficult to evaluate as clinical trial data are lacking, and proof of overall improvements in health and longevity is scanty. According to the American Medical Association (AMA), the long-term consequences of weight loss surgery remain uncertain. To establish the overall safety and efficacy of such surgery, more research and stringent clinical trials are needed.

—Sue Tarjan

See also Digestion; Eating disorders; Gastrectomy; Gastroenterology; Gastrointestinal system; Hyperadiposis; Liposuction; Malabsorption; Malnutrition; Nutrition; Obesity; Obesity, childhood; Plastic surgery; Weight loss and gain; Weight loss medications.

For Further Information:

American Society for Bariatric Surgery (ASBS). http://www.asbs.org/.

Flancbaum, Louis, Erica Manfred, and Deborah Flancbaum. *The Doctor's Guide to Weight Loss Surgery: How to Make the Decision That Could Save*

Your Life. West Hurley, N.Y.: Fredonia Communications, 2001.
Hart, Dani. *I Want to Live: Gastric Bypass Reversal*. Fort Collins, Colo.: Mountain Stars, 2002.
Inabnet, William B., Eric J. DeMaria, and Sayeed Ikramuddin, eds. *Laparoscopic Bariatric Surgery*. Philadelphia: Lippincott Williams & Wilkins, 2005.
Mitchell, James E., and Martina de Zwaan, eds. *Bariatric Surgery: A Guide for Mental Health Professionals*. New York: Routledge, 2005.
U.S. Department of Health and Human Services. Public Health Service. National Institutes of Health. Office of Medical Applications of Research. *Gastrointestinal Surgery for Severe Obesity: A Consensus Development Conference*. Bethesda, Md.: Author, 1991.

Basal cell carcinoma. *See* Skin cancer.

Batten's disease

Disease/disorder

Also known as: Neuronal ceroid lipofuscinoses (NCLs), Spielmeyer-Vogt-Sjögren-Batten disease, Santavouri-Haltia disease, Jansky-Bielchowsky disease, Spielmeyer-Vogt disease, Kufs' disease, Parry's disease

Anatomy or system affected: Brain, cells, eyes, nervous system, skin

Specialties and related fields: Genetics, neurology, ophthalmology, pediatrics

Definition: A progressive neurological disruption and deterioration of intellectual and physical development caused by mutated genes.

Causes and Symptoms

An umbrella term for neuronal ceroid lipofuscinoses (NCLs), Batten's disease occurs in four types that are distinguished by the patient's age when symptoms first appear. Batten's disease is associated with defective genes and usually is transmitted as a recessive trait. The prevalence of this disease in the United States is approximately 1 per 25,000 births. Variations of the disease share similar symptoms associated with lipopigment accumulation in tissues. These excess proteins and fats disrupt cellular functioning, particularly in the brain and eyes. Abnormal enzyme activity alters metabolism and body chemistry.

Infantile type, sometimes referred to as Finnish or Santavouri-Haltia type, usually is evident when children are between six months and two years old. A defective palmitoyl protein thioesterase (PPT) gene on chromosome 1 causes this type of Batten's disease. The patient's physical and mental development and growth, particularly head size, cease to follow normal patterns. Most patients with this type die by age six.

Information on Batten's Disease

Causes: Genetic mutation leading to excess proteins and fats in tissues

Symptoms: Seizures, sight impairment, diminished motor skills and intellect, behavioral extremes, unbalanced movement, dementia

Duration: Lifelong

Treatments: Medications to prevent seizures and minimize motor difficulties, institutionalization

Children with late infantile type, or Jansky-Bielchowsky type, seem normal until two to four years of age. They then suffer seizures, sight impairment, and diminished motor skills and intellect. Death often occurs by age twelve. This type is linked to the ceroid-lipofuscinosis, neuronal 2 (CLN2) gene on chromosome 11.

Juvenile NCL, or Spielmeyer-Vogt, type appears in children at approximately five to ten years of age. The ceroid-lipofuscinosis, neuronal 3 (CLN3) gene on chromosome 16 is associated with this type. Symptoms occur at a slower rate than with the first two types. Patients sometimes become paralyzed.

Kufs' or Parry's disease is the rare adult type of Batten's disease. Sometimes this type is inherited as a dominant disease, and people with one defective gene are affected. Unlike with other types, adult patients do not have convulsions or impaired eyesight. Behavioral extremes and unbalanced movement characterize this type. Progressive mania can result in dementia.

Physicians diagnose Batten's disease by studying the patient's skin tissues for lipopigment deposits. An eye examination may reveal the cell depletion associated with Batten's disease. Additional tests, imaging, X rays, and electroencephalograms can verify the diagnosis.

Treatment and Therapy

Because Batten's disease cannot be prevented or cured, treatment focuses on the alleviation of symptoms. Physicians prescribe medications to prevent seizures and to minimize motor difficulties and loss of balance. Nutritional strategies and various therapies can also ease symptoms. Sometimes, patients need to be institutionalized as a result of their mental and visual incapacities.

Perspective and Prospects

Dr. Christian Stengel's 1826 medical article is credited as the first clinical report of patients with Batten's disease symptoms. Dr. Frederick E. Batten observed several types of this disease in patients in 1903, differentiating it from Tay-Sachs disease. Dr. Karl Sjögren initiated genetic investigations. By the 1990's, researchers linked specific genes to Batten's disease.

The Batten's Disease Support and Research Association distributes information, while the National Batten's Disease Registry and designated tissue banks compile data.

—*Elizabeth D. Schafer, Ph.D.*

See also Balance disorders; Brain; Brain disorders; Eyes; Genetic diseases; Mental retardation; Nervous system; Neuralgia, neuritis, and neuropathy; Neuroimaging; Neurology; Neurology, pediatric; Seizures; Vision disorders.

For Further Information:

Batten Disease Support and Research Association (BDSRA). http://www.bdsra.org/.

Mole, Sara E. "Batten's Disease: Eight Genes and Still Counting?" *Lancet* 354, no. 9177 (August 7, 1999): 443-445.

Opitz, John M., ed. *Ceroid-Lipofuscinoses: Batten Disease and Allied Disorders*. New York: A. R. Liss, 1988.

U.S. Department of Health and Human Services. Public Health Service. National Institutes of Health. *Batten Disease*. Bethesda, Md.: Author, 1992.

Wisniewski, Krystyna E., and Nanbert Zhong, eds. *Batten Disease: Diagnosis, Treatment, and Research*. San Diego, Calif.: Academic Press, 2001.

Bed-wetting

Disease/disorder

Also known as: Enuresis

Anatomy or system affected: Bladder, muscles, musculoskeletal system, urinary system

Specialties and related fields: Family medicine, pediatrics, psychology, urology

Definition: A condition characterized by an inability of the bladder to contain the urine during sleep, often a developmental condition in children.

Information on Bed-Wetting

Causes: Immature development of the phrenic reflex, physical illness, disease, anatomical defect

Symptoms: Passage of urine during sleep

Duration: Often chronic until phrenic reflex matures

Treatments: Alarm therapy, chiropractic manipulation, drug therapy

Key terms:

alarm therapy: the practice of utilizing mechanical or electronic devices to detect bed-wetting as it occurs

bladder: a membranous sac in the body that serves as the temporary retention site of urine

diaphragm: a body partition of muscle and connective tissue separating the chest and abdominal cavities

enuresis: an involuntary discharge of urine; incontinence of urine

nervous system: the bodily system that receives and interprets stimuli and transmits impulses to the organs

neurophysiological: pertaining to the nervous system in the human body

phrenic: of or relating to the diaphragm

sphincter: a muscle surrounding and able to contract or close a bodily opening (such as the opening to the bladder)

Causes and Symptoms

Primary enuresis is defined medically as the inability to hold one's urine during sleep. The condition is quite common and occurs most often in children; approximately 20 percent of children under the age of six suffer from the condition. These percentages decrease to about 5 percent at age ten, 2 percent at age fifteen and only about 1 percent of adults. Secondary enuresis is bed-wetting in a child who had previously achieved bladder control. (These terms do not apply, however, to urination problems caused by physical illness, disease, or anatomical defect.) The condition is more common in boys than in girls. Bed-wetting usually occurs during the first third of sleep, although it can occur during all sleep stages and without relation to awakening periods.

It is important to realize that enuresis is considered to be a developmental concern rather than an emotional, behavioral, or physical one. Donald S. Kornfeld and Philip R. Muskin report in *The Columbia University College of Physicians and Surgeons Complete Home*

Medical Guide (Rev. ed., 1989) that "enuresis is due to a lag in development of the nervous system's controls on elimination." Many parents fail to understand this neuropsychological element and thus punish the child for a wet bed. Punishing, ridiculing, or shaming the child does not correct the situation; in fact, in many cases, it may prolong the problem as well as cause other unnecessary and undesirable psychological problems. Emotional problems have resulted from enuresis, as the child may be too embarrassed to partake in normal childhood activities such as camping or sleepovers.

Treatment and Therapy

Techniques for helping the enuretic child achieve dryness range from withholding liquids near bedtime to alarm systems to medical intervention. Generally, restriction of liquid intake after dinner is the first course of action. This treatment method, however, does not have a very high success rate. Should this treatment fail after a trial period of a few weeks, other methods may be employed.

Alarm therapy can help a child achieve control within four months, sometimes in only a few weeks. A beeper- or buzzer-type alarm sounds when moisture touches the bedding or underwear; the desired result is that the child, while sleeping, will eventually recognize the need to urinate and awaken in time to get to the bathroom. Electronic alarms are generally of two types. The first is a wired pad, consisting of two screens, which is placed under the sheets to detect wetness; when the child wets, the moisture activates the battery-operated alarm. The second is a device worn on the body, either in the underpants and connected by a wire to an alarm or a wristwatch-type alarm; the underwear serves as a separating cloth for the contact points. In either case, as wetness occurs, the alarm sounds, thus wakening the child; the child can then be directed to the bathroom to complete urination.

Barry G. Powell and Lynda Muransky cite several case histories in which alarm therapy proved to be effective in stopping enuresis. For example, a six-year-old who never had a dry bed achieved dryness within a week through the use of an alarm. In another case, a fifteen-year-old had been trying to overcome his bed-wetting problem for ten years. Several trips to the doctor showed that he had no physical cause for enuresis. His parents labeled him "lazy, inconsiderate, and difficult." His desire to join his hockey team in overnight travel gave him the impetus to seek help. Powell and Muransky found his problem to be primary enuresis aggravated by family ridiculing. Through the use of his alarm, he achieved dryness within two weeks.

A case involving secondary enuresis is described as well. A child who had suffered through primary enuresis, then achieved dryness, was found to be wetting again. This second bout of bed-wetting seems to have been the result of his parents' marital separation. After a medical examination revealed no physical problems, it appeared the problem was psychological, caused by emotional upset. He resumed dryness in three weeks (although an alarm system on his bed for six months gave him more confidence). It is important to note, however, that alarms can take up to several months' time before a child feels comfortable in stopping its use. Also, parental supervision is imperative in order for this type of therapy to work properly.

Chiropractic spinal manipulation has been found to be effective in the treatment of some cases of enuresis. Some believe that a spinal reflex is involved in bed-wetting. As nighttime breathing slows down (a normal reaction), carbon dioxide builds up in the body. When the carbon dioxide buildup reaches a certain level, a breathing mechanism called the phrenic reflex is triggered. This mechanism normally causes the diaphragm to return breathing to its normal pattern. If the mechanism does not work properly, however, the carbon dioxide continues to increase, resulting in an involuntary relaxation of the sphincter muscle at the opening to the bladder. Fluid (urine) is released and leaks out of the bladder. A child in a deep state of sleep does not recognize that the bed has been wet. Generally, chiropractors believe that the bed-wetting child sleeps in a state of high carbon dioxide intoxication.

While immature development of the phrenic reflex is the most common cause of bed-wetting, in some children a misalignment of the bones in the neck and spine (referred to as "subluxation" by chiropractors) is thought to cause pressure on the nerves that are related to the phrenic reflex. Through chiropractic adjustments, it is argued, the subluxation can be corrected, thus relieving pressure on the nerves. With the spine realigned and bodily functions working normally, enuresis can be eliminated. One child had never had a dry bed in his first ten years of life; after only two spinal adjustments by a licensed chiropractor, the child stopped wetting immediately. Chiropractors usually recommend a series of adjustments in order to realign the spine and nerves and keep them in the proper position.

Drug therapy solely for the treatment of enuresis is controversial. However, when an illness such as diabetes mellitus is the underlying cause of the bed-wetting, the use of drugs may be indicated. The drug imipramine hydrochloride (an antidepressant agent) has been studied to assist in contraction of the sphincter; however, because of the high toxicity and limited effectiveness of such antidepressants, its use is not widespread. Relapse rates are high, and a cure rate of only 25 percent is seen. More success has been achieved with desmopressin acetate, an antidiuretic drug. There is an immediate improvement in 70 percent of treated children. Relapse rates are lower than those associated with imipramine but higher than with the use of bed-wetting alarms, probably because the sphincter muscle is not fully developed in the enuretic child. In general, drug therapy yields a final success rate of 25 percent.

Perspective and Prospects

The history of bed-wetting is probably a lengthy one. The term "enuresis" was coined around 1800, and the condition has plagued children from every ethnic background and socioeconomic level around the world. It continues to be a problem for many children today and probably will be so in the future as well.

Most enuretics are deep sleepers who are usually quite active during their waking hours. This sleeping pattern, combined with urinary systems that are not yet fully developed, is generally the main cause of bed-wetting. There are some indications that enuresis is hereditary; many children who suffer from the condition have a parent who was enuretic as a child. It is reassuring to know that almost all affected children outgrow the problem by adulthood. While no immediate cure is available, continued experiments with alarm systems and drugs will certainly alleviate the discomfort and embarrassment until the body's lag in development corrects itself.

—*Carol A. Holloway*

See also Anxiety; Incontinence; Psychology; Sleep disorders; Stress; Urinary disorders; Urinary system; Urology; Urology, pediatric.

For Further Information:

"Alarm Bells for Enuresis." *The Lancet* 337 (March 2, 1991): 523. Alarm therapy is discussed as a treatment for enuresis (nocturnal bed-wetting) in children. Attention is given to the importance of parental supervision, family stress, environmental obstacles, and behavioral problems that can contribute to bed-wetting.

American Medical Association. *American Medical Association Family Medical Guide*. 4th rev. ed. Hoboken, N.J.: John Wiley & Sons, 2004. Medical myths concerning the problem are discussed. Related articles covering such topics as urinary infections in children and nephritis are conveniently located in the same chapter of the book.

"Defining Enuresis." *FDA Consumer* 23 (May, 1989): 10. This article, written for the layperson, is easy to understand and even offers a helpful pronunciation guide for difficult terms. The links between enuresis and sleep patterns, sleepwalking, and nightmares are examined.

Kemper, Kathi J. *The Holistic Pediatrician: A Pediatrician's Comprehensive Guide to Safe and Effective Therapies for the Twenty-five Most Common Ailments of Infants, Children, and Adolescents*. 2d ed. New York: HarperCollins, 2002. A comprehensive guide to integrative medicine for children, which includes good information and recommendations for bed-wetting.

Kornfeld, Donald S., and Philip R. Muskin. "Enuresis, or Bed-Wetting." In *The Columbia University College of Physicians and Surgeons Complete Home Medical Guide*, edited by Donald Tapley et al. Rev. 3d ed. New York: Crown, 1995. A well-written article explaining the causes, effects, and treatments of bed-wetting in children. Offers the encouraging suggestion that even if all treatments fail, the problem is usually outgrown by adulthood.

Morison, Moya J. "Living with a Young Person Who Wets the Bed: The Families' Experience." *British Journal of Nursing* 9, no. 9 (May 11-24, 2000): 572. An ethnographic study in which family members describe the practical and social consequences of bed-wetting, both for themselves and for the family, and the methods that they have employed to encourage cessation of bed-wetting.

Rogers, June. "Child Centered Approach to Bed-Wetting." *Community Practitioner* 76, no. 5 (May, 2003): 163-165. A pediatric continence adviser explores the role that nurse-led community enuresis services play in effectively diagnosing and treating the underlying causes of childhood bed-wetting.

Behçet's disease

Disease/disorder

Also known as: Mucocutaneous ocular syndrome, Silk Road disease

Anatomy or system affected: Eyes, genitals, mouth, nervous system, skin

Specialties and related fields: Internal medicine, ophthalmology, rheumatology

Definition: A multisystem disease characterized by recurrent oral and genital ulcers.

Causes and Symptoms

Behçet's disease usually appears in early adulthood with painful aphthous ulcers (similar to canker sores) in the mouth and genitals. These ulcers generally subside after one to two weeks, but they recur throughout the course of the disease. Some patients also have painful skin nodules known as erythema nodosum. Brief periods of joint pain are also common. Rarely, the ulcers of Behçet's disease are found in the gastrointestinal tract. Involvement of the central nervous system causes a variety of symptoms ranging from mild confusion to paralysis. However, the most serious complication of Behçet's disease is involvement of the eyes, since this may progress to blindness. Patients also have an increased predisposition for the formation of blood clots, usually in the venous system. These clots can be life-threatening if they migrate to the lungs.

The common factor underlying these diverse manifestations of Behçet's disease is inflammation of the small blood vessels, but it remains unclear what environmental or genetic factors trigger this inflammation. Rare reports have been made of familial forms of the disease, raising the possibility of a genetic basis, but this remains under investigation. Diagnosis is made on clinical grounds.

Treatment and Therapy

Behçet's disease is a chronic condition, but the severity of the disease generally lessens over time. Ulcers are first treated with topical glucocorticoids, in the form of either mouthwash or paste. Refractory cases may require thalidomide, a drug that must be used with extreme caution because of its ability to cause birth defects. Because of the risk of blindness, ocular and central nervous system disease is managed more aggressively with oral steroids (such as prednisone), along with azathioprine or cyclosporine.

Apart from the above complications, the long-term prognosis of Behçet's disease is quite good, and the life expectancy of patients is comparable with that of the general population.

Perspective and Prospects

The first description of Behçet's disease appears in the writings of Hippocrates in the fifth century B.C.E., but it was first recognized in the modern era by the Turkish physician Dr. Hulusi Behçet in 1937. Although Behçet's disease is seen throughout the world, the highest prevalence is in countries along the ancient Silk Road, a trading route extending from the Far East to the Mediterranean Sea.

—Ahmad Kamal, M.D.

See also Blindness; Eyes; Genital disorders, female; Genital disorders, male; Nervous system; Neurology; Ophthalmology; Rheumatology; Thrombosis and thrombus; Ulcers; Vascular medicine; Vascular system; Vision disorders.

Information on Behçet's Disease

Causes: Unknown

Symptoms: Inflammation of small blood vessels, oral and genital ulcers, painful skin nodules, joint pain; complications may include mild confusion, paralysis, blindness, blood clots

Duration: Chronic, with episodes lasting one to two weeks

Treatments: Topical glucocorticoids, thalidomide, oral steroids (prednisone), immunosuppressive agents (azathioprine, cyclosporine)

For Further Information:

Lee, Sungnack, et al., eds. *Behçet's Disease: A Guide to Its Clinical Understanding*. New York: Springer, 2001.

Parker, James N., and Philip M. Parker, eds. *The Official Patient's Sourcebook on Behcet's Disease*. San Diego, Calif.: Icon Health, 2002.

Plotkin, Gary R., John J. Calabro, and J. Desmond O'Duffy, eds. *Behçet's Disease: A Contemporary Synopsis*. Mount Kisco, N.Y.: Futura, 1988.

Zeis, Joanne. *Essential Guide to Behçet's Disease*. Uxbridge, Mass.: Central Vision Press, 2002.

Bell's palsy

Disease/disorder

Anatomy or system affected: Ears, eyes, head, mouth, muscles, nerves

Specialties and related fields: Family medicine, neurology, nutrition

Definition: A weakening or paralysis of facial muscles caused by damage to the seventh cranial nerve.

Causes and Symptoms

The most likely cause of Bell's palsy is a weakened immune system produced by the common cold virus or herpesviruses. The condition has also been associated with chronic middle ear infection, sarcoidosis, Lyme disease, high blood pressure, tumors, and trauma to the head. A diagnosis of Bell's palsy is made from facial appearance and weakness, blood tests, electromyography to confirm nerve damage, and magnetic resonance imaging (MRI) or computed tomography (CT) to assess any pressure on the facial nerve.

In 99 percent of cases, Bell's palsy produces paralysis on only one side of the face. Other symptoms may include an inability to close the eye on the affected side, frequent tearing from that eye, dryness of the affected eye, drooping of the eyelid and mouth, drooling, increased sensitivity to sound and ringing in the affected ear, impairment of taste, jaw pain, impaired speech, headache, and dizziness. Typically, the symptoms appear rather suddenly and peak within the first forty-eight hours after onset. Most patients experience dramatic improvement within two weeks, and most recover totally within three to six months after onset.

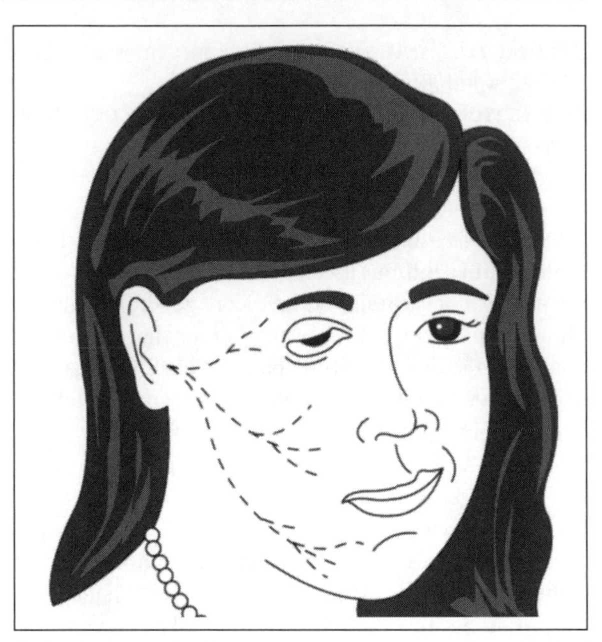

Bell's palsy results in a temporary sagging and paralysis of one side of the face; dashed lines show the main neural pathways affected.

Treatment and Therapy

Various treatments can be effective if administered within seven days after onset. Antiviral drugs such as acyclovir, famciclovir, or valacyclovir cause the virus to run its course faster by binding viral enzymes so that the harmful cells cannot replicate. Prednisone, a synthetic hormone that mimics the natural steroid cortisol produced by the body, is also administered to help reduce swelling and the inflammation compressing the seventh cranial nerve.

The application of moist heat can help reduce pain and discomfort. The affected eye should be kept moist to protect it from debris and injury. Facial massage and exercise may help prevent the permanent shrinkage of facial muscles. Since vitamins B_1, B_6, and B_{12} are essential for proper nervous system functioning, a B-complex vitamin is often prescribed. Ample rest is necessary to restore the immune system.

Information on Bell's Palsy

Causes: Damage to seventh cranial nerve, immune system weakness from common cold or herpes, chronic middle ear infection, sarcoidosis, Lyme disease, high blood pressure, tumors, head trauma

Symptoms: Weakening or paralysis of facial muscles on one side, with inability to close eye, frequent tearing and dryness of eye, drooping eyelid and mouth, drooling, increased sensitivity to sound, ringing in ear, taste impairment, jaw pain, impaired speech, headache, dizziness

Duration: Improvement within two weeks, total recovery within three to six months

Treatments: Antiviral drugs (acyclovir, famciclovir, valacyclovir), prednisone, moist heat, facial massage and exercise, B vitamins

Perspective and Prospects

First described in the nineteenth century by Scottish surgeon Sir Charles Bell, Bell's palsy affects approximately 40,000 Americans each year. It can occur at any age but is more common before age fifteen and after age sixty. Diabetics are particularly susceptible to the condition, as are pregnant women, particularly during the last trimester.

No cure has been found for Bell's palsy. Research focuses on achieving a better understanding of how the nervous system works, developing methods of repairing damaged nerves and restoring full use of injured areas, and finding ways to prevent nerve damage. Methylcobalamin, an essential component in the process of building nerve tissue, shows promise for treating Bell's palsy.

—Alvin K. Benson, Ph.D.

See also Muscle sprains, spasms, and disorders; Muscles; Nervous system; Neuralgia, neuritis, and neuropathy; Neuroimaging; Neurology; Neurology, pediatric; Palsy; Paralysis.

For Further Information:

Matthews, Gary G. *Cellular Physiology of Nerve and Muscle*. 4th ed. Malden, Mass.: Blackwell Science, 2003.

Standring, Susan, et al., eds. *Gray's Anatomy*. 39th ed. New York: Elsevier Churchill Livingstone, 2005.

Waxman, Bruce. *Electrotherapy for Treatment of Facial Nerve Paralysis (Bell's Palsy)*. Rockville, Md.: U.S. Department of Health and Human Services, 1984.

Benign prostatic hyperplasia. *See* Prostate enlargement.

Beriberi

Disease/disorder

Also known as: Thiamine deficiency, vitamin B_1 deficiency

Anatomy or system affected: Gastrointestinal system, heart, muscles, nervous system

Specialties and related fields: Family medicine, pediatrics

Definition: A nutritional disease resulting from thiamine deficiency.

Information on Beriberi

Causes: Thiamine deficiency from chronic alcoholism, malnutrition, diuresis, dialysis, high carbohydrate intake

Symptoms: Weakness, irritability, nausea, vomiting, tingling, loss of sensation in hands and feet, confusion, difficulty speaking or walking; may progress to coma and death

Duration: Chronic, sometimes fatal

Treatments: Thiamine hydrochloride, dietary changes

Causes and Symptoms

Thiamine, one of the B vitamins, plays an important role in energy metabolism and tissue building. When there is not enough thiamine in the diet, these basic energy functions are disturbed, leading to problems throughout the body. There are two major manifestations of thiamine deficiency, cardiovascular disease (wet beriberi) and nervous system disease (dry beriberi). Each can be caused by chronic alcoholism, malnutrition, diuresis, dialysis, and high carbohydrate intake.

The accompanying symptoms of thiamine deficiency may include weakness, irritability, nausea, vomiting, tingling, or loss of sensation in the hands and feet (peripheral neuropathy). Progressed symptoms include mental confusion and difficulties speaking or walking; these are often the precursor symptoms leading to coma and/or death.

Treatment and Therapy

Thiamine hydrochloride is the initial treatment of choice for beriberi. Successful treatment reverses the deficiency and alleviates most of the symptoms. Severe deficiencies may be treated with high doses of thiamine given by muscular injection.

Alternative treatments stress a diet rich in foods that provide thiamine and other B vitamins, such as brown rice, whole grains, raw fruits and vegetables, legumes, nuts and seeds, and yogurt. Additional supplements of B vitamins, a multivitamin and mineral complex, and vitamin C are also recommended. A balanced diet containing all essential nutrients will prevent thiamine deficiency and the development of beriberi. People who consume large quantities of soda, pretzels, chips, candy, and high-carbohydrate foods made with unenriched flours may also need vitamin supplements to avoid thiamine deficiency.

Perspective and Prospects

The first clinical descriptions of beriberi were conducted by the Dutch physician Nicolaas Tulp around 1652. Tulp treated a young Dutchman who, upon returning from the East Indies, suffered from what the natives of the Indies called beriberi, or "the lameness." Not until the early 1900's did scientists discover that rice bran, the outer covering of white rice, actually contains something that prevented the disease, thiamine. In the 1920's, extracts of rice polishings were used to treat the disease.

Beriberi is fatal if left untreated. Most symptoms can be reversed, and full recovery is possible when thiamine levels are returned to normal and maintained with a balanced diet and vitamin supplements as needed.

—Jason A. Hubbart, M.S.

See also Alcoholism; Malnutrition; Nutrition; Vitamins and minerals.

FOR FURTHER INFORMATION:

Anderson, Jean, and Barbara Deskins. *The Nutrition Bible*. New York: William Morrow, 1997.

Behrman, Richard E., Robert M. Kliegman, and Hal B. Jenson, eds. *Nelson Textbook of Pediatrics*. 17th ed. Philadelphia: Saunders, 2004.

Rivlin, Richard. "Vitamin Deficiency." In *Conn's Current Therapy*, edited by Robert E. Rakel. Philadelphia: W. B. Saunders, 1996.

Williams, Sue Rodwell, and Eleanor D. Schlenker. *Essentials of Nutrition and Diet Therapy*. 8th ed. St. Louis: Mosby, 2003.

BIOFEEDBACK

PROCEDURE

ANATOMY OR SYSTEM AFFECTED: Brain, circulatory system, endocrine system, glands, heart, muscles, musculoskeletal system, nerves, nervous system, psychic-emotional system

SPECIALTIES AND RELATED FIELDS: Alternative medicine, cardiology, exercise physiology, family medicine, internal medicine, neurology, occupational health, physical therapy, preventive medicine, psychology, sports medicine, vascular medicine

DEFINITION: The learned self-regulation of the autonomic nervous system through monitoring of the physiological activity occurring within an individual.

KEY TERMS:

biodisplay: audio or visual information about the physiological activity within an organism displayed by various instruments and processes

biofeedback: the provision of information about the biological or physiological processes of an individual to him or her, with the objective of empowering the individual to make conscious changes in the processes being monitored; it can be instrumental (using devices that monitor physiological or biological processes) or noninstrumental (using bodily sensations)

biofeedback instrument: a device (usually electronic) that is capable of measuring and displaying information about a physiologic process in a way that allows an individual to monitor the physiologic activity through his or her own senses

electrodermal response (EDR) biofeedback: the monitoring and displaying of information about the conductivity of the skin; used for anxiety reduction, asthma treatment, and the treatment of sleep disorders

electroencephalographic (EEG) biofeedback: the monitoring and displaying of brain wave activity; used for the treatment of substance abuse disorders, epilepsy, attention-deficit disorders, and insomnia

electromyograph (EMG): an instrument that is capable of monitoring and displaying information about electrochemical activity in a group of muscle fibers

neuromuscular rehabilitation: the process of employing electromyographic biofeedback to correct physiological disorders that have both muscular and neurological components, such as the effects of strokes and fibromyalgia; also called myoneural rehabilitation

physiological autoregulation: the process by which an individual utilizes information about a physiological activity to effect changes in that activity in a direction that contributes to normal (or desirable) functioning

INDICATIONS AND PROCEDURES

Biofeedback has been utilized in both research and clinical applications. The term itself denotes the provision of information (feedback) about a biological process. It has been found that individuals (laboratory animals included), when given feedback that is reinforcing, are able to change physiological processes in a desired direction; homeostatic processes being what they are, these changes are in a positive direction. In the case of humans, the feedback is provided about a physiological function of which the individual would not otherwise be aware if it were not for the provision—via a biodisplay—of information about that process.

It has been observed that for persons employing biofeedback, the equipment used serves as a kind of a sixth sense. Quoting from the publication *Biofeedback*, by the National Institute of Mental Health,

> This sixth sense allows the person to "see" or "hear" activity inside of their bodies—activity that they would otherwise be unaware of. For the individual who now knows what the physiological activity actually is (and knowing in what direction the physiological process should be heading) the biofeedback equipment now serves as a "mirror." The "mirror" provides the feedback which the individual uses in order to make corrections (physiological autoregulation) in the given physiological process in the desired direction.

Human maladies range from the purely structural to the purely functional, with various gradations. An example of a structural disorder is a broken bone, while an example of a functional disorder might be a person who manifests symptoms of blindness for which there is no known or identifiable organic cause. Looking at the spectrum of human maladies, one can consider the continuum as "structural," "psychophysiological," "mental-emotional," "hysterical," and "feigned." The category of psychophysiological lies midway between structural and mental-emotional. A psychophysiological disorder has elements of both mind and body interactions; it is a physiological disorder brought about by thoughts, feelings, and emotions. There are those who take the position that all human maladies and disorders have a mental-emotional component to them, that there can be no change in the mental-emotional state without a corresponding change in the physiological state and no change in the physiological state without a corresponding change in the mental-emotional state.

It is currently the preference of many scientifically and technologically oriented practitioners to deal with the more structural disorders (or to treat the disorder as if it were mostly structural). It is also the case that many mental health practitioners prefer to deal with disorders that fall more into the mental-emotional category. A growing number of practitioners, however, have an interest in and training for dealing with psychophysiological disorders. This emerging field is referred to as behavioral medicine, and a large percentage of the practitioners in this field employ biofeedback as a modality.

A classic example of biofeedback being used to correct a physiological problem would be the employing of electromyograph (EMG) biofeedback for the correction of a simple tension (or psychophysiologic) headache. The headache is caused by inappropriately high muscle tension in the neck, head, or shoulders. In surface electromyographic biofeedback, the biofeedback practitioner attaches electronic sensors to the muscles of the forehead, neck, or shoulders of the patient. The electronic sensors pick up signals from electrochemical activity at the surface of the skin in the area of the involved muscle groups. The behavior of the muscles being monitored is such that minute changes in the electrochemical activity in the muscles—tension and relaxation—occur naturally.

The sensitivity of the biofeedback instrument (the magnification of the signal may be as high as one thousand times) and the display of the signal make the individual aware of these changes via sound or visual signals (biodisplays). When the biofeedback signal indicates that the muscle activity is in the direction of relaxation, the individual makes an association between that muscle behavior and the corresponding change in the strength of the signal. The individual can then increase the duration, strength, and frequency of the relaxation process. Having learned to relax the involved muscles, the individual is able to prevent or abort headache activity.

It is axiomatic that any physiological process (behavior) that is capable of being quantified, measured, and displayed is appropriate for biofeedback applications. The following are some of the more commonly used biofeedback instruments.

An electromyograph is an instrument that is capable of monitoring and displaying information about electrochemical activity in a group of muscle fibers. Common applications of surface electromyography (in which sensors are placed on the surface of the skin, as opposed to the insertion of needles into the muscle itself) include stroke rehabilitation. Surface electromyography is also used in the treatment of tension headaches and fibromyalgia.

An electrodermal response (EDR) biofeedback instrument is capable of monitoring and displaying information about the conductivity of the skin. An increase in the conductivity of the skin is a function of moisture accumulating in the space recently occupied by blood. The rate of blood flow depends on the amount of autonomic nervous system arousal present within the organism at the time of measurement. The higher the level of autonomic nervous system arousal, the greater the amount of skin conductivity. Common applications of EDR biofeedback are the reduction of anxiety caused by phobic reactions, the control of asthma (especially in young children), and the treatment of sleep disorders. For example, many insomniacs are unable to drop off to sleep because of higher-than-appropriate autonomic nervous system activity.

An instrument that is capable of monitoring and displaying the surface temperature of the skin, as correlated with an increase in vascular (blood flow) activity in the area of the skin in question, can also be used for biofeedback. Such an instrument is helpful in treatment for high blood pressure and migraine headaches.

Electroencephalographic (EEG) biofeedback involves the monitoring and displaying of brain wave activity as a correlate of autonomic nervous system activity. Different brain waves are associated with different levels of autonomic nervous system arousal. Common applications of EEG biofeedback are in the treatment of substance abuse disorders, epilepsy, attention-deficit disorders, and insomnia.

Uses and Complications

Biofeedback is gaining in popularity because of a number of factors. One of the principal reasons is a growing interest in alternatives to the lifetime use of medications to manage a disorder.

To understand the rationale for biofeedback in a clinical setting, it is essential to discuss the types of disorders for which it is commonly employed. As pointed out in the publication *Biofeedback*, the more common usages of biofeedback treatment techniques include "migraine headaches, tension headaches, and many other types of pain; disorders of the digestive system; high blood pressure and its opposite, low blood pressure; cardiac arrhythmias (abnormalities, sometimes dangerous, in the rhythm of the heartbeat); Raynaud's disease (a circulatory disorder that causes uncomfortably cold hands); epilepsy; paralysis and other movement disorders."

Thus, biofeedback can be safely and effectively employed in the alleviation of numerous disorders. One example worth noting—in terms of the magnitude of the problem—is the treatment of cardiovascular disorders. Myocardial infarctions, commonly known as heart attacks, are one of the major health problems in the industrialized world and an area of special concern to those practitioners with a psychophysiological orientation. In the United States alone, approximately 700,000 persons die of heart attacks each year.

One of the principal causes of heart attacks is hypertension (high blood pressure). Emotions have much to do with the manifestation of high blood pressure (hypertension), which places this condition in the category of a psychophysiological disorder. Researchers have demonstrated that biofeedback is an effective methodology to correct the problem of high blood pressure. The data reveal that many individuals employing biofeedback have been able to decrease (or eliminate entirely) the use of medication to manage their hypertension. Studies also show that these individuals maintain normal blood pressure levels for as long as two years following the completion of biofeedback training.

Because of its noninvasive properties and its broad applicability in the clinical setting, biofeedback is also increasingly becoming one of the more commonly utilized modalities in many fields, such as behavioral medicine. Researchers have provided documented evidence showing that biofeedback is effective in the treatment of so-called stress-related disorders. It is recognized that the four major causes of death and disability in the United States fall into the "stress-related" category. Research has also shown that biofeedback has beneficial applications in the areas of neuromuscular rehabilitation (working with stroke victims to help them develop greater control and use of afflicted muscle groups) and myoneural rehabilitation (working with victims of fibromyalgia and chronic pain to help them obtain relief from debilitating pain).

Research in the 1960's pointed to the applicability of EEG biofeedback for seizure disorders (such as epilepsy). Advanced technology and later research findings, however, have demonstrated EEG biofeedback to be effective in the treatment of attention-deficit disorder, hyperactivity, and alcoholism as well.

Biofeedback appears to have particular applicability for children. Apparently, there is an innate ability on the part of the young to learn self-regulation skills much more quickly than older persons, such as the lowering of autonomic nervous system activity. Since this activity is highly correlated with respiratory distress, biofeedback is often used in the treatment of asthma in prepubescent children. Biofeedback is also being successfully used as an alternative to prescription medications (such as Ritalin) for youngsters with attention-deficit disorder.

The use of biofeedback is also found in the field of athletics and human performance. Sports psychologists and athletic coaches have long recognized that there is an inverted "U" pattern of performance where autonomic nervous system activity and performance are concerned. In the field of sports psychology, this is known as the Yerkes-Dobson law. The tenets of this law state that as the level of autonomic nervous system arousal rises, performance will improve—but only to a point. When autonomic nervous system arousal becomes too high, a corresponding deterioration in performance occurs. At some point prior to an athletic competition, it may be desirable for an athlete to experience an increase (or a decrease) in the level of autonomic nervous system activity (the production of adrenaline, for example). Should adrenaline levels become too high, however, the athlete may "choke" or become tense.

To achieve physiological autoregulation (often referred to in this athletic context as self-regulation), athletes have used biofeedback to assist them with establishing better control of a variety of physiologic processes. Biofeedback applications have ranged from hand-warming techniques for cross-country skiers and mountain climbers to the regulation of heartbeat for sharpshooters (such as biathletes and archers) to the lowering of adrenaline levels for ice-skaters, gymnasts, and divers.

Biofeedback, apart from empirical studies or research on both animal and human subjects, is seldom used in isolation. In most treatment protocols, it is employed in combination with such interventions as behavioral management, lifestyle counseling, exercise, posture awareness, and nutritional considerations. In most biofeedback applications, the individual is also taught a number of procedures that he or she is encouraged to use between therapy sessions. The conscientious and effective practice of these recommended procedures has been proven to be a determining factor in the success rate of biofeedback. The end aim of biofeedback is self-regulation, and self-regulation must extend to situations outside the clinical setting.

Biofeedback (when employed as a part of a behavioral medicine program) is usually offered as a component of a treatment team approach. The biofeedback practitioner commonly interfaces with members of other disciplines to design and implement a treatment protocol implemented to correct the presenting problem (for example, fibromyalgia) for which the referral was made.

One commonly found model of biofeedback is for the patient, the biofeedback practitioner, and the primary medical care provider to constitute a team. The team concept applies even to the extent that the biofeedback practitioner (in many ways acting as a coach) will give the patient a number of procedures to follow between treatment sessions and will then evaluate, with the patient and the medical practitioner, the effectiveness of the procedure. Modifications in the modalities and in the interventions follow from these evaluations. Biofeedback interventions are dynamic and measurable so that the effectiveness of the protocol can be adjusted to meet the needs of the patient.

PERSPECTIVE AND PROSPECTS

Biofeedback, as a treatment modality, is relatively new. The history of biofeedback as a research tool, however, dates back to early attempts to quantify physiological processes. From the time of Ivan Pavlov and his research on the salivary processes in canines, both psychologists and physiologists have long been interested in the measurement of human behavior (including physiological processes).

Early in the twentieth century, the work of Walter B. Cannon, with his book *The Wisdom of the Body* (1932), helped to set the stage for the field of self-regulation. Another landmark was the 1929 publication of Edmund Jacobson's *Progressive Relaxation*. More recently, the work of such pioneers as John V. Basmajian, Neal Miller, Elmer Green, Joseph Kamiya, and many others spawned research and development efforts that by 1975 produced more than twenty-five hundred literature references utilizing biofeedback as a part of a study.

The evolution of biofeedback as a treatment modality has its historical roots in early research in the areas of learning theory, psychophysiology, behavior modification, stress reactivity, electronics technology, and biomedical engineering. The emerging awareness—and acceptance by the general public—that individuals do in fact have the potential to promote their own wellness and to facilitate the healing process gave additional impetus to the development of both the theory and the technology of biofeedback treatment. Several other factors have combined to produce the climate within which biofeedback has gained recognition and acceptance. One of these was widespread recognition that many of the disorders that afflict humankind today have, as a common basis, some disruption of the natural feedback processes. Part of this recognition is attributable to the seminal work of Hans Selye on stress reactivity.

Developments in the fields of electronics, physiology, psychology, endocrinology, and learning theory produced a body of knowledge which spawned the evolution and growth of biofeedback. Further refinement and an explosion of technology have resulted in procedures and techniques that have set the stage for the use of biofeedback as an effective intervention with wide applications in the treatment of numerous disorders.

A new version of biofeedback has promising hope for people with brain damage due to injury, paralysis, or stroke. Known as neuroprosthetics, nanobiotechnology, or occasionally as brain interface chips, this technology is in the early stages of research but is enabling people to control machinery with their thoughts.

In 2005, the Food and Drug Administration (FDA) approved a biotechnology company, Cybernetics Neurotechnology Systems, to test a new system that involves implanting electrodes into disabled people who are unable to use the muscles necessary to complete a task. Some research and clinical trial studies have shown that quadriplegic people can learn to use a computer, manipulate a robotic arm, or play video games. Cyberkinetics inserts a microchip into the motor cortex that has one hundred tiny needles composed of silicon electrodes. Signals from the chip are sent to an analog-to-digital converter, which processes the simultaneous firings of one hundred neurons into digital data. For example, if a person thinks about turning off a computer, the analog information translates this into an actual motion, controlling the cursor on the computer screen. Other research has utilized noninvasive methods of assimilating neuronal activity. In some research studies, quadriplegic persons, and persons with no neuromuscular impairment, could control a cursor by controlling their EEG patterns. Participants are able to do this by learning to identify, over time, feedback from brain-wave activity.

Both electrode implants and EEG methods have their positives and negatives. EEGs are a bit cumbersome, due to the wires and electronic equipment; however, wireless technology in the future is possible. Implanted electrodes may provide more precise information, but this approach requires surgery and is expensive and potentially risky.

Neither method directly affects actual movement; that is, it does not read minds but instead enables the mind to act directly on an external object. The futuristic prospect of controlling machinery with thoughts has many psychological, medical, and ethical implications that will need to be uncovered as research progresses.

The practice of biofeedback has extended to a number of disciplines. Included in the membership of the Association of Applied Psychophysiology and Biofeedback (formerly the Biofeedback Society of America) are representatives from the fields of medicine, psychology, physical therapy, social work, occupational therapy, and chiropractic. The professional journal of the association is *Biofeedback and Self-Regulation*, published by Plenum Press. The accrediting arm of the Association of Applied Psychophysiology and Biofeedback is the Biofeedback Certification Institute of America.

—Ronald B. France, Ph.D.; updated by LeAnna DeAngelo, Ph.D.

See also Alternative medicine; Anxiety; Arrhythmias; Asthma; Attention-deficient disorder; Brain; Cardiac rehabilitation; Cardiology; Electrocardiography (ECG or EKG); Electroencephalography (EEG); Epilepsy; Exercise physiology; Headaches; Heart attack; Hypertension; Hypnosis; Meditation; Nervous system; Neurology; Pain management; Paralysis; Phobias; Physical rehabilitation; Physiology; Preventive medicine; Respiration; Sleep disorders; Sports medicine; Stress; Stress reduction.

For Further Information:

Blumstein, Boris, et al., eds. *Brain and Body in Sport and Exercise: Biofeedback Applications in Performance Enhancement*. New York: Wiley, 2002. Notes that technical advances in biofeedback have made it a vital method of training athletes in order to increase individual awareness and control over the body and reduce habitual physiological tensions. Brings together current research and applications and shows how different biofeedback approaches can be used in various sports.

Constans, A. "Mind Over Machines." *The Scientist* 19, no. 3 (2005): 27. This article gives a good overview of the neuroprosthetics field.

Olton, David S., and Aaron R. Noonberg. *Biofeedback: Clinical Applications in Behavioral Medicine*. Englewood Cliffs, N.J.: Prentice Hall, 1980. A practical overview of the applicability of biofeedback in the practice of behavioral medicine. This reference contains a basic overview of the development of biofeedback, as well as fundamental clinical applications in the treatment of various disorders.

Phillips, Nelson, et al., eds. *Handbook of Mind-Body Medicine for Primary Care*. Thousand Oaks, Calif.: Sage, 2003. Introduces a mind-body approach to the medical and behavioral problems of primary care patients and includes discussions of biofeedback and neurofeedback.

Robbins, Jim. *A Symphony in the Brain: The Evolution of the New Brain Wave Biofeedback*. New York: Atlantic Monthly Press, 2000. This work discusses brain-wave biofeedback (or neurofeedback), in which an electroencephalograph measures brain waves, and patients are trained to control them consciously. Robbins interviewed many key researchers for this book.

Schwartz, Mark S., and Frank Andrasik, eds. *Biofeedback: A Practitioner's Guide*. 3d ed. New York: Guilford Press, 2003. One of the more recent references in the field of biofeedback. The chapters contain updated information concerning the fundamentals of and state-of-the-art methodologies concerning biofeedback.

BIOINFORMATICS

SPECIALTY

ANATOMY OR SYSTEM AFFECTED: None

SPECIALTIES AND RELATED FIELDS: Genetics

DEFINITION: A rapidly growing area of quantitative, mathematical, and computational biology that is coming to resemble physics and chemistry in the detail and rigor of the science.

KEY TERMS:

genomics: the study of genetic material, such as the deoxyribonucleic acid (DNA) sequences of chromosomes

microarray: a technique used to measure the amount of ribonucleic acid (RNA) that each gene makes

molecular evolution: how genomes and regulatory networks change over time

phylogenetics: the building of evolutionary trees, such as to describe accurately the base-by-base changes in a particular protein from different species

proteomics: studying the results after RNA translation, such as the amounts of protein in different forms

sequence alignment: lining up (with gaps if necessary) the same sites in the same gene from different species or different genes

structural biology: the study of how proteins fold into a three-dimensional shape and how they interact with one another to form larger complexes

systems biology: the study of how systems of molecules, subcellular structures, and cells work together

INTRODUCTION

The answer to the question "What is bioinformatics?" is not straightforward, yet in addressing this question the richness and extent of the field become clear. Part of the reason that it is difficult to give a concise definition of bioinformatics is that, as researchers publishing in the field realize, the definition is somewhat artificial and its boundaries are still expanding. This is not surprising as bioinformatics might also be called mathematical/computational molecular biology, which points to large parts of biology taking on the aspects of a "hard" science such as physics or chemistry.

The creation of bioinformatics was triggered by a combination of factors in the 1990's. Key elements were progress in computing power, the existence of much larger data sets, and increasingly quantitative approaches to molecular biology, including molecular evolutionary studies. The large data sets came from a number of sources, including long individual DNA sequences (for example, genomes), large between-species comparative or evolutionary alignments, microarray-generated gene expression data, proteomics data from two-dimensional gel electrophoresis and mass spectroscopy techniques, and structural information—broadly speaking, the fields of comparative, functional, and structural genomics. It was also increasingly recognized that quantitative molecular biology required vast amounts of computer power not only to assemble genomes but also to complete fundamental analyses, such as aligning related DNA sequences or building a tree from such an alignment. For example, with just twenty sequences there are more different trees relating these sequences than Avogadro's number (approximately 6×10^{23}), and every tree must be checked to ensure that the optimal solution has been found.

THE SCOPE OF RESEARCH

Bioinformatics itself touches on other areas of science such as biomedical informatics, computer science, statistical analysis, molecular biology, and mathematical modeling. In turn, each of these fields contributes uniquely to the progress of bioinformatics toward a mature science. Equally definitive of bioinformatics is recognizing those areas wholly or partly subsumed by an approach mixing computing power with mathematical and statistical modeling to solve biological questions based on molecular data. These areas include genomics, evolutionary biology, population genetics, structural biology, microarray gene expression analysis, proteomics, and the modeling of cellular processes plus systems biology (for example, modeling a neurological pathway in which individual neurons respond to molecular events).

In bioinformatics, as in chemistry and physics, there is a fundamental split between empirical/experimental and theoretical science. At one extreme may be a laboratory focusing on generating large amounts of microarray data with relatively little analysis, and at the other extreme may be a mathematician working alone to solve a theorem with an application to better analyze that microarray data. It is clear that both approaches are needed for science to develop. However, it is not uncommon to find researchers actively tackling both problems (for example, gathering large data sets and seeking better methods to analyze them). Increasingly, the scale and cost of major bioinformatics projects call for a new model of interdisciplinary biological research, in which biologists, statisticians, computer scientists, chemists, mathematicians, physicians, and physicists interact closely together.

The nature of bioinformatics research highlights the need for interdisciplinary skills in modern biology. Some universities issue bioinformatics degrees based on their own formulas. A more direct approach is to require a quadruple major in statistics, computer science, mathematics, and biology. The importance of such a background is that, for example, someone who is not the best mathematician still needs to know how to ask the best mathematicians for help with the problems that inevitably crop up in research in this area. A good example of this interdependence arose in the Celera Genomics effort to complete the human genome, in which mathematicians with a specialty in tiling algorithms were essential to reassembling the millions of sequenced fragments.

In the future, bioinformatics will be increasingly involved with projects, the magnitude of which are technically and intellectually as challenging as anything previously faced in science. For example, a key problem might be a complete computer model of a single cell. Perfection would be achieved only when a biologist could not tell the difference between real and experimental data when the cell experienced a change internally or externally. The science to achieve this result is probably decades off, yet key elements are at the forefront of bioinformatics research today.

A current example of a single element in this bigger picture is the Blue Gene project at International Business Machines (IBM). Blue Gene aims to use a new generation of supercomputer to model protein folding accurately. In this endeavor, computer scientists will undoubtedly be key to assembling the machine and programming it. However, a mathematician, physicist, biologist, or statistician may improve the accuracy of the mathematical model of folding, which may ultimately make the predictions as good as structural biologists currently obtain from experimental work using methods such as X-ray crystallography. It may even be that Blue Gene stumbles, and it is the input of an evolutionary model of the same protein in different organisms that gives the folding algorithm the power to identify the correct solution from trillions of others.

Perspective and Prospects

The implications of bioinformatics for medicine are enormous. The strictly informatics side is already central to medical genetics. Databases of human characteristics, including detailed medical histories and biochemical profiles, are matched up with millions of genetic markers within each individual. Only through such enormous databases can statistical sleuths uncover the basis of most diseases that are caused by multiple genes. This is the population genetics of humans on a vast scale. Elsewhere, medical research such as cancer modeling is rapidly becoming a branch of bioinformatics, driven by the fact that cancer is caused by many interacting genes.

The overall prospect is that bioinformatics will make possible a different sort of medicine in the twenty-first century in which fundamental research leads to pharmaceutical intervention, which leads to treating a disease at its root cause in a way that avoids the need for surgical intervention. Treatments of tomorrow, from diagnosis to cure, will involve processing large amounts of data via computers, with doctors remaining the key to ensuring an appropriate treatment regime with the consent and comfort of the patient foremost.

In short, one answer to the question "What is bioinformatics?" is the development of virtual molecular biology. As time passes, this scientific endeavor will propagate upward and outward to meet other major areas of biology, such as physiology and ecology. Eventually, much of biology and medicine may come to rest solidly on the same principles as chemistry and physics, yet require major computational resources because of the complexity of the models needed to approximate reality reliably.

—Peter J. Waddell, Ph.D.

See also Biophysics; Biostatistics; DNA and RNA; Genomics.

For Further Information:

Campbell, A. Malcolm, and Laurie J. Heyer. *Discovering Genomics, Proteomics, and Bioinformatics*. 2d ed. San Francisco: Pearson/Benjamin Cummings, 2007. An introductory book that gives basics in an accessible manner.

Davidson, Eric H. *The Regulatory Genome: Gene Regulatory Networks in Development and Evolution*. Boston: Elsevier/Academic Press, 2006. One of the areas where bioinformatics has a huge future, in elucidating gene regulatory networks.

International Human Genome Sequencing Consortium. "Initial Sequencing and Analysis of the Human Genome." *Nature* 409, no. 6822 (2001): 860-921. Example of a major bioinformatics collaboration in the area of genomics.

Biological and chemical weapons

Anatomy or system affected: All

Specialties and related fields: Bacteriology, emergency medicine, environmental health, epidemiology, immunology, public health, toxicology, virology

Definition: The use of chemicals, living organisms, or toxins produced by living organisms as weapons in warfare or in attacks on noncombatant populations in an effort to advance political, social, or military causes.

Key terms:

biological warfare: also called biowarfare; warfare using biological agents or toxins produced by biological agents

biological weapon: also called a bioweapon; a biological agent or toxin produced by a biological agent used as a weapon

chemical warfare: warfare using synthetic chemical agents and devices that spread chemical agents

chemical weapon: a synthetic chemical agent used as a weapon, or a device used to disseminate a chemical weapon

preparedness: being prepared, in terms of having sufficient training and materiel to respond to emergencies

risk assessment: the science of determining the potential risks posed by exposure to biological or chemical agents

terrorist: a person who uses force or threats of force to intimidate others and achieve a political, social, or military goal

Introduction

During the Cold War, which began at the end of World War II in 1945, the world's major military powers prepared for biological and chemical warfare. Scourges that once inflicted a dreadful toll on humankind were being harnessed in the name of national defense. Chemical agents that terrorized Allied and Axis troops in World War I were mass-produced and stockpiled. As the superpowers and their allies backed away from the brink of nuclear annihilation, however, they also began to rethink the possible use of biological and chemical weapons. When the Soviet Union collapsed in 1989—thus eliminating one of the major perceived enemies of the West—fear of biological and chemical attacks subsided.

The terrorist attacks of September 11, 2001, on the World Trade Center and Pentagon, and the deadly anthrax-by-mail attacks against media and political figures in the United States that followed shortly afterward, refocused the world's attention on the possibility of biological and chemical terrorism. As the world's major military powers dismantle their biological and chemical warfare capabilities, terrorist groups have begun to show interest in the potential of biological and chemical weapons.

The political upheavals that toppled the Soviet Union and affiliated governments in the 1980's and the 1990's were followed by economic upheavals—nations that could no longer afford to run command economies likewise could not afford to maintain a large military infrastructure. As a result, by 2003, security around many biological and chemical warfare research facilities had become weakened or disappeared altogether. Control over biological and chemical weapons stocks was nonexistent in some cases, leaving some of the world's most feared killers unguarded—easily stolen or easily sold by unemployed or underemployed scientists and staff. With the proliferation of organized terrorist and criminal networks worldwide, the demand for such weapons was disturbingly high. Intelligence and news reports showed that terrorist groups such as al-Qaeda, the group that carried out the September 11 attacks, were actively seeking, and possibly testing, these weapons.

The History of Biological and Chemical Warfare

Biological warfare has a long history. Scythians as early as 400 B.C.E. used arrows tipped with a mixture of blood, manure, and decomposing bodies. The great Carthaginian general Hannibal, outnumbered in a battle against King Eumenes II of Pergamum in 184 B.C.E., hurled jars containing poisonous snakes onto the enemy ships. Hannibal won. Dead bodies have long been used to poison enemy water supplies, such as when Barbarossa used the tactic against Tortona in 1155 or when Confederate forces did so against Union troops in the American Civil War.

Dead bodies have also been weapons of choice during sieges, when the remains of those who had died from some dreaded disease were catapulted over the walls of besieged citadels. In one such example, a Tartar army flung the bodies of plague victims over the walls of the Genoese citadel of Caffa (now Feodosiya, Ukraine) in 1346. Fleeing Genoese mariners may have unwittingly brought the Black Death from Caffa to Europe, triggering one of the most devastating epidemics in history. Contaminated clothing or other items have been used to equally deadly effect, as in the French and Indian War (1754-1763), when British forces under Sir Jeffrey Amherst distributed smallpox-contaminated blankets to American Indians. The native population was devastated.

Japan tested biological weapons against the Chinese in the years following the Japanese invasion of Manchuria in 1931. The Epidemic Prevention and Water Purification Department of the Kwantung Army, otherwise known as Unit 731, tested various ways of infecting the local population with typhoid, plague, anthrax, cholera, and other diseases. The death toll from Japan's biowarfare activities is unknown.

Chemical warfare has a similarly ancient history. The Chinese reportedly used arsenic-laden smoke as far back as 1000 B.C.E. The Spartans similarly used noxious smoke and flames against their enemies during the Peloponnesian War between 429 and 424 B.C.E. Water supplies have frequently been targeted in chemical attacks.

Advances in chemistry and in weapons technology in the nineteenth century led to the development of chemical warfare as most people conceive it today. The use of hollow artillery shells laden with liquid chlorine, which would release chlorine gas upon detonation, was first suggested by a New York City schoolteacher during the U.S. Civil War. Picric acid-filled shells were used by the British in the Boer War, and arsenical rag torches were used by the Japanese in the Russo-Japanese War.

Chemical warfare reached its zenith during World War I. Both sides unsuccessfully experimented with several agents in the first few months of the war. The first successful large-scale attack, using chlorine gas, was launched by the Germans at Ypres in April, 1915. By the time the war was over, phosgene, diphosgene, cyanide, mustard gas, and several other compounds had been deployed as chemical weapons.

Most biological and chemical weapon attacks throughout history were carried out in times of war, but terrorists took up the mantle in the twentieth century. One of the more infamous bioterror attacks occurred in 1984 in The Dalles, Oregon. Residents of a commune led by the Bhagwan Shree Rajneesh tried to poison diners at ten city restaurants with *Salmonella typhimurium*, the bacterium that causes salmonella, by spreading it in salad bars. The goal of the attack was purely political: By sickening area residents, commune members hoped to make it easier for commune advocates to be elected to the local county commission. More than seven hundred were poisoned during the attacks.

Aum Shinrikyo repeatedly tried to carry out biological weapons attacks using *Clostridium botulinum*, the bacteria that produces botulinum toxin. Cult members even went to Zaire to try to obtain samples of the Ebola virus. None of the cult's biological weapon efforts proved successful. However, the cult carried out two successful chemical attacks, in an apartment complex in Matsumoto, Japan, in 1994 and in a Tokyo subway station in 1995. In both cases, sarin gas, a powerful chemical weapon, was released, killing nearly twenty victims and injuring nearly six thousand.

Biological Agents of Choice

Several biological agents have shown potential for use as biological weapons. Bacteria such as *Bacillus anthracis* (anthrax), *Yersinia pestis* (plague), *Francisella tularensis* (tularemia), *Brucella* spp. (brucellosis), and *Coxiella burnetii* (Q fever), or toxins produced by bacteria (botulinum toxin, staphylococcal enterotoxin B, and other pyrogenic toxins), are the primary type of agent evaluated for use as bioweapons. Viruses, such as those that cause smallpox, several forms of viral encephalitis, and viral hemorrhagic fevers, have been evaluated and used as well. Other major sources of toxins include fungi (trichothecene mycotoxins), plants (ricin, derived from the castor plant, *Ricinis communis*), and marine microorganisms (saxitoxin, produced by dinoflagellates). Three of these agents have caught the public's attention in recent years: smallpox, anthrax, and ricin. Even though smallpox has been eradicated in the wild, samples of the virus survive in a few research laboratories. Anthrax has been used in a terrorist attack, and ricin has been sent through the mail and found in the hands of terrorists.

Smallpox, caused by *Variola* virus, would at first seem like an unlikely threat. The World Health Organization (WHO) declared it eradicated in the wild in 1980. However, the specter of the disease, one of the most feared in history, looms. Despite the fact that there are only two WHO-approved repositories, at the Centers for Disease Control in the United States and at Vector Laboratories in Russia, unapproved stocks may exist. Viable virus may be found in cadavers buried in permafrost or dry crypts. In addition, since the genetic sequence of the virus is known, it may be possible for the virus to be remade using its deoxyribonucleic acid (DNA) blueprint.

Smallpox was eradicated as a result of an aggressive global vaccination program, but immunity does not last forever. Much of the world's population would be vulnerable to the disease should it reemerge, and supplies of the vaccine are limited. The United States, in response to the September 11 terrorist attacks and subsequent anthrax attacks, ordered enough vaccine—made from a live form of a related virus, *Vaccinia*—to inoculate every citizen. Debate raged, however, over whether a mass vaccination campaign should be implemented in response to an attack, much less whether such a campaign should be implemented in the absence of an attack. Because of well-established concerns over potential side effects of the vaccine, response to a campaign to inoculate health care and emergency response workers was poor.

Bacillus anthracis is a naturally occurring bacteria that typically infects animals, particularly those of agricultural importance. Anthrax can infect humans, however, spreading by direct contact or by inhalation of bacterial spores. Inhalational anthrax, first described among woolsorters in the late nineteenth century, spreads easily and has a high mortality rate. Those two qualities make anthrax a potentially fearsome weapon. Anthrax comes in two other forms, cutaneous and gastrointestinal, both of which also cause significant mortality.

Even so, some experts found comfort in the fact that only a handful of people died from the anthrax attacks of 2001. However, the psychological and economic toll—the attacks shut down the postal system and affected other shipping services in parts of the United States—cannot be underestimated. It should not be forgotten that the goals of terrorists include more than causing casualties—in fact, casualties are usually merely the means to other ends.

Castor oil, the often-dreaded cure for constipation and vomiting, is made from the beans of the castor plant. Ricin is a by-product of castor oil production. While ricin is not nearly as toxic as botulinum toxin, it is stable and easily made from a readily available source. Less than 1 milligram is lethal.

Ricin has never been used in warfare, but it has been used in several high-profile murders, such as the assassination of Bulgarian defector Georgi Markov in London in 1978. Markov, waiting for a bus, was injected—using a modified umbrella—with a tiny, hollow metal pellet 1.5 millimeters in diameter. The sphere, containing ricin, contained two holes that allowed the toxin to seep out. Markov died four days after the attack. Bulgarian agents had tried unsuccessfully to use ricin pellets to assassinate another defector, Vladimir Kostov, earlier that year.

In 2003, traces of ricin were discovered in an apartment used by an alleged terrorist cell, and ricin was mailed to the U.S. Senate and the White House, although no injuries occurred. Some experts doubt that it can be used in a large-scale terrorist attack, since it needs to be inhaled, ingested, or injected to work. Given the ease with which ricin can be manufactured, however, it remains a compound of concern. If used in a well-planned attack, ricin could cause significant casualties in a confined area.

Disturbingly, a new generation of bioweapons may be developed within the next decade. These new weapons are not organisms or toxins produced by organisms, but compounds that disrupt gene expression, or the function of the immune, neurological, or endocrine systems. Some of the specific mechanisms of concern include ribonucleic acid (RNA) interference, which blocks the expression of specific genes and synthetic biology, or the engineering of gene networks to make novel proteins.

Chemical Agents of Choice

The U.S. Army recognizes seven basic classes of chemical weapons: cyanides, nerve agents, lung toxicants, vesicants, incapacitating agents, tear gases, and vomiting gas.

Cyanide, present in low levels in many foods, has been used as a poison for millennia, but it was most widely used as a weapon in World War I. High doses can kill a victim quickly—cyanide is a major component of Zyklon B, the agent used by the Nazis to dispatch millions of concentration camp victims in World War II. Cyanide-containing agents may have been used in alleged chemical attacks in Syria and Iraq in the 1980's.

Nerve agents, such as the organophosphate compounds sarin, tabun, soman, and VX, are particularly fearsome. They cause seizures and respiratory failure by inhibiting acetylcholinesterase enzyme activity. Nerve agents intended for chemical warfare were first synthesized between the two world wars. While never used in combat, many weapons containing these compounds were produced and are still stockpiled.

Lung toxicants, such as chlorine, phosgene, and diphosgene, damage lung tissue, causing pulmonary edema and possibly death. Despite the ancient history of lung toxicants in warfare, the most widespread use was in World War I. Chlorine and phosgene are readily available because they are can be used in civilian as well as military applications. Consequently, they are of considerable concern because of the ease with which they could be acquired by terrorists.

Vesicants (blistering agents), such as mustard gas and Lewisite, irritate the skin and mucous membranes, such as those of the eyes and respiratory tract. No symptoms may be noted for several hours after exposure, but once the blisters develop, the victim is incapacitated. Hospitalization may be required for months afterward. Vesicants were first used in World War I and remain a significant threat today.

Incapacitating agents, tear gases, and vomiting gases are rarely lethal, but they can incapacitate a victim for a number of hours. The long-term effects of exposure to these compounds are not well known.

PERSPECTIVE AND PROSPECTS

Preparedness is key to responding to—or even better, preventing—terrorist attacks. One way to reduce the risk of attack by some bioterror agents would be to vaccinate the population against them, but vaccines are not always available and some vaccines have potentially dangerous side effects. In the arguably fuzzy math of risk assessment, there is little guarantee that the benefits of a vaccination program, such as that for smallpox, would outweigh the risks.

Recognizing a biological or chemical weapon attack can be difficult as well, particularly when the symptoms mimic those of more common ailments. At least one of the victims of the 2001 anthrax attacks in the United States was diagnosed with something other than anthrax. The victim, a postal worker employed at a facility that processed some of the anthrax-contaminated mail, recognized that he might be the victim of a bioterror attack before his doctors did. The misdiagnosis proved fatal in his case.

Even if the cause of the illness is ascribed to the proper biological or chemical agent, it may be difficult to determine whether the exposure was accidental or intentional. The Oregon salmonella attacks carried out by the Rajneeshee cult were initially thought to be isolated cases of food poisoning. An accidental chemical release at a plant in Bhopal, India, in 1984 killed thousands of nearby residents. Accidents—or attacks—involving tanker trucks, rail cars, or ships could be devastating to a surrounding region, but without a claim of responsibility it might take weeks or months to determine whether the release was accidental or otherwise.

Medical professionals and emergency responders are not the only ones who need to be able to recognize a biological or chemical attack. The aforementioned postal worker who died of anthrax realized only hours before his death the cause of his illness. The panic caused by the attacks would not have been as widespread had the public been better informed. An educated public that is not easily frightened thus denies terrorists their most powerful weapon—fear.

—David M. Lawrence

See also Anthrax; Bacterial infections; Bacteriology; Botulism; Emergency medicine; Environmental health; Epidemiology; Food poisoning; Parasitic diseases; Plague; Poisoning; Poisonous plants; Salmonella infection; Smallpox; Toxicology; Tularemia; Viral infections.

FOR FURTHER INFORMATION:

Alibek, Ken, and Stephen Handelman. *Biohazard: The Chilling True Story of the Largest Covert Biological Weapons Program in the World, Told from the Inside by the Man Who Ran It*. New York: Random House, 1999. Alibek, who used to run the Soviet Union's biological weapons program, offers insights into the minds of those who develop weapons that could easily wipe out millions of their fellow humans.

Bartlett, John G., et al., eds. *Bioterrorism and Public Health: An Internet Resource Guide*. Montvale, N.J.: Thomson/Physicians' Desk Reference, 2002. A guide to more than five hundred Web sites—prepared by government agencies, research centers, nongovernmental organizations, and others—that contain information about bioterrorism and what people can do to protect themselves against it.

Broad, William, Judith Miller, and Stephen Engelberg. *Germs: Biological Weapons and America's Secret War*. New York: Simon & Schuster, 2001. Three reporters for *The New York Times* discuss the recent history of biological warfare and the risk of a biological attack today.

Carus, W. Seth. *Bioterrorism and Biocrimes: The Illicit Use of Biological Agents Since 1900*. Washington, D.C.: Center for Counterproliferation Research, National Defense University, 2002. Reviews documented terrorist and other criminal acts of bioterrorism from 1900 to 2000.

Committee on Advances in Technology and the Prevention of Their Application to Next Generation Biowarfare Threats. National Research Council. *Globalization, Biosecurity, and the Future of the Life Sciences*. Washington, D.C.: National Academies Press, 2006. This report describes the challenges in defending against bioterrorism posed by advances in the biological sciences.

Darling, Robert G., Jerry L. Mothershead, Joseph F. Waeckerle, and Edward M. Eitzen, eds. *Emergency Medicine Clinics of North America: Bioterrorism.* Philadelphia: W. B. Saunders, 2002. This book has been called an essential desk reference for those who must plan for and possibly respond to a bioterror attack.

Frist, William H. *When Every Moment Counts: What You Need to Know About Bioterrorism from the Senate's Only Doctor.* Lanham, Md.: Rowman & Littlefield, 2002. This book, written by the Senate Majority Leader, is an accessible discussion of bioterrorism and the United States' preparedness, or lack thereof, to respond to a bioterror attack.

Henderson, Donald A., Thomas V. Inglesby, and Tara Jeanne O'Toole. *Bioterrorism: Guidelines for Medical and Public Health Management.* Chicago: American Medical Association, 2002. This compilation contains updated versions of papers about bioterrorism originally published in the *Journal of the American Medical Association.*

Novick, Lloyd F., and John S. Marr. *Public Health Issues in Disaster Preparedness: Focus on Bioterrorism.* Gaithersburg, Md.: Aspen, 2001. This compilation includes articles and a book chapter on various facets of bioterrorism and on the steps necessary to reduce the risks posed by potential attack.

Sidell, Frederick R., and Ernest T. Takafuji. *Medical Aspects of Chemical and Biological Warfare.* Washington, D.C.: Borden Institute, Walter Reed Army Medical Center, 1997. An extensive review of chemical and biological weapons, with chapters on a number of bioterror agents, including smallpox, anthrax, and plague.

BIONICS AND BIOTECHNOLOGY

PROCEDURES

ANATOMY OR SYSTEM AFFECTED: All

SPECIALTIES AND RELATED FIELDS: Biotechnology, cytology, genetics, immunology, microbiology

DEFINITION: The integration and application of biological and engineering knowledge to the medical sciences; bionics applies this knowledge to the design of artificial systems that act in the place of natural systems, while biotechnology applies this knowledge at the molecular and genetic levels of these natural systems in order to diagnose, treat, cure, or learn more about diseases.

KEY TERMS:

bioengineering: the combination of biological principles and engineering concepts and/or methodology to improve knowledge in both areas

biological principles: knowledge concerned with living organisms and their natural systems, particularly at the cellular, molecular, and genetic levels

biological systems: any of several levels of life, from that of the individual organism to the functional level (for example, the circulatory system, respiratory system, or musculoskeletal system), the organ level (such as the heart or liver), the cellular level, and the molecular level; also called natural systems

cybernetics: a field of study, closely associated with bionics, which is concerned with communication and control in living systems and their application to artificial systems

engineering concepts and methodology: an analysis of how systems work (in particular, the step-by-step processes involved) and how these systems can be duplicated

gene: a segment of deoxyribonucleic acid (DNA) that provides information to make a protein

genomic DNA: the complete sequence of an organism's DNA

monoclonal antibodies: antibodies (proteins that protect the body against disease-causing foreign bodies such as bacteria and viruses) produced in large quantities from cloned cells

protein: a biological macromolecule that performs a specified function within a living cell

recombinant DNA technology: manipulation of the genetic material DNA whereby pieces are separated and interchanged in order to obtain a desired result

INDICATIONS AND PROCEDURES

Bionics and biotechnology are part of the larger arena of bioengineering. This broad interdisciplinary field integrates the many disciplines of biology, physics, and engineering for use in the medical sciences, as well as in other areas such as agriculture, chemical manufacturing, environmental studies, and mining. Because of the interdisciplinary nature of these studies, an often-confusing array of terms may be used, such as biochemical engineering, bioelectronics, biofeedback, biological modeling, biomaterials, biophysics, biomechanics, environmental health engineering, genetic engineering, human engineering, and medical engineering. When applied to the medical sciences, these various areas of knowledge can be integrated under the headings of bionics and biotechnology when considering the diagnosis, investigation, prevention, or treatment of diseases and damaged biological systems.

Within the medical sciences, bionics is concerned with applying physics and engineering concepts and methodology to constructing artificial systems, such as organs or limbs, in order to replace damaged or diseased natural systems. In order to duplicate biological systems and replace them successfully, knowledge of how these systems function biologically, chemically, and mechanically is required. Creating artificial systems has evolved from the making of crude imitations, such as an artificial kidney machine, to the making of sophisticated replicas of the natural system, with the replacement being made in the living organism. While it is necessary to apply physics and engineering knowledge to duplicate these natural systems, the fact that these are natural systems requires the application of biological knowledge to the engineering effort. Some animals have the ability to regenerate lost or destroyed limbs; humans, however, must rely on their ingenuity. Biotechnology is an interdisciplinary field that seeks to replace, if not re-create, nature.

Within the medical sciences, biotechnology is concerned with the manipulation and study of biological systems at the molecular and genetic level. In addition to a basic understanding of how these systems function at these levels, biotechnology is used for practical purposes as well, including noninvasive diagnostic methods, cardiovascular measurements, bio-optics, medical imaging, modeling in physiology, and microsurgical techniques. A significant application is the synthesis of biological products, such as antibiotics, biochemicals used in diagnostic tests, drugs, enzymes, vaccines, and vitamins. This field is also concerned with the manipulation of genetic material to improve this synthetic process, as well as the study of genetic diseases and the manipulation of the associated genes to prevent or cure these diseases. These kinds of syntheses and studies involve the use of molecules, cells, or genes as raw materials in biological processes that are duplicated under artificial conditions in order to improve or increase the quantities of needed biological products. The techniques and methodologies used to achieve these results are the basis of the technology. So, once again, a thorough knowledge of biology and engineering is needed to understand the natural system and to improve the process by which the natural system works in order to accomplish an imposed artificial result.

Much of this work has been carried out through the use of recombinant DNA technology. Since genes provide the instructions controlling those processes by which biological products are made, it is possible to change the processes, or the rate of the processes, by changing the genes. Through genetic engineering, cell cloning, and other techniques, it is possible to make naturally produced antibiotics, vaccines, vitamins, and other needed biological products rather than duplicating these products with artificial materials using artificial means. Also, the rate at which these products are naturally produced can be increased so that large quantities can be obtained (under natural conditions, these products are produced in extremely small amounts). Another aspect of recombinant DNA technology has to do with diseases that result from biological processes that are improperly controlled by genes at critical points. Genetic engineering is used to replace or correct the genetic structure in order to replace or correct the instructions used to guide the biological process.

There is still much to be learned about biological processes and about the genetic material. It is estimated that there are about 100,000 genes constructed from some 3 billion base pairs. Discovering how these genes interact and the biological processes that each controls is a formidable task. In June, 2000, it was announced that the comprehensive effort known as the Human Genome Project had successfully mapped the entire human genetic structure from which all biological processes are controlled, including the flawed ones that cause diseases. Eventually, studies of other genomes, such as those of bacteria and viruses, will treat or prevent diseases and illnesses caused by them as well. This study of genetic material and the use of the tools of proteomics, whereby proteins produced from this genetic material are identified and their functions are elucidated, along with the ongoing study of genetic diseases and of other diseases at the molecular level, will have an increasingly important impact on the overall diagnosis, prevention, and treatment of diseases.

Biotechnology has contributed much to the medical sciences in a relatively short time. It has provided a better understanding of human physiology and an improved fundamental knowledge of disease itself. Knowledge has been gained about the physiological control networks (in part resulting from related studies in cybernetics), the key regulatory agents and processes, the target molecules needed for therapeutic intervention, and the molecular and genetic causes of disease.

With rapid advances in biotechnology, however, the scientific and medical professions are entering sensitive and controversial areas that have raised legal and regulatory concerns. The alteration of genes, the creation of modified organisms, the development of new drugs, the safety and side effects of new biochemicals, the detection of genetic diseases in the fetus, experimental therapies, the ability to clone, the ability to enhance brain functions, and the national and international competition to produce pharmaceuticals are some of the concerns facing medical practitioners, the biomedical industry, government, society, and the individual. These concerns will escalate as biotechnological advances delve even deeper into the molecular and genetic basis of life in order to achieve improved health benefits.

Uses and Complications

Most of the applications of bionics have been centered on replacing damaged or diseased natural systems. Bionic implants, either in development or commercially available, include retinal implants, urinary implants, cochlear implants, hippocampus replacements, larynx implants, and advanced hand replacements.

For example, the learning retinal implant system includes an implant that replaces the function of a defective retina in individuals with retinal degeneration, including, for example, those with retinitis pigmentosa and macular degeneration. A normal retina includes cells that are stimulated by light to produce a signal that is transmitted to the brain and converted into a visual perception. When such cells do not function, vision is affected. The newest system includes a retinal stimulator implanted in the eye, a pocket processor, and glasses that contain a small camera. The processor includes a microcomputer responsible for translating image data into retinal stimulation commands. Initial studies with four patients using a prototype system, which included all the above components except the camera, have been positive in that the patients were able to see light as well as simple patterns. A thirty-person clinical trial in Europe with the newest system is scheduled.

The urinary implant is an implantable pacemaker for the bladder. It will be marketed for bladder dysfunctions caused by spinal cord injury. The device allows for urine storage and full bladder control without the use of catheters.

The cochlear implant is commercially available and consists of an implant that delivers electrical signals to an electrode array. Unlike hearing aids, which act to amplify sound, the cochlear implant sends sound signals directly to the auditory nerve, thus bypassing the damaged portion of the ear.

A neural interface system is being developed that allows severely motor-impaired individuals to communicate with a computer through their thoughts. The system includes a sensor that attaches to a portion of the brain and a device that analyzes brain signals. The signals are translated and allow an individual to control a computer cursor. In the future, it is hoped that the device will allow an individual to control other devices, including lights, telephones, and television sets.

Yet another brain implant being developed is a hippocampus replacement. The hippocampus is a portion of the brain that is important, among other things, in learning and memory; it is the first portion of the brain damaged in Alzheimer's disease. The silicon hippocampus replacement is considered the first prosthesis to replace a damaged area of the brain. As of 2007, it was being tested in rats, although tests in humans were projected to take place in the next five years.

A further application being developed is the implantable artificial electrolarynx communication system. The system is designed for patients who have had a complete laryngectomy. Approaches will be used to attempt to approximate normal voice and speech production.

The Cyberhand Project is developing a cybernetic prosthesis that is controlled by brain signals. Therefore, the hand will allow amputees to use their thoughts to move it and use it to grasp objects naturally. Additionally, the user will also be able to feel objects with which the device comes in contact.

While there are many applications of biotechnology, some of the more significant ones include the production of pharmaceuticals and biochemicals, the production of monoclonal antibodies, the improved understanding and control of complex diseases such as cancer and acquired immunodeficiency syndrome (AIDS), and the improved understanding of genetic diseases. Many of the biotechnology techniques and methodologies are still experimental, as are the resulting products (for example, antibodies, drugs, enzymes, vaccines, vitamins, cloned cells, and recombinant DNA). Some are considered useful and practical, but are not yet approved for use.

The production of pharmaceuticals and biochemicals has been one of the most practical outgrowths of biotechnology research. It has produced both the knowledge of what needs to be done to correct a certain disease process and the ability to make the needed corrections. Some diseases result from deficiencies in particular proteins, as is the case with diabetes, hemophilia, and dwarfism. Others result from deficiencies in enzymes that would normally break down other chemicals, thus resulting in an accumulation of these chemicals, such as in Fabry's, Gaucher's, and Tay-Sachs disease. Still others result from a lack of cellular control, such as cancers.

It has been possible to produce proteins (insulin for diabetes, factor VIII for hemophilia, and growth hormone for dwarfism), enzymes, and bioregulatory proteins (interferon for cancer). This is done by learning how these proteins are produced naturally and then engineering the cells or biochemical processes that can produce these proteins in quantity. In addition to these various kinds of proteins, other biochemical products can be made, including antibiotics, vaccines, and vitamins. Scientists may produce natural, unaltered biochemicals; altered biochemicals (for improved results); or synthetic versions of the biochemicals.

Monoclonal antibodies are a significant group of naturally produced, unaltered biochemicals. They are highly specific biochemicals used for the diagnosis of infectious diseases, for monitoring cancer therapy, for determining the blood concentrations of therapeutic drugs and hormones, for use in some pregnancy tests, for suppressing immune responses, and, to some extent, for disease therapy (for example, to kill cancer cells). Examples of monoclonal antibodies that have been approved by the Food and Drug Administration (FDA) include those used to treat transplant rejection, macular degeneration, multiple sclerosis, inflammatory diseases (including inflammatory bowel disease, rheumatoid arthritis, psoriasis, and allergy-related asthma), and a wide variety of cancers (including non-Hodgkin's lymphoma, breast cancer, acute myelogenous leukemia, chronic lymphocytic leukemia, colorectal cancer, head and neck cancers, and non-small cell lung cancer). While much of this work is still experimental, there is a great potential for the development of highly specific vaccines and for reagents used in diagnostic tests. In addition to being highly specific, these vaccines and reagents would be free of any biological contamination and tend to be reliably stable at room temperature. The vaccines would also be safer since their production would not require the handling of large quantities of the pathogenic agent (which is how vaccines have traditionally been obtained). Possible uses could involve immunological protection against hepatitis B, herpes simplex, polio myelitis, rabies, and malaria.

Molecular pharmacologists also develop biochemicals from nonhuman sources. In fact, the diversity of animal and plant life in the world is a natural pharmacy of potentially useful biochemicals. Many medicinal plants are already known, and systematic studies of other species are under way. Animals also contribute useful biochemicals. For example, excretions from the skin of tropical frogs have been used to treat skin diseases, diabetic ulcers, eye infections, and cancers. Through the study of fifty species of poison arrow frogs, scientists have discovered more than three hundred chemicals. Only about 5 percent of the world's frog species have been studied, and this is only one group in the world's great biodiversity. Biotechnology has made it possible to study natural biochemicals in small amounts and at the molecular level and has provided the necessary techniques and methodologies for using these biochemicals in the study of diseases.

Cancers form a complex group of diseases that continue to defy the best attempts to understand them. A cancer is composed of cells that have proliferated uncontrollably. This response may be caused by a mutated gene, by carcinogenic agents (for example, chemicals or ultraviolet light), or by viruses. Cancers develop in multiple stages that involve different physiological mechanisms. Understanding these mechanisms and the genes and biochemicals that are involved has been possible in large part because of the techniques and methodologies of biotechnology research. Gene therapy is showing great promise for curing some types of cancer.

The same can be said of the efforts to study AIDS. This syndrome is caused by a virus that infects and kills certain kinds of T lymphocytes that are needed to initiate and maintain normal immune system responses; therefore, AIDS is characterized by the occurrence of unusual infections or by Kaposi's sarcoma (a rare cancer). The nucleotide sequence of the viral genome has been determined through recombinant DNA technology, and the functions of the genes are being characterized. Diagnostic tests to determine if blood is contaminated by the virus have been developed, and efforts are under way to develop a vaccine. The proteins used in these immunological investigations are made in large quantities by genetically engineered microorganisms. Other vaccine studies are concerned with using recombinant DNA technology to disable the AIDS virus genetically (by removing or altering its genes) so that it will infect and generate protective immunity without actually causing the disease.

Genetic diseases are also beginning to be understood as a result of biotechnology. Many of these diseases are caused by gene mutations that cause the absence of a protein or the production of a defective protein, affecting biochemical processes. Recombinant DNA technology is providing methods of detecting these defects, as well as providing therapies for correcting or replacing them. Many of these defects can even be diagnosed in the fetus and in previously undetectable carriers. Some of the commonly known genetic diseases include Alzheimer's disease, cystic fibrosis, hemophilia, Huntington's disease, muscular dystrophy, sickle cell disease, and thalassemia. There are approximately three thousand genetic diseases resulting from single-gene mutations. In addition to studying these numerous mutations, efforts are being made to study diseases associated with specific normal genes (such as the susceptibility for heart attacks by individuals with genes producing specific cholesterol-carrying proteins) and to cure genetic disorders by replacing the mutated gene with a normal gene. This normal DNA acts as a template for production of a certain type of ribonucleic acid (RNA), messenger RNA (mRNA), which acts as a template for production of the normal protein.

One advantage of learning more about common genetic diseases is that more can be learned about normal genomes by comparing them with mutated genomes. These diseases are few in number, however, and much remains to be done. With a map of the human genome (as well as the genome of other animals, plants, bacteria, and viruses), biotechnology, and its usefulness to the medical sciences, will advance significantly. The Human Genome Project has essentially produced a map of the entire human genetic structure, including every gene in the twenty-three chromosome pairs. This accounts for about 100,000 genes with about 3 billion base pairs. In addition, there are about 3 million differences per genome from one individual to another. These differences are responsible for such things as personality differences and inherited diseases. In order to find and understand some of the rarest disease-causing genes, it is estimated that the differences between the genomes of some 4 billion individuals will need to be studied. This resulting database would strain even state-of-the-art computers, not to mention the researchers who will compile the database.

Study of the differences between the genomes of individuals, and in particular the differences in genes involved in drug metabolism, will be a starting place to provide researchers with a way to overcome adverse reactions to drugs from selected portions of the population by applying the tools of pharmacogenomics, the study of how a person's genetic makeup (genotype) affects the response to drug treatment. It is estimated that more than 100,000 people die each year from various reactions to medications that help others. Another 2.2 million people experience severe reactions to medications while others are not affected either positively or negatively. After correlating the differences in the

IN THE NEWS: NANOBOTS

Robots the size of the period at the end of this sentence are being developed to capture and transport single cells and bacteria. These minuscule robots, also known as microbots or nanobots, are fewer than seven hundred millionths of a meter tall and approximately two hundred millionths of a meter wide. Some of these tiny robots are being constructed from layers of polymers and gold. Resembling a human arm, the nanobots have flexible elbow and wrist joints. They are being made in a variety of forms with "hands" containing two to four digits.

Because nanobots are being constructed to work while submerged in liquids, including blood, urine, and cell-culture media, they have many biotechnical applications. Since the joints contain conducting polymers, the nanobots can either absorb ions from the surrounding liquid or lose ions to the liquid. The resulting swelling or shrinking of the robot joints causes them to bend. As they do so, the nanobot arm flexes, causing the wrist to bend and the fingers to open and close.

Future nanobots might be able to repair the human body by picking up cells and moving them about for detailed analysis or assemblage into needed microstructures. By placing them at the end of a catheter, surgeons may be able to probe deeper inside the human body. Other possible applications include using them to create images directly on the human retina and implanting them in the brain to substitute for brain functions in the event of a stroke.

—Alvin K. Benson, Ph.D.

genes with a specific negative response, researchers will then need to determine the genotype of a specific individual and use that information to determine the treatment regime that will be most effective for that individual. Alternatively, such information will allow drugs to be developed that are customized for the population to which the individual belongs.

Although many therapeutic strategies involve replacing a mutated gene with a normal gene, other strategies that are currently being developed use short pieces of DNA, called oligonucleotides, to correct the underlying mutation in the DNA of an individual. For example, single-stranded oligonucleotides that include the correct sequence of nucleotides (the basic components of DNA) are introduced into a living cell and, through a process known as homologous recombination, are exchanged with the defective portion of the genomic DNA. Other methods include use of RNA of the proper sequence to substitute for defective RNA formed from defective DNA. Although these methods ensure a properly functioning protein will be produced, in some cases it is advantageous to stop production of selected proteins in various disease states, such as in various viral infections, cardiovascular disease, or cancer.

RNA may be used to prevent production of specified proteins. For example, using antisense technology, single-stranded RNA or DNA (called the antisense strand) is administered to an individual and binds to a portion of the mRNA that will produce a specified protein. Once bound, it will physically block production of the protein, and the double-stranded molecule formed will then be degraded. Other methods to prevent protein synthesis utilizing RNA include RNA interference. In this method, double-stranded RNA is administered to an individual and it ultimately causes the target mRNA to be degraded, thereby preventing protein production, by a different mechanism than found in antisense technology. Vitravene (fomivirsen) is the first, and presently the only, antisense drug that the FDA has allowed to be marketed. It is used to treat a particular viral infection, cytomegalovirus retinitis, in individuals with AIDS. Many other antisense drugs are currently in various stages of development to treat a variety of other viral infections, cardiovascular diseases, or cancers, including cancer of the colon, skin, lung, and prostate.

PERSPECTIVE AND PROSPECTS

Artificial limbs have been in use for centuries, but no attempt was made to duplicate natural limbs except in the crudest sense. The use of microorganisms for the production of fermented beverages (such as beer, wine, and vinegar) and food (such as bread) goes back many centuries. Likewise, folk medicine made use of natural biochemicals to treat diseases for many centuries. These traditional processes, however, did not involve an understanding of what was occurring and may only be considered biotechnology by default. The knowledge needed for biotechnology required the development of several scientific disciplines, all of which only occurred after the 1950's, when scientifically understood and controlled processes were developed to produce biological products. It was not until the 1970's that recombinant DNA technology allowed significant advances in the understanding of many molecular and genetic processes.

The advancement of bionics and biotechnology after the 1950's was the result of advances made in related scientific fields during earlier decades, primarily after 1900. These developments included the discovery that enzymes were proteins and the theory of enzyme action; the discovery of the structure and function of vitamins; the discovery of the composition of nucleic acids; the discovery of the structure of carbohydrates; the development of a better understanding of the cellular infrastructure; work on natural and experimentally induced mutation; the study of hereditary metabolic errors; a better understanding of immunology, viral and bacterial diseases, tumors, and cell pathology; the realization that genes were found in the chromosomes; early studies concerning chromosome recombinations and the mechanisms of genetic expression; the ultraviolet analysis of DNA and RNA; the increased use of electron microscopy; the development of the technology involved in the large-scale production of penicillin; and the further development and integration of studies in genetics, biochemistry, and physiology.

The 1950's and 1960's saw important advances in the discovery of the structure of DNA, the breaking of the genetic code, the discovery of how gene actions were regulated, the structure of the gene and of numerous proteins, the discovery and study of numerous hereditary diseases, the development of medical procedures for organ transplants, the evolution of the branch of science known as molecular biology, and the continuing synthesis of discoveries and theories from a variety of scientific disciplines. The 1970's saw the development of technologies that further developed these areas of study, in particular recombinant DNA technology and monoclonal antibody technology. The future will see an increased refinement of these technologies and further developments resulting from the success of the Human Genome Project.

—Vernon N. Kisling, Jr., Ph.D.; updated by Jason J. Schwartz, Ph.D., J.D.

See also Amputation; Biofeedback; Biophysics; Cloning; Computed tomography (CT) scanning; Dialysis; DNA and RNA; Electrocardiography (ECG or EKG); Electroencephalography (EEG); Gene therapy; Genetic engineering; Genetics and inheritance; Heart transplantation; Heart valve replacement; Magnetic resonance imaging (MRI); Mutation; Pacemaker implantation; Pharmacology; Physical rehabilitation; Plastic surgery; Positron emission tomography (PET) scanning.

For Further Information:

Albertini, Alberto, Claude Lenfant, and Rodolfo Paoletti, eds. *Biotechnology in Clinical Medicine*. New York: Raven Press, 1987. A technical review of specific applications of biotechnology in various areas of medicine.

Borem, Aluizo, et al. *Understanding Biotechnology*. Englewood Cliffs, N.J.: Prentice Hall, 2003. Provides good introductory discussions of topics such as cloning, gene therapy, pharmacogenomics, molecular markers, forensic DNA, bioremediation, biodiversity, and bioterrorism.

Glick, Bernard, and Jack Pasternak. *Molecular Biotechnology: Principles and Applications of Recombinant DNA*. Rev. ed. Washington, D.C.: ASM Press, 2003. Explores the scientific principles of recombinant DNA technology and its wide-ranging use in industry, agriculture, and the pharmaceutical and biomedical sectors.

Human Genome Program. U.S. Department of Energy. *Genomics and Its Impact on Science and Society: A 2003 Primer*. http://www.ornl.gov/sci/techresources/Human_Genome/publicat/primer/index.shtml/. A basic primer of molecular biology, the history of the Human Genome Project and information obtained therefrom, the anticipated benefits of genetic research, future directions in the field, and further resources for more detailed study.

Murray, Thomas H., and Maxwell J. Mehlman, eds. *Encyclopedia of Ethical, Legal, and Policy Issues in Biotechnology*, New York: John Wiley & Sons, 2000. A reference providing articles by experts in the field relating to the ethical, legal and policy issues in biotechnology

Rehm, Hans-Jürgen, and Gerald Reed, eds. *Biotechnology*. Rev. 2d ed. 8 vols. Deerfield Beach, Fla.: Verlag Chemie, 1991-2001. An eight-volume set covering microbial fundamentals, biochemical engineering, microbial products, food and feed production with microorganisms, biotransformations, enzyme technology, and gene technology.

Vasil, Indra K. *Biotechnology: Science, Education, and Commercialization*. New York: Elsevier, 1990. Broad overviews of several areas of biotechnology, in particular the regional and international efforts to overcome problems in education and commercial development.

Walker, Sharon. *Biotechnology Demystified*. New York: McGraw Hill, 2007. Provides a primer of biology, including genetics and immunology, and discusses medical and agricultural applications of biotechnology.

Biophysics

Specialty

Anatomy or system affected: All

Specialties and related fields: Audiology, biotechnology, neurology, nuclear medicine, ophthalmology, optometry, radiology

Definition: The scientific field that applies the laws, methods, and instrumentation of physics to study the structures, systems, and processes of biological organisms.

Key terms:

atom: the smallest chemically and biologically active unit of matter; composed of electrons enclosing an atomic nucleus containing protons and neutrons

cell: the basic unit of living matter; composed of a cell membrane, a cell nucleus containing DNA, and many other specialized, complex units

charge: the quantity of electricity responsible for attraction and repulsion among atoms and molecules

current: the flow of electrical charges through space or a material

deoxyribonucleic acid (DNA): the helical genetic material of plants, animals, and many lower organisms

electron: the negatively charged, fundamental particle that gives atoms their structure and their chemical and biological activity

energy: a measure of a system's capacity to do work

momentum: the product of mass and velocity for a particle; inverse with wavelength (the distance between peaks of a wave) *photon:* the smallest unit of an electromagnetic wave; energy increases with the frequency of wave peaks

quantum theory: the theory that energy, momentum, and other physical quantities appear in indivisible units of finite quantity

voltage: energy per unit charge; typical biological voltages range from hundredths to tenths of a volt

Science and Profession

A young boy skips a stone across a still pond, and a startled frog jumps into the water. Physics studies nature in the arc of the stone, the rippling of the water, the sound of the splash, and the surprising motions of the atoms and molecules within the stone and the water of the pond. Biology, on the other hand, studies the boy and the frog—their cells, nerves, muscles, and senses—which are very different from the dead mass of the stone and the still water of the pond. Despite their immense differences, the boy, the frog, the stone, and the pond have the same atoms and obey the same basic laws of nature. Biophysics enters, for example, when the boy hears the sound of the splash, one of many meeting grounds between biology and physics as they merge into one knowledge. Since biological systems are chemical and mathematics is the language of physics, biophysics has significant overlap with biochemistry and biomathematics.

Biology is the scientific investigation of the laws of life. In particular, biology studies both the structure and function of cells and organisms such as viruses, bacteria, plants, and animals, including their communities. It studies the means by which life nourishes and maintains itself and by which it perpetuates itself by genetic transmission, reproduction, and evolution. Medical science applies this knowledge in the service of humankind. Physics is the scientific investigation of the laws of nature. Physics has two major divisions, experimental and theoretical physics. Instruments are the tools of the experimental physicist, and mathematics is the tool of the theoretical physicist. Distinct from biology, physics restricts its investigations to inanimate objects. At the human level, nature appears as matter and waves; physics studies the properties of both and their interactions. For the arena of biophysics, the most useful branches of physics are atomic, energetic, fluid, and electromagnetic physics.

Broadly taken, atomic physics studies atoms and their nuclei and molecules (which are isolated atom groups) and their formation into solids, liquids, and gases. Atoms consist of electrons circulating around a tiny nucleus of protons and neutrons. Electrons have negative charges and give the atoms their distinctive shapes and chemical, biological, and medical properties. Protons and neutrons are similar except that protons have a positive charge and neutrons have no charge. The protons hold the electrons within the atoms by electrical forces, while nuclear forces bind protons and neutrons within the nucleus. The exchange of electrons between and among atoms determines the chemical properties of materials, including biological and medical materials.

Most atoms are neutral, with an equal number of electrons and protons. Hydrogen, with one electron and one proton, is the smallest atom and a common biological constituent, along with carbon, nitrogen, and oxygen, which possess six, seven, and eight electrons, respectively. When an electron is missing from an otherwise neutral atom, the atom becomes a positive ion. Adding an electron converts a neutral atom to a negative ion. Ions are abundant in biological fluids. The hydrogen positive ion, along with calcium, potassium, and sodium positive ions and the chlorine negative ion, are important biological atomic ions. In most electronic devices, electrons produce electrical activity, but in living organisms and humans, ions govern this activity.

Since atomic nuclei do not play a significant role within living organisms, the smallest matter particles of biological importance are atoms. Groups of atoms make biological molecules, deoxyribonucleic acid (DNA), carbon dioxide, water, and bones, for example. Some atomic nuclei are unstable and release energetic particles and waves. These radioactive products are usually damaging to cells and their DNA, but under controlled conditions, they are useful, for example, as radioactive tracers.

Energetic physics studies the basic forces of nature. The electromagnetic force, together with gravity and the nuclear forces, is one of the known fundamental forces of nature. In biological materials, other forces, such as the osmotic force, are complex manifestations of the electrical force. These forces allow matter to interact—to hold, pull, and push other matter and to exchange energy and momentum. While the prime biological interaction among matter is electrical, the major interaction between matter and waves is electromagnetic. An example is the absorption of the electromagnetic wave—light—by the eye to form visual images.

Fluids are groups of atoms or molecules that move easily; included in this definition are both liquids and gases. Biological fluids are important for the transportation of materials across cell membranes, for blood circulation, and for respiration. Fluid physics investigates fluid motions under the influence of various forces. Confined fluids develop pressures as a result of the forces between the fluid particles. Under a pressure difference, fluids flow toward the lower pressure. Thus, blood flows because of the blood pressure generated by the heart and arteries.

Electromagnetic physics studies electrical, magnetic, and electromagnetic fields in detail. Charge motion occurs when an electrical voltage acts across conducting materials, whether in an electronic device or in a biological system. In the body, biochemical activity generates voltages across nerve cell membranes, allowing the nerves to serve as the body's electronic network.

Oscillating electric charges produce electromagnetic waves. Thus nuclei produce gamma rays and atoms generate X rays and ultraviolet, visible, and infrared waves; electronic devices generate a variety of microwave and radio waves. Individual electromagnetic waves appear as packets, called photons, which carry both energy and momentum. Photon energy and momentum decrease dramatically in going from gamma rays to radio waves. Gamma rays and X rays carry high energy and momentum and are very destructive if encountered by molecules within cells. Both of these radiations easily penetrate soft tissues, so that their damage may permeate an entire organism. (Low X-ray dosages, however, give safe images of the body's structure.) Even ultraviolet rays carry sufficient energy to damage biological organisms. Since ultraviolet rays are not very penetrating, they mainly damage skin cells.

Visible photons carry enough energy to be useful to life as it has evolved on Earth and not so much as to be damaging. Infrared photons produce heat. Individual microwave and radio photons have essentially no biological effects, but both can cause damage if the total energy that they carry creates excess heat, as with a defective microwave oven, or if the electric or magnetic fields in the waves produce undesirable biological effects. The level at which such effects occur has not been clearly established.

Senses are the means by which organisms know their surroundings. Light (an electromagnetic wave) and sound (a matter wave in air) are two physical stimuli. Vision and hearing are the biological responses to these stimuli. Biophysics of the senses studies vision, hearing, and other senses, including the orientational, chemical, somatic, and visceral senses.

Color vision is an extraordinary phenomenon. The human eye evolved under direct and reflected sunlight. Light absorbed differently by three color pigments in the retina signals to the brain the colors of an illuminated scene. Lack of one or two of the pigments produces different forms of color blindness. Normal humans can distinguish roughly twenty thousand different colors. The response of the eye peaks at yellow green, where sunlight has its maximum energy at the earth surface. Matching detector response to source output is characteristic of any efficient electronic detector. Indeed, evolution has made the eye so efficient that a dark-adapted eye can respond to perhaps only one visible photon. This superb detector is at the limit allowed by the laws of physics.

The ear is another exquisite sense organ fashioned by evolution. Hearing picks up sound waves. Speech is one prime source for sound, so human hearing matches the human vocal range. Although human hearing extends over a very wide range, from about 20 to 20,000 cycles per second, it is so precise that the ear can tune in to single tones. A possible explanation for this paradoxical behavior is that evolution has shaped the ear as a mechanical traveling wave amplifier.

Perceived sensations move from a sense organ, such as the eye, by electrical signals conducted over the nervous system to the animal brain. The response to these signals triggers other nerve impulses to the muscles, which contract and move the animal, such as a frog jumping into a pond. This is the arena of electrical biophysics, which investigates the effects of electrical and magnetic fields in living organisms.

Nerve impulses are electrical signals within the nerve. A stimulus at the end of a nerve initiates chemical changes that produce the electrical motion of ions. Tunnel-like proteins on the membrane surface channel the ions across the membrane. The resulting local change in charge propagates along the length of the nerve; in this way, for example, sound in the ear sends signals to the brain. This electrical activity produces low-frequency electrical waves that can be detected in various parts of the body, such as by brain wave monitors and electrocardiograms (EKGs or ECGs).

Typical nerve voltages occur in pulses somewhat smaller than one hundredth of a volt, lasting several thousandths to hundredths of a second. These pulses involve the conduction of sodium and potassium positive ions across the membrane through the protein ion channels. The result is ionic communication in the nervous system. The human brain is part of that system and generates electrical waves with frequencies of about 0.5 to 50.0 cycles per second, with voltages of hundredths to tenths of a volt when picked up by external electrodes attached to the scalp.

Electrocardiograms pick up electrical activity in the heart. The beating heart displays time traces with narrow spikes of uniform height. These spikes represent electrical signals that trigger the heart muscle to contract at a continuous, seemingly rhythmic beat of about once a second. The electrical stimulus, however, is decidedly not rhythmic but is instead a staccato beating. A mathematical technique called Fourier analysis shows that such spikes have a wide range of rhythmic frequencies, from zero to about 10 cycles per second.

Danger would ensue if the electrical activity of the heart became a pure rhythm. If this happens, the frequency range collapses to around 6 cycles per second, too fast for the heart to follow. Deadly ventricular fibrillations may follow. The heart beats in shallow, spasmodic pulses, and sudden cardiac arrest results. Here medical physics saves lives in the form of heart pacemakers and defibrillators. A pacemaker delivers mild electrical current to speed up a chronically slow heart rate, while a defibrillator provides a sharp electrical jolt to restore the normal heartbeat when fibrillation threatens cardiac arrest. Without treatment, patients identified as candidates for sudden cardiac arrest have only a 60 percent change of living a full year. The odds rise to 90 percent, however, for those who receive jolts from a defibrillator.

The latest generation of defibrillators is quite sophisticated. They can coax ventricular tachycardia back to a slower, normal beat by delivering mild electrical currents but also deliver ever-stronger stimulation and, if needed, a sharp jolt to prevent cardiac arrest. Some devices deliver a positive pulse immediately followed by a negative one. This requires less energy from the power source and produces less tissue damage in the patient.

DIAGNOSTIC AND TREATMENT TECHNIQUES

Perhaps the most obvious example of the influence of physics upon biology and medicine is in instruments. Physicists and engineers continually fashion new instruments based on novel developments in physics, and many of these find important applications in biology and medicine. This area of biophysics changes continually. As the complexity of instrumentation is reduced to the routine, the necessity for the involvement of physicists disappears. Biology and medicine take over the new tool.

The optical microscope is an example of a valuable instrument taken into biology and medicine. E. B. Wilson (1856-1939) used a microscope to draw the first primitive pictures of the cell in 1922. Only six cell constituents were clearly shown. Today, advanced instruments such as the electron microscope have provided a more detailed picture of the cell, with its dozens of specialized structures. Microscopes have long been a staple of medicine and are now supplemented by fiber-optic technology. Thin fibers guide light inside the patient's body and allow a physician to heal lesions and diseased sections with lasers.

X-ray analysis is another valuable tool of the biophysicist. X rays have wavelengths that match the distances between atoms in molecules. Thus, molecules produce distinctive X-ray patterns. Computational analysis allows a scientist to determine molecular structure from these patterns. In 1953, James D. Watson and Francis Crick used X-ray analysis to determine the double helix structure of DNA, allowing the genetic code to be cracked.

Sophisticated computer analysis of a patient's three-dimensional X-ray patterns provides startling and accurate imaging of the body's interior without intrusion. Magnetic resonance imaging (MRI) provides complementary three-dimensional internal images, using microwave resonance in a high magnetic field produced by superconducting magnets. MRI produces images by picking up radio signals from the hydrogen atoms that permeate all body tissues. The spinning hydrogen nuclei are aligned by the strong magnetic field. A pulse of radio waves disorients the nuclei, which emit a distinctive radio signal as they reorient to the magnetic field. In comparison, ultrasonography is a surprisingly simple tool, creating images with high-frequency sound.

The use of lasers in medicine has become widespread. A medical laser is created by choosing a suitable laser wavelength to offer desirable penetration and absorption within the human tissue involved in a given procedure, along with an effective beam delivery and tissue removal systems. A partial list of medical laser applications includes retinal attachment, corneal alterations to adjust vision, dental drilling, the removal of surface lesions and stains on the skin, pulsed lithotripsy to break kidney stones into fragments, laser angioplasty to repair and unclog blood vessels, gynecological surgery, and bloodless incision for all types of procedures. Of importance to the physician are ease of operation of the laser equipment, reliability, reasonable cost, and, above all, effectiveness.

Body tissues are mainly composed of water. The water molecule absorbs strongly in the infrared spectrum and is transparent to the visible spectrum. Hemoglobin (in the blood) and melanin (in the skin) play important roles in laser-tissue interactions. Both absorb strongly, but differently, in the visible and near infrared ranges. The bulk of medical procedures that use lasers rely on rapid, selective heating of the target body tissue. For example, bloodless laser surgery requires rapid heating and vaporization of body tissue in the cut. The pulse duration is adjusted so that a thin layer of nearby tissue is heated to cause coagulation and stop bleeding.

An exciting, but experimental, cancer treatment that involves lasers is photodynamic therapy. Safe, light-sensitive dyes, such as the porphyrins, are injected into animals that have tumors. The dyes are absorbed by the tumors, and the tumor is exposed to intense laser light. The dyes alter to a toxic form, and tumor destruction is produced.

Lasers also make possible many research activities. One extraordinary application is the use of the laser's intense beam to act as optical tweezers. The beam can capture one living cell for study and can move organelles within the cell.

A final application is within molecular biophysics, which deals with the molecular constituents of living cells. Here biophysics applies quantum physics to determine the physical structure and biological behavior of the molecules that make up the human body.

Individually, all the molecules studied are inanimate and dead. With the aid of modern computers, physics accurately describes the behavior of the smaller cell constituents. In principle, quantum theory appears to be capable of describing the most complex molecules, including DNA, the basis of the genetic code. This code instructs the assembly of amino acids and proteins, and therefore the structure of an organism. In this task, quantum theory appears to be limited only by computational complexity.

When these dead molecules assemble as a cell, life begins. Viruses are such an assembly, but they inhabit the border region between large, inanimate molecules and the smallest living cells. The *Escherichia coli* (*E. coli*) virus is about a hundred atoms across and contains approximately one hundred thousand atoms. With the virus, dead physics meets live biology and medicine has its most elementary protagonist. Here all the sciences are challenged with the unanswered question of how life arises and survives.

Perspective and Prospects

Physics has both enriched biology and profited greatly from the discoveries of many scientists educated in medical colleges and universities. These pioneers include Copernicus, Galileo, and at least a dozen other noted scientists who practiced from the fifteenth century to the nineteenth century. During this period, medicine was the major scientific profession—and before the seventeenth century the only one—at universities.

Nicolaus Copernicus (1473-1543), who proposed that the sun was the center of the solar system, studied medicine briefly in Padua, Italy. Galileo Galilei (1564-1642) was a medical student at Pisa, Italy, but finished in canon law. He used one of the first telescopes to help verify Copernicus's ideas, constructed some of the first microscopes, and laid the foundations for the present understanding of the laws of motion.

The list of medical doctors who made significant scientific contributions is long. William Gilbert (1544-1603), physician to Queen Elizabeth I, pioneered the study of electricity and magnetism. Luigi Galvani (1737-1798), for twenty years a doctor, investigated animal electricity. The physician William Wollaston (1766-1828) discovered palladium and rhodium and was the first to observe ultraviolet light. Thomas Young (1773-1829) practiced medicine unsuccessfully, but he made important contributions to the understanding of energy and developed the three-color theory of vision. Julius Robert Mayer (1814-1878), a medical practitioner for ten years, presented the law of energy conservation five years before its more widely known introductions by James P. Joule (1818-1889) and surgeon Hermann von Helmholtz (1821-1894). Helmholtz was the first to determine nerve pulse speed, and he developed the cochlear theory of hearing and did important work in electromagnetism.

The broad education favored by the early medical schools fostered pioneering scientific discoveries by its students and physicians, uniquely merging physics and biology at the beginnings of biophysics.

—Peter J. Walsh, Ph.D.

See also Anatomy; Audiology; Bioinformatics; Computed tomography (CT) scanning; Ears; Electrocardiography (ECG or EKG); Eyes; Imaging and radiology; Laser use in surgery; Magnetic field therapy; Magnetic resonance imaging (MRI); Microscopy; Nervous system; Neurology; Optometry; Physiology; Sense organs.

For Further Information:

Bergethon, Peter R. *The Physical Basis of Biochemistry: The Foundations of Molecular Biophysics*. New York: Springer, 1998. This comprehensive introductory text describes the philosophy and foundations of molecular biophysics. It is aimed at advanced undergraduates or beginning graduate students in biochemistry.

Campbell, Gaylon S., and John M. Norman. *An Introduction to Environmental Biophysics*. 2d ed. New York: Springer-Verlag, 1998. This book describes some aspects of the physical microenvironment and presents an introduction to models of heat and mass transfer between organisms and their microenvironments. It also provides excellent examples of these models in real systems.

Cotteril, Rodney M. J. *Biophysics: An Introduction*. New York: Wiley, 2002. An accessible text that introduces the subject and explores such topics as biopolymers, biomembranes, biological energy, protein folding, DNA/RNA conformations, molecular motors, and the biological origins of consciousness and intelligence.

Davidovits, Paul. *Physics in Biology and Medicine*. 2d ed. New York: Elsevier Science, 2001. An accessible text that requires no science background and relates important concepts in physics to living systems.

Marion, Jerry B. *General Physics with Bioscience Essays*. New York: John Wiley & Sons, 1985. A physics text with twenty-seven simple, readable bioscience essays sprinkled throughout. The essays apply physics to biology using only elementary math.

Sybesma, Christiaan. *Biophysics: An Introduction*. Rev. ed. Boston: Kluwer Academic, 1989. An introductory text on biophysics tilted toward the theoretical side of the science. More abstract than the other references listed here, requiring a good science background.

Biopsy

Procedure

Anatomy or system affected: Cells

Specialties and related fields: Cytology, dermatology, general surgery, gynecology, histology, oncology, pathology, radiology

Definition: The removal and examination of tissue and cells from the body, which is performed to establish a precise diagnosis and to determine proper treatment and prognosis.

Key terms:

cytology: the study of cells, their morphologic changes, and pathology

endoscopy: the visual inspection of body cavities and hollow structures and organs through the use of a tubelike instrument that can be introduced through any body orifice (for example, the mouth or anus) or through small cuts into the skin leading to a cavity

excisional biopsy: biopsy by incision to excise and completely remove an entire lesion, including adjacent portions of normal tissue

frozen section: an extremely thin tissue section cut by a specially designed instrument called a microtome from tissue that has been rapidly frozen, for the purpose of microscopic evaluation and rendering a diagnosis

incisional biopsy: biopsy of a selected sample of lesion

needle biopsy: the obtaining of tissue fragments by the puncture of a tumor, through a larger caliber needle, syringe, and plunger; the tissue within the lumen of the needle is obtained through the rotation and withdrawal of the needle

oncology: the branch of medicine concerned with the study and treatment of cancer

pathology: the branch of medicine that treats the essential nature of disease, especially of the structural and functional changes in cells, tissues, and organs of the body that cause or are caused by disease

staining: the artificial coloring of tissue sections and cells to facilitate their microscopic study

surgical pathology: the branch of pathology that deals with the interpretation of biopsies

Indications and Procedures

Biopsy is one of the most common diagnostic tools in medicine. Illness or disease can be caused by biological agents (such as viruses, bacteria, fungi, and parasites), by physical agents (such as radiation, heat, extreme cold, and trauma), by genetic and metabolic abnormalities (such as diabetes), or by cancer, which is a new, abnormal growth commonly called a tumor. Often, however, the cause of an illness or disease may not be known. Nevertheless, the structural changes caused by the disease are characteristic enough so that the study of these alterations can give a clear picture of the nature and course of the disease. Diseases may primarily affect one organ at a time, such as hepatitis (the inflammation of the liver), or may involve many organ systems at once, as in acquired immunodeficiency syndrome (AIDS).

The signs and symptoms of disease are not specific and are often shared by many conditions. For example, all diseases of the liver can result in jaundice, or yellowing of the skin, and abnormal blood tests. The clinician, who may be an expert in liver disease, may not be able to tell for certain whether the underlying liver condition is caused by a virus, by a toxic substance such as alcohol, or by both. A needle biopsy of the liver may then be obtained. The sample is examined by an expert surgical pathologist, and a specific diagnosis is rendered.

Similarly, a lump in the breast may be innocuous (benign) or cancerous (malignant). Only a biopsy of such a lesion can determine this conclusively. Such a biopsy can be obtained by fine needle aspiration, which is a simple procedure that can be performed in a clinic, or by excision in the operating room. A frozen section is then made for the purpose of rapid diagnosis and management.

Once a biopsy is obtained, it is placed in a special fixative, such as formalin. This solution will preserve—or fix—the internal structure of the tissue and its cells. Expert technicians in histology, called histotechnologists, will then embed the tissue in waxlike paraffin to obtain a "block." The tissue block is then placed in a microtome, and extremely thin pieces (about 5 micrometers thick in width) are cut from it. The slices are placed on glass slides and stained with different dyes, the most common of which is hematoxylin and eosin (H & E), to delineate the cellular substructures. The slides are examined by a surgical pathologist, who renders a pathology report in which the gross and microscopic features are described, and a diagnosis is made. A differential diagnosis may also be made, in which other possible causes of disease that may give a similar histologic picture are discussed. In addition to the routine study described above, a much more extensive and expensive workup of the biopsy may be done, depending on the anticipated complexity of the condition and organ.

The study of a biopsy requires diligent preparation and staining of the tissue, which is the realm of histotechnologists. Staining refers to the application of artificial dyes to tissue sections and cells to facilitate their microscopic study. Certain tissues and cell parts have different chemical and biological affinities for dyes which, when properly applied, help demarcate and differentiate the properties of these cells. A huge battery of special stains exists that can be used to examine every aspect of cell function in both health and disease. For example, specific enzymes can be evaluated; this technique is called enzyme histochemistry.

Immunologic stains, which help evaluate the status of immune system cells, are expensive and extremely tedious, and their proper interpretation requires considerable expertise. Many antibodies are commercially available for such testing. When directed against specific antigenic cell markers, they form immune complexes that can be targeted with immunological stains. Such stains can then be evaluated by immunofluorescence or immunoperoxidase techniques. Both types employ as their principle of action the forming of complexes between antigens and antibodies and the staining of these complexes. Immunofluorescence staining techniques involve the use of special stains that cause the tissue to shine when it is viewed under a fluorescent microscope; such procedures are performed on frozen section tissues. With immunoperoxidase stains, fixed tissues are used, and the stains are permanent.

Tissue samples can also be studied with an electron microscope, in which electron beams greatly magnify subcellular structures. In this way, the alterations of specific cellular components such as cell membranes, mitochondria, and intracellular viruses can be visualized and analyzed. This ultrastructural study is especially valuable in needle biopsies of the kidneys, as well as in the study of certain unusual cancer cells.

Another highly sophisticated method used to evaluate tissue and cell function in a biopsy is the application of molecular genetics and molecular biopsy techniques. The polymerase chain reaction (PCR) involves the splitting (splicing) of a specific section of genetic material in a cell and its amplification through a chemical chain reaction into innumerable folds, so that it can be visualized through a light microscope. This type of evaluation allows for the examination of specific microorganisms in a cell and can determine the presence of certain genetic markers of unusual diseases or cancer.

Another way to study the properties of cells is by examining their genetic makeup. Karyotyping is a technique in which the actual chromosomes in a cell are photographed during mitotic divisions; the chromosomes appear as patterns of bands. Genetic abnormalities can be identified by the number of chromosomes and their appearance. This procedure is often used in the study of cancer cells. An even more sophisticated study of cellular genetic makeup is called gene rearrangement, in which the order of gene stacking is examined for specific markers of certain cancerous growths, especially of white blood cells. Other techniques that are used to evaluate cell functions and morphology are cellular imaging, in which the contours of cell membranes and surfaces are compared using computers, and the use of flow cytometers, in which cells are targeted immunologically and then counted. Both techniques are employed in cancer studies, and the second is also used for patients with abnormal immune systems, such as those with AIDS.

The aforementioned studies are expensive and available only at large medical centers and research institutes. The diagnostic workup in most hospitals, however, does not require the use of these sophisticated methods. Usually, routine H & E stains are applied. The Papanicolaou stain is commonly used with fine needle aspiration biopsies.

A department of pathology in a large medical center usually has one or more surgical pathologists, who are closely affiliated with the clinical and surgical departments and with their many branches and specialties. Interpreting biopsies obtained by any of the surgical or medical specialties is the most important duty of the surgical pathologist, and it requires great expertise and diligence. Because of the complexity of this task, specialized experts in pathology are becoming the norm. For example, a dermatopathologist is a surgical pathologist trained to interpret skin biopsies. Similarly, hematopathologists, neuropathologists, and nephropathologists are experts in the interpretation of blood-related, nerve- and brain-related, and kidney-related biopsies, respectively.

In incisional biopsies, only a portion of the lesion is sampled, and the procedure is strictly of a diagnostic nature. In excisional biopsy, the entire lesion is removed, usually with a rim of normal tissue, and therefore the procedure serves both a diagnostic and a therapeutic function. The decision whether to perform an incisional or an excisional biopsy depends primarily on the size and location of the lesion; the smaller the lesion, the more logical it is to remove it completely. It is preferable, however, to sample a deeply seated large tumor first because the type and extent of the excision varies considerably depending on the tumor type. For example, a small skin mole is usually excised com-

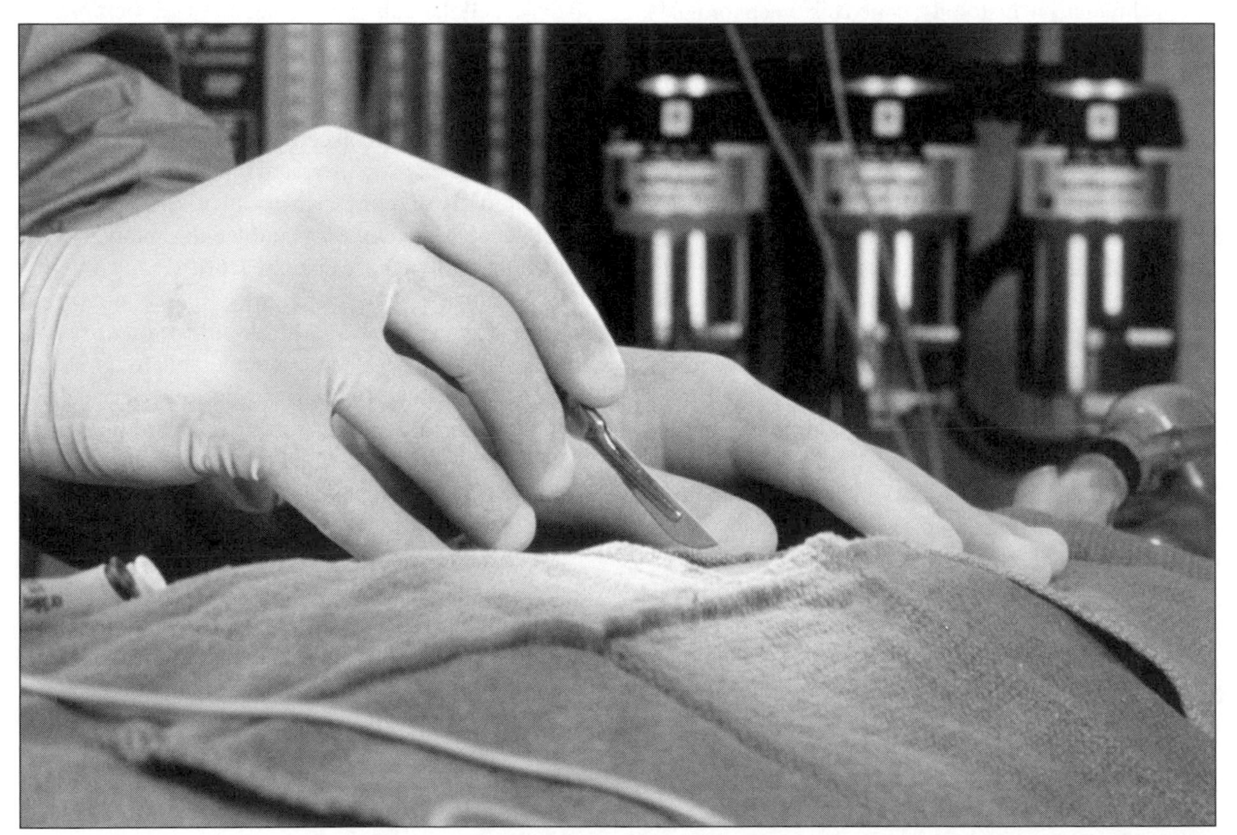

A biopsy is performed when diagnosis requires a sample of cells, tissue, or fluid for further analysis in the laboratory. The gathering of such a sample can be done with a scalpel (shown here), needle, curette, or syringe. (PhotoDisc)

pletely, whereas a large soft tissue or bone tumor should be sampled.

Biopsies are also classified according to the instrument used to obtain them: cold knife versus cautery, needle, or endoscope. Of these the one usually least suitable for microscopic study is that obtained with a cautery, which uses a hot knife that burns, chars, and distorts tissue.

An endoscope is a tubelike fiber-optic instrument that is inserted into an orifice or small incision in order to view the contents of a body cavity. The instrument can be rigid or flexible and is equipped with a light source (usually a laser) and a small cutting tool at its tip to allow for the removal of small samples of tissue. Endoscopic biopsies are frequently used to obtain tissue and cell samples from the lungs and the airways, mainly to diagnose laryngeal and lung cancers; this procedure is usually done by a lung specialist. The endoscope is also used to sample lesions in the esophagus, stomach, intestines, and the rest of the intestinal tract, including the rectum. Such procedures are usually performed by a gastroenterologist, a specialist in the stomach and the gastrointestinal tract. Endoscopic biopsies of the urinary bladder and the prostate are done by urologists.

Needle biopsies are commonly used to obtain samples from superficial or deep-seated lumps. A slender, cylindrical core of tissue, corresponding to the open diameter of the needle, is obtained. The needle biopsy is commonly used to obtain tissue samples from kidneys, bone, and the deep viscera such as the liver. The modified technique of aspiration cytology, commonly called fine needle aspiration, employs a fine-caliber needle (0.6 to 0.9 millimeter in open diameter) and is widely used to obtain cytologic and minute tissue samples, especially for lesions of the lymph glands, breasts, thyroid gland, salivary glands, lungs, and prostate. Fine needle aspiration is often inexpensive, safe, quick, and, when performed and interpreted by experienced workers, quite accurate. Because of the ready availability and relative inexpense of the endoscopic and fine needle aspiration biopsy techniques, they have become popular; almost every part of the body is now within reach of one or another of these two techniques.

Frozen section biopsy requires great expertise because this biopsy is usually a form of consultation done during surgery. A tissue sample is instantly frozen, sectioned, stained, and examined—all within about fifteen minutes—in order to render a specific diagnosis. The implications of this diagnosis are far reaching and will influence the surgical procedure and the long-term therapy and outcome for the patient. A frozen section report, for example, may determine whether an organ such as a breast, lung, or kidney must be removed and whether long-term radiation therapy or chemotherapy will be administered; such would be the case if the diagnosis is read as malignant.

There are two indications, other than establishing a diagnosis, for performing a frozen section: determining the adequacy of the margins of surgical excision (for example, to remove a malignant tumor completely) and establishing whether the tissue obtained contains an ample diagnosable sample to carry out other specialized tissue studies.

Uses and Complications

The following examples illustrate the practical use of the various biopsy techniques.

An excisional biopsy is performed on a pigmented dark lesion on a sun-exposed surface of the body of a young man and is diagnosed as malignant melanoma, which is a tumor of the pigment-producing cells of the body. This diagnosis is confirmed through the use of specialized immunological stains employing specific antibodies against melanin. The pathologist also comments that surgical margins of excision of that tumor are safe and do not contain tumor, and that the tumor is only superficial in nature and does not show deep invasion into the tissue. These two points imply that the patient will probably have a complete cure.

A fine needle aspiration biopsy is applied on a lump on the breast of a young woman. The material obtained is spread on slides, stained with a Papanicolaou stain, and evaluated within hours of its removal. The lump is diagnosed as a fibroadenoma, which is a benign tumor that is completely innocuous and of no further consequence to the young patient.

An elderly patient has an endoscopic biopsy of a visualized mass in the colon, which proves to be cancer. The patient is taken to the operating room, and the colon is resected. A frozen section is performed on the margin on the surgical excision to make sure that it contains no tumor. The stains used in this example are the simple and routine H & E stains.

A liver biopsy is performed on a patient with jaundice (yellowing of the skin), and a diagnosis of viral hepatitis B is made. This diagnosis is made following the study of the liver biopsy by routine stains and by stains that use immunological antibodies against the viral antigen. This is a specific and highly accurate diagnostic study.

A lymph gland excisional biopsy is performed on a patient who feels lumps all over his body. The biopsy is examined with routine and special stains, immunological marker studies, and gene rearrangement. Such extensive studies are performed to make sure that his condition is completely benign and is not neoplastic—that is, that he does not have malignant lymphoma (cancer of lymph tissue).

The biopsy, in its varied forms and techniques, has become an essential component of quality medical care. The biopsy report is both a medical and a legal document. Tissue slides and blocks are often stored for many years, in some places indefinitely. Peer slide reviews and consultations are common and are used as gauges for quality control and management. There are some limitations with histologic diagnosis, which mainly revolve around recognizing a specialist's own limitations and the need to seek a consultation by another expert pathologist as needed.

Perspective and Prospects

The first attempts to affirm the role of biopsy in medical practice were made by Carl Ruge and Johann Veit of the University of Berlin, who in the 1870's introduced surgical biopsy as an essential diagnostic tool. Despite the inevitable controversies that followed, Johann F. A. von Esmarch, a professor of surgery and a leading military surgeon of his time, presented forceful arguments at the German Surgical Congress of 1889 on the need to establish a microscopic diagnosis before operating in suspected cases of malignant tumors requiring extensive mutilating procedures. Shortly thereafter, the freezing microtome was introduced for the purpose of creating frozen sections, which hastened the acceptance of this recommendation. In the United States, the specialty of surgical pathology, which deals with biopsy interpretations, was created by a collaboration between surgeons and a gynecologist.

It is said that the first full-fledged American surgical pathologist was Joseph Colt Bloodgood, in the division of surgical pathology created by W. S. Halsted of The Johns Hopkins Hospital in Baltimore, Maryland. The founders of modern American surgical pathology and biopsy interpretation are Arthur Purdy Stout of Columbia Presbyterian Hospital in New York, James Ewing and his successors Fred Stewart and Frank Foote of Memorial Hospital in New York City, and Pierre Masson of the University of Montreal, Canada.

The biopsy remains the cornerstone for modern medical management, especially in cancer therapy. It will continue to enjoy that role in diagnostics as more venues become established to obtain, study, and evaluate minute tissue and cytologic samples.

—Victor H. Nassar, M.D.

See also Breast biopsy; Breast cancer; Colon and rectal polyp removal; Colon cancer; Cyst removal; Cysts; Cytology; Cytopathology; Dermatology; Dermatopathology; Endometrial biopsy; Endoscopy; Histology; Immunopathology; Invasive tests; Laboratory tests; Mastectomy and lumpectomy; National Cancer Institute (NCI); Oncology; Pap smear; Pathology; Skin; Skin cancer; Skin disorders; Skin lesion removal; Tumor removal; Tumors.

For Further Information:

Bancroft, John D., and Marilyn Gamble, eds. *Theory and Practice of Histological Techniques*. 5th ed. New York: Churchill Livingstone, 2002. A standard text on tissue preparation and the various methods of staining, used mostly by histologists and technicians. A somewhat technical book.

Koss, Leopold G., Stanisław Woyke, and Włodzimierz Olszewski. *Aspiration Biopsy: Cytologic Interpretation and Histologic Basis*. 2d ed. New York: Igaku-Shoin, 1992. The definitive treatise on the subject of fine needle aspiration biopsy.

Mills, Stacey E., et al., eds. *Sternberg's Diagnostic Surgical Pathology*. 4th ed. 2 vols. Philadelphia: Lippincott Williams & Wilkins, 2004. An authoritative treatise written by recognized experts on the various fields in biopsy interpretation. Frequently used by surgical pathologists and students of the discipline.

Rosai, Juan. *Rosai and Ackerman's Surgical Pathology*. 9th ed. 2 vols. New York: Mosby, 2004. This standard text on surgical pathology contains chapters on biopsy interpretation of all body organs. Written by a foremost authority on the subject matter and richly illustrated.

Sloan, John P. *Biopsy Pathology of the Breast*. 2d ed. New York: Oxford University Press, 2001. A practical guide to diagnosing breast pathology. The second edition examines the way in which advances in mammographic screening, more treatment options, greater involvement by pathologists in clinical management, and the expansion of molecular pathology have affected the field.

Yazdi, Hossein M., and Irving Dardick. *Diagnostic*

Immunocytochemistry and Electron Microscopy: Guides to Clinical Aspiration Biopsy. New York: Igaku-Shoin, 1992. A resource on highly technical and specialized methods in biopsy interpretation.

BIOSTATISTICS

PROCEDURE

ANATOMY OR SYSTEM AFFECTED: None

SPECIALTIES AND RELATED FIELDS: All

DEFINITION: The application of statistical concepts to biology and medicine in order to summarize the characteristics of samples and to test predictions about the populations from which the samples were taken.

KEY TERMS:

correlation: a number between −1 and +1 that describes the strength of the relationship between two variables

descriptive statistics: the use of numbers to summarize the characteristics of samples

inferential statistics: the making and testing of numerical statements about populations

null hypothesis: a statement about a population that can be tested numerically

population: all the people, research animals, or other items of interest in a particular study

probability: a number varying between 0 (for an impossible event) to 1 (for an absolutely certain event)

random sample: a sample in which every member of the population has the same probability of being included

regression: an equation that allows one variable to be predicted from another

sample: the members of a population that are actually studied or whose characteristics are measured

variable: any quantity that varies, such as height or cholesterol level

THE METHODOLOGY OF STATISTICS

The aim of every study in the field of biostatistics is to discover something about a population—all patients with a particular disease, for example. Populations are usually much too large to be studied in their entirety: It would be very impractical to round up all the patients with diabetes in the world for a study, and the researcher would still miss those who lived in the past or who have yet to be born. For this reason, most research focuses on a sample drawn from the population of interest—for example, those diabetics who were studied at a particular hospital over a two-year period. Ideally, the sample would be a random sample, one in which each member of the population has an equal chance of being included. In practice, a random sample is hard to achieve: The patients with diabetes at a hospital in Chicago, for example, will differ in various ways from those at hospitals in London, Hong Kong, or rural Mexico.

Descriptive statistics are statistics that describe samples. The most commonly used statistics are mean, median, mode, and standard deviation. The mean of *n* values is simply the sum of all the values divided by *n*, or, symbolically, $\overline{X} = \Sigma x/n$, where $\overline{X}$ (pronounced "*x*-bar") stands for the mean, *n* stands for the number of observations, and Σx (pronounced "sum of *x*") stands for the sum obtained when all the diffent values of *x* (*n* of them) are added together. The median of a series of values is the middle value; it must always be the case that half of the values are above the median and half are below. The mode is simply the most common value, the value that occurs most often.

The mean, median, and mode are all "typical" values that characterize the center of distribution of all the values. The standard deviation, which is always positive, is a measure of variation that describes how close all the values cluster about a central value. The formula for the standard deviation is

$$s = \sqrt{\frac{\Sigma (x - \overline{X})^2}{n - 1}}$$

The numerator is calculated by subtracting the mean ($\overline{X}$) from each value, squaring the difference, and adding together all these squared differences. After the sum is divided by $n - 1$, the square root of the entire quantity is taken to determine the standard deviation. A small standard deviation indicates that the values differ very little from one another; a large standard deviation indicates greater variability among the values.

When two quantities vary, such as height and weight, correlation and regression coefficients are also calculated. A correlation coefficient is a number between −1 and +1. A correlation near +1 shows a very strong relationship between the two variables: When either one increases, the other also increases. A correlation near −1 is also strong, but when either variable increases, the other decreases. A correlation of 0 shows independence, or no relationship, between the variables: An increase in one has no average effect on the value of the other. Correlations midway between 0 and 1 show that an increase in one variable corresponds only to an average increase in the other, but not a dependable increase in each value. For example, taller people are generally heavier, but this is not true in every case.

Regression is a statistical technique for finding an equation that allows one variable to be predicted from the value of the other. For example, a regression of weight on height allows a researcher to predict the average weight for persons of a given height.

Inferential statistics, the statistical study of populations, begins with the study of probability. A probability is a number between 0 and 1 that indicates the certainty with which a particular event will occur, where 0 indicates an impossible occurrence and 1 indicates a certain occurrence. If a certain disease affects 1 percent of the population, then each random sampling will be subject to a .01 probability that the next person sampled will have the disease. For a larger sample than only one individual, the so-called binomial distribution describes the probability that the sample will include no one with the disease, one person with the disease, two people with the disease, and so on.

A variable such as height is subject to so many influences, both genetic and environmental, that it can be treated mathematically as if it were the sum of thousands of small, random variations. Characteristics such as height usually follow a bell-shaped curve, or normal distribution (see figure), at least approximately. This means that very few people are unusually tall or unusually short; most have heights near the middle of the distribution.

Each study using inferential statistics includes four major steps. First, certain assumptions are made about the populations under study. A common assumption, seldom tested, is that the variable in question is normally distributed within the population. Second, one or more samples are then drawn from the population, and each person or animal in the population is measured and tested in some way. Most studies assume that the samples are randomly drawn from the populations in question, even though true randomness is extremely difficult to achieve. Third, a particular assumption, called the null hypothesis, is chosen for testing. The null hypothesis is always an assumption that can be expressed numerically and that can be tested by known statistical tests. For example, one might assume that the mean height of the population of all diabetics is 170 centimeters (5.5 feet). Fourth, each statistical procedure allows the calculation of a theoretical probability, often a calculated value from a table. If the calculated probability is moderate or high, the null hypothesis is consistent with the observed results. If the calculated probability is very small, the observed results are very unlikely to occur if the null hypothesis is true; in these cases, the null hypothesis is rejected.

Some common types of inferential statistics are *t*-tests, chi-square tests, and the analysis of variance (also called ANOVA).

THE APPLICATION OF STATISTICS TO MEDICINE

Nearly all medical research studies include biostatistics. Descriptive statistics are often presented in tables of data or in graphic form.

In the following example, height and weight data were gathered from a sample of six diabetic patients, and height was also measured in a sample of six nondiabetic patients (see table 1). The mean height of these diabetic patients is (166 + 171 + 157 + 161 +

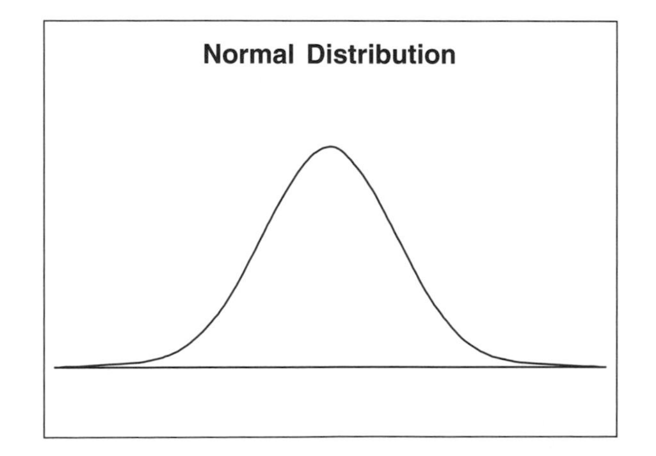

TABLE 1. A COMPARISON BETWEEN DIABETICS AND NONDIABETICS

Diabetics		*Nondiabetics*
Height (cm)	*Weight (kg)*	*Height (cm)*
166	78	172
171	90	180
157	72	184
161	82	187
179	92	166
186	82	173

179 + 186) ÷ 6 = 1,020 ÷ 6 = 170 centimeters. In order to calculate the standard deviation, this mean is subtracted from each of the six values, to yield differences of −4, 1, −13, −9, 9, and 16. Squaring these differences and adding them up gives a numerator of 16 + 1 + 169 + 81 + 81 + 256 = 604. Dividing this by $n - 1 = 5$ (n is 6) and taking the square root reveals that the standard deviation is 11.0 centimeters (rounded to the nearest tenth). Similar calculations show that the mean height of the nondiabetic sample is 177 centimeters, with a standard deviation of 8.0 centimeters.

In this example, the nondiabetic sample averaged 7 centimeters taller than the diabetic sample. Inferential statistics can be used to find out if this difference is a meaningful one. In this case, a technique known as a *t*-test can compare the means of two samples to determine whether they might have come from the same population (or from populations with the same mean value). The assumptions of this test (not always stated explicitly) are that the six diabetic patients were randomly drawn from a normally distributed population and that the six nondiabetic patients were randomly drawn from another normally distributed population. The null hypothesis in this case is that the populations from which the two samples were drawn have the same mean height. The value of t calculated in this test is 1.141; this value is looked up in a table to reveal that the probability is larger than .1 (or 10 percent). In other words, if the null hypothesis is true, then this value of t (or a larger value) is expected to arise by chance alone more than 10 percent of the time. Under the usual criterion of a test at the 5 percent level of significance, one would keep or accept the null hypothesis. This means that the difference between the above sample means is not large enough to demonstrate a difference between the two populations from which these samples are derived. There may in fact be an average difference in height between diabetic and nondiabetic populations, but samples this small cannot detect such a difference reliably. In general, when differences between populations are small, larger sample sizes are required to demonstrate their existence.

A *t*-test similar to the one above can also be used in drug testing. A drug is given to one set of patients, and a placebo (a fake medicine lacking the essential drug ingredient being tested) is given to a second group. Some relevant measurement (such as the drug's level of an important chemical that the patients normally lacked) is then compared between the two groups. The null hypothesis would be that the groups are the same and that the drug makes no difference. Rejection of the null hypothesis would be the same as demonstrating that the drug is effective.

For the diabetic patients in the above sample, a correlation coefficient of .60 can be calculated. This moderate level of correlation shows that, on the average, the taller among these patients are also heavier and thus the shorter patients are also lighter. Despite this average effect, however, individual exceptions are likely to occur. The square of the correlation coefficient, .36, indicates that about 36 percent of the variation in weight can be predicted from height. The equation for making the prediction in this case is "weight = 13.99 + .404 (height)," where the numbers 13.99 and .404 are called regression coefficients. The variable being predicted (weight in this example) is sometimes called the dependent variable; the variable used to make the prediction (in this case, height) is called the independent variable. A high positive correlation signifies that the regression equation offers a very reliable prediction of the dependent variable; a correlation near zero signifies that the regression equation is hardly better than assigning the mean value of the dependent variable to every prediction.

To illustrate another type of inferential statistics, consider the following data on the diseases present among elderly patients who own pets, compared to a comparable group who do not. This type of table is called a contingency table.

As illustrated in table 2, 90 ÷ 240, or three-eighths of the patients sampled, are pet owners. Thus, if there were no relationship between the diseases and pet ownership (which is the null hypothesis), one would expect three-eighths of the eighty arthritis patients (or 30) to be pet owners and five-eighths of the eighty (or 50) to be nonowners. Calculating all the expected frequencies

TABLE 2. A CONTINGENCY TABLE COMPARING PET OWNERS AND NON-OWNERS

	Pet owners	*Non-owners*	*Totals*
Arthritis	22	58	80
Heart Disease	11	29	40
Cancer	21	9	30
Other	36	54	90
TOTALS	90	150	240

in this way, one can compare them with the actual observations shown above.

The result is a statistic called chi-square, which in this problem has a value of 18.88. A table of chi-square values shows that, for a 2 × 4 contingency table, a chi-square value this high occurs by chance alone much less than 1 percent of the time. Thus, something has been observed (a chi-square value of 18.88) that is extremely unlikely under the null hypothesis of no relationship between disease and pet ownership, so the null hypothesis is rejected and one must conclude that there is a relationship. This conclusion applies only to the population from which the sample was drawn, however, and it does not reveal the nature of the relationship. Further investigation would be needed to discover whether pet ownership protected people from arthritis, whether people who already had arthritis were less inclined to take on the responsibility of pet ownership, or whether people who had pets gave them up when they became arthritic. All these possibilities (and more) are consistent with the findings.

The analysis of variance (also called ANOVA) is a very powerful technique for comparing many samples at once. Suppose that overweight patients were put on three or four different diets; one diet might be better than another, but there is also much individual variation in the amount of weight lost. Analysis of variance is a statistical technique that allows researchers to compare the variation between diets (or other treatments) with the individual variation among the people following each diet. The null hypothesis would be that all the diets are the same and that individual variation can account for all the observed differences. Rejecting the null hypothesis would demonstrate that a consistent difference existed and that at least one diet was better than another. Further tests would be required to pinpoint which diet was best and why.

Perspective and Prospects

The historical foundations of biostatistics go back as far as the development of probability theory by Blaise Pascal (1623-1662). Karl Friedrich Gauss (1777-1855) first outlined the characteristics of the normal (also called Gaussian) distribution. The chi-square test was introduced by Karl Pearson (1857-1936). The greatest statistician of the twentieth century was Ronald A. Fisher (1890-1962), who clearly distinguished descriptive from inferential statistics and who developed many important statistical techniques, including the analysis of variance.

Although medicine existed long before statistics, it has become a nearly universal practice for every research study to use statistics in some important way. New medical procedures and new drugs are constantly being evaluated by using statistical techniques to compare them to other procedures or older drugs.

—Eli C. Minkoff, Ph.D.

See also Bioinformatics; Epidemiology; Screening.

For Further Information:

Brase, Charles Henry, and Corrinne Pellillo Brase. *Understandable Statistics*. 8th ed. Boston: Houghton Mifflin, 2006. A good introduction, with many helpful examples that are carefully explained.

Daniel, Wayne W. *Biostatistics: A Foundation for Analysis in the Health Sciences*. 8th ed. Hoboken, N.J.: John Wiley & Sons, 2005. A good reference specific to problems of drug testing and similar medical applications.

Hebel, J. Richard, and Robert J. McCarter. *A Study Guide to Epidemiology and Biostatistics*. 6th ed. Sudbury, Mass.: Jones and Bartlett, 2006. Introduces basic principles in epidemiology and biostatistics and provides study notes, exercises, and multiple-choice tests.

Le, Chap T. *Health and Numbers: Problems-Based Introduction to Biostatistics*. 2d ed. New York: Wiley, 2001. Introductory text that takes a problems-based approach to statistical methods, using real-life examples with real data, and emphasizes descriptive statistics.

Phillips, John L. *How to Think About Statistics*. 6th ed. New York: Henry Holt, 2002. A very simple introduction to the subject.

Sokal, Robert R., and F. James Rohlf. *Biometry*. 3d ed. San Francisco: W. H. Freeman, 1995. A good advanced reference, especially with respect to various types of ANOVA.

Walpole, Ronald E. *Elementary Statistical Concepts*. New York: Macmillan, 1976. Gently eases the reader into some moderately advanced concepts.

Zar, Jerrold H. *Biostatistical Analysis*. 4th ed. Englewood Cliffs, N.J.: Prentice Hall, 1999. A good, very thorough, but somewhat technical account.

BIOTECHNOLOGY. *See* BIONICS AND BIOTECHNOLOGY.

Bipolar disorders

Disease/disorder

Anatomy or system affected: Psychic-emotional system

Specialties and related fields: Psychiatry, psychology

Definition: Affective (mood-related) illness characterized by periods of depressed and elevated mood.

Key terms:

anticonvulsants: drugs typically used to manage conditions involving brain seizures and sometimes used to treat bipolar disorders

bipolar I: less formally known as manic-depressive disorder; a condition that involves both severe symptoms of mania and depression and includes at least one episode of mania

bipolar II: a condition that involves both hypomania (milder symptoms of mania) and severe symptoms of depression and includes at least one episode of hypomania

dual diagnosis: a broad term used among professionals to indicate that an individual has two disorders needing integrated care and often used in psychiatry to indicate that an individual has received the diagnosis of a substance use disorder and another major clinical syndrome, such as a bipolar disorder

lithium: a drug composed of lithium carbonate used in the treatment of bipolar disorders

mood disorders: a group of disorders characterized by disturbance of mood and including symptoms of depression and/or mania that are not caused by any other physical or mental disorder

mood stabilizers: drugs that decrease the frequency and intensity of mood fluctuation, including drugs such as lithium and anticonvulsants

psychosis: a symptom associated with a variety of mental disorders and characterized by faulty perceptions and thinking that may be short-lived or enduring, being out of touch with reality, and lacking awareness of these problems; often includes hallucinations and delusions

unipolar depression: a term used by professionals to indicate that a person has the condition of depression with no evidence of having experienced a manic or hypomanic episode

unipolar mania: a very rare condition in which a person experiences periods of mania but has no experience of depression; is not caused by another disorder or condition

Causes and Symptoms

Although the causes of bipolar disorders are not known definitively, research indicates that some persons may be genetically predisposed to respond readily with manic or depressive episodes to internal and external influences. While changes in brain metabolism are thought to be significant in the development of bipolar disorders, both psychological and nonpsychological stresses are known to precipitate the onset of problems. It is often not possible to find one precipitating factor, however, because there is presumably a complex interaction between the effects of internal and external influences in persons suffering from this illness.

Bipolar disorders are illnesses that often occur in attacks, or episodes, lasting several days to a week or longer. They may be attacks of mania (periods of extreme elation and increased activity), hypomania (notably elevated mood and heightened activity), or depression (periods of abnormal sadness and melancholy). Recent work indicates that many variants of this disorder exist. Bipolar I is a variant of bipolar disorder in which individuals experience at least one episode of depression and one episode of mania. Bipolar II is a variant in which individuals experience at least one episode of depression and one episode of hypomania. For some individuals, these episodes signifying the presence of a disorder may be time limited and singular occurrences. For others, there may be repeated bouts of depression, mania, and hypomania or even times when symptoms appear to be a mix of all three. Further, these episodes may be interspersed with periods of normal behavior, with no mood problems at all, which can vary in length from brief amounts of time to years. In addition, a condition called cyclothymia refers to the presence of hypomania and a milder form of depression than is seen in bipolar disorders. These disorders are distinguished from unipolar depression (in which there is no mania or hypomania), the very rare condition of unipolar mania, and a more chronic but less severe form of depression known as dysthymia.

Bipolar disorders occur in about 1 percent of the population as a whole. They may occur in both adults and children and are diagnosed more often in women than in men. For persons over the age of eighteen, they are diagnosed in about two to three persons out of every one hundred. They also may occur in adolescence and childhood.

The onset of the disease frequently occurs between the ages of twenty and fifty, but it may appear for the first time in childhood or in later life, even beyond age sixty. Bipolar episodes manifest themselves differently in different persons. They can also vary within a particular person from one time to another. Further, although depression, mania, and hypomania have characteristic features, not all features are present during each episode.

Prominent features of manic episodes are elation, easily aroused anger, and increased mental activity. The elation varies from unusual vigor to uninhibited enthusiasm. The anger most often takes the form of irritability. Manic patients become annoyed if other people are unable to keep up with their racing thoughts. Intellectual activity takes place with lightning speed, ideas race through the mind, and speech flows with great rapidity and almost uninterruptedly.

During a manic episode, individuals are often excessively self-confident and lacking in self-criticism and insight into their behavior. This accompanies previously unknown energy, and when that energy is combined with racing thoughts, indefatigability, and lack of inhibition, the consequences are often disastrous. During manic episodes, individuals may destroy their relationships, ruin their reputations, create financial disasters, and engage in behavior that is not characteristic for them, such as indiscriminant sexual behavior, substance use, or even criminal activity. They may even demonstrate signs of psychosis. Despite reduced sleep, they also rarely feel tired and are usually kept awake by the rapid flow of ideas. Sexual activity may be greatly increased. Manic individuals may neglect to eat, and so they may lose considerable weight. The combination of activity, decreased food intake, and an inadequate amount of sleep may lead to dangerous physical exhaustion.

Hypomanic episodes are distinguished from manic episodes primarily in terms of being less intense, having fewer symptoms, and being less disruptive. The elevated mood also never reaches the point where psychosis is present. In fact, individuals may be highly functional during hypomanic episodes and may experience these times as pleasant and productive. The primary disruption is likely to be related to the driven nature of the behavior and how it may affect social interactions. Generally, though, any problems caused are not severe in nature.

Depressed episodes are in many respects the opposite of manias. They are characterized by sadness, a lack of self-confidence, and decreased mental activity. The sadness may vary from a slight feeling of being "down" to the bleakest despair. Ideas are few, thoughts move slowly, and memory function is impaired. Frequently, depressed individuals feel tired and emotionally drained; they feel the need to cry but are unable to do so. Weighed down by feelings of guilt and self-reproach, they may contemplate or even commit suicide. The depressed individual's self-confidence often is eroded, and, as a result, they may withdraw socially, lack initiative and energy, feel that obstacles are insurmountable, and have difficulty making even trivial decisions. Because of accompanying low self-esteem and feelings of inadequacy, individuals suffering from depression often fear social interaction and become anxious, agitated, and restless in a crowd. Sleep disturbances are also frequent. Occasionally, there is an increased need for sleep, and often individuals have difficulty sleeping, such as with insomnia. Some individuals find it difficult to fall asleep, others wake up frequently during the night, and others wake up early with feelings of anxiety. Depressed individuals also often experience variations in mood over the course of a day. The desire to stay in bed is overwhelming, and during the first hours of the day, they may experience basic daily activities as an extraordinary challenge.

Depressive episodes are often accompanied by physical transformations. The muscles may give the impression of being slack, the facial expression static, and movement slowed. There may be constipation, menstruation may stop, and sexual interest and activity may decrease or disappear completely for a time. Appetite may decrease and may result in loss of weight. Alternatively, eating may increase or remain the same,

Information on Bipolar Disorders

Causes: Unknown; possibly genetic factors, changes in metabolism of brain, stress

Symptoms: Episodes of mania (increased mental activity, heightened emotions, excessive self-confidence and feelings of invincibility, sleeplessness) and depression (extreme sadness, lack of self-confidence, decreased mental activity, feeling tired and emotionally drained, fear of social interaction, anxiety and agitation)

Duration: Chronic

Treatments: Medications (lithium, antidepressants, neuroleptics), psychotherapy, electroconvulsive therapy

but because of decreased activity, weight gain may be experienced.

In addition to manic, hypomanic, and depressed episodes, bipolar disorders may manifest as mixed states during which signs of mania, hypomania, and depression are present concurrently. Individuals who experience mixed states may be sad and without energy but also irritable, or they may be manic and restless yet feel an underlying melancholy. Mixed states may occur as independent episodes, but they are seen more often during transitions between episodes. During these periods of transition, the condition may alternate between mood states several times a day.

Treatment and Therapy

Lithium is the drug frequently used for the treatment of bipolar disorders. A metallic element discovered by a Swedish chemist in 1818, lithium is produced from minerals such as spodumene, amblygonite, lepidolite, and petalite. As a drug, lithium is always used in the form of one of its salts—for example, lithium carbonate or lithium citrate. It is the lithium portion of these salts that is effective medically. Lithium was introduced into medicine in 1850 for the treatment of gout, and during the following century many medical uses of the element were proposed. It was used as a stimulant, as a sedative, for the treatment of diabetes, for the treatment of infectious diseases, as an additive to toothpaste, and for the treatment of malignant growths. The efficacy of lithium in these conditions was not proved, however, and lithium treatment never became widespread.

In 1949, an Australian psychiatrist, John Cade, published an article that forms the basis of all later lithium treatment. The prophylactic action of lithium in manic-depressive type illnesses was debated in the psychiatric literature for some years, but extensive trials in many countries have fully documented the efficacy of the drug. Its prophylactic action is exerted against both manic and depressive relapses. One of the characteristic features of lithium is that it removes manic symptoms without producing sedation, unlike treatment with neuroleptics, which are also effective in the treatment of mania but which exert sedative action. Lithium may occasionally produce side effects, such as nausea, stomachache, tremor of the hands, and muscle weakness, but these symptoms are usually neither severe nor incapacitating. The greatest drawback of the treatment is that the full antimanic effect is usually not seen until after six to eight days of treatment, and sometimes it is necessary to supplement lithium with a neuroleptic drug.

Until the 1950's, the condition commonly described as manic depression, and now known as the varied conditions of bipolar disorders, had remained intractable, frustrating the best efforts of clinical practitioners and their predecessors. This long history ended abruptly with the discovery of the therapeutic effects of lithium. In an ironic turn of events, the pharmacologic revolution then initiated a renaissance in the psychotherapy of manic-depressive patients. Substantially freed from the severe disruptions of mania and the profound withdrawal of depression, these individuals, with the help of their therapists, focused on the many psychological issues related to the illness and confronted what was needed for them to maintain health. Unfortunately, lithium and the psychotherapy approaches available at that time did not help everyone every time, and so the search for helpful treatments continued. Part of this was because not all individuals who need to take lithium will adhere to their prescribed drug regimen. Also, some individuals cannot take lithium because of its toxicity to the body or because of physical conditions they may have.

Electroconvulsive therapy (ECT) is one alternative to medications in treating bipolar disorders. This therapy is particularly useful for individuals who have failed to respond to drugs, who may not be able to tolerate drugs such as lithium because of other physical conditions, or who need immediate relief from their mood symptoms in order to avoid suicide or life-threatening conditions. In ECT, following narcosis (an unconscious state induced by narcotics), certain parts of the patient's brain are stimulated electrically through electrodes placed on the skin. This stimulation elicits a seizure, but since the drug relaxes the muscles, the seizure manifests as muscle twitching only. The individuals do not feel the treatment, but during the hours following the treatment, they may have headaches and feel tenderness of the muscles. Short-term memory impairment may also occur. Treatment often occurs two to four times a week for three to four weeks at a hospital or on an outpatient basis and leads to amelioration of symptoms in most patients.

For treatment of symptoms such as agitation related to bipolar conditions, drugs referred to as antipsychotic medications, or neuroleptics, are often used. These are sedative drugs such as chlorpromazine (Largactil, Thorazine) and haloperidol (Haldol). Neuroleptics exert a powerful tranquilizing effect on anxiety, restlessness, and tension. They also attenuate or relieve hallucinations and delusions. Neuroleptics are not specific for any single disease. They may be used, possibly in conjunction with lithium, in the treatment of mania, and they may be used in depressions that are accompanied by delusions. Neuroleptics may, however, produce side effects involving the muscles and the nervous system.

Antidepressants act, as the name indicates, on depression, but only on abnormal depression. They do not affect the normal ups and downs that people without these conditions might experience, and they do not make people experience a "drug high" or become happy. They instead work to bring individuals back from a depressed state to normal. Drugs that fit in this group have included substances such as imipramine (Tofranil), amitriptyline (Elavil, Tryptizol), and fluoxetine (Prozac), among others. The side effects of antidepressants may include tiredness, mouth dryness, tremor, constipation, difficulty in urinating, and a tendency to faint. Changes in heart rate and rhythm may also occur, and careful evaluation is necessary in patients with cardiac disease. As new drugs are developed, drug makers often work hard to reduce such side effects. Also, some of these side effects may lessen over time as the person's body becomes habituated to the drug.

Where antidepressants do work, however, treatment is often continued for some time after disappearance of the symptoms. For example, continuing treatment for three, six, twelve, or even twenty-four months would not be uncommon.

Bipolar disorder is treated most effectively with a combination of lithium or other medications and adjunctive psychotherapy. Drug treatment, which is primary, relieves most patients of the severe disruptions of mood episodes. Psychotherapy can assist them in coming to terms with the repercussions of past episodes and in comprehending the practical implications of living with bipolar disorder. It may also be useful for helping to identify life stressors that may cause or exacerbate their mood-related symptoms.

Although not all patients require psychotherapy, most can benefit from individual, group, and/or family therapy. Moreover, participation in a self-help group is often useful in supplementing or supplanting formal psychotherapy. Psychotherapeutic issues are dictated by the nature of the illness for the specific individual. What this means is that the way in which their therapy will progress depends on what other issues of importance may be present. Additional problems related to suicide, violence, alcohol and drug use, and other mental health concerns may be present. It is also important to remember that although reactions vary widely, some individuals will feel angry and ambivalent about both the illness and its treatment. They may deny its existence, its severity, or its consequences, and they are often concerned about issues such as relationships and the possibility of genetically transmitting the illness to their children.

No one technique has been shown to be superior in the psychotherapy of individuals with bipolar disorder. The therapist is guided by knowledge of both the illness itself and its manifestation in the individual patient. In style and technique, the therapist must remain flexible in order to adjust to the patient's fluctuating levels of dependency and mood change, cognition, and behavior. The therapist must be especially alert to their reactions to working with these types of individuals, which may pose special challenges for the therapist. In addition, educating patients and their families is essential because it helps them to recognize new episodes.

Perspective and Prospects

Bipolar disorders are among the most consistently identifiable of all mental disorders, and among the oldest. They are discernible in descriptions in the Old Testament, and they were recognized in clinical medicine almost two thousand years ago. The medical writers of ancient Greece (the Hippocratic school) conceived of mental disorders in terms that sound remarkably modern. They believed that melancholia was a psychological manifestation of an underlying biological disturbance—specifically, a perturbation in brain function. Early conceptions of "melancholia" and "mania" were, however, broader than those of modern times. These two terms, together with "phrenitis," which roughly corresponds to an acute organic delirium, comprised all mental illnesses throughout most of the ancient period.

As they did with other illnesses, the Hippocratic writers argued forcefully that mental disorders were not caused by supernatural or magical forces, as primitive societies had believed. Their essentially biological explanation for the cause of melancholia, which survived until the Renaissance, was part of the prevailing understanding of all health as an equilibrium of the four humors—blood, yellow bile, black bile, and phlegm—and all illness as a disturbance of this equilibrium. First fully developed in the Hippocratic work *Nature of Man* (c. 400 B.C.E.), the humoral theory linked the humors with the seasons and with relative moistness. An excess of black bile was seen as the cause of melancholia, a term that literally means "black bile." Mania, by contrast, was usually attributed to an excess of yellow bile.

Reflections on the relationship between melancholia and mania date back at least to the first century B.C.E. and Soranus of Ephesus. Aretaeus of Cappadocia, who lived in the second century C.E., appears to have been the first to suggest that mania was an end-stage of melancholia, a view that was to prevail for centuries to come. He isolated "cyclothymia" as a form of mental illness with phases of depression alternating with phases of mania. Though this term is no longer used in this way, he provided an early record of problems similar to bipolar disorders. Although Aretaeus included syndromes that in the twentieth century would be classified as schizophrenia, his clear descriptions of the spectrum of mood conditions involving depression and mania are impressive even in modern times.

The next significant medical writer, Galen of Pergamum (129-c. 199 C.E.), firmly established melancholia as a chronic condition. His few comments on mania included the observation that it can be either a primary disease of the brain or secondary to other diseases. His primary contribution was his all-encompassing elaboration of the humoral theory, a system so compelling that it dominated medical thought for more than a millennium.

Medical observations in succeeding centuries continued to subscribe to the conceptions of depression and mania laid down in classical Greece and Rome. Most authors wrote of the two conditions as separate illnesses yet suggested a close connection between them. Yet where mania and depression are considered in the historical medical literature, they are almost always linked.

The explicit conception of manic-depressive illness as a single disease entity dates from the mid-nineteenth century. Jean Pierre Falret and Jules Baillarger, French "alienists," independently and almost simultaneously formulated the idea that mania and depression could represent different manifestations of a single illness. In 1854, Falret described a circular disorder that he expressly defined as an illness in which the succession of mania and melancholia manifested itself with continuity and in an almost regular manner. That same year, Baillarger described essentially the same thing, emphasizing that the manic and depressive episodes were not two different attacks, but two different stages of the same attack. Despite the contributions of Falret, Jeanne-Étienne-Dominique Esquirol, and other observers, however, most clinical investigators continued to regard mania and melancholia as separate chronic entities that followed a deteriorating course.

It was left to the German psychiatrist Emil Kraepelin (1856-1926) to distinguish psychotic illnesses from one another and to draw the perimeter clearly around manic-depressive illness. He emphasized careful diagnosis based on both longitudinal history and the pattern of current symptoms. By 1913, in the eighth edition of Kraepelin's textbook of psychiatry, virtually all of melancholia had been subsumed into manic-depressive illness.

Wide acceptance of Kraepelin's broad divisions led to further explorations of the boundaries between the two basic categories of manic-depressive illness and dementia praecox, the delineation of their similarities, and the possibility that subgroups could be identified within two basic categories. Kraepelin's synthesis was a major accomplishment because it formed a solid and empirically anchored base for future developments.

During the first half of the twentieth century, the views of Adolf Meyer (1866-1950) gradually assumed a dominant position in American psychiatry, a position that they maintained for several decades. Meyer believed that psychopathology emerged from interactions between an individual's biological and psychological characteristics and his or her social environment. This perspective was evident in the label "manic-depressive reaction" in the first official American Psychiatric Association diagnostic manual, which was published in 1952. When the Meyerian focus, considerably influenced by psychoanalysis, turned to manic-depressive illness, the individual in the environment became the natural center of study, and clinical descriptions of symptoms and the longitudinal course of the illness were given less emphasis.

Eugen Bleuler (1857-1939), in his classic contributions to descriptive psychiatry, departed from Kraepelin by conceptualizing the relationship between manic-depressive (affective) illness and dementia praecox (schizophrenia) as a continuum without a sharp line of demarcation. Bleuler also broadened Kraepelin's concept of manic-depressive illness by designating several subcategories and using the term "affective illness." His subcategories of affective illness anticipated the principal contemporary division of the classic manic-depressive diagnostic group—the bipolar-unipolar distinction. The bipolar-unipolar distinction represents a major advance in the classification of affective disorders primarily because it provides a basis for evaluating genetic, pharmacological, clinical, and biological differences rather than representing a purely descriptive subgrouping. As research on this disorder continues, it is likely that the relationship of bipolar disorder to substance use disorders will increase. In 1997, it was estimated that at least 50 percent of individuals affected by one are affected by the other. As such, common mechanisms of problems related to these two types of disorders may lead to more specific treatments designed to address situations when there is a dual diagnosis.

—Genevieve Slomski, Ph.D.; updated by Nancy A. Piotrowski, Ph.D.

See also Antidepressants; Anxiety; Depression; Psychiatric disorders; Psychiatry; Psychiatry, child and adolescent; Psychiatry, geriatric; Psychoanalysis; Psychology; Shock therapy; Sleep disorders.

For Further Information:

Castle, Lana R., and Peter C. Chybrow. *Bipolar Disorder Demystified: Mastering the Tightrope of Manic Depression*. New York: Avalon, 2003. A layperson's guide to the disorder, written by a bipolar disorder patient. Provides an understanding of the true nature of bipolar disorder, the factors that complicate its diagnosis, and numerous strategies for successfully coping with the illness.

Depression and Bipolar Support Alliance. http://www.ndmda.org/. Offers information on mood disorders, support groups, referrals for mental health professionals, research links, and discussion forums.

Geller, Barbara, and Melissa P. DelBello, eds. *Bipolar Disorder in Childhood and Early Adolescence*. Rev. ed. New York: Guilford, 2005. An examination of the little-studied occurrence of the disorder in children, including its epidemiology, diagnosis, natural history, neurobiology, genetics, and treatment.

Goodwin, Frederick K., and Kay Redfield Jamison. *Manic-Depressive Illness*. 2d ed. New York: Oxford University Press, 2007. Drawing on their extensive clinical and research experience, the authors have analyzed and interpreted the literature on manic-depressive illness and presented a unique synthesis of information for the acute and chronic management of manic-depressive patients.

Jamison, Kay Redfield. *An Unquiet Mind: A Memoir of Moods and Madness*. New York: Alfred A. Knopf, 1998. This book articulately describes the personal experiences of a prominent psychiatric researcher with her bipolar condition. The highs and lows of the condition are well illustrated, as is the importance of consistent medication with lithium.

Mondimore, Francis M. *Depression: The Mood Disease*. 3d ed. Baltimore: Johns Hopkins University Press, 2006. In this excellent scholarly work, the author discusses the biological basis of and medical treatment for depression, mood swings, and other affective disorders. Contains a bibliography.

Rosenthal, Norman E. *Winter Blues: Everything You Need to Know to Beat Seasonal Affective Disorder*. New York: Guilford Press, 2006. An insightful popular account of depression originally titled *Seasons of the Mind*. The author discusses the etiology of the "winter blues" and what can be done about it. Charting moods to obtain an objective pattern of moods and treatment responses is one useful technique suggested by Rosenthal. Contains a useful reading list.

Birth. *See* Childbirth; Childbirth complications.

Birth defects

Disease/Disorder

Anatomy or system affected: All bodily tissues

Specialties and related fields: Embryology, genetics, neonatology, obstetrics, pediatrics, perinatology

Definition: Congenital malformations or structural anomalies and their accompanying functional disorders that originate during embryonic development; they are involved in up to 6 percent of human live births.

Key terms:

deletion: the loss of a portion of a chromosome as a result of induced or accidental breakage

multifactorial inheritance: the interaction of genetic and environmental factors, which leads to certain congenital malformations

mutation: a change in the deoxyribonucleic acid (DNA), which may lead to the occurrence of congenital malformations

nondisjunction: the failure of chromosomes to separate during cell division, resulting in new cells that either lack a chromosome or have an extra chromosome

organogenetic period: the period of embryonic development, from approximately fifteen to sixty days after fertilization, during which most body organs form

spina bifida: a birth defect involving malformation of

vertebrae in the lower back, often resulting in paralysis and lower-body organ impairment

teratogen: an environmental factor that can induce the formation of congenital malformations

teratology: the study of congenital malformations

translocation: the structural chromosomal defect that occurs when a piece of one chromosome attaches to another

INFORMATION ON BIRTH DEFECTS

CAUSES: Genetic factors (chromosomal abnormalities, gene mutations), environmental factors (drugs, disease, radiation)

SYMPTOMS: Varies widely; can include missing limbs or body parts, reduced mental capacity, developmental delays, speech impediments, metabolic disorders

DURATION: Varies widely; some temporary and treatable in utero or shortly after birth, others lifelong

TREATMENTS: Preventive measures (genetic counseling, healthy diet during pregnancy), specialized and intense medical treatment (surgery, drug therapy)

CAUSES AND SYMPTOMS

As the human embryo develops, it undergoes many formative stages from the simple to the complex, most often culminating in a perfectly formed newborn infant. The formation of the embryo is controlled by genetic factors, external influences, and interactions between the various embryonic tissues. Because genes play a vital role as the blueprint for the developing embryo, they must be unaltered and the cellular mechanisms that allow the genes to be expressed must also work correctly. In addition, the chemical and physical communications between cells and tissues in the embryo must be clear and uninterrupted. The development of the human embryo into a newborn infant is infinitely more complex than the design and assembly of the most powerful supercomputer or the largest skyscraper. Because of this complexity and the fact that development progresses without supervision by human eye or hand, there are many opportunities for errors that can lead to malformations.

Errors in development can be caused by both genetic and environmental factors. Genetic factors include chromosomal abnormalities and gene mutations. Both can be inherited from the parents or can occur spontaneously during gamete formation, fertilization, and embryonic development. Environmental factors, called teratogens, include such things as drugs, disease organisms, and radiation.

Chromosomal abnormalities account for about 6 percent of human congenital malformations. They fall into two categories, numerical and structural. Numerical chromosomal abnormalities are most often the result of nondisjunction occurring in the germ cells that form sperm and eggs. During the cell division process in sperm and egg production, deoxyribonucleic acid (DNA) is duplicated so that each new cell receives a complete set of chromosomes. Occasionally, two chromosomes fail to separate (nondisjunction), such that one of the new cells receives two copies of that chromosome and the other cell none. Both of the resulting gametes (either sperm or eggs) will have an abnormal number of chromosomes. When a gamete with an abnormal number of chromosomes unites with a normal gamete, the result is an individual with an abnormal chromosome number. The missing or extra chromosome will cause confusion in the developmental process and result in certain structural and functional abnormalities. For example, persons with an extra copy of chromosome number 21 suffer from Down syndrome, which often includes mental deficiency, heart defects, facial deformities, and other symptoms and can be caused by nondisjunction in one or more cells of the early embryo. Abnormal chromosome numbers may also result from an egg's being fertilized by two sperm, or from failure of cell division during gamete formation.

Structural chromosomal abnormalities result from chromosome breaks. Breaks occur in chromosomes during normal exchanges in material between chromosomes (crossing over). They also may occur accidentally at weak points on the chromosomes, called fragile sites, and can be induced by chemicals and radiation. Translocations occur when a broken-off piece of chromosome attaches to another chromosome. For example, an individual who has the two usual copies of chromosome 21 and, as the result of a translocation, carries another partial or complete copy of 21 riding piggyback on another chromosome will have the symptoms of Down syndrome. Deletions occur when a chromosome break causes the loss of part of a chromosome. The cri du chat syndrome is caused by the loss of a portion of chromosome number 5. Infants affected by this disorder have a catlike cry, are mentally retarded, and have cardiovascular defects. Other structural chromosomal abnormalities include inversions (in which segments of chromosomes are attached in reverse order), duplications (in which portions of a chromosome are present in multiple copies), and isochromosomes (in which chromosomes separate improperly to produce the wrong configuration).

Gene mutations (defective genes) are responsible for about 8 percent of birth defects. Mutations in genes occur spontaneously because of copying errors or can be induced by environmental factors such as chemicals and radiation. The mutant genes are passed from parents to offspring; thus certain defects may be present in specific families and geographical locations. Two examples of mutation-caused defects are polydactyly (the presence of extra fingers or toes) and microcephaly (an unusually small cranium and brain). Mutations can be either dominant or recessive. If one of the parents possesses a dominant mutation, there will be a 50 percent chance of this mutant gene being transmitted to the offspring. Brachydactyly, or abnormal shortening of the fingers, is a dominantly inherited trait. Normally, the parent with the dominant gene also has the disorder. Recessive mutations can remain hidden or unexpressed in both parents. When each parent possesses a single recessive gene, there is a 25 percent chance that any given pregnancy will result in a child with a defect. Examples of recessive defects are the metabolic disorders sickle cell disease and hemophilia.

Environmental factors called teratogens are responsible for about 7 percent of congenital malformations. Human embryos are most sensitive to the effects of teratogens during the period when most organs are forming (organogenetic period), that is, from about fifteen to sixty days after fertilization. Teratogens may interfere with development in a number of ways, usually by killing embryonic cells or interrupting their normal function. Cell movement, communication, recognition, differentiation, division, and adhesion are critical to development and can be easily disturbed by teratogens. Teratogens can also cause mutations and chromosomal abnormalities in embryonic cells. Even if the disturbance is only weak and transitory, it can have serious effects because the critical period for development of certain structures is very short and well defined. For example, the critical period for arm development is from twenty-four to forty-four days after fertilization. A chemical that interferes with limb development, such as the drug thalidomide, if taken during this period, may cause missing arm parts, shortened arms, or complete absence of arms. Many drugs and chemicals have been identified as teratogenic, including alcohol, aspirin, and certain antibiotics.

Other environmental factors that can cause congenital malformations include infectious organisms, radiation, and mechanical pressures exerted on the fetus within the uterus. Certain infectious agents or their products can pass from the mother through the placenta into the embryo. Infection of the embryo causes disturbances to development similar to those caused by chemical teratogens. For example, German measles (rubella virus) causes cataracts, deafness, and heart defects if the embryo is infected early in development. Exposure to large doses of radiation—such as those released by the accident at the Chernobyl nuclear power plant in 1986 or by the atomic bombs dropped on Hiroshima and Nagasaki, Japan, during World War II—can result in death and damage to embryonic cells. There was an increase of about 10 to 15 percent in birth defects in children born to pregnant women exposed to atomic bomb radiation in Japan. Diagnostic X rays are not known to be a cause of birth defects. Some defects such as hip dislocation may be caused by mechanical forces inside the uterus; this could happen if the amnion is damaged or the uterus is malformed, thus restricting the movement of the fetus. About 25 percent of congenital defects are caused by the interaction of genetic and environmental factors (multifactorial), and the causes of more than half (54 percent) of all defects are unknown.

Treatment and Therapy

Because many birth defects have well-defined genetic and environmental causes, they often can be prevented. Preventive measures need to be implemented if the risk of producing a child with a birth defect is higher than average. Genetic risk factors for such defects include the presence of a genetic defect in one of the parents, a family history of genetic defects, the existence of one or more children with defects, consanguineous (same-family) matings, and advanced maternal age. Prospective parents with one or more of these risk factors should seek genetic counseling in order to assess their potential for producing a baby with such defects. Also, parents exposed to higher-than-normal levels of drugs, alcohol, chemicals, or radiation are at risk of producing gametes that may cause defects, and pregnant women exposed to the same agents place the developing embryo at risk. Again, medical counseling should be sought by such prospective parents. Pregnant women should maintain a well-balanced diet that is about 200 calories higher than normal to provide adequate fetal nutrition. Women who become anemic during pregnancy may need an iron supplement, and the U.S. Public Health Service recommends that all women of childbearing age consume 0.4 milligram of folic acid (one of the B vitamins) per day to reduce the risk of spina bifida and other neural tube defects. Women at high risk for producing genetically defective offspring can undergo a screening technique whereby eggs taken from the ovary are screened in the laboratory to select the most normal appearing ones prior to in vitro fertilization and then returned to the uterus. Some couples may decide to use artificial insemination by donor if the prospective father is known to carry a defective gene.

The early detection of birth defects is crucial to the health of both the mother and the baby. Physicians commonly use three methods for monitoring fetal growth and development during pregnancy. The most common method is ultrasound scanning. High-frequency sound waves are directed at the uterus and then monitored for waves that bounce back from the fetus. The return waves allow a picture of the fetus to be formed on a television monitor, which can be used to detect defects and evaluate the growth of the fetus. In amniocentesis, the doctor withdraws a small amount of amniotic fluid containing fetal cells; both the fluid and the cells can be tested for evidence of congenital defects by growing the cells in tissue culture and examining their chromosomes. Amniocentesis generally cannot be performed until the sixteenth week of pregnancy. Another method of obtaining embryonic cells is called chorionic villus sampling and can be done as early as the fifth week of pregnancy. A tube is inserted into the uterus in order to retrieve a small sample of placental chorionic villus cells, identical genetically to the embryo. Again, these cells can be tested for evidence of congenital defects. The early discovery of fetal defects and other fetal-maternal irregularities allows the physician time to assess the problem and make recommendations to the parents regarding treatment. Many problems can be solved with therapy, medications, and even prenatal surgery. If severe defects are detected, the physician may recommend termination of the pregnancy.

Children born with defects often require highly specialized and intense medical treatment. For example, a child born with spina bifida may have lower-body paralysis, clubfoot, hip dislocation, and gastrointestinal and genitourinary problems in addition to the spinal column deformity. Spina bifida occurs when the embryonic neural tube and vertebral column fail to close properly in the lower back, often resulting in a protruding sac containing parts of the spinal meninges and spinal cord. The malformation and displacement of these structures result in nerve damage to the lower body, causing paralysis and the loss of some neural function in the organs of this area. Diagnostic procedures including X rays, computed tomography (CT) scans, and urinalysis are carried out to determine the extent of the disorder. If the sac is damaged and begins to leak cerebrospinal fluid, it needs to be closed immediately to reduce the risk of meningitis. In any case, surgery is done to close the opening in the lower spine, but it is not possible to correct the damage done to the nerves. Urgent attention must also be given to the urinary system. The paralysis often causes loss of sphincter muscle control in the urinary bladder and rectum. With respect to the urinary system, this lack of control can lead to serious urinary tract infections and the loss of kidney function. Both infections and obstructions must be treated promptly to avoid serious complication. Orthopedic care needs to begin early to treat clubfoot, hip dislocation, scoliosis, muscle weakness, spasms, and other side effects of this disorder.

The medical treatment of birth defects requires a carefully orchestrated team approach involving physicians and specialists from various medical fields. When the abnormality is discovered (before birth, at birth, or after birth), the primary physician will gather as much information as possible from the family history, the medical history of the patient, a physical examination, and other diagnostic tests. This information is interpreted in consultation with other physicians in order to classify the disorder properly and to determine its possible origin and time of occurrence. This approach may lead to the discovery of other malformations, which will be classified as primary and secondary. When the physician arrives at a specific overall diagnosis, he or she will counsel the parents about the possible causes and development of the disorder, the recommended treatment and its possible outcomes, and the risk of recurrence in a subsequent pregnancy. Certain acute conditions may require immediate attention in order to save the life of the newborn.

In addition to treating the infant with the defect, the physician needs to counsel the parents in order to answer their questions. The counseling process will help them to understand and accept their child's condition. In order to promote good parent-infant bonding, the parents are encouraged to maintain close contact with the infant and participate in its care. Children born with severe chronic disabilities and their families require special support. When parents are informed that their child has limiting congenital malformations, they may react negatively and express feelings of shock, grief, and guilt. Medical professionals can help the parents deal with their feelings and encourage them to develop a close and supportive relationship with their child. Physicians can provide a factual and honest appraisal of the infant's condition and discuss treatments, possible outcomes, and the potential for the child to live a happy and fulfilling life. Parents are encouraged to learn more about their child's disorder and to seek the guidance and help of professionals, support groups, family, and friends. With the proper care and home environment, the child can develop into an individual who is able to interact positively with family and community.

Perspective and Prospects

Birth defects have been recognized and recorded throughout human history. The writer of the Old Testament book of 2 Samuel (21:20) describes the defeat of a giant with six fingers and six toes. Defects were recorded in prehistoric art, and the cuneiform records of ancient Babylon considered birth defects to be omens of great significance. Aristotle described many common human birth defects such as polydactyly. Superstitions about birth defects abounded during the Middle Ages. People believed that events occurring during pregnancy could influence the form of the newborn; for example, deformed legs could be caused by contact with a cripple. Mothers of deformed children were accused of having sex with animals. In a book written about birth defects in 1573, *Monstres et prodiges*, Ambroise Paré describes many human anomalies and attempts to explain how they occur. Missing body parts such as fingers or toes were attributed to a low sperm count in the father, and certain characteristics such as abnormal skin pigmentation, body hair, or facial features were said to be influenced by the mother's thoughts and visions during and after conception.

With advances in science and medicine these superstitions were swept aside. Surgery for cleft palate was performed as early as 1562 by Jacques Honlier. William Harvey, a seventeenth century English physician, recognized that some birth defects such as cleft lip are normal embryonic features that accidentally persist until the time of birth. The study of embryology, including experiments on bird and amphibian embryos, blossomed as a science during the nineteenth century, leading to a better understanding of how defects arise. At the same time, physicians were developing improved ways to treat birth defects. By 1816, Karl von Graefe had developed the first modern comprehensive surgical method for repairing cleft palate. The modern technique for repairing congenital pyloric stenosis (narrowing of the junction between the stomach and small intestine) was developed by Conrad Ramstedt in 1912. The principles of genetic inheritance developed by Gregor Mendel in the mid-1800's were rediscovered by biologists at the beginning of the twentieth century and soon were applied to the study of human heredity, including the inheritance of birth defects. Geneticists realized that defects such as hemophilia and Down syndrome are inherited diseases. Beginning in the 1930's, other scientists began to show that congenital defects could be induced in experimental animals by such factors as dietary deficiencies, hormone imbalances, chemicals, and radiation. In some cases, lack of complete testing of environmental factors such as drugs has led to tragedies but also a better understanding of the nature of birth defects. The tranquilizer thalidomide caused limb malformations in more than seven thousand children in Europe before it was withdrawn from the market in 1961. Pregnant women treated for cervical cancer in the 1960's with large doses of radiation bore children with defects and mental retardation.

Indeed, much of the medical and environmental health research today centers on the effects of drugs, toxic chemicals, radiation, and other factors on human health and development. Genetic counseling and testing of parents at risk for inherited defects has become an accepted part of medical practice. In addition, there have been many advances in the treatment of congenital defects since the 1950's. Modern orthopedic and plastic surgery is used to correct such problems as clubfoot and cleft palate. Transplants are used to correct deficiencies of the liver, kidneys, and other organs. Biomedical engineers have developed improved prosthetic devices to replace lost limbs and to aid in hearing, speaking, and seeing. An understanding of metabolic disorders such as phenylketonuria (PKU) has led to better treatment that utilizes special diets and medications. Because it is difficult to undo the damage of congenital defects fully, the most promise seems to be in the areas of prevention and protection. Prospective parents and their medical care providers need to be alert to potential hereditary problems, as well as to exposure to hazardous environmental agents. Pregnant women need to maintain a healthy diet and check with their physicians before taking any drugs. With advances in preventive medicine, diagnosis, and treatment, the future is much brighter for reducing the health toll of congenital malformations.

—*Rodney C. Mowbray, Ph.D.; updated by Alexander Sandra, M.D.*

See also Amniocentesis; Cardiology, pediatric; Cerebral palsy; Childbirth; Childbirth complications; Chorionic villus sampling; Cleft lip and palate; Cleft lip and palate repair; Color blindness; Congenital heart disease; Cornelia de Lange syndrome; Cystic fibrosis; Diabetes mellitus; DiGeorge syndrome; DNA and RNA; Down syndrome; Dwarfism; Embryology; Endocrinology, pediatric; Enzymes; Fetal alcohol syndrome; Fetal surgery; Gene therapy; Genetic counseling; Genetic diseases; Genetics and inheritance; Gigantism; Hemophilia; Hydrocephalus; Mental retardation; Metabolic disorders; Multiple sclerosis; Muscular dystrophy; Mutation; Obstetrics; Phenylketonuria (PKU); Porphyria; Pregnancy and gestation; Premature birth; Rubinstein-Taybi syndrome; Screening; Sickle cell disease; Spina bifida; Tay-Sachs disease; Teratogens; Thalassemia; Thalidomide.

For Further Information:

Heyman, Bob, and Mette Henriksen. *Risk, Age, and Pregnancy: A Case Study of Prenatal Genetic Screening and Testing*. New York: Palgrave, 2001. Examines prenatal testing in the context of a British hospital, exploring the perspectives of pregnant women, hospital doctors, and midwives, and the way in which the decision for prenatal testing is made.

March of Dimes. http://www.marchofdimes.com/. Web site offers a range of excellent fact sheets on myriad birth defects, information about prenatal testing, and special sections for pregnant women and researchers and professionals.

Moore, Keith L., and T. V. N. Persaud. *The Developing Human*. 7th ed. Philadelphia: W. B. Saunders, 2003. An outstanding textbook on human embryonic development, with specific information about the causes of congenital malformations and common defects occurring in each of the body's systems.

Nixon, Harold, and Barry O'Donnel. *The Essentials of Pediatric Surgery*. 4th ed. Boston: Butterworth Heinemann, 1992. Describes in accessible terms the surgical treatment of many congenital abnormalities, including birth injuries, imperforate anus, spina bifida, hydrocephalus, pyloric stenosis, birthmarks, cleft lip and palate, and hernias.

Sadler, T. W. *Langman's Medical Embryology*. 10th ed. Philadelphia: Lippincott Williams & Wilkins, 2006. Text that covers the fundamentals of embryology with a chapter devoted to birth defects.

Sherwood, Lauralee. *Human Physiology: From Cells to Systems*. 6th ed. Belmont, Calif.: Thomson/Brooks/Cole, 2007. This college textbook contains useful biological information about pregnancy and genetic defects, as well as facts useful to understanding amniocentesis and its advantages and disadvantages. Provides many valuable definitions and diagrams.

Stray-Gundersen, Karen, ed. *Babies with Down Syndrome*. Rev. ed. Kensington, Md.: Woodbine House, 1995. A complete guide for parents with a Down syndrome child, written by doctors, nurses, educators, lawyers, and parents. The book includes a complete medical description of the disorder and extensive coverage of care concerns, child development, education, and legal rights.

Birthmarks

Disease/disorder

Anatomy or system affected: Skin

Specialties and related fields: Dermatology, family medicine, pediatrics, plastic surgery

Definition: Spots or marks on the skin that are present at birth or shortly thereafter.

Key terms:

angioma: from *angio*, meaning "blood vessel," and *oma*, meaning "tumor"; a localized swelling or tumor caused by the proliferation of blood vessels that may or may not be dilated

hemangioma: a blood-filled malformation of the skin; a type of birthmark composed of a cluster of dilated blood vessels

nevus: a congenital mole; a round, pigmented region of skin that can be flat or raised

Causes and Symptoms

Many different types of birthmarks may be present on an infant, such as hemangiomas, stork bites, strawberry marks, port-wine stains, moles, and Mongolian spots. They range in color, size, shape, and longevity.

Hemangiomas (blood-filled birthmarks) ensue when a particular area of the skin receives an abnormal blood supply during fetal or neonatal (newborn) life. As a result, the tissue in this area enlarges over a period of several weeks to months and becomes reddish blue. A hem-

Information on Birthmarks

Causes: Changes in blood supply to skin during fetal or neonatal life
Symptoms: Colored or raised areas of skin
Duration: Ranges from several months to lifelong
Treatments: None (spontaneous disappearance), surgical removal, shrinking by injection

angioma is classified according to the type of blood vessels supplying it, which determine its appearance.

The most common birthmark in infants is the stork bite (flat angiomata), a patch of deep pink located on the bridge of the nose, lower forehead, upper eyelids, back of the head, or neck. Most often, stork bites occur in light-skinned babies. They are not considered serious and usually disappear early in an infant's life.

Strawberry marks or hemangiomas are caused by dilated capillaries (the smallest blood vessels) in the top layers of the skin. A strawberry mark is a raised dot with a rough texture that may be white during the first week of life before it turns red. Thus, this birthmark may not be noticeable at birth but is apparent within the first month of life. It may be located on the face, head, neck, or trunk. Most often, a baby has only one strawberry mark, but occasionally these birthmarks are scattered over different parts of the body. In very rare instances, strawberry marks appear in large numbers on the face and upper trunk and may also be present on organs inside the body. Strawberry hemangiomas typically grow quite rapidly for six months, which is alarming to parents, then gradually shrink and disappear without treatment. Virtually all these birthmarks fade by the time that the child reaches age nine, and most reduce in size at age two to three years.

Port-wine stains (flat hemangiomas) are large, flat, irregularly shaped red, pink, or purple areas caused by a surplus of blood vessels under the skin. They are typically present at birth and enlarge as a child ages. They are found on the face or limbs and are usually located on only one side of the body. Port-wine stains generally remain for life, although in some cases they fade over time.

Dark-pigmented birthmarks, termed nevi or moles, are composed of cells that produce melanin. Nevi range in color from yellow brown to dark brown to black. They are small and relatively common in light-skinned babies, occurring in one of every hundred white newborns. Large nevi, ranging in size from a coin to a square measuring 8 by 11 inches, are rare (occurring in one of every 20,000 births) and more serious, as they may develop into melanoma, a serious skin cancer. These birthmarks can be flat or raised, may have hair growing from them, and can cover the entire limb of a newborn.

Mongolian spots are large, flat spots containing extra pigment that resemble bruises. They commonly occur in dark-skinned babies and are usually located on the back or buttocks. These birthmarks disappear by the time a child enters school and are of no clinical significance.

Treatment and Therapy

While most birthmarks do not require treatment, certain types must be monitored carefully and treated if they develop further.

Although parents may want to have strawberry marks removed immediately, especially after witnessing their rapid growth in a newborn, it is generally best to leave them untreated. Few complications or cosmetic problems are associated with strawberry hemangiomas that are left alone.

In certain cases, however, intervention is required, such as the presence of the mark near a vital structure such as the eye, ear, throat, or mouth. Treatment of these hemangiomas is also initiated if they grow faster than usual, become infected, or bleed profusely. These cases require evaluation and management by a pediatrician and a dermatologist.

In addition, treatment may be undertaken if a child is particularly self-conscious about the mark. Because there is a greater risk for complications and an undesirable change in appearance with intervention, this step must be considered carefully. Cases in which the presence of strawberry marks on internal organs is suspected require tests and monitoring under the supervision of a pediatrician. If therapy is deemed necessary, steroids may be utilized to shrink these birthmarks. The disadvantage of this treatment is the side effects of the steroids. Hemangiomas may also be removed with traditional surgery, which causes scarring.

Port-wine stains rarely cause any problem in an infant or growing child. If they are located in certain areas, however, there is potential for serious sequelae. A flat hemangioma on the upper eyelid or forehead may be associated with Sturge-Weber syndrome, a related problem in the underlying brain structure. Port-wine stains located next to an eye may influence the development of glaucoma, a degenerative disease that leads to blindness if left untreated. In such cases, the birthmark may be removed by surgery or shrunk by injections. Regular monitoring for signs of glaucoma is essential.

Surgery is not recommended for port-wine stains if they simply pose a cosmetic problem; reassurance and a covering makeup is the treatment of choice. Plastic surgery can be performed when the child is older.

Small nevi tend to grow slightly as the child ages and are usually not associated with any adverse sequelae. Nevertheless, a small percentage of these moles develop into melanoma, a serious skin cancer, usually during or just after adolescence. Thus, nevi should be checked periodically by a pediatrician and observed carefully for any change in appearance (color, size, or shape). In such cases, the mole should be removed by a pediatric dermatologist.

PERSPECTIVE AND PROSPECTS

The most recent development in the treatment of birthmarks and skin lesions is laser therapy. Although laser therapy is not widely used on hemangiomas, it has shown remarkable success in the shrinking of strawberry hemangiomas and has been used to remove certain types of port-wine stains. This method causes less scarring than conventional surgical procedures. Most patients need a single five- to ten-minute session under general anesthesia. About a third of patients require one or more subsequent treatments. In some cases, plastic surgery may be needed to tighten loose skin following laser treatment.

—Lee Williams

See also Dermatology; Dermatology, pediatric; Klippel-Trenaunay syndrome; Moles; Plastic surgery; Skin; Skin disorders; Sturge-Weber syndrome; Warts.

FOR FURTHER INFORMATION:

Karlsrud, Katherine, and Dodi Schultz. "What to Do About Birthmarks." *Parents* 68, no. 9 (September, 1993): 70-72. "Nevus" is the term for any circumscribed malformation of the skin, especially one that is congenital—in other words, a birthmark. Information on the most common types of birthmarks seen in newborns and on moles is presented.

"Lifelong Companions: Birthmarks." *Current Health 2* 18, no. 8 (April, 1992): 30-31. A birthmark is a skin

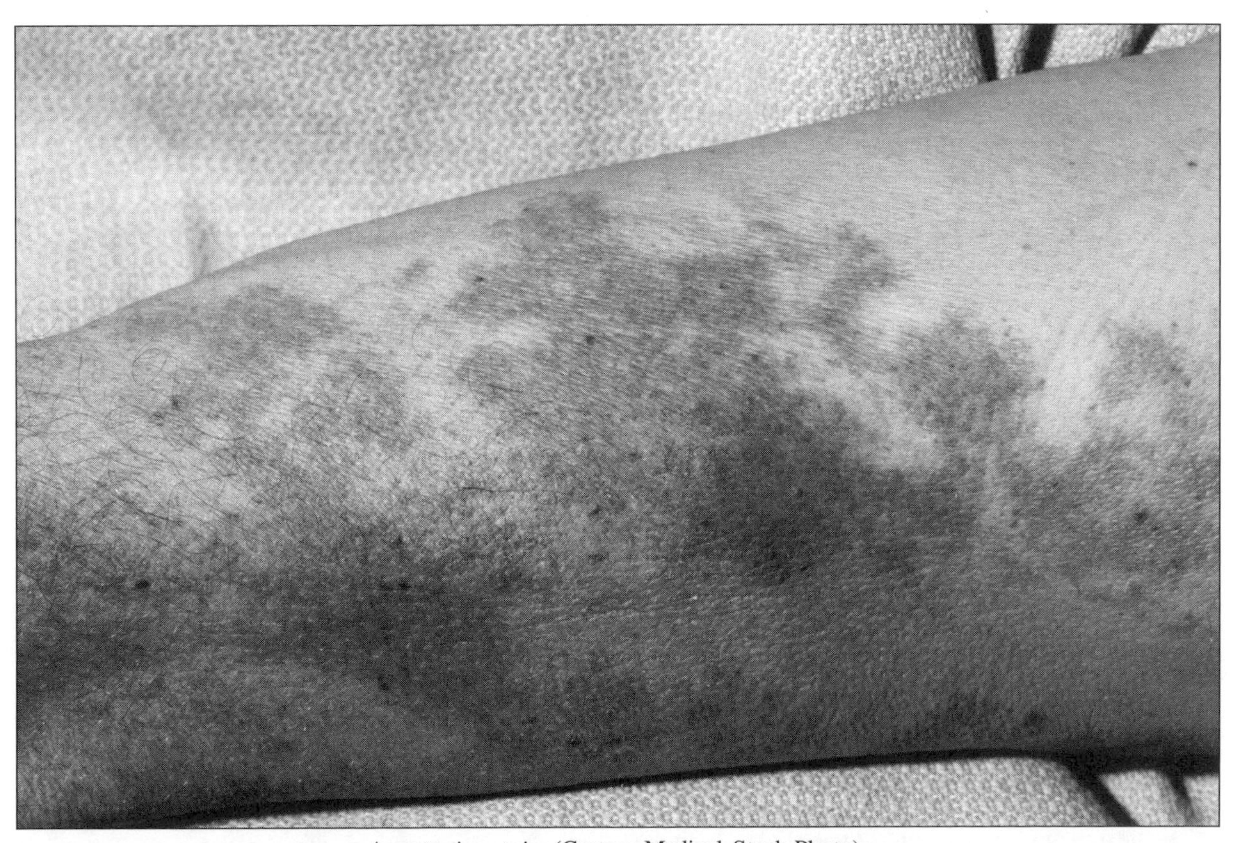

A port-wine stain. (Custom Medical Stock Photo)

blemish or coloration that is present at birth or appears shortly thereafter as the result of some abnormality in the development of the skin. Treatment options for birthmarks and moles are discussed.

Shelov, Steven P., et al. *Caring for Your Baby and Young Child: Birth to Age Five*. 4th ed. New York: Bantam Books, 2004. Offers a discussion of birthmarks.

Thompson, June. *Spots, Birthmarks, and Rashes: The Complete Guide to Caring for Your Child's Skin*. Toronto: Firefly Books, 2003. Guide for identifying and treating skin disorders with special attention to birthmarks and growths. Text accompanied by clear, color photographs.

Bites and stings

Disease/disorder

Anatomy or system affected: Heart, immune system, skin

Specialties and related fields: Emergency medicine, immunology, toxicology

Definition: Injuries from animals or insects.

Information on Bites and Stings

Causes: Bite or wound from an organism
Symptoms: Bleeding, swelling, infection, allergic response
Duration: Temporary or acute
Treatments: Immunization, drug therapy (antivenin, adrenaline, antihistamines)

Bites and stings cause four major types of damage to the victim's body: physical damage, the introduction of disease-causing organisms, the introduction of poisons (toxins, venoms), and allergic responses, including anaphylactic shock. Often, more than one form of damage is associated with a bite or sting. Alone or in combination, they can be life-threatening, but usually the damage from a bite or sting is minor. A wide variety of organisms can bite or sting, but the most important among them are mammals, reptiles (snakes and lizards), some fish (sharks, rays, moray eels), arthropods (including insects, centipedes, spiders, mites, ticks, and scorpions), and cnidarians (jellyfish, Portuguese man-of-wars, and their relatives).

Bites causing physical damage. Bites delivered by a mammal (most often a dog or cat) are likely to cause the most extensive physical damage. The specialized teeth of mammals, especially carnivores, in combination with powerful jaw muscles, can produce a serious wound. If wounding is in a vulnerable spot or is very extensive, or if the bleeding is not stopped, the physical damage can be fatal. A bite that causes physical damage is almost certain to introduce bacteria, viruses, or other infectious agents. An important example is the rabies virus, but many kinds of organism are dangerous if introduced into the bloodstream, or into the bone marrow of bones broken by the bite. Most mammalian bites do not introduce toxins into the victim. Some shrews have a venom in their saliva, but their small size and secretive habits minimize their threat to human health. Bites from mammals are also of minimal concern with respect to dangerous allergic responses. Physical damage is also the most serious problem in shark and moray eel bites.

Prevention, by avoiding animals prone to bite, is usually readily accomplished. Treatment involves stopping the bleeding, repairing the damage, and preventing infection.

Bites introducing infectious agents. Bites that cause serious physical damage are not the only ones that can introduce infectious agents. Any bite or sting can introduce infection to the victim because it penetrates the first line of defense, the skin. The arthropods are the most important disease vectors. Malaria is caused by a parasitic protozoan (single-celled, animal-type organism) transferred from one host to another by mosquitoes. Lyme disease is caused by a bacterium and is transported between hosts by ticks. Viruses cause yellow fever, and mosquitoes transport the virus to new hosts. Insects and ticks are vectors for a number of other diseases, most of which are introduced to the victim by a bite (including the stabs of blood-sucking arthropods such as mosquitoes).

Prevention of these diseases involves avoiding and/or eliminating the vectors; neither is always possible. Active immunization (stimulating the host to form antibodies against the disease-causing organism) is also used when available. Treatment involves drugs that destroy the disease organism or the use of passive immunization (the injection of preformed antibodies against the disease organism).

Bites and stings introducing toxins. Toxins or poisons are introduced to the victim most often by arthropods (scorpion stings, spider bites), cnidarians (stings), or reptiles (bites). Some mollusks—the cone shell snails, for example—can also inject toxins into a victim. The chemicals involved include enzymes that destroy tissue, neurotoxins that interfere with appropriate nerve cell responses (blocking or stimulating nerve cell signals), and others that interfere with the normal functions of the victim's body chemistry. Rattlesnakes and their relatives, coral snakes, and the Gila monster (a large lizard) are examples of poisonous reptiles. The brown recluse and black widow spiders are dangerous examples of their group. The sea wasp (a jellyfish) and the Portuguese man-of-war are the best known, but by no means the only, dangerous cnidarians in coastal waters off North America.

Prevention involves avoiding the animals that inject the toxin, which is easily accomplished much, but not all, of the time. Treatment involves injection of antivenin, a solution of antibodies that neutralize a specific toxin. Research on snake antivenin indicates that it might be possible to create a single antivenin that inactivates several snake venoms.

Bites and stings causing allergic reactions. Any bite or sting can cause an allergic response in the victim, because all introduce large foreign molecules, called antigens. These are often proteins, and they stimulate a response in the victim's immune system. If the response is more than that needed to destroy the antigen, it is called an allergic response and the foreign protein is called an allergen. The allergic response may simply be a nuisance causing minor inflammation, but it is exceptionally dangerous if it escalates into anaphylaxis. Anaphylaxis is a hyperreaction to a foreign substance in which the heart rate increases; bronchioles in the lungs constrict, making breathing difficult; and blood pressure drops. If symptoms continue, the victim may go into shock and even die. The toxins introduced by venomous arthropods, reptiles, cnidarians, and mollusks are often allergenic, even causing anaphylaxis, but even nonpoisonous or minimally toxic materials such as the venom introduced in a bee or wasp sting can cause life-threatening anaphylactic shock in sensitive people. A painful sting for people not sensitized to the foreign material becomes a threat to the life of a sensitized, hypersensitive person.

Prevention, by avoiding the allergen, is the preferred defense against allergic reactions. If avoidance is not possible or cannot be assured, the injection of small amounts of the substance to which an individual is hypersensitive, followed by increasingly larger doses, is sometimes effective in desensitizing the individual. Treatment of severe anaphylactic reactions involves the injection of adrenaline. Antihistamines, taken orally or injected, are used in less severe situations.

—*Carl W. Hoagstrom, Ph.D.*

See also Allergies; Chagas' disease; Emergency medicine; Encephalitis; Epidemiology; Immune system; Infection; Insect-borne diseases; Leishmaniasis; Lice, mites, and ticks; Lyme disease; Malaria; Parasitic diseases; Plague; Poisoning; Rabies; Shock; Sleeping sickness; Snakebites; Toxicology; Tropical medicine; Yellow fever; Zoonoses.

FOR FURTHER INFORMATION:

Dossenbach, Hans D. *Beware! We Are Poisonous! How Animals Defend Themselves.* Woodbridge, Conn.: Blackbirch Press, 1999. Dossenbach examines some of the world's most poisonous animals and shatters some myths about creatures long perceived as dangerous. Includes a bibliography.

Foster, Steven, and Roger A. Caras. *A Field Guide to Venomous Animals and Poisonous Plants: North America, North of Mexico.* Boston: Houghton Mifflin, 1994. Containing excellent information and bright color pictures, and written for an easy understanding, this book should be in any nature enthusiast's library.

Halstead, Bruce W., and Paul S. Auerbach. *Dangerous Aquatic Animals of the World: A Color Atlas.* Princeton, N.J.: Darwin Press, 1992. Spectacular gallery of animals as diverse as polar bears and sea anemones. A natural history of the envenomation, or wounding apparatus, with slight detail on range, and none on life cycles. The excellent color photos are augmented by fine drawings of the anatomy of the dangerous parts of animals.

Harvey, Alan L., ed. *Snake Toxins.* New York: Pergamon Press, 1991. Discusses various topics, such as immunology of snake toxins, dendrotoxins, the structure and pharmacology of elapid cytotoxins, the influence of snake venom proteins on blood coagulation, and amino acid sequences and toxicities of snake venom components. Includes an index.

Krohmer, Jon R., ed. *American College of Emergency Physicians First Aid Manual.* 2d ed. New York: DK, 2004. A comprehensive guide that details the treatment and techniques, in text and photographically, of a range of emergencies. Bites and stings are covered specifically.

Nagami, Pamela. *Bitten: True Medical Stories of Bites and Stings.* New York: St. Martin's Press, 2004. Nagami describes strange and often gruesome true cases of bites and stings, resulting infections, and treatments.

Silverstein, Alvin, et al. *Bites and Stings.* New York:

Scholastic, 2002. A young adult book that covers information about bites and stings from insects, pets, wild animals, sea creatures, and plants. Body reactions, transmittable diseases, treatment, and protection are also covered.

Spiders and Other Arachnids. http://spiders.ucr.edu. Site provides links to information about the spider, scorpion, bee, wasp, and ant species worldwide whose bites cause morbidity and mortality.

Tu, Anthony T., ed. *Reptile Venoms and Toxins*. New York: Marcel Dekker, 1991. In twenty-four contributed chapters, thirty-seven international specialists describe the latest developments in research on snake venom—including different types of venoms and toxins, actions, antidotes, and applications—and summarize what is known to date on Gila monster and frog toxins.

Bladder cancer

Disease/disorder

Also known as: Bladder malignancy, bladder carcinoma, urothelial cancer, urothelial carcinoma

Anatomy or system affected: Bladder, urinary System

Specialties and related fields: Oncology, urology

Definition: Cancer that forms in tissues of the bladder, including transitional cell carcinomas (cancers that form in cells in the innermost tissue layer of the bladder), which account for about 90 percent of all bladder cancer cases; squamous cell carcinomas (cancers that begin in flat cells lining the bladder); and adenocarcinomas (cancers that begin in cells that release fluids). In 2002, 357,000 new cases and 145,000 deaths were attributed to the disease worldwide.

Key terms:

Bacille Calmette-Guérin (BCG): an inactive strain of *Mycobacterium bovis* that stimulates the immune system in nonspecific ways

bladder: the muscular, membranous, hollow organ that stores urine and is located in the front of the pelvic cavity; also called the vesica urinaria

cystoscope: a thin, tubelike instrument used to look inside the bladder and urethra; has a light and a lens for viewing and usually equipped with a tool to remove tissue

cystoscopy: examination of the bladder and urethra using a cystoscope inserted through the urethra and into the bladder

urothelial: pertaining to a layer of cells that line the bladder and some other organs of the urinary system

Information on Bladder Cancer

Causes: Unknown; factors include advanced age, carcinogens (smoking, radiation), chronic or frequent bladder infections

Symptoms: Blood in the urine, pain and burning during urination, frequent urination, pelvic pain, and the presence of tumor(s)

Duration: Chronic

Treatments: Depends on severity; may include tumor removal, chemotherapy, Bacillus Calmette-Guérin bacterium, bladder removal

Causes and Symptoms

The symptoms of bladder cancer are the presence of blood in the urine, pain and burning during urination, frequent urination, and pelvic pain. Urinary tract infections create the same symptoms, but the presence of a tumor or tumors distinguishes bladder cancer from an infection. Tumors can be imaged by cystography, ultrasound, computed tomography (CT) or magnetic resonance imaging (MRI) scans, and cystoscopy. Occasionally, a mass is conspicuous upon manual examination. If any of these procedures suggest the presence of a tumor, then cystoscopy can confirm the diagnosis. During cystoscopy, a doctor looks inside the bladder with a cystoscope passed through the urethra and removes material for biopsy to determine whether malignant cells, which are diagnostic for cancer, are present. Frequently, malignant cells can be seen by microscopic examination of urine from patients with bladder cancer.

Although the precise cause of bladder cancer is not known, age, gender, and several environmental factors contribute to its occurrence. Bladder cancer affects mainly elderly people, with an average age at diagnosis of sixty-five to seventy years, and males account for about 77 percent of all cases. Cigarette smoking is reported to be the primary risk factor for the disease, and exposure to other carcinogens such as radiation, aromatic amines, and polycyclic aromatic hydrocarbons also increases risk. Chronic or frequent bladder infections can increase the risk of bladder cancer. Additionally, it appears that diets high in meat and fat increase the risk of bladder cancer. All these risk factors taken together suggest that irritations of the interior walls of the bladder play an important role in the development of this disease.

Treatment and Therapy

Appropriate treatment of bladder cancer depends on the severity of the disease. In the vast majority of cases, the tumors are superficial and can be removed completely by cystoscopic procedures. Even with complete removal, recurrences are likely, so patients are usually given an anticancer agent, which is instilled directly into the bladder. This can be a chemotherapeutic agent such as mitomycin C or doxorubicin, but often Bacillus Calmette-Guérin (BCG) is used. This inactivated bacterium stimulates the immune system and is thought to be the most effective preventative for future occurrences. Some studies have indicated, however, that high doses of vitamins A, B_6, and C and zinc are more effective at delaying recurrences than BCG treatment.

Patients with tumors that have invaded the muscles of the bladder wall usually require partial or total surgical removal of the bladder. A patient without a bladder will be provided with an alternate means of storing and removing urine. Some patients are given an external bag connected by a piece of intestine. Increasingly, patients whose bladders have been removed are provided with a neobladder, an internal reservoir built from intestinal tissue. These patients learn how to control the shape of this reservoir with their abdominal muscles in order to regulate the flow of urine. In this way, the neobladder works almost like a normal bladder.

Patients with inoperable cancers or whose cancer has spread to other parts of the body may benefit from chemotherapy, depending on their ability to tolerate the toxicity of the treatments. Doctors and patients evaluate the probable benefits to each individual before starting such a drug regimen.

Perspective and Prospects

The introduction of the cystoscope in 1877 by the German scientist Maximilian Nitze, who is called the father of urology, initiated the first scientific studies of bladder cancer. This instrument allowed the first accurate morphological descriptions of tumors within the bladder and led directly to the ability to remove bladder tumors without invasive surgery. Although the yearly number of new cases of bladder cancer has been increasing in the past three decades, the number of deaths has declined. This is in part a tribute to Nitze's genius.

Studies with bladder cancer in the 1890's were the first to show an association between environmental toxins and any cancer. These studies showed that people who worked with aniline dyes were more likely to develop bladder cancer.

Although smoking may be the primary risk factor for bladder cancer, and although the number of smokers is declining, the number of new cases of bladder cancer continues to increase. This leaves researchers with the idea that other environmental risk factors are becoming more important.

This increase in new cases of bladder cancer while treatment continues to improve has motivated an increasing emphasis on prevention. Many studies are underway to look at ways of preventing both the initial occurrence and recurrences of bladder cancer. Various studies have suggested that selenium supplementation and high-fiber diets, as well as megadoses of the vitamins mentioned above, may be beneficial. Other studies have pointed to environmental assaults to be avoided.

—Lorraine Lica, Ph.D.

See also Bladder removal; Cancer; Carcinogens; Chemotherapy; Cystoscopy; Oncology; Tumor removal; Tumors; Urinalysis; Urinary disorders; Urinary system; Urology.

For Further Information:

Dunetz, Gary N. *Bladder Cancer: A Resource Guide for Patients and Their Families*. Bloomington, Ind.: AuthorHouse, 2006. A recent book for general audiences.

Gillenwater, Jay Y., et al., eds. *Adult and Pediatric Urology*. 4th ed. Baltimore: Lippincott Williams & Wilkins, 2002. A comprehensive textbook on urology.

Grossman, H. Barton, ed. "Contemporary Diagnosis and Management of Urothelial Carcinoma." *Urology* 67, no. 3, supp. S1 (March, 2006): 1-72. A special supplement devoted to bladder cancer, with eight articles by leading authorities. Technical but worthwhile for patients who want to read about the latest research. Also available through http://www.goldjournal.net/issues/contents.

Schoenberg, Mark P. *The Guide to Living with Bladder Cancer*. Baltimore: Johns Hopkins University Press, 2000. A book for general audiences written by a urologist from one of the top medical centers in the United States.

Wein, Alan J., et al. *Campbell-Walsh Urology*. 9th ed. Philadelphia: Saunders, 2007. The bible of urology.

BLADDER INFECTIONS. ***See*** **URINARY DISORDERS.**

BLADDER REMOVAL

PROCEDURE

ANATOMY OR SYSTEM AFFECTED: Abdomen, bladder, urinary system

SPECIALTIES AND RELATED FIELDS: General surgery, gynecology, proctology, urology

DEFINITION: The surgical removal of the bladder and accompanying structures or organs.

INDICATIONS AND PROCEDURES

Cystectomy (bladder removal) is often the treatment of choice in cases of bladder cancer, which may be treated with chemotherapy or radiation in combination with surgery. The procedure, usually performed under general anesthesia, is carried out by making an incision in the abdomen, after which the ducts that carry urine from the bladder, called ureters, are cut and tied. The affected bladder is removed and, in men, the prostate gland is also excised. In women, the uterus, Fallopian tubes, and ovaries are removed along with the diseased bladder.

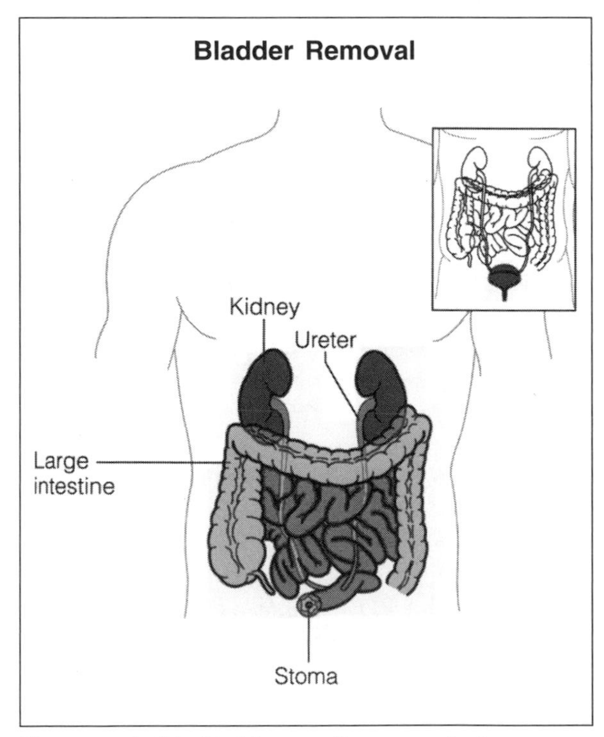

The removal of the bladder, usually as a result of cancer, necessitates the creation of a stoma, in which the ureters are connected to a section of small intestine, through which urine is voided from the body.

If an external bag will be used for urine storage, then a permanent opening is made in the abdomen. The two ureters are joined to a tiny section of small intestine that has been removed from the rest of the intestines, formed into a loop, and inserted through the abdominal wall. Urine is excreted through this opening, called a stoma. If an internal reservoir, called a neobladder, is to be created, then intestinal tissue will be used.

USES AND COMPLICATIONS

A cystectomy has serious consequences. In men, the result is usually impotence because the nerve tracts that permit penile erections are usually damaged severely by the surgery. In women, the outcome is infertility as a result of the combination of cystectomy and hysterectomy. Because most women who undergo the procedure have already experienced menopause, however, this consequence usually does not affect them adversely.

In addition to the complications from infection and systemic shock that can accompany any major surgery, cystectomy poses another problem: Following surgery and for the remainder of a patient's life, either urine must be collected in a pouch that is worn externally or patients must learn to control the internal neobladder with their abdominal muscles. It takes some patients considerable time to adapt to such complications. Enterostomy therapists teach patients how to care for a stoma; patients are usually referred to these specialists following a cystectomy.

Some patients also experience problems with proper intestinal function in the days immediately following a cystectomy. This difficulty is overcome through the regular administration of a solution of saline fluids and glucose intravenously beginning soon after the surgery.

—*R. Baird Shuman, Ph.D.*

See also Bladder cancer; Cancer; Cystoscopy; Hysterectomy; Oncology; Prostate gland removal; Urinalysis; Urinary disorders; Urinary system; Urology.

FOR FURTHER INFORMATION:

Chalker, Rebecca, and Kristene E. Whitmore. *Overcoming Bladder Disorders*. New York: HarperCollins, 1990.

Droller, Michael J. *Bladder Cancer: Current Diagnosis and Treatment*. Totowa, N.J.: Humana Press, 2001.

Ellsworth, Pamela, and Brett Carswell. *One Hundred Questions and Answers About Bladder Cancer*. Sudbury, Mass.: Jones and Bartlett, 2006.

Guyton, Arthur C., and John E. Hall. *Textbook of Medical Physiology*. 11th ed. Philadelphia: Elsevier Saunders, 2006.

Humes, H. David, et al., eds. *Kelley's Textbook of Internal Medicine*. 4th ed. Philadelphia: Lippincott Williams & Wilkins, 2000.

Schoenberg, Mark P., et al. *The Guide to Living with Bladder Cancer*. Baltimore: Johns Hopkins University Press, 2001.

Wallace, Robert A., Gerald P. Sanders, and Robert J. Ferl. *Biology: The Science of Life*. 4th ed. New York: HarperCollins, 1996.

Walsh, Patrick C., and Darracott Vaughan. *Campbell's Urology*. 8th ed. New York: Elsevier, 2002.

BLADDER STONES. *See* STONE REMOVAL; STONES.

BLEEDING

DISEASE/DISORDER

ANATOMY OR SYSTEM AFFECTED: Blood, blood vessels, circulatory system

SPECIALTIES AND RELATED FIELDS: Emergency medicine, family medicine, hematology, internal medicine, vascular medicine

DEFINITION: Damage or disruption to hemostasis (the normal absence of bleeding)—the appropriate interactions among blood cells, proteins in the blood, and blood vessels—resulting in loss of blood or abnormal clotting.

KEY TERMS:

coagulation: the sequential process by which multiple, specific factors (predominantly proteins in plasma) interact, ultimately resulting in the formation of an insoluble clot made of fibrin

fibrin: the insoluble protein that forms the essential portion of a blood clot; the soluble protein in plasma converted to fibrin is called fibrinogen

fibrinolysis: the process of dissolving clots; the fibrinolytic system dissolves fibrin through enzymatic action

hemostasis: the arrest of bleeding from injured blood vessels, confining circulating blood to those vessels; blood vessels, platelets, the coagulation system, and the fibrinolytic system contribute to the process of hemostasis

plasma: the fluid portion of blood in which the particulate components are suspended; the majority of coagulation factors are proteins in plasma

platelets: disk-shaped structures in blood that are vital for the maintenance of normal hemostasis

vitamin K: a group of fat-soluble vitamins that play an integral role in the production of multiple, properly functioning coagulation factors by the liver

CAUSES AND SYMPTOMS

Patients with bleeding abnormalities are commonly encountered in medicine. Such patients may be evaluated because of previous bleeding episodes, a family history of bleeding, or sometimes abnormalities detected during preliminary studies before surgery or other invasive procedures. Bleeding episodes are often described as local (the source of bleeding is pinpointed to a specific part of the body) or generalized (abnormal bleeding occurring at multiple, distinct anatomic sites). It is important to distinguish between these two possibilities because treatment may differ markedly. Localized bleeding disorders may be correctable with surgery, while the treatment of generalized bleeding disorders may be more complex and long-term. The evaluation of patients with suspected bleeding disorders includes a detailed medical history, a thorough physical examination, and appropriate screening tests for hemostatic functioning. Subsequently, more specific laboratory tests are usually required to define the nature of a bleeding abnormality. Abnormal bleeding may result from blood vessel abnormalities (vascular defects), low platelet counts (thrombocytopenia), excessively high platelet counts (thrombocytosis), platelet function abnormalities, deficiencies or abnormalities of plasma coagulation factors, excessive breakdown of blood clots (excessive fibrinolysis), or a combination of these abnormalities. Bleeding disorders may be inherited or acquired.

Generalized bleeding abnormalities are suggested by several characteristics. Bleeding from multiple sites, bleeding in the absence of a known causative event (often termed spontaneous bleeding), and bleeding following trauma that is much more severe than expected for the degree of injury are all characteristics of generalized bleeding defects. An unexplained increase in bleeding severity may be a sign of a newly acquired generalized bleeding abnormality.

Inherited disorders. There are numerous inherited disorders of hemostasis. Fortunately, most are quite rare. The two most common inherited bleeding disorders are von Willebrand's disease and hemophilia A.

Inherited bleeding disorders usually become evident in infancy or early childhood. There is often a family history of abnormal bleeding, and abnormal bleeding may have been experienced in association with surgery or trauma. Bleeding from the umbilical cord at birth or bleeding following circumcision may provide evidence of inherited hemostatic disorders. In contrast, a lack of abnormal bleeding following surgery such as tonsillectomy or dental procedures such as tooth extraction lowers the likelihood that even a mild inherited hemostatic disorder is present. There are, however, exceptions to such trends. Inherited disorders of hemostasis such as Ehlers-Danlos syndrome or hereditary hemorrhagic telangiectasia may not become evident until later in life. Idiopathic (or immune) thrombocytopenic purpura (ITP) is an acquired hemostatic abnormality that may occur in childhood, usually as a result of an infection. Hemorrhagic disease of the newborn is a short-lived bleeding abnormality caused by a transient deficiency of coagulation factors (known as the vitamin K dependent factors) in the newborn period.

INFORMATION ON BLEEDING

CAUSES: Injury, disease, inherited disorders, medications, nutritional deficiency
SYMPTOMS: Local (bleeding pinpointed to specific body part) or generalized (abnormal bleeding at multiple, distinct sites)
DURATION: A few minutes to chronic
TREATMENTS: Surgery, drug therapy

Family history is helpful in the evaluation of hemostatic disorders because a pattern of bleeding among family members may be revealed. If only male members of a family are affected, this suggests an X-linked recessive pattern of inheritance (transmitted by the X sex chromosome). Such diseases are usually transmitted from females who are carriers of the trait. Hemophilia A, hemophilia B, and Wiskott-Aldrich syndrome are transmitted as X-linked recessive traits. Inherited bleeding disorders such as von Willebrand's disease occur in both sexes through non-sex-linked, or autosomal, transmission. Some bleeding disorders occur because of a gene mutation. Some individuals, therefore, are the first members of their family to have an inherited bleeding disorder.

Acquired disorders. These may first become evident in adulthood. A negative family history for bleeding may exist, and diseases may be present that are associated with bleeding abnormalities, such as kidney or liver disease. Liver disease may lead to abnormal bleeding for numerous reasons. Causes of abnormal bleeding include decreases in plasma coagulation factors (most coagulation factors are manufactured by the liver), low platelet counts, platelet function abnormalities, production of abnormal coagulation factors (such as abnormal fibrinogen), vulnerability to a condition called disseminated intravascular coagulation (DIC), and abnormal lysis (breakdown) of blood clots. Platelet function abnormalities are associated with kidney failure and many blood diseases (for example, dysproteinemias, leukemias, and myeloproliferative disorders). Vitamin K is necessary for the production of numerous functional plasma coagulation factors. A deficiency of vitamin K, therefore, may lead to abnormal bleeding. Poor nutrition or antibiotic therapy may lead to vitamin K deficiency, which may also occur in newborns. One source of vitamin K is bacteria located in the gastrointestinal (GI) tract. Because the newborn GI tract is sterile, newborns have no bacterial source of vitamin K. Some medical conditions, such as sprue or biliary obstruction, may lead to inadequate absorption of vitamin K from the GI tract.

Numerous drugs and medications may cause abnormal bleeding. Drugs or medications may cause low platelet counts or platelet dysfunction or may affect coagulation factors. Oral anticoagulant therapy (warfarin therapy), which is used in the treatment of blood clots in the legs, causes a reduction of functional vitamin K dependent coagulation factors and is a common cause of drug-induced bleeding.

Nutritional deficiency, a major problem in many parts of the world, may result in bleeding disorders. One example is severe protein deficiency, a syndrome known as kwashiorkor, which produces severe liver damage. Vitamin C deficiency may cause scurvy, which may result in skin hemorrhages, bleeding gums, and bleeding beneath the lining of the bones (subperiosteal bleeding).

Evaluating hemostatic functioning. Dental extractions are a good measure of hemostatic functioning because bleeding occurs over rigid bone. The bleeding sites, therefore, are not easily compressible. Persistent and excessive bleeding after incisor removal is more significant as a diagnostic indicator than such bleeding following molar removal. (Even patients with normal hemostasis may experience persistent bleeding after molar extractions.) Tonsillectomy is evaluated in a similar manner. Because tonsillectomy may lead to persistent bleeding in the setting of normal hemostasis, the significance of excessive bleeding following tonsillectomy may be difficult to interpret. The lack of bleeding following tonsillectomy, however, implies normal hemostasis.

Investigation of trauma-related bleeding is an important component of hemostatic evaluation. When considering trauma-related bleeding, it is important to determine other details related to the events: Were blood transfusions required? What methods were used to bring bleeding under control? How easily was bleeding brought under control? Was there clearly a local cause of bleeding? Were any medications being taken which could lead to abnormal bleeding? A lack of abnormal bleeding with prior trauma does not absolutely exclude inherited bleeding disorders. Patients with milder forms of hemophilia may bleed abnormally only following severe trauma. Oral contraceptives or pregnancy influence the hemostatic reaction to a degree that may mask von Willebrand's disease in women.

Diagnosis by type of bleeding. In diagnosis, the type of abnormal bleeding may provide important clues. In vascular or platelet abnormalities, bleeding typically occurs in the skin or mucous membranes. Bleeding usually starts within seconds of the time of injury and may continue for hours; however, once the bleeding stops it may not recur. Posttraumatic bleeding in coagulation disorders may be delayed for many hours after a traumatic episode; recurrent episodes of bleeding following trauma are also a characteristic of such disorders.

Petechiae, small, red spots about the size of a pinhead, represent tiny hemorrhages from small blood vessels, such as capillaries. These spots are a sign of platelet or vascular abnormalities. Petechiae caused by vasculitis (the inflammation of blood vessels) are often elevated lesions that are distinct to the touch (palpable) as well as being evident visually. Petechiae associated with low platelet counts or abnormalities of platelet function are not palpable and, while often widespread, may first appear on the lower extremities, such as the ankles, or on mucous membranes, such as in the mouth.

Ecchymoses (bruises) are larger lesions caused by the leakage of blood into tissue of the skin or mucous membranes, usually as the result of trauma. Ecchymoses can be seen with all hemostatic disorders. Spontaneous ecchymoses, bruises appearing in the absence of prior trauma, may be a sign of a hemostatic problem. The location of the ecchymoses may provide diagnos-

First Aid for Trauma-Related Bleeding

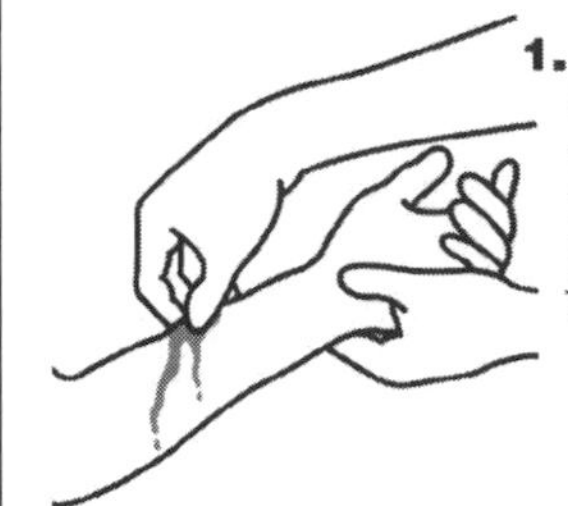

1. Press hard over the wound. If necessary, pinch the wound edges together with fingers and thumb. Maintain pressure for at least 10 minutes.

2. Lay the patient down to elevate the bleeding area (this reduces the area blood flow).

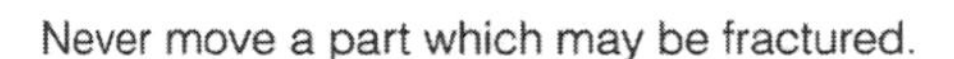
Never move a part which may be fractured.

3. Replace the hand pressure with pressure from a pad held firmly in place by a tight bandage or by whatever is at hand: stockings, belts, socks, handkerchiefs, ties.

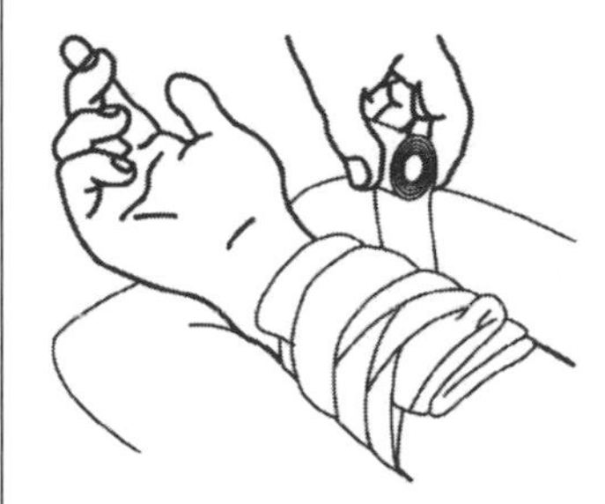

4. If blood appears to be oozing through, do not investigate by removing the bandage already applied; instead apply additional pressure with more padding and bandage. Continue this procedure until control is achieved.

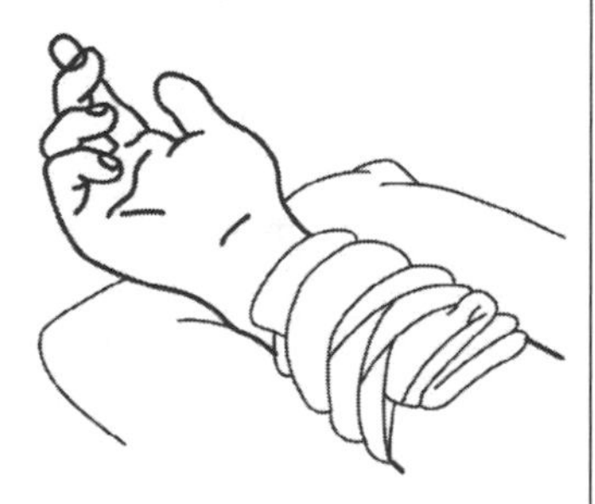

5. Apply antishock measures, as necessary. Get medical aid.

tic information. Bruises occurring only on the limbs, which are at greater risk for minor trauma, are less indicative of a possible bleeding abnormality than bruising that occurs on the trunk. Women frequently have one or two bruises, which may be normal. More than a half dozen bruises on a woman, however, warrants further evaluation. Easy bruising in a man also warrants further study.

Hematomas are collections of blood that accumulate in organs, body spaces, or tissues. They produce deformity of the area in which they develop and may be quite painful. Hematomas tend to be associated with abnormalities in the coagulation mechanism, such as hemophilia. Bleeding into joint spaces is known as hemarthrosis. Hemarthroses are characteristic of severe coagulation disorders such as hemophilia. Telangiectases and angiomata, caused by vascular malformations, are red spots or patches caused by the presence of blood in abnormally dilated vessels. Unlike the other lesions previously discussed, these vascular lesions blanch with pressure.

Epistaxis (nose bleeding) is most frequently caused by mild trauma (for example, nose blowing) to dilated vessels of the nose in individuals with normal hemostasis. Epistaxis in the setting of bleeding disorders is often associated with low platelet counts, the vascular abnormality called hereditary hemorrhagic telangiectasia, and von Willebrand's disease. Epistaxis consistently occurring on one side may be the result of a local abnormality, as opposed to a generalized hemostatic defect.

Abnormal bleeding may also be seen in other areas. Gingival bleeding (gum bleeding) may be caused by gum disease; however, it is also seen in association with low platelet counts, platelet dysfunction, and scurvy, and in conditions where there are abnormally high levels of proteins in the blood (hyperviscosity syndrome). Hematuria (blood in the urine) may be caused by low platelet counts, platelet dysfunction, coagulation factor abnormalities, and oral anticoagulant therapy. Hematuria is a serious medical symptom that requires medical investigation to determine the cause. Bleeding from the GI tract can be seen with all types of hemostatic disorders. GI bleeding must be completely investigated to determine whether there is local cause for the bleeding or the bleeding is part of a generalized hemostatic defect. Menorrhagia (abnormal bleeding during menstrual periods) is associated with low platelet counts, platelet dysfunction, von Willebrand's disease, and coagulation factor abnormalities. Information such as the number and type of sanitary pads or tampons needed, period duration, the necessity of sanitary pad changes at night, the passage of clots, and the requirement of iron for anemia may be helpful in quantifying menstrual blood loss.

Laboratory tests. Laboratory evaluation of hemostatic functioning consists of screening tests, to aid in the detection of abnormalities, and confirmatory tests, to characterize the disorders. Microscopic examination of a blood smear is a simple screening procedure that may provide valuable information. A disease process associated with abnormal bleeding, such as leukemia, may be detected. Numerous red cell fragments may be present in hemostatic disorders such as DIC or thrombotic thrombocytopenic purpura (TTP). An estimate of the number of platelets and an evaluation of their size and shape can be made. Abnormally low and high platelet counts can lead to abnormal bleeding. Large platelets can be seen in conditions in which they are being destroyed rapidly, such as ITP. Large platelets are also seen in Bernard-Soulier syndrome, an inherited platelet function disorder.

The automated platelet count and bleeding time are screening tests for the evaluation of platelets. A normal interaction between platelets and damaged blood vessels is a necessary first step to control bleeding. This step is often termed primary hemostasis. An adequate number of normally functioning platelets are necessary to provide normal primary hemostasis. A representative normal range for the platelet count is 150,000 to 400,000 platelets per microliter of blood. In the absence of platelet dysfunction, spontaneous bleeding is rare when the platelet count is greater than 20,000 per microliter. The risk of life-threatening hemorrhage does not markedly increase until the platelet count drops below 10,000 per microliter. The bleeding time is primarily used to screen for platelet dysfunction, although it may also indicate some vascular abnormalities. The bleeding time measures the interval required for bleeding to cease following a standard skin incision on the forearm. A blood pressure cuff on the arm is inflated to a pressure of 40 millimeters of mercury during the procedure. A representative normal range for the bleeding time is four to seven minutes. A prolonged bleeding time may be a sign of a platelet or vascular abnormality.

The plasma coagulation system is composed primarily of a set of proteins that interact to produce clotting of blood (fibrin clots). This system is often referred to as secondary hemostasis. Most plasma coagulation factors are identified by a roman numeral (for example coagulation factor VIII). For ease of analysis, the plasma coagulation system has been divided into groups of proteins known as the intrinsic pathway, the extrinsic pathway, and the final common pathway. Screening tests for the plasma coagulation system include the thrombin time (TT), the prothrombin time (PT), and the activated partial thromboplastin time (aPTT). The screening tests detect significant deficiencies or abnormalities of plasma coagulation factors and help localize the defects within the pathways.

Specific, and often more complex, laboratory studies of hemostasis are performed based on information derived from the medical history, physical examination, and screening laboratory tests. The goal of specific tests is to pinpoint the diagnosis of hemostatic abnormalities.

Platelet disorders. Thrombocytopenia, a low platelet count in the blood, has numerous causes. Platelets are produced in the bone marrow and subsequently released into the blood. Bone marrow damage may result in inadequate numbers of platelets. Drugs, toxins, radiation, and infections may damage the bone marrow. Certain diseases, such as leukemia or other cancers, may lead to the replacement of bone marrow cells with abnormal cells or fibrous tissue. Some diseases result in inadequate release of platelets from the bone marrow. Inadequate platelet release may be the result of nutritional deficiencies, such as vitamin B_{12} or folic acid deficiencies, or it can be seen in some rare hereditary disorders, such as May-Hegglin anomaly or Wiscott-Aldrich syndrome. Individuals with an enlarged spleen may develop thrombocytopenia because of the pooling of platelets within the organ. Massive transfusion may result in thrombocytopenia when the blood volume is replaced with transfused solutions that do not contain platelets.

Certain disorders result in the rapid destruction or consumption of platelets. If the production of platelets by the bone marrow does not compensate for the rate of destruction, thrombocytopenia occurs. Platelet consumption with resultant thrombocytopenia is a component of DIC. Thrombocytopenia caused by accelerated destruction may also occur with prosthetic heart valves, blood infections (sepsis), and vascular defects called hemangiomas. The development of antibodies against one's own platelets (such as with ITP) causes platelet consumption. ITP can be a self-limited disorder with a complete return to normal (acute ITP) or a prolonged thrombocytopenic condition (chronic ITP). Acute ITP is seen most frequently in children between two and six years of age. The disease is preceded by a viral infection in about 80 percent of cases. The platelet count returns to normal within six months in more than 80 percent of patients; the usual period of thrombocytopenia is four to six weeks. Mortality from acute ITP occurs in about 1 percent of cases. Chronic ITP typically occurs in young and middle-aged adults, and the disorder is about three times more common in females than in males. As many as 50 percent of children born to mothers with ITP have thrombocytopenia at birth as a result of the transfer of antiplatelet antibodies across the placenta. Isoimmune neonatal thrombocytopenia and post-transfusion purpura are other conditions in which thrombocytopenia is caused by antiplatelet antibodies.

Numerous drugs have been associated with thrombocytopenia. Examples of such drugs include gold salts, quinine, quinidine, sulfonamide drugs, and heparin. Thrombocytopenia may occur within twenty-four hours following exposure to an offending drug. All nonessential medications should be discontinued in patients suspected of having drug-induced thrombocytopenia.

Platelet function defects may be inherited or acquired. They may occur without evidence of an associated disease or be secondary to a recognizable clinical disorder. Platelet function defects are suspected when there is abnormal skin or mucous membrane bleeding, a prolonged bleeding time, and a normal platelet count. Bleeding disorders caused by the inability of platelets to stick to damaged blood vessel walls in a normal manner are called platelet adhesion defects; Bernard-Soulier syndrome and von Willebrand's disease are examples of such defects.

Certain molecules necessary for normal platelet function are contained within platelets (that is, in the storage pool). Deficiencies or defects of these molecules lead to platelet dysfunction and are called storage pool defects. Examples of storage pool defects include gray platelet syndrome and dense granule deficiency. Platelet release defects occur when there is a failure to release storage pool contents normally. Hereditary deficiency of the enzymes cyclooxygenase or thromboxane synthetase causes platelet release defects. Aspirin causes a platelet release defect by inactivating cyclooxygenase.

Disorders that render platelets unable to interact with one another to form large clumps at the site of vascular injury are known as platelet aggregation defects.

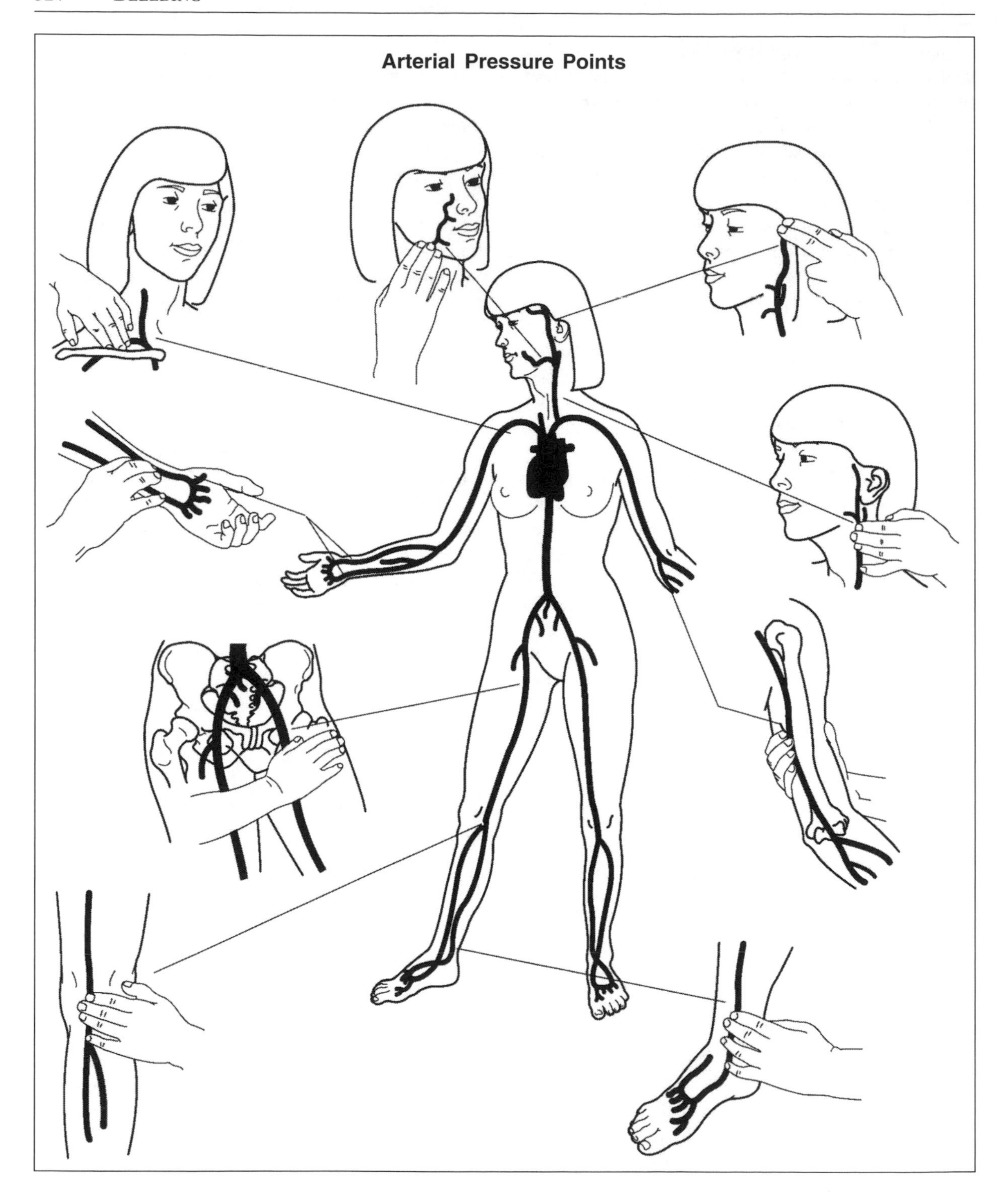

Ganzmann's thrombasthenia and hereditary afibrinogenemia are examples of such defects.

Platelets also play a key role in secondary hemostasis by providing a surface on which many coagulation factors can interact. A bleeding disorder results if the platelet surface is incapable of supporting secondary hemostasis. Hereditary bleeding disorders caused by this type of platelet defect are quite rare.

Acquired platelet dysfunction is quite common. Renal failure (uremia) may cause acquired platelet dysfunction. Liver disease can cause multiple bleeding abnormalities, including platelet dysfunction. A vast number of drugs and medications, such as aspirin and penicillin, cause platelet dysfunction. Acquired platelet function defects are seen with cardiopulmonary bypass procedures and in association with numerous blood diseases.

Coagulation disorders. The overall incidence of inherited coagulation factor disorders is about 1 in 10,000. In such conditions, either there is a failure to make a sufficient amount of a coagulation factor (quantitative disorder) or a dysfunctional factor is made (qualitative disorder). An inherited disorder exists for every coagulation factor, although most are quite rare. Symptoms range from serious spontaneous bleeding, which occurs in the severe forms of hemophilia A (factor VIII disorder) or hemophilia B (factor IX disorder), to an absence of abnormal bleeding in other inherited conditions (factors XII, prekallikrein, and high molecular weight kininogen). In general, for disorders which cause bleeding, the more profound the coagulation factor defect, either quantitatively or qualitatively, the more severe the bleeding. Severe disorders are usually easily identified. Moderate or mild disorders are more common and may go undetected until there is a significant hemostatic challenge, such as surgery.

Von Willebrand's disease is probably the most common inherited bleeding disorder. It is caused by deficiencies or defects in a vital group of hemostatic proteins known collectively as von Willebrand factor. Manifestations include epistaxis, menorrhagia, prolonged bleeding after trauma or surgery, frequent ecchymoses, and persistent gum bleeding. Severe episodes of epistaxis may occur during childhood, and such episodes may cease during puberty. In women, epistaxis may recur after the menopause. Important diagnostic clues include a family history of abnormal bleeding, affected members in every generation (males and females), and marked worsening of bleeding following the ingestion of aspirin or other drugs that impair platelet function. Von Willebrand's disease consists of a very diverse spectrum of abnormalities: At least twenty-one distinct subtypes of von Willebrand's disease have been recognized.

Hemophilia A and hemophilia B are clinically indistinguishable; laboratory testing is required for their diagnosis. Hemophilia A is described here. Hemophilia A is an inherited disorder of a portion of coagulation factor VIII. Hemophilia A is typically seen in males, while females are carriers of the abnormal gene and can transmit the disease. Twenty percent of affected individuals have a negative family history and likely developed their disease because of a mutation of the factor VIII gene. Once the abnormal gene is established in a family, the severity of the disease is the same for all affected males. Hemophilia A is divided into severe, moderate, and mild subtypes based on the amount of functional factor VIII present. Bleeding in hemophiliacs may be spontaneous or posttraumatic. Spontaneous bleeding tends to occur only in severe hemophilia. It characteristically affects joints and muscles, and it may lead to crippling injury without prompt and adequate treatment. Posttraumatic bleeding may occur in mild, moderate, or severe hemophilia A. Such episodes are often prolonged and dangerous. Bleeding into the head (intracranial bleeding) remains a common cause of severe disability and death in hemophilia A. Modern treatment, however, has reduced the incidence of this severe complication. Antibodies (inhibitors) directed against factor VIII develop in approximately 12 to 15 percent of patients who require transfusions to provide factor VIII. The development of inhibitors is a serious complication which may compromise the effectiveness of therapy. Factor VIII inhibitors may occur in nonhemophiliacs, leading to serious bleeding in affected males and females.

Acquired coagulation factor disorders may be caused by reduced or absent factor production (for example, in liver disease), the production of defective or inactive factors (such as in liver disease or vitamin K deficiency), factor inhibitors, or accelerated consumption or clearance of factors. Examples in the latter group include DIC (accelerated consumption), kidney disease (factors lost in the urine), and the attachment of factors to abnormal tissue, which occurs in a disease called amyloidosis.

DIC is a hemostatic disorder which arises as part of a disease or medical condition. Examples of associated conditions include obstetrical accidents, abnormal destruction of red blood cells within blood vessels, infections, malignancies, burns, severe injuries, liver disease, and diseases of blood vessels. DIC may be an explosive, life-threatening syndrome (high-grade DIC) or a troublesome, less dramatic feature of a disease (low-grade DIC). Conditions associated with DIC cause abnormal activation of the hemostatic response, resulting in the widespread formation of blood clots in the vascular system. The clots obstruct the blood supply to vital organs (the kidneys, heart, lungs, and brain), leading to impaired organ function. Abnormal bleeding may develop if coagulation factors and platelets become depleted because of their incorporation into widespread blood clots. The breakdown of blood clots may also become inadequately controlled and contribute further to abnormal bleeding.

Perspective and Prospects

The existence of bleeding disorders has been known for many centuries. Abnormal bleeding observed in the males of certain families was described in the Jewish Talmud in the second century. Interest in such disorders increased markedly with the discovery of hemophilia in the royal families of Europe. In 1853, Queen Victoria gave birth to her fifth son, Leopold. She was a carrier of hemophilia, and Leopold had the disease. He died of a brain hemorrhage following a minor blow to the head at the age of thirty-one. Two of Victoria's daughters gave birth to affected sons. Her granddaughter, Alexandra, became the czarina of Russia, and Alexandra's only son, Alexis, suffered from hemophilia.

The transformation of fluid blood to a solid mass has fascinated investigators since ancient times. Aristotle noted that blood contained fibers and, upon cooling, solidified. He also observed that "diseased" blood did not solidify. The realization that blood clotting minimized blood loss from wounds occurred in the early eighteenth century. In the late eighteenth century, William Hewson described the clotting time of whole blood. He found it to be shortened in some diseases and infinite in one woman after delivering a baby. In 1863, work published by Lord Joseph Lister laid the foundation for the discovery of the intrinsic pathway of coagulation. In 1905, Paul Morawitz, aided by the discoveries of such investigators as Alexander Schmidt and Olof Hammarsten, proposed what is now called the classic theory of blood coagulation. This led to the characterization of the extrinsic pathway of coagulation. In 1964, the "cascade" (by Robert Macfarlane) and "waterfall" (by Earl Davie and Oscar Ratnoff) hypotheses of coagulation were proposed. These discoveries paved the way for much of the current understanding of coagulation.

Alfred Donné is credited with the first description of platelets, reported in 1842. In 1881, Giulio Bizzozero became the first author to use the term "blood platelets." Shortly thereafter, discoveries in the late nineteenth century highlighted the importance of platelets in normal hemostasis. In recent times, the study of platelets has intensified. A large volume of information on platelets and platelet function has accumulated since the 1960's.

The study of the cells lining blood vessels (endothelium) and their role in hemostasis is a relatively young discipline. Much has already been learned about these cells, and much more information is anticipated. The future promises great advances in the study of hemostasis and hemostatic disorders. Further definition of the interrelationships of endothelium, platelets, and coagulation factors in normal and abnormal hemostasis is expected. There is hope for a greater understanding of inherited hemostatic disorders. Additional studies on the processes that keep blood from clotting (anticoagulants) and those that break down clots (fibrinolysis) are expected. The effect of diseases such as cancer on hemostasis awaits clarification, as does the effect of hemostasis on other processes, such as the spread of cancer.

—James R. Stubbs, M.D.

See also Anemia; Blood and blood disorders; Circulation; Concussion; Disseminated intravascular coagulation (DIC); Ebola virus; Emergency medicine; Healing; Hematology; Hematology, pediatric; Hemophilia; Intraventricular hemorrhage; Nosebleeds; Shock; Thrombocytopenia; Transfusion; Vascular medicine; Von Willebrand's disease; Wiskott-Aldrich syndrome.

For Further Information:

Bick, Roger L. *Disorders of Thrombosis and Hemostasis: Clinical and Laboratory Practice*. 3d ed. Philadelphia: Lippincott Williams & Wilkins, 2002. An excellent introduction to the diagnosis and management of clotting and bleeding disorders.

Colman, Robert W., et al., eds. *Hemostasis and Thrombosis: Basic Principles and Clinical Practice*. 5th ed. Philadelphia: Lippincott Williams & Wilkins, 2006. This is the bible in the study of hemostasis. An extensive and comprehensive reference textbook that deserves a spot on the bookshelf of all those involved with hemostasis.

Dahlback, Bjorn. "Blood Coagulation." *The Lancet* 355, no. 9215 (May 6, 2000): 1627-1632. Discusses the coagulation pathway and the role of thrombin in the clotting cascade. Also covers disturbances of the natural balance between the procoagulant and anticoagulant systems due to genetic or acquired factors.

Grogan, Tracy A. "Bringing Bloodless Surgery into the Mainstream." *Nursing* 29, no. 11 (November, 1999):

58-61. Grogan discusses how bloodless surgery can benefit a patient who objects to transfusions for religious reasons. Bloodless surgery means that surgeons use all available alternatives to minimize blood loss, salvage as much of the patient's blood as possible, and treat the patient with pharmaceuticals to maximize blood production.

Harmening, Denise M., ed. *Clinical Hematology and Fundamentals of Hemostasis*. 4th ed. Philadelphia: F. A. Davis, 2002. A technical work designed for professionals in the field.

Lichtman, Marshall L., et al. *Williams Manual of Hematology*. 6th ed. New York: McGraw-Hill, 2002. An accessible handbook that covers the pathogenetic, diagnostic, and therapeutic essentials of blood cell and coagulation protein disorders.

Owen, Charles A., E. J. Walter, and John H. Thompson. *The Diagnosis of Bleeding Disorders*. 2d ed. Boston: Little, Brown, 1975. A classic in the field of hemostasis. Although this is a somewhat older work, much vital information on hemostasis can still be obtained from the text. The extensive chapter on the history of hemostasis is interesting reading.

Portyansky, Elena. "Drug Offers New Clotting Factor for Hard-to-Treat Hemophilia." *Drug Topics* 143, no. 9 (May 3, 1999): 25. A recently approved product, Novoseven (recombinant coagulation factor VIIa) from Novo Nordisk, holds promise for hemophilia A or B patients with inhibitors to coagulation factors VIII or IX.

Ratnoff, Oscar D., and Charles D. Forbes, eds. *Disorders of Hemostasis*. 3d ed. Philadelphia: W. B. Saunders, 1996. A comprehensive textbook edited by two giants in the field of hemostasis. Although this is a detailed textbook, the authors cover various aspects of hemostasis in an organized and understandable manner.

Rodak, Bernadette, ed. *Hematology: Clinical Principles and Applications*. 2d ed. Philadelphia: W. B. Saunders, 2002. A comprehensive textbook covering all aspects of hematology and hemostasis.

Voet, Donald, and Judith G. Voet. *Biochemistry*. 3d ed. Hoboken, N.J.: John Wiley & Sons, 2004. An excellent general biochemistry book that contains a few sections on blood and blood components, their properties, and functions.

BLEPHAROPLASTY. *See* FACE LIFT AND BLEPHAROPLASTY.

BLINDNESS

DISEASE/DISORDER

ANATOMY OR SYSTEM AFFECTED: Eyes

SPECIALTIES AND RELATED FIELDS: Geriatrics and gerontology, ophthalmology

DEFINITION: The absence of vision, or its extreme impairment to the extent that activity is limited; about 95 percent of all blindness is caused by eye diseases, the rest by injuries.

KEY TERMS:

glaucoma: excessive pressure inside the eye that can damage the optic nerve

laser: an intense light beam used in eye surgery

macular degeneration: a deterioration of vision in the most sensitive, central region of the retina

retina: a paper-thin membrane lining the inside surface of the eyeball, where light is transformed into nerve impulses

trachoma: a contagious eye infection primarily found in Third World countries

CAUSES AND SYMPTOMS

The major cause of blindness among older adults in the Western world is glaucoma. The aqueous fluid produced inside the eye fails to drain properly and causes pressure to build up. In extreme cases, the eyeball becomes hard. Without prompt treatment, the outer layer of the optic nerve starts to deteriorate. The patient can still see straight ahead but not off to the side. When the cone of forward vision has narrowed to less than 20 degrees (called tunnel vision), the patient is considered legally blind.

Cataracts are another common defect of vision among the elderly. The lens of the eye develops dark spots that interfere with light transmission. Cataracts are not caused by an infection or a tumor but instead are a normal part of the aging process, like gray hair. There is no known treatment to retard or reverse the growth of cataracts.

Macular degeneration and diabetes mellitus can cause blindness as a result of hemorrhages from tiny blood vessels in the retina. The macula is a small region in the middle of the retina where receptor cells are tightly packed together to obtain sharp vision for reading or close work. With aging, blood circulation in the macula gradually deteriorates until the patient develops a black spot in the center of the field of view. Advanced diabetes also causes blood vessel damage in the eye. In serious cases, fluid can leak behind the retina, causing it to become detached. The resulting visual effect resembles a dark curtain that blacks out part of the scene.

Trachoma is a blinding eye disease that afflicts millions of people in poor parts of the world. It is a contagious infection of the eyelid similar to conjunctivitis (commonly known as pinkeye). If untreated, it causes scarring of the cornea and eventual blindness. Trachoma is caused by a virus that is spread by flies, in water, or by direct contact with tears or mucus.

Many kinds of injuries may cause blindness. Car accidents, sports injuries, chemical explosions, battle wounds, and small particles that enter the eye all can result in a serious loss of vision.

Treatment and Therapy

An indispensable tool in the treatment of serious eye problems is the laser. Its intense light focused into a tiny spot, the laser's heat can burn away a ruptured blood vessel or weld a detached retina back into place. For glaucoma patients, medication to reduce fluid pressure in the eye may be effective for a while. Eventually, a laser can be used to burn a small hole through the iris in order to improve fluid drainage. The laser can be used only to prevent blindness, however, and not to restore sight.

Cataracts formerly were a major cause of blindness among older people. Once the eye lens starts to become cloudy, nothing can be done to clear it. Cataract surgery to remove the defective lens and to insert a permanent, plastic replacement has become common. In the United States, more than a million cataract surgeries are performed annually, with a success rate that is greater than 95 percent.

The infectious eye disease called trachoma has been known for more than two thousand years. Effective modern treatment uses sulfa drugs taken orally, combined with antibiotic eyedrops or ointments. Unfortunately, reinfection is common in rural villages where most people have the disease and sanitation is poor. The World Health Organization has initiated a public health program to teach parents about the importance of cleanliness and frequent eye washing with sterilized water for their children.

In the News: New Drugs for Age-Related Macular Degeneration and Other Visual Impairments

At the annual meeting of the Association for Research in Vision and Ophthalmology (ARVO) held in May, 2003, several research groups reported their research findings for promising new drugs being tested as possible treatments for neovascular macular degeneration (also called wet macular degeneration), a condition that has previously been resistant to drug therapy.

Angiogenesis is the growth of new blood vessels, and when new blood vessels grow into regions of the eye where they are normally absent, visual impairment follows. Abnormal blood vessel growth specifically has been implicated in neovascular macular degeneration, diabetic retinopathy, neovascular glaucoma, and the retinopathy of prematurity. Angiogenesis is a multistep process with many regulatory points and thus provides many possible targets for drug action. Several different approaches that take advantage of recent advances in the understanding of the process of angiogenesis are being used to devise antiangiogenesis drugs to treat wet macular degeneration.

One treatment approach makes use of an antibody that binds specifically to a growth factor called vascular endothelial growth factor (VEGF), which is required for blood vessel formation. One such antibody, called rhuFAB, has been tested on humans by injecting it into the vitreous. When it binds to VEGF, it should theoretically inactivate it and thus stop the growth of blood vessels that would interfere with vision. At the ARVO annual meeting, researchers at Genentech, where rhuFAB was developed, reported that in their clinical trials, rhuFAB was well tolerated and effective at improving vision or stabilizing vision loss in approximately 90 percent of patients with newly developed wet macular degeneration.

Other approaches that treat impaired vision caused by new blood vessel formation include inhibiting the action of VEGF with RNA molecules called aptamers; inhibiting the production of VEGF by antisense RNA; inhibiting enzymes required for angiogenesis, such as matrix metalloproteinases; preventing cell-cell interactions needed for angiogenesis; inhibiting angiogenesis with thalidomide; and making use of steroids, such as anecortave acetate, that block blood vessel formation.

—Lorraine Lica, Ph.D.

INFORMATION ON BLINDNESS

CAUSES: Eye injury, disease (especially glaucoma), aging process
SYMPTOMS: Tunnel vision, black spots, pain, eventual loss of sight
DURATION: Temporary to chronic
TREATMENTS: Laser therapy, medication, surgery

PERSPECTIVE AND PROSPECTS

Various techniques have been developed for helping sightless people to live a self-reliant lifestyle. Using a white cane or walking with a trained dog allows a blind person to get around. Biomedical engineers have designed a miniature sonar device built into a pair of glasses that uses reflected sound waves to warn the wearer about obstacles.

The Braille system of reading, using patterns of raised dots for the alphabet, was invented in 1829 and is still widely used. For blind students, voice recordings of textbooks, magazines, and even whole encyclopedias are available on tape. A recent development is an optical scanner connected to a computer with a voice simulator that can read printed material aloud.

The National Federation of the Blind was founded in 1940. Its goals are to assist the blind to participate fully in society and to overcome the still-prevalent stereotype that the blind are helpless. Blind men and women hold jobs as engineers, teachers, musical performers, ministers, insurance agents, computer programmers, and school counselors. As society becomes more sensitive to all forms of disability, opportunities for blind people continue to expand.

—*Hans G. Graetzer, Ph.D.*

See also Behçet's disease; Blurred vision; Cataract surgery; Cataracts; Color blindness; Diabetes mellitus; Eye infections and disorders; Eye surgery; Eyes; Glaucoma; Macular degeneration; Refractive eye surgery; Trachoma; Vision disorders.

FOR FURTHER INFORMATION:

American Foundation for the Blind. http://www.afb.org/. Site of the American Foundation for the Blind (AFB), which publishes materials about blindness for professionals and consumers through AFB Press, and maintains and preserves the Helen Keller Archives, housed at the M. C. Migel Memorial Library, one of the world's largest collections of print materials on blindness. AFB also maintains the Careers Technology Information Bank (CTIB), a network of individuals who are blind from all fifty states and Canada.

Buettner, Helmut, ed. *Mayo Clinic on Vision and Eye Health: Practical Answers on Glaucoma, Cataracts, Macular Degeneration, and Other Conditions.* Rochester, Minn.: Mayo Foundation for Medical Education and Research, 2002. A helpful handbook on all the medical, social, and emotional facets of vision impairment.

Johnson, Gordon J., et al., eds. *The Epidemiology of Eye Disease*. 2d ed. New York: Oxford University Press, 2003. Designed for professionals in the field, this work covers many of the basics of eye disease.

Maurer, Marc. "Reflecting the Flame." *Vital Speeches of the Day* 57 (September 1, 1991): 684-690. A speech by the president of the National Federation of the Blind. He criticizes the media, government agencies, and educators for perpetuating false stereotypes of helplessness. Maurer is a forceful spokesperson for the blind.

Morrison, John C., and Irvin P. Pollack. *Glaucoma: A Clinical Guide*. New York: Thieme Medical, 2003. Chapters examine topics related to genetics, gonioscopy, perimetry, childhood glaucoma, retinal disorders, neuroprotection, and ocular hypotony.

National Federation of the Blind. http://www.nfb.org/. The site of the National Federation of the Blind (NFB), which provides public education about blindness, information and referral services, scholarships, literature and publications about blindness, aids and appliances and other adaptive equipment for the blind, advocacy services and protection of civil rights, job opportunities for the blind, development and evaluation of technology, and support for blind persons and their families.

Peninsula Center for the Blind. *The First Steps: How to Help People Who Are Losing Their Sight*. Palo Alto, Calif.: Peninsula Center, 1982. A pamphlet designed to help people cope with the emotional trauma of blindness and the process of adjustment. Highly recommended.

Sardegna, Jill, et al. *Encyclopedia of Blindness and Vision Impairment*. 2d ed. New York: Facts On File, 2002. All aspects of vision impairment are covered in five hundred entries, including health and social issues, surgery and medications, adaptive aids, education, and helpful organizations. Twelve appendixes provide myriad resources for research, support, and services.

Westcott, Patsy. *Living with Blindness*. Austin, Tex.: Raintree Steck-Vaughn, 2000. Designed for children in grades three through five, this volume explains how people with disabilities go about their everyday lives. Westcott offers a brief explanation of how the eye normally functions and looks at some of the causes of visual impairment.

Blisters

Disease/disorder

Also known as: vesicles (small), bullae (large)

Anatomy or system affected: Skin

Specialties and related fields: Dermatology, family medicine, pediatrics

Definition: A local swelling of the skin that contains watery fluid and is usually caused by burning or irritation.

Causes and Symptoms

Blisters are fluid-filled lesions that can be caused by a variety of medical conditions or problems. They can be viral in origin, as in the case of chickenpox (also known as varicella), or they can arise because of irritants such as hot water or oil splashing on the skin. Blisters can also be caused by the friction of something rubbing against the skin, as in the case of an improperly fitting shoe.

A blister can range from painless to very painful. An individual with a blister will notice an area of the skin that is raised and filled with a clear liquid. The liquid inside of the blister is typically sterile, which means that it does not contain bacteria. In some instances, as in chickenpox, the fluid may carry a virus. If the blister contains a virus, the virus spreads once the blister has ruptured or opened. Blisters can also contain blood, generally as the result of trauma that has caused a blood vessel to break. A blister can be singular, or they can occur in groups or clusters. If a group of blisters forms one larger blister, it is often referred to as a bulla.

Blisters are commonly located on the arms or legs. However, depending on the cause, they can be found on any part of the body.

Blisters that are very painful are usually associated with herpes 1 (cold sores), herpes 2 (genital herpes), and shingles (varicella-zoster virus). Other common causes of blisters are insect or spider bites, improperly fitting shoes, exposure to plants such as poison ivy or poison oak, trauma from heat or electrical burns, and hives resulting from allergic contact.

Impetigo is a staphylococcal (bacterial) infection of the skin that occurs commonly in children and is highly contagious. When the fluid within a blister becomes cloudy, this means that there is most likely a bacterial infection that needs to be treated with an antibiotic (by mouth or topical).

Information on Blisters

Causes: Viruses (varicella, herpes), irritation (hot liquids, friction), insect or spider bites, poisonous plants, trauma (heat or electrical burns), allergic contact (hives)

Symptoms: Raised area of skin filled with clear liquid and sometimes blood; may become red, warm, and painful

Duration: Acute

Treatments: None; if rupture occurs, topical antibiotic

Treatment and Therapy

Prevention is the first step in the management of blisters. Blisters on the feet can be prevented by wearing properly fitting shoes and all-natural fiber (cotton or wool) socks, which minimizes friction. Since the fluid inside blisters is generally sterile, the best management is not to open the blister and instead to let it reabsorb into the skin. If the blister spontaneously opens, then it is best to keep the area clean and dry. A topical antibiotic can be used. If infection develops, then the area will become red, warm, and painful. Medical treatment, such as the administration of an antibiotic, should be sought. In the case of insect bites, an anti-itch medicine such as caladryl and/or an oral antihistamine (Benadryl) is useful to alleviate the itch. Scratching blisters or lesions can lead to a secondary infection, which may require an oral and/or topical antibiotic. Keeping the area clean and dry is another component of ensuring that the lesion will heal.

—Rosslynn S. Byous, D.P.A., PA-C

See also Abscess drainage; Abscesses; Acne; Antibiotics; Bacterial infections; Boils; Burns and scalds; Chickenpox; Cold sores; Cysts; Dermatitis; Dermatology; Dermatopathology; Eczema; Frostbite; Gangrene; Hand-foot-and-mouth disease; Herpes; Impetigo; Insect-borne diseases; Lice, mites, and ticks; Plague; Poisonous plants; Rashes; Scabies; Skin; Skin disorders; Smallpox; Staphylococcal infections; Sunburn.

For Further Information:

Graedon, Joe, and Theresa Graedon. *The People's Pharmacy Guide to Home and Herbal Remedies*. New York: St. Martin's Press, 2002.

Lanternier, Matthew L., and Karen Brannon. "Dermatology." In *The Family Practice Handbook*, edited by Lanternier, Mark A. Graber, and the University of Iowa. Philadelphia: Saunders Elsevier, 2006.

Wolff, Klaus, Richard Allen Johnson, and Dick Suurmond. *Fitzpatrick's Color Atlas and Synopsis of Clinical Dermatology*. 5th ed. New York: McGraw-Hill Medical, 2005.

Blood and blood disorders

Biology

Anatomy or system affected: Blood vessels, circulatory system, immune system, liver, lymphatic system

Specialties and related fields: Hematology, immunology, serology

Definition: The fluid that circulates in the veins and arteries, carrying oxygen and nutrients through the body, transporting waste materials to excretory channels, and participating in the body's defense against infection.

Key terms:

blood: the fluid that circulates through the cardiovascular system; composed of a fluid fraction and a cellular fraction consisting of erythrocytes, leukocytes, and thrombocytes

blood group system: a classification of individuals into groups on the basis of their possession or nonpossession of specific blood substances

blood typing: the identification of the blood group substances of an individual so as to classify him or her in a specific blood group

erythrocytes: red blood cells; the nonnucleated, disk-shaped blood cells that contain hemoglobin

hemoglobin: the oxygen-carrying red pigment present in red blood cells that is responsible for oxygen exchange in cells and tissues

leukocytes: white blood cells; any of the white or colorless nucleated cells occurring in blood

plasma: the protein-containing fluid portion of the blood in which the blood cells are normally suspended

serum: the clear, yellowish fluid obtained from blood after it has been allowed to clot

thrombocytes: platelets; small, irregularly shaped cells in the blood that participate in blood clotting

Structure and Functions

Blood provides a common communication channel for all organs in the body. It is responsible for the transport of oxygen, enzymes, hormones, drugs, and many other substances, as well as for the transfer of heat produced by chemical reactions in the body. The average-sized adult has about 10 pints of blood. At rest, 10 pints a minute (and up to 40 pints during exercise) are pumped by the heart via the arteries to the lungs and all other tissues. This blood then returns to the heart through the veins, in a continuous circuit.

About half the volume of blood consists of cells, which include red blood cells (erythrocytes), white blood cells (leukocytes), and platelets (thrombocytes). The remainder is a fluid called plasma, which contains dissolved proteins, sugars, fats, and minerals.

All types of blood cells are formed within the bone marrow by a series of divisions from a single type of cell called a stem cell. Red blood cells, or erythrocytes (from the Greek *eruthros*, "red"), are very small, have no nucleus, and consist almost completely of hemoglobin. Very little oxygen is needed for the survival of these cells. They have a large surface relative to their volume, which allows oxygen and carbon dioxide to diffuse in and out of the cell rapidly. This large surface also allows the cell to swell and shrink and to be squashed through narrow capillaries without its surface being subjected to shearing or bursting. Red blood cells cannot repair themselves, and after three or four months in circulation they are eliminated and replaced. Their main function is to act as containers for hemoglobin; as such, they are among the most highly specialized cells in the body.

Hemoglobin, the red, iron-containing pigment responsible for the color of blood, has a great affinity for oxygen. It will release the oxygen in a situation where free oxygen is scarce, as it is among the live cells of working tissues. Hemoglobin gives blood an oxygen-carrying capacity eighty times greater than if the oxygen were merely dissolved in plasma. When hemoglobin gives up its oxygen, it becomes capable of taking up carbon dioxide, which it carries to the lungs. Thus this substance provides a sophisticated oxygen delivery system that provides the proper amount of oxygen to the tissues under a wide variety of circumstances. Hemoglobin occupies 33 percent of the volume of the red cell and accounts for 90 percent of its dry weight.

Leukocytes, or white blood cells (from the Greek *leukos*, meaning "clear" or "white"), are larger and less plentiful than red blood cells and can also be found outside the blood. Their purpose is to clean the system of wastes and foreign material and to act as defense against living germs. They travel through the circulatory system and can pass through the walls of blood vessels to do their work in the surrounding tissues. White blood cells play an important role in the defense against infection by viruses, bacteria, fungi, parasites, and inflammation of any cause. There are three main types: granulocytes, monocytes, and lymphocytes. Granulocytes, or polymorphonuclear leukocytes, contain granules and have an oddly shaped nucleus; they are themselves of three types: neutrophils, basophils, and eosinophils. The most important are the neutrophils, which are responsible for isolating and killing invading bacteria (pus consists largely of neutrophils). They are also called phagocytes ("engulfing cells") because of their capability to swallow bacteria and other foreign materials. They normally remain in the blood for only six to nine hours and then travel to the tissues, where they spend a few more days and then move to sites of infection. Eosinophils are involved in allergic reactions. Monocytes circulate in the blood for six to nine days and are also a type of phagocyte important in the immune system.

Lymphocytes are the entities responsible for immune response, such as the production of antibodies and the rejection of tissue grafts. They direct the activity of all other cells in the immune response. Many of them are formed in the lymph nodes rather than in the bone marrow. Their lifetime is between three months and ten years. Unlike granulocytes and monocytes, they do not engulf solid particles but instead play a part in antibody production. An antibody is a protein that may dissolve freely in the blood plasma or in other body fluids and may affix to other cells. Antibodies can be regarded as disinfectants, since they kill or specifically mark foreign material so that it is more readily noticed, caught, digested, or swept away by scavenger cells. There are many different types of lymphocytes, each of which has a different function. T lymphocytes are responsible for delayed hypersensitivity phenomena and produce substances called lymphokines, which affect the function of many cells. They also moderate the activity of other lymphocytes called B lymphocytes. These cells form the antibodies that protect against a second attack of a disease. Most of these cells are in a state of patrol, forming an early warning system that moves out of the circulation, into the tissue fluids, and back to the blood. If these cells encounter foreign material that fits a specific molecular pattern in their structure, or receive such material from another cell, they move to a lymph node or similar area. There they

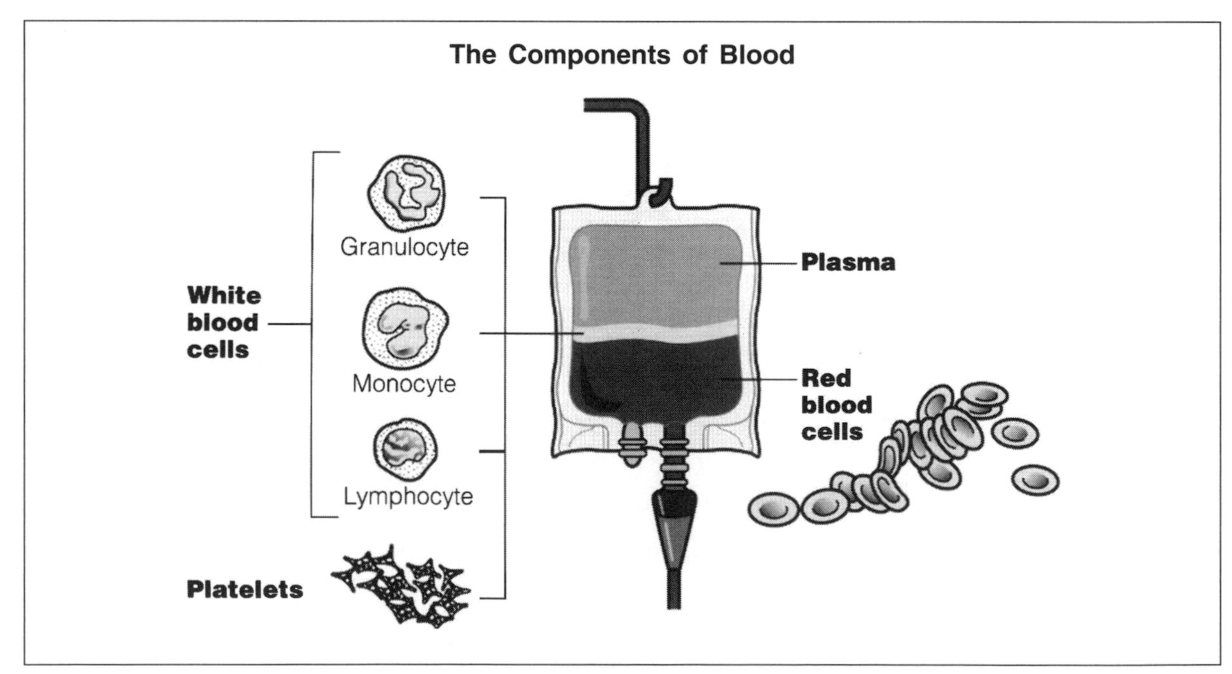

Blood consists of cells floating in a fluid called plasma. Red blood cells contain hemoglobin, an important substance that carries oxygen; platelets are involved in clotting mechanisms; and white blood cells, which are divided into granulocytes, monocytes, and lymphocytes, are responsible for the immune response to foreign matter.

divide to produce a line of daughter cells, all of which manufacture an antibody specifically active against that foreign or irregular material.

Platelets, or thrombocytes, are the smallest cells in blood; they can survive there for about nine days. They circulate in the blood in an inactive state, but under certain circumstances they begin to adhere to blood vessels and one another, producing and releasing chemicals that begin the process of blood clotting. Thus they are critical in hemostasis (the arresting of bleeding).

Plasma is the straw-colored fluid in which blood cells are suspended. It is composed mainly of water (95 percent), with a salt content that is similar to salt water. Some of its other important constituents are nutrients, waste products, proteins, and hormones. Nutrients are transported to the tissues after absorption from the intestinal tract or following release from storage places such as the liver. They include sugars, fats, vitamins, minerals, and the amino acids required to make proteins. The main waste product of tissue metabolism is urea, which is transported in the plasma to the kidneys. The waste product from the destruction of hemoglobin is a yellow pigment called bilirubin, which is normally removed from the plasma by the liver and turned into bile. Among the proteins in plasma are substances such as fibrinogen (involved in the process of coagulation and clotting), immunoglobulins and their complements (bacteria fighters that are part of the immune system), and albumin. Hormones are chemical messengers transported from various glands to their target organs.

The term "blood group" refers to the classification of blood according to differences in the makeup of its red blood cells. The ABO system consists of three blood group substances, the A, B, and H antigens (substances that induce the production of an antibody when injected into an animal), which are components of erythrocyte surface substances. Individuals with type A cells carry anti-B antibodies in their serum; those with type B cells carry anti-A antibodies; those with type AB cells (which bear both A and B antigens) carry neither anti-A nor anti-B antibodies; and type O individuals, whose cells bear neither antigen, carry both anti-A and anti-B antibodies. The transfusion of type A blood into a type B individual, for example, clumps together the transfused erythrocytes and results in an often fatal blockage of blood vessels, which indicates the importance of blood typing before a transfusion is performed.

Another blood group system is based on the rhesus (or Rh) factor. The system involves several antigens, but the most important is called factor D. It is found in 85 percent of the population; those individuals are called Rh positive. If it is not present, the person is classified as Rh negative. Based on this system, individuals are therefore classified as O positive or AB negative, for example, on the basis of their ABO and Rh blood groups. The main importance of the Rh group is during pregnancy. An Rh-negative women who is pregnant with an Rh-positive baby may form antibodies against the baby's blood. Such women are given antibodies directed against factor D after delivery to prevent the development of anti-D antibodies, which would cause hemolytic disease of the newborn in successive Rh-positive infants. The transfusion of Rh-positive blood into an Rh-negative patient can cause a serious reaction if the patient has had a previous blood transfusion that contained the Rh antigen.

About four hundred other antigens have been discovered, but they are widely scattered throughout the population and rarely cause transfusion problems. Only the ABO and the Rh blood group systems have major clinical importance.

Blood typing is used to categorize blood for transfusion. Knowledge of blood group substances and of their inheritance has been useful for legal, historical, and medical purposes. The ABO blood groups are found in all people, but the frequency of each group varies with race and geographical distribution. This fact can aid anthropologists who are involved in investigating, for example, early population migrations. The blood group of an individual is determined by the genes inherited from his or her parents. Identification of a blood group can be used in a paternity case to establish that a man could not have been the father of a particular child, although it cannot be shown positively that a man is the father by blood grouping. Blood found at the scene of a crime can be typed and used to exclude suspects if the type does not match. Some blood groups are associated with particular disorders. For example, blood group A has been found to be more common in people suffering from cancer of the stomach, while group O is found more often in people suffering from peptic ulcers.

DISORDERS AND DISEASES

Blood tests can be used to check on the health of major organs as well as respiratory functions, hormonal balance, the immune system, and metabolism. They can reveal not only the blood cell abnormalities characteristic of some diseases but also healthy variations in blood induced by response to infections. Blood tests can be classified into three categories. Hematological tests involve studying the components of blood itself by looking at the number, shape, size, and appearance of its cells, as well as by testing the function of clotting factors. The most important tests of this type are the blood count, blood smear, and blood-clotting tests. Biochemical tests look at chemicals in the blood such as sodium, potassium, uric acid, urea, vitamins, gases, and drugs. In microbiological tests, blood is examined for microorganisms, such as bacteria, viruses and viral particles, fungi, and parasites, and for antibodies that form against them.

Known causes of blood disorders include genetic reasons (an inherited abnormality in the production of some blood component), nutritional disorders (such as a vitamin deficiency), infections by microorganisms, tumors (such as bone marrow cancer), poisons (carbon monoxide, lead, and snake and spider venoms), drugs (which can produce blood abnormalities as a side effect), and radiation.

Abnormalities can occur in any of the components of blood, including some constituents of plasma. Leukemias are disorders in which the number of white blood cells is abnormally high. In acquired immunodeficiency syndrome (AIDS), the T lymphocytes are infected by a virus, resulting in dysfunction and an increased risk for certain types of infections and cancers. Abnormal platelets or the lack of platelets can lead to some types of bleeding disorders, such as hemophilia (an inability of the blood to clot properly). Unwanted clot formation (thrombosis) can occur from circumstances that overactivate the blood's clotting mechanisms. Anemia results from a deficiency of hemoglobin and a corresponding reduction in the blood's oxygen-carrying capacity; this is the most common blood disorder. Deficiencies of the proteins in blood plasma include albuminemia (albumin deficiency).

Perspective and Prospects

Blood is a liquid of complex structure and vital functions that has been considered the essence of life for centuries. There is no shortage of irrational or unscientific ideas about the supposed properties of human blood—one can speak of "blood brotherhood," "blood feuds," "blood relations," and of someone being "bloodthirsty."

The present medical understanding of blood has developed over the past two or three thousand years. The study of blood began in Egypt and Mesopotamia, around 500 B.C.E., and it moved to the countries around the Mediterranean that had become intellectually active. Ancient Greek thinkers noted that there were differences between arteries and veins, and that the blood moved through them. According to whether the heart, the liver, or the brain was thought to be the prime organ controlling the rest of the body, various functions were tentatively ascribed to blood, such as its relation to sleep, the distribution of heat, and the animation of the body.

The Greek school of medicine became personified in Hippocrates. He denied the widely accepted theory of the existence of spirits and proposed that the body followed natural laws. He presented the concept of body juices, or humors. There were four of them: blood, lymph or phlegm, yellow bile (or choler), and black bile (or melancholy), with blood being the most important one. The philosopher Aristotle accepted the humoral hypothesis. One of his pupils was Alexander the Great, whose military conquests spread Greek influence widely. A notable medical school developed in Alexandria, Egypt, and the ideas of Hippocrates and Aristotle were taught there. There was, however, a variation in regard to blood; namely, the theory of plethora, in which it was postulated that an excess of blood in the circulatory system or one organ caused illness.

Four hundred years later, Galen, a product of the Alexandria School of Medicine, denied the doctrine of plethora and went back to the humoral approach. Health and disease were thought to occur as a result of an upset in the equilibrium of these humors. Bloodletting to restore the balance of the humors by purging the body of its contaminated fluids was practiced from the time of Hippocrates until the nineteenth century. During Galen's time, animal dissection was widely practiced and provided a better concept of blood and its functions. It was proposed that the liver changed food to blood, which was distributed to the body along the veins. At the same time, impurities from the body were thought to be absorbed into the venous blood and to be returned to the liver and then to the right side of the heart, where they supposedly ascended in the pulmonary artery to the lungs to be exhaled.

The weakening of medieval ideas set the stage for English doctor William Harvey's discovery of the circulation of blood. He used the analogy of the heart as a pump and veins and arteries as pipes, where blood is moving around and is being driven in some kind of continuous circuit. Four years after Harvey died in 1661, the Italian anatomist Marcello Malpighi observed the capillary blood vessels with the aid of the microscope. The cellular composition of blood was also recognized with the aid of this device, as Antoni van Leeuwenhoek, a Dutch naturalist, accurately described and measured red blood cells. The discovery of white blood cells and platelets followed after microscope lenses were improved. William Hewson first observed leukocytes in the eighteenth century. He thought that these cells came from the nucleated cells in the lymph and that they eventually emerged from the spleen as red blood cells. In the nineteenth century, the interest in leukocytes intensified with studies on inflammation and microbial infection.

In 1852, Karl Vierordt published the first quantitative results of blood cell analysis, after several attempts were made to correlate blood cell counts with various diseases. The observation of crystalline hemoglobin was first reported in 1849. In 1865, Felix Hoppe-Seyler discovered the oxygen-carrying capacity of the red pigment (hemoglobin) in the cells. The early history of protein chemistry is essentially that of hemoglobin, because it was one of the first molecules to have its molecular weight accurately determined and the first to be associated with a specific physiological function (that of carrying oxygen).

In 1900, the German pathologist Karl Landsteiner began mixing blood taken from different people and found that some mixtures were compatible and others were not. This incompatibility resulted in illness and sometimes death after transfusions. He discovered two types of marker proteins, or antigens, on the surface of red blood cells, which he called A and B. According to whether a person's blood contains one or the other antigen, both, or neither, it is classified as type A, B, AB, or O. He also discovered the Rh factor in 1940 during experiments with rhesus monkeys. Improved methods of blood examination in the 1920's and the growth of knowledge of blood physiology in the 1930's allowed anemias and other blood disorders to be studied on a rational basis.

Modern hematology recognizes that alterations in the components of blood are a result of disease, and research is conducted continually for a better understanding of this relationship and of blood itself.

—*Maria Pacheco, Ph.D.*

See also Anemia; Angiography; Bleeding; Blood banks; Blood testing; Bone marrow transplantation; Cholesterol; Circulation; Cyanosis; Dialysis; Disseminated intravascular coagulation (DIC); Ebola virus; Ergogenic aids; Fluids and electrolytes; Forensic pathology; Heart; Hematology; Hematology, pediatric; Hemochromatosis; Hemolytic disease of the newborn; Hemophilia; Histiocytosis; Hypercholesterolemia; Hyperlipidemia; Hypoglycemia; Immunization and vaccination; Ischemia; Jaundice; Laboratory tests; Leukemia; Liver; Marburg virus; Nephrology; Nephrology, pediatric; Pathology; Pharmacology; Rh factor; Septicemia; Serology; Sickle cell disease; Thalassemia; Thrombocytopenia; Thrombolytic therapy and TPA; Toxicology; Transfusion; Von Willebrand's disease; Wiskott-Aldrich syndrome.

FOR FURTHER INFORMATION:

Bick, Roger L. *Disorders of Thrombosis and Hemostasis: Clinical and Laboratory Practice*. 3d ed. Philadelphia: Lippincott Williams & Wilkins, 2002. An excellent introduction to the diagnosis and management of clotting and bleeding disorders.

Leiken, Jerrold B., and Martin S. Lipsky, eds. *American Medical Association Complete Encyclopedia of Medicine*. New York: Random House, 2003. An excellent presentation on blood—its components, illnesses, and treatments.

Lichtman, Marshall L., et al. *Williams Manual of Hematology*. 6th ed. New York: McGraw-Hill, 2002. An accessible handbook that covers the pathogenetic, diagnostic, and therapeutic essentials of blood cell and coagulation protein disorders.

Litin, Scott C., ed. *Mayo Clinic Family Health Book*. 3d ed. New York: HarperResource, 2003. Good presentation of blood; concentrates on illnesses, their causes and treatments.

Loscalzo, Joseph, and Andrew I. Schafer, eds. *Thrombosis and Hemorrhage*. 3d ed. Philadelphia: Lippincott Williams & Wilkins, 2003. Covers an array of relevant topics including the basic elements of hemostasis, the normal function and response of platelets, and specific clinical disorders and laboratory approaches, thrombotic disorders, and management of patients with hemorrhagic and thrombotic conditions.

Provan, Drew, and John Gribben, eds. *Molecular Haematology*. 2d ed. Malden, Mass.: Blackwell, 2005. Targeted at the medical professional, this resource discusses diseases of the blood at the molecular level.

Rodak, Bernadette, ed. *Hematology: Clinical Principles and Applications*. 2d ed. Philadelphia: W. B. Saunders, 2002. A comprehensive textbook covering all aspects of hematology and hemostasis.

Voet, Donald, and Judith G. Voet. *Biochemistry*. 3d ed. Hoboken, N.J.: John Wiley & Sons, 2004. An excellent general biochemistry book that contains a few sections on blood and blood components, their properties and functions.

Zucker-Franklin, D., et al. *Atlas of Blood Cells: Function and Pathology*. 2d ed. Philadelphia: Lea & Febiger, 1988. Great pictorial presentation of blood components in different stages of function and disease.

Blood banks

Organizations

Definition: Temporary storehouses of blood, kept at reduced temperatures, for transfusions into persons needing an additional supply; such transfers are vital in surgery and in unexpected emergency procedures.

Key terms:

cardiology: the study of the heart and its action, as well as the diagnosis and treatment of its diseases

cardiovascular: relating to or involving the heart and blood vessels

corpuscle: a minute particle; a protoplasmic cell floating free in the blood

erythrocyte: a red blood cell

hematosis: the formation of blood

hemophilia: a tendency (usually hereditary) to profuse bleeding, even from slight cuts

leukocyte: a white or colorless blood corpuscle

phagocyte: any leukocyte active in ingesting and destroying waste and harmful material

phlebotomy: the act or practice of opening a vein for letting blood

serology: the science of serums, their reactions, preparation, and use

The Study of Blood Throughout History

For centuries, blood was thought to be a simple liquid, but it is actually a body tissue. The cells, instead of being joined together as in solid body tissues, are suspended in a fluid called plasma, which is more than half of blood composition. The cellular portion of blood is largely red blood cells and smaller numbers of white blood cells and platelets. Blood itself is the final functioning tool of the circulatory system, which helps to transport the blood to where it is needed in the body. Blood is an extremely complicated substance, and more things are being learned about it every year.

Some ancient civilizations, such as that of the Greeks, recognized that blood was an important fluid in the body, but they thought that it was motionless in certain areas. Between 300 and 250 B.C.E., some Egyptians were studying the anatomy of corpses. About 300 B.C.E., the Greek physician Praxagoras showed that there were tubes connected to the heart. Some were filled with blood; others were empty, filled with air. One of the physician's students, Herophilus, found that arteries gave a beat or pulse. When dissection was outlawed in Egypt, progress in learning about blood was stopped for a thousand years.

Galen, the Greek physician who served five Roman emperors over thirty years to 200 C.E., believed that the arteries originated in the heart and pumped blood. Contrary to later Egyptian medical thought, Galen theorized that the heart was one pump, not two. Around 1300, doctors in Italy began to dissect bodies again, and in 1316, Mondino de Luzzi wrote the first book dealing entirely with anatomy, in which he supported Galen's teachings. In 1543, Belgian anatomist Andreas Vesalius wrote a much-improved book on anatomy which did not improve, however, on Galen's theories about the heart.

In 1242, a Syrian surgeon named Ibn an-Nafīs had written a book in which he theorized about how blood moved from the right ventricle to the left and that a double pump was involved in moving it. Ironically, his writings were not discovered by Europeans until 1924.

Meanwhile, Spanish physician Michael Servetus published a treatise in 1553 describing how circulation of blood to the lungs and back (often called the lesser circulation) might occur. Unfortunately, because he also included religious views, all copies of his writings that could be found were destroyed, and he was burned at the stake. Eventually, in 1694, a copy of his book was found; his circulation theory matched later findings.

In 1559, an Italian anatomist, Realdo Colombo, also thought of lesser circulation and published a book on it. Colombo's work was so widely read that he is credited with discovering lesser circulation. In 1574, another Italian, Girolamo Fabrici, observed little valves on veins that opened in only one direction. The importance of this discovery was deducted by a student of Fabrici, the English doctor William Harvey, when he determined that blood in the leg veins could move only to the heart. His laboratory work proved that the heart pumped blood into the arteries and that the blood returned by way of the veins. Further, Harvey showed that the blood had a double circulation, returning to both ventricles. His continued experimentation showed that the same blood had to circulate and be used repeatedly.

All these medical pioneers were hampered by the inability to see more than the human eye would permit—until the development of lenses and microscopes. In 1661, Italian anatomist Marcello Malpighi was able to see, with the aid of a microscope, very fine blood vessels that connected the smallest arteries and veins: capillaries. With the discovery of capillaries, the concept of the circulation of blood was complete. In the eighteenth century, the English scientist Stephen Hales was the first to measure blood pressure.

The microscope also enabled scientists to observe some components of blood. Malpighi saw reddish objects in a clear, faintly yellow fluid. Dutch scientist Jan Swammerdam, with the aid of a microscope, was able to describe them further. In 1674, the renowned Dutch scientist Antoni van Leeuwenhoek, using the best of these early microscopes, was able to describe the red cells as flat disks with depressions in the center. He even tried to measure them; his calculations were refined in 1852 by German scientist Karl Vierordt. Leeuwenhoek was able to study the path of red blood cells in tadpoles, frogs, and other animals and determined that, without doubt, blood traveled in an entirely closed circle, proving Harvey's contention. Soon, in 1669, English doctor Richard Lower noted that blood coming through arteries was red and that blood flowing toward the heart in veins was bluish.

English chemist Joseph Priestley discovered the gas oxygen in 1774, and French chemist Antoine-Laurent Lavoisier was able to show in 1778 that air consisted (mainly) of two gases, oxygen (one-fifth) and nitrogen (four-fifths). A German chemist, Julius Lothar Meyer, showed in 1857 that oxygen did not generally mix with the liquid part of the blood, combining instead with red blood cells.

The scientific detective work on blood continued with the aid of improved microscopes. It was learned that the cells of the body contained complicated substances called proteins, each of which was made up of groups of atoms called molecules. German scientists were among the first to examine the composition of blood. Otto Funke obtained a protein from red blood cells in 1851. Then Felix Hoppe-Seyler purified it, studied it, and named it hemoglobin ("blood protein"). The secrets of this precious commodity continued to unfold. In 1747, Italian chemist Vincenzo Antonio Menghini found that there was a small quantity of iron in blood, apparently in red blood cells.

Gradually, these findings led to the transfusion of blood from one person to another. In the seventeenth century, blood transfusions were attempted between animals. In 1666, Richard Lower unsuccessfully tried to transfuse blood from an animal to a human being. Sometimes the operation helped, but occasionally people died after such a transfusion, so doctors largely abandoned the practice. Then, in 1818, James Blundell, an English physician who theorized that the blood of a particular kind of animal would help only that particular kind, transfused blood from healthy human beings to other human beings who needed blood. While often successful, the procedure sometimes caused agglutination, in which red blood cells clumped together and would not function properly.

In 1901, an Austrian doctor named Karl Landsteiner solved the problem by observing that there were four kinds of blood cells. Depending on the chemical content, the blood was typed A, B, AB, and O. Continuing practice showed that not all blood types work well with one another; some tend to agglutinate when introduced to the wrong type.

Although red blood cells are by far the most numerous objects that float in the bloodstream, they are not the only ones. In 1850, French physician Casimir-Joseph Davaine noticed cells, pale and uneven in shape, that were much larger than red blood cells. By 1869, he noticed that these cells would absorb bits of foreign matter in the blood. In 1875, German doctor Paul Ehrlich, interested in using dyes on these white cells, found that he was able to classify them into different types.

In the late nineteenth century, Russian scientist Élie Metchnikoff (also known as Ilya Ilich Mechnikov), while studying bacteria, noticed that whenever there was a cut, white cells were carried to it in great numbers by the blood. So much blood went to the injured part that it grew red and inflamed and was painful from the pressure exerted by the blood on the vessel walls. Metchnikoff called the bacteria-eating cells phagocytes. He had become interested in the study of bacteria following the pioneering work of France's Louis Pasteur in the 1860's.

The clotting of wounds became more interesting to the medical community. In 1842, French scientist Alfred Donne had reported a new type of object floating in the bloodstream. An Italian physician, Giulio Cesare Bizzozero, concluded that the foreign objects had something to do with clotting. He called them platelets because their shape resembles tiny plates. What was to be learned about them much later is that they have a life span of about nine days and that they break down when exposed to air after bleeding starts. As they begin to break down, platelets release a substance that starts a long chain of chemical changes that ends in clotting.

While many scientists were concentrating on the study of red blood cells, white blood cells, and platelets, attention was also being paid to plasma, the colorless liquid that is a vehicle for objects floating in it. Eventually, it was learned that plasma carries red blood cells to the lungs to take up oxygen and then to all the rest of the body to deliver the oxygen. Plasma carries white blood cells to any part of the body where they are needed to fight bacteria. It also carries platelets to any part of the body where blood loss must be stopped. Furthermore, the watery plasma absorbs heat at the liver and delivers it to the skin, so that the body stays warm.

More recent studies show that about 8 percent of plasma is composed of dissolved substances that are important in keeping conditions in the body even. Some chemicals in the plasma neutralize acids and bases, which could threaten cells. The plasma also carries glucose molecules and fatty acids to specific destinations in order to produce energy in the body. Furthermore, it dissolves wastes such as carbon dioxide and delivers urea to the kidneys for disposal. Hormones, which were first discovered in 1902, are also carried by the plasma to any part of the body where they are needed.

More than half the weight of substances dissolved in plasma are proteins. Proteins fall into two groups, albumins and globulins. Some proteins combine easily with substances that the body needs in small amounts. Gammaglobulins have the capacity to neutralize foreign molecules—viruses or the poisonous toxins produced by bacteria—by combining with them. Gammaglobulins that act in this way are called antibodies.

All these discoveries and many others (such as the existence of fibrinogen, fibrin, the Rh factor, and enzymes) have combined to improve the procedures for storing and transfusing blood. Safeguarding blood for transfusion has always been a problem. The precious liquid is unstable, and a fresh supply has always been needed in any emergency.

In the late 1930's, Russian scientists discovered that citrated blood can be stored if refrigerated at a temperature of about 4.5 degrees Celsius (40 degrees Fahrenheit). Then, in 1936, a Canadian doctor, Norman Bethune, made large-scale use of a blood bank with antifascist forces during the Spanish Civil War. During World War II, the noted American blood bank pioneer Charles Drew, who had made a special study of ways to store and ship blood plasma, organized a nationwide "Blood for Britain" campaign in which thousands of lives were saved.

Before blood banks could evolve, a number of additional discoveries had to be made. Before the discovery of agglutinins and blood typing, blood was transfused directly from donor to patient. The two lay side by side, and the blood flowed from the artery of the donor to the vein of the recipient. There was no way of measuring the amount of blood being transfused. It became dangerous for the donor if he or she changed from rosy-colored and talkative to pale or unconscious. There was also danger that a blood clot in the tube might enter the patient's blood vessels. In addition, the blood might be flowing too fast and overload the patient's heart.

A new tube to facilitate blood transfusion more safely was developed in 1909. Then, in 1914, Argentine doctor Luis Agote discovered that sodium citrate could stop the clotting of blood, permitting blood to be kept in a bottle while it was slowly directed into a patient's vein. Physicians could finally control the amount and speed of transfusions.

The use of stored blood began in 1918 by Oswald H. Robertson, a World War I physician, who found it could be kept virtually intact for several days by storing it at low temperatures, from 2 to 4 degrees Celsius. The first large blood bank was established at the Cook County Hospital in Chicago in 1937.

The Role of Blood Banks

A blood bank is an organizational unit responsible for collecting, processing, and storing blood to be used for transfusion and other purposes. It is usually a subdivision of a laboratory in a hospital and is often charged with the responsibility for all serologic testing. Although blood can be withdrawn from one person and transfused directly into another, the usual practice is for hospitals and authorized agencies to select donors, draw blood (phlebotomy), screen the specimens, arrange them into blood groups, and store the blood until it is needed.

The storage of blood was once short-lived because of clotting and too-high temperature levels. A blood bank can now store blood for much longer periods of time, sometimes a year or two. It is stored with an anticoagulant, generally an acid-citrate-dextrose (ACD) solution composed of trisodisum citrate, citric acid, dextrose, and sterile water. Red blood cells from blood stored in an ACD solution will survive in the recipient for one hundred days. Blood banks consider blood unsuitable

In the News: Blood Banks and Antigerm Screening

Blood banks in the early twenty-first century faced growing challenges as new diseases threatened the purity of their blood supplies. In response to such threats, researchers attempted to design improved methods for blood banks to screen donors and blood for protection against contamination.

West Nile virus, a mosquito-borne disease, was first identified in the United States in 1999. In the fall of 2002, health officials discovered that organ transplant recipients had become infected with the virus through blood transfusions. The majority of West Nile victims display no visible symptoms and had unintentionally donated contaminated blood. In November of that year, the Food and Drug Administration (FDA) called for the development of a test before the outbreak of the 2003 mosquito season. Although some experts doubted that a screening method could be produced so quickly, two tests that detected minute fragments of the West Nile virus genes were in use by July 1, 2003. The tests also revealed the presence of viruses responsible for Japanese, St. Louis, and Murray encephalitis, permitting blood banks to reject blood contaminated with these diseases as well.

Although no conclusive evidence proved that either Creutzfeldt-Jakob disease (the human form of mad cow disease) or severe acute respiratory syndrome (SARS) were in fact transmissible through blood transfusions, blood banks used verbal screening of potential donors to defend against these recent disease outbreaks. FDA guidelines mandated rejection or deferral of blood donations from people who might have been exposed to either disease.

In 2002, the FDA approved nucleic acid amplification tests (NAT) for the hepatitis C virus (HCV) and the human immunodeficiency virus 1 (HIV-1). Unlike existing tests for the presence of antibodies, which do not develop in the earliest stages of a disease, the NAT reacts to small fragments of virus deoxyribonucleic acid (DNA) and can detect infections before the appearance of symptoms. The West Nile virus tests use similar methods.

Ongoing research into improved techniques for detecting bacteria and other blood pathogens, and into ways of using physical or chemical methods to destroy these organisms, may further improve blood supply safety.

—*Milton Berman, Ph.D.*

for transfusion if it is retained more than twenty-one days. After that, stored blood may be reduced to plasma by centrifuging it to eliminate the red blood cells.

All chemical changes in blood are slowed by refrigeration. It has been found that prolonged storage of blood can be achieved by freezing and maintaining it at extremely low temperatures—below –70 degrees Celsius (–94 degrees Fahrenheit). While freezing and thawing of whole blood does not harm plasma, it can damage red blood cells unless glycerol or dimethyl sulfoxide solutions are used to minimize the damage and permit red cells to be maintained in a frozen state for months without significant injury.

After Karl Landsteiner discovered that blood could be classified into four major blood groups, safer transfusions could be attempted. Landsteiner also worked with the American pathologist Alexander S. Wiener to discover another system of blood grouping known as the Rh system. The name was derived from the rhesus monkeys with which the scientists experimented.

It was found that a person with type A blood (having "A" agglutinogens in the red blood cells and "b" agglutinins in the blood plasma) cannot successfully give blood to a person with type B blood (having "B" agglutinogens and "a" agglutinins) because the clumping of blood cells will occur.

Successful blood transfusions depend on the type of agglutinogens in the donor's red blood cells, not on the type of agglutinin in the plasma, because the recipient's blood cells greatly outnumber the agglutinin in the donor's blood, and serious clumping could not occur. A donor's red blood cells, however, are few enough in number that all of them can be agglutinated by the recipient's agglutinins. These clumps could then plug the capillaries, reducing and eventually cutting off the flow of blood. This reaction is serious and can cause death.

A person with type AB blood, who has both "A" and "B" agglutinogens in the red blood cells and no agglutinins in the plasma, can receive the red blood cells of any other group. A type O person (a universal donor) has no agglutinogens and can donate blood to any person but can receive only type O blood. In practice, however, physicians use donors having the same type as their recipients.

The ABO system of grouping blood types has led to further refinements. Ten major and minor blood groupings have been identified from the variety of proteins also found in blood cells. The most important is the Rh system. There are two Rh blood types, Rh positive and Rh negative. A person with the Rh-positive factor has the protein, while a person with Rh-negative blood does not have the protein. Infusing an Rh-negative person with Rh-positive blood causes special agglutinins to be formed in the blood of the recipient. A later transfusion of Rh-positive blood would result in the agglutination of the red blood cells received.

This reaction is especially important when incompatibility occurs between the blood of a pregnant woman and her baby. This happens only if the mother has Rh-negative blood and the baby has Rh-positive blood because it has inherited Rh-positive genes from the father. When such a baby is born, some of the baby's blood enters the mother's circulation system, causing her body to produce antibodies to combat the "foreign material." Since this intrusion of blood almost always happens as a delayed reaction after the baby is born, the first baby is probably unharmed, but a subsequent baby could be the victim of these antibodies, which the mother's body continues to produce. Such a developing baby could suffer the destruction of its red blood cells if it has Rh-positive blood, unless preventive steps such as a blood transfusion for the baby are taken. Another medical development is a serum for protective vaccination that has almost eliminated the dangers of Rh incompatibility.

Blood transfusions are regularly used in crises such as accidents or life-threatening illnesses. Most commonly, they are used to restore the volume of circulating blood lost by acute hemorrhaging. They are also used to restore the large volume of plasma that is often lost after severe burns. In acute or chronic anemia cases, such as with acquired immunodeficiency syndrome (AIDS), they are used to maintain hemoglobin and red blood cells at adequate levels. Transfusions are also used to provide platelets for coagulation in order to counteract various bleeding disorders or acute hemorrhaging.

The technique of blood transfusion has become routinely simple. Blood withdrawn by hypodermic needle from an arm vein of a healthy donor is passed through plastic tubing into a sterile glass bottle or plastic bag that contains sodium citrate or another solution that prevents coagulation. The blood is then transfused into the arm of the recipient through a second plastic tube connection which contains a gauze filter. About 500 milliliters (about 1 pint) are drawn and infused slowly, except in emergency cases.

Blood transfusions are being used more extensively—and more safely—than ever before. Many more surgeries are possible with transfusions: organ implants, heart repair, limb reconstruction, grafting for severe burn cases, and bone grafts. Blood transfusions are also important in the treatment of anemia and AIDS.

Perspective and Prospects

In the United States, the work of blood banks comes under the ultimate supervision of the Food and Drug Administration (FDA) and federal agencies, as well as the Oversight and Investigations Subcommittee of the House Energy and Commerce Committee. Also interested in their function are the congressionally funded Public Health Service and the Centers for Disease Control. The largest United States blood bank is that of the Red Cross, which provides, through its local affiliates, about half of the 18 million units of blood donated each year. The Red Cross, as well as individual nonprofit and commercial agencies, is striving for improved health and safety procedures in blood donation.

The American Association of Blood Banks gathers and interprets data each year. It has found that there have been relatively few transfusion-induced cases of viral infection. Almost all the transfusion-related AIDS cases, for example, developed in 1985, before tighter screening of donors, safer procedures, and strict testing were instituted. Only fifteen cases of AIDS from blood transfusion were reported between 1985 and 1992. This contrasts with the pre-1985 figure of 3,425 transfusion-associated cases of AIDS reported to the Centers for Disease Control.

Concern about other viral infections transmitted through blood transfusions has increased vigilance against blood impurities and has improved sanitary procedures. Governmental agencies, the Red Cross, and private corporations have intensified their efforts to protect the quality of the blood supply. The International Society of Blood Transfusion continues to examine new threats.

Steps are continually reviewed to improve record keeping, blood collection, tracking, and distribution by all organizations. The FDA has a comprehensive inspection program which focuses on all phases of the collection-dispersal program of all blood banks, as well as on their training of workers and updating of procedures. It looks closely at procedures for donor screening, the testing for hepatitis and AIDS virus antibodies, and the quarantine and destruction of unsuitable blood products.

The American Red Cross complies with these regulations and works with the FDA to create the safest blood supply possible. It has a state-of-the-art computerized information system. It keeps track of all its donors and retains files on all persons disqualified from giving blood and the reasons. This information is available throughout the United States. The computerized program is also being expanded internationally because there is a growing import-export business between countries in need of new supplies. Data banks are being developed with lists of disqualified would-be donors, types and quantities of blood in storage, location of hospitals and distribution centers, and other information vital to the prompt, efficient, and safe distribution of blood.

The Blood Center, a nonprofit blood bank that serves eighty-five hospitals across a sixteen-country area, uses an automatic tracking software system to help send the right blood or blood components to those in need and to guard against contaminated blood entering the supply. The system collects 47,000 units a year.

Blood safety begins with screening. Only healthy individuals are allowed to give blood. Blood samples undergo extensive screening designed to detect any blood-borne infectious agent. Some collection agencies are developing lists of unwanted donors, persons with a high risk of having been exposed to the AIDS virus or to other dangerous viruses or bacteria, such as those that cause hepatitis or syphilis. The goal is to reduce the chance of contagion as much as possible.

Four million patients a year receive blood, largely in emergency cases. Many are in need of emergency surgery for an internal disorder, but many others are victims of social violence, earthquakes, and hurricanes. Large-scale devastation often comes close to depleting the blood supply in an area. New and repeat donors, therefore, are always in demand. New ways of storing blood safely and for longer periods of time are constantly being researched. Some components can be frozen, for example, to give them a longer usable life.

Currently, there is a possible sequence of seven tests to screen blood donations. A polymerase chain reaction (PCR) test almost always amplifies and detects human immunodeficiency virus (HIV). Other tests are sophisticated efforts to detect HIV-1, HIV-2, and hepatitis C viruses. A test with the acronym ELISA, for enzyme-linked immunosorbent assay, is often supported by the Western blot, which conclusively demonstrates specific antibodies to specific viral proteins. It is an expensive set of procedures, and hospitals, clinics, and other medical institutions are working on how to reduce these costs.

Many viruses are elusive, including the dreaded HIV, which takes time to develop. To hasten its identification, scientists have developed the technique of "pooling" by combining blood known to contain infected cells with samples of blood with uninfected normal lymphocytes in an effort to stimulate HIV replication and make the HIV come to light faster. It has been found that the most reliable mix is a pool of fifty donors. The concept of pooling is scientifically valid and economically feasible.

While the risk of acquiring a hepatitis infection has been reduced from a possibility of 33 percent to less than 1 percent, there is growing concern among the public that individuals might be susceptible to specific blood diseases.

—*Walter Appleton*

See also Bleeding; Blood and blood disorders; Blood testing; Cytology; Emergency medicine; Hematology; Hematology, pediatric; Rh factor; Screening; Serology; Transfusion.

For Further Information:

Hillier, Christopher D., et al., eds. *Blood Banking and Transfusion Medicine: Basic Principles and Practice*. 2d ed. Philadelphia: Churchill Livingstone/Elsevier, 2007. Draws data from basic, transnational, and clinical studies; explores the latest advances in the use of blood products, new methods of disease treatment, and stem cell transplantation; and addresses a range of controversies in practice.

McCullough, Jeffrey. *Transfusion Medicine*. 2d ed. Philadelphia: Elsevier Churchill Livingstone, 2005. Transfusion medicine, a young science, is continuously growing and changing. The result is a great body of knowledge about the practical aspects of blood collection and transfusion, and an incomparably better understanding of the blood groups and of the unintended effects of transfusion at the molecular level.

Schaub Di Lorenzo, Marjorie, and Susan King Strasinger. *Blood Collection in Healthcare*. Philadelphia: F. A. Davis, 2001. Details all phlebotomy issues important in collecting a quality blood specimen and includes excellent photographs that clearly demonstrate the preferred techniques, supplies, and collection procedures.

Starr, Douglas P. *Blood: An Epic History of Medicine and Commerce*. New York: Knopf, 1998. Starr reflects on the societal role of blood as it transformed from a mythical enigma to a scientific entity to a product of industry. He examines the past racism of blood banks, the spread of the AIDS epidemic among hemophiliacs, and the role of blood in helping the Allies win World War II.

Wailoo, Keith. *Drawing Blood: Technology and Disease Identity in Twentieth-Century America*. Baltimore: Johns Hopkins University Press, 1999. The author, a medical historian, traces the way in which physicians throughout the twentieth century used medical technology to define disease, establish medical specialties, and shape political agendas.

Blood poisoning. *See* Septicemia.

Blood testing

Procedure

Anatomy or system affected: Blood, blood vessels, circulatory system, skin

Specialties and related fields: Cytology, forensic medicine, hematology, pathology, public health, serology, toxicology

Definition: The withdrawal of blood from an individual and its analysis for one of many purposes, including blood typing and a search for acquired or genetic disease indicators.

Key terms:

antibody: a protein synthesized in response to a specific antigen; antibodies physically combine with antigens as part of the immune process

antigen: a molecule which induces the production of antibodies

antiserum: the fluid portion of blood that contains specific antibodies

Rh factor: a specific antigen present on 85 percent of an individual's red blood cells; also called Rhesus factor

Indications and Procedures

Most blood tests require a substantial sample of blood. A sample of several milliliters or more is withdrawn from a vein using a syringe. The sample is transported to a diagnostic laboratory for the appropriate analysis.

Red blood cells are marked on their surface with the protein antigens designated A, B, AB (both A and B), or O (no antigen). Individuals possess antibodies, found in the liquid or serum portion of the blood, to the antigens that they themselves do not possess. In ABO typing, red blood cells are isolated from the blood sample and mixed with antisera with a known antibody type. Cells marked with antigen A will clump when mixed with antibody A, cells with B antigen will clump when exposed to antibody B, AB antigens clump with either, and O clumps with neither. The type of positive clumping reaction determines blood type. Rh type is determined in the same manner, with Rh-positive blood exhibiting a clumping reaction with Rh antibodies. Histocompatibility leukocyte antigen (HLA) typing is performed similarly but uses white blood cells as the antigenic material. HLA typing is more complex and time consuming because more than forty different HLAs are known to exist.

Deoxyribonucleic acid (DNA) analysis requires isolating DNA from white blood cells and amplifying certain regions with a procedure called polymerase chain reaction (PCR). The amplified DNA is cut with enzymes and run through an electric field in a gel matrix, thus separating the pieces of DNA by size. Specific patterns are visually analyzed. When this technique is repeated across many different regions of a person's DNA, a pattern unique to that individual can be obtained. This information can be used to answer questions of paternity and relatedness or to help convict or exonerate suspects in murder and rape cases. A similar analysis is used to determine the presence of certain genetic diseases or the possibility of transmitting a genetic disease.

The use of blood tests to diagnose diseases covers a wide range, and the test is matched to the analysis requested. Abnormal levels of red blood cells can indicate anemia, while abnormal white cell counts may suggest a severe infection. Inappropriate enzyme levels could signal organ malfunction, and abnormal hormone levels indicate an endocrine disease. High levels of particular antibodies herald an infection with the corresponding antigenic agent.

Uses and Complications

Blood testing may be performed for a variety of reasons. If an individual has suffered a large loss of blood and/or requires surgery that may necessitate a blood transfusion, ABO and Rh factor blood typing is performed. Pregnant women need to know their own Rh

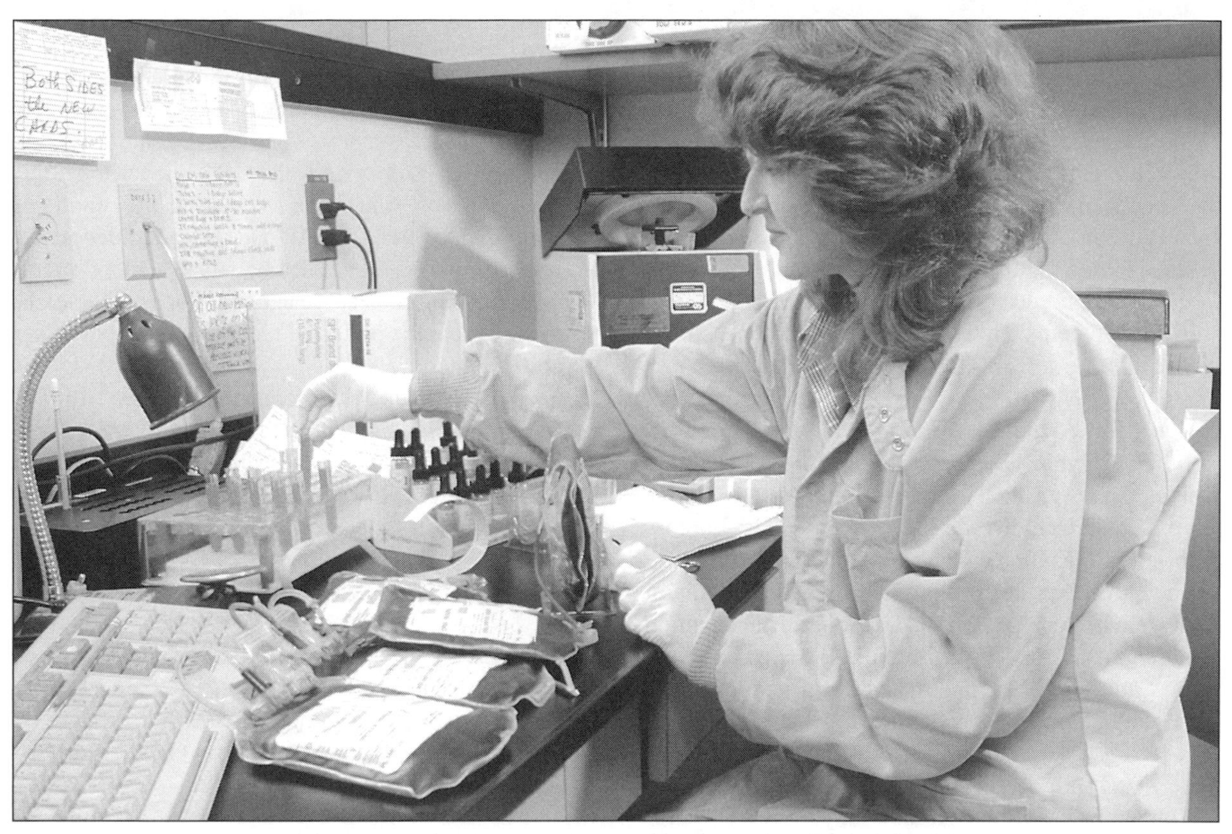

A laboratory technician runs tests on blood samples. (Digital Stock)

status and that of their fetus in order to prevent gestational complications from Rh incompatibility. If an organ transplant is required, the HLAs present on all cells except red blood cells must be matched as closely as possible to prevent graft rejection. In the event of paternity determination or forensic analysis, the DNA sequences found in white blood cells can be analyzed for proper identification. Some genetic diseases in an affected individual, a fetus, or unaffected individuals who may transmit the genetic disease to their offspring can be detected with blood DNA analysis. Many types of disorders and diseases are diagnosed through a determination of the presence of abnormal levels of blood cell types, enzymes, hormones, and electrolytes (sodium, potassium, phosphate, magnesium, and calcium) or the presence of infectious agents in the blood, such as bacteria and viruses. Not all genetic diseases can be tested using DNA analysis. A partial list of those that can be detected includes hemophilia, Huntington's disease, cystic fibrosis, and sickle cell disease. Others, such as Tay-Sachs disease, can be detected with an enzyme test of the blood.

Should proper ABO typing not be performed and an individual be given an incompatible blood transfusion, the antibodies in the individual's blood would destroy the newly transfused cells, causing a life-threatening condition. Failure to diagnose and treat an Rh-incompatible pregnancy could result in death of the fetus or a baby born with severe hemolytic disease and jaundice because of the destruction of fetal blood cells by the mother's immune system.

In modern hospitals with standard precautions, there are only minor side effects to blood withdrawal with a syringe. Some pain from puncturing the vein wall may occur, as well as localized bruising. If the procedure is done under unsanitary conditions or if needles are used repeatedly, the risk of transmitting bacterial infections or viral infections such as hepatitis and acquired immunodeficiency syndrome (AIDS) increases dramatically.

Perspective and Prospects

DNA analysis is rapidly providing new and better diagnostic tools for the identification of genetic disease and its carriers as well as for the prediction of an individual's tendency to develop certain cancers, such as of the breast and colon, and heart disease. Such predictive tests could save millions of lives through close monitoring and early treatment.

Such advances of technology, however, are not without consequences. Since genetic testing became routine in the 1980's, there has been great concern about the access of employers and insurance companies to such potentially damaging information. For many years, lack of regulation of DNA testing laboratories frequently resulted in incorrect or ambiguous test results. Movements toward regulation and licensing of these laboratories are alleviating these problems.

—*Karen E. Kalumuck, Ph.D.*

See also Acquired immunodeficiency syndrome (AIDS); Anemia; Blood and blood disorders; Blood banks; Cholesterol; Circulation; Dialysis; DNA and RNA; Endocrine disorders; Ergogenic aids; Forensic pathology; Genetic counseling; Genetic diseases; Genetics and inheritance; Grafts and grafting; Hematology; Hematology, pediatric; Hormones; Human immunodeficiency virus (HIV); Immune system; Laboratory tests; Pathology; Pregnancy and gestation; Rh factor; Screening; Serology; Transfusion.

For Further Information:

Feldman, Eric A., and Ronald Bayer. *Blood Feuds: AIDS, Blood, and the Politics of Medical Disaster.* Oxford: Oxford University Press, 1999. Discusses the effect of the emergence of HIV on the medical establishment, the history of blood screening, and the plight of hemophiliacs who have contracted the virus through blood products. Advocates a safer blood supply and addresses the limitations of public policy.

Hillier, Christopher D., et al., eds. *Blood Banking and Transfusion Medicine: Basic Principles and Practice.* 2d ed. Philadelphia: Churchill Livingstone/Elsevier, 2007. Draws data from basic, transnational, and clinical studies; explores the latest advances in the use of blood products, new methods of disease treatment, and stem cell transplantation; and addresses a range of controversies in practice.

Pagana, Kathleen Deska, and Timothy J. Pagana. *Mosby's Diagnostic and Laboratory Test Reference.* 7th ed. St. Louis: Elsevier Mosby, 2005. A clinical handbook that gives alphabetically organized laboratory and diagnostic tests for easy reference. Each listing includes such things as alternate or abbreviated test names; type of test; normal findings; possible critical values; test explanation and related physiology; and potential complications.

Rodak, Bernadette, ed. *Hematology: Clinical Principles and Applications.* 2d ed. Philadelphia: W. B. Saunders, 2002. A comprehensive textbook covering all aspects of hematology and hemostasis.

Schaub Di Lorenzo, Marjorie, and Susan King Strasinger. *Blood Collection in Healthcare.* Philadelphia: F. A. Davis, 2001. Details all phlebotomy issues important in collecting a quality blood specimen and includes excellent photographs that clearly demonstrate the preferred techniques, supplies, and collection procedures.

Youngson, Robert M. "Blood Transfusion." In *The Surgery Book: An Illustrated Guide to Seventy-three of the Most Common Operations.* New York: St. Martin's Press, 1993. A chapter in an atlas of common surgeries. Includes an index.

Blood transfusion. *See* Transfusion.

Blue baby syndrome

Disease/disorder

Also known as: Tetralogy of Fallot

Anatomy or system affected: Circulatory system, heart

Specialties and related fields: Cardiology, embryology, neonatology

Definition: A congenital heart disease consisting of four distinct defects that result in poorly oxygenated blood being delivered to the tissues, thereby causing a bluish discoloration of the skin and mucous membranes upon birth.

Causes and Symptoms

Most congenital heart defects are thought to arise from maternal infections or the intake of certain drugs during pregnancy. The developing fetal heart is particularly susceptible to these effects during the second month of pregnancy, when major developmental changes are taking place.

Four distinct defects, called the tetralogy of Fallot, occur in infants suffering from blue baby syndrome. The first is a narrowing (stenosis) of the pulmonary trunk that takes blood to the lungs, where it is oxygenated. Narrowing of the pulmonary trunk is accompanied by a narrowing of the pulmonary semilunar valve, which resides in the pulmonary trunk. These two defects decrease blood flow to the lungs, resulting in a decreased oxygenation of the blood. Second, the wall that separates the left and right ventricles of the heart fails to form completely, thereby allowing the poorly oxygen-

INFORMATION ON BLUE BABY SYNDROME

CAUSES: Congenital heart defects resulting in poorly oxygenated blood delivered to body tissue
SYMPTOMS: Bluish discoloration of skin and mucous membranes upon birth, breathlessness after exertion
DURATION: Temporary, once corrected
TREATMENTS: Surgery

ated blood in the right ventricle to mix with the well-oxygenated blood in the left ventricle and decreasing oxygen delivery to tissues. Third, the aorta, which typically opens from the left ventricle and carries oxygenated blood to the tissues, is misaligned such that it opens from both the left and right ventricle. Fourth, the right ventricular muscle is thickened, as this muscle must work harder to push blood through the narrowed pulmonary semilunar valve and pulmonary trunk.

The first three defects result in poorly oxygenated blood being delivered to tissues, causing the skin and mucous membranes to appear bluish within minutes after birth, a condition called cyanosis. Children with uncorrected blue baby syndrome suffer from breathlessness after any form of exertion.

TREATMENT AND THERAPY

The tetralogy of Fallot is relatively rare, occurring in about 1 in every 1,500 births. Most defects can be corrected surgically. Successful correction of these defects early in the child's life prevents delayed growth and other complications of poor oxygen delivery.

—David K. Saunders, Ph.D.

See also Apgar score; Birth defects; Cardiology, pediatric; Cardiovascular system; Circulation; Congenital heart disease; Cyanosis; Heart; Neonatology; Surgery, pediatric.

FOR FURTHER INFORMATION:

Gersh, Bernard J., ed. *The Mayo Clinic Heart Book*. 2d ed. New York: William Morrow, 2000.

Koenig, Peter, Ziyad M. Hijazi, and Frank Zimmerman, eds. *Essential Pediatric Cardiology*. New York: McGraw-Hill, 2004.

Levin, Daniel L., and Frances C. Morriss, eds. *Essentials of Pediatric Intensive Care*. 2d ed. New York: Churchill Livingstone, 1997.

MacDonald, Mhairi G., Mary M. K. Seshia, and Martha D. Mullett, eds. *Avery's Neonatology: Pathophysiology and Management of the Newborn*. 6th ed. Philadelphia: Lippincott Williams & Wilkins, 2005.

Neill, Catherine A., Edward B. Clark, and Carleen Clark. *The Heart of a Child: What Families Need to Know About Heart Disorders in Children*. 2d ed. Baltimore: Johns Hopkins University Press, 2001.

Nixon, Harold, and Barry O'Donnel. *The Essentials of Pediatric Surgery*. 4th ed. Boston: Butterworth Heinemann, 1992.

Park, Myung K. *Pediatric Cardiology Handbook*. 3d ed. New York: Mosby, 2003.

BLURRED VISION

DISEASE/DISORDER

ANATOMY OR SYSTEM AFFECTED: Eyes

SPECIALTIES AND RELATED FIELDS: Emergency medicine, environmental health, family medicine, geriatrics and gerontology, gynecology, internal medicine, occupational health, ophthalmology, optometry, pediatrics, pharmacology, preventive medicine, sports medicine

DEFINITION: A decrease in clarity of vision (visual acuity).

CAUSES AND SYMPTOMS

Blurred vision can result from any disturbance in the pathway of light as it travels from the cornea (the front of the eye) to the retina. By far the most common causes, however, are myopia (nearsightedness), hyperopia (farsightedness), astigmatism (failure of the eye to focus light evenly), and presbyopia (age-related difficulty in keeping near objects in focus). With nearsightedness and astigmatism, distance vision tends to be blurred. With farsightedness, near vision is blurred. Presbyopia is first noticed as middle-aged persons find difficulty in reading small type, such as that in telephone directories. Common, too, are incidents of blurred vision caused by improper prescription lenses or by improperly fitted or misused contact lenses.

Viral conjunctivitis (pinkeye) may produce blurred vision. It may be a symptom of infections of the retina by viruses, fungi, or parasites (often seen in AIDS patients) and of many other eye disorders including cataracts, glaucoma, and macular degeneration.

Blurred vision may also be a symptom of an underlying disease or disorder. Diabetes is a common cause; blurred vision can also result from the fluctuations in blood sugar level common to women in pregnancy.

Information on Blurred Vision

Causes: Myopia, hyperopia, astigmatism, presbyopia, viral conjunctivitis, retinal infections, disease, injury, environmental factors, medications
Symptoms: Difficulty reading small type, lack of visual acuity or focus
Duration: Temporary to chronic
Treatments: New or corrected lens prescription, medications, surgery

Blurred vision has been connected with kidney and nerve disease and with hypertension; it may be a warning sign or symptom of a stroke. Blurred vision has been associated with migraine headaches and brain tumors.

Environmental factors may also produce blurred vision. The most common environmental cause is extended exposure to the glare of computer monitors. Blurred vision can also result from injuries to the eye and head, exposure to chemical spills, and reactions to pollen, wind, sunlight, soaps, lotions, or cosmetics. Welders' exposure to ultraviolet radiation can produce blurred vision. Many prescription medicines, including some antibiotics, antihistamines, antidepressants, appetite suppressants, hormonal supplements, and blood pressure medications can cause difficulty in focusing. Steroids, which can lead to glaucoma, may also cause a swift rise in blood sugar, producing blurred vision.

Treatment and Therapy

Therapy and treatment depend on quick and reliable diagnosis of the cause, so examination by an ophthalmologist is advisable; adults should regularly schedule such examinations. Injuries to the eye or head and blurred vision in conjunction with any other symptom of retinal detachment require emergency care. Problems with prescription lenses may be taken either to opticians or ophthalmologists. Persons suffering from computer-screen glare may benefit from antireflective coatings on eyeglasses or glare-cutting filters that fit over computer monitors.

—Betty Richardson, Ph.D.

See also Astigmatism; Brain disorders; Cataracts; Conjunctivitis; Diabetes mellitus; Eye infections and disorders; Eye surgery; Eyes; Glaucoma; Hypertension; Macular degeneration; Migraine headaches; Myopia; Occupational health; Ophthalmology; Optometry; Optometry, pediatric; Sense organs; Sjögren's syndrome; Steroids; Strokes; Vision disorders.

For Further Information:

Beers, Mark H., et al., eds. *The Merck Manual of Medical Information, Second Home Edition.* Whitehouse Station, N.J.: Merck Research Laboratories, 2003.

Buettner, Helmut, ed. *Mayo Clinic on Vision and Eye Health: Practical Answers on Glaucoma, Cataracts, Macular Degeneration, and Other Conditions.* Rochester, Minn.: Mayo Foundation for Medical Education and Research, 2002.

Cassel, Gary H., Michael D. Billig, and Harry G. Randall. *The Eye Book: A Complete Guide to Eye Disorders and Health.* Baltimore: Johns Hopkins University Press, 1998.

Komaroff, Anthony, ed. *Harvard Medical School Family Health Guide.* New York: Free Press, 2005.

National Foundation for Eye Research (NFER). http://www.nfer.org/. Provides consumers and professionals with access to developing technology for treating impaired vision.

Sardegna, Jill, et al. *Encyclopedia of Blindness and Vision Impairment.* 2d ed. New York: Facts On File, 2002.

Boils

Disease/disorder

Also known as: Skin abscesses

Anatomy or system affected: Immune system, skin

Specialties and related fields: Dermatology, family medicine, pediatrics

Definition: A localized bacterial infection deep in the skin.

Causes and Symptoms

Boils are skin lesions most often caused by *Staphylococcus aureus*, a common skin bacterium. A boil begins as a hard red nodule at an opening of the skin, the base of a hair follicle, or plugged sweat gland. During the next three to four days, inflammatory white cells invade the skin tissue, changing the hard nodule into a small pustular lesion often called a furuncle. On occasion, a large furuncle develops multiple pustules and forms a carbuncle. Other lesions formed by this same process are cystic acne, and boils in the glandular tissue under the arms and in the groin are called hidradenitis suppurativa.

Anyone can develop a boil, but people with an impaired immune system or a chronic illness such as dia-

Information on Boils

Causes: Staphylococcal infection at skin opening, hair follicle, or plugged sweat gland
Symptoms: Hard red nodule that changes into small pustular lesion (furuncle); may develop multiple pustules (carbuncle)
Duration: Acute
Treatments: Hot compresses or soaks, lancing by a health care provider

betes or kidney disease have an increased risk. Also, many medications can suppress the normal immune response and increase the risk of developing boils. These medications include steroids such as cortisone and drugs used to treat cancer.

Treatment and Therapy

The initial treatment for most boils is the application of heat. Hot compresses or hot soaks will increase the circulation and bring antibodies and white blood cells to the site of infection. It is not recommended to lance or drain a boil until it becomes soft and forms a pustule. Often with very large boils it is necessary to have them lanced by a health care provider. A pilonidal cyst or hidradenitis suppurativa often requires the surgical removal of sweat glands.

Antibiotics are not immediately necessary unless there is infection of the surrounding skin or high fever or the patient is in poor health or has a compromised immune system. A health care provider should be contacted if the boil worsens, does not resolve in two weeks, or is accompanied with fever or if red lines radiate from the boil.

A serious complication occurs if the boil is infected with methicillin-resistant *Staphylococcus aureus* (MRSA). This bacterium is resistant to penicillin and other drugs commonly used to treat boils. Once mainly confined to hospitals, MRSA now affects many people in the community. It is highly contagious and spreads rapidly in crowded conditions. Serious MRSA infections respond well to several antibiotics, however if treated with the wrong medications, the infection can be difficult to control. To prevent the spread of this disease, it is important for people to keep skin lesions well covered, wash their hands after touching wounds or dressings, and talk to their health care provider if their condition is not improving.

—*Jane Blood-Siegfried, R.N., D.N.Sc., C.P.N.P.*

See also Abscess drainage; Abscesses; Acne; Antibiotics; Bacterial infections; Blisters; Burns and scalds; Chickenpox; Cold sores; Cysts; Dermatitis; Dermatology; Dermatopathology; Eczema; Frostbite; Gangrene; Hand-foot-and-mouth disease; Herpes; Impetigo; Lice, mites, and ticks; Plague; Rashes; Scabies; Skin; Skin disorders; Smallpox; Staphylococcal infections; Sunburn.

For Further Information:

American Medical Association. *American Medical Association Family Medical Guide*. 4th rev. ed. Hoboken, N.J.: John Wiley & Sons, 2004.
Beers, Mark H., et al. *The Merck Manual of Diagnosis and Therapy*. 18th ed. Whitehouse Station, N.J.: Merck Research Laboratories, 2006.
Professional Guide to Diseases. 8th ed. Ambler, Pa.: Lippincott Williams & Wilkins, 2005.

Bonding

Development

Anatomy or system affected: Psychic-emotional system
Specialties and related fields: Neonatology, psychiatry, psychology
Definition: The formation of an attachment; specifically, the developing relationship between infants and their parents that begins immediately after birth.

Key terms:

attachment: the development of a nurturing relationship between an infant and its caretaker(s)
failure to thrive: a lack of healthy growth that may result from the absence of a nurturing presence and support, both emotionally and physically

Physical and Psychological Factors

Bonding is usually associated with neonates (newborns), but it is an ongoing relationship that occurs between infants, toddlers, or children and their caretakers.

After the initial cry, the neonate calms down and uses its first touch with the mother to relax. This experience may occur in a brightly lit hospital room with medical attendants or in a semidark birthing room at home with nurses or midwives attending. The sense of wonder that surrounds the birth process is often overwhelming for the mother and father, as well as for other relatives who may be present. Usually, the infant is placed on the mother's abdomen for contact to begin. The initial moments of connection may include the parents touching, rubbing, and stroking the baby's cheeks, fingers, toes, abdomen, and back. Research reports that even in these early moments, an infant may be engaged in limited imitations of the parents by moving the head, opening and closing the mouth, and responding to the facial gestures of the parents.

These first touches begin the relationship that may initiate a successful bonding attachment with the primary caregivers and the extended family. Some circumstances, however, may start a process that does not lead to successful attachment. The process of bonding between a newborn and caregivers is an essential part of normal development. The care that the infant receives at this point, as well as through the subsequent early stages of life, is vital to his or her healthy development. Some infants, however, may need ancillary medical care that removes the child from the mother's touch and postpones connecting immediately after birth.

As the infant begins to grow, the early stages of development should be supported, sharpened, and enhanced during the continuing developmental and bonding process. Babies are born with the desire to survive. They actively seek stimulation. The first week of life involves hearing, seeing, smelling, and touching. Distinguishing sounds is a learning process. Soft noises, lullabies, and soft music are soothing. Basic visual powers exist that are important for communication and learning. Infants are sensitive to the intensity of light. They can discriminate shapes and patterns. Feeding involves smelling food, distinguishing tastes, and becoming aware of the presence of the mother or primary caregiver. The infant can feel changes in temperature and respond to skin contact and touch.

While most bonding tends to be associated with the mother-infant relationship, the attachment and bonding process also includes the relationship with the father, siblings, and other relatives who come into frequent contact with the developing baby. The interaction within this social network creates a variety of relationships and opportunities for positive and responsive stimulation, support, and encouragement. Connections with grandparents, aunts, uncles, and cousins can provide strong supportive bonds that help infants thrive. The strength of these relationships can make up for limitations with the primary caregivers.

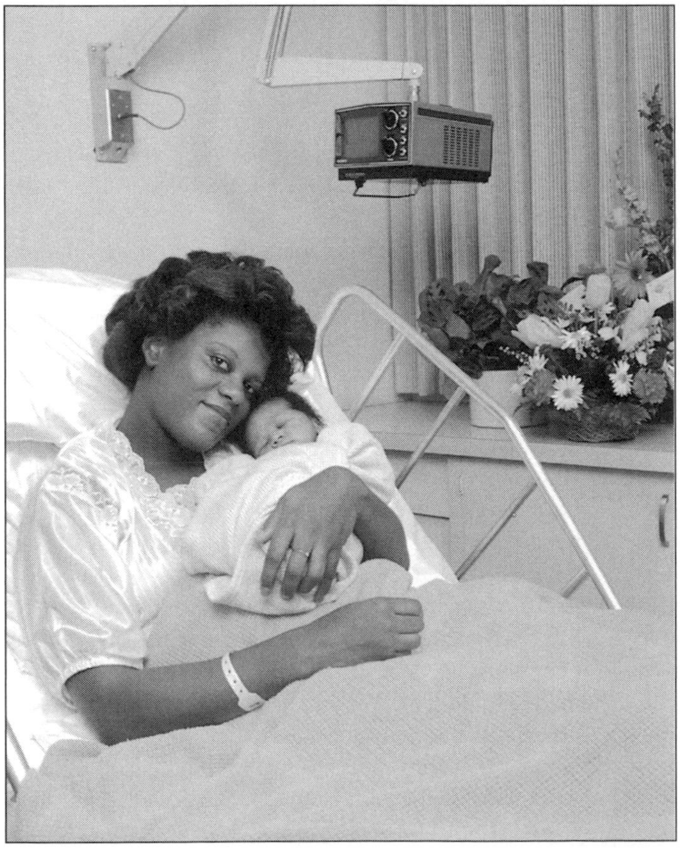

Bonding is an emotional and physiological process that begins at birth. (Digital Stock)

Disorders and Effects

The relationship between some caregivers and infants may encounter serious problems as they try to establish attachment. Bonding disorders such as failure to thrive can occur with infants who are abused or neglected. One of the major reasons that babies in institutions do not do well is the infrequent handling and touching that they receive.

Infants exhibiting failure to thrive show a variety of symptoms. They are usually quite small. They appear ill, listless, and immobile and may be unable to digest food. Other symptoms of failure to thrive include low birth weight, eye contact avoidance, and evidence of developmental retardation. Improvements can occur with appropriate feeding and care. Failure to thrive may also occur due to purely physical causes, such as congenital genetic disorders. Such disorders are generally not reversible, unless the specific defect can be corrected medically.

If a mother had early developmental experiences of abuse and neglect, these experiences may appear as obstacles to the development of her own infant. The mother of a failure-to-thrive infant may be using drugs or alcohol. She may be depressed, physically or mentally ill, or unable to cope well enough to provide a positive bonding experience for her child. She may have recently been involved in a significant crisis that was emotionally draining.

Significant variables may precede the attachment phase, or environmental forces may impede the infant's maternal attachment as the bonding process proceeds. If the infant does not have a positive experience with the mother during the first months of life, developmental problems may begin. When the mother or infant must remain in a hospital for a prolonged period of time, the mother may be unavailable; nurturing can be delayed or occur only for short periods. A mother may be psychologically unable to be close to her infant because of other young children or her own psychological problems or disorders. Some mothers experience postpartum depression as a result of hormonal imbalances and overwhelming demands. Economic and social circumstances may create situations that dampen the joy of the maternal process.

Establishing warm, comforting relationships through interactions between babies, parents, caregivers, and other family members in the earliest weeks is critical to forming secure attachments and developing successful bonding.

—Gwenelle S. O'Neal, D.S.W.; updated by Alexander Sandra, M.D.

See also Breast-feeding; Cognitive development; Developmental stages; Failure to thrive; Psychiatry, child and adolescent.

For Further Information:

Caplan, Theresa. *The First Twelve Months of Life: Your Baby's Growth Month by Month*. New York: Bantam, 1995. This reference book is the product of the Princeton Center for Infancy and Early Childhood's compilation of current research and ideas regarding infant and toddler development.

Cohen, Lawrence. *Playful Parenting*. New York: Random House, 2002. The author, a child psychologist, argues that play helps children communicate deep feelings, get close to those they care about, work through stressful situations, and ultimately, build strong bonds between parents and children.

Craig, Grace J., Marguerite D. Kermis, and Nancy Digdon. *Children Today*. 2d ed. Toronto: Pearson Education Canada, 2002. This text provides a comprehensive description of the prenatal and early stages of infant and child development.

Leach, Penelope. *Your Baby and Child: From Birth to Age Five*. 3d ed. New York: Alfred A. Knopf, 1997. This book pools the common experiences of different family types and their needs for information about raising children.

Mercer, Jean. *Understanding Attachment: Parenting, Child Care, and Emotional Development*. Westport, Conn.: Praeger, 2006. A valuable work designed for parents, child care providers, teachers, nurses, social workers, attorneys, therapists, students, and counselors. Defines attachment over the course of development and discusses attachment disorders.

Parker, DeAnsin Goodson, and Karen W. Bressler. *Yoga Baby: Exercises to Help You Bond with Your Baby, Physically, Emotionally, and Spiritually*. New York: Broadway Books, 2000. This book takes parents to the next step in baby bonding. Parker, a licensed child psychologist and certified yoga instructor, here outlines yoga positions that will benefit newborns to toddlers, revealing the results of her work with babies and their parents at New York's Goodson Parker Wellness Center.

Sears, William, and Martha Sears. *The Attachment Parenting Book: A Commonsense Guide to Understanding and Nurturing Your Baby*. New York: Little, Brown, 2001. The authors, the founders of the attachment parenting movement, advocate what they call "the six Baby B's": bonding, breast-feeding, babywearing, bedding close to baby, belief in the language value of baby's cry, and beware of baby trainers. This guide answers common parenting questions from their unique perspective.

Bone cancer

Disease/disorder

Anatomy or system affected: Bones, musculoskeletal system

Specialties and related fields: Immunology, oncology, orthopedics, radiology

Definition: Cancer of the bone, which may have originated there or have spread from another site in the body.

Key terms:

adjuvant therapy: the use of multiple treatments for cancer, such as chemotherapy and/or radiation, following surgery to prevent metastasis

biopsy: the removal of tissue from a suspected cancer

site in order to identify abnormal cells under microscopic examination by a pathologist

bone scan: a diagnostic technique using a radioactive tracer that is strongly absorbed by a tumor, whose location then can be detected by radiation counters

computed tomography (CT) scanning: a method of displaying the outline of a tumor, utilizing a computer to combine information from multiple X-ray beams

magnetic resonance imaging (MRI): a diagnostic technique used to see the outline of an internal organ or a tumor without using X rays

medullary cavity: the interior of a bone, where new blood cells are formed by the bone marrow, surrounded by a hard outer cortex

metastasis: the spread of cancer cells from an original tumor site to other parts of the body

palliative treatment: the use of drugs or radiation to suppress a tumor and to provide relief from pain when a cure is not possible

sarcoma: a malignant tumor originating in bone or connective tissue

staging: a numerical classification system used by physicians to describe how far a cancerous growth has advanced

Causes and Symptoms

Out of about one million new cancers that are diagnosed annually in the United States, less than 1 percent are primary bone cancer. Most of these cases arise in children under the age of twenty. If diagnosis is made before the bone cancer has spread to the lungs or other sites in the body, prompt treatment by surgery, radiation, or chemotherapy can provide a good prognosis for recovery.

In older adults, most cases of so-called bone cancer actually are secondary tumors that have spread from other parts of the body, especially from the breast, prostate, thyroid, lung, or kidney. Such metastasized tumors consist of cells that are characteristic of their original, primary site. Secondary bone cancers are far more common than those which start in the bone.

The first symptom of bone cancer in children usually is a localized swelling followed by persistent, dull pain. It is easily mistaken for a sprain or a bruise that might come from a minor injury. Additional symptoms are fatigue, fever, loss of appetite, and other signs of general illness. Unfortunately, early symptoms may be ignored until the disease has already spread to other parts of the body. Before chemotherapy became available in the 1970's, the spread of bone cancer to the lungs occurred within two years for about 80 percent of patients.

Information on Bone Cancer

Causes: Gene mutations in bone cells, metastasized tumors from other sites
Symptoms: Localized swelling followed by persistent, dull pain; fatigue, fever, loss of appetite, other signs of general illness
Duration: Acute or long-term
Treatments: Surgery, radiation, chemotherapy

A variety of diagnostic techniques are available to the physician if the examination of a patient arouses the suspicion of bone cancer. Blood tests, including a study of liver and kidney functions, have become increasingly useful because of improvements in analytical procedure. X-ray photography and computed tomography (CT) scanning will give pictorial evidence of any lesions or excess bony growth. Magnetic resonance imaging (MRI) provides the best visualization of tumors extending into soft tissue. Finally, the most important diagnostic procedure is biopsy. Usually, the bone is opened surgically and a sample of tissue is taken. Sometimes, a hollow needle inserted through the bone cortex can be used to withdraw a small sample. A pathologist who specializes in oncology examines the tissue under a microscope to confirm if cancer cells are present and to identify their type.

Magnetic resonance imaging as a diagnostic technique was developed in the 1980's, giving remarkable picture clarity for soft tissue. A strong magnetic field and radio waves are used to determine the concentration of hydrogen in a region of the body. Since tissue is mostly water (which contains hydrogen) and bone is dry, the image will show bright areas for tissue or soft organs against a dark background. Also, MRI shows contrast between normal tissue and a denser, tumorous mass.

Another diagnostic technique, the bone scan, is used to investigate whether a tumor has metastasized to other bones in the body. A small amount of radioactive tracer, usually technetium, is injected into the patient. It circulates in the bloodstream and gradually accumulates in the bone marrow. After several hours, radiation counters are used to scan the entire skeleton from head to foot. Regions of rapid cell growth, which may signal a tumorous mass, are indicated by a relatively high counting rate. If secondary tumors are detected by the bone scan, their shape and size can be investigated further using MRI.

Several kinds of bone cancer have been identified. One type is called osteosarcoma. It occurs most frequently during puberty, when a child's bones are growing rapidly. The tumor is likely to develop inside the long bones of the arms, in the legs near the knee, or in the pelvis. As its size increases and the surrounding bone material becomes soft, the bone may fracture because of internal pressure in the bone. Osteosarcomas also may grow on the exterior surface of bones, producing hard spikes that radiate outward. Another type of bone cancer is called Ewing's sarcoma. MRI and CT scans commonly exhibit a "moth-eaten" appearance where bone destruction has taken place. Both the inner (medullary) cavity and the outer cortex of the bone can be affected. Subsequently, a tumorous mass develops within the covering of tissue that surrounds the bone. This abnormal growth tends to form concentric layers, like the skin of an onion. The localized swelling expands in size, causing soreness and eventually impeding motion at the joints.

Bone cancer can take a variety of other forms. For example, a tumor may invade the bone from the outside and then penetrate into the medullary cavity. In order to make an accurate diagnosis and institute the best possible treatment for bone cancer, particularly for children, it is important for patients and their families to find an oncologist and supporting staff with specialized experience in this relatively rare condition. In general, the orthopedic surgeon who does the biopsy should be a specialist who is trained to do the ultimate bone surgery, so that any cancer cell contamination at the site of the biopsy will be completely removed.

Treatment and Therapy

In order to develop an appropriate treatment plan for a patient with bone cancer, all the relevant diagnostic information must be brought together. A medical team consisting of a radiologist, pathologist, radiation therapist, orthopedic surgeon, and medical oncologist will assess how far the cancer has advanced. This is called staging, that is, classifying its stage of growth.

Three designations commonly are used to characterize a cancer: G for its grade (based on the microscopic tissue analysis), T for tumor size and penetration, and M for evidence of metastasis. For example, (G1) (T2) (M0) would describe a low-grade tumor (G1) that has broken out of its bone compartment (T2) but has not metastasized (M0) to the lungs or elsewhere.

Before 1970, treatment of a cancerous bone normally meant amputation. The prognosis for recovery was less than 20 percent, however, because microscopic, invisible metastases to the lungs and other organs usually were already present. The experimental search for drugs that can fight cancer cells started in the 1930's. Dr. Charles B. Huggins discovered that the female sex hormone estrogen could halt the growth of prostate cancer in men. He received the Nobel Prize in Medicine in 1966 for his work. Since that pioneering success, several hundred thousand drugs have been tested, with less than a hundred showing any substantial benefit. The anticancer drugs also can have severe side effects on healthy cells. Fortunately, a rapidly growing tumor has a higher rate of metabolism, so drugs will kill the cancer cells at a lower dose and spare most normal cells.

An effective method of treating bone cancer in children is to use chemotherapy or radiation even before surgery, in order to shrink the size of a tumor. Instead of complete amputation, the surgeon may need to remove only part of a bone, thus saving the limb. Even when a bone joint must be amputated, it may still be possible to salvage the limb by inserting an artificial joint or one from an organ donor.

In older adults, cancer of the bone almost invariably is caused by metastasis from another location in the body. The tumor in the bone may be very painful. Radiation to the affected area can provide palliative treatment, while more aggressive action is taken against the primary cancer site.

A wide range of medications is available to help control pain and to counteract the disagreeable side effects of radiation or chemotherapy. Special attention is given to the diet of cancer patients to prevent weight loss and to maintain body strength. Loss of appetite and digestion problems are common symptoms during therapy. Strong painkilling drugs such as codeine and morphine sometimes are necessary. The dose should be limited, however, so that the patient's ability to interact socially is not completely lost.

Vigorous research to find more effective therapies for cancer is widely supported. The goal is to find procedures that are less mutilating, less expensive, and less painful for the patient. Promising new drugs must be tested to determine how large a dose is needed and how serious the side effects are. Therefore, patients may be asked to become volunteers in a clinical trial of an experimental treatment. Although people have a justified sense of reluctance to become "guinea pigs" in an untested therapy, clinical trials with human subjects have been essential in the development of successful medical procedures. Firm guidelines have been established for testing new therapies, such as the requirement to obtain the informed consent of patients and their families. In addition, doctors in the United States are responsible to a medical oversight committee and are obligated to submit their results for professional review. Cancer treatment can make progress through willing participation by patients in the carefully planned clinical trials.

Perspective and Prospects

Bone cancer first came to the attention of the American public in the 1920's through a notorious case of industrial poisoning. A manufacturing company in New Jersey was utilizing radioactive radium to make watch dials that would glow in the dark. The women workers who were hired to apply the luminous paint would twirl the paint brushes between their lips to make a fine tip. The ingested radium, being chemically similar to calcium, became concentrated in bones, especially of the jaw and neck. Eventually, more than forty workers died of bone cancer, including the company's chief chemist.

After this incident, it became clear that radiation has a particularly damaging effect on bone marrow. In fact, any rapidly dividing cells in the body are especially radiosensitive. This would include hair, skin, and the reproductive system. It is unfortunate that it took until the 1950's before X-ray fluoroscopes were removed from shoe stores. Parents were fascinated to see the bones of their child's foot inside a new shoe without realizing that the radiation was harmful.

Until 1970, the outlook for a child who developed bone cancer was very poor. In spite of amputation of the affected limb, 80 percent of the young patients died within two years. In 1972, Norman Jaffe and Emil Frei in Boston made a major breakthrough in therapy by giving their patients large doses of a drug called methotrexate after limb surgery. It was a new approach in chemotherapy to stop the cancer from spreading even though no metastasis was visible yet. The experimental drug was so powerful that other antidote drugs were given to control side effects. The first trial with seventeen children was very successful, with all of them still surviving after twenty-one months.

However, an article written in 1994 by Tim Beardsley summarizing the status of cancer in the United States came to a rather pessimistic conclusion. The cancer rate was higher and the likelihood of cure had not improved for most types of adult cancer since the "war on cancer" was initiated by President Richard M. Nixon in 1971. The cumulative effects of smoking, poor diet, and continuing exposure to harmful chemicals may help to explain this lack of progress. The good news was that the death rate from childhood cancer fell by almost half in that period. Early diagnosis and improved therapy have helped greatly. The family of a child with cancer can now look forward with substantial hope for a cure without recurrence.

—Hans G. Graetzer, Ph.D.

See also Bone disorders; Bones and the skeleton; Cancer; Chemotherapy; Ewing's sarcoma; Fracture and dislocation; Fracture repair; Malignancy and metastasis; National Cancer Institute (NCI); Nuclear radiology; Oncology; Orthopedic surgery; Orthopedics; Orthopedics, pediatric; Radiation therapy; Sarcoma; Stem cells; Tumors.

For Further Information:

American Cancer Society (ACS). http://www.cancer.org/. Designed for patients, family, and friends; health information seekers; ACS supporters; and professionals. Information on all cancers is wide ranging.

Cady, Blake, ed. *Cancer Manual*. 7th ed. Boston: American Cancer Society, 1986. A collection of forty essays on various aspects of cancer management, written for health care professionals. The article that discusses sarcomas of the bone requires some knowledge of medical terminology. One interesting chapter deals with worthless cures.

Dollinger, Malin, et al. *Everyone's Guide to Cancer Therapy*. 4th rev. ed. Kansas City, Mo.: Andrews & McMeel, 2002. An excellent source of medical information about cancer, written for the general public. Various cancer sites in the body are described, and one essay focuses on sarcomas of the bone. A helpful glossary of medical terminology is provided.

Dorfman, Howard D. and Bogdan Czerniak. *Bone Tumors*. St. Louis: Mosby, 1998. This volume represents one of the most complete and definitive pathology texts dealing with benign and malignant bone tumors. Its contents are drawn from the author's personal consultation experience plus the experience of the M.D. Anderson Hospital and the U.S. National Cancer Institute's surveillance epidemiology statistics.

Eyre, Harmon J., Dianne Partie Lange, and Lois B. Morris. *Informed Decisions: The Complete Book of Cancer Diagnosis, Treatment, and Recovery*. 2d ed.

Atlanta: American Cancer Society, 2002. This text from the American Cancer Society is intended for the layperson. It is exemplary in its discussion of cancer.

Janes-Hodder, Honna, and Nancy Keene. *Childhood Cancer: A Parent's Guide to Solid Tumor Cancers.* 2d ed. Cambridge, Mass.: O'Reilly and Associates, 2002. Covers a range of helpful information for parents with children suffering from cancer, including medical information about solid tumor childhood cancers such as bone sarcomas, liver tumors, and soft tissue sarcomas. Procedures, hospitalization, and educational, social, and financial issues are additional topics covered, among others.

Bone disorders

Disease/disorder

Anatomy or system affected: Back, bones, legs, musculoskeletal system

Specialties and related fields: Geriatrics and gerontology, oncology, orthopedics, rheumatology

Definition: The various traumatic events that can occur to the bones and the tissues surrounding them, such as fractures, dislocations, degenerative processes, infections, and cancer.

Key terms:

acute: referring to the sudden onset of a disease process

cartilage: connective tissue between bones that forms a pad or cushion to absorb weight and shock

chronic: referring to a lingering disease process

pathogen: any disease-causing microorganism

Causes and Symptoms

Bones are usually studied in combination with their surrounding structures because many of the disorders to which bones can be subjected also involve muscular, cartilaginous, and other tissues to which they are connected. Hence, a common term for this medical category is "musculoskeletal and connective tissue disorders."

There are 206 bones in the human body that serve three functions. Some form protective housing for body organs and structures; these include the skull, which encloses the brain, and the rib cage, which encloses the heart and lungs. Some support the body's posture and weight, including the spine and the bones of the hips and legs. The third function is motion: Most of the bones in the body are involved in movement. These bones include those of the hands, wrists, arms, hips, legs, ankles, and feet.

Bone consists of three sections: an outer layer called the periosteum; the hard bony tissue itself, consisting of mineral compounds that form rigid skeletal structures; and the interior, a spongy mass of cancellous (chambered) tissue, where blood marrow is manufactured and some fat cells are stored. Bone is living tissue. It is a depository for calcium, phosphate, and other minerals that are vital to many body processes. Calcium and phosphate in particular are constantly being deposited in and withdrawn from bone tissue to be used throughout the body.

Bones can be attacked in many ways: They can be broken or dislocated; the processes by which they form, grow, and maintain themselves can be compromised; they can be attacked by pathogens; they can be subject to a series of degenerative diseases that impede function and even destroy bone tissue; and they can become cancerous.

Dislocations take place when the bones of a joint are forced out of alignment. They may occur in the elbows of young children whose arms are forcibly pulled. Fractures are more common. They arise from sports activities, accidents, falls, or hundreds of possible causes, including various disease conditions.

Osteoporosis and other diseases can destroy bone structure to the point where fractures occur with minimal stress. This condition is common in elderly women. The supply of calcium within the bones is gradually drained, leaving the bones porous and brittle. Hip fractures occur often in these people. Also, compression fractures occur in the vertebrae (the bones of the spine), causing the spine to bend forward. A hump develops, and the patient may not be able to raise his or her head.

Osteomalacia is similar to osteoporosis. Called rickets in children, this disease is caused by a deficiency in

Information on Bone Disorders

Causes: Fractures, dislocations, degenerative processes, infections, cancer

Symptoms: Varies widely; may include porous and brittle bones, impaired movement, pain, inflammation, numbness and tingling

Duration: Acute to chronic

Treatments: Setting and immobilization of bones in cast or splint, surgery, medications (antirheumatic drugs, corticosteroids), supplements (vitamin D, calcium, hormone therapy), orthopedic support, lifestyle changes

vitamin D, which impairs the absorption of calcium by the bone. In this condition, bones become soft and pliable. In children, leg bones do not develop correctly and may become bowed. The chest and stomach may protrude.

Bone infection is called osteomyelitis; it occurs most often in children. Infection can be introduced to the bone by fracture or other exposure, or it can be carried to the bone in the blood.

By far the most prevalent long-term bone disorders are those in the general class of diseases called arthritis. Osteoarthritis, a common form, is sometimes called "wear-and-tear arthritis" because it usually surfaces in older people after years of work have constantly challenged certain joints. It occurs often in contact sports such as football, where its progression can be accelerated by years of rough-and-tumble activity. Joints are cushioned by pads of cartilage. Eventually, this cartilage can wear down and become rough. It cannot protect the bones of the joint, and little nodes form at the ends of the bones. Bones of the neck and back are often affected, as are the hips and knees.

Osteoarthritis is painful and debilitating, but it is rarely crippling. More painful and far more serious is rheumatoid arthritis, a progressive disease. It often starts with inflammation in the joints of the hands or feet and is usually bilateral, for example affecting both hands, both feet, or both knees. While rheumatoid arthritis may start with relatively mild inflammation, it can progress to severe deformity and even total destruction of the joint. Fingers and toes can become grossly twisted; the joint can become completely fused and immobile.

There are other relatively common forms of arthritis. People with the skin condition psoriasis can develop psoriatic arthritis. Reiter's syndrome is a form of arthritis that can be transmitted through sexual contact. Ankylosing spondylitis is a form of arthritis that can affect any of the joints in the torso, such as the shoulders and hips, but is most often found in the neck and spine. Patients with inflammatory bowel disease (IBD) may also develop a concomitant arthritis in the joints of the hands or feet.

The bone condition called gout can affect many joints, but it appears most often in the big toe. The body produces a substance called uric acid. If, for any reason, too much is produced, or if it is not properly eliminated, uric acid crystals can form around joints and trigger inflammation. Gout is extremely painful, and an attack may last for weeks.

The spine is subject to a wide range of disorders. One of the most common is the prolapsed (slipped) disk. The individual vertebrae of the spine are separated and cushioned by pads of cartilage called disks. For various reasons, a disk can bulge out and impinge on the nerves of the spinal column. The result can be severe pain, numbness, and loss of movement. In some individuals, the spine fails to grow correctly or becomes misaligned, or curved. This condition is called scoliosis. The curvature of the spine can cause the ribs on one side of the body to separate as those on the other side are pushed together. Over time, this separation can cause severe heart and lung problems.

Many cases of joint pain are attributable to inflammation of the tissues surrounding the bony structures. An example is bursitis, in which the bursa, a saclike membrane enclosing many joints, becomes inflamed. Repetitive activities, such as throwing a baseball, hitting a tennis ball, or scrubbing the floor on one's knees, can irritate the membrane and cause inflammation.

Bone cancers or tumors can be benign or malignant. Cancer rarely begins in the bone; it usually spreads there from a tumorous site elsewhere in the body. Of the cancers that arise directly within bone tissue, the most common are multiple myeloma and osteosarcoma.

Treatment and Therapy

In treating a fractured bone, the most important thing is to realign the segments and keep them immobile until they can fuse. Most often, the physician will X-ray the fracture, set the bones correctly, and immobilize the limb in a cast. If injury to the spinal column is suspected, the physician may also order computed tomography (CT) scanning. Surgery is sometimes required in order to set the bones, and the surgeon may join the bone segments together with pins, plates, or screws. In some cases, it is possible to cement bone fragments together with a special glue. Broken arms, legs, fingers, and toes can usually be easily immobilized with appropriate casts or splints. In cases of accidents, falls, or other trauma, if there is any suspicion of injury to the spinal column, it is critical not to move the patient. Movement can worsen the injury and even cause permanent paralysis.

Dislocations, like fractures, should be X-rayed. If the spinal column appears to be involved, CT scanning may be required. The misaligned bones are put back in their proper positions, and the joint is immobilized, often with a splint.

Osteoporosis requires both preventive and therapeutic care. If the physician recognizes that an individual, usually a postmenopausal woman, is at high risk for osteoporosis, supplementary calcium will be prescribed and, in some patients, estrogen replacement therapy. When osteoporosis has begun, supplementary calcium, vitamin D, and hormone therapy may check the progress of the disease.

A patient may suffer from acute back pain because of crushed vertebrae in the spine. Pain relievers such as aspirin may be required, and the patient may need orthopedic support. Gentle exercise is recommended to strengthen back muscles.

In osteomalacia, vitamin D, phosphorus, and calcium supplements are the mainstays of therapy. In osteomyelitis, antibiotics will usually eradicate the infection, but in some cases, surgery is required in order to remove infected tissue. In other cases, amputation is the only option.

The first line of therapy for osteoarthritis and rheumatoid arthritis is the relief of pain and inflammation. The physician may recommend rest and immobilization of the joint; heating pads and hot baths may give some relief. Exercise can maintain motility in the joints and help the patient avoid stiffness. Most patients are given over-the-counter pain relievers such as aspirin, ibuprofen, or acetaminophen. In a large number of patients, however, these drugs are either not adequate to manage the pain or, as in the case of aspirin, ibuprofen, and others, may be irritating to the gastrointestinal tract. Gastrointestinal disturbances are also common with the drugs proscribed for arthritis. Gastric and duodenal ulcers are often reported and are sometimes so severe that the patient requires surgery. In a small but significant number of patients who develop such ulcers, the outcome is fatal.

Because rheumatoid arthritis is a crippling disease that worsens over the years, the physician has an additional goal: to prevent the progress of the disease, avoiding bone deterioration and degeneration. In these patients, a group of drugs called disease-modifying antirheumatic drugs (DMARDs) may be used in conjunction with pain relievers. Corticosteroids are also used to alleviate acute episodes of pain and inflammation. They can be very effective, but they cannot be used over the long term and may have severe side effects.

Surgery is often required for arthritis patients. Synovectomy is a procedure in which part or all of the synovial membrane that surrounds the diseased joint is removed. It gives temporary relief in inflammation and may help preserve joint function. When a joint has deteriorated severely, the physician may recommend joint replacement therapy. In this procedure, the degenerated bone and joint structures are surgically removed and replaced with an orthopedic device of metal and/or plastic. This procedure is most effective in hip replacement, although it is also used in the knee.

Relief of pain is the main goal of therapy in other arthritic conditions such as psoriatic arthritis and Reiter's syndrome. In ankylosing spondylitis, exercise is also an important facet of treatment, to help avoid stiffening of the spine.

Gout has a tendency to recur. Therefore there are medications for acute episodes, such as pain relievers, and others to control levels of uric acid and prevent attacks.

Benign bone tumors sometimes require surgery. Malignant tumors can be treated surgically and may also require radiation and chemotherapy.

Perspective and Prospects

Radical new therapies for bone disorders are evolving, with exciting possibilities: bone regeneration, bone cements, and glues to knit fractures and replace bone destroyed by disease.

Osteoarthritis, rheumatoid arthritis, and other forms of arthritis continue to afflict vast populations around the world. Current medical treatment is significantly flawed by the incidence of side effects, especially gastrointestinal effects, from the medications used. The search for safer medications is ongoing, as is the search for treatment modalities that will halt the degenerative processes of rheumatoid arthritis.

Orthopedic implants are now quite successful in the hip, sometimes successful in the knee, but otherwise not universally useful in elbows, fingers, toes, and other joints that can be destroyed by disease. This is an area that is being addressed.

Operating techniques and instrumentation improve constantly. Many procedures are now done with the aid of arthroscopic instruments. Rather than an extensive incision to reveal the joint and surrounding tissues, the surgeon works through a tiny hole, through which he or she can inspect the inflamed joint and even perform minor surgery.

Operations on prolapsed spinal disks once entailed long incisions and laborious, careful removal of disk tissue. Fusion of the involved vertebrae was often necessary, limiting spinal movement. Healing time could be extensive. Today, simpler, less painful procedures may be as successful and far less traumatic. In one procedure, an enzyme is injected into the prolapsed disk, causing it to shrink and reducing pressure on nearby nerves. In another procedure, disk material is removed with a needle inserted through the skin into the disk.

Overall, progress in the treatment of bone disorders has been significant: Many people who would have lived with deformities and disability are being helped with modern medical and surgical techniques, medications, and instrumentation.

—C. Richard Falcon

See also Amputation; Arthritis; Bone cancer; Bone grafting; Bone marrow transplantation; Bones and the skeleton; Bowlegs; Bunions; Cerebral palsy; Chiropractic; Ewing's sarcoma; Feet; Flat feet; Foot disorders; Fracture and dislocation; Fracture repair; Hammertoe correction; Hammertoes; Head and neck disorders; Heel spur removal; Hip fracture repair; Hip replacement; Jaw wiring; Kneecap removal; Knock-knees; Kyphosis; Lower extremities; Orthopedic surgery; Orthopedics; Orthopedics, pediatric; Osgood-Schlatter disease; Osteochondritis juvenilis; Osteogenesis imperfecta; Osteomyelitis; Osteonecrosis; Osteoporosis; Paget's disease; Pigeon toes; Rheumatology; Rickets; Sarcoma; Scoliosis; Slipped disk; Spina bifida; Spinal cord disorders; Spine, vertebrae, and disks; Upper extremities.

For Further Information:

Hodgson, Stephen F., ed. *Mayo Clinic on Osteoporosis: Keeping Bones Healthy and Strong and Reducing the Risk of Fractures*. Rochester, Minn.: Mayo Clinic, 2003. A comprehensive overview of the disorder.

Hunder, Gene G. *Mayo Clinic on Arthritis*. Rev. ed. Rochester, Minn.: Mayo Clinic, 2002. Bones, muscles, and connective tissues are discussed, with disease conditions, symptoms, treatment, and outlook clearly explained. The text and illustrations are complete and easy to understand.

Lane, Nancy E., and Daniel J. Wallace. *All About Osteoarthritis: The Definitive Resource for Arthritis Patients and Their Families*. New York: Oxford University Press, 2002. Two leading doctors discuss a range of relevant topics, including how diagnosis is made, how the body is affected, methods to alleviate pain, good exercise regimens, and how to find the best resources to cope with the disorder.

Lenarz, Michael, and Victoria St. George. *The Chiropractic Way*. New York: Bantam, 2003. Explores the healing qualities of a rapidly growing alternative health field. Basic principles of spinal health, chiropractic techniques, and complementary diet, exercise, and stress-relief programs are covered.

National Institutes of Health. Osteoporosis and Related Bone Diseases National Resource Center. http://www.niams.nih.gov/bone/. Comprehensive site with newsletters, research bibliographies, and fact sheets, among other features.

Nelson, Miriam E., and Sarah Wernick. *Strong Women, Strong Bones: Everything You Need to Know to Prevent, Treat, and Beat Osteoporosis*. New York: G. P. Putnam, 2001. Basics of osteoporosis, adopting a therapeutic lifestyle, treatment and prevention, and research resources are covered.

Neuwirth, Michael, and Kevin Osborn. *The Scoliosis Sourcebook*. 2d ed. New York: McGraw-Hill, 2001. Origins of the disease, early detection and treatment, the pros and cons of braces, and surgery preparation are topics covered, as well as a comprehensive list of scoliosis organizations and associations.

Rosen, Clifford J., Julie Glowacki, and John P. Bilezikian. *The Aging Skeleton*. San Diego, Calif.: Academic Press, 1999. Although the target audience of this book is clinicians working in the area of osteoporosis, there is a sound coverage of the underlying biology, including recent developments in bone-cell biology and a useful description of animal models of osteoporosis.

Schommer, Nancy. *Stopping Scoliosis*. Rev. ed. New York: Putnam, 2002. Schommer covers the condition of scoliosis with thoroughness and clarity.

Yates, George, and Michael B. Shermer. *Meeting the Challenge of Arthritis*. Los Angeles: Lowell House, 1990. A good treatment of the arthritic diseases, covering their causes and treatment. Concentrates on helping patients to help themselves.

Bone fractures. *See* Fracture and dislocation.

Bone grafting

Procedure

Anatomy or system affected: Bones, immune system, musculoskeletal system

Specialties and related fields: Hematology, immunology, orthopedics

Definition: The transplantation of a section of bone from one part of the body to another, or from one individual to another.

Indications and Procedures

Ideally, the grafting procedure involves the transfer of bone tissue from one site to another on the same individual, which is termed an autogenous graft. This method eliminates the chance of rejection, allowing the transplantation of entire functional units of tissue: arteries, veins, and even nerves, as when a toe is used to replace a finger or thumb (toe-digital transfer). Autogenous rib or fibula grafts may be utilized for the reconstruction of the face or extremities.

Often, bone grafts are used during situations in which a bone fracture is not healing properly. A fracture that fails to heal in the usual time is considered to be a delayed union. Cancellous material from the bone (the spongy inner material), usually obtained from the iliac crest of the pelvis or from the ends of the long bones, is placed around the site. The fracture must then be immobilized for several months, allowing the grafted material to infiltrate and repair the fracture.

Uses and Complications

The grafting of bone tissue is carried out to correct a bone defect, to provide support tissue in the case of a severe fracture, or to encourage the growth of new bone. The source of the skeletal defect may be congenital malformation, disease, or trauma. For example, reconstruction may be necessary following cancer surgery, particularly for the jaw or bones elsewhere in the face.

If the autogenous bone supply is inadequate to fill the need, allogeneic bone grafts, the transplantation of bone from an individual other than an identical twin, may be necessary. Such foreign tissue is more likely to undergo rejection, reducing the chance of a successful procedure; the more closely the tissues of the two persons are matched, the less likely rejection will be a problem.

If the graft is able to vascularize quickly and to synthesize new tissue, the procedure is likely to be successful. The graft itself may provide structural support, or it may gradually be replaced by new bone at that site, completing the healing process.

—Richard Adler, Ph.D.

See also Amputation; Bone cancer; Bone disorders; Bones and the skeleton; Fracture and dislocation; Fracture repair; Grafts and grafting; Lower extremities; Oncology; Orthopedic surgery; Orthopedics; Osteonecrosis; Transplantation; Upper extremities.

For Further Information:

Bentley, George, and Robert B. Greer, eds. *Orthopaedics*. 4th ed. Oxford, England: Linacre House, 1993.

Callaghan, John J., Aaron Rosenberg, and Harry E. Rubash, eds. *The Adult Hip*. 2d ed. Philadelphia: Lippincott Williams & Wilkins, 2007.

Doherty, Gerard M., and Lawrence W. Way, eds. *Current Surgical Diagnosis and Treatment*. 12th ed. New York: Lange Medical Books/McGraw-Hill, 2006.

Eiff, M. Patrice, Robert L. Hatch, and Walter L. Calmbach. *Fracture Management for Primary Care*. 2d ed. Philadelphia: Saunders, 2003.

Lindholm, T. Sam. *Advances in Skeletal Reconstruction Using Bone Morphogenetic Proteins*. London: World Scientific, 2002.

Tapley, Donald F., et al., eds. *The Columbia University College of Physicians and Surgeons Complete Home Medical Guide*. Rev. 3d ed. New York: Crown, 1995.

Tierney, Lawrence M., Stephen J. McPhee, and Maxine A. Papadakis, eds. *Current Medical Diagnosis and Treatment 2007*. New York: McGraw-Hill Medical, 2006.

Bone marrow transplantation

Procedure

Anatomy or system affected: Back, blood, bones, immune system, musculoskeletal system

Specialties and related fields: General surgery, genetics, hematology, immunology, oncology

Definition: The replacement of diseased or inadequate bone marrow with healthy marrow.

Key terms:

bone marrow: the material in the center of bones that produces red blood cells (which carry oxygen), platelets (which stop bleeding), and white blood cells (which are the functional units of the immune system)

stem cell: a master cell from which other blood cells develop; these cells are primarily located in the bone marrow

Indications and Procedures

Bone marrow transplantation is used when the immune and blood-forming systems of the body are malfunctioning or have been severely damaged. Without adequate white blood cells, a person will soon die from infection. Transplantation is an attempt to cure or arrest diseases such as leukemia, cancer, and sickle cell disease and conditions such as brain tumors and hereditary

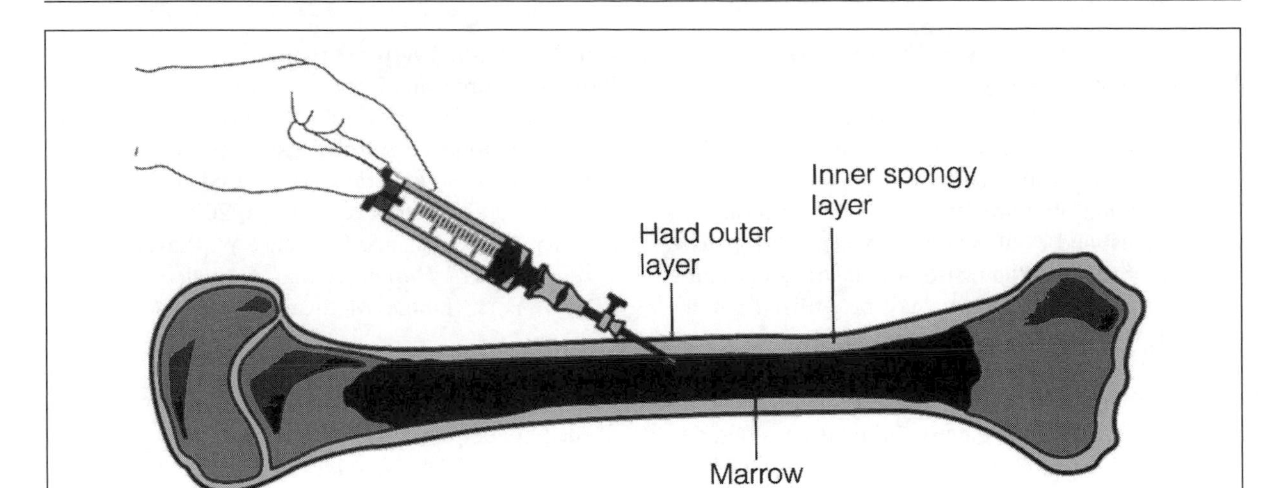

Bone marrow transplantation is used to treat several types of cancer. Marrow can be extracted from a donor or from the patient and reintroduced at a later time, usually after chemotherapy or radiation therapy.

diseases. Bone marrow transplantation is used when all other methods of treatment have failed. The procedure is usually performed on patients who are younger than fifty years old, with the greatest success rates found in children.

Before the procedure can be performed, a suitable donor must be found. The donor can be the patient (autologous transplantation) or someone else (allogeneic transplantation). Once the donor is identified, the bone marrow is harvested. This procedure is usually done under general anesthesia and takes one to two hours. A needle is inserted in the hip, and marrow is sucked out from different locations in the pelvic bone. Approximately 1 to 3 pints of marrow are taken. The donor usually stays overnight in the hospital and may be sore for one or two weeks following the operation.

The marrow, which contains the stem cells necessary to reestablish the blood-producing and immune systems of the patient, is processed and stored until the patient is prepared for the transplantation. During the hospital stay, the patient is kept in a sterile room to prevent infection. If the surgery is being performed on a cancer patient, the patient receives extensive chemotherapy and/or radiation before the donor marrow is transplanted; this action destroys any cancer cells in the patient, as well as his or her immune system.

The patient then receives the bone marrow transplantation in a manner similar to a blood transfusion: The donor cells are introduced through the veins and into the bloodstream. Until the transplanted cells begin to function (usually two to four weeks), the patient receives blood and platelet transfusions, as well as antibiotics to fight infection. The patient is usually discharged from the hospital in a month but must take antibiotics and antiviral medications for six months to two years after the transplantation because the recovery of the immune system is slow.

Uses and Complications

Bone marrow transplantation is a risky procedure with a success rate that ranges from 10 to 90 percent. One of the greatest obstacles is finding a suitable donor. The best possible match is between siblings, but even here the probability of a correct match is only 25 percent. Unrelated donor and patient matches made with marrow from donor banks increase the risk of a mismatch.

Finding a suitable donor is imperative because of the risk of graft-versus-host disease (GVHD). GVHD occurs when the donor cells recognize the host's body as foreign and react against it. This reaction may occur within a hundred or more days after the transplant and can vary in severity from a mild rash to the fatal destruction of tissue and organs. For correctly matched donors and recipients, the risk of life-threatening GVHD is 10 to 20 percent. For mismatched donors and recipients, the risk rises to 80 percent. In some cases, especially with leukemia and cancerous blood diseases, patients who suffer mild GVHD have an improved chance of survival because part of GVHD is a graft-versus-leukemia (GVL) effect. In these cases, the transplanted immune system acts against any remaining leukemia cells.

When the patient does not have a condition that damages the bone marrow, transplantation can be performed with his or her own marrow. After marrow has been collected from the patient, radiation and/or chemotherapy can be used to destroy the remaining immune system. Autologous transplantation eliminates the need to find a compatible donor and the risk of GVHD. This method can be used for treating solid tumors and has shown promise in curing brain tumors that were once considered fatal, with a success rate of 20 percent.

PERSPECTIVE AND PROSPECTS

Research on bone marrow transplantation began in the early 1950's, with the first successful transplantations performed on children in 1968. By the 1990's, more than five thousand bone marrow transplantations were being performed worldwide every year. The development of drugs that work to suppress the immune system has increased the chances for survival for these patients.

Several areas of research promise even better results in the future. A growing understanding of disease at the genetic level offers the possibility of separating unhealthy bone marrow cells from healthy ones. Methods of growing cells outside the body for use in transplantation are being developed. Progress has also been made in increasing the donor pool. National and international programs actively seek potential donors. Healthy people may begin storing their own bone marrow for a possible need in the future.

Perhaps one of the most promising potential sources of donor bone marrow is umbilical cord blood, which is rich in stem cells. Transplants using umbilical cord blood were first used in 1989 and have proven very successful. If established, umbilical cord blood banks could greatly increase the quantity of available donor marrow.

—*Virginia L. Salmon*

See also Blood and blood disorders; Blood banks; Bones and the skeleton; Cancer; Chemotherapy; Immune system; Immunology; Immunopathology; Leukemia; Oncology; Radiation therapy; Sickle cell disease; Stem cells; Transfusion; Transplantation.

FOR FURTHER INFORMATION:

Blood and Marrow Transplant Information Network. http://www.bmtinfonet.org/. Site contains resource directory, information on transplant centers in the United States and Canada, a drug database, and news bulletin, among other features.

Bolwell, Brian J., ed. *Current Controversies in Bone Marrow Transplantation.* Totowa, N.J.: Humana Press, 2000. This work provides useful insights about the most common clinical questions that are still being debated by physicians who work in the field of hematopoietic stem cell transplantation. The topics range from transplant strategies to the complications of bone marrow transplantation.

Bone Marrow Transplantation and Peripheral Blood Stem Cell Transplantation. Rev. ed. Bethesda, Md.: U.S. Department of Health and Human Services, Public Health Service, National Institutes of Health, 1994. A research report from the NIH that includes bibliographic references.

Marget, Madeline. *Life's Blood.* New York: Simon & Schuster, 1992. Presents basic information on bone marrow transplantation, supplemented by interviews with doctors and the stories of patients and their families.

Marshak, Daniel R., David Gottlieb, and Richard L. Gardner, eds. *Stem Cell Biology.* Cold Spring Harbor, N.Y.: Cold Spring Harbor Laboratory Press, 2002. Text that provides a broad foundation for understanding stem cell biology, with topics that include human adult bone marrow, the ovary as a stem cell system, and embryonal carcinoma cells as embryonic stem cells.

National Research Council. *Stem Cells and the Future of Regenerative Medicine.* Washington, D.C.: National Academy Press, 2002. A lay exploration of the scientific and ethical debate surrounding stem cell research, as well as an overview of medical advances and leading recommendations for the use of stem cells.

Stewart, Susan K. *Autologous Stem Cell Transplants: A Handbook for Patients.* Highland Park, Ill.: Blood and Marrow Transplant Information Network, 2000. Explains the procedure with solid medical and pharmaceutical information and tells the stories of people who have gone through the experience.

Swerdlow, Joel L. "A New Kind of Kinship." *National Geographic* 180, no. 3 (September, 1991): 64-92. This article addresses advances in transplantation and research, as well as the need for organ and tissue donors.

Bones and the skeleton

Anatomy

Anatomy or system affected: Back, feet, hips, legs, musculoskeletal system

Specialties and related fields: Exercise physiology, orthodontics, orthopedics, osteopathic medicine, podiatry, sports medicine

Definition: Bones are hard tissues that form the skeleton, the structure underlying the softer tissues of the body; they provide support while allowing flexibility.

Key terms:

calcitonin: a hormone made and released by the thyroid gland that lowers the level of calcium in the blood by stimulating the formation of bone

collagen: a protein found in bone and other connective tissues; collagen fibers are well suited for support and protection because they are sturdy, flexible, and resist stretch

hormones: molecules made in the body and released into the blood that act as chemical messengers for the regulation of specific body functions

matrix: in bone, the matrix is a solid nonliving material that is a composite of protein fibers and mineral crystals

osteoblast: a bone cell that can produce and form bone matrix; osteoblasts are responsible for new bone formation

osteoclast: a large bone cell that can destroy bone matrix by dissolving the mineral crystals

osteocyte: the primary living cell of mature bone tissue

tissue: a collection of similar cells that perform a specific function

Structure and Functions

Bones are active throughout life: The 206 bones of the skeleton establish the size and proportions of the body and interact with all other organ systems. Disorders of the skeleton can have profound effects on the other organ systems and serious health consequences for the organism.

Bone, or osseous tissue, contains specialized cells and a solid, stony matrix. The unique hardened quality of the matrix results from layers of calcium salt crystals such as calcium phosphate, which is responsible for about two-thirds of a bone's weight, and calcium carbonate. The living cells found in bone account for less than 2 percent of the total bone mass.

Despite the great strength of the calcium salts, their inflexible nature means that they can fracture when exposed to sufficiently great bending or twisting forces, or to sharp impacts. Because the calcium crystals exist as minute plates positioned on a framework of collagen protein fibers, the resulting composite structure does lend a certain degree of flexibility to the bone matrix.

Based on the internal organization of its matrix, bone is classified as either compact (dense) bone or cancellous (spongy) bone. Compact bone is internally more solid, while cancellous bone is made from bony filaments (trabeculae) whose branching interconnections form a three-dimensional network. The cavities of the cancellous bone network are filled usually by bone marrow, the primary location for blood cell formation in adults.

Both types of bone contain bone cells (osteocytes) living in small chambers called lacunae, found periodically between the plates of the matrix. Microscopic channels (canaliculi) connect neighboring lacunae and permit the exchange of nutrients and wastes between osteocytes and accessible blood vessels. Osteocytes provide the collagen fibers and the conditions for proper maintenance of the mineral crystals of the matrix.

A typical skeletal bone has a central marrow cavity that is bordered by cancellous bone. This is enclosed by compact bone, and the outer surface is covered by periosteum. Periosteum consists of a fibrous outer layer and a cellular inner layer. The periosteum plays an important part in the growth and repair of bone, and it is the attachment site for muscles. Collagen protein fibers from the periosteum interconnect with the collagen fibers of the bone.

The marrow cavity inside the bone is lined by endosteum. Endosteum is an incomplete layer covering the trabeculae of cancellous bone and contains a variety of different types of cells. The endosteum also plays important roles during bone growth and repair.

The bone matrix is not an unchanging, permanent structure. During the life of a person, the bone matrix is being constantly dissolved while new matrix is synthesized and deposited. Approximately 18 percent of the protein and mineral constituents of bone are replaced each year. Such bone remodeling can result in altered bone shape or internal rearrangement of the trabeculae. It may also result in a change in the total amount of minerals stored in the skeleton. These processes of bone demineralization (osteolysis) and new bone production (osteogenesis) are precisely regulated in the healthy individual.

The type of bone cell responsible for dissolving the

mineralized matrix is called an osteoclast. The cells that produce the materials that later become the bony matrix are called osteoblasts. The activities of these cells are influenced by several hormones as well as by the physical stress forces to which a bone may be exposed, such as when a particular muscle becomes stronger as the result of weight training and pulls more strongly on the bones to which it is attached. Increased stress forces on a bone result in that bone becoming thicker and stronger, thereby allowing the bone to withstand better the stresses and reducing the risks of bone fracture. When bones are not subjected to ordinary stresses, such as in persons confined to bed or in astronauts living in microgravity conditions during space flight, there is a corresponding loss of bone mass, with the unstressed bones becoming thinner and more brittle. After several weeks in an unstressed state, a bone can lose nearly a third of its mass. Following the resumption of normal loading stresses, the bone can regain its mass just as quickly.

The skeleton has five major functions: support for the body; protection of the soft tissues and organs; leverage to change the direction and size of the muscular forces; blood cell production, which occurs within the red marrow residing in the marrow cavities of many bones; and storage of both minerals (to maintain the body's important reserves of calcium and phosphate) and fats (in yellow marrow to serve as an important energy reserve for the body).

The human skeleton contains 206 bones. These are distributed between two subdivisions of the skeleton: the axial skeleton and the appendicular skeleton. The axial skeleton contains 80 bones distributed among the skull (29 bones), the chest, or thoracic, cage (25 bones), and the spinal (vertebral) column (26 bones). The remaining 126 bones are found in the appendicular skeleton's components: 4 bones in the shoulder (pectoral) girdles, 60 bones in the arms (including the 54 bones located in both of the hands and wrists), 2 bones in the hip (pelvic) girdle, and 60 bones in the legs (including the 52 bones found in the ankles and feet).

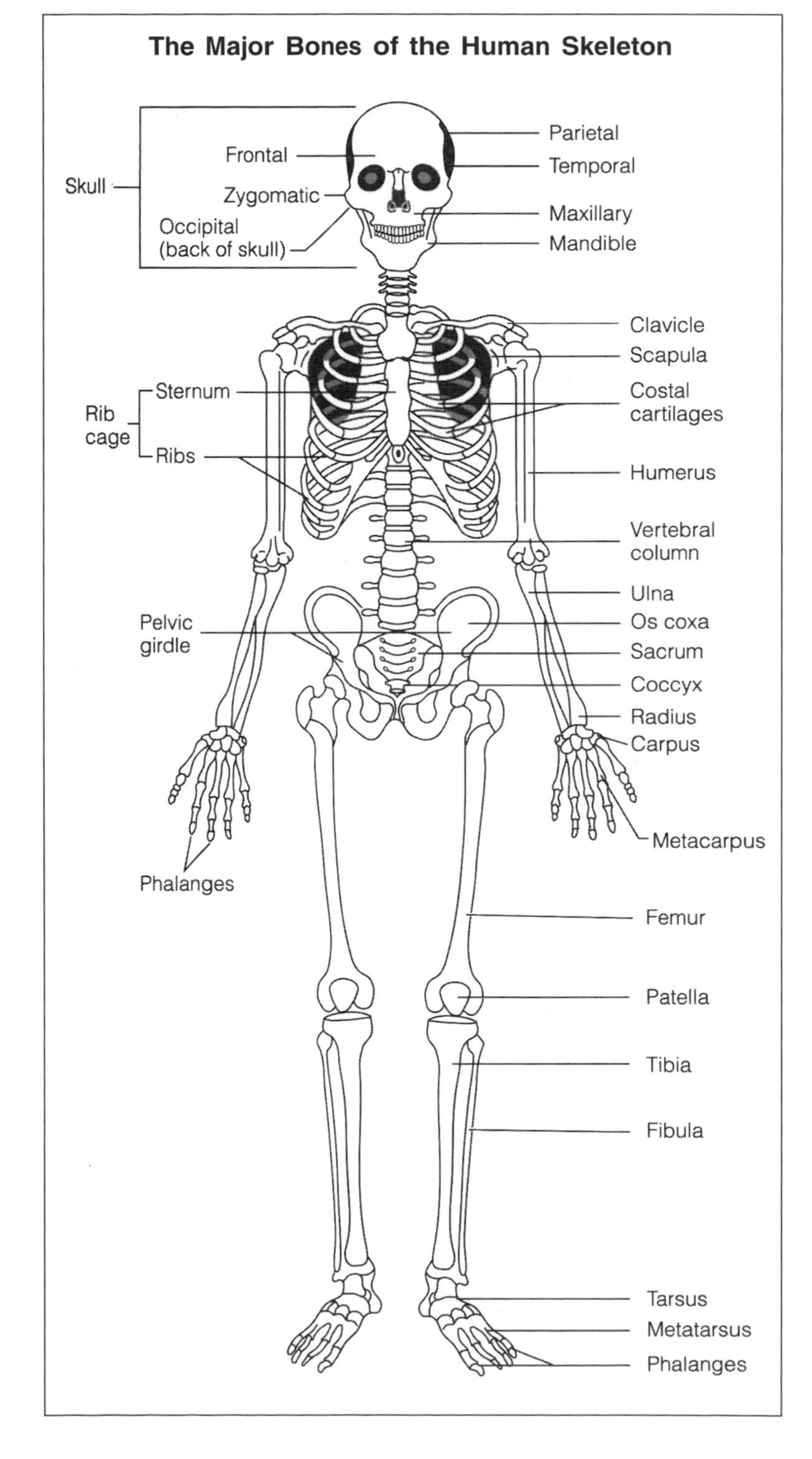

Skeletal bones are classified according to their shape. Long bones occur in the upper arm, the forearm, the thigh, the lower leg, the palm, the fingers, the sole of the foot, and the toes. Short bones are cuboid in shape and are found in the wrist and the ankle. Flat bones form the top of the skull, the shoulder blade, the breastbone, and the ribs. Sesamoid bones are typically small, round, and flat. They are found near some joints, such as the kneecap on the front of the knee joint. Irregular bones have shapes that are difficult to describe because of their complexity. Examples of irregular bones are found in the spinal column and the skull.

Learning to name the bones solely by their appearance is made somewhat easier by the fact that each one has a definitive form and distinctive surface features. The places where blood vessels and nerves enter into a bone, or lie along its surface, are commonly discernible as indentations, grooves, or holes. The locations where muscles are connected to bones by tendons, or where a bone is tethered to another bone by ligaments, are often clearly visible as elevations, projections, or ridges of bony matrix, or as roughened areas on the surface of the bone. Finally, the areas of the bone that are involved in forming joints (articulations) with other bones have characteristic shapes that impart particular properties to the joint. Various specialized terms are used to name these features.

Articulations are found wherever one bone meets another. The amount of motion permitted between the bones forming an articulation ranges from none (for example, between the skull bones) to considerable (as at the shoulder joint). The anatomy of the joint determines its functional capability, and the parts of the bones that form the joint have distinctive structural features.

Disorders and Diseases

Among the disorders of the skeleton, a number of them occur during the growth and development of the bones. The problems usually result in abnormal (most often decreased) stature or abnormal shape of the bones. The aberrations may alter the entire skeleton or be restricted to a portion of it. The basis of the pathology is to be found in a disruption of the normal, orderly sequence of events that take place during the growth and remodeling of the bones.

Osteopetrosis belongs to this class of disturbance. It is an inherited condition in which abnormal remodeling results in increased bone density. This seems to result from a reduced level of activity by the cells responsible for dissolving the bone matrix—the osteoclasts. In healthy, normal individuals, there is a precisely regulated relationship between osteoclast and osteoblast activity. Depending on the current needs of the body, or merely those of a single bone, the rate of bone matrix formation by osteoblasts may be greater than, equal to, or less than the rate of bone resorption by osteoclasts.

Osteoclasts are derived from cells that are made in the bone marrow. For this reason, bone marrow transplantation has been tried as a treatment for osteopetrosis; however, only a few patients have been successfully cured by this approach. There has also been some improvement in the condition of at least one osteopetrosis patient following treatment with a hormone related to vitamin D. This particular hormone can increase bone resorption and thereby may prevent the increase in bone density that characterizes this condition.

Another member of this category of disturbance is commonly referred to as cretinism. The basic problem in cretinism is underactivity of the thyroid gland during the development of the fetus, resulting in a decrease in the production of thyroid hormones in the fetus. This condition can be caused by an insufficient supply of the element iodine in the pregnant mother, or it may result from inherited errors in the production of the thyroid hormones.

Among the organ systems seriously affected by this condition is the skeleton. The bones do not develop correctly and show retarded growth in length. Consequently, the bones are shorter and thicker than normal, with corresponding changes in the appearance of the child. Early diagnosis of the condition and timely treatment with drug forms of the thyroid hormones can halt the disease. Otherwise, the adult skeleton has the form referred to as a dwarf, with stubby arms and legs, a somewhat flattened face, and disproportionately large chest and head.

A disorder of the pituitary gland can result in skeletal development abnormalities that are opposite to those observed in cretinism: namely, excessive growth in the length of bones. This condition is called giantism (or gigantism) and results from the overproduction of growth hormone by the pituitary gland before normal adult stature has been achieved. The most common cause of this situation is a tumor in the pituitary gland. Cases are known of people attaining heights of more than eight feet tall. Unfortunately, because of complications involving other organ systems as a result of the excessive production of growth hormone, the persons suffering from this disorder usually die before the age of thirty.

Surgical removal of the pituitary tumor is often attempted. If the tumor is successfully removed, then the overproduction of growth hormone will be stopped. In other cases, radiation treatments are used to destroy the tumor. It is also possible to combine both of these treatment techniques. Drug therapy is also possible. Because of the high doses necessary and the accompanying side effects of high drug dosages, however, the reduction of growth hormone levels through drug treatment is usually applied only in conjunction with one or both of the other therapies.

There are also disorders that afflict adult bone. Most of the remodeling disorders involve a loss of bone mass. The group of disorders known as osteoporosis (porous bone) is a rather common example that affects approximately 29 percent of women and 18 percent of men between the ages of forty-five and seventy-nine in the United States. The reduction in bone mass is sufficient to result in increased fragility and ease of breakage. There is also slower healing of bone fractures. In advanced cases, bones have been known to break when the person sneezes or simply rolls over in bed.

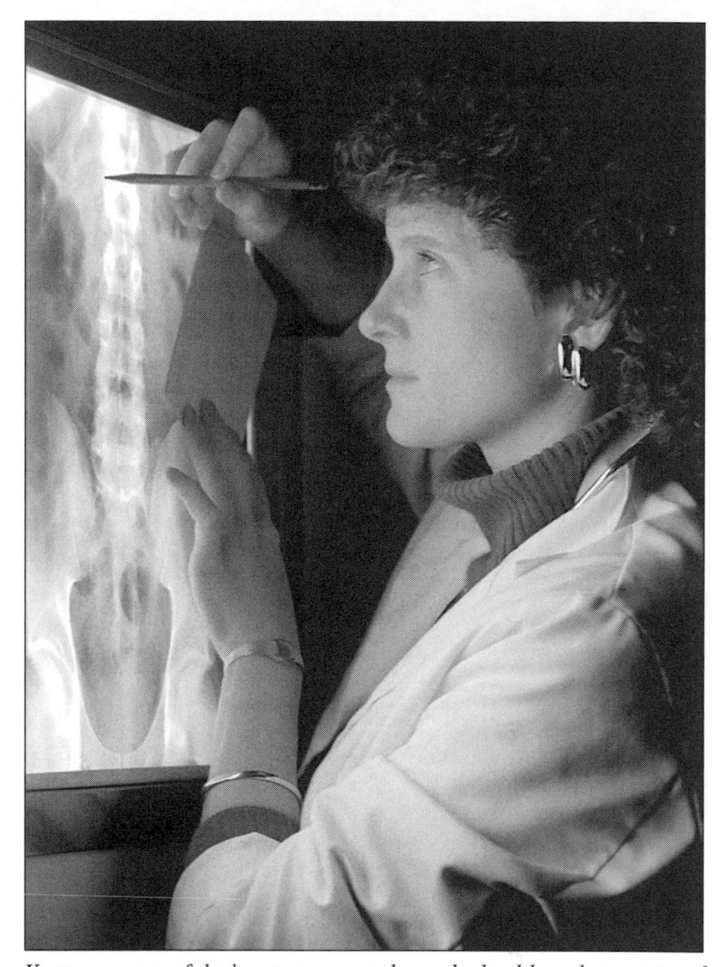

X rays are one of the best ways to evaluate the health and structure of the skeleton. (Digital Stock)

Loss of bone mass is a normal feature of aging, becoming quite marked after the age of seventy-five, particularly in the hip and leg bones. Because of the normal decrease in bone mass with aging, there is not a clear distinction to be made between normal, age-related skeletal changes and the clinical condition of osteoporosis. The occurrence of excessive fragility at a relatively early age is an indication that osteoporosis is developing. Normally, between the ages of thirty and forty, the activity of the osteoblast cells (those that form bone matrix) begins to decrease while the osteoclast cells (those that dissolve the matrix) maintain their previous level of activity. This results in the loss of about 8 percent of the total bone mass each decade for women and about 3 percent for men. Because of unequal loss in the different regions of the skeleton, the outcome is a gradual reduction in height, the loss of teeth, and the development of fragile limbs.

Osteoporotic bones are indistinguishable from normal bones with respect to their bone composition. The problem is simply too little of the strength-imparting matrix, with both compact and spongy bone being affected.

There are multiple causes of osteoporosis. Some cases have no known cause (idiopathic osteoporosis), some are inherited, and others are brought about as a result of hormonal (endocrine) disorders, vitamin or mineral deficiency, or effects of the long-term use of certain drugs.

The fact that women are more often affected than men, and that the process is most conspicuous in women beyond the age of the menopause, has implicated the female sex hormones (and, specifically, their decreased production) in the initiation of the osteoporotic process. One form of therapy is the administration of certain female sex hormones (specifically estrogens) to postmenopausal women (who have decreased production of estrogens). This treatment slows their loss of bone mass. While hormone replacement therapy (HRT) has been the mainstay of osteoporosis treatment for many years, controversy regarding the risks of hormone replacement therapy has caused many women to stop using this treatment altogether. In 2002, two major studies found that the risks associated with HRT outweigh the benefits. Following these studies, doctors began to look closer at the roles that high-impact exercise and the use of calcium and vitamin D play in decreasing bone density loss.

Other treatments of osteoporosis include administering the hormone calcitonin and increasing the dietary intake of the mineral calcium. The hormone calcitonin, produced by the thyroid gland, is sometimes used to treat osteoporosis because it stimulates the production of bone matrix by increasing the activity of the osteoblasts. At the same time, calcitonin inhibits the breakdown of bone by decreasing the activity of osteoclasts. Although this treatment theoretically should produce the desired result of preventing the accelerated loss of bone mass characteristic of osteoporosis, actual clinical results are not always positive.

For those cases of osteoporosis that are the result of endocrine gland disturbances, the appropriate treatment depends on the specific glandular disorder that is present. In some instances, hormone replacement therapy can produce improvement in the patient's condition.

Regular exercise is a means both of preventing the onset of osteoporosis and of slowing its progression. Because muscular activity is critical for the maintenance of bone mass, extended periods of inactivity or immobilization can actually induce osteoporosis. For women, it is known that the amount and regularity of their exercise during the teenage years is strongly associated with their chances of developing osteoporosis thirty and more years later. The exercise need only be of moderate intensity in order to decrease significantly the risk of developing osteoporosis. Indeed, exercise that is at a level of intensity so high that it interferes with the normal female menstrual cycle (stopping the occurrence of menstruation completely or causing irregular cycle lengths) can actually increase the risk of developing osteoporosis later in life.

Perspective and Prospects

Bone has, as one of its primary functions, the protection of softer, more vulnerable tissues and organs. The physical properties of bone—it is as strong as cast iron but only weighs as much as an equally large piece of pine wood—make it ideally suited for this job. This combination of strength and lightness derives from the bony matrix of mineral crystals and the architecture of the bone, which unites compact and spongy bone.

The physical and chemical properties of the mineral crystals also result in the permanency of bone following death. Often the only trace of a dead body is the skeleton. Because of the resistance of bone to the processes of decomposition that befall the other tissues of the body following death, investigators are often able to determine the sex of the person whose skeleton has been found even though all other tissues have long since disappeared. This is possible because of the characteristic differences between male and female adult skeletons. Racial differences in the detailed structure of the skull and pelvis, age-related changes in the skeleton, signs of healed bone fractures, and the prominence of ridges where muscles attach (giving clues about the degree of muscular development) are also valuable sources of information when attempting to identify skeletal remains.

The sexual differences in the human skeleton are most obvious in the adult pelvis. These are genetically determined differences that are structural adaptations for childbearing. For example, the pelvis is smoother and wider in the female than in the male. Other differences include a lighter and smoother female skull, a more sloping male forehead, a larger and heavier male jawbone, and generally heavier male bones that also typically possess more prominent markings.

Among the common age-related changes found in skeletons are a general reduction in the mineral content and less prominent bone markings, both of which become more obvious after about age fifty. Various bones in the skull fuse together at characteristic ages ranging from one to thirty years of age. Other bones throughout the body can also be examined to achieve more accurate estimates of the age of a skeleton at the time of death.

Another consequence of the permanent nature of bone is that it provides a record of the changes in the skeletal anatomy of humans that have occurred during the hundreds of thousands of years of human evolution. Expert examination of skeletal remains can actually reveal an amazing wealth of information concerning the health and even the lifestyle of the deceased.

—*John V. Urbas, Ph.D.*

See also Amputation; Anatomy; Arthritis; Arthroplasty; Arthroscopy; Bone cancer; Bone disorders; Bone grafting; Bone marrow transplantation; Bowlegs; Bunions; Cerebral palsy; Chiropractic; Cleft lip and palate; Cleft lip and palate repair; Disk removal; Dwarfism; Ewing's sarcoma; Feet; Flat feet; Foot disorders; Fracture and dislocation; Fracture repair; Gigantism; Hammertoe correction; Hammertoes; Head and neck disorders; Heel spur removal; Hip fracture repair; Hip replacement; Jaw wiring; Kneecap removal; Knock-knees; Kyphosis; Laminectomy and spinal fusion; Lower extremities; Orthopedic surgery; Orthopedics; Orthopedics, pediatric; Osgood-Schlatter disease; Osteochondritis juvenilis; Osteogenesis imperfecta; Osteomyelitis; Osteonecrosis; Osteopathic medicine; Osteoporosis; Paget's disease; Physical rehabilitation; Pigeon toes; Podiatry; Rheumatology; Rickets; Sarcoma; Scoliosis; Slipped disk; Spinal cord disorders; Spine, vertebrae, and disks; Sports medicine; Temporomandibular joint (TMJ) syndrome; Tendon disorders; Tendon repair; Upper extremities.

For Further Information:

Ballard, Carol. *Bones*. Chicago: Heinemann Library, 2002. An excellent book for young people that covers myriad topics as they relate to the musculoskeletal system, including types of bone, bone structure and marrow, bone injuries and diseases, joints, arthritis, and spinal functions and injuries.

Currey, John D. *Bones: Structures and Mechanics*. Princeton, N.J.: Princeton University Press, 2002. Very accessible overview of a range of information related to whole bones, bone tissue, and dentin and enamel. Topics include stiffness, strength, viscoelasticity, fatigue, fracture mechanics properties, buckling, impact fracture, and properties of cancellous bone.

Joyce, Christopher, and Eric Stover. *Witnesses from the Grave: The Stories Bones Tell*. Boston: Little, Brown, 1991. This book presents a fascinating account of the work of Clyde Snow, a forensic anthropologist. Snow has reported on new findings about what lies under the ground at Custer's Last Stand at the Little Bighorn. He has also identified the victims of serial killer John Wayne Gacy.

Marieb, Elaine N., and Katja Hoehn. *Human Anatomy and Physiology*. 7th ed. San Francisco: Pearson Benjamin Cummings, 2007. Nonscientists at the advanced high school level or above will be able to understand this fine textbook. The chapters titled "Bones and Bone Tissue," "The Skeleton," and "Joints" are very well illustrated and include many applications in the fields of physical education and medical science.

Seeley, Rod R., Trent D. Stephens, and Philip Tate. *Anatomy and Physiology*. 7th ed. New York: McGraw-Hill, 2006. A beautifully illustrated text for readers at the advanced high school level and above. Three chapters are concerned with bone, skeleton, and joints. There are numerous essays on sports medicine, pathologies, clinical applications, and more.

Van De Graaff, Kent M., and Stuart Ira Fox. *Concepts of Human Anatomy and Physiology*. 5th ed. Dubuque: Iowa: Wm. C. Brown, 2000. Chapters 8 through 11 present a first-rate introduction to bones, the skeleton, and joints. The many clear illustrations, photographs, clinical commentaries, and X rays, as well as a pronunciation guide, a complete index, and a glossary, make this a very accessible book for the nonspecialist reader.

Botox

Treatment

Also known as: Botulinum toxin

Anatomy or system affected: Eyes, head, muscles, neck

Specialties and related fields: Neurology, ophthalmology, plastic surgery

Definition: A neurotoxin produced by bacteria that causes botulism in very high doses and is also used as a therapeutic agent for a variety of conditions.

Indications and Procedures

Botulinum toxin has found wide applications as an effective treatment for a variety of conditions associated with excessive muscle contractions. A protein produced by the bacterium *Clostridium botulinum*, botulinum toxin is a potent neurotoxin, causing botulism in very high doses. Botulism is a syndrome of paralysis associated with gastrointestinal symptoms including abdominal cramps and ultimately with respiratory failure from the paralysis of respiratory muscles. As a therapeutic agent, botulinum toxin is injected into muscles and blocks the release of the neurotransmitter acetylcholine from nerve terminals, thus causing paralysis. There are seven different types of botulinum toxin. Two types, botulinum A and B, are available in the United States for clinical use. Botulinum A is also known under the brand name Botox.

Botulinum toxin is available as a purified, vacuum-dried toxin and is reconstituted by the addition of sterile, preservative-free saline. The toxin is then injected into targeted muscles to produce a localized muscle paralysis effect.

Uses and Complications

The utility of botulinum toxin was first demonstrated clinically for the treatment of strabismus, a disorder of abnormal alignment of the eyes. Other disorders treated with botulinum toxin include blepharospasm, a condition of forceful eyelid closure, and focal dystonias, which are syndromes of sustained muscle contractions associated with abnormal postures. Examples of focal dystonias treated with botulinum toxin include cervical torticollis (involuntary neck turning), laryngeal dystonia (abnormal movements of the vocal cords), and oromandibular dystonia (abnormal muscle spasms of the jaw and lower facial muscles). Hemifacial spasm, a disorder of involuntary contractions of the face, also responds well to toxin treatment. Botulinum toxin is also used to treat spasticity, which refers to an excessive increase in muscle tone in the extremities. Hyperhidrosis (excessive sweating) and sialorrhea (hypersalivation) have also been treated with botulinum toxin, with good results reported. Botulinum toxin has achieved much public attention for its cosmetic use as a treatment for facial wrinkles.

The onset of effect of the injection occurs within several days and generally causes weakness and muscle atrophy for approximately several months, with the effect wearing off gradually. Side effects of botulinum toxin treatment are generally transient and may be the result of a local effect of injection, such as bruising, or related to diffusion of the toxin to nearby muscles. The potential side effect encountered depends on the location of injection. For example, injection into neck muscles has the potential side effects of excessive weakness or dysphagia (difficulty swallowing). Over time, some patients may develop resistance to the effects of the medication, which may be associated with the development of neutralizing antibodies.

—*Winona Tse, M.D.*

See also Botulism; Face lift and blepharoplasty; Head and neck disorders; Hyperhidrosis; Muscle sprains, spasms, and disorders; Muscles; Nervous system; Neuralgia, neuritis, and neuropathy; Neurology; Neurology, pediatric; Paralysis; Plastic surgery; Strabismus; Sweating; Torticollis; Wrinkles.

For Further Information:

Blitzer, Andrew, and Lucian Sulica. "Botulinum Toxin: Basic Science and Clinical Uses in Otolaryngology." *Laryngoscope* 111 (2001): 218-226.

Childers, Martin K., Daniel J. Wilson, and Diane Simison. *The Use of Botulinum Toxin Type A in Pain Management*. New York: Demos Medical, 1999.

Klein, Arnold W., ed. *The Clinical Use of Botulinum Toxin*. Philadelphia: Saunders, 2004.

Thant, Zin-Soe, and Eng-King Tan. "Emerging Therapeutic Applications of Botulinum Toxin." *Medical Science Monitor* 9, no. 2 (2003): RA40-48.

Botulism

Disease/disorder

Anatomy or system affected: Nervous system

Specialties and related fields: Bacteriology, critical care, emergency medicine

Definition: A paralytic illness caused by a powerful neurotoxin produced by the bacterium *Clostridium botulinum*.

Causes and Symptoms

Clostridium botulinum is a bacillus that produces spores. Both bacteria and spores can be found in the intestines of humans and other animals as well as in contaminated soil and water. The spores are highly resistant to heat and can survive boiling and other measures employed to kill bacteria and destroy toxins for safe food preparation. Under appropriate anaerobic conditions (those lacking oxygen), the spores germinate into the toxin-producing vegetative bacilli. The exotoxin is a protein synthesized within the bacteria and released only after the death and lysis (disintegration) of the bacteria. When ingested, the toxin resists the acid and enzymes of the stomach by creating complexes with other bacterial proteins. This allows the toxin to reach the intestines, where it is absorbed into the bloodstream and carried to nerve endings. The toxin is bound and internalized into the presynaptic nerve endings, preventing release of the neurotransmitter acetylcholine. The binding is irreversible, and recovery can occur only after nerve endings regenerate.

Human illness is caused by toxin ingestion or the entry of toxin-producing bacteria into the host. Improper processing of food, especially home canning, can result in the germination of contaminating spores, with subsequent toxin production. Food poisoning occurs when toxin-containing food is ingested, unless it has has been heated sufficiently to denature the protein toxin.

The symptoms of descending paralysis usually begin twelve to thirty-six hours after ingestion. Blurred vision, slurred speech, and difficulty swallowing are followed by labored breathing and weakness of the upper and then the lower extremities. Spores may also contaminate a wound and then germinate and form

Information on Botulism

Causes: Infection with bacterial spores through ingestion or wound contamination
Symptoms: Descending paralysis, with blurred vision, slurred speech, difficulty swallowing, labored breathing, weakness in extremities
Duration: Acute
Treatments: Antitoxin, intubation and mechanical ventilation

toxin within the host, producing symptoms similar to food poisoning. Botulism is diagnosed by identification of the toxin and/or bacteria in the patient's serum, stool, or wound or in ingested food. The specific type of botulinum toxin is verified using the mouse neutralization test.

Treatment and Therapy

The outcome of botulism has improved with the development of critical care and supportive measures. Intubation and mechanical ventilation is vitally important until neuromuscular control of breathing is regained. Specific treatment with botulism antitoxin may be used in severe or progressive cases. Because this antitoxin is of equine origin, however, a high incidence of hypersensitivity reactions (9 to 20 percent) occurs in human patients.

Perspective and Prospects

In 1820, a German named Justinus Kerner first noted the association between sausage consumption and paralytic disease. The term "botulism" is derived from *botulus*, the Latin word for "sausage." Wound botulism was first recognized in 1943. Infant botulism, which is caused by swallowed spores rather than preformed toxin, was first noted in 1976. The most common form of human botulism in the United States, infant botulism can be contracted from exposure to honey, but most cases seem to be related to spores found in soil and dust.

Despite these insights, however, the epidemiology of many botulism cases remains obscure. A diagnostic test more rapid and widely available than the mouse neutralization test, which takes forty-eight hours, is needed. Antitoxin, perhaps from deoxyribonucleic acid (DNA) hybridization technology, would improve therapy over the scarce and dangerous equine product.

—H. Bradford Hawley, M.D.

See also Bacterial infections; Bacteriology; Biological and chemical weapons; Botox; Food poisoning; Nervous system; Neuralgia, neuritis, and neuropathy; Neurology; Neurology, pediatric; Paralysis; Poisoning; Toxicology.

For Further Information:

Evans, Alfred S., and Philip S. Brachman, eds. *Bacterial Infections of Humans: Epidemiology and Control*. 3d ed. New York: Plenum, 1998.

Mandell, Gerald L., John E. Bennett, and Raphael Dolin, eds. *Mandell, Douglas, and Bennett's Principles and Practice of Infectious Diseases*. 6th ed. New York: Elsevier/Churchill Livingstone, 2005.

Pommerville, Jeffery C. *Alcamo's Fundamentals of Microbiology*. 7th ed. Sudbury, Mass.: Jones and Bartlett, 2004.

Bowlegs

Disease/disorder

Also known as: Genu varum

Anatomy or system affected: Bones, feet, hips, joints, knees, legs, ligaments, muscles

Specialties and related fields: Orthopedics, pediatrics, physical therapy

Definition: A deformity of the legs that can be temporary or persistent, depending on causation.

Causes and Symptoms

Bowlegs describes a condition in which a person standing with ankles and feet together has knees that do not touch and tibias and femurs that curve away from the body's axis. Because of the compression of limbs in the uterus, babies are born with flexed hips and knee capsules with contracted fibers. Infants have rotated feet and legs, with tibias curving inward and femurs outward. As children mature, knee angles gradually acquire normal alignment because ligament fibers stretch and bones rotate to correct positions. If the legs do not straighten, a child's movement will be hindered. These children may be susceptible to falling and walking pigeon-toed. Some children exhibit a single bowleg, with the other leg appearing straight.

Bone diseases, genetic conditions, injuries, tumors, and deformities can cause bowlegs to persist beyond childhood. Some babies are born with misshapen leg bones that curve. Blount's disease (tibia vara) alters tibia growth in the plate adjacent to the knee, causing bowing. Environmental factors include inadequate nutrition resulting in rickets and conditions associated

INFORMATION ON BOWLEGS

CAUSES: Compression of limbs in uterus, bone diseases, genetic diseases, injuries, tumors, deformities, rickets, repetitive motions
SYMPTOMS: Curving leg bones
DURATION: Temporary or chronic
TREATMENTS: Muscle exercises, vitamin D supplements, orthotic braces and shoes, surgical straightening

with deficient vitamins and minerals that are essential to healthy bone growth. Weak bones are more vulnerable to curve unnaturally. Repetitive motions such as kicking can change the strength and length of leg muscles. As a result, muscles can become uneven. When movement exerts pressure on knees and imbalanced legs, curvature is exacerbated.

TREATMENT AND THERAPY

Physicians assess the degree of a patient's bowlegs by measuring the space between the legs while standing. They also observe the patient's movement. Most mild cases occurring temporarily during normal childhood development do not require treatment. Legs can be manipulated to stretch fibers and rotate bones gradually to desired angles. Muscle exercises can prevent imbalances that make people susceptible to bowlegs. Vitamin D supplements can resolve bowlegs caused by rickets.

Doctors use X rays to detect knee and leg bone structural flaws in older children whose bowlegs have not naturally straightened or have worsened. Braces and shoes are sometimes used to correct bowlegs. Most Blount's disease patients constantly wear a corrective knee-ankle-foot orthosis (KAFO) to aid normal bone growth by reducing joint pressure. Surgical bone straightening occasionally is required for extreme cases of bowlegs. Pins are used to inhibit leg bone growth where it is abnormal. The osteotomy procedure adjusts the upper tibia. Some Blount's disease patients require osteotomy if the KAFO does not alleviate their condition.

PERSPECTIVE AND PROSPECTS

Philipp Erlacher documented Blount's disease by 1922. Fifteen years later, Walter Blount differentiated between the infantile and adolescent types of that condition. Later researchers expanded knowledge of this condition and bowlegs, and using radiographic images, Anders Langenskiold and E. B. Riska classified six stages of Blount's disease deformity.

—*Elizabeth D. Schafer, Ph.D.*

See also Bone disorders; Bones and the skeleton; Braces, orthopedic; Growth; Lower extremities; Orthopedic surgery; Orthopedics; Orthopedics, pediatric; Rickets; Vitamins and minerals.

FOR FURTHER INFORMATION:

England, Stephen P., ed. *Common Orthopedic Problems*. Philadelphia: W. B. Saunders, 1996.
Hensinger, Robert N., ed. *The Pediatric Lower Extremity*. Philadelphia: W. B. Saunders, 1987.
Herring, John A., ed. *Tachdjian's Pediatric Orthopaedics*. 3d ed. 3 vols. Philadelphia: W. B. Saunders, 2002.
Morrissy, Raymond T., and Stuart L. Weinstein, eds. *Lovell and Winter's Pediatric Orthopaedics*. 6th ed. Philadelphia: Lippincott Williams & Wilkins, 2006.

BRACES, ORTHOPEDIC

TREATMENT

ANATOMY OR SYSTEM AFFECTED: Back, bones, joints, knees, musculoskeletal system, neck
SPECIALTIES AND RELATED FIELDS: Orthopedics, sports medicine
DEFINITION: A device to aid a joint by immobilization, restriction of movement, movement assistance, weight-bearing support or postural maintenance.

INDICATIONS AND PROCEDURES

Orthopedic braces have been developed for virtually any joint of the human body. Braces are used to prevent injury, maintain function, or enhance rehabilitation. They are often used in sports-related activities. Individuals who are considered susceptible to a specific injury are be given a brace to reduce the chances of injury. Some individuals may have had a previous injury that affects performance or the ability to perform day-to-day activities. These people would be given braces to help them function normally or obtain closer-to-normal function. People who are recovering from an injury may also use braces to help speed up the recovery process and protect against further injury.

When professionals choose a specific brace, several factors must be considered, including type of shoes worn, type of playing surface, type of activity, previous injuries, weather, and the individual's attitude about wearing braces. Selecting the appropriate brace is critical for protecting the body part or decreasing recovery time.

In order for orthopedic braces to perform well, they must be positioned properly, securely fastened, easy to put on, comfortable, and durable. Improper placement may increase the chances of injury. Adjustments to the brace during activity may also be necessary if the brace becomes loose and moves around. Many athletes do not like wearing braces because they find them uncomfortable, do not like to spend time putting them on, and believe they can negatively affect performance. Therefore, good braces generally are easy to apply and are made of comfortable, light materials. Durability of materials used in brace construction is also important because braces are often exposed to sweat, environmental elements, and impact with other objects during normal use.

USES AND COMPLICATIONS

Braces fall in to one of two broad types, prophylactic and rehabilitative. Prophylactic braces are used to protect joints from injuries during various activities, many of which fall in the category of competitive sports. These braces stabilize the joint to protect it against contact forces, lateral movements, falls, or repetitive movements. Rehabilitative braces are used after an injury or surgery to support joints or limit movements and assist the healing process.

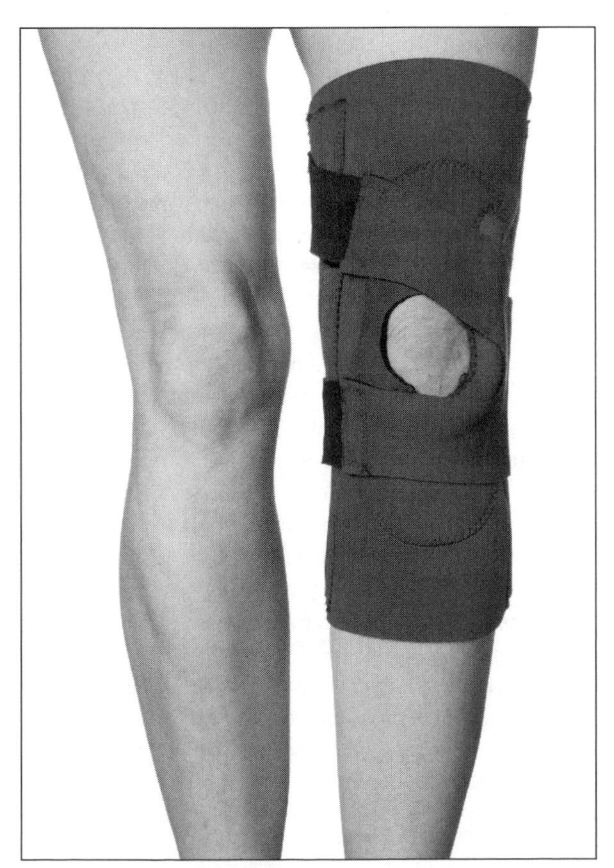

An orthopedic brace can be used to support the knee after injury. (© Suzanne Tucker/Dreamstime.com)

The most commonly injured joint is the ankle. There are numerous ankle braces on the market, such as lace-up braces, elastic braces, and semirigid braces. Still, it is common to see standard ankle taping as an injury prevention technique. Despite these numerous options, professionals do not agree about which method of ankle bracing is best.

Another common joint injury is to the knee, especially the anterior cruciate ligament (ACL). Many different knee braces have been designed, ranging from simple neoprene to more elaborate hinged braces. Although these braces cannot completely protect the knee, they do help to stabilize the joint.

Upper extremity braces are also used. Specialized braces are made for the shoulder, elbow, wrist, hand, and fingers. These braces include casts, cuffs, and splints as well as basic taping. By limiting some movements at specific joints, the joints are protected from some injuries or reinjuries.

Braces can be used to protect the core of the body as well, as with neck, back, abdominal, and rib braces. Neck or cervical collars are used to stabilize the neck and in some cases to limit movement. Back braces help to reduce back pain by supporting the back and abdominal muscles. Abdominal binders are generally used to compress the abdominal muscles, which may have been weakened by incisions from surgery or childbirth. Rib belts are used to compress the chest area and restrict the expansion of the rib cage. This is beneficial for individuals with chest injuries such as broken ribs or chest infections.

In general braces are noninvasive and present few complications to the individual as long as they are put on appropriately. They have been successfully used to prevent injuries and assist in rehabilitation without major risks to the individuals using them.

PERSPECTIVE AND PROSPECTS

Advances om orthopedic braces are due in part to better materials and enhanced designs. A common brace many years ago was the plaster cast. These casts are very effective at immobilizing body parts, but they are not commonly used for athletes because of its greater weight, limited durability, and hardness, which poses a danger to other athletes. Silicone rubber splints are used in competitive contact sports because they are rigid enough to stabilize the body part but soft enough that the injured athlete or opponents or are not put at risk of injury from contact with the device.

Thermoplastics are materials that can be shaped when heated to fit a specific body part. Upon cooling, the material hardens to the shape of the limb and helps to protect it. However, the thickness is less than other braces, and thermoplastics cannot be used for recent fractures. One of the more common materials used in the construction of orthopedic braces is neoprene. Neoprene works well because it compresses the joint, which reduces pain, helps warm the joint (which aids healing), and helps train the body to react to external forces. Since neoprene is soft and light, it is comfortable to wear.

By combining new materials with better designs, orthopedic braces will continue to improve. They will be lighter, stronger, softer, easy to put on, and more durable. Most important, they will better protect the body parts from injury.

—Bradley R. A. Wilson, Ph.D.

See also Back pain; Bones and the skeleton; Exercise physiology; Fracture and dislocation; Fracture repair; Head and neck disorders; Kinesiology; Muscle sprains, spasms, and disorders; Muscles; Orthopedic surgery; Orthopedics; Orthopedics, pediatric; Physical rehabilitation; Preventive medicine; Rotator cuff surgery; Spine, vertebrae, and disks; Sports medicine; Tendinitis; Tendon disorders; Tendon repair; Whiplash.

For Further Information:

Perrin, David H. *Athletic Taping and Bracing*. Champaign, Ill.: Human Kinetics, 2005.

Prentice, William E. *Arnheim's Principles of Athletic Training*. 12th ed. Boston: McGraw-Hill, 2006.

Street, Scott, and Deborah Runkle. *Athletic Protective Equipment: Care, Selection, and Fitting*. New York: McGraw-Hill, 2000.

Brain

Anatomy

Anatomy or system affected: Head, nerves, nervous system, psychic-emotional system

Specialties and related fields: Neurology, psychiatry, psychology

Definition: The most complex organ in the body, which is used for thinking, learning, remembering, seeing, hearing, and many other conscious and subconscious functions.

Key terms:

action potential: an electrochemical event that nerve cells use to send signals along their cellular extensions in the nervous system

axon: a nerve cell extension used to carry action potentials from one place to another in the nervous system

dendrite: a branching nerve cell extension that receives and processes the effects of action potentials from other nerve cells

dyskinesia: a neurologic disorder causing difficulty in the performance of voluntary movements

nucleus: in reference to brain structure, a collection of nerve cell bodies separable from other groups by their cellular form or by surrounding nerve cell extensions

soma: the body of a cell, where the cell's genetic material and other vital structures are located

synapse: an area of close contact between nerve cells that is the functional junction where one cell communicates with another

tract: a collection of nerve fibers (axons) in the brain or spinal cord that all have the same place of origin and the same place of termination

Structure and Functions

The human brain is a complex structure that is composed of two major classes of individual cells: nerve cells (or neurons), and neuroglial cells (or glial cells). It has been estimated that the adult human brain has around one hundred billion neurons and an even larger number of glial cells. An average adult brain weighs about 1,400 grams and has a volume of 1,200 milliliters. These values tend to vary directly with the person's body size; therefore, males have a brain that is typically 10 percent larger than that of females. There is no correlation of intelligence with brain size, however, as witnessed by the fact that brains as small as 750 milliliters or larger than 2,000 milliliters still show normal functioning.

Neurons process and transmit information. The usual structural features of a neuron include a cell body (or soma), anywhere from several to several hundred branching dendrites that are extensions from the soma, and a typically longer extension known as the axon with one or several synaptic terminals at its end.

The information that is processed and transmitted in the brain takes the form of very brief electrochemical

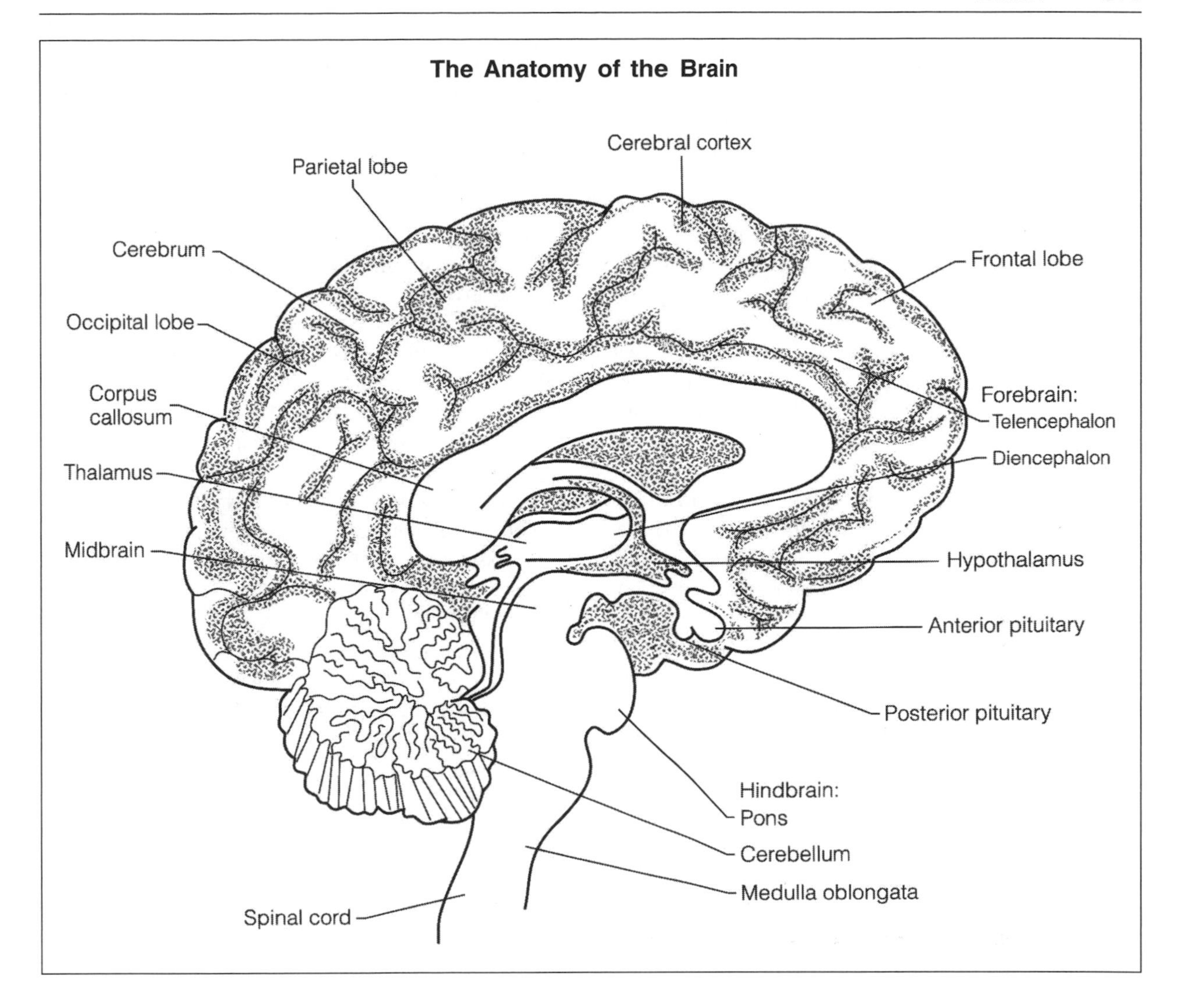

events (with a typical duration of less than 2 milliseconds) called action potentials or nerve impulses. These impulses most often originate near the point at which the axon and soma are joined and then travel at speeds of up to 130 meters per second along the axon to the synaptic terminals.

It is at the synaptic terminals that one neuron communicates its information to other neurons in the brain. These specialized structural points of neuron-to-neuron communication are called synapses. Most synapses are found on the dendrites and soma of the neuron that is to receive the nerve signal. A neuron may have as many as fifty thousand synapses on its surface, although the average seems to be around three thousand. It is thought that as many as three hundred trillion synapses may exist in the adult brain.

The neuroglia function as supporting cells. They have a variety of important duties that include acting as a supporting framework for neurons, increasing the speed of impulse conduction along axons, acting as removers of waste or cellular debris, and regulating the composition of the fluid environment around the neurons in order to maintain optimal working conditions in the brain. Neuroglia actually make up about half of the brain's total volume.

The brain can be divided into two major components: gray matter and white matter, both named for their general appearance. The gray matter is composed primarily of neural soma, dendrites, and axons that transmit information at relatively slow speeds. The white matter is made of collections of axons that have layers of specialized glial cells wrapped around them. This enables much faster information transfer along these axons.

The brain has six major regions. Beginning from the top of the spinal cord and moving progressively upward, these regions are the medulla oblongata, the pons, the cerebellum, the mesencephalon (or midbrain), the diencephalon, and the cerebrum.

The initial lower portion of the medulla oblongata resembles the spinal cord. The medulla has a variety of functions besides the simple relaying of various categories of sensory information to higher-brain centers. Within the medulla there are a number of centers that are important for the execution and regulation of basic survival and maintenance duties. These duties are called visceral functions and include jobs such as regulating the heart rate, breathing, digestive actions, and blood pressure.

The term "pons" comes from the Latin word meaning bridge. The pons serves as a bridge from the medulla oblangata to the cerebellum, which is actually situated on the backside of the brain stem. The pons contains tracts and nuclei that permit communication between the cerebellum and other nervous system structures. Some pontine nuclei facilitate the control of such voluntary and involuntary muscle actions as chewing, breathing, and moving the eyes; other nuclei process information related to the sense of balance.

The cerebellum is a small brain in itself. The two main functions of the cerebellum are to make adjustments, quickly and automatically, to the muscles of the body that assist in maintaining balance and posture and to coordinate the activities of the skeletal muscles involved in movements or sequences of movements, thereby promoting smooth and precise actions. These functions are possible because of the input of sensory information to the cerebellum from position sensors in the muscles and joints; from visual, touch, and balance organs; and even from the sense of hearing. There are also many communication channels to and from the cerebellum and other brain areas concerned with the generation and control of movements. While the cerebellum is not the origin of commands that initiate movements, it does store the memories of how to perform patterns of muscle contractions that are used to execute learned skills, such as serving a tennis ball.

The mesencephalon, or midbrain, is located just above the pons. The midbrain contains pathways carrying sensory information upward to higher-brain centers and transmitting motor signals from higher regions down to lower-brain and spinal cord areas involved in movements.

Two important pairs of nuclei, the inferior and superior colliculi, are found on the backside of the mesencephalon. They coordinate visual and acoustic reflexes involving eye and head movements, such as eye focusing and orienting the head and body toward a sound source. The nucleus known as the substantia nigra operates with nuclei in the cerebrum to generate the patterns and rhythms of such activities as walking and running. Additional mesencephalic nuclei are important for the involuntary control of muscle tone, posture maintenance, and the control of eye movements.

The diencephalon, located above the midbrain, contains the two important brain structures known as the thalamus and hypothalamus. The thalamus is the final relay for all sensory signals (except the sense of smell) before they arrive at the cerebral cortex (the cerebrum's outer covering of gray matter). The hypothalamus is important for regulating drives and emotions, and it serves as a master link between the nervous and endocrine systems.

The thalamus is a collection of different nuclei. Some cooperate with nuclei in the cerebrum to process memories and generate emotional states. Other nuclei have complex involvement in the interactions of the cerebellum, cerebral nuclei, and motor areas of the cerebral cortex.

The relatively small hypothalamus plays many crucial roles that help to maintain stability in the body's internal environment. It regulates food and liquid intake, blood pressure, heart rate, breathing, body temperature, and digestion. Other significant duties encompass the management of sexual activity, rage, fear, and pleasure.

The final major brain region is the cerebrum, which is the largest of the six regions and the seat of higher intellectual capabilities. Sensory information that reaches the cerebrum also enters into a person's conscious awareness. Voluntary actions originate in the cerebral neural activities.

The cerebrum is divided into two cerebral hemispheres, each covered by the gray matter known as the cerebral cortex. Below the cortex is the white matter, which consists of massive bundles of axons carrying signals between various cortical areas, down from the cortex to lower areas, and up into the cortex from lower areas. Embedded in the white matter are also a number of cerebral nuclei.

The cerebral cortex has areas that are the primary sensory areas for each of the senses, and other areas whose major duties deal with the origin and planning of motor activities. The association areas of the cortex integrate and process sensory signals, often resulting in the initiation of appropriate motor responses. Cortical integrative centers receive information from different association areas. The integrative centers perform complex analyses of information (such as predicting the consequences of various possible responses) and direct elaborate motor activities (such as writing).

The cerebral nuclei, also called the basal nuclei or basal ganglia, form components of brain systems that have complex duties such as the regulation of emotions, the control of muscle tone and the coordination of learned patterns of movement, and the processing of memories.

The electrochemical signal that constitutes an action potential in a neuron, and that is sent along the neuron's axon to the synaptic contacts formed with other neurons in the brain, is the basic unit of activity in neural tissue. Although the electrical voltage generated by a single action potential is very small and difficult to measure, the tremendous number of neurons active at any moment results in voltages large enough to be measured at the scalp with appropriate instruments called electroencephalographs. The recorded signals are known as an electroencephalogram (EEG).

Although interpreting an EEG can be compared to standing outside of a football stadium filled with screaming fans and trying to discern what is happening on the playing field by listening to the crowd noises, it still provides clinically useful information and is used regularly in clinics around the world each day. The typical EEG signal appears as a series of wavy patterns whose size, length, shape, and location of best recording on the head provide valuable indications concerning the conditions of brain regions beneath the recording electrodes placed on the scalp.

Disorders and Diseases

One of the most useful applications of the EEG is in the diagnosis of epilepsy. Epilepsy is a group of disorders originating in the brain. There are multiple possible causes. Epilepsy is characterized by malfunctions of the motor, sensory, or even psychic operations of the brain, and there are often accompanying convulsive movements during the attack.

The most common type is known as idiopathic epilepsy, so called because there is no known cause of the attacks. The usual episode occurs suddenly as a large group of neurons begins to produce action potentials in a very synchronized fashion (called a seizure), which is not the typical mode of action in neural tissue. There may be no impairment of consciousness or a complete loss of consciousness, and the seizure may be restricted to a localized area of brain tissue or may spread over the entire brain. When areas of the brain that generate or control movements become involved, the patient will exhibit varying degrees of involuntary muscle contractions or convulsions.

Some cases of epilepsy can be traced to definite causes such as brain tumors, brain injuries, drug abuse, adverse drug reactions, or infections that have entered the brain. Regardless of the cause, the diagnosis is often made through examination of the EEG whereby a trained examiner can quickly identify the EEG abnormalities characteristic of epilepsy.

The usual treatment is directed toward preventing the synchronized bursts of neural activity. This is most often achieved by administering anticonvulsive drugs such as phenobarbital or phenytoin. These agents block the transmission of neural signals in the epileptic regions, and thereby suppress the explosive episodes of synchronized neuronal discharges that induce the seizures. Many epileptics are successfully treated by this approach and are able to lead normal, productive lives, free from the uncontrollable seizures. In some cases, the medication can eventually be discontinued and the patient will never again suffer a seizure.

Unfortunately, there are also cases where even the strongest medications do not prevent the seizures, or only do so at the expense of debilitating drug effects. In the most severe cases, the patients may have dozens of seizures each day, making any form of normal existence impossible. In addition, the large number of seizures eventually can lead to permanent brain damage. For some of these patients, the most drastic form of treatment has been used: surgical removal of the brain tissue responsible for the seizures. This technique is accompanied by great risk because of the danger that removing a portion of brain tissue may leave the patient unable to speak or to speak intelligently, unable to understand spoken words, unable to interpret visual information, or suffering from any of a wide variety of behavioral disturbances, depending on the precise area of the brain that has been removed.

Although this approach is not appropriate in all cases, it has been successful in many. For these patients, success is usually defined as the possibility, following surgery, to control or prevent future seizures through the use of anticonvulsive drugs and to resume a normal life or a life that is much more normal than it was before surgery.

A varied group of disorders known as dyskinesias causes difficulty in the performance of voluntary movements. The movements actually look like normal body movements or portions of normal movements. Dyskinesia often results from problems involving the basal nuclei. When the basal nuclei are affected, the dyskinesic movements usually do not occur during sleep and are reduced during periods of emotional tranquillity. Anxiety, emotional tension, and stressful conditions, however, cause the dyskinesia to become worse. These observations can be explained by the fact that neural pathways are known to connect the brain centers involved with the generation of emotional states to the basal nuclei.

One example of a dyskinesia affecting the basal nuclei is the inherited condition of Huntington's disease (or Huntington's chorea), for which no treatment exists. A chorea is a dyskinesia in which the patient's movements are quick and irregular. Huntington's chorea first makes its appearance when the patient is in middle age. It results in the progressive degeneration of the basal nuclei, known as the corpus striatum, that are located in the cerebrum. Some of the common symptoms are involuntary facial grimacing, jaw and tongue movements, twisting and turning movements of the torso, and speaking difficulties. As the brain atrophy (degeneration) progresses, the patients become totally disabled. Death usually results ten to fifteen years following the appearance of the first symptoms.

A category of generalized disturbances of higher-brain function is known as dementia, more commonly referred to as senility. The term "senile" is derived from the Latin word meaning "old age," and its use reflects the fact that senility was previously considered to be an inevitable consequence of aging. Senility, or dementia, is characterized by a generalized deficiency of intellectual performance (often referred to as being "feeble-minded"), mental deterioration, memory impairment, and limited attention span. These are often accompanied by changes in personality such as increased irritability and moodiness.

Various diseases can cause dementia. One of the most frequently observed is known as Alzheimer's disease; it is progressive and usually develops between the ages of forty and sixty. The disease is marked by the death of neurons in the cerebral cortex and the deep cerebral regions known as the nucleus basalis and the hippocampus. The exact cause of neural death in Alzheimer's disease is unknown. While some cases are inherited, other instances seem to appear without any family history of the disease. Death usually occurs within ten years after the appearance of the first symptoms, and no cure exists.

The areas of the brain showing neural degeneration also have abnormal collections of a specific type of protein. The appearance of this protein in the blood and the fluids that surround the brain is a clinical sign for Alzheimer's disease. The areas of the brain that deteriorate during the progression of this disease illustrate the functional roles played by these regions. The hippocampus, in particular, is crucial for learning, the storage of long-term memories, memory of recent events, and the sense of time. Therefore, the death of hippocampal neurons helps to explain the memory disturbances and related behavioral changes seen in Alzheimer's disease patients.

Perspective and Prospects

Given the complexity of the human brain, understanding its structure and function is the ultimate challenge to medical science. The challenge exists because, in order to rationally treat brain disorders, it is necessary to know how a normal brain functions. An appreciation of this can be gleaned by studying the history of some approaches used through the ages to treat brain disorders.

For example, in the Middle Ages it was a common practice to treat people suffering from epilepsy by cutting open the patient's scalp and pouring salt into the wound (all of which was performed without anesthesia, since anesthetics were not yet known). The purpose of this treatment was to poison the spirits possessing the patient, forcing them to leave.

As modern science discovered the cellular basis of life, such draconian measures were gradually replaced with treatments directed toward the biochemical imbalances, infections, or interruptions of blood flow that were found to be the cause of many brain disorders. The development of nonsurgical techniques permitting the visualization of the brain regions that are active, or inactive, during various tasks or illnesses greatly advanced the understanding of brain function and improved diagnosis, the planning of effective treatments, and the tracking of either the improvement or the deterioration of patients.

Late in the 1970's, the disease known as acquired immunodeficiency syndrome (AIDS) attracted the attention of the world's scientists. AIDS is caused by the human immunodeficiency virus (HIV). Nearly 60 percent of AIDS patients experience various neurological problems, including difficulties of movement, loss of memory, and cognitive disturbances. In some cerebral cortical areas, as many as half of the neurons may die. In order to understand how the AIDS virus causes these effects, it is necessary to analyze how the brain's components function when infected by the virus, and then to form a clear explanation of the consequences of viral infection.

HIV actually infects certain classes of neuroglial cells. Infection of these glial cells causes them to release distinct types of chemicals that can be toxic to neurons. One type of glial cell, known as the astrocyte, can begin to appear in abnormally large numbers as a result of these chemicals being released. In turn, the presence of large numbers of astrocytes provokes the release of even more of the toxic chemicals. This sort of effect is referred to as a positive feedback loop. The significance of this cascade of mutually stimulating events (neurotoxic chemicals causing astrocytes to appear in greater numbers, and increased numbers of astrocytes causing more production of neurotoxic chemicals) is that only a few HIV-infected cells can trigger extensive neural damage.

Additionally, a protein part of the virus, called gp120, can stimulate release of the same neurotoxic chemicals and can disrupt the normal functioning of the astrocytes. One important function of astrocytes is to regulate the chemical environment of neurons by removing certain types of chemicals. One of these chemicals, called glutamate, is normally present and used by some neurons to send signals to other neurons at their synaptic contacts. When glutamate is not promptly removed from the environment of the target neurons, however, it becomes toxic to the neurons and kills them. The HIV protein gp120 disrupts the ability of astrocytes to remove glutamate, thereby increasing the death of neurons in the brain as they become exposed to toxic levels of glutamate.

—John V. Urbas, Ph.D.

See also Abscess drainage; Abscesses; Addiction; Alcoholism; Altitude sickness; Alzheimer's disease; Amnesia; Anatomy; Aneurysmectomy; Aneurysms; Angiography; Aphasia and dysphasia; Biofeedback; Brain damage; Brain disorders; Brain tumors; Chronic wasting disease (CWD); Cluster headaches; Coma; Computed tomography (CT) scanning; Concussion; Craniotomy; Creutzfeld-Jakob disease (CJD); Dementias; Dizziness and fainting; Dyslexia; Electroencephalography (EEG); Embolism; Emotions: Biomedical causes and effects; Encephalitis; Endocrinology; Endocrinology, pediatric; Epilepsy; Fetal tissue transplantation; Hallucinations; Head and neck disorders; Headaches; Huntingdon's disease; Hydrocephalus; Hypnosis; Intraventricular hemorrhage; Learning disabilities; Leukodystrophy; Light therapy; Memory loss; Meningitis; Mental retardation; Migraine headaches; Narcolepsy; Narcotics; Neuroimaging; Neurology; Neurology, pediatric; Neurosurgery; Parkinson's disease; Positron emission tomography (PET) scanning; Psychiatric disorders; Psychiatry; Psychiatry, child and adolescent; Psychiatry, geriatric; Psychology; Seizures; Shock therapy; Shunts; Sleep disorders; Strokes; Systems and organs; Thrombosis and thrombus; Toxicology; Transient ischemic attacks (TIAs); Trembling and shaking; Tumor removal; Tumors; Unconsciousness.

For Further Information:

Bear, Mark F., Barry W. Connors, and Michael A. Paradiso. *Neuroscience: Exploring the Brain*. 3d ed. Philadelphia: Lippincott Williams & Wilkins, 2007. Undergraduate text that introduces the topics of neuroscience, neurobiology, and physiological psychology.

Bloom, Floyd E., M. Flint Beal, and David J. Kupfer, eds. *The Dana Guide to Brain Health*. New York: Simon & Schuster, 2003. An easy-to-understand health guide to the brain from neuroscience, neurology, and psychiatry perspectives. More than seventy psychiatric and neurological disorders, their diagnoses, and their treatments are covered.

Davis, Joel. *Mapping the Mind: The Secrets of the Human Brain and How It Works*. Bridgewater, N.J.: Carol, 1999. An easy-to-read book on the brain and mind that gives details about different structures and functions.

Edelman, Gerald M. *Bright Air, Brilliant Fire*. New York: Basic Books, 1992. The author is a winner of the 1972 Nobel Prize in Physiology or Medicine and a leading brain scientist. This book is accessible to the nonscientist because of the importance that the author places on the subject of understanding the brain and how it gives rise to the mind.

Marieb, Elaine N., and Katja Hoehn. *Human Anatomy and Physiology*. 7th ed. San Francisco: Pearson Benjamin Cummings, 2007. Several chapters explore the fundamentals of the nervous system and nervous tissue, the central nervous system, and neural integration. Well illustrated and includes many applications in the fields of physical education and medical science.

Nolte, John. *Human Brain: An Introduction to Its Functional Anatomy*. 5th ed. St. Louis: Mosby, 2002. Text covering major concepts and structure-function relationships in the human neurological system.

Scientific American 267 (September, 1992). A special issue titled *Mind and Brain*. This outstanding collection of articles by leading scientists, edited by Jonathan Piel, presents information on a wide range of topics such as the development of the brain, age-related changes in the brain, sex differences in the brain, major disorders of the brain and the mind, and others.

Seeley, Rod R., Trent D. Stephens, and Philip Tate. *Anatomy and Physiology*. 7th ed. New York: McGraw-Hill, 2006. A beautifully illustrated text with drawings, photographs and summary tables. Four chapters are concerned with the brain and nervous tissue.

Van De Graaff, Kent M., and Stuart Ira Fox. *Concepts of Human Anatomy and Physiology*. 5th ed. Dubuque, Iowa: Wm. C. Brown, 2000. Chapters 14 and 15 present a first-rate introduction to the brain and nervous tissue. Other aspects of the nervous system are treated in chapters 16 through 19.

Woolsey, Thomas A., Joseph Hanaway, and Mokhtar Gado. *Brain Atlas: A Visual Guide to the Human Central Nervous System*. 2d ed. New York: Wiley, 2002. Excellent text whose sections include "Background Information," "The Brain and Its Blood Vessels," "Brain Slices," "Histological Sections," and "Pathways."

Brain damage

Disease/disorder

Anatomy or system affected: Brain, nervous system

Specialties and related fields: Neurology, psychiatry, psychology

Definition: Mild, moderate, or traumatic brain injury, which occurs when cells that make up the brain die.

Key terms:

closed head injury: an injury to the brain that arises from a problem within the cranium

cognitive functions: mental functions such as reasoning, language, memory, and problem-solving

computed tomography (CT) scan: a visual diagnostic technology using X rays that can detect brain abnormalities

glucose: a simple sugar that is the primary source of fuel brain cells

magnetic resonance imaging (MRI): a visual diagnostic technology that can create high-resolution pictures of brain structures

paralysis: inability to move a particular part of the body

stroke: temporary loss of blood flow to the brain

Information on Brain Damage

Causes: Accidents (automobile collisions, falls, sports injuries); strokes

Symptoms: Motor control problems, paralysis, balance and sensory problems; often speech and language difficulties, memory loss, concentration and attention problems; if extensive, loss of consciousness, coma, and death

Duration: Acute

Treatments: Depends on cause; may include surgery (hemorrhage, tumor) or drug therapy (swelling, blockage, infection)

Causes and Symptoms

Brain damage can occur as a result of several causes. Therefore, physicians have found it helpful to categorize the types of injuries that most often lead to the death of brain cells. The most common type that leads to brain damage is the closed head injury. It occurs when a problem, such as the disruption of blood flow to the brain, prevents vital oxygen and nutrients from reaching the cells that make up the brain. If the brain is deprived of oxygen and glucose for more than six or seven seconds, then a person usually becomes unconscious and brain cells begin to die.

Accidents such as automobile collisions, falls, and sports injuries can lead to brain damage by causing the brain to bleed inside the cranium. This kind of closed head injury frequently results in brain swelling that puts pressure on delicate structures, preventing them from working properly and sometimes leading to permanent damage. Strokes also result in brain damage either by blocking normal blood flow within the arteries that feed the brain or by causing a blood vessel to break and leak blood into surrounding tissue.

When brain damage occurs, symptoms may include motor control problems, paralysis, and difficulty with balance and the integration of sensory information. In the case of an accident that leads to brain damage, it would not be uncommon to see cognitive functions affected, creating speech and language difficulties, memory loss, and problems with concentration and attention. Problems with motivation and the expression of emotions may develop, and to some degree a person's personality can be altered because of brain damage. In cases of extensive damage, the result could be loss of consciousness, coma, and even death.

TREATMENT AND THERAPY

Treatment for brain damage begins with an assessment of the cause and extent of the injury. Several distinct technologies can be used to image not only the structures of the brain but the functioning of specific areas as well. If bleeding or swelling of the brain is suspected, then a computed tomography (CT) scan can be used to provide pictures of the brain to assess which structures are implicated. If a tumor or areas of localized damage is suspected, then magnetic resonance imaging (MRI) is more helpful because of its ability to create a clear, well-defined image.

The extent of deficits in cognitive, sensory, or motor functioning is evaluated by specialized tests that assess reflexes, muscle tone, functioning of the nerves that exit the base of the head, level of consciousness, language processing, memory, and decision-making abilities. With all these tests, behaviors are used to determine the extent and location of the brain damage.

Since there are several different causes of brain damage, treatments can vary. Drug therapy can be used in instances where the brain is being damaged by swelling or when an artery inside the brain is partially blocked. High doses of antibiotics can be used when damage occurs as a result of a bacterial infection. If a weakened artery is found that is leaking blood into the brain or a tumor is detected using an MRI, then surgery could be recommended. In instances where no immediate treatment can be performed, specific rehabilitation therapies are used to stimulate surviving brain tissue that is near the injury to take over some of the functioning of the damaged tissue.

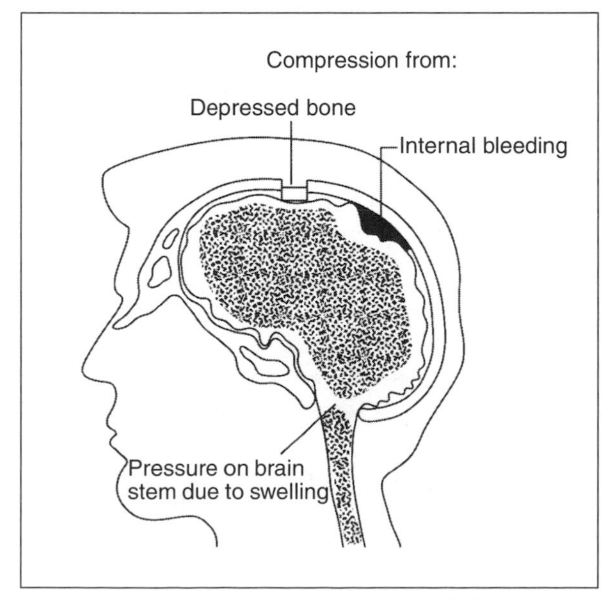

Head trauma may result in compression of the brain, consequent distortions, and severe neurological reactions.

PERSPECTIVE AND PROSPECTS

Although brain injuries have occurred since the beginning of humankind, the question of what the brain does and how it contributes to behavior has only been partially answered. There is evidence from human skull remains that small holes were drilled as a form of crude brain surgery as far back as 2000 B.C.E. The purpose of the procedure is unknown; however, it could have helped an injured person by relieving brain swelling. Prior to the first century C.E., it was not widely accepted that the brain was the center for reasoning, emotions, and movement. During early human history, the heart was believed to control the thoughts and emotions. Galen of Pergamum (130-201 C.E.), a Roman physician, was influential in bringing forth the notion that the brain, and not the heart, gave rise to behavior. He learned much about the brain and its impact on behavior by observing injured gladiators who survived fierce battles in the Roman coliseum.

Prospects for future therapies to compensate for brain damage include stem cell tissue transplantation to stimulate new brain cell development. Better drugs are being developed for stroke victims whose blood has leaked into the brain and had begun killing nearby cells. Also, brain imaging technologies are continuing to be refined to produce clearer pictures that allow practitioners to make more accurate diagnoses.

—*Bryan C. Auday, Ph.D.*

See also Accidents; Brain; Brain disorders; Coma; Computed tomography (CT) scanning; Concussion; Craniotomy; Critical care; Critical care, pediatric; Dizziness and fainting; Emergency medicine; Emergency medicine, pediatric; Emotions: Biomedical causes and effects; Fetal tissue transplantation; Head and neck disorders; Intraventricular hemorrhage; Magnetic resonance imaging (MRI); Memory loss; Neuroimaging; Neurology; Neurology, pediatric; Neurosurgery; Sports medicine; Strokes; Unconsciousness.

For Further Information:

Cooper, Paul R., and John G. Golfinos, eds. *Head Injury*. 4th ed. New York: McGraw-Hill, 2000.

Gronwall, Dorothy, Philip Wrightson, and Peter Waddell. *Head Injury: The Facts*. 2d ed. New York: Oxford University Press, 1998.

Landau, Elaine. *Head and Brain Injuries*. Berkeley Heights, N.J.: Enslow, 2002.

Brain disorders

Disease/disorder

Anatomy or system affected: Brain, head, nervous system, psychic-emotional system

Specialties and related fields: Embryology, geriatrics and gerontology, neurology, psychiatry

Definition: Disorders of the brain can interfere with its role in the control of body functions, behavior, learning, and expression, while defects can also threaten life itself.

Key terms:

anencephaly: a fatal congenital condition in which tissues that should have differentiated to form the brain failed to do so

coma: a condition of unconsciousness that may or may not be reversible; various degrees of coma are assessed by the presence or absence of reflex responses, such as pupil dilation when a light is shone into the eyes

dementia: a diseased state in which intellectual ability is ever decreasing; personality changes, decreased interest or ability to care for one's self, and long-term and short-term memory loss can indicate dementia

embolus: a clot or other piece of matter that may travel through the circulatory system to tiny blood vessels (as in the brain) and block the path that normally allows blood flow

hydrocephalus: a painful condition caused by excess cerebrospinal fluid within the spaces of the brain

ischemia: an inadequate blood flow to a region; may be caused by an incomplete blockage in or constriction of a blood vessel (as may occur with atherosclerosis or a blood clot)

seizure: a misfiring of cortical neurons that alters the patient's level of consciousness; the seizure may or may not involve muscular convulsions

stroke: a complete loss of blood flow to a region of the brain that is of sudden onset and causes abrupt muscular weakness, usually to one side of the body

thrombus: a blood clot that is attached to the interior wall of a blood vessel

Causes and Symptoms

The cerebral cortex acts as a processor for sensory information and as an integrator of memory, interpretation, creativity, intellect, and passion. Disorders of the brain or brain defects can disrupt these processing or integrating functions. Disorders of the brain include such commonly heard terms as stroke, ischemia, dementia, seizure, and coma. Brain disorders may also occur as a result of infection, various tumors, traumas leading to blot clots (hematomas) or lack of oxygen (hypoxia), and cancer. Brain defects include anencephaly, a congenital defect in which a newborn lacks a brain, and hydrocephaly, commonly called "water on the brain."

A stroke is any situation in which the blood supply to a region of the brain is lost. This can occur as a result of a cerebral hemorrhage, during which blood escapes from blood vessels to surround and compress brain tissue; cerebral thrombosis, whereby a clot attached to the wall of a blood vessel restricts the amount of blood flowing to a particular region; or an embolus, a foreign substance which may be a clot that migrates in the bloodstream, often to lodge in a smaller vessel in the brain. The embolus will block blood flow to some area. An embolus can originate from substances other than a blood clot, which is why health care staff often squirt fluid out of a needle before administering a shot or other therapy: to ensure that no air embolus, which could induce a stroke or prove fatal if it enters the brain, is injected.

Transient ischemic attacks (TIAs) are often thought of as small strokes, but, technically, ischemia simply means that oxygen is not reaching the cells within a tissue. Basically, the mechanism is similar to a stroke, in that blood flow to a portion of the brain is compro-

Information on Brain Disorders

Causes: Congenital disorders, age-related degeneration, traumas leading to blood clots or restricted blood flow to brain, disease, infection, seizure, stroke, psychological disorders

Symptoms: Varies widely; may include forgetfulness, sudden sharp pain, impaired movement, dementia, lethargy, headache, dullness, blurred vision, nausea, vomiting

Duration: Acute to chronic

Treatments: Surgery, medications

mised. Although blood actually reaches the brain tissue during ischemia, there is not a sufficient flow to ensure that all cells are receiving the oxygen necessary to continue cellular life. This condition is called hypoxia (low oxygen). If hypoxia is sustained over a sufficient period of time, cellular death occurs, causing irreversible brain damage.

The important differences between a stroke and a TIA are the onset and duration of symptoms, as well as the severity of the damage. Persons with atherosclerosis actually have fat deposits along the interior walls of their blood vessels. These people are vulnerable to experiencing multiple TIAs. Many TIAs are small enough to be dismissed and ignored; others are truly inapparent, causing no symptoms. This is unfortunate because TIAs often serve as a warning of an impending full-scale stroke. Action and treatments could be implemented, if medical advice is sought early, to decrease the likelihood of a stroke. Repeated TIAs also contribute to dementia.

Dementia is not the normal path for the elderly, nor is it a sign of aging. Dementia is a sign of neurological chaos and can be caused by diseases such as Alzheimer's disease or acquired immunodeficiency syndrome (AIDS). Although most elderly are not afflicted with dementia, nearly all have a slowing of reaction and response time. This slowing is believed to be associated with chemical changes within nerve cell membranes as aging occurs; slowing of reaction times is not necessarily indicative of the first steps on a path to dementia. In addition, forgetfulness may not be a sign of dementia, since it occurs at all ages. Forgetfulness is such a sign, however, if it is progressive and includes forgetting to dress or forgetting one's name or date of birth.

While it is incorrect to say that dementia is caused by aging, it is correct to say that dementia is age-related. It may first appear in a person any time between the late thirties and the mid-nineties, but it usually begins to appear in the late seventies. Patients with Alzheimer's disease are believed to account for about 20 percent of all cases of dementia. Other diseases cause dementia, including an autosomal-dominant genetic disease called Huntington's disease. Huntington's disease manifests itself with a distinct chorea, or dance, of the body that is neither solicited nor controlled. This genetic disease is particularly cruel in that its symptoms appear in midlife, often after the adult has had offspring and passed on the gene. The disease continues to alter the intellect and personality of the afflicted one and progresses to the point of complete debilitation of the body and mind.

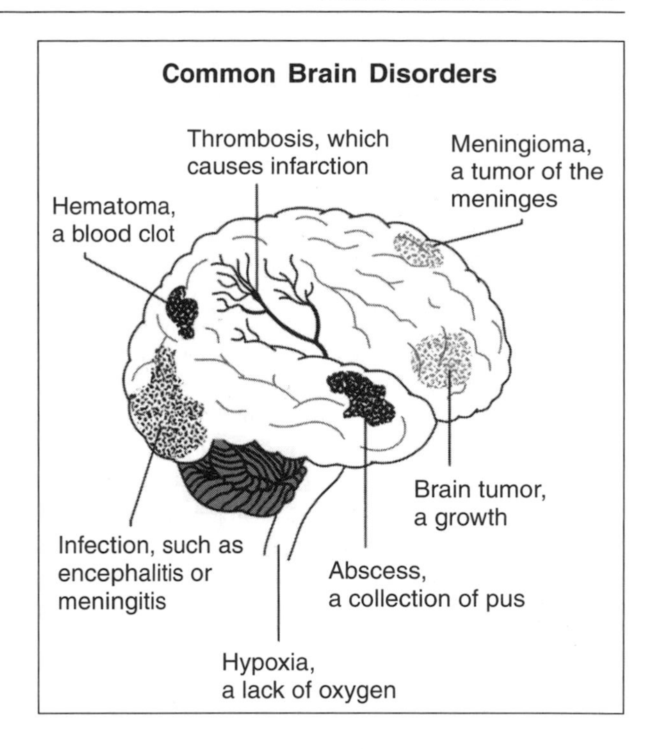

A seizure occurs when a collection of neurons misfires, sending nerve impulses that are neither solicited nor controllable. In the everyday use of the term, seizure describes a condition of epilepsy or convulsion. Medically speaking, a seizure is a sign of an underlying problem within the gray matter of the brain; it is the most common neurological disorder. Epilepsy is a term used to describe a condition of repeated seizures, while convulsion is a term generally applied to describe an isolated seizure. A seizure may occur as a consequence of extreme fever or a violent blow to the head. Seizures are also associated with metabolic disorders, such as hypoglycemia (low blood sugar); trauma causing a loss of blood or oxygen to a region, such as in a newborn after a traumatic birth; toxins, as seen in drug abuse or withdrawal; or bacterial or viral encephalitis or meningitis. In addition, about one-third of those persons who survive a gunshot wound to the head will experience seizures afterward. In closed head trauma, which can occur in a sporting or automobile accident, there is a 5 percent chance of post-trauma seizures.

Loss of consciousness can be caused by a violent impact to the head, a lack of oxygen or blood flow to the head, a metabolic imbalance, or the presence of a toxin such as alcohol. Usually, this is a transient event, but it may become a permanent condition. When this happens, a person is said to be in a coma. A comatose person exists in a nonresponsive state and may be assessed for brain death. Brain death is a legally defined term which means that no electrical activity in the brain is seen on an electroencephalogram (EEG). Thus some comatose patients may be determined to be brain-dead, particularly if the condition is deemed irreversible.

Brain defects are not common, but they do occur. One particularly tragic defect is the absence of a brain in a newborn, called anencephaly. Death usually occurs within a few hours of birth. Although anencephaly is rare and generally associated with a genetic factor, there have been cases in population clusters, such as one in the Rio Grande area of south Texas, suggesting that an environmental factor may contribute to these defects.

Another defect that may appear in newborns or in an infant's first months of life is hydrocephalus. Although the descriptive term "water on the brain" is often used, the condition does not involve a collection of water in the cranium; rather, it involves an accumulation of cerebrospinal fluid (CSF). CSF is the fluid that insulates the brain and allows it to "float" under the bony cranial encasement. As the ventricles, or spaces, in the brain fill with CSF, bulging occurs and pressure builds to the point of compressing the surrounding brain tissue. This can be very painful and is fatal if untreated. Hydrocephalus can be caused by an overproduction of CSF or a blockage of the CSF drainage from the ventricles of the brain. The symptoms often include a protrusion or abnormal shape of the cranium. In newborns, the skull bones have not yet sutured (fused) to one another, so the soft bones are pushed apart, causing unusual head shapes. This is a warning sign. Another sign is observed if a newborn's head has a circumference greater than 35.5 centimeters (14 inches); if that is the case, the newborn must be immediately checked for hydrocephalus. Adolescents and adults may also experience hydrocephalus. This can be a response to head trauma, infection, or the overproduction of CSF. The symptoms include lethargy, headache, dullness, blurred vision, nausea, and vomiting.

Treatment and Therapy

TIAs can progress to strokes. In fact, about 30 percent of those diagnosed with TIA will have a major stroke within the subsequent four years. One of the most prevalent causes of TIAs is hypertension. Hypertension is known as the "silent killer" because many persons with this problem ignore the subtle symptoms of fatigue, headache, and general malaise. Hypertension is also known as a good predictor of major strokes if left untreated. Thus, hypertensive persons need to be diagnosed as such in order to control their blood pressure. This allows them to avoid or delay either a major stroke or multiple TIAs. Management for the hypertensive's blood pressure may include taking diuretics and hypotensive drugs (to lower the blood pressure). If taken diligently, these drugs offer longevity and quality of life to the sufferer. Aside from hypertension, TIAs may be induced in some metabolic disorders, which should be corrected if possible, or by constricted blood vessels. Sometimes, surgery on such vessels can stop the ischemic attacks and prevent or delay the onset of a stroke.

Although TIAs lead to strokes, strokes are not necessarily preceded by a TIA. Nearly 90 percent of all major strokes occur without a TIA warning. Sadly, hypertension is the main contributor to this number. Measures can be taken to avoid strokes. This includes maintaining cardiovascular health by exercising, not smoking, and managing hypertension, diabetes mellitus, or other problems that may place stresses on the body's chemical balance.

Dementia is so poorly understood in terms of causes that a rational probe of drug therapy or a cure is nearly impossible. The drugs most often used in dementia treatment, the ergoloid mesylates, are used to manage the symptoms; namely, the confused mind. These drugs, however, do not stop or prevent the unexplained cellular degeneration associated with dementia. It is interesting to note that a tiny subgroup within those persons suffering from Alzheimer's disease have greatly improved in mental status with the drug tacrine. It is unfortunate that all patients are not responsive to this drug—a fact which suggests that Alzheimer's disease is a complex condition.

Seizures are treated pharmacologically according to type. Carbamazepine, phenobarbitol, phenytoin, and valproate are some of the drugs available to treat seizure disorders. Barbiturates may also be used in certain cases. Most of these drugs are highly effective when taken as prescribed, and patient noncompliance is the main cause of drug failure. Sometimes, two drugs are combined in therapy. It should be mentioned that pregnant women with epilepsy are urged to continue taking antiepilepsy drugs during pregnancy since a maternal seizure may be more damaging to the fetus than the drug itself.

Some forms of hydrocephalus can be corrected surgically by performing a CSF shunt from the cranium to the peritoneal (abdominal) region, where the fluid can be eliminated from the body as waste. This is not without risk, and the introduction of infection into the brain is a major concern.

Perspective and Prospects

The therapies in use for brain diseases and disorders have been derived from the practical experience of physicians, the laboratory research of scientists, and the hopes of multitudes of doctors, patients, families, and friends. Medical science has done much to improve the lives of those who suffer with seizures, to reduce the risk of strokes to the hypertensive person and those with TIAs, and is making great progress in treating certain kinds of dementia. Yet much remains to be done.

While one can argue that much is known about the human brain, it would be erroneous to argue that the human brain is fully understood. Despite centuries of research, the brain, as it functions in health, remains largely a mystery. Since the healthy brain is yet to be understood, it is not surprising that the medical community struggles to determine what goes wrong in dementia, seizure, or mental illness or to discover drug therapies that can cross the blood-brain barrier. Thus, the human brain is the uncharted frontier in medicine. As technology improves to support researchers and medical practitioners in their pursuits of cures and treatments for brain diseases and disorders, one can only remain hopeful for the future ability to restore health to the damaged human brain.

—*Mary C. Fields, M.D.*

See also Abscess drainage; Abscesses; Alzheimer's disease; Amnesia; Aphasia and dysphasia; Brain; Brain damage; Brain tumors; Cerebral palsy; Chronic wasting disease (CWD); Cluster headaches; Concussion; Creutzfeldt-Jakob disease (CJD); Dementias; Dyslexia; Embolism; Encephalitis; Epilepsy; Guillain-Barré syndrome; Hallucinations; Headaches; Hemiplegia; Huntington's disease; Hydrocephalus; Intraventricular hemorrhage; Lead poisoning; Learning disabilities; Leukodystrophy; Memory loss; Meningitis; Migraine headaches; Motor neuron diseases; Multiple sclerosis; Nervous system; Neuralgia, neuritis, and neuropathy; Neuroimaging; Neurology; Neurology, pediatric; Neurosurgery; Numbness and tingling; Palsy; Paralysis; Parkinson's disease; Pick's disease; Seizures; Shock therapy; Tics; Unconsciousness.

For Further Information:

American Medical Association. *American Medical Association Family Medical Guide*. 4th rev. ed. Hoboken, N.J.: John Wiley & Sons, 2004. An excellent reference for the beginner. The scientific accuracy of the text is not compromised by its accessibility.

Bannister, Roger. *Brain and Bannister's Clinical Neurology*. 7th ed. Oxford, England: Oxford University Press, 1992. Several chapters are dedicated to the topics of seizures, dementia, hydrocephalus, and loss of consciousness. Because the writing can be fairly technical, it is best used by someone with a background in human anatomy and physiology.

Bloom, Floyd E., et al., eds. *The Dana Guide to Brain Health*. New York: Simon & Schuster, 2003. An easy-to-understand health guide to the brain from neuroscience, neurology, and psychiatry perspectives. More than seventy psychiatric and neurological disorders, their diagnoses, and their treatments are covered.

Castle, Lana R., and Peter C. Chybrow. *Bipolar Disorder Demystified: Mastering the Tightrope of Manic Depression*. New York: Avalon, 2003. A layperson's guide to the disorder, written by a bipolar disorder patient. Provides an understanding of the true nature of bipolar disorder, the factors that complicate its diagnosis, and numerous strategies for successfully coping with the illness.

Dana.org. http://www.dana.org/. A nonprofit organization of neuroscientists, which was formed to provide information about the personal and public benefits of brain research. The Web site is research oriented and gives excellent information and links on current brain studies, new diagnosis and treatment technology, and brain-related news stories.

Freeman, John M., Eileen P.G. Vining, and Diana J. Pillas. *Seizures and Epilepsy in Childhood: A Guide*. 3d ed. Baltimore: Johns Hopkins University Press, 2002. Designed for parents, an overall guide to the symptoms, diagnosis, and treatment of children with epilepsy. Third edition includes new chapters on alternative therapies and medicines, routine health care, insurance issues, and research resources.

Heilman, Kenneth M. *Matter of Mind: A Neurologist's View of Brain-Behavior Relationships*. New York: Oxford University Press, 2002. A leading researcher in behavioral and cognitive neurology uses case studies to explore brain functions such as speaking, reading, writing, emotion, skilled movement, perception, attention, and motivation that have been gained from the study of patients with diseases of or damage to the brain. An excellent, accessible examination of neurological disorders.

Mace, Nancy L., and Peter V. Rabins. *The Thirty-Six-Hour Day: A Family Guide to Caring for Persons with Alzheimer Disease, Other Dementias, and Memory Loss in Later Life*. 4th ed. Baltimore: Johns Hopkins University Press, 2006. Provides a wealth of information for families coping with Alzheimer's disease, including topics such as the evaluation of persons with dementia, hospice care, assisted living facilities and financing care, and the latest findings on eating and nutrition.

Parsons, Malcolm, and Michael Johnson. *Diagnosis in Color: Neurology*. New York: Mosby, 2001. An excellent atlas that allows the pictures to tell the story. The color photographs and brief descriptions capture the essence of brain disorders.

Wiederholt, Wigbert C. *Neurology for Non-neurologists*. 4th ed. Philadelphia: W. B. Saunders, 2000. This small volume is a clear, concise, and useful summary of clinical neurology for physicians who are not specialists in neurology. It emphasizes the recognition and treatment of the usual neurological conditions, ranging from vascular to degenerative to neoplastic.

Woolsey, Thomas A., Joseph Hanaway, and Mokhtar Gado. *Brain Atlas: A Visual Guide to the Human Central Nervous System*. 2d ed. New York: Wiley, 2002. Excellent text whose sections include "Background Information," "The Brain and Its Blood Vessels," "Brain Slices," "Histological Sections," and "Pathways."

Brain tumors

Disease/disorder

Anatomy or system affected: Brain, head, nervous system, spine

Specialties and related fields: General surgery, neurology, oncology, radiology

Definition: An abnormal growth in or on the brain.

Key terms:

glioma: a cancer arising from and in brain substance

hydrocephalus: excessive cerebrospinal fluid within the cranial cavity; commonly called water on the brain

metastasis: the spread of cancer cells

Causes and Symptoms

The earliest symptom of a brain tumor may be a persistent headache, although this symptom does not necessarily stem from a brain tumor. Nevertheless, when headaches occur regularly, it is essential that the cause be investigated as early as possible and a diagnosis made.

> **Information on Brain Tumors**
>
> **Causes:** Possible genetic factors, radiation or carcinogen exposure, metastasis from other cancers (particularly lung cancer)
>
> **Symptoms:** May include headaches, muscle weakness, dizziness, vision and hearing loss, nausea, speech problems, emotional problems, disorientation, seizures, uncharacteristic behavior, memory loss, and hydrocephalus
>
> **Duration:** Progressive
>
> **Treatments:** Surgical removal, radiation, chemotherapy, corticosteroids

As brain tumors continue to grow and crowd the brain, other symptoms become evident. Even though such tumors are frequently benign, they can become disabling. As brain tissue and the nerve tracks inside the skull are compressed by the incursion that such tumors make on them, patients may suffer muscle weakness, dizziness, loss of vision, reduction of hearing, nausea, speech problems, emotional problems, disorientation, and sometimes seizures.

A reduction of mental functions that often accompanies developing brain tumors may result in uncharacteristic behavior. Loss of memory can occur. Unexplained mood swings often accompany brain tumors. If the encroaching tumor obstructs the flow of cerebrospinal fluid, then hydrocephalus may develop.

The incidence of brain tumors is small, representing about 1.3 percent of cancers diagnosed in the United States in a given year. Two age groups are at greater risk than the general population. Adult males between fifty-five and sixty-five years of age seem to be vulnerable to primary brain tumors, and children between three and twelve also have a higher incidence of this condition.

The causes of brain tumors have not been fully determined. It has been noted that genetic factors may play a role in the development of such tumors in young people, particularly those with a parent who has had colon cancer or cancer of the salivary glands or nervous system. Children exposed to high energy radiation applied to the head in the treatment of leukemia or who develop neck or facial cancers suffer an increased risk of developing brain tumors.

Among adults, those whose work exposes them to vinyl chloride have a high incidence of brain tumors, as do those whose work involves exposure to lead in such industries as mining, printing, and chemical industries. Those who suffer from epilepsy are at higher risk of developing gliomas, tumors arising from brain substance, some 60 percent of which are malignant. The risk seems less in people whose diets include little fat and refined sugar and plentiful fresh fruits and vegetables.

Many brain tumors develop from tissues within the skull, but others result from the metastasis, or spread of cancer cells from malignancies elsewhere in the body, often the lungs or breasts. Of the 170,000 Americans who develop lung cancer annually, about 55,000 will also develop brain tumors. Adults who have had organ transplants are also at increased risk.

Treatment and Therapy

Where a brain tumor—malignant or benign—exists, the preferred treatment is surgical removal by opening the skull. Such delicate surgery is performed by a neuro-oncological surgeon who understands the brain's contours and their relationship to the nervous system and spinal cord.

Such diagnostic tools as computed tomography (CT) scanning and magnetic resonance imaging (MRI) can determine the extent of a brain tumor before a decision is made about how to treat the condition. Sometimes surgery is not indicated because the tumor is embedded in vital areas of the brain that would be irreparably damaged by removal.

In such cases, radiation may be used initially to shrink the tumor, sometimes to the point that eventually it can be removed surgically. In other cases, it may be possible to remove part of the tumor, thereby releasing the pressure that it exerts on the brain. Partial removal is usually followed by a course of radiation and/or chemotherapy, generally with the expectation that additional surgical removal will occur if the tumor decreases in size.

Corticosteroids have in some cases succeeded in controlling the swelling of tumors so that pressure on the brain is reduced and symptoms are mitigated.

Perspective and Prospects

In the United States, brain tumors do not occur frequently. About six new cases of primary brain tumors occur every year for every hundred thousand people in the population. Of these, four eventually cause death. The life of one child in every three thousand in the population ends before age ten because of a primary brain tumor. Some fifteen hundred children are diagnosed every year with brain tumors, most located in the cerebellum, the midbrain, or the optic nerve.

There has been an increase in primary brain tumors among the elderly since 1980, while the percentage of resulting deaths has decreased. In viewing such statistics, one must remember that with advances in medical technology, more people are achieving old age and are developing diseases when, fifty years ago, they would not have still been living.

Advances in cell research and in the development of drugs that control and, in some cases, eliminate specific cancer cells provide encouragement that medical progress is being made consistently. Neuro-oncological surgery has undergone great advances and will likely substantially reduce the threat of human error as sophisticated robotic surgical procedures are developed. Although cancer is still a scourge, recent medical research offers realistic hope of controlling it.

—R. Baird Shuman, Ph.D.

See also Brain; Brain disorders; Cancer; Chemotherapy; Head and neck disorders; Headaches; Hydrocephalus; Imaging and radiology; Malignancy and metastasis; Neuroimaging; Neurology; Neurology, pediatric; Neurosurgery; Oncology; Plastic surgery; Radiation therapy; Tumor removal; Tumors.

For Further Information:

Register, Cheri. *The Chronic Illness Experience: Embracing the Imperfect Life*. City Center, Minn.: Hazelden, 1999.

Roloff, Tricia Ann. *Navigating Through a Strange Land: A Book for Brain Tumor Patients and Their Families*. 2d ed. Minneapolis: Fairview Press, 2001.

Shiminski-Maher, Tania, Patsy Cullen, and Maria Sansalone. *Childhood Brain and Spinal Cord Tumors: A Guide for Families, Friends, and Caregivers*. Sebastopol, Calif.: O'Reilly & Associates, 2002.

Stark-Vance, Virginia, and M. L. Dubay. *100 Questions and Answers About Brain Tumors*. Sudbury, Mass.: Jones and Bartlett, 2004.

Zeltzer, Paul M. *Brain Tumors: Leaving the Garden of Eden*. Encino, Calif.: Shilysca Press, 2004.

Breast biopsy

Procedure

Anatomy or system affected: Breasts (female)

Specialties and related fields: General surgery, gynecology

Definition: The surgical removal of a lump or tissue from the breast to determine whether it is malignant.

Indications and Procedures

Among American women, breast cancer is the most common malignancy. (While men can have breast cancer, such cases are relatively rare.) Women have learned the importance of regular self-examination of their breasts and the need to report suspicious lumps and other changes to a physician. Women finding suspicious lumps is the most common indication for breast biopsy to be done. Mammography (an X ray of the breasts) is also used as a cancer screening tool, and suspicious findings often lead to biopsy. Some physicians use breast ultrasound to determine whether biopsy is needed.

Many techniques are used to conduct a breast biopsy. The physician can use a thin needle and syringe to collect cells from suspicious areas (fine needle aspiration). Often, draining a cyst (a fluid-filled sac) is the only treatment needed. Surgeons can conduct a core needle biopsy, using a needle with a cutting edge to cut out a small piece of tissue. Small lumps are often removed in an excisional biopsy (lumpectomy). When lumps are larger, the surgeon may do an incisional biopsy to remove part of the lump for further examination. When no lump is present but suspicious tissue has been revealed by mammography, the surgeon can use the X ray to place small needles in order to remove tissue samples.

Pathologists examine the lump, tissue, or cells removed from the breast to determine whether cancer is present. If cancer is found, the patient has several treatment options, including removal of part or all of the breast, lumpectomy with radiation therapy, chemotherapy, and/or hormone therapy.

—Russell Williams, M.S.W.

See also Biopsy; Breast cancer; Breast disorders; Breast surgery; Breasts, female; Cancer; Cyst removal; Cysts; Gynecology; Mammography; Mastectomy and lumpectomy; Mastitis; Oncology; Pathology; Plastic surgery; Tumor removal; Tumors; Women's health.

For Further Information:

Carter, Darryl. *Interpretation of Breast Biopsies*. 4th ed. Philadelphia: Lippincott Williams & Wilkins, 2003. Updates medical advances in the field and examines such topics as the anatomy and physiology of the breast, changes that occur, types of biopsies, intraductal lesions, skin adnexa or salivary gland-like tumors, and invasive carcinomas.

DeVita, Vincent, Jr., Samuel Hellman, Steven A. Rosenberg, et al., eds. *Cancer: Principles and Practice of Oncology*. 7th ed. Philadelphia: Lippincott Williams & Wilkins, 2005. Four sections present the essentials of molecular biology, signal transduction, and immunology; updated information on the cell cycle, cytogenetics, the metastatic process, causes of cancer, and the principles of chemotherapy, radiation therapy, and surgery.

Elk, Ronit, and Monica Marrow. *Breast Cancer for Dummies*. New York: Wiley, 2003. An excellent resource that covers diagnosis to prognosis to treatment and recovery for those diagnosed with the disease. Helps set expectations for chemotherapy, hormone therapy, and surgery, and offers resources for coping and support.

Mulholland, Michael W., et al., eds. *Greenfield's Surgery: Scientific Principles and Practice*. 4th ed. Philadelphia: Lippincott Williams & Wilkins, 2006. The contributors represent the various specialties of surgery, including gastrointestinal, vascular, pediatric, trauma, plastic and reconstructive, cardiothoracic, and surgical oncology. Most are from respected academic medical centers in the United States.

Sloane, John P. *Biopsy Pathology of the Breast*. 2d ed. New York: Oxford University Press, 2001. A practical guide to diagnosing breast pathology. Second edition examines the way in which advances in mammographic screening, more treatment options, greater involvement by pathologists in clinical management, and the expansion of molecular pathology have affected the field.

U.S. Department of Health and Human Services, Public Health Service, and National Institutes of Health. *Breast Biopsy: What You Should Know*. Bethesda, Md.: Author, 1990. This publication is designed to educate patients on the risks and benefits of biopsy as a treatment for cancer.

Breast cancer

Disease/disorder

Anatomy or system affected: Breasts, cells, glands, lymphatic system

Specialties and related fields: General surgery, genetics, gynecology, histology, oncology, pathology, preventive medicine, radiology

Definition: A general term for a group of solid tumor malignancies arising in the tissues of the breast.

Key terms:

carcinoma: a solid tumor malignancy occurring in cells of the epithelium or tissues surrounding the major organ systems of the body *metastasis:* the unique property of cancer cells that permits them to spread to multiple sites within the body

mutation: a change in gene structure that disrupts the normal functions of the encoded protein

Causes and Symptoms

Breast cancer is the most common malignancy in women (besides skin cancer) and the second leading cause of cancer deaths in women (behind lung cancer). Approximately 200,000 new cases are diagnosed each year in the United States alone, and more than 40,000 deaths occur yearly as a consequence of this disease. A diagnosis of breast cancer may strike a profound sense of fear in a patient, but this fear can be alleviated somewhat through a better understanding of its causes and the treatment options and preventive strategies that show promise in countering this disease.

To understand breast cancer, it is first necessary to know the anatomy and structures that constitute the breast tissue from which cancer arises. Breast tissue consists of fatty tissue and the functional tissue of the breast: the lobes and ducts that are involved in the production and secretion of milk. The arrangement of the lobes and ducts of the breast resembles the spokes of a wheel around the nipple area. Inside each lobe are multiple lobules in which the milk is produced. The milk then travels down the ducts and is released through the nipple. Most important, the growth and development of the breast tissue is under hormonal control and begins at the time of puberty. The sex hormones progesterone and estrogen, produced by the ovaries, are largely responsible for the development of breast tissue.

This information is important to an understanding of how cancer arises in the breast. The majority of breast cancers occur in the ductal tissue (80 percent), and most of the remaining breast cancers originate in the lobular tissue (10 to 15 percent). Moreover, many cancers are hormonally responsive, meaning that the sustained growth of the abnormal tissue is stimulated by the presence of the female sex hormones. Cells of the breast may undergo growth changes during the process of tissue renewal and differentiation that ultimately may give rise to cancer.

Thus, in many ways tumor formation in the breast may reflect aspects of the normal proliferation of newly forming ductal or lobular cells, including hormonal sensitivity. In breast cancer, however, the process goes awry to produce abnormal cells with proliferative and invasive properties that may become life-threatening. Thus, to understand how breast cancer arises it is necessary to understand the developmental pathways of the tissue and its responses to the hormones and growth factors that regulate tissue development.

Information on Breast Cancer

Causes: Hormonal, genetic, environmental, and lifestyle factors

Symptoms: Tumor, which may or may not be palpable

Duration: Chronic

Treatments: Surgical removal of tumor and sometimes surrounding tissues and structures, radiation, chemotherapy (selective estrogen receptor modulators, aromatase inhibitors, monoclonal antibodies, etc.)

The nature of the cellular abnormalities responsible for the development of breast cancer has been the object of intense research for many years. Although the process by which malignant tumors of the breast develop remains unclear, scientists have learned a great deal about the profound cellular transformation that results in breast cancer. Tumors originate in the individual cells within the breast tissue that begin to proliferate abnormally as a direct result of genetic changes within the breast cells and/or in response to abnormal proliferative stimuli, such as hormones or other growth factors in the local environment of the breast.

Approximately 5 to 10 percent of women who develop breast cancer have mutations in genes that are inherited and predispose them to develop this disease. The first gene to be identified was BRCA1. Carriers of mutations in this gene have a 90 percent chance of developing breast cancer or ovarian cancer during their lifetime. Inherited mutations in a second gene, BRCA2, also produce significantly greater risks for the development of this disease. Mutations in BRCA1 and BRCA2 appear to promote the development of cancer as a result of their growth-promoting effects on breast tissue.

In the vast majority of women, however, breast cancer develops in the absence of any known predisposing genetic factor. The original lesion in those cases may involve a spontaneous mutation that alters the cells' proliferative capacity and/or sensitivity to hormonally induced signals. For patients without a family history (approximately 90 percent of women), a number of risk factors have been identified. The disease is linked to advancing age, with 77 percent of cases occurring in women over age fifty. Additional factors which may increase the risk of developing breast cancer are first menstruation before age twelve, first childbirth after age thirty, and menopause after age fifty. These risk factors are linked to the exposure of breast tissue to the circulating reproductive hormones estrogen and progesterone. In fact, breast cancers can generally be divided into two groups depending on whether they display sensitivity to hormonal stimulation of tumor cell growth.

To understand further this process of malignant cell transformation, it is necessary to follow the fate of a cell along the path of malignancy. Cancer begins at the level of individual cells within a tissue that proliferate abnormally as a direct result of genetic changes and/or in response to abnormal proliferative stimuli. The most common type of cancer arises in the ductal tissue of the breast and is termed ductal carcinoma in situ (DCIS) in its earliest, curable stages. This type of breast cancer originates in the milk ducts and may progress to invasive infiltrating ductal carcinoma as the tumor breaks through the lining of the milk ducts and invades the fatty tissue of the breast. In the normal process of development during puberty, the ductal tissue develops in response to the hormone estrogen that is produced by the ovaries. Similarly, the growth of lobular tissue in the breast is stimulated by the hormone progesterone. Tumors that arise in this tissue are called lobular carcinoma in situ (LCIS). This type of cancer begins in the lobules that produce milk and may progress to infiltrating invasive lobular carcinoma.

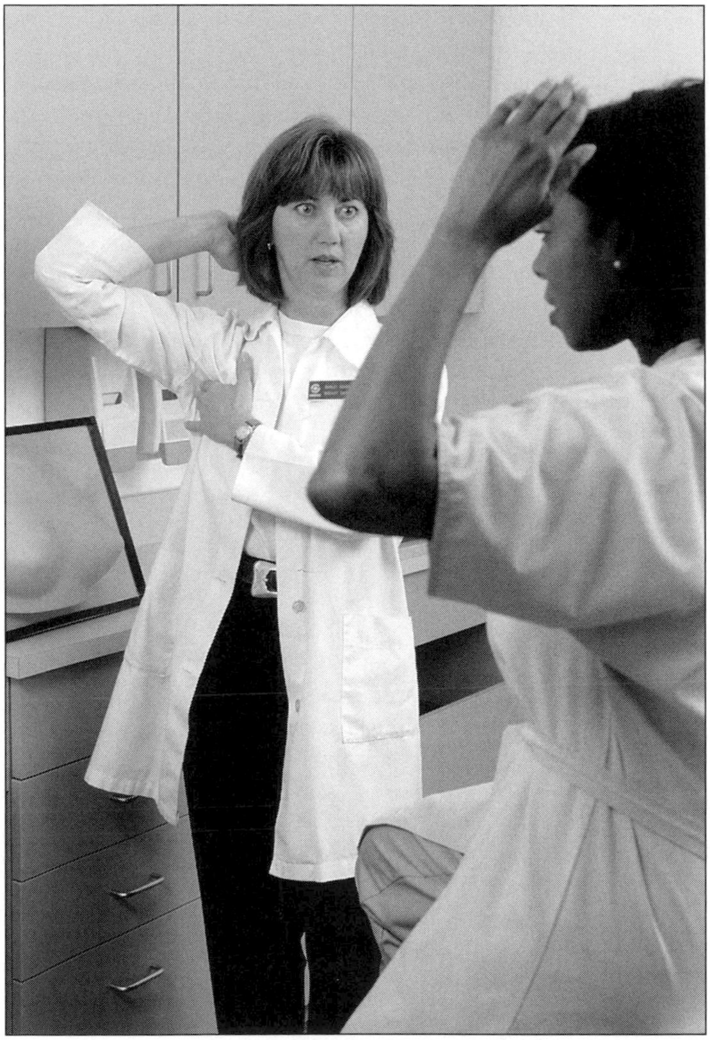

A doctor shows a woman how to perform a breast self-examination. Combined with periodic mammograms, such screening procedures can catch many cases of breast cancer. (PhotoDisc)

Cells of the breast may undergo genetic changes during the process of development or tissue renewal that ultimately give rise to cancer. Breast cancer may take years to develop, silently progressing from a small group of abnormal cells that are no longer responsive to the "rules" governing normal cell cycle proliferation. Over a long period, these cells may accumulate added mutations that render them even more capable of unrestricted proliferation. Target genes that frequently appear to be involved in this process include members of the epidermal growth factor receptor (EGFR) family and the estrogen receptor (ER).

By the time that a tumor is palpable and can be detected as a lump by breast self-examination, the tumor may be defined as malignant based on the results of a number of diagnostic procedures. The vast majority of breast cell abnormalities are benign, meaning that the abnormal tissue is localized in the breast and will not spread further. For example, fluid-filled cysts represent benign breast lesions, as do the cysts characteristic of fibrocystic breast disease. Mammography, a procedure involving radiography of the soft tissue of the breast, and ultrasonography, which uses sound waves to explore tissue structure, are common diagnostic tests useful in detecting the presence of small tumors in the breast and distinguishing between benign and malignant lesions. The definitive test for malignancy is the microscopic examination of affected breast tissue. This examination requires a biopsy, a procedure that involves the removal of a small amount of tissue from the breast.

Cells comprising a benign tumor generally appear very similar in morphology and appearance to normal cells of the same tissue type. In contrast, malignant cells may deviate significantly in structure, morphology, and staining properties, to the extent that the tissue of origin may not even be identifiable in tumors designated "high grade."

At the time of diagnosis, a malignant tumor may be restricted to its site of origin, defined as a carcinoma in situ, or may have spread within the breast or possibly to other tissues and organs of the body, such as the lungs or bones, by a process termed metastasis. Metastasis occurs when tumor cells travel first to the local lymph nodes in the area of the breast and then are disseminated to other sites within the body, where secondary tumors may develop. The diagnosis of metastatic tumor spread, made through lymph node analysis, is of concern since breast cancer is significantly more difficult to treat once it has spread to other sites within the body.

Treatment and Therapy

The hallmarks of malignancy—tumor size, appearance, local invasiveness, and lymph node involvement as evidence of possible metastasis—are all critical components of treatment recommendations and long-term prognosis. Although much research has been directed toward a more molecular diagnostic and therapeutic approach to breast cancer, the BRCA1 and BRCA2 mutations are the only genetic lesions that have been definitively linked to the occurrence of this disease.

Surgical removal of the tumor is the primary treatment for breast cancer. For small, localized tumors that show no evidence of spread within the tissue or lymph node involvement, simple removal of the tumor and surrounding tissues by a procedure termed lumpectomy is the general treatment choice. Even for more advanced breast malignancies, radical mastectomy, a procedure that involves complete removal of the breast, associated lymph nodes, and underlying chest muscles, is seldom performed any longer, since the operation causes disfigurement and similar results can usually be obtained using less extensive surgery. For example, for tumors that have spread within the breast, a portion of the breast may be removed without significant disfigurement. In cases where complete breast removal is required for tumor resection, simultaneous breast reconstruction often accompanies the surgical procedure in order to reduce the physical and psychological effects of mastectomy.

If any evidence exists that a cancer has spread, either locally within the breast tissue or lymph nodes or systemically to other sites within the body, then radiation and chemotherapy may be useful adjuvants to surgical removal of the tumor. Localized treatment involves the use of external beam high-energy radiation that is directed locally to the target tissue to avoid damaging other organs and tissues in the body. The principle underlying the use of radiation to treat cancer involves the fact that high-energy ionizing radiation damages deoxyribonucleic acid (DNA) and destroys dividing cells within the body.

Similarly, conventional chemotherapy involves the use of drugs that interfere with the process of DNA duplication or replication in dividing cells by producing changes in the structure or integrity of the DNA molecule. Unlike radiation, chemotherapy is a systemic form of cancer treatment that is directed at metastatic tumors and cancer cells that may have spread to various sites within the body. Many chemotherapeutic drugs have been used in the treatment of breast cancer. Some of the more commonly used are cyclophosphamide, methotrexate, 5-fluorouracil, and cisplatin. These drugs may be administered intravenously, either individually or in combinations, over a period of weeks to months in an attempt to destroy any remaining cancer cells following surgery or radiation. Another chemotherapeutic drug that has been used successfully to treat breast cancer is paclitaxel, better known as Taxol, a drug originally obtained from the Pacific yew tree which blocks the process of cell division. Taxol targets a specific stage in the cell division cycle involving the separation of chromosomes by threadlike fibers called microtubules in newly forming cells. Taxol binds to the microtubules, thereby arresting the cell division process.

Both radiation and chemotherapy may produce significant side effects, such as anemia, hair loss, nausea and vomiting, fatigue, weight loss, and mouth sores. These side effects occur because radiation and chemotherapeutic drugs target not only cancer cells but also all cells within the body that are actively dividing.

In many patients, chemotherapy and radiation may block the progress of disease within the body, resulting in long-term survival. However, each year many

IN THE NEWS: NEW TREATMENTS

According to the National Cancer Institute, the results of a twenty-year follow-up to the British Columbia randomized radiation trial indicated that when radiation therapy is used in addition to chemotherapy after surgery, breast cancer survival rates increase by nearly one-third. Patients involved in this study were women who had lymph node involvement, prompting the American Cancer Society to state that the use of radiation to the breast and the lymph nodes after surgery (mastectomy or lumpectomy) should improve the survival rates of breast cancer patients who either had lymph node involvement or a tumor larger than five centimeters.

Radiation therapy, which today exists in many different forms, typically is not begun until about a month after surgery in order to allow the tissue to heal. The most common type of radiation used to treat breast cancer is external beam radiation. With this approach, the entire breast (and chest wall) receives radiation. A newer technique undergoing clinical trials is partial breast irradiation. With this technique, the patient receives radiation to only part of the breast and for a shorter period of time (five days). Results from this study are eagerly awaited.

The alternative to external radiation therapy is brachytherapy or internal (interstitial) radiation. With this technique, radioactive isotopes are implanted in the breast tissue next to the cancer site. Another method of internal radiation used following lumpectomy is mammosite. This involves the insertion of a balloon filled with saltwater solution into the lumpectomy space. Over a period of five days, a radioactive material is inserted and removed twice a day and then treatment is terminated. Additional evaluation of internal radiation is ongoing. Newer radiation techniques also minimize side effects. Since radiation is avoided with these techniques, no increase in heart disease is seen. Remaining side effects are fatigue, decreased sensation in the radiated tissue, and dermatological problems in the treated area.

Just as chemotherapy paired with radiation has led to increased survival, so have two new chemotherapy techniques. "Dose dense" chemotherapy involves chemotherapy administered with a reduced time period between successive doses. Patients can tolerate this "dose dense" schedule thanks to a new drug, filgrastin, which helps prevent the decrease in white blood cells (neutropenia) that usually accompanies chemotherapy. A second technique, involving the use of Herceptin (a genetically engineered drug) along with individual chemotherapy to advanced breast cancer patients, also leads to increased survival.

—Robin Kamienny Montvilo, Ph.D.

women continue to die of breast cancer despite aggressive treatment. The reasons that cancer treatments fail are as mysterious as the disease process itself. Tumor cells may not respond to chemotherapy and radiation even at very high doses as a result of the phenomenon of drug resistance, which is characteristic of many cancers, especially at advanced stages. For example, very high dose chemotherapy, which removes cells of the immune system, followed by stem cell replacement therapy has been shown to have negligible benefits in patients with advanced metastatic disease. Though the molecular basis of drug resistance remains unclear, mutations in certain genes, such as the multidrug resistance gene 1 (MDR1), have been identified. Moreover, the complexities of tumor structure and behavior may overwhelm the potential cytotoxic (cell-killing) effects of drugs commonly used to treat this disease.

New treatments for breast cancer have been developed as a consequence of an increased understanding of the biology of breast cancer neoplasms. For example, a significant percentage of breast cancers have been shown to be hormonally responsive, meaning that their growth is stimulated by the female sex hormones estrogen or progesterone. These tumors are classified as estrogen-responsive (ER) or progesterone-responsive (PR). A class of drugs that targets the estrogen receptor in ER-positive breast cancers, called selective estrogen receptor modulators (SERMs), has shown great clinical promise in the treatment of breast cancer as well as in preventing recurrences of the disease.

Tamoxifen is the oldest and most prominent member of this group; this drug specifically targets the estrogen receptor in breast tissue and blocks the growth-promoting effects of estrogen in estrogen-sensitive breast cancers. Tamoxifen has been used therapeutically to treat metastatic breast disease and also to prevent breast cancer recurrences, with significant success. A number of clinical studies have shown that patients receiving this drug have dramatically lower recurrence and mortality rates than patients who do not receive this drug. For example, a major study conducted in 1998 by the National Cancer Institute demonstrated a 50 percent reduction in breast cancer occurrence in high-risk women treated with tamoxifen. Moreover, the study showed that this drug also arrested the progression of DCIS and LCIS to invasive disease. These clinical trials have shown significant benefits from tamoxifen taken over periods of up to five years to prevent the recurrence of breast cancer in high-risk patients. It is not surprising, however, that this drug is ineffective against breast cancers that are not estrogen-responsive. Tamoxifen has also been used in combined chemotherapy with conventional chemotherapeutic drugs such as cyclophosphamide, methotrexate, and 5-fluorouracil, with varying results.

Unfortunately, tamoxifen does have significant side effects, including an increased risk of developing uterine cancer, since the drug stimulates the growth of ER-positive endometrial cells in the uterus. For this reason, patients taking this drug should be monitored carefully by a physician. Tamoxifen use has also been linked to vascular disease, including blood clots and strokes in some patients.

Another SERM called raloxifene hydrochloride, marketed under the name Evista, is an antiestrogen that has also shown significant clinical benefit, with results similar to those obtained using tamoxifen. For example, clinical trials have indicated that raloxifene use decreases the risk of breast cancer in high-risk postmenopausal women by as much as 70 percent. An important difference between these two drugs, however, is that raloxifene blocks estrogen receptors in both the breast and the uterus, thereby decreasing the risk of developing uterine cancer for patients taking this drug. However, additional long-term studies will be needed to assess more fully the risks and benefits obtained by using raloxifene versus tamoxifen.

A newer class of antiestrogens are the aromatase inhibitors (AI). These drugs block the formation of estrogen within the body and are especially beneficial to older, postmenopausal women. This class of drugs works by blocking the conversion, or aromatization, of androgens produced by the adrenal glands to estrogen. This reaction is carried out by enzymes called aromatases and occurs in fatty tissues throughout the body, significantly contributing to estrogen production in postmenopausal women. These aromatase inhibitors, marketed under the names Arimidex and Femara, have shown clinical promise in the treatment of postmenopausal women with advanced breast cancer. However, clinical studies on the combined use of AIs with SERMs such as tamoxifen have shown no significant clinical benefit so far over the use of these drugs individually.

As a means of reducing the potential side effects associated with tamoxifen, clinical studies published since 2002 have demonstrated the increased effectiveness of adjuvant chemotherapy in treating certain forms of breast cancer in postmenopausal women. For example, anastrozole (Arimidex), an aromatase inhibitor, when used in conjuction with tamoxifen during long-term treatment, produced fewer side effects and was as effective in reducing metastasis.

In addition to hormone therapy, drugs that target abnormal genes in breast cancer cells have also been used successfully to treat breast cancer and to prevent its recurrence. For example, approximately 25 percent of breast cancer patients show overexpression of the HER2/neu gene product as a consequence of genetic rearrangements that increase the number of copies of this gene by a process called gene amplification in the tumor cells. The HER2/neu gene is a member of a family of genes that encode cell surface receptors for epidermal growth factor, a growth-promoting protein that stimulates cell cycle proliferation. The overexpression of the HER2/neu receptor in breast cancer cells therefore renders these cells inordinately sensitive to growth factor stimulation of cell division, which directly contributes to the growth of the malignant breast tissue. The drug trastuzumab, better known as Herceptin, is a humanized monoclonal antibody that specifically targets and binds to the HER2/neu receptor, thereby blocking its interaction with epidermal growth factor and the resulting stimulation of cell proliferation. Herceptin has shown positive clinical benefit in patients with HER2/neu-positive tumors, both in the treatment phase and in long-term use in the prevention of breast cancer recurrence.

Perspective and Prospects

The ultimate goal of breast cancer research is prevention. To achieve this goal, it will be necessary to identify more clearly the risk factors that contribute to the development of this disease and to design preventive strategies for counteracting genetic changes and/or hormonal changes within the body that may ultimately give rise to malignant tumors of the breast tissue. Women with an inherited genetic predisposition to breast cancer, such as mutations in the BRCA1 and BRCA2 genes, would receive the greatest benefit from these preventive approaches. Currently, some women that carry BRCA1 or BRCA2 mutations undergo preventive bilateral mastectomy in a desperate attempt to avoid overlooking precancerous lesions that cannot be detected by existing diagnostic technologies.

Early detection methods aimed at identifying and removing precancerous breast lesions such as DCIS and LCIS represent an important preventive strategy whose benefits have not yet been fully realized. Currently, mammography and breast self-examination are the most common means of breast cancer detection. Although useful, these methods may fail to detect small tumors before they have become invasive. Ultrasonography, used in conjunction with other detection methods, may improve the likelihood of detecting premalignant lesions and early-stage cancers. Better methods of breast cancer detection need to be developed, a goal that may become increasingly possible given the increased understanding of the molecular basis of breast cancer. Molecular methods may also be useful in the development of diagnostic tests that identify additional genetic predispositions to the development of breast cancer, so that aggressive preventive approaches can be taken in women identified as higher risk that may prevent the occurrence of this disease.

Clinical studies using hormone therapy approaches have shown that, under certain conditions, breast cancer can be prevented by drugs that target hormone and growth factor receptor signal pathways in tumor cells. These data provide further evidence in support of many epidemiological studies suggesting that the lifetime exposure of breast tissue to estrogen is associated with an increased risk of developing breast cancer. For this reason, women who take oral estrogen/progesterone in the form of oral contraceptives or hormone replacement therapy (HRT) need to be aware of potential risks associated with the use of these drugs. Many studies have shown that oral contraceptive use in women under age thirty-five who do not smoke does not appear to produce a significantly elevated risk of breast cancer or other complications. However, recent well-documented clinical data on HRT in perimenopausal or postmenopausal women suggest that its use may contribute to a significantly elevated risk of aggressive breast cancers that are difficult to detect by mammography. In addition, HRT has been associated with side effects that may result in an increased risk of blood clots, strokes, and heart attacks. For these reasons, it appears that current forms of HRT should be used only for limited duration under the careful supervision of a physician.

Many studies have been carried out to assess the role of diet in breast cancer prevention. For example, epidemiological studies have shown repeatedly that Japanese women have a far lower incidence of breast cancer than do American women. This decreased incidence in Japanese women has been attributed in part to dietary differences in the amount of fat consumption, as well as to the extensive use of soy products in Japanese cooking. Soy contains an estrogen receptor binding substance called genistein. It is believed that the genistein in soy binds to estrogen receptors to block their binding to the growth-promoting hormone estrogen. The role of diet in the prevention of breast cancer is unclear, as study results range from reduced risk associated with low-fat diets to no effects at all. Some of the confusion may be the result of the complexity of breast cancer. Low-fat, high-fiber (vegetarian) diets have been demonstrated to reduce the levels of estrogen and other reproductive hormones, and it may be in this manner that the risk of certain forms of cancer is reduced.

Although the goal of eliminating breast cancer still remains elusive, those who conduct breast cancer research and those whose lives have been touched by this disease may find it comforting to realize that so much progress has been made in understanding the cellular and molecular basis of this disease.

—Sarah Crawford, Ph.D.; updated by Richard Adler, Ph.D.

See also Breast biopsy; Breast disorders; Breast surgery; Breasts, female; Cancer; Chemotherapy; Gynecology; Malignancy and metastasis; Mammography; Mastectomy and lumpectomy; Oncology; Radiation therapy; Women's health.

For Further Information:

Arnot, Bob. *Breast Cancer Prevention Diet*. Boston: Little, Brown, 1999. A practical description of healthful dietary habits that may reduce the risks of developing breast cancer.

Canfield, Jack, et al. *Chicken Soup for the Soul Healthy Living Series: Breast Cancer*. Deerfield Beach, Fla.: Hci, 2005. A collection of stories by cancer survivors, as well as suggestions for seeking treatment, creating a diet, and dealing with the side effects of treatment.

Link, John. *Breast Cancer Survival Manual*. Rev. 2d ed. New York: Henry Holt, 2000. Counsels how to manage breast cancer from a medical and psychological perspective.

Love, Susan, with Karen Lindsey. *Dr. Susan Love's Breast Book*. Rev. 4th ed. Cambridge, Mass.: Da Capo Press, 2005. Provides a sensitive woman's perspective to understanding and managing this disease.

Narod, Steven, and William Foulkes. "BRCA1 and BRCA2: 1994 and Beyond." *Nature Reviews/Cancer* 4 (September, 2004): 665-676. Discusses the role of specific mutations behind the genetic predisposition for breast cancer.

Breast disorders

Disease/disorder

Anatomy or system affected: Breasts, glands, lymphatic system

Specialties and related fields: Cytology, general surgery, gynecology, histology, neonatology

Definition: A variety of benign breast conditions, including fibrocystic disease and mastitis, which cause discomfort and anxiety and can make self-examination and diagnosis of cancer difficult.

Key terms:

biopsy: the removal of sample tissue for microscopic inspection and analysis by a pathologist

cyst: a fluid-filled, enclosed sac in the body

fine needle aspiration: a surgical procedure in which a thin, hollow needle is used to withdraw tissue from the body

necrosis: cell death, usually involving the rupture of the cell membrane and the release of cell contents into the surrounding tissue

Causes and Symptoms

Because of fear of breast cancer and discomfort, noncancerous breast disorders often cause women a great deal of anxiety and distress. The most common noncancerous breast disorder is fibrocystic breast condition, also known as mammary dysplasia, a condition in which the breast tissue is lumpy and tender. Other, less common breast disorders include mastitis, fat necrosis, and a variety of benign breast tumors.

Common symptoms of fibrocystic breast condition include a dense and lumpy texture, which is usually more evident in the upper and outer quadrants of the breast. Intermittent or persistent dull pain, tenderness, and itching of the nipples often occur premenstrually, lessening after menstruation begins. This condition is so common, occurring in an estimated 60 percent of women between thirty and fifty years old, that it is considered a variation of normal. The lumpy tissue often causes significant discomfort, and its presence can terrify women checking for cancer during breast self-examination and make the diagnosis of cancer more difficult.

The cause of fibrocystic breasts is unknown, although the associated discomfort fluctuates with the menstrual cycle and rarely occurs after menopause, so ovarian hormones are likely involved. A family history of the disorder increases risk, and excessive dietary fat and caffeine intake may exacerbate the condition.

After breast lumps and pain, nipple discharge is the third most common breast complaint. Clear, milky, yellow, or green discharge occurring from both nipples does not usually indicate cancer, and a significant percentage of women will experience such discharge at some point while performing a self-examination. Women should see a doctor if the nipple discharge is bloody, watery, sticky, persistent, occurs on one side, or appears spontaneously without squeezing the nipple, although only about 10 percent of such discharges are the result of cancer.

Mastitis is an infection caused when the *Staphylococcus aureus* bacteria found normally on the skin enters the breast and causes swelling in the fatty breast tissue. It is most common in breast-feeding women. The symptoms include pain; lumps; irregular breast enlargement; breast swelling, redness, or warmth; nipple discharge and itching; enlarged lymph nodes; and fever. In rare cases, severe infections may cause abscesses.

Four types of benign tumors commonly occur in the breast. Galactoceles are noncancerous cysts filled with breast milk that occur in pregnant and lactating women. Fibroadenomas are round tumors comprised of con-

Information on Breast Disorders

Causes: Hormones, bacterial infection, trauma

Symptoms: Swelling and tenderness, lumps or cysts, pain, infection and inflammation, nipple discharge, fibroadenomas

Duration: Acute to chronic

Treatments: Surgery, antibiotics, hormonal treatment

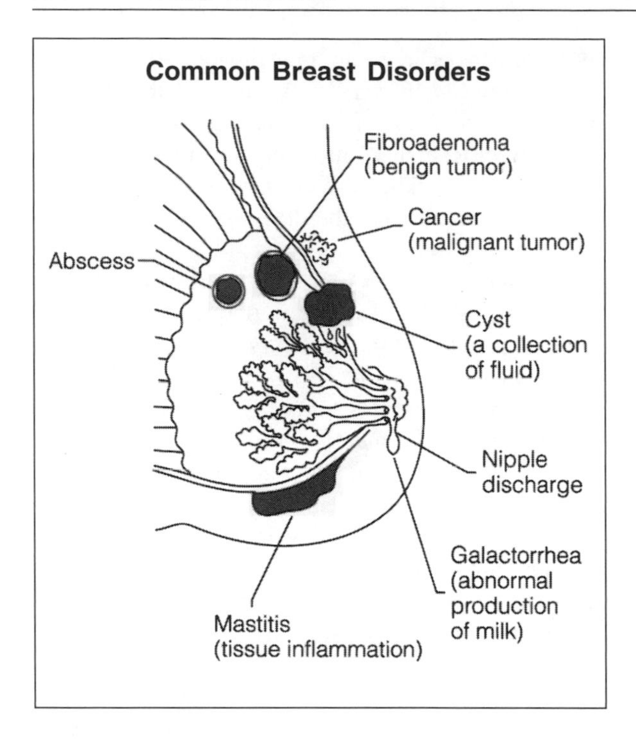

nective and glandular breast tissue that develop in young adult women, most commonly African Americans. They occur singly and in clusters, are marblelike, and are diagnosed by needle biopsy. Intraductal papillomas are branching, stalklike growths in the milk ducts near the nipple. They can cause bloody nipple discharge. Duct ectasia, which typically affects women aged forty to sixty, is a hardening of the milk duct that can cause a thick, dark green discharge. A lump can develop around the duct and be mistaken for cancer.

Fat necrosis often occurs after the breast has been injured and the injured area is replaced with firm scar tissue or oil-filled cysts.

Treatment and Therapy

The diagnosis of fibrocystic breast disorder is made by physical examination. Fibrocystic lumps are usually rounded, smooth, and malleable, although they can mimic hard and stationary cancerous lumps. The density of fibrocystic tissue makes physical examinations and mammography less effective, and ultrasound scans and needle biopsies are often necessary to rule out cancer. Although synthetic androgen (male) hormone therapy can be prescribed in severe cases and oral contraceptives can lessen symptoms, reducing dietary fat and caffeine intake are good first steps. Homeopathic treatments such as soy, vitamin E, vitamin B_6, and evening primrose oil are controversial.

For mastitis, application of a hot, moist compress to the infected area can relieve symptoms, and the infection usually responds well to antibiotics. Lactating women should continue to breast-feed or pump while undergoing treatment. For women who are not breast-feeding, mastitis should be differentiated from a rare form of breast cancer through mammography or biopsy.

Galactoceles are generally left untreated unless they cause discomfort. They can be drained by fine needle aspiration if necessary. Fibroadenomas usually stop growing without treatment, but they need to be surgically removed if they continue to grow. Intraductal papillomas are treated by removing the affected duct. Duct ectasia can be treated with heat compresses, by antibiotics, or, in severe cases, by removal of the duct.

For fat necrosis, fine needle aspiration, often used for diagnosis, usually relieves the symptoms and serves as the primary treatment.

Perspective and Prospects

Like most disorders that primarily affect women and are associated with sex differentiation, noncancerous breast disorders were rarely discussed and were not well understood before the mid-twentieth century. In the nineteenth century, breast disorders were surrounded by myth and social stigma, and mastitis often went untreated for weeks, causing tremendous discomfort. The invention of mammography in the mid-1960's, as well as that decade's increased sexual openness, made it easier to talk about breast disorders as well as to diagnose them accurately. Fibrocystic breast condition, originally called fibrocystic disease, is now accepted as normal for many women, and testing procedures are beginning to adapt to this norm. Over time, mammography, the collection of data from two generations of women, and the generally increased awareness of women's health issues have improved the diagnosis and treatment of these disorders.

—Caroline M. Small

See also Breast biopsy; Breast cancer; Breast-feeding; Breasts, female; Cyst removal; Cysts; Gynecomastia; Mastitis.

For Further Information:

Chinyama, Catherine N. *Benign Breast Disease: Radiology, Pathology, Risk Assessment.* New York: Springer, 2004.

Dixon, J. Michael, ed. *ABC of Breast Diseases.* 3d ed. Malden, Mass.: Blackwell Science, 2006.

Love, Susan M., and Karen Lindsey. *Dr. Susan Love's Breast Book*. Rev. 4th ed. Cambridge, Mass.: Da Capo Press, 2005.

McGinn, Kerry Anne. *Informed Woman's Guide to Breast Health: Breast Changes That Are Not Cancer*. 3d ed. Palo Alto, Calif.: Bull, 2001.

Breast-feeding

Biology

Anatomy or system affected: Breasts, glands, reproductive system

Specialties and related fields: Gynecology, nutrition, obstetrics, perinatology

Definition: The preferred feeding method for infants, providing optimal nutrition for the infant (including immunologic protection), mother-infant bonding, and enhanced maternal health.

Key terms:

alveoli: the milk-producing cells of the mammary gland

bifidus factors: factors in colostrum and breast milk that favor the growth of helpful bacteria in the infant's intestinal tract

bonding: a process in which a mother forms an affectionate attachment to her infant immediately after birth

colostrum: the secretion from the breast before the onset of milk

foremilk: the milk released early in a nursing session, which is low in fat and rich in nutrients

hindmilk: the milk released late in a nursing session, which is higher in fat content

lactoferrin: a breast milk factor that binds iron, preventing it from supporting the growth of harmful intestinal bacteria; it may also promote the ability to absorb dietary iron

let-down reflex: the reflex that forces milk to the front of the breast

oxytocin: the hormone secreted from the posterior pituitary gland that stimulates the mammary glands to eject milk; it also stimulates the uterus to contract after birth

prolactin: a hormone secreted from the anterior pituitary gland that signals the breast to start and sustain milk production

Process and Effects

The terms "breast-feeding," "nursing," and "lactation" all refer to the best method of infant feeding. Although there are a few rare exceptions, almost every mother can breast-feed and thereby provide low-cost, nutritional support for her infant. Although it is often thought otherwise, the size of the mother's breast has no relationship to successful lactation. In fact, the physiology of successful lactation is determined by the maturation of breast tissue, the initiation and maintenance of milk secretion, and the ejection or delivery of milk to the nipple. This physiology is dependent on hormonal control, and all women have the required anatomy for successful lactation unless they have had surgical alteration of the breast.

Hormonal influence on breast development begins in adolescence. Increased estrogen causes the breast ducts to elongate and duct cells to grow. (The ducts are narrow tubular vessels that run from the segments of the breast into the tip of the nipple.) More fibrous and fatty tissue develops, and the nipple area matures. As adolescence progresses, regular menstrual cycle hormones cause further development of the alveoli, which are the milk-producing cells.

The elevated levels of estrogen present during pregnancy promote the growth and branching of milk ducts, while the increase in progesterone promotes the development of alveoli. Throughout pregnancy and especially during the first three months, many more milk ducts are formed. Clusters of milk-producing cells also begin to enlarge, while at the same time placental hormones promote breast development.

Shortly before labor and delivery, the hormone prolactin is produced by the pituitary gland. Prolactin, which is necessary for starting lactation and sustaining milk production, reaches its peak at delivery. Another hormone, oxytocin, which is also produced by the pituitary, stimulates the breast to eject milk. This reaction is called the "let-down reflex," which causes the milk-producing alveoli to contract and force milk to the front of the breast. Oxytocin serves an important function after delivery by causing the uterus to contract. Initially, the let-down reflex occurs only when the infant suckles, but later on it may be initiated simply by the baby's cry. An efficient let-down reflex is critical to successful breast-feeding. Emotional upset, fatigue, pain, nervousness, or embarrassment about lactation can interrupt this reflex; these psychological factors, rather than breast size or physiology, are predictive of successful lactation.

Not only is breast-feeding a natural response to childbirth, but the nutrient content is tailor-made for the human infant as well. More than one hundred constituents of breast milk, both nutritive and nonnutritive, are known. Although the basic nutrient content is a solution of protein, sugar, and salts in which fat is suspended, those concentrations vary depending on the period of lactation and even within a given feeding.

Colostrum, often called "first milk," is produced in the first few days after birth. It is lower in fat and Calories (kilocalories) and higher in protein and certain minerals than is mature breast milk. Colostrum is opaque and yellow because it contains a high concentration of the vitamin A-like substances called carotenes. It also has a high concentration of antibodies and white blood cells, which pass on immunologic protection to the infant.

Within a few days after birth, the transition is made from colostrum to mature milk. There are two types of mature milk. Foremilk is released first as the infant begins to suckle. It has a watery, bluish appearance and is low in fat and rich in other nutrients. This milk accounts for about one-third of the baby's intake. As the nursing session progresses, the draught reflex helps move the hindmilk, with its higher fat content, to the front of the breast. It is important that the nutrient content of breast milk be determined from a sample of both types of milk in order to make an adequate assessment of all nutrients present.

Breast milk best meets the infant's needs and is the standard from which infant formulas are judged. Several nutrient characteristics make it the ideal infant food. Lactose, the carbohydrate content of breast milk, is the same simple sugar found in any milk, but the protein content of breast milk is uniquely tailored to meet infant needs. An infant's immature kidneys are better able to maintain water balance because breast milk is lower in protein than cow's milk. Most breast milk protein is alpha-lactalbumin, whereas cow's milk protein is casein. Alpha-lactalbumin is easier to digest and provides two sulphur-containing amino acids that are the building blocks of protein required for infant growth.

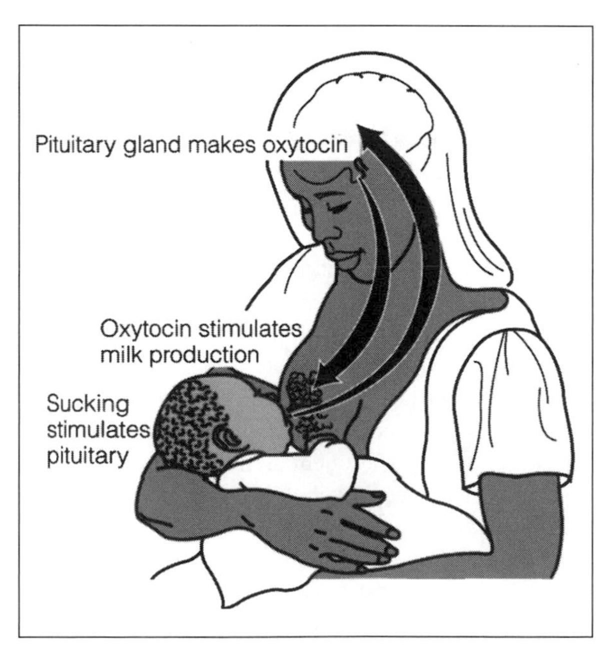

Breast-feeding involves a hormonal feedback loop that encourages milk production.

The fat (lipid) content of breast milk differs among women, and even from the same woman, from day to day. The types of fatty acids that make up most of the fat component of the milk may vary in response to maternal diet. Mothers fed a diet containing corn and cottonseed oil produce a milk with more polyunsaturated fatty acids, which are the predominant fatty acids in those oils. Breast milk is higher in the essential fatty acid called linoleic acid than is cow's milk, and it also contains omega-3 fatty acids. About 55 percent of human milk Calories come from fat, compared to about 49 percent of Calories found in infant formulas. In addition, enzymes in breast milk help digest fat in the infant's stomach. This digested fat is more efficiently absorbed than the products that result from digesting cow's milk.

Breast milk contains more cholesterol than cow's milk, which seems to stimulate development of the enzymes necessary for degrading cholesterol, perhaps offering protection against atherosclerosis in later life. Cholesterol is also needed for proper development of the central nervous system.

The vitamin and mineral content of breast milk from healthy mothers supplies all that is needed for growth and health except for vitamin D and fluoride, and these are easily supplemented. Breast milk and the infant's intestinal bacteria also supply all the necessary vitamin K, but since no bacteria are present at birth, an injection of vitamin K should be given to prevent deficiencies.

Breast milk mineral content is balanced to promote growth while protecting the infant's immature kidneys. Breast milk has a low sodium content, which helps the immature kidneys to maintain water balance. No type of milk is a good source of iron. Although breast milk contains relatively small amounts of iron, about 50 percent of this iron can be absorbed by the body, compared to only 4 percent from cow's milk. This phenomenon is called bioavailability. Because of the high bioavailability of breast milk iron, the introduction of solids, which are given to replace depleted iron stores, can be delayed until six months of age in most infants; this delay may help to reduce the incidence of allergies in susceptible infants. There is also evidence that zinc is better absorbed from breast milk.

The vitamin content of milk can vary and is influenced by maternal vitamin status. The water-soluble vitamin content of breast milk (the B vitamins and vitamin C) will change more because of maternal diet than the fat-soluble vitamin content (vitamins A, E, and K). If women have diets that are deficient in vitamins, their levels in breast milk will be lower. Yet even malnourished mothers can breast-feed, although the quantity of milk is decreased. As the maternal diet improves, the level of water-soluble vitamins in the milk increases. There is a level, however, above which additional diet supplements will not increase the vitamin content of breast milk.

There are many nonnutritive advantages to breast-feeding. A major advantage is the immunologic protection and resistance factors that it provides to the infant. Bifidus factors, found in both colostrum and mature milk, favor the growth of helpful bacteria in the infant's digestive tract. These bacteria in turn offer protection against harmful organisms. Lactoferrin, another resistance factor, binds iron so that harmful bacteria cannot use it. Lysozyme, lipases, and lactoperoxidases also offer protection against harmful bacteria.

Immunoglobulins are present in large amounts in colostrum and in significant amounts in breast milk. These protein compounds act as antibodies against foreign substances in the body called antigens. Generally, the resistance passed to the infant is from environmental antigens to which the mother had been exposed. The concentration of antibodies in colostrum is highest in the first hour after birth. Secretory IgA is the major immunoglobulin that provides protection against gastrointestinal organisms. Breast milk also contains interferon, an antiviral substance which is produced by special white blood cells in milk. Protection against allergy is another advantage of breast-feeding. It is not known, however, whether less exposure to the antigens found in formula or some substance in the breast milk itself provides this protection. Normally, a mucous barrier in the intestine prevents the absorption of whole proteins, the root of an allergic reaction. In the newborn, this barrier is not fully developed to allow whole immunologic proteins to be absorbed. The possibility that whole food proteins will be absorbed as well is greater if cow's milk or early solids are given, and this absorption increases the potential for allergic reactions.

Other possible benefits of breast-feeding are protection against the intestinal disorders Crohn's disease and celiac sprue, and insulin-dependent diabetes. The reasons for this protection are not clear.

Breast-feeding encourages infant bonding, a process in which the mother forms an affectionate attachment to her baby. It is a matter of controversy whether breast-feeding mothers bond better than bottle-feeding mothers. If a mother has early and prolonged contact with her baby, however, the mother is more likely to breast-feed and to nurse her baby for more months.

Milk from mothers delivering preterm infants is higher in protein and nonprotein nitrogen, calcium, IgA, sodium, potassium, chloride, phosphorus, and magnesium. It also has a different fat composition and is lower in lactose than mature milk of mothers delivering after a normal term. These concentrations support more rapid growth of a preterm infant.

Breast-feeding is not only good for the baby but also good for the mother. There is an association between reduced breast cancer rates and breast-feeding, although the reason is not known. In addition, the hormonal influences caused by suckling the infant help to contract the uterus, returning it to prepregnancy size and controlling blood loss. Breast-feeding also helps to reduce the mother's weight. Calories required to make milk are drawn from the fat stores that were deposited during pregnancy. Nevertheless, breast-feeding should be viewed not as a quick weight loss program but as a healthful, natural weight loss process.

If a woman breast-feeds completely, which means that no supplements or solid foods are given until the baby is six months of age, often she will not menstruate. Many women find this lack of menstrual periods psychologically pleasant while not realizing the physiological benefit of restoring the iron stores that were depleted during pregnancy and delivery. An important advantage to breast-feeding in developing countries is that it can help to space pregnancies naturally. Most infant malnutrition occurs when the second child is born, because breast-feeding is stopped for the first child. The first child is weaned to foods that do not supply enough nutrients. By spacing pregnancies out, the first child has a chance to nurse longer.

Breast-feeding is very convenient and does not require time to mix and prepare formula or sterilize bottles. Breast milk is always sterile and at the proper temperature. The money needed for the extra food required to produce breast milk is much less than that required to purchase commercial formula. This can be a major benefit for women with low incomes and is critically important for the health of those babies born in developing countries.

Complications and Disorders

Some special problems or circumstances can make breast-feeding difficult. The breasts may become engorged—so full of milk that they are hard and sore—making it difficult for the baby to latch onto the nipple. Gentle massaging of the breasts, especially with warm water or a heating pad, will allow release of the milk and reduce pain in the breast. This situation is common during the first few weeks of nursing but will occasionally recur if a feeding is missed or a schedule changes.

Sometimes a duct will become plugged and form a hard lump. Massaging the lump and continuing to nurse will remedy the situation. If influenza-like symptoms accompany a plugged duct, the cause is probably a breast infection. Since the infection is in the tissue around the milk-producing glands, the milk itself is safe. The mother must apply heat, get plenty of rest, and keep emptying the breast by frequent feedings. Stopping nursing would plug the duct further, making the infection worse.

Of concern to many mothers are reports of contaminants in breast milk. Drugs, environmental pollutants, viruses, caffeine, alcohol, and food allergens can be passed to the infant through breast milk. Drug transmission depends on the administration method, which influences the speed with which it reaches the blood supply to the breast. Whether that drug can remain functional after it is subjected to the acid in the baby's digestive tract varies. Large amounts of caffeine in breast milk can produce a wakeful, hyperactive infant, but this situation is corrected when the mother stops her caffeine consumption. Large amounts of alcohol produce an altered facial appearance which is reversible; however, some psychomotor delay in the infant may remain even after the mother's drinking has stopped. Nicotine also enters milk, but the impact of secondhand smoke may pose more of a health threat than the nicotine content of breast milk. Since the human immunodeficiency virus (HIV), the virus that causes acquired immunodeficiency syndrome (AIDS), can also pass through breast milk, HIV-positive mothers should not breast-feed their infants.

Of greater concern is the presence of contaminants that cannot be avoided, such as pesticide residues, industrial waste, or other environmental contaminants. Polychlorinated biphenyls (PCBs) and the pesticide DDT have received the most attention. Long-term exposure to contaminants promotes their accumulation in the mother's body fat, and the production of breast milk is one way to rid the body of these contaminants. Concentrations present in the breast milk vary. Ordinarily, these substances are in such small quantities that they pose no health risk. Women who have consumed large amounts of fish from PCB-contaminated waters or have had occupational exposure to this chemical, however, need to have their breast milk tested. It is also possible for these substances to enter the infant's food supply from other sources.

Perspective and Prospects

Although breast-feeding is the best method of infant feeding, many women choose not to breast-feed. Before the 1700's, human milk was the only source for infant feeding. If a mother did not breast-feed, a woman called a wet nurse fed her baby. At the end of the nineteenth century, formula feeding became popular when bottles were developed and water sanitation improved. Breast-feeding declined to less than 20 percent by 1970 but dramatically increased to nearly 70 percent in the early twenty-first century. More than 32 percent of mothers continue breast-feeding until their infants are six months of age.

Breast-feeding used to be more prevalent among more-educated, higher-income mothers. Increased employment of women outside the home, however, has dramatically altered trends in breast-feeding. Although mothers may opt to breast-feed in the hospital, many quit because they are returning to work and believe that it would be too difficult to continue. A working mother needs four to six weeks at home to establish successful breast-feeding.

Formula use has increased in developing countries. Because formula is very expensive, it is often diluted with water and therefore does not provide enough nutritional support to the infant. The quality of water is often so poor in these countries that the infant is exposed to disease-causing organisms. In addition, formula-fed infants do not receive the immunologic protection of breast milk. The result is a higher infant mortality rate.

There are very few instances in which a woman should not breast-feed her infant. Babies with a rare genetic disorder called galactosemia cannot nurse, since they lack the enzyme to metabolize milk sugar. Phenylketonuria (PKU), another genetic disorder, requires close monitoring of the infant's blood phenylalanine level, but the infant can be totally or at least partially breast-fed. Breast-feeding is contraindicated for women suffering from AIDS, alcoholism, drug addiction, malaria, active tuberculosis, or a chronic disease that results in maternal malnutrition. The presence of other conditions, from diabetes to the common cold, are not reasons to avoid breast-feeding.

Lactation, the secretion of milk, is a physiological process, but breast-feeding is a learned practice, a philosophy about nurturing an infant that goes beyond nutritional support. Society needs to foster this practice. Unfortunately, the etiquette of nursing in public areas is not clearly defined, often resulting in embarrassment that inhibits mothers from nursing their babies. The only remedy is for society to recognize that the normal function of breasts is to nurture infants. Breast-feeding represents a vital resource that improves the health and nutritional status of children, especially in underdeveloped countries.

—*Wendy L. Stuhldreher, Ph.D., R.D.*

See also Breast disorders; Breasts, female; Glands; Hormones; Mastitis; Nutrition; Perinatology; Phenylketonuria (PKU); Pregnancy and gestation.

For Further Information:

Bennett, Peter N., ed. *Drugs and Human Lactation*. 2d ed. New York: Elsevier, 1996. This is a useful book on the health aspects of breast-feeding.

Hillis, Anne, and Penelope Stone. *Breast, Bottle, Bowl: The Best Fed Baby Book*. New York: HarperCollins, 2003. Examines breast-feeding from a nutritional perspective.

Huggins, Kathleen. *The Nursing Mother's Companion*. 5th ed. Boston: Harvard Common Press, 2005. This personable book provides comprehensive information about breast-feeding. Topics include preparation, special situations, returning to work, and nursing the older infant.

La Leche League International. *The Womanly Art of Breastfeeding*. 7th rev. ed. New York: Plume, 2004. This bible of breast-feeding covers preparation, the advantages of breast-feeding, and how to overcome problems. This illustrated manual provides the most up-to-date, comprehensive information, supported by an advisory board of medical experts.

Mason, Diane, and Diane Ingersoll. *Breastfeeding and the Working Mother*. Rev. ed. New York: St. Martin's Griffin, 1997. This book, written by women who have personal experience in the area, provides a host of practical tips for the working mother who wishes to breast-feed her baby. How-to basics as well as suggestions for practically every job situation are addressed.

Meek, Joan Younger, and Sherill Tippins, eds. *American Academy of Pediatrics New Mother's Guide to Breastfeeding*. New York: Bantam, 2006. Excellent overview of breast-feeding, which includes information about mastitis and plugged ducts.

Riordan, Jan, ed. *Breastfeeding and Human Lactation*. 3d ed. Sudbury, Mass.: Jones and Bartlett, 2005. Designed for lactation consultants. Discusses the physiology of breastfeeding, milk supply, positioning, the management of breastfeeding, and the role of the lactation consultant.

Rolfes, Sharon Rady, Linda Kelly DeBruyne, Eleanor Noss Whitney. *Life Span Nutrition: Conception Through Life*. 2d ed. St. Paul, Minn.: West, 1998. Chapter 5 of this textbook contains a comprehensive section on breast-feeding. Covers societal support, special medical conditions, physiology, the nutritional characteristics of breast milk, and the nutrient requirements for nursing mothers.

Stanway, Penny, and Andrew Stanway. *Breast Is Best*. 4th rev. ed. London: Pan Books, 2005. Written by two doctors who are also parents, this book provides practical, yet medically sound information about many aspects of breast-feeding. Chapters on etiquette, working, special situations, and readers' questions and answers cover issues not discussed in other books.

Breast surgery

Procedures

Anatomy or system affected: Breasts, glands

Specialties and related fields: General surgery, plastic surgery, psychiatry

Definition: Procedures performed on the breast to diagnose or treat benign and malignant breast disease or for reconstructive and cosmetic purposes.

Key terms:

abscess: a collection of infected fluid, which may be treated with antibiotics and drainage

areola: the pigmented tissue immediately surrounding the nipple

augmentation: an increase in the volume or size of the breast

axillary dissection: removal of lymph nodes found in the armpit (also known as axilla) to determine the spread of breast cancer; this procedure helps in planning therapy and in preventing spread of the cancer

lumpectomy: removal of a breast mass without removal of the noninvolved areas of the breast
mastectomy: surgical removal of the breast
reduction: a decrease in the total volume or mass of breast tissue

Indications and Procedures

The indications for breast surgery can be grouped into benign disease, malignant disease, reconstructive purposes, and cosmetic purposes. Indications for breast surgery in benign disease include persistent breast cysts which are not responsive to aspiration, such as in fibrocystic breast disease. In women who have a solid breast mass, excision of the lump to determine whether it is cancerous would be another indication for breast surgery. In this situation, the breast surgery would be diagnostic as well as potentially curative (for example, if the mass is benign). Another indication for breast surgery would be a breast abscess refractory to drainage; in this situation, excision of the abscess would offer the best chance of a cure.

Breast cancer is another indication for breast surgery. The surgery is usually performed after clinical breast examination, mammogram, and biopsy have confirmed the malignancy. The extent of disease and its aggressiveness determine to a large extent the type of breast surgery performed. In early-stage breast cancer, a modified radical mastectomy may be performed. This involves removal of the entire breast and the axillary lymph nodes. Alternatively, a lumpectomy with axillary node dissection (followed by radiation therapy) may be performed. Which procedure a patient receives also depends on the tumor size, tumor location, and the patient's breast size.

When a breast is completely removed, the patient may opt for reconstructive surgery. One common type of reconstructive surgery involves fashioning a new breast using a saline implant and a piece of the rectus abdominis muscle (a muscle on the anterior abdominal wall) called a transverse rectus abdominis myocutaneous (TRAM) flap. The areola may be reconstructed using a darker piece of skin taken from another part of the body, and tattooing may also be performed to give the nipple a more natural appearance.

Cosmetic breast surgery is indicated in cases where the patient is not satisfied with the appearance or size of her breasts. Most commonly, this cosmetic surgery takes the form of breast augmentation or breast reduc-

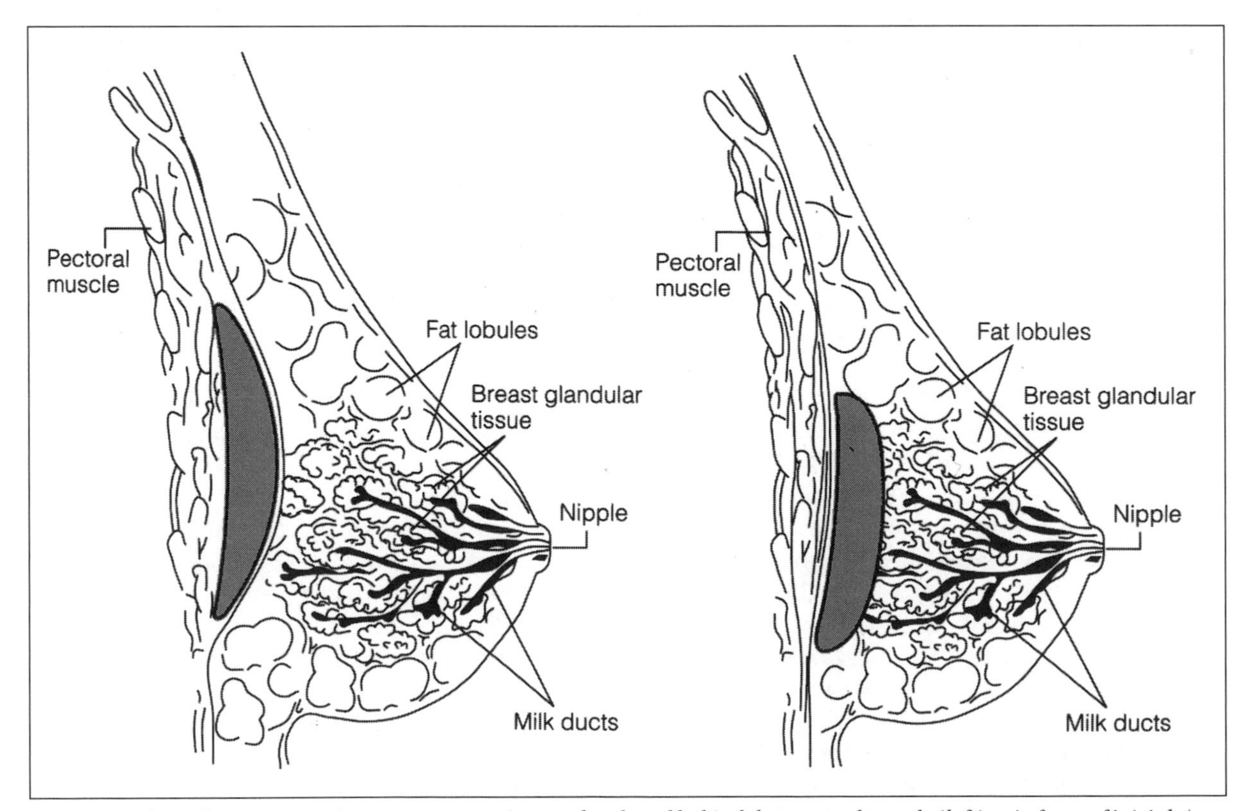

Breast implants for augmentation or reconstruction can be placed behind the pectoral muscle (left) or in front of it (right).

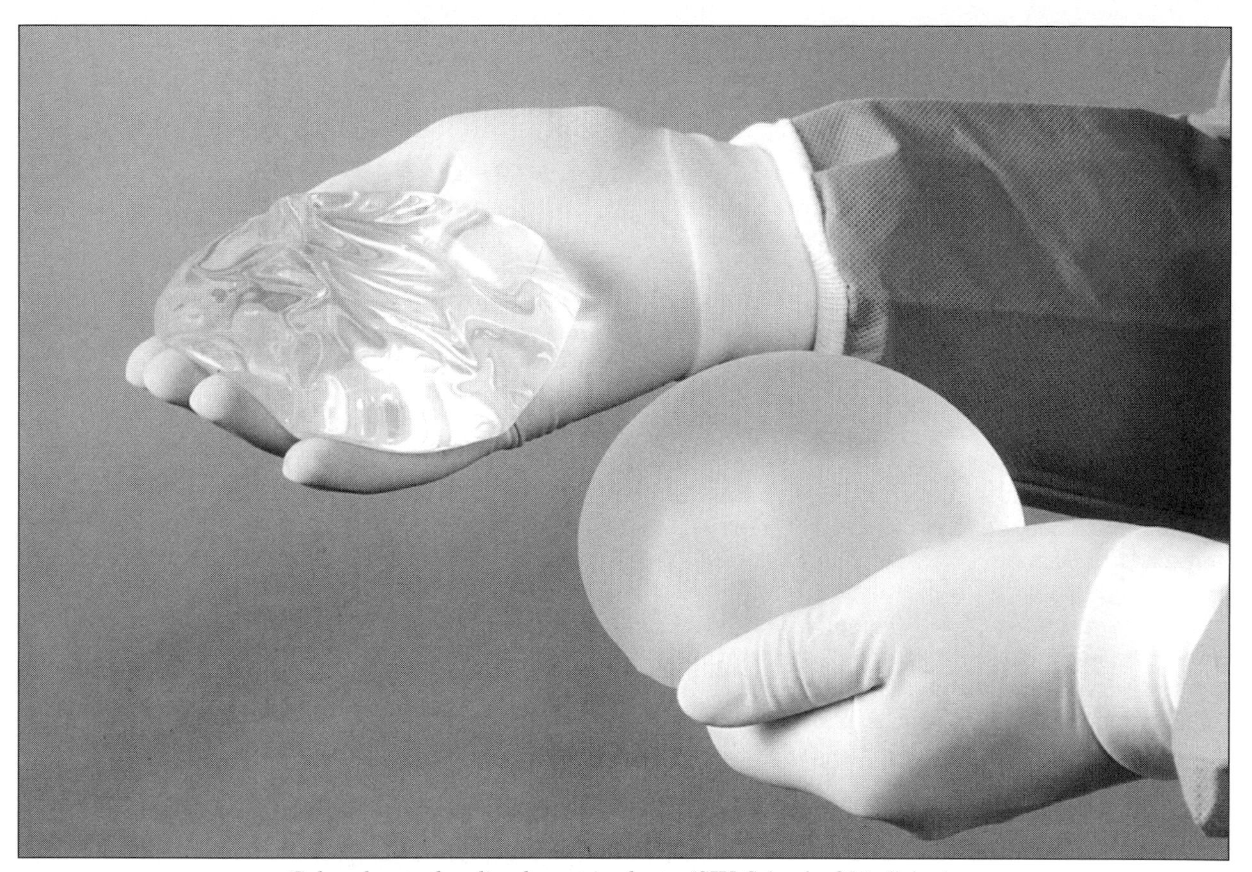

Gel and smooth saline breast implants. (SIU School of Medicine)

tion. In breast augmentation, implants are introduced under or over the pectoralis major muscle that lies underneath the existing breast. This is accomplished through an incision under the armpit, from the underside of the breast, or in the margin around the areola. The procedure may be done under local anesthesia as an outpatient procedure or under general anesthesia. The latter option is generally used when the implants are placed underneath the pectoralis muscle.

Breast reduction surgery, also called reductive mammoplasty, can be indicated when the patient suffers from back, shoulder, or neck pain from large breasts. It is also indicated when the patient is not satifisfied with the appearance of her breasts. A patient with large breasts often suffers from ptosis, or drooping of the breasts (which can also occur with aging or pregnancy and lactation). Reductive mammoplasty will correct the ptosis as well as reduce the overall size of the breasts. Commonly, tissue is removed from the most dependent (lowest) portion of the breast using vertical incisions, preserving the nipple and the underlying structures (nerves and lactic ducts). After the excess breast tissue is removed, the incision is then closed, with care taken for optimal cosmetic appearance. The breasts are wrapped in bandages to support the tissue while they heal. General anesthesia is almost always used, and blood loss can be greater than for breast augmentation. Drains may be placed temporarily in the breasts to prevent infection and the buildup of fluid. The patient is usually hospitalized for several days.

Uses and Complications

The uses of breast surgery include the diagnosis and treatment of benign and malignant breast disease, reconstruction after trauma or mastectomy, and the alteration of breast size and appearance for cosmetic or functional purposes.

Potential complications of all breast surgery include infection, scarring, and bleeding. Infections are infrequent but must be treated aggressively with antibiotics when they occur. If a prosthesis is involved, then it may be removed and reinserted three to six months later. Scarring is of concern because breast surgery is most often undertaken for cosmetic or aesthetic reasons. The placement of incisions along skin folds and careful skin closure help to minimize scarring. Restricting immediate postoperative activities, especially those that require stretching, also reduces scarring. As with all surgical procedures, bleeding is a risk of breast surgery. Blood loss from breast surgery can be minimized with careful inspection prior to closing incisions and the cauterization of any bleeding areas.

Although most patients who receive breast augmentation maintain normal breast function and can breastfeed after the surgery, many patients who have undergone breast reduction have difficulty with lactation. In addition, a larger number of women who have undergone breast reduction report loss of sensation than do women who have undergone breast augmentation. Also, scarring in women who have undergone breast reduction tends to be more extensive than in women who have undergone breast augmentation.

When implants are used, complications such as contracture and leakage may occur. Contracture occurs when the tissue immediately surrounding the prosthesis scars and shrinks, leading to an unnatural breast appearance. In rare cases, saline implants may leak. In the past, implants filled with silicone leaked, and a number of patients claimed that these leaks led to a number of medical problems. Although the connection between silicone leakage and medical disease remains controversial, the legal climate led to the withdrawal of silicone breast implants in North America.

Perspective and Prospects

The number of breast surgeries performed in the United States continues to rise. In particular, cosmetic breast augmentation procedures increased despite the ban on silicone breast implants in 1992. According to the American Society of Plastic Surgeons, more than 132,000 women in the United States underwent breast augmentation procedures in 1998, and the total number of women with implants in the United States is in the millions. As the number of women who have had breast augmentation grows, health care providers will probably deal more with the problems particular to breast implants, such as the increased difficulty in detecting breast masses and breast cancers.

—L. Fleming Fallon, Jr., M.D., Ph.D., M.P.H.; updated by Anne Lynn S. Chang, M.D.

See also Breast biopsy; Breast cancer; Breast disorders; Breasts, female; Grafts and grafting; Mammography; Mastectomy and lumpectomy; Oncology; Plastic surgery; Sex change surgery; Women's health.

For Further Information:

Berger, Karen, and John Bostwick III. *A Woman's Decision: Breast Care, Treatment, and Reconstruction*. 3d rev. ed. St. Louis: Quality Medical Publishing, 1998. Discusses various treatment options with regard to quality of life; combines physicians' perspectives with those of patients. Especially valuable is a section detailing surgical options for breast reconstruction.

Bostwick, John, III. *Plastic and Reconstructive Breast Surgery*. 2d ed. St. Louis: Quality Medical Publishing, 2000. This textbook presents an excellent discussion of cosmetic and reconstructive breast surgery.

Doherty, Gerard M., and Lawrence W. Way, eds. *Current Surgical Diagnosis and Treatment*. 12th ed. New York: Lange Medical Books/McGraw-Hill, 2006. A concise medical text that outlines major indications for breast surgery.

Georgiade, Nicholas G., Gregory S. Georgiade, and Ronald Riefkohl, eds. *Aesthetic Surgery of the Breast*. Philadelphia: W. B. Saunders, 1990. This book describes procedures for cosmetic breast surgery. It is written by internationally recognized authorities and well illustrated.

Guthrie, Randolph, and Doug Podolsky. *The Truth About Breast Implants*. New York: John Wiley & Sons, 1994. This book helps to clear away the confusion and anxiety surrounding the silicone implant controversy. The author is a plastic surgeon who details the safest techniques available to women and tells how to find the right doctor.

Stewart, Mary White. *Silicone Spills: Breast Implants on Trial*. Westport, Conn.: Praeger, 1998. Stewart details the trials and tribulations of the many women who suffered devastating (and sometimes fatal) consequences of silicone breast implants at the hands of doctors and manufacturers seeking monetary gain.

Breasts, female

Anatomy

Anatomy or system affected: Endocrine system, glands, muscles, musculoskeletal system, reproductive system

Specialties and related fields: Endocrinology, gynecology, obstetrics, oncology, plastic surgery

Definition: The female mammary glands and their surrounding muscles and tissues.

Key terms:

alveolar cell: also known as an acinar cell; the fundamental secretory unit of the mammary glandular tissue

colostrum: thin, yellow milky secretions of the mammary gland just a few days before and after childbirth; it contains more proteins and less fat and carbohydrates than does milk

Cooper's ligament: projections of breast parenchyma covered by fibrous connective tissue that extend from the skin to the deep layer of superficial fascia

lactiferous duct: a single excretory duct from each lobe of mammary glandular tissue that converges yet opens separately at the tip of the nipple; the mammary gland has fifteen to twenty lactiferous ducts

milk line: a line that originates as a primitive milk streak on each front side of the fetus; it extends from axilla to vulva, where rudimentary breast tissues or nipples could be located

myoepithelial cell: a cell that is anatomically located next to the alveolar cells and contractile in nature to aid in the movement of milk from the alveoli into the ducts

Structure and Functions

Mammogenesis—the growth and differentiation of the mammary gland—begins early in fetal life. By the sixth week of fetal development, the primitive milk streak can be identified as an ectodermal thickening along the ventrolateral aspect on each side of the fetus. In the ensuing weeks, this milk streak regresses, leaving normally only one pair of mammary glands in the thoracic region; however, multiple nipples and breast tissue may occasionally continue to develop anywhere along the milk line, extending from the armpit to the groin.

During the second trimester, projections of the ectoderm from the primary sprouts—usually between fifteen and twenty—will eventually elongate and arborize (branch out) to form the lactiferous ducts. Canalization of the ducts occurs late in fetal life and requires placental hormones for stimulation. Once the ducts canalize, two layers of epithelial cells are identified: the inner layer of cells, which forms the secretory component, and the outer layer of cells, which forms the myoepithelium, constituting the contractile elements for the expulsion of milk.

Between approximately four and seven days after birth, 80 to 90 percent of newborns have breast secretions (so-called witches' milk). Such secretions have been noted with equal frequency in male and female infants, and they usually last for three or four weeks. After the first neonatal month, the breast tissue reverts to an undifferentiated state and remains quiescent until puberty. Minimal ductal growth occurs during childhood, and there is no lobuloalveolar development.

At puberty, the surge of female hormones initiates lactiferous duct proliferation, along with deposition of fat and connective tissue. These changes produce a rapid increase in the size and density of the breast and are coordinated by the action of multiple hormones (prolactin, cortisol, growth hormone, insulin, and thyroxin) in addition to estrogen and progesterone. Estrogen encourages ductal proliferation and maturation, while progesterone stimulates lobuloalveolar growth. Ovarian steroids appear necessary for mammary development, as breast enlargement fails to occur at puberty in girls with gonadal dysgenesis. By the time of breast enlargement, the areola becomes more pigmented and the nipple enlarges. In adult women, size, density, and nodularity of the breast are dependent on the build of the individual, because much of the breast tissue consists of fat.

During the menstrual cycle, the breasts undergo a cyclic change. The rising estrogen and progesterone levels cause an increase in blood flow and interlobular edema. The engorgement, along with increase in density and nodularity, is particularly noticeable late in the menstrual cycle. In the week preceding menstruation, hormonal changes can bring about breast discomfort, tenderness, and a sensation of fullness. This increased sensitivity, often accompanied by marked nodularity, makes the clinical breast examination difficult. It is therefore important to examine the breasts seven to ten days following the onset of menstruation, as only during this time can tumors be differentiated from physiological nodularity. At menses, the breast decreases in size, the result of a reduction in the number and size of glandular cells with loss of edema.

During pregnancy, the breast undergoes final maturation in preparation for lactation. In the early weeks, the breast begins to enlarge, and marked histological changes take place. There is concurrent enlargement, pigmentation, and increased vascularity of the nipple. The earliest histological change within the acinar epithelial cells is cytoplasmic vacuolation. Lymphocytes, plasma cells, and eosinophils collect in the interstitial spaces. During the second trimester, the lobules enlarge and there is increase in the number and size of the constituent acini. The mammary blood supply is

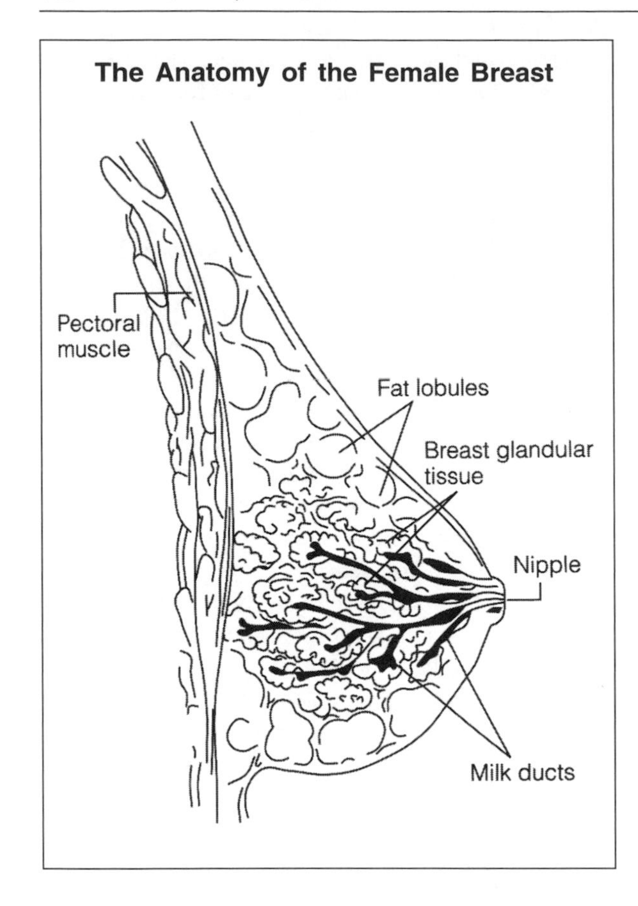

enhanced by increasing vascular luminal diameters and by formation of new capillaries around the lobules. During the last trimester, the secretory cells fill with fat droplets, and the alveoli are distended with a proteinaceous secretion termed colostrum.

Within three to four days postpartum, estrogen and progesterone levels rapidly decline. Prolactin can now, unrepressed by estrogen and progesterone, activate lactation, which is maintained by the infant's suckling. This stimulates further release of prolactin and oxytocin, which activate the myoepithelial cells, leading to expulsion of the alveolar secretion. During the first few days of lactation, only colostrum is produced. Once the colostrum has been expelled, normal production of milk ensues. Prolactin sustains milk production. Each nursing episode makes prolactin increase fivefold to tenfold, but, as weeks go by, prolactin levels gradually return to normal until even the nursing-induced rise is negligible. For unknown reasons, however, successful lactation can be maintained for months.

Changes of involution occur in the breast with increasing age and also after lactation. Between the ages of thirty-five and forty-five, the glandular tissue begins to disappear and alveoli and lobules shrink. These changes are not uniform throughout the breast; some lobules remain prominent, while others become more atrophic. At the menopause, the breasts decrease in size and become less dense. There is an increase in the elastic tissue component of the breast.

Anatomically, the extent of the normal female breast is approximately from the second to the sixth rib. The medial border touches the sternum, and the lateral border extends to the mid-portion of the armpit (axilla). The majority of the glandular tissue is in the upper outer quadrant and often extends deep into the axilla. The most important factor controlling the variation in breast size, shape, and density is obesity.

The mammary gland is enclosed between the superficial and deep layers of the superficial fascia. The superficial layer is a thin and delicate structure that is thicker at the inferior portion of the breast and becomes thinner as it approaches the clavicle. The deeper layer splits off the superficial fascia and extends deep into the mammary gland. Between this deep layer and the pectoral fascia, there is a well-defined space, termed retromammary space, that contains loose tissue, allowing the breast to glide freely over the chest wall. Portions of the deep layer of the superficial fascia form connective tissue extensions that pass through the retromammary space and join with the pectoral fascia. These extensions help support the breast. The breast is firmly fixed to the skin in the area of the nipple, and the remainder of the lobules are attached to the skin by dense fibrous bands termed Cooper's ligaments. Involvement of these ligaments with cancer gives rise to the physical sign of skin dimpling.

The breast is composed of glandular tissue, blood vessels, nerves, lymphatics, and varying amounts of fat. The glandular tissue is composed of between fifteen and twenty lactiferous ducts radially arranged around the nipple, each separated by fibrous septa. The terminal portion of the lactiferous duct dilates, forming the lactiferous sinus before it empties into the nipple. The functional unit of the breast is the terminal duct lobular unit, which consists of between ten and one hundred alveoli with the intralobular terminal duct and extralobular terminal duct.

The arteries supplying the breast are derived from the thoracic branches of the internal mammary artery, the axillary artery, and the intercostal arteries. The chief blood supply to the breast is from perforating branches of the internal mammary artery. The venous drainage of the breast is through the superficial subcutaneous veins, which drain either through the superficial veins into the lower neck or via medial connections into the internal mammary veins. There are also three groups of deep venous drainage. Although there appears to be some cross-drainage from one breast to the other, it is highly unlikely that this is a significant route for metastatic spread of carcinoma to the opposite breast.

Innervation of the breast skin is separated by quadrants. The upper quadrants receive their innervation from the third and fourth branches of the cervical plexus, while the lower quadrants are supplied by the thoracic intercostal nerves. The nipple's sensitivity is derived from the lateral cutaneous branch of the fourth intercostal nerve.

Lymphatic drainage of the breast can be divided into a superficial system draining the skin and a deeper system draining the lobules. The drainage from the upper quadrants passes to the axilla, as does drainage from the lower medial quadrant and adjacent abdominal wall. The breast's lymphatic drainage is primarily to the axilla, with lesser drainage occurring along the internal mammary chain.

Disorders and Diseases

Congenital anomalies of the breast are relatively rare. The most common are accessory breast tissue (polymastia) and accessory nipples (polythelia) along the milk line. A complete lack of one or both breasts (amastia) or nipples (athelia) is very rare; however, underdeveloped rudimentary breasts are not uncommon. Accessory breasts or nipples occur in approximately 2 percent of the population. Their most frequent location is just below the normal breast. This accessory breast tissue is of little clinical significance, although it is subject to the same disease processes that occur in normal breasts.

Hypertrophy, or overgrowth, of the breast is another development variation that affects young women, especially adolescents. The most frequent type of true hypertrophy of the breast occurs in adolescence following a normal puberty. The breasts fail to cease enlargement as they reach their normal limits. The excessive growth is the result of increased deposition of fibrous and adipose tissue. Little abnormality is to be found in the glandular elements of the breast. The breasts may gain massive size and require surgical reduction.

The pathology of benign breast lesions can be broadly categorized into inflammatory, hyperplastic, and neoplastic groups. The inflammatory conditions of the breast may be acute or chronic and can be caused by various factors, including infectious agents, foreign bodies, or trauma. Acute mastitis is usually the result of spread of microorganisms from the nipple, particularly during lactation. The breast shows acute inflammation with swelling, warmness, and redness. An abscess, or collection of pus, may form in the subareolar or deep glandular tissue. Diffuse cellulitis occasionally develops as the infection spreads into the adjacent soft tissue. Acute mastitis usually resolves following appropriate antibiotic treatment. Chronic mastitis may follow acute mastitis, or its onset may be insidious. The causative organisms are similar to those responsible for acute mastitis.

Fat necrosis within the breast tissue may follow trauma or a breast augmentation procedure using silicone or other materials. It may also be associated with necrosis developing in a malignant tumor. A history of trauma with surrounding bruises and pain is found in only about half the cases. Fat necrosis often manifests itself as a small, firm nodular mass of insidious onset. The consistency, adhesion to skin, and lack of pain, as well as the presence of calcifications on mammography, add to the confusion with carcinoma. In chronic cases, extensive fibrosis is seen. Careful microscopic sampling of different areas of the lesion is necessary, since malignant tumors could be associated with the foci of fat necrosis.

Almost all women are affected by a benign condition called fibrocystic change of breast at some time in their lives. Many other terms have been used for fibrocystic change in the medical literature, such as mammary dysplasia, fibrocystic disease, and chronic cystic mastitis, but these terms are no longer considered appropriate. This condition primarily affects women between twenty and forty-five years of age. Symptoms include nodularity in the breasts that may be associated with pain and tenderness, particularly around menses. Although the pathogenesis is not clear, fibrocystic changes appear to be the result of a hormonal imbalance of estrogen and progesterone. Oral contraceptives reduce the incidence of some types of fibrocystic changes. Genetic makeup, age, parity, and lactational history, as well as psychosomatic factors, may also play a role. The majority of fibrocystic changes are not premalignant.

The most common benign neoplasm of the breast is fibroadenoma, with most cases occurring between fifteen and thirty years of age. It is estimated that 10 to 25 percent of women have one or more of these tumors, which are thought to be of lobular origin. These neoplasms are estrogen-dependent, are often associated with menstrual irregularities, and can enlarge significantly during pregnancy. Clinically, fibroadenomas are usually well-defined, rounded lesions that have a firm or rubbery consistency. They are freely mobile, since there are no attachments between the tumor and the adjacent tissue. Fibroadenomas vary in size, with the majority being between 1 and 3 centimeters in diameter. Some tumors, however, can be as large as 10 to 12 centimeters and are termed giant fibroadcnoma; these are more common in adolescents, particularly blacks in their second decade of life. The large size of these tumors may be intimidating, but they have no malignant potential. Local excision with nipple preservation is adequate and allows subsequent normal development of the breast.

Breast cancer has been the major cause of death for several decades among women in the United States. In 1991 alone, 175,000 women were afflicted with breast cancer. It is the second leading cause of cancer mortality after lung carcinoma. As of 1992, it was estimated that one of nine American women has a lifetime risk of developing breast cancer. The incidence of this disease has increased at a 2 to 4 percent rate per year since 1980. The underlying reason for this continual growth in breast cancer cases remains unclear.

The initial physical signs and symptoms of breast carcinoma are varied. The most common clinical manifestation is a discrete lump. Swelling, nipple retraction, skin dimpling, axillary lumps, and occasionally bloody nipple discharge make up the remainder of the local physical signs. In general, nipple discharge is not often associated with cancer. When it is, it is usually a persistent, spontaneous bloody discharge. In women younger than fifty years of age, the presence of a bloody discharge is usually associated with an intraductal papilloma, which is not a malignant breast lesion. Skin retraction is caused by shortening of the Cooper's ligaments; its presence classically raises strong suspicion of a breast carcinoma. Other benign breast lesions can produce similar changes, however, the most common of which are plasma cell mastitis, fat necrosis, and Mondor's disease. Women with distant metastasis may experience general malaise, weight loss, bone pain, and headaches.

The site of the breast lump in most cases is in the upper outer quadrant or in the retroareolar area, just beneath the nipple. This is likely attributable to the fact that the majority of mammary glandular tissue occupies the upper outer quadrant of the breast. Approximately 5 percent of breast cancers occur in both breasts.

There are several different histopathological subtypes of breast cancer. Their recognition by the pathologist is crucial, since some have different prognostic implications. Most breast malignancies are primarily epithelial in origin, with only a small number of sarcomas and metastatic tumors reported. Although the terminal duct lobular unit is probably the location of origin of almost all cancers, neoplasms are traditionally classified into ductal and lobular carcinomas.

The most common malignant neoplasm of the breast is a nonspecific type of infiltrating ductal carcinoma, which is reported in 75 percent of breast cancer cases. It is presumed to be ductal in origin, and there may be coexistent areas of intraductal carcinoma, although this component is not always obvious. There is a poorly defined area of firmness that can often be palpated within the breast. At the time of surgical biopsy, most of these cancers range between 1 and 3 centimeters in diameter. Tumors less than 1 centimeter in diameter are not usually detected, although the increased use of screening mammography has brought some of these early lesions to light. Other tumors may reach a massive size, greater than 10 centimeters, before the patient seeks medical advice, often because of the patient's denial or lack of knowledge. The mass has a hard consistency and gives a gritty resistance when the specimen is cut. The outer margin of the mass is irregular with numerous fibrous bands, which can cause retraction of the nipple and dimpling of the overlying skin. The neoplasm may also be fixed to the underlying chest wall. Ulceration of the nipple or other parts of the skin is uncommon, except in advanced cases.

Invasive lobular carcinoma is the second most common breast malignancy, accounting for less than 10 percent of all breast cancers. These tumors tend to be multifocal and bilateral. When the opposite or "uninvolved" breast is sampled, about one-third show areas of carcinoma. Nodules of invasive lobular carcinoma are frequently difficult to localize, and occasionally no masses are encountered.

PERSPECTIVE AND PROSPECTS

Perhaps the diseases and treatment of no other organ have had more significance for human culture than those of the breast. Breast cancer has been described in many cultures and can even be found recorded in early Egyptian hieroglyphics. Breast cancer is important not only because of its frequency but also because of its psychosocial implications. In certain contexts, the breast symbolizes motherhood and nourishment, while in others it represents beauty and femininity.

In recent years, the investigation of breast diseases has blossomed. The normal physiological conditions of the breast, various benign diseases, and breast cancer have been clearly separated. The significance, prognosis, relation to breast cancer, and treatment of these diseases have been elucidated. Epidemiological studies have shown marked differences in the incidence of breast cancer within populations. These findings have suggested hypotheses as to the etiology and natural history of breast cancer. Increased patient awareness and continued advancement of screening mammography have resulted in earlier diagnosis of the disease.

Throughout the nineteenth century and in the early twentieth century, the prognosis for breast cancer was dismal because of the advanced stage of the disease at the usual time of its initial manifestation. In 1894, William Halsted and Willy Meyer each published, independently and for the first time, a description of the radical mastectomy procedure, including the resection of the entire breast, pectoral muscles, axillary lymph nodes, and associated skin and subcutaneous tissue. It was not until the late 1930's, however, that the Halsted radical mastectomy was beginning to be questioned by other surgeons. Enthusiasm for more conservative management—simple mastectomy with adjuvant radiation therapy—was ignited.

In the early 1950's, newer concepts emerged for the management of benign and malignant breast diseases. For example, the concept that breast cancer was a systemic disease and potentially unaffected by local treatment had risen. For the first time, a staging system was devised. Several studies confirmed that the most important prognostic indicator was the presence or absence of axillary nodal metastasis. In the 1960's and 1970's, hormonal therapy and adjuvant chemotherapy gradually gained acceptance.

Developments in the understanding of breast diseases and the variety of treatments available have provided major roles for the surgeon, medical oncologist, radiation oncologist, diagnostic radiologist, and pathologist. The multidisciplinary approach necessitates a coordinated, multidisciplinary team of experts to achieve the most optimal outcome of patient care.

—Stan Liu, M.D., and Lawrence W. Bassett, M.D.

See also Anatomy; Biopsy; Breast biopsy; Breast cancer; Breast disorders; Breast-feeding; Breast surgery; Cancer; Cyst removal; Cysts; Glands; Gynecology; Mammography; Mastectomy and lumpectomy; Mastitis; Muscles; Oncology; Pathology; Plastic surgery; Reproductive system; Sex change surgery; Systems and organs; Tumor removal; Tumors; Women's health.

For Further Information:

Bland, Kirby I., and Edward M. Copeland III. *The Breast: Comprehensive Management of Benign and Malignant Diseases*. 2d ed. Philadelphia: W. B. Saunders, 1998. The authors cover a number of diseases of the breast, with special emphasis on breast cancer and treatment.

Boston Women's Health Collective. *Our Bodies, Ourselves: A New Edition for a New Era*. 35th anniversary ed. New York: Simon & Schuster, 2005. This book was written by women for women and is one of the best reference works available on women's bodies and health for the general reader.

Elk, Ronit, and Monica Marrow. *Breast Cancer for Dummies*. New York: Wiley, 2003. An excellent resource that covers diagnosis to prognosis to treatment and recovery for those diagnosed with the disease. Helps set expectations for chemotherapy, hormone therapy, and surgery, and offers resources for coping and support.

Isaacs, John H. *Textbook of Breast Disease*. St. Louis: Mosby Year Book, 1992. This text, a summation of significant efforts from multiple physicians predominantly in the field of obstetrics and gynecology, offers a concise and clear description of the management of breast problems.

Love, Susan M., and Karen Lindsey. *Dr. Susan Love's Breast Book*. Rev. 4th ed. Cambridge, Mass.: Da Capo Press, 2005. This easy-to-read paperback is one of the most influential books in women's health written for a general audience. The splendidly well written guide explains with exceptional clarity and details breast development, changes with age, and breast cancer detection and treatment.

Mitchell, George W., Jr., and Lawrence W. Bassett, eds. *The Female Breast and Its Disorders*. Baltimore: Williams & Wilkins, 1990. This comprehensive text offers the expertise of multiple representatives from diverse fields, including obstetrics and gynecology, diagnostic radiology, pathology, surgery, medicine, therapeutic radiology, and psychiatry.

Oktay, Julianne S., and Carolyn A. Walter. *Breast Cancer in the Life Course: Women's Experience*. New

York: Springer, 1991. Deals with the emotional and psychological impact of having breast cancer at different phases of adulthood. Using multiple case studies and vignettes, the authors provide readers with easy-to-understand discussions of how women of different ages adapt to and cope with breast cancer.

Olson, John Stuart. *Bathsheba's Breast: Women, Cancer, and History*. Baltimore: Johns Hopkins University Press, 2002. Examines breast cancer from a historical and cultural perspective, discussing famous women in history with the disease, medicine's evolving understanding of its pathology and treatment options, and the rise of patient activism, among other topics.

Rogers, Kenneth, and A. J. Coup. *Surgical Pathology of the Breast*. London: Butterworth, 1990. This book contains multiple histopathologic illustrations of both malignant and benign breast diseases. In addition, many color photographs are provided to highlight the important physical signs of malignancy.

Tagliaferri, Mary, and Isaac Cohen, eds. *Breast Cancer: Beyond Convention, the World's Foremost Authorities on Complementary and Alternative Medicine Offer Advice on Healing*. New York: Atria Books, 2002. A team of breast cancer experts contribute their knowledge and experience to this book and explore alternative approaches to breast cancer treatment.

Breathing difficulty. *See* Pulmonary diseases; Respiration; Respiratory distress syndrome.

Bronchiolitis

Disease/disorder

Anatomy or system affected: Chest, lungs, respiratory system

Specialties and related fields: Family medicine, internal medicine, pediatrics, pulmonary medicine

Definition: An inflammation of the bronchioles that affects breathing and the transfer of oxygen to the bloodstream.

> **Information on Bronchiolitis**
>
> **Causes:** Viral or bacterial infection
> **Symptoms:** Sudden breathing difficulty (rapid, shallow breathing), wheezing, fever, dehydration, retractions of chest and abdomen
> **Duration:** Temporary, sometimes chronic
> **Treatments:** Moist air, antibiotics, antiviral medications, bronchodilators

Causes and Symptoms

Bronchiolitis is caused by a viral or bacterial infection, or a combination of the two, which infects and narrows the bronchioles, the smallest branches in the respiratory system that carry air from the large bronchial tubes to microscopic air sacs in the lungs. Some young children develop this disorder after a cold; it is contagious and may become epidemic. Symptoms include sudden breathing difficulty characterized by rapid, shallow breathing, wheezing, fever, dehydration, and retractions of the chest and abdomen. In severe cases, the skin or nails may turn blue.

Treatment and Therapy

The general treatment of bronchiolitis involves keeping the child's room as humid as possible with a cool-mist humidifier, or by running cold or hot water in the shower with the windows and doors closed. Breathing cool outside air may also help. In the case of bacterial infections, a doctor can prescribe antibiotics, and antiviral medications may be helpful in severe cases of viral infection. In addition, bronchodilators, drugs that widen the airways in the lungs, may prove helpful. The infected child should drink clear fluids—such as water, carbonated drinks, lemonade, weak bouillon, diluted fruit juice, or gelatin—frequently to help thin mucus secretions and avoid dehydration. Diagnostic measures include parental observation of symptoms, physical examination by a doctor, laboratory blood studies, and X rays of the lungs. With proper treatment, the disorder is typically curable within seven days.

Perspective and Prospects

Bronchiolitis is usually a disease of early infancy, with almost 90 percent of the patients being less than one year of age. It is important that bronchiolitis be diagnosed and treated properly because it can lead to chronic bronchitis, collapse of a small portion of a lung, repeated bouts of pneumonia, and in some cases, chronic obstructive pulmonary disease. Studies also indicate that infants who have two or more episodes of bronchiolitis prior to age two are more prone to developing allergies and asthma.

—Alvin K. Benson, Ph.D.

See also Antibiotics; Bacterial infections; Bronchitis; Childhood infectious diseases; Common cold; Pneumonia; Pulmonary medicine, pediatric; Respiration; Viral infections; Wheezing.

FOR FURTHER INFORMATION:

Mason, Robert J., et al., eds. *Murray and Nadel's Textbook of Respiratory Medicine*. 4th ed. Philadelphia: Elsevier Saunders, 2005.

Myers, Adam. *Respiratory System*. Philadelphia: Mosby/Elsevier, 2006.

Niederman, Michael S., George A. Sarosi, and Jeffrey Glassroth. *Respiratory Infections*. 2d ed. Philadelphia: Lippincott Williams & Wilkins, 2001.

Parker, Steve. *The Lungs and Breathing*. Rev. ed. London: Franklin Watts, 1989.

Pennington, James E. *Respiratory Infections: Diagnosis and Management*. 3d ed. Hoboken, N.J.: Raven Press, 1994.

West, John B. *Pulmonary Pathophysiology: The Essentials*. 6th ed. Baltimore: Lippincott Williams & Wilkins, 2003.

BRONCHITIS

DISEASE/DISORDER

ANATOMY OR SYSTEM AFFECTED: Chest, lungs, respiratory system

SPECIALTIES AND RELATED FIELDS: Family medicine, internal medicine, pulmonary medicine

DEFINITION: An inflammation of the bronchial tree of the lungs.

CAUSES AND SYMPTOMS

The inflammation associated with bronchitis may be localized or diffuse, acute or chronic, and it is usually caused by infections or physical agents. In its infectious form, acute bronchitis is part of a general, acute upper respiratory infection, sometimes brought on by the common cold. It can also develop from a viral infection of the nasopharynx, throat, or tracheobronchial tree. Acute bronchitis is most prevalent in winter. Factors contributing to the onset of the disease include exposure, chilling, malnutrition, fatigue, or rickets. The inflammation may be serious in debilitated patients and those with chronic pulmonary disease, and the real danger rests in the development of pneumonia. Certain physical and chemical irritants can bring on acute bronchitis. Such agents as mineral and vegetable dusts, strong acid fumes, volatile organic compounds, and tobacco smoke can trigger an attack.

> **INFORMATION ON BRONCHITIS**
>
> **CAUSES:** Upper respiratory infection, chronic pulmonary disease, physical and chemical irritants
>
> **SYMPTOMS:** Swollen mucous membranes, bronchial spasms, shortness of breath
>
> **DURATION:** Acute
>
> **TREATMENTS:** Antibiotics, bed rest, exposure to warm, moist air

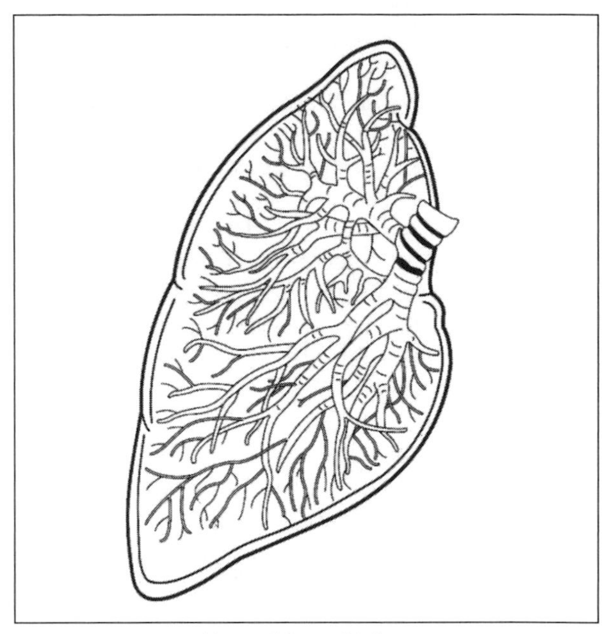

Normal bronchioles.

The disease causes thickening of the bronchi and a loss of elasticity in the bronchial tree. Changes in the mucous membranes occur, leukocytes infiltrate the submucosa, and a sticky, mucopurulent exudate is formed. The normally sterile bronchi are invaded by bacteria and cellular debris. A barking cough is often present, and this serves as an essential mechanism for eliminating bronchial secretions.

Chronic bronchitis is characterized by swollen mucous membranes, tenacious exudate, and spasms in the bronchiolar muscles. The result is dyspnea, the ventilatory insufficiency known as shortness of breath.

TREATMENT AND THERAPY

Acute bronchitis is treated with bed rest and medication to counteract the symptoms of inflammation. The room air should be kept warm and humid. Steam inhalation and cough syrup sometimes give relief from the severe, painful cough.

All surveys have demonstrated a high incidence of bronchitis in cigarette smokers when compared with nonsmokers, thus providing a good reason for the cessation of smoking.

—*Jane A. Slezak, Ph.D.*

See also Asbestos exposure; Chronic obstructive pulmonary disease (COPD); Coughing; Inflammation; Lungs; Oxygen therapy; Pneumonia; Pulmonary diseases; Pulmonary medicine; Pulmonary medicine, pediatric; Respiration; Wheezing.

For Further Information:

American Lung Association. http://www.lungusa.org/. Includes in-depth information and recent research findings, a guide to local events and programs, and a section to share personal stories, among other features.

Goldman, Lee, and Dennis Ausiello, eds. *Cecil Textbook of Medicine*. 22d ed. Philadelphia: W. B. Saunders, 2004. A comprehensive textbook covering the diagnosis and treatment of diseases.

Niederman, Michael S., et al. *Respiratory Infections*. 2d ed. Philadelphia: Lippincott Williams & Wilkins, 2001. Text that covers a range of respiratory problems, including bronchitis.

Shayevitz, Myra, and Berton R. Shayevitz. *Living Well with Chronic Asthma, Bronchitis, and Emphysema*. Yonkers, N.Y.: Consumer Reports Books, 1991. A book written to help those suffering from chronic lung disease. Provides an agenda for living with the disease.

Smolley, Laurence A., and Debra Fulghum Bruce. *Breathe Right Now: A Comprehensive Guide to Understanding and Treating the Most Common Breathing Disorders*. New York: W. W. Norton, 1998. Realizing that often breathing disorders may be linked to other medical problems or behavior (such as smoking), Smolley and Bruce provide perspective on the physiology of the respiratory system and the factors that can trigger its malfunction.

West, John B. *Pulmonary Pathophysiology: The Essentials*. 6th ed. Baltimore: Lippincott Williams & Wilkins, 2003. Examines lungs afflicted with obstructive, restrictive, vascular, and environmental diseases. Bronchoactive drugs, the causes of hypoventilation, and the pathogenesis of asthma and pulmonary edema are new topics covered in this edition.

Bruises

Disease/disorder

Also known as: Ecchymoses, contusions, hematomas

Anatomy or system affected: Blood vessels, lymphatic system, skin

Specialties and related fields: Emergency medicine, hematology, family medicine, pediatrics, vascular medicine

Definition: A bruise is an area of skin that has become discolored, usually as a result of trauma (a fall or hit to the affected area).

Causes and Symptoms

A bruise is a usually benign condition that happens when an individual has some type of injury. It may be a fall or a direct blow to any part of the body. As a result of the trauma, the affected body part undergoes various changes. A bruise can also occur spontaneously (a more serious illness or disease state) or from an allergic reaction. In most cases, bruises are not serious and resolve without any medical treatment.

Bruises occur when small blood vessels that are just beneath the skin are broken. They then begin to leak their contents (blood) into the surrounding soft tissue underneath the skin, which produces the characteristic black-and-blue discoloration. There are three types of bruises: subcutaneous (just beneath the skin), intramuscular (in the underlying muscle), and periosteal (in the bone). Bruises can last from several days to months. The typical black-and-blue mark begins to fade as the blood that leaked into the surrounding tissue is reabsorbed. The discoloration turns to a light yellowish-green and then fades completely.

Treatment and Therapy

The initial treatment of bruises should include decreasing the bleeding, minimizing any swelling, and controlling the pain. Ice is very effective and should be applied to the affected area for thirty to sixty minutes at a time. This can be done several times a day for two to three days. The ice should be in a container and covered by a towel to prevent damage to the skin. If possible, the affected area should be elevated above heart level. This helps in minimizing the swelling, which also helps decrease pain. If there is still discomfort after this period, then heat can be applied for twenty minutes at a time. The application of heat will help the blood to be reabsorbed into the tissue, then follow with cold. The last component of the treatment regimen should include

Information on Bruises

Causes: Bleeding under the skin following injury; sometimes an allergic reaction or clotting disorder
Symptoms: Black-and-blue skin discoloration, pain, swelling
Duration: Acute
Treatments: Ice, analgesics, sometimes heat

pain control. Pain can be easily controlled by using acetaminophen (Tylenol) or ibuprofen (Advil or Motrin).

Medical care should be sought if there is increased pain, a decrease in function (the affected part can no longer be used), headache, dizziness, fever (101 degrees Fahrenheit or more), or a noticeable change in vision, or if the symptoms continue.

Perspective and Prospects

Bruises are benign conditions that usually resolve without treatment. Simple self-care therapies will generally decrease discomfort and aid in a complete return to normal. Bruises are significant, however, in an individual experiencing bruising without any clear reason for the occurrence. In this case, bruises can be indicative of something more serious, such as clotting disorders or other diseases.

—Rosslynn S. Byous, D.P.A., PA-C

See also Accidents; Bleeding; Blood and blood disorders; Dermatology; Dermatology, pediatric; Emergency medicine; Emergency medicine, pediatric; Hematology; Hematology, pediatric; Safety issues for children; Safety issues for the elderly; Skin; Skin disorders.

For Further Information:

Gottleib, William. *Alternative Cures: The Most Effective Natural Home Remedies for 160 Health Problems*. Emmaus, Pa.: Rodale, 2000.

Griffith, H. Winter. *Complete Guide to Sports Injuries: How to Treat Fractures, Bruises, Sprains, Strains, Dislocations, Head Injuries*. Rev. and updated ed. New York: Body Press/Perigee, 1997.

Prevention Magazine, editors of. *The Doctors Book of Home Remedies*. Rev. ed. New York: Bantam Books, 2003.

Bulimia

Disease/disorder

Also known as: Bulimia nervosa

Anatomy or system affected: Blood, brain, gastrointestinal system, gums, heart, intestines, musculoskeletal system, nerves, psychic-emotional system, teeth

Specialties and related fields: Biochemistry, family medicine, gastroenterology, nutrition, psychiatry, psychology

Definition: An eating disorder that is characterized by repeated, uncontrollable episodes of overeating followed by induced vomiting or laxative abuse to eliminate the undigested food.

Causes and Symptoms

Bulimia is typically regarded as a psychologically based disorder caused by childhood experiences, family influences, and social pressures, particularly on young women to be thinner than natural. Many people who develop bulimia have been overweight in the past and suffer from poor self-image and depression. Body weight is often within normal limits, but persons with bulimia perceive themselves as fat and are often obsessed with their body image. Others may have a history of sexual or physical abuse or of alcohol or drug abuse. Medical research suggests that bulimia may be partially caused by impaired secretion of cholecystokinin (CKK), a hormone that normally induces a feeling of fullness after a meal, or by depletion of the chemical serotonin in the brain, which contributes to a craving for carbohydrates.

Intense preoccupation with food and weight are invariably present, and eating binges are followed with self-induced vomiting or the ingestion of laxatives to rid the body of the consumed food. Depression and suicidal feelings sometimes accompany bulimia. The disorder can cause nutritional deficiencies, dehydration, hormonal changes, gastrointestinal problems, changes in metabolism and blood chemistry, heart disorders, persistent sore throat, and teeth and gum damage as a result of the acidic nature of regurgitated food.

Treatment and Therapy

Treatment of bulimia requires a combination of nutritional counseling, medication, and psychotherapy. Psychotherapists try to get to the root of any underlying psychological problems and resolve them. Various modes of group and cognitive behavioral therapy have proven effective.

INFORMATION ON BULIMIA

CAUSES: Emotional and psychological disorders pertaining to body image
SYMPTOMS: Intense preoccupation with food and weight, eating binges followed by self-induced vomiting or ingestion of laxatives, depression, suicidal feelings, nutritional deficiencies, dehydration, hormonal changes, gastrointestinal problems, heart disorders, persistent sore throat, tooth and gum damage
DURATION: Chronic
TREATMENTS: Psychotherapy, nutritional counseling, medication

Cognitive therapy usually includes confronting people with bulimia about their inaccurate perceptions of body weight and making contracts with them to shift their focus to nutrition rather than weight gain in exchange for rewards. Group therapy has helped many bulimics stop their binge eating, while treatment with antidepressant drugs, especially fluoxetine (Prozac), has helped many bulimic patients gain partial or full relief from their symptoms. Hospitalization is common treatment and is virtually always necessary if body weight is more than 30 percent below ideal.

PERSPECTIVE AND PROSPECTS

Bulimia was classified as a distinct disorder by the American Psychiatric Association in 1980; the name was officially changed to bulimia nervosa in 1987. The disorder occurs mostly in adolescent and young adult females, with only about 10 percent of cases in males. Many cases of bulimia end after a few weeks or months but may reoccur. Other cases last for years without interruption.

In 2006, researchers developed a new test that analyzes carbon and nitrogen in hair, which is suggestive of eating disorders. This technique is beneficial because eating disorders are difficult to diagnose, in part because sufferers sometimes do not know that they have an eating disorder or do not want to be honest. By analyzing just five strands of hair, researchers were able to diagnose anorexia and bulimia accurately 80 percent of the time. This test may hasten treatment and prove an effective and objective method of monitoring recovery.

—Alvin K. Benson, Ph.D.;
updated by LeAnna DeAngelo, Ph.D.

See also Anorexia nervosa; Eating disorders; Hyperadiposis; Malnutrition; Nausea and vomiting; Nutrition; Obesity; Phobias; Psychiatric disorders; Psychiatry, child and adolescent; Puberty and adolescence; Weight loss and gain; Weight loss medications; Women's health.

FOR FURTHER INFORMATION:

Brownell, Kelly D., and Christopher G. Fairburn, eds. *Eating Disorders and Obesity: A Comprehensive Handbook*. 2d ed. New York: Guilford Press, 2002.

Maj, Mario, et al., eds. *Eating Disorders*. New York: Wiley, 2003.

National Association of Anorexia Nervosa and Associated Disorders. http://www.altrue.net/site/anadweb/.

National Eating Disorders Association. http://www.nationaleatingdisorders.org/.

Parker, James M., and Philip M. Parker, eds. *The 2002 Official Patient's Sourcebook on Binge Eating Disorder*. San Diego, Calif.: Icon Health, 2002.

Reindl, Shiela M. *Sensing the Self: Women's Recovery from Bulimia*. Cambridge, Mass.: Harvard University Press, 2001.

Swain, Pamela I., ed. *Anorexia Nervosa and Bulimia Nervosa: New Research*. New York: Nova Science, 2006.

BUNIONS

DISEASE/DISORDER

ANATOMY OR SYSTEM AFFECTED: Bones, feet

SPECIALTIES AND RELATED FIELDS: Family medicine, general surgery, orthopedics, podiatry

DEFINITION: An enlargement which develops on the joint of the big toe, producing deformity, pain, and discomfort.

CAUSES AND SYMPTOMS

A bunion, or hallux valgus, is a swelling on the foot, usually at the joint of the big toe, that is caused by a misaligned bone in the joint. Bunions often develop with aging as a result of widening of the feet, arthritic conditions, or the wearing of improperly fitted shoes. Typically, the misaligned bone protrudes outward at the joint of the big toe, giving the bunion its bulging appearance. The bursa, a fluid-filled sac in the joint, becomes inflamed and swells, often twisting the big toe toward the second toe. Since the big toe supports most of the body's weight every time an individual pushes off the ground, a bunion can cause severe pain and discomfort. In addition, because bunions can change the shape of the feet, it becomes much harder for an aging sufferer to find shoes that fit properly.

While bunions themselves cannot be inherited, an individual can inherit the tendency to develop bunions by being born with extra bone near a toe joint. The risk of developing bunions can be reduced by exercising daily to keep the muscles of the feet and legs in good condition and by wearing wide-toed shoes that fit well. Women tend to develop bunions more than men do, possibly because many women wear shoes that are too small or narrow. Symptoms of bunions include pain, redness, stiffness, swelling, thickness of the skin over the bunion, fluid accumulation under the thickened skin, and the eventual development of osteoarthritis that impairs the joint's flexibility.

TREATMENT AND THERAPY

If a bunion is not severe, greater comfort can come from simply wearing a different style of shoe, including those that have been stretched in the big toe area, that are made of soft leather, or that have cushioned insoles. Sandals with cross straps and athletic shoes are best for providing maximum comfort for people with bunions. Other ways to relieve the pain include using shoe inserts called bunion pads, using a moist heating pad on the bunion at night, applying an ice pack to reduce swelling, and taking an over-the-counter anti-inflammatory medication such as aspirin or ibuprofen (Advil or Motrin). Aging persons with medical conditions should read product labels carefully and consult their doctor or a pharmacist before taking pain-relieving medications. If home care measures do not provide relief, a podiatrist (foot doctor) may prescribe a special shoe insert known as an orthotic device.

INFORMATION ON BUNIONS

CAUSES: Misaligned bone joint from aging, arthritic conditions, improperly fitting shoes
SYMPTOMS: Toe deformity, pain, discomfort, redness, stiffness
DURATION: Acute to chronic
TREATMENTS: Well-fitting shoes, bunion pads, moist heating pad or ice pack, anti-inflammatory medication, outpatient surgery

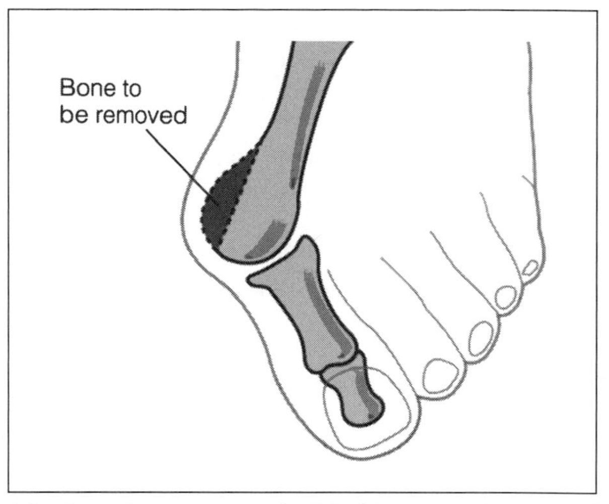

A bunion, a bony overgrowth of the big toe, can be removed surgically by cutting off the excess segment of bone, thus reshaping the foot.

For severe bunions, outpatient surgery may be required. The most common surgery reduces the angle between the big and second toes. Bones in the big toe are realigned, and the bunion is shaved away. Ligaments and tendons on the outside of the toe may be tightened to hold the joint properly, while any tight tendons on the inside of the toe are released. Bunion surgery can reduce pain and improve the appearance of the feet. Recovery involves the use of crutches to keep weight off the foot, and the majority of healing typically occurs within a few weeks. After surgery, pain will gradually subside and deformity of the foot will improve. However, tight shoes must still be avoided.

—Alvin K. Benson, Ph.D.

See also Bones and the skeleton; Fallen arches; Feet; Foot disorders; Hammertoe correction; Hammertoes; Orthopedic surgery; Orthopedics; Podiatry.

FOR FURTHER INFORMATION:

Bentley, George, and Robert B. Greer, eds. *Orthopaedics*. 4th ed. Oxford, England: Linacre House, 1993.

Copeland, D. P. M. Glenn, and Stan Solomon. *The Foot Doctor: Lifetime Relief for Your Aching Feet*. Emmaus, Pa.: Rodale Press, 1986.

Lippert, Frederick G., III, and Sigvard T. Hansen, Jr.. *Foot and Ankle Disorders: Tricks of the Trade*. New York: Thieme, 2003.

Lorimer, Donald L., et al., eds. *Neale's Disorders of the Foot*. 7th ed. New York: Elsevier Churchill Livingstone, 2006.

Burkitt's lymphoma

Disease/disorder

Anatomy or system affected: All, especially lymphatic system

Specialties and related fields: Family medicine, hematology, internal medicine, oncology, pediatrics

Definition: A highly aggressive lymphoma often presenting in extranodal sites or as an acute leukemia.

Causes and Symptoms

The three different clinical variants of Burkitt's lymphoma—endemic, sporadic, and immunodeficiency-associated—have varying clinical manifestations and epidemiologies. Endemic Burkitt's lymphoma occurs in equatorial Africa and Papua, New Guinea, most commonly in children. In this form, the jaws and other facial bones are the site of presentation in about half of the cases. Other extranodal sites may be involved, such as the distal ileum, cecum, omentum, ovaries, kidneys, and breasts, as well as the central nervous system. Sporadic Burkitt's lymphoma occurs throughout the world and mainly in children and young adults. In this form, jaw tumors are less frequent, and the majority of these cases present with abdominal masses. Immunodeficiency-associated Burkitt's lymphoma is seen primarily in association with human immunodeficiency virus (HIV) infection.

Epstein-Barr virus (EBV) plays an important role in endemic Burkitt's lymphoma, and the EBV genome is present in the majority of the neoplastic cells of these patients. In sporadic Burkitt's lymphoma, however, the frequency of EBV association is much lower (less than 30 percent of cases). In immunodeficiency-associated Burkitt's lymphoma, EBV is identified in only 25 to 40 percent of cases. While the exact relationship of EBV to the pathogenesis of Burkitt's lymphoma is not understood, it is known that genetic abnormalities involving chromosome 8 play an essential role in Burkitt's lymphoma.

Information on Burkitt's Lymphoma

Causes: Unknown; may be related to Chromosomal abnormalities, infection with HIV or Epstein-Barr virus

Symptoms: Jaw and facial tumors, abdominal masses, acute leukemia, bone marrow and central nervous system involvement

Duration: Chronic or acute

Treatments: Chemotherapy

Treatment and Therapy

In endemic and sporadic Burkitt's lymphoma, the tumor is highly aggressive but potentially curable. Endemic Burkitt's lymphoma is highly sensitive to intensive combination chemotherapy and results in high cure rates (up to 90 percent) in patients with low-stage disease and significant cure rates (60 to 80 percent) in patients with advanced disease. Bone marrow and central nervous system involvement are associated with a poor prognosis, especially in sporadic Burkitt's lymphoma. If Burkitt's disease presents as an acute leukemia, the treatment consists of very intensive chemotherapy of relatively short duration, which differs substantially from the current treatment of acute lymphoblastic leukemia.

Perspective and Prospects

Burkitt's lymphoma is one of the first human cancers in which characteristic chromosomal translocations have been shown to be related to the development of the malignancy. This finding may be an important clue to the basic mechanism of the development of this cancer and hopefully will result in the prevention and complete cure of the disease.

—*Cherie H. Dunphy, M.D.*

See also Cancer; Chemotherapy; Lymphadenopathy and lymphoma; Lymphatic system; Malignancy and metastasis; Oncology; Radiation therapy.

For Further Information:

Gorczyca, Wojciech, with James Weisberger and Foxwell N. Emmons. *Atlas of Differential Diagnosis in Neoplastic Hematopathology*. New York: Taylor & Francis, 2005.

Jaffe, Elaine S., et al., eds. *Pathology and Genetics of Tumours of Haematopoietic and Lymphoid Tissues*. Oxford, England: Oxford University Press, 2001.

Knowles, Daniel M., ed. *Neoplastic Hematopathology*. 2d ed. Philadelphia: Lippincott Williams & Wilkins, 2001.

Lymphoma Focus. http://www.lymphomafocus.org/.

BURNS AND SCALDS

DISEASE/DISORDER

ANATOMY OR SYSTEM AFFECTED: Skin, other tissues in severe cases

SPECIALTIES AND RELATED FIELDS: Critical care, dermatology, emergency medicine, physical therapy, plastic surgery

DEFINITION: Injury to skin and other tissues caused by contact with dry heat (fire), moist heat (steam or hot liquid), chemicals, electricity, lightning, or radiation.

KEY TERMS:

burn: an injury to tissues caused by contact with dry heat (fire), moist heat (steam or a hot liquid), chemicals, electricity, lightning, or radiation

burn degrees: system of classification for burns based on the depth of damage to the skin

major (or severe) burn: a burn covering more than 20 percent of the body and any deep burn of the hands, face, feet, or perineum

minor burn: a superficial burn of less than 5 percent of the body that can be treated without hospitalization

moderate burn: a burn that requires hospitalization but not specialized care

rule of nines: a system used to designate areas of the body, represented by various body parts; used in determining the extent of a burn

skin graft: a surgical graft of skin from one part of the body to another or from one individual to another

CAUSES AND SYMPTOMS

Burns are injuries to tissues caused by contact with dry heat (fire), moist heat (steam or a hot liquid, also called scalds), chemicals, electricity, lightning, or radiation. The word "burn" comes from the Middle English *brinnen* or *brennen* (to burn) and from the Old English *byrnan* (to be on fire) combined with *baernan* (to set afire). Each year in the United States, more than two million people are burned or scalded badly enough to need medical treatment, and about 70,000 require admission to a hospital. Burns are most common in children and older people, and many are caused by accidents in the home that are usually preventable.

The depth of the injury is proportional to the intensity of the heat of the causative agent and the duration of exposure. Burns can be classified according to the agent causing the damage. Some examples of burns according to this classification are brush burns, caused by friction of a rapidly moving object against the skin or ground into the skin; chemical burns, caused by exposure to a caustic chemical; flash burns, caused by very brief exposure to intense radiant heat (the typical burn of an atomic explosion); radiation burns, caused by exposure to radium, X rays, or atomic energy; and respi-

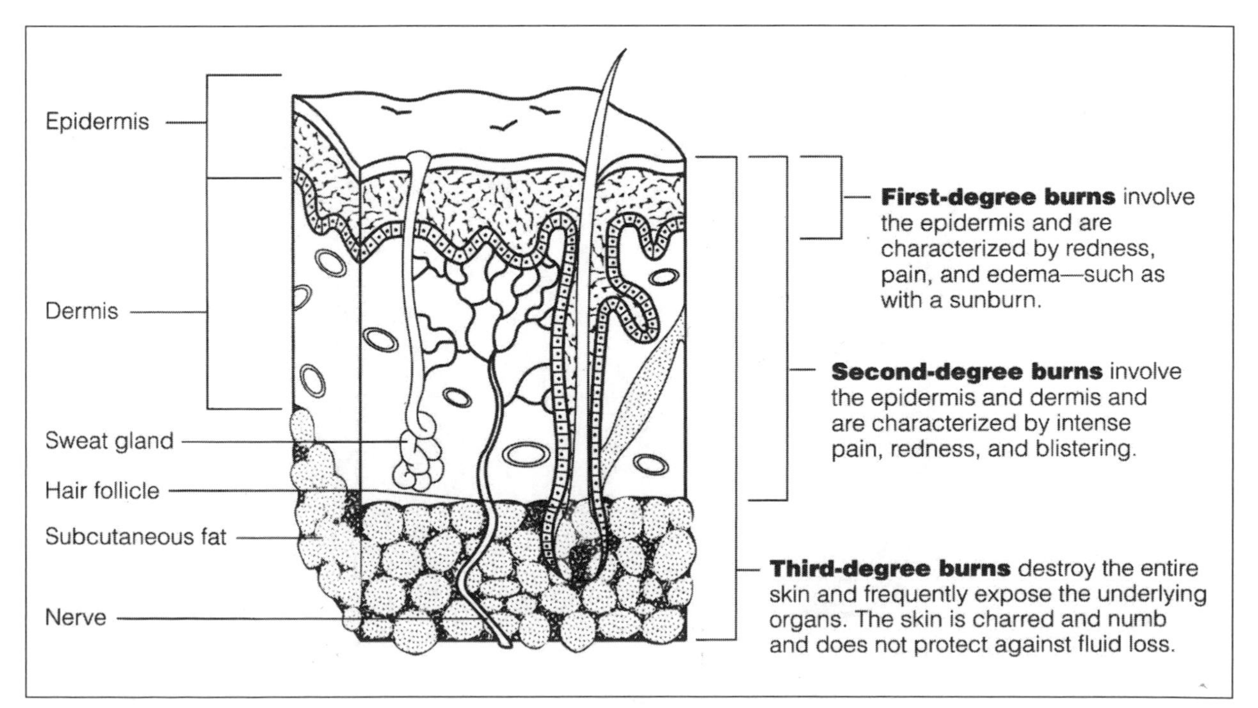

Burns are measured by the layer(s) of skin affected.

ratory burns, caused by inhalation of steam or explosive gases.

Burns can also be classified as major or severe (involving more than 20 percent of the body and any deep burn of the hands, face, feet, or perineum), minor (a superficial burn involving less than 5 percent of the body that can be treated without hospitalization), and moderate (a burn that requires hospitalization but not specialized care, as with burns covering 5 to 20 percent of the body but without deep burns of hands, face, feet, or perineum).

While many domestic burns are minor and insignificant, more severe burns and scalds can prove to be dangerous. The main danger for a burn patient is the shock that arises as a result of loss of fluid from the circulating blood at the site of the burn. This loss of fluid leads to a fall in the volume of the circulating blood in the area. The maintenance of an adequate blood volume is essential to life, and the body attempts to compensate for this temporary loss by withdrawing fluid from the uninjured areas of the body into the circulation. In the first forty-eight hours after a severe burn is received, fluid from the blood vessels, salt, and protein pass into the burned area, causing swelling, blisters, low blood pressure, and very low urine output. The body loses fluids, proteins, and salt, and the potassium level is raised. Such low-fluid levels are followed by a shift of fluid in the opposite direction, resulting in

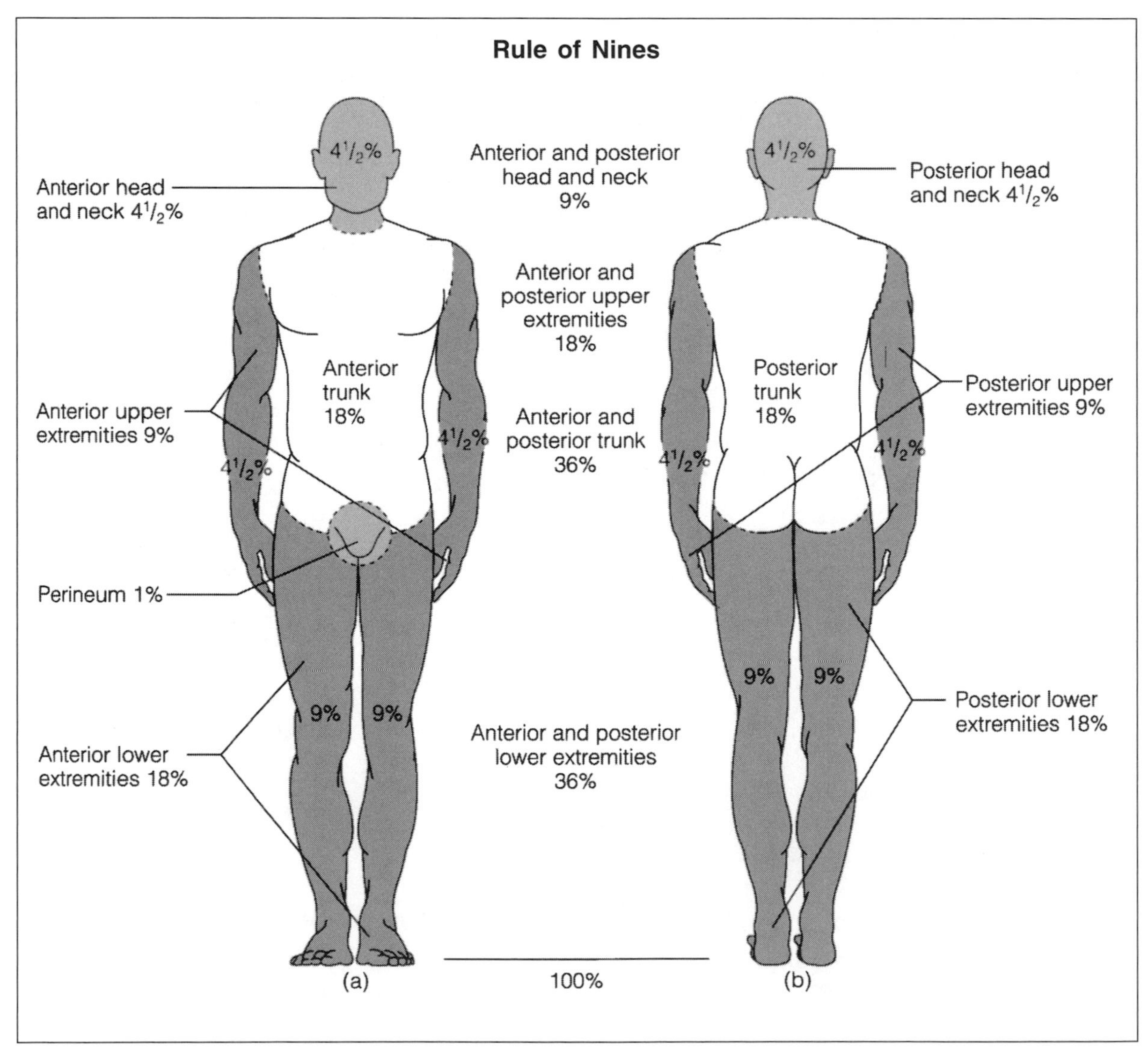

The "rule of nines" specifies the extent and hence seriousness of a burn in relation to the body's surface area.

excess urine, high blood volume, and low concentration of blood electrolytes. If carried too far, this condition begins to affect the viability of the body cells. As a result, essential body cells such as those of the liver and kidneys begin to suffer, eventually causing the liver and kidneys to cease proper function. Liver and renal failure are revealed by the development of jaundice and the appearance of albumin in the urine. In addition, the circulation begins to fail, with a resultant lack of oxygen in the tissues. The victim becomes cyanosed, restless, and collapsed, and in some cases death ensues. Other possible problems related to burns include collapse of the circulatory system, shutdown of the digestive and excretory systems, shock, pneumonia, and stress ulcers.

In addition, particularly with severe burns, there is a strong risk of infection. This type of burn can leave a large area of raw skin surface exposed and extremely vulnerable to any microorganisms. The infection of extensive burns may cause fatal complications if effective antibiotic treatment is not given. The combination of shock and infection can often be life-threatening unless expert treatment is immediately available.

The immediate outcome of a burn is more determined by its extent (amount of body area affected) than by its depth (layers of skin affected). The "rule of nines" is used to assess the extent of a burn in relation to the surface of a body. The head and each of the arms cover 9 percent of the body surface; the front of the body, the back, and each leg cover 18 percent; and the crotch accounts for the remaining 1 percent. The greater the extent of a burn, the more seriously ill the victim will become from loss of fluid. The depth of the burn (unless it is very great) is mainly of importance when the question arises as to how much surgical treatment, including skin grafting, will be required. An improvement over the rule of nines in the evaluation of the seriousness of burns is the Berkow formula, which takes into account the age of the patient.

A burn caused by chemicals differs from a burn caused by fire only in that the outcome of the chemical burn is usually more favorable, since the chemical destroys the bacteria on the affected part and reduces the chance of infection. Severe burns can also be caused by contact with electric wires. As current meets the resistance in the skin, high temperatures are developed and burning of the victim takes place. Exposure to 220 volts burns only the skin, but higher voltage can cause severe underlying damage to any tissue in its path. Electrical burns normally cause minimal external skin damage, but they can cause serious heart damage and require evaluation by a physician. Explosions and the action of acids and other chemicals also cause burns. Severe and extensive fire burns are most frequently produced by the clothes catching fire.

Information on Burns and Scalds

Causes: Fire, steam or hot liquid, chemicals, electricity, lightning, radiation

Symptoms: Swelling, blisters, low blood pressure, very low urine output, infection, shock

Duration: Temporary and acute; may be followed by long-term rehabilitation

Treatments: Varies widely; ranges from cooling agents and antiseptic medication, to antibiotics and pain relief, to skin grafts, fluid and electrolyte maintenance, and high-protein diet

Treatment and Therapy

General treatment of a burn injury includes pain relief, the control of infection, the maintenance of the balance of fluids and electrolytes in the system, and a good diet. A high-protein diet with supplemental vitamins is prescribed to aid in the repair of damaged tissue. The specific treatment depends on the severity of the burn. Major burns should be treated in a specialized treatment facility, while minor burns can be treated without hospitalization. A moderate burn normally requires hospitalization but not specialized care.

In the case of minor burns or scalds, all that may be necessary is to hold the body part under cold running water until the pain is relieved, as cooling is one of the most effective ways of relieving the pain of a burn. If the burn involves the distal part of a limb—for example, the hand and forearm—one of the most effective ways of relieving the pain is to immerse the burned part in lukewarm water and add cold water until the pain disappears. If the pain does not return when the water warms up, the burn can be dressed in the usual way (a piece of sterile gauze covered by cotton with a bandage on top). The part should be kept at rest and the dressing dry until healing takes place. Blisters can be pierced with a sterile needle, but the skin should not be cut away. No ointment or oil should be applied, and an antiseptic is not always necessary. Even this type of burn can be serious if it covers as much as two-thirds of the body area. On a child, such burns are dangerous on an even smaller area of the skin, and special attention should be given to the patient.

In the case of moderate burns or scalds, it is advisable to use antiseptics (such as chlorhexidine, bacitracin, and neomycin), and the patient should be taken to a doctor. Treatment may consist of using a dressing impregnated with a suitable antibiotic or of applying a cream containing antiseptic and pain-relieving creams and covering the burn with a dressing sealed at the end. This dressing is left on for four to five days and removed if there is evidence of infection or if pain occurs.

For severe burns and scalds, the only sound rule is to go to the hospital. Unless there is a need for resuscitation, or attention to other injuries, nothing should be done on the spot except to make sure that the patient is comfortable and warm and to cover the burn with a clean or sterile cloth. Clothing should be removed from the burned area only if this does not traumatize the skin further. Burned clothing should be sent to the burn center, as it may help determine the chemicals and other substances that either caused or entered the wound. Once the victim is in the hospital, the first thing to check is the extent of the burn and whether a transfusion is necessary. If the burn covers more than 9 percent of the body surface, a transfusion is required. It is essential to prevent infection or to bring it under control. A high-protein diet with ample fluids is needed to compensate for the protein that has been lost along with the fluid from the circulation. The process of healing is slow and tedious, including careful nursing, physiotherapy, and occupational therapy. The length of hospital stay can vary from a few days in some cases to many weeks in the case of severe and extensive burns.

In some cases depending on the extent of the burn, it will be necessary to consider skin grafting, in which a graft of skin from one part of the body (or from another individual) is implanted in another part. Skin grafting is done soon after the initial injury. The donor skin is best taken from the patient, but when this is not possible, the skin of a matched donor can be used. Prior to grafting, or in some cases as a substitute for it, the burn may be covered with either cadaver or pig skin to keep it moist and free from exogenous bacterial infection. Newly de-

IN THE NEWS: TREATING BURNS WITH ARTIFICIAL SKIN

Since the end of the twentieth century, surgeons have been using biosynthetic skin substitutes (sometimes called artificial skin or cellular wound dressings) to manage extensive or deep burns. Integra and TransCyte, approved by the Food and Drug Administration (FDA) in 1996 and 1997, respectively, are common substitutes. Both are layered products composed of synthetic silicone and a biologically active, collagen-based composite that promotes healing. TransCyte also has a nylon mesh between the two layers. Integra is produced by the Integra LifeSciences Corporation in Plainsboro, New Jersey; TransCyte is produced by Advanced Tissue Sciences in La Jolla, California.

TransCyte is a temporary skin substitute for partial thickness or less serious burns; it is removed after the wound heals or in preparation for a skin graft. Integra is a permanent skin substitute for full thickness or deep burns; however, after the patient's dermal layer regenerates, the silicone layer is replaced with a thin skin graft. As of 2003, a "one-step" skin substitute did not exist for deep burn wounds.

In the past, surgeons relied exclusively on biological skin to cover burn wounds or to promote wound closure. Typically, surgeons used xenografts from other species, such as pig skin, allografts from the same species, such as cadaver skin, or autografts from the patient's own skin.

Biosynthetic substitutes were developed to meet the needs both of increasing numbers of serious burn survivors and of survivors of extensive burns where fewer donor sites for autografts exist. Biosynthetic substitutes adhere to cleaned wounds, serve as a protective barrier, and minimize pain as well as length of hospital stay. For deep burns, substitutes promote regeneration of the survivor's own dermis and minimize scarring. Ideally, a skin substitute should look and feel like the patient's healthy skin. In reality, artificial skin may not match the patient's skin color and texture. Also, biosynthetic substitutes may transmit disease via the biological component or may seal in deep infection at the wound site. Although the development of biosynthetic skin substitutes is an important medical advance, bioengineering of skin tissue in the early twenty-first century is a relatively new science.

—Tanja Bekhuis, Ph.D.

veloped artificial skin holds great promise for treating severe burns.

In the case of chemical burns, treatment can be specific and depends on the chemical causing the burn. For example, phenol or lysol can be washed off promptly, while acid or alkali burns should be neutralized by washing with sodium bicarbonate or acetic acid, respectively, or with a buffer solution for either one. In many cases, flushing with water to remove the chemical is the first method of action.

Victims who have inhaled smoke may develop swelling and inflammation of the lungs, and they may need special care for burns of the eyes. People who have suffered an electrical burn may suffer from shock and may require artificial respiration, which should begin as soon as contact with the current has been broken.

PERSPECTIVE AND PROSPECTS

Burns have been traditionally classified according to degree. The French surgeon Guillaume Dupuytren divided burns into six degrees, according to their depth. A first-degree burn is one in which there is simply redness; it may be painful for a day or two. This level of burn is normally seen in cases of extended exposure to X rays or sunlight. A second-degree burn affects the first and second layers of skin. There is great redness, and the surface is raised up in blisters accompanied by much pain. Healing normally occurs without a scar. A third-degree burn affects all skin layers. The epidermis is entirely peeled off, and the true skin below is destroyed in part, so as to expose the endings of the sensory nerves. This is a very painful form of burn, and a scar follows on healing. With a fourth-degree burn, the entire skin of an area is destroyed with its nerves, so that there is less pain than with a third-degree burn. A scar forms and later contracts, and it may produce great deformity in the affected area. A fifth-degree burn will burn the muscles as well, and still greater deformity follows. In a sixth-degree burn, a whole limb is charred, and it separates as in gangrene.

In current practice, burns are referred to as superficial (or partial thickness), in which there is sufficient skin tissue left to ensure regrowth of skin over the burned site; and deep (or full thickness), in which the skin is totally destroyed and grafting will be necessary. It is difficult to determine the depth of a wound at first glance, but any burn involving more than 15 percent of the body surface is considered serious. As far as the ultimate outcome is concerned, the main factor is the extent of the burn—the greater the extent, the worse the outlook.

Unfortunately, burns are most common in children and older people, those for whom the outcome is usually the worst. Many of the burns are caused by accidents in the home, which are usually preventable. In fact, among the primary causes of deaths by burns, house fires account for 75 percent of the incidents. Safety measures in the home and on the job are extremely important in the prevention of burns. Severe and extensive burns most frequently occur when the clothes catch fire. This rule applies especially to cotton garments, which burn quickly. Particular care should always be exercised with electric fires and kettles or pots of boiling water in houses where small children or elderly people are present.

In the United States, most severely burned patients are given emergency care in a local hospital and are then transferred to a large burn center for intensive long-term care. The kind of environment provided in special burn units in large medical centers varies, but all have as their main objective avoiding contamination of the wound, as the major cause of death in burn victims is infection. Some special units use isolation techniques and elaborate laminar air flow systems to maintain an environment that is as free of microorganisms as possible.

The patient who has suffered some disfigurement from burns will have additional emotional problems in adjusting to a new body image. Burn therapy can be long and tedious for the patient and for family members. They will need emotional and psychological support as they work their way through the many problems created by the physical and emotional trauma of a major wound.

—Maria Pacheco, Ph.D.

See also Blisters; Critical care; Critical care, pediatric; Dermatology; Electrical shock; Emergency medicine; Grafts and grafting; Healing; Heat exhaustion and heat stroke; Radiation sickness; Shock; Skin; Wounds.

FOR FURTHER INFORMATION:

Glanze, Walter D., Kenneth N. Anderson, and Lois E. Anderson, eds. *The Signet Mosby Medical Encyclopedia*. New York: Signet, 1996. Excellent general reference for the layperson. Offers a concise but clear presentation of numerous medical topics.

Landau, Sidney I., ed. *International Dictionary of Medicine and Biology*. New York: John Wiley & Sons, 1986. Contains a brief presentation of medical and biological terms. A good, easy-to-comprehend general reference.

Leikin, Jerrold B., and Martin S. Lipsky, eds. *American Medical Association Complete Medical Encyclopedia*. New York: Random House Reference, 2003. A concise presentation of numerous medical terms and illnesses. A good general reference.

Marcovitch, Harvey, ed. *Black's Medical Dictionary*. 41st ed. Lanham, Md.: Scarecrow Press, 2006. An excellent presentation of the topic can be found in this general medical reference work.

Miller, Benjamin F., Claire Brackman Keane, and Marie T. O'Toole. *Miller-Keane Encyclopedia and Dictionary of Medicine, Nursing, and Allied Health*. Rev. 7th ed. Philadelphia: W. B. Saunders, 2005. A good, concise presentation of the topic of burns.

Burping

Disease/disorder

Also known as: Belching

Anatomy or system affected: Abdomen, gastrointestinal system, stomach

Specialties and related fields: Family medicine, internal medicine

Definition: The mouth release of gas that is brought up from the stomach

Causes and Symptoms

Burping or belching is the act of releasing air from the stomach with a characteristic sound. Depending on the cause, belching may change in duration and intensity.

Gas is often trapped or created in the digestive tract and is created either from swallowing air or the breakdown of certain foods by bacteria. Air swallowing, also known as aerophagia, is usually caused by drinking or eating rapidly, as well as by chewing gum, drinking carbonated beverages, smoking, or even wearing loose dentures. Most of the swallowed air is released by burping while still in the stomach. Any leftover gas is either partially absorbed in the small intestine or released through the rectum together with the gases produced by the breakdown of undigested foods.

The movement of gases in the gastrointestinal tract leads to the characteristic sounds known as borborygmi. The volume of these gases in the whole gastrointestinal tract is about 200 milliliters (half a quart) and is mostly nitrogen (up to 90 percent), oxygen (up to 10 percent), hydrogen (up to 50 percent), methane (up to 10 percent), and carbon dioxide (up to 30 percent).

> **Information on Burping**
>
> **Causes:** Trapped gas in digestive tract, air swallowing, upper gastrointestinal disorder
> **Symptoms:** Nausea, dyspepsia, heartburn
> **Duration:** Temporary to chronic
> **Treatments:** Dietary changes, slower pace while eating, medications

Treatment and Therapy

Burping during or after meals is normal, but people who belch frequently may be swallowing too much air and releasing it before it reaches the stomach. Chronic belching may also be indicative of an upper gastrointestinal disorder, such as peptic ulcer disease, gastroesophageal reflux, or even gastritis.

According to the National Institute of Diabetes and Digestive and Kidney Diseases, chronic incidents of belching include the Meganblase syndrome and the gas-bloat syndrome. In the first case, an enlarged air bubble is trapped in the stomach, especially after a heavy meal, and leads to fullness and shortness of breath that may mimic a heart attack. Gas-bloat syndrome occurs after surgery to correct gastrointestinal disorders. Usually the taking of X rays to review the esophagus, stomach, and upper small intestine allows for identification of the problems associated with chronic belching.

Young babies also appear to undergo air swallowing when they eat, whether via breast-feeding or bottle-feeding, as they express the discomfort of entrapped air by crying. Normally patting the child's back for a few minutes, followed by running a hand up and down the child's belly, is effective in releasing the gas. Holding the baby upright over the caregiver's shoulder allows the air bubbles to rise to the mouth, where they are expelled.

Perspective and Prospects

Burping may alleviate symptoms such as nausea, dyspepsia, and heartburn. Although not life threatening, gas entrapment is uncomfortable and, if possible, should be expelled from the digestive tract. The most common ways to reduce the discomfort of gas include changes in the diet and reduction of swallowed air, which is achieved via a slower pace while eating. The role of meditation also appears to have a positive effect on the reduction of belching.

—Soraya Ghayourmanesh, Ph.D.

See also Acid reflux disease; Digestion; Gastroenterology; Gastroenterology, pediatric; Gastrointestinal disorders; Gastrointestinal system; Heartburn; Nausea and vomiting; Ulcers.

For Further Information:

American Medical Association. *American Medical Association Family Medical Guide*. 4th rev. ed. Hoboken, N.J.: John Wiley & Sons, 2004.

Bonci, Leslie. *American Dietetic Association Guide to Better Digestion*. New York: Wiley, 2003.

Margolis, Simeon, et al. *Johns Hopkins White Papers 2003: Arthritis, Coronary, Depression and Anxiety, Diabetes, Digestive Disorders, Hypertension and Stroke*. Vol. 1. New York: Rebus, 2002.

Minocha, Anil, and David Carroll. *Natural Stomach Care: Treating and Preventing Digestive Disorders with the Best of Eastern and Western Healing Therapies*. New York: Avery, 2003.

Peikin, Steven R. *Gastrointestinal Health: A Self-Help Nutritional Program to Prevent, Cure, or Alleviate Irritable Bowel Syndrome, Ulcers, Heartburn, Gas, Constipation, and Many Other Digestive Disorders*. Rev. ed. New York: HarperCollins, 1999.

Bursitis

Disease/disorder

Anatomy or system affected: Hands, joints, knees, legs

Specialties and related fields: Internal medicine, rheumatology

Definition: An inflammation of a bursa, one of the membranes that surround joints.

Causes and Symptoms

Bursas are flattened, fibrous sacs that minimize friction on adjacent structures during activity involving a joint. The most well known bursas are around the knees, elbows, and shoulders. These protective joint sacs are lined with a fluid-producing membrane called the synovial membrane. Bursas are common in sites where ligaments, muscles, skin, or tendons overlie and may rub against bone. Most bursas are present at birth, but false bursas may develop at any site where there is excessive motion.

Bursitis is inflammation of a bursa, causing it to become warm, painful, and often swollen. Bursitis is usually caused by the inappropriate or excessive use of a joint. For example, pressure, friction, infections, or injury to a joint and surrounding tissues can cause membranes of the bursa to become inflamed.

Information on Bursitis

Causes: Inappropriate or excessive joint use, pressure, friction, infections, injury

Symptoms: Warm, painful, swollen joints

Duration: Temporary to chronic

Treatments: Rest, avoidance of pain-inducing activity, ice packs, anti-inflammatory medications, antibiotics, surgery, physical therapy

Bursitis of the kneecap (prepatellar bursitis, or "housemaid's knee") is commonly caused by prolonged kneeling on a hard surface such as the floor. Similarly, olecranon bursitis ("student's elbow") is caused by pressure of the elbow against a table or desk. Perhaps the most common type of bursitis is of the shoulder joint, called subdeltoid bursitis.

Treatment and Therapy

The treatment for bursitis caused by overuse is usually rest and avoidance of the activity that resulted in the condition. Several days of rest is typically all that is needed for the swelling to subside. Ice packs may help relieve some of the minor pain and inflammation. If the inflammation does not subside after a few days, a physician may prescribe anti-inflammatory drugs such as ibuprofen or naproxen to reduce the inflammation and pain. Occasionally, a doctor will inject the inflamed bursa with a corticosteroid such as triamcinolone. In rare cases, where the symptoms are recurrent, a physician may remove the bursa (bursectomy). If the bursitis is caused by an infection, the most appropriate treatment is antibiotic therapy. During and after medical or surgical treatment, physical therapy may be recommended to improve the strength and mobility of the joint.

—*Matthew Berria, Ph.D.*

See also Arthritis; Gout; Inflammation; Osteoarthritis; Rheumatoid arthritis; Rheumatology.

For Further Information:

Leikin, Jerrold B., and Martin S. Lipsky, eds. *American Medical Association Complete Medical Encyclopedia*. New York: Random House Reference, 2003. A concise presentation of numerous medical terms and illnesses. A good general reference.

Marieb, Elaine N., and Katja Hoehn. *Human Anatomy*

and Physiology. 7th ed. San Francisco: Pearson Benjamin Cummings, 2007. Nonscientists at the advanced high school level or above will be able to understand this fine textbook. It includes a complete glossary, index, pronunciation guide, and other helpful features.

Parker, James N., and Philip M. Parker, eds. *The Official Patient's Sourcebook on Shoulder Bursitis*. San Diego, Calif.: Icon Health, 2002. Draws from public, academic, government, and peer-reviewed research to provide a wide-ranging handbook for patients with bursitis.

Bypass surgery

Procedure

Anatomy or system affected: Abdomen, blood vessels, circulatory system, chest, gastrointestinal system, heart, intestines, legs

Specialties and related fields: Cardiology, gastroenterology, general surgery

Definition: Surgical provision of an additional or alternative channel to divert blood or the contents of the digestive system around an obstruction or narrowing.

Key terms:

angina: severe chest pains caused by insufficient blood supply to the heart.

angiography: the injection of radiopaque dye into the arteries to make narrowing and blockages visible in X rays

angioplasty: the insertion of an inflatable probe into an artery, followed by inflation of a balloon to clear obstructions to blood flow

ischemia: a decrease in the blood supply to a body organ caused by a constriction or obstruction of blood vessels

laparoscope: a fiber-optic tube which can be used to examine internal organs

Indications and Procedures

Coronary artery bypass surgery is needed when angiography reveals a narrowing or blockage in heart arteries causing angina that cannot be controlled by medication or relieved by angioplasty. The traditional method of open chest bypass surgery, which first became popular in the 1970's, requires that the patient be fully anesthetized. The surgeon cuts open the patient's chest, saws through the breastbone, and spreads the halves of the ribcage to expose the heart. The heart is stopped and cooled, and the major heart vessels are attached to a heart-lung machine, which oxygenates and circulates the blood. At the same time, another surgeon removes a leg vein and prepares grafts to be sewn around blockages in the heart arteries. Mammary arteries are also employed to redirect blood flow around obstructed arteries. After the bypasses are satisfactorily implanted, the heart-lung machine is disconnected and the heart resumes pumping on its own. The two halves of the breastbone are reattached with stainless steel wire, and the incision is sewn closed. Patients are taken to a cardiac intensive care unit overnight and are normally discharged from the hospital within a week. They recover fully in one to three months.

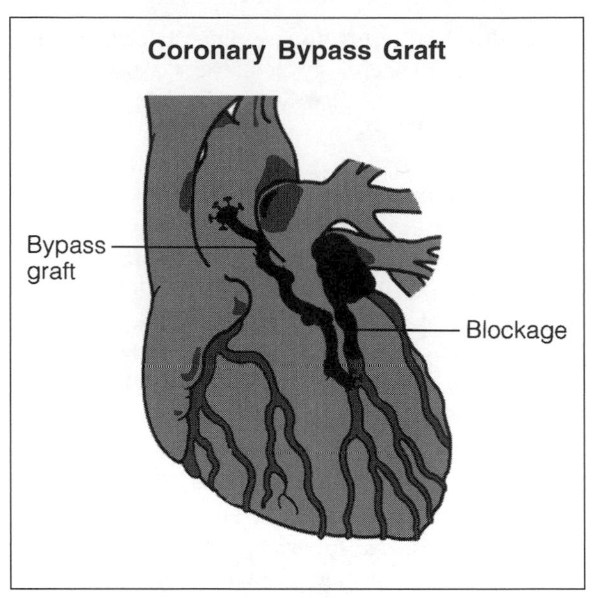

Bypass surgery can be performed in any part of the body where a blood vessel has become blocked; a common location for such a procedure is the heart, where from one to four arteries may require the placement of bypass grafts.

Bypass surgery of the peripheral arteries, usually those of the legs, is indicated when ischemia causes severe pain. Sections of leg veins and grafts made of synthetic material, such as Dacron, are used to bypass obstructions and to open blood flow to the legs.

An obstruction in the intestines can be treated surgically by removing the blocked region and sewing together the healthy portions of the gut. Severe problems may require creating an opening for the digestive tract through the abdominal wall, called a stoma, through which its contents can empty into a removable plastic bag. The procedure may be permanent or temporary, to allow the affected gut to heal. After successful healing, the bypass and bag are removed and the intestine segments are reattached.

Removal of part of the stomach or small intestine is sometimes used to treat cases of extreme obesity. The operation improves the patient's quality of life and may also extend its duration.

Uses and Complications

Traditional coronary artery bypass surgery is profoundly invasive. The heart-lung machine can create problems, even though newer machines are less stressful than the original models. The action of the pump is more powerful than that of a normal heart and can generate turbulence that damages blood cells and other organs. The machines have been blamed for blood clot formation, causing strokes and heart attacks during an operation. Patients, especially the elderly, often experience memory loss and confusion following surgery; though usually temporary, the problem can last for years. Surgeons, therefore, have been seeking less stressful and invasive methods of treating coronary artery disease.

Neither peripheral artery surgery nor intestinal bypass surgery involves using heart-lung machines, but the large incisions commonly used in such operations can also lead to complications by exposing extensive body areas to possible infection. Although traditional surgery is highly successful, innovators continue to seek the development of less invasive procedures.

Perspective and Prospects

The goal of research is minimally invasive surgery. Intestinal surgeons led the way with the development of laparoscopic gallbladder and kidney stone surgery in the 1980's. Only small circular incisions are needed to insert a fiber-optic instrument that transmits enlarged images of the surgical site to a screen. Laparoscopic tools are introduced though several additional small incisions. Segments of bowel can then be removed though tubes and their ends joined without opening the abdomen. The use of laparoscopic techniques reduces the tissue damage caused by traditional surgery. The patient feels less pain after the operation, experiences a shorter hospitalization, returns to normal activity sooner, and develops a smaller scar.

To avoid use of the heart-lung machine, and its medical complications, cardiac surgeons have experimented with open chest surgery on a beating heart. This very delicate operation involves temporarily immobilizing the area of the heart where the surgeon intends to attach a graft, slowing the heartbeat with drugs, and stitching the bypass into place between heartbeats. Only the most skilled surgeons succeed in mastering this difficult technique.

In the 1990's, cardiac surgeons, following intestinal surgeons, adopted the use of fiber-optic tubes that permit so-called keyhole surgery. Incisions of 3.0 inches in the chest and holes 0.5 inch in diameter under the armpit are sufficient to gain entry to the heart, thereby eliminating any need to open the chest cavity. Immobilizing segments of the heart and sewing grafts to the rhythm of the heartbeat, however, is considerably more difficult when done through a tube while viewing a television screen. In the twenty-first century, surgeons have begun using computer-controlled robots to carry out the intricate maneuvers needed to repair ailing hearts.

—Milton Berman, Ph.D.

See also Angina; Angioplasty; Arteriosclerosis; Bariatric surgery; Cardiology; Cardiology, pediatric; Circulation; Gastrectomy; Gastroenterology; Gastrointestinal system; Gastrostomy; Heart; Heart disease; Heart valve replacement; Ileostomy and colostomy; Intestines; Obesity; Vascular medicine; Vascular system.

For Further Information:

Doherty, Gerard M., and Lawrence W. Way, eds. *Current Surgical Diagnosis and Treatment*. 12th ed. New York: Lange Medical Books/McGraw-Hill, 2006.

Emery, Robert W., ed. *Techniques for Minimally Invasive Direct Coronary Artery Bypass (MIDCAB) Surgery*. Philadelphia: Hanley & Belfus, 1997.

Klaidman, Stephen. *Saving the Heart: The Battle to Conquer Coronary Disease*. New York: Oxford University Press, 2000.

Youngson, Robert. *The Surgery Book: An Illustrated Guide to Seventy-three of the Most Common Operations*. New York: St. Martin's Griffin, 1997.

Caffeine

Biology

Anatomy or system affected: Blood vessels, brain, heart, nervous system

Specialties and related fields: Biochemistry, family medicine, neurology, preventive medicine

Definition: An addictive chemical substance found in foods such as coffee, tea, chocolate, and some soft drinks.

Structure and Functions

Caffeine, known chemically as trimethylxanthine, is a substance found naturally in coffee beans, cocoa beans, and tea leaves. Caffeine renders significant physiological effects on its consumers, and individuals often use it in an effort to boost energy or wake up in the morning. In addition to its natural occurrences, caffeine is added by food processors to a variety of foods, including select soft drinks. Pills formulated to combat fatigue that are available without a prescription usually contain high doses of caffeine. A 6-ounce cup of drip-brewed coffee contains around 100 milligrams of caffeine, while an equal volume of tea contains 70 milligrams. A 12-ounce can of cola has about 50 milligrams of caffeine, while a 50-gram chocolate bar can contain between 5 and 60 milligrams.

In the brain, the chemical compound adenosine binds to adenosine receptors, which leads to drowsiness and decreased firing of neurons. Adenosine also interacts with blood vessels to dilate them. Caffeine has an appearance similar to that of adenosine, and it will bind to adenosine receptors, thus preventing adenosine from doing so. As a result, adenosine cannot initiate drowsiness, and alertness is increased. Under the influence of caffeine, blood vessels constrict and neurons fire rapidly. The brain responds to these cues by releasing the hormone adrenaline, commonly referred to as the "fight or flight" hormone. Adrenaline causes the pupils of the eyes to dilate, increases heart rate and blood pressure, constricts blood flow to the body surface and increases blood flow to the muscles, and releases sugar from the liver into the bloodstream, among other physiological effects.

Disorders and Diseases

Caffeine is the most widely used psychoactive chemical in the world. In moderate doses, caffeine can increase alertness, but it may also cause insomnia, nervousness, and decreased fine motor coordination. While alertness is perceived by the consumer, caffeine does not increase energy. Instead, the body experiences stress, which leads to the physical sensations described above.

Caffeine is addictive. It is believed that caffeine acts similarly to heroin on the pleasure centers of the brain. Caffeine withdrawal is associated with headaches and irritability.

One of the most serious consequences of caffeine consumption is insomnia. The amount of time that it takes half of the caffeine consumed to leave the body is about six hours. It may take up to twelve hours for the body to process caffeine and permit normal sleep.

Caffeine consumption has also been associated with depletion of B vitamins, increased calcium loss and an accompanying risk of osteoporosis, and decreased ability to absorb iron from food. Caffeine has also been shown to raise the blood level of the amino acid homocysteine, which is associated with an elevated risk of heart attack.

—*Karen E. Kalumuck, Ph.D.*

See also Addiction; Anxiety; Biofeedback; Brain; Ergogenic aids; Headaches; Metabolism; Nervous system; Neurology; Nicotine; Osteoporosis; Psychiatry; Psychology; Sleep disorders; Smoking; Stress; Stress reduction; Vitamins and minerals; Weight loss medications.

For Further Information:

Cherniske, Stephen. *Caffeine Blues: Wake Up to the Hidden Dangers of America's Number One Drug*. New York: Warner Books, 1998.

Exploratorium Magazine: Coffee and Tea 25, no. 3 (Fall, 2001).

Weinberg, Bennett Alan, and Bonnie K. Bealer. *The World of Caffeine: The Science and Culture of the World's Most Popular Drug*. New York: Routledge, 2001.

Calculi. *See* Stones.

Cancer

Disease/disorder

Anatomy or system affected: All

Specialties and related fields: Cytology, histology, immunology, oncology, orthopedics, radiology

Definition: Inappropriate and uncontrollable cell growth within one of the specialized tissues of the body, threatening normal cell and organ function and in serious cases traveling via the bloodstream to other areas of the body.

Key terms:

carcinogen: a cancer-causing substance; usually a chemical that causes mutations

cell: the basic functional unit of the body, each of which contains a set of genes and all the other materials necessary for carrying out the processes of life

cell cycle: a step-by-step process whereby one cell duplicates itself to form two cells; it is the way in which most growth occurs, and the cycle leads to cancer if it becomes defective

gene: a master molecule that encodes the information needed for the body to carry out one specific function; many thousands of genes working together are needed to sustain normal human life

immortalized: the state of a cancer cell that allows it to divide an unlimited number of times

initiation: the first abnormal change that starts a cell along the pathway to cancer

messenger RNA: The messenger ribonucleic acid molecule is encoded from DNA in a process called transcription; this molecule is then translated into protein.

metastasis: the process whereby tumor cells spread from one part of the body to another

mutation: damage to a gene that changes how it works

oncogene: a gene that functions normally to allow cells to progress through the cell cycle; when mutated, such genes can cause cancer

promotion: the second step in tumor development, which causes initiated cells to begin growing into tumors

telomerase: the enzyme that synthesizes the repeated sequences called telomeres at the ends of chromosomes

telomere: the repeated sequences at the end of chromosomes

transformation: genetic change in cancer cells which results in loss of growth control and often immortalization

tumor suppressor genes: genes that normally keep cell division in check, orderly, and properly timed; when mutated, they can cause cancer

Causes and Symptoms

Cancer is a disease of abnormal cellular growth. Growth is a feature of all living things, but it must be precisely regulated for development to occur properly. All growing cells pass through a strictly regulated series of events called the cell cycle, where most cellular structures are duplicated. At the end of the cycle, one cell is separated into two "daughter cells," each receiving one copy of the duplicated structures. The most important structures to be duplicated are the genes, which govern all cellular activities.

Information on Cancer

Causes: Genetic, environmental, or lifestyle factors; viruses

Symptoms: Varies widely; may include tumor growth, headaches, lethargy, fever, bloating, pain, swelling

Duration: Chronic, possibly recurrent

Treatments: Surgery, chemotherapy, radiation

Human life begins as a fertilized egg which divides again and again; the adult human body is composed of a trillion cells, each with a specific job to perform. At adulthood, most cells stop duplicating. Some cells, however, must continue dividing to replace worn-out cells in places like the blood, skin, and intestine. Such growth is accurately controlled so excess cells are not produced. Sometimes, however, a mutation arises in one or more genes, resulting in needless cell duplication and ultimately loss of growth control: a malignant transformation. This is the start of cancer.

At first, these cells resemble their neighbors. For example, newly altered blood cells look like normal blood cells, and in most respects are. However, cancer cells differ in a number of ways from "normal" cells. First, cancer cells grow uncontrollably. They may or may not grow faster than normal cells, but cancer cells do not cease growth. If placed in a laboratory cell culture dish, cancer cells will pile upon one another in a manner analogous to formation of a tumor. By contrast, normal cells grow in a single layer (monolayer) and stop replicating when they reach the edges of their dish when cellular signals instruct them to halt. Second, cancer cells often grow independently of hormones and growth factors, like insulin, required by other cells. They become "growth factor independent." Third, cancer cells are immortal. Normal cells are able to replicate themselves a regulated number of times, usually approximately fifty divisions, while cancer cells have no such limit. For example, HeLa cells, originally obtained from a woman with cervical cancer in the mid-1950's, have been cultured in laboratories for more than fifty years. Fourth, cancer cells in later stages change shape and size compared to normal cells. They may look very different. Oncologists (cancer specialists) use this information to identify cancer types and make prognoses.

The first event triggering cancer is initiation, precipitated by a mutation in one of the genes controlling some feature of the cell cycle. There are several hundred such genes regulating different aspects of the cell cycle and cellular growth. These genes have mundane jobs governing the life of the cell until they become damaged. When there is a mutation in a controlling gene, it functions improperly. It does not govern the cell cycle correctly, and the cell cycle proceeds when it should be halted. Such cancer-causing genes are called oncogenes.

After initiation, additional mutations and defects begin to accumulate, and the defective cells become increasingly abnormal. Tumor suppressor genes, normally functioning to keep cell division from becoming disorganized, are the site of these second-stage mutations. Those cells whose division and growth genes have mutated (oncogenes) and whose division and growth inhibitor genes (tumor suppressor genes) have also mutated will become cancer cells. Typically, a further change, "promotion," must take place before cancer cells begin growing freely. Promotion allows cells to escape the monitoring activity of the body. For example, various hormones instruct cells how to behave; a change of the promotion type may allow a cell to ignore such instructions. Both initiation and promotion occur randomly. Many initiated cells fail to grow into tumors. It is only those few cells that happen to acquire both defects that cause a problem. Fortunately, few cells have both their oncogenes turned "on" and their tumor suppressor genes turned "off."

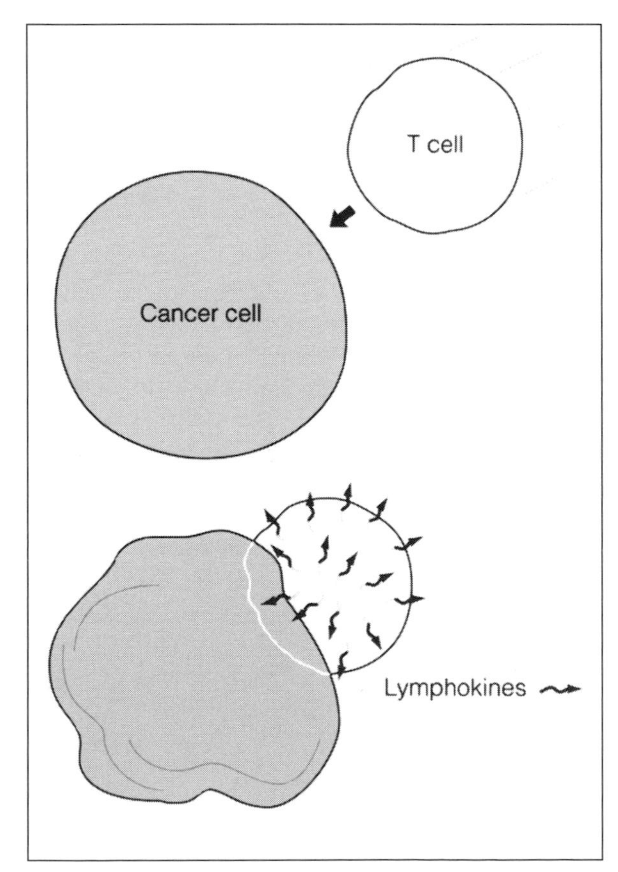

Cancer cells are fast-growing, irregular cells; normally, the body releases killer T cells that interact with antigens on the surface of the cancer cell, releasing lymphokines that are toxic to the cancer cell.

At this point in the process, the new cancer cell is dividing and producing larger numbers. These cells grow into a mass called a tumor—except in blood and lymph tissues, where cancer cells circulate individually. Nevertheless, these cells look normal at this early stage and are relatively easy to control with surgery. The excess cells may not cause much harm. Warts, for example, result from underlying skin cells exhibiting abnormal growth control. Such harmless tumors are called benign.

Unfortunately, as cells continue to replicate uncontrollably, more mutations develop. The most harmful changes result in complete loss of growth control. Cancer cells spread, resulting in damage to other parts of the body. For example, cancer cells may acquire the ability to digest their way through nearby tissues, a process called invasion. Eventually, the functioning of organs containing such cells becomes impaired. Other cancer cells may break loose from the tumor and travel to other parts of the body in the circulatory or lymphatic systems. This process is called metastasis. In advanced stages, a cancer patient may actually have dozens or hundreds of tumors, all of which developed from a single tumor cell. Cells that can invade or metastasize are called malignant. It becomes increasingly difficult to eradicate cancer cells as they become more malignant. Because each event leading to tumor development is rare, it may take years for the several acquired mistakes to aggregate in a single cell, resulting in a malignant tumor. The idea that the incidence of cancer is increasing in the general population is mostly myth; most cancers are primarily diseases of older persons.

Cancer-causing mutations occur when outside forces cause oncogenes and tumor suppressor genes to function abnormally. For example, genes may be chemically damaged by a number of highly active and dangerous chemicals known as carcinogens. Additionally, several kinds of radiation can damage genes: ultraviolet radiation, gamma radiation, nuclear radiation, and possibly electromagnetic field radiation. Finally, several kinds of viruses, including certain strains of the human papillomavirus or human herpesviruses, can cause oncogenes to function improperly. In most cancers, however, the origin of the disease is unknown and may result simply from a genetic mistake which takes place during gene duplication.

TREATMENT AND THERAPY

The most common cancer treatments fall into three categories: surgery, chemotherapy, and radiotherapy. The oldest treatment, going back several hundred years, is the surgical removal of tumors. If performed at an early stage, before metastasis, this method can be highly successful. Even so, surgery is much easier and less dangerous for some cancers (like that of the skin) than others (like that of the brain, which can be difficult to reach and remove). Surgery is not an option for blood and lymph cancers that are widely distributed.

The second most common type of cancer treatment for tumors is radiotherapy. The radiation of choice is X rays, which can penetrate the body to reach a tumor in very high dosages using modern equipment. X rays can be focused on a specific small area or be administered over the whole body in the case of metastasized cancer. Therapeutic radiation damages genes to such an extent that they become physically fragmented and nonfunctional, ending the life of the target cell.

Radiotherapy has major drawbacks. The most serious problem is that normal cells in the path of the radiation will also be killed. Bone marrow, the source of blood cells, is destroyed with whole-body cancer treatments. This problem can be overcome after radiotherapy by transplanting new bone marrow into the patient, so that a treated patient can begin to manufacture new blood cells. Ironically, radiation designed to kill cancer cells can also cause malignant mutations in normal cells. Recent innovations in radiotherapy include instrumentation such as the gamma knife, a method to direct radiation precisely into the center of a tumor. In this manner, damage to surrounding cells may be minimized.

If a patient has metastasized tumor cells, radiation and surgery are not the treatments of choice. Neither of these therapies acts systemically. The most common systemic treatment used that can reach everywhere in the body is chemotherapy. Patients are treated with chemicals that prevent cells from duplicating or slow the process. Such drugs reach all parts of the body much more effectively than surgery when cancer has reached a later stage of distribution.

Different kinds of chemicals work in different ways to achieve this result. These chemicals can be divided into four major categories. First are chemicals that react directly with the substances required for cells to survive and function. Many such agents directly attack a cell's genes, preventing them from passing along information required for a cancer cell to stay alive. Second are "antimetabolites," which prevent the chemical reactions that allow cells to produce the energy needed to live. The third category consists of steroid hormones. Cancer cells in some tissues respond to these hormones, which can therefore be used to regulate growth. Thus estrogens, the female steroid hormones, are often used for treatment of breast cancer, while the male steroids, androgens, may influence prostate cancer. Fourth are miscellaneous drugs that affect cancer cells in various ways. For example, drugs called vinca alkaloids stop the mechanical process of cell division and prevent growth. A derivative of the insecticide DDT (dichloro-diphenyl-tricholorethane) prevents unwanted steroid-hormone production and has been useful for treating tumors of the adrenal gland.

The newest class of anticancer drugs are known as taxanes. Taxol, isolated from the bark of the yew tree, is the best known of these drugs. Taxanes are active, poisonous constituents that can induce tumor cell death. This class of drug promotes the polymerization of the tubulin protein, which is needed to move chromosomes during cell division. By stabilizing the tubulin in the cancer cells, the equilibrium in the cell is disrupted, leading ultimately to cell death. The drugs paclitaxel and docetaxel are used frequently in ovarian and breast cancer and often in conjunction with one another.

The most common and difficult problem with the chemotherapeutic approach to cancer management is that normal cells are also affected by the same drugs that halt the growth of cancer cells. This reaction causes many difficulties for patients. Probably the most serious problems are with the immune system. Growth of the white blood cells that make antibodies is necessary to fight an infectious disease. Chemotherapy often depresses the immune system so it functions inefficiently; therefore patients in chemotherapy are more vulnerable to bacterial and viral illnesses. Red blood cells do not carry oxygen optimally during chemotherapy, making patients breathless and "sickly." Skin often becomes pale and unhealthy looking. The digestive tract cells stop dividing, causing weight loss and digestive problems. Finally, a less serious irritant for such patients is hair loss, since hair follicles are also prevented from growing.

Accordingly, cancer surgery is inefficient. Radiation therapy may cause as many problems as it solves, and chemotherapy, despite its anticancer efficiency, is toxic and can make the patient very ill. The problems for a cancer sufferer seem to have only just begun with their diagnosis since many of the cures seem, in the short term, as potentially harmful as the disease. Chemotherapy has developed such an unwholesome reputation that some patients refuse treatment, preferring death to the "indignities" of chemotherapy's effects. Oncologists are presently experimenting with a whole series of promising new treatments that may be less harmful to patients while being more efficacious.

Antisense therapy is one method in the new arsenal of treatments emerging from advances in biotechnology. Oncogenes, like other genes, are read (transcribed) by the machinery of the cell so that cellular messages called messenger ribonucleic acid (mRNA) are made. The mRNA is then itself read (translated) by the ribosomes of the cell to make proteins. Proteins are the major component of every enzyme and structural part of a cell. The problem with oncogenes is that they have been turned on and cannot be turned off, so the cancer cells continue growing. One type of antisense cancer therapy works by injection into the cancer cells of a "backward" (complementary) copy of the mRNA molecule made from the active oncogene. This "backward" copy interferes with the oncogene's "forward" mRNA message, causing it not to be made into an oncogenic protein. Consequently, this treatment stops the cancer cells from growing, because the cells are no longer encouraged to grow by the oncogenic protein. The advantages of this treatment are that it is very specific to cancer cells and has few side effects. The major disadvantages are that the physician must know precisely what oncogene is causing the disease in order to design the antisense treatment and that the treatment must be individualized in most cases, making a single "magic bullet" cure for all unavailable. University of Illinois oncologist Herbert Engelhard reports that this method has been successfully used to keep glial tumor cells (gliomas) of the brain from growing.

A related cancer treatment scheme is gene replacement therapy. In this method, an additional gene is introduced into the tumor cell with a laboratory-designed virus. This gene moves into the nucleus of the cell, becomes expressed as mRNA, and is translated into a protein. This protein is usually engineered to replace a missing or nonfunctioning gene. For example, the introduced factor may restore a missing tumor suppressor protein to the cancer cells, inducing them to become "normal" again.

A third biotechnologic approach to cancer treatment is gene-directed enzyme prodrug ("suicide gene") therapy. In this method, the cancer cells are treated with viral DNA containing a special suicide gene. When an inactive antibiotic drug is later given to the cancer patient, the drug is converted into a toxic form by the gene. This kills only the tumor cells making the enzyme. Other cells without the suicide gene are unaffected. The chief advantages of this treatment are high cancer-cell specificity, few side effects, and effectiveness with a wide variety of tumor types.

Yet another approach, oncolytic virus therapy, holds a great deal of promise. Genetically engineered viruses are made "safe" by deleting essential genes but are left with the ability to replicate. They are also given the ability to target and bind only cancer cells. Cancer cells are treated with these viruses. Viral replication occurs within the cells. Many viruses are made within the cancer cell; it bursts open (lyses) and dies. More viruses are then released that have the ability to infect and destroy adjacent cancer cells. The herpes simplex virus 1 (HSV1) has become a popular virus for oncolytic therapy. The "wild" HSV1 is usually quite virulent and induces illness in humans, but researchers have produced a genetically modified virus with low binding capacity to normal cells but high affinity for tumor cells.

Another new therapeutic method is photodynamic therapy (PDT). Cancer cells are treated with certain photosensitive dyes. In the presence of light, the dyes react to make molecular oxygen radicals. These radicals are poisonous and specifically kill any cancer cells treated with the dye.

Finally, a series of new types of anticancer drug treatments are being developed that do not simply kill cancer cells but prevent them from proliferating and growing. These new drugs are called cytostatic therapies and have a variety of functions. Some inhibit the formation of new blood vessels (angiogenesis) essential to tumor tissue growth. Other drugs inhibit the proteases used by certain tumors to dissolve the proteins that hold the normal tissues together. Without these proteases, tumor cells could not invade tissues, gain access to blood vessels, and colonize distant sites. Still other treatments inhibit growth by interfering with the signals that tell cancer cells to keep proliferating.

Perspective and Prospects

In the mid-1990's, evidence of a potential new basis for cancer emerged. The hypothesis suggested that overproduction of the enzyme telomerase, which synthesizes the telomeres at the ends of chromosomes, may cause uncontrolled growth in cells.

In normal human cells, the telomeres, long DNA repeats of TTAGGG, are slowly shortened and erode away as the cells age. The lengthening enzyme telomerase is not active in normal cells, so the ends of the chromosomes shorten more and more over a lifetime; in fact, these chromosomal changes have been postulated as one possible cause of cellular aging. When the telomeres become short enough, cell senescence is induced as the cells stop dividing. Tumor cells have active telomerase and do not lose their chromosomal ends. One source of immortality in cancer cells may be their long telomeres.

It is not clear whether lengthening of telomeres is an oncogenic event causing cells to become cancerous or whether these events are simply crucial in tumor formation. The importance of the telomerase activity in inducing cancer is quite controversial. Mice who have had telomerase genes turned off permanently show no ill effects and age normally. Although researchers have shown that oncogenes become operative if the telomerase is active in cell culture, it is unclear what role telomerase plays in actual biological systems. Researchers have suggested that perhaps the loss of that enzyme activity could be a protective mechanism against cancer. However, that is unlikely, since a phenomenon that usually occurs at the end of an organism's lifetime, and after reproduction, such as cancer, would not be evolutionarily selected against.

Telomerase offers another possible avenue of treatment for cancer as a therapeutic agent. It may turn out that treatments that shut off the telomerase activity in cancer cells will slow or stop their growth. Pharmacological treatments may induce cancer cells to become normal cells once again. Once the mechanism of telomerase activity is understood, medical treatments may even induce cancer cells to destabilize and die.

Earlier detection and treatment has significantly improved the prognosis for those diagnosed with cancer. Nevertheless, since 1999, cancer has surpassed heart disease as the leading cause of death among Americans younger than eighty-five. Nearly 1.4 million cancer cases are diagnosed each year, with some 575,000 deaths. Improved diagnosis and treatment, however, have resulted in decreased mortality from the three most common forms of cancer among men: colon/rectal, lung, and prostate. Likewise, mortality has decreased among women with the two most common forms: breast and colon/rectal. Distribution of such cancers among ethnic or racial lines continues to show significant differences, as African Americans are far more likely to be diagnosed with advanced stage disease than are Caucasians.

—Howard L. Hosick, Ph.D.;
Connie Rizzo, M.D., Ph.D.,
and James J. Campanella, Ph.D.;
updated by Richard Adler, Ph.D.

See also Antioxidants; Biopsy; Bladder cancer; Bladder removal; Bone cancer; Bone marrow transplantation; Brain tumors; Breast biopsy; Breast cancer; Burkitt's lymphoma; Carcinogens; Carcinoma; Cells; Cervical, ovarian, and uterine cancers; Chemotherapy; Colon and rectal polyp removal; Colon and rectal surgery; Colon cancer; Colonoscopy and sigmoidoscopy; Cytology; Cytopathology; Dermatopathology; Endometrial biopsy; Epstein-Barr virus; Gallbladder cancer; Gastrectomy; Genomics; Hodgkin's disease; Hysterectomy; Imaging and radiology; Immunology; Immunopathology; Kaposi's sarcoma; Kidney cancer; Laryngectomy; Leukemia; Liver cancer; Lung cancer; Lung surgery; Lymphadenopathy and lymphoma; Malignancy and metastasis; Mammography; Mastectomy and lumpectomy; Melanoma; Mouth and throat cancer; National Cancer Institute (NCI); National Institutes of Health (NIH); Oncology; Plastic surgery; Prostate cancer; Prostate gland removal; Radiation therapy; Sarcoma; Screening; Skin cancer; Skin lesion removal; Stem cells; Stomach, intestinal, and pancreatic cancers; Terminally ill: Extended care; Testicular cancer; Tumor removal; Tumors.

For Further Information:

American Cancer Society (ACS). http://www.cancer.org/docroot/home/index.asp. Web site is divided into sections for patients, family, and friends; survivors; health information seekers; ACS supporters; and professionals. Information on all cancers is wide ranging.

Bognar, David, et al. *Cancer: Increasing Your Odds for Survival: A Resource Guide for Integrating Mainstream, Alternative, and Complementary Therapies.* Alameda, Calif.: Hunter House, 1998. This is a resource guide for cancer patients and their families, covering the emotional shock and disorientation at diagnosis and how to deal with it.

Cairns, John. *Matters of Life and Death.* Princeton, N.J.: Princeton University Press, 1998. Cairns is a prominent molecular biologist who has turned his attention to cancer. He writes eloquently but nontechnically about the biology and medical implications of cancer.

Cancer Care. http://www.cancercare.org. Site provides information, including links and resources, to help people who have cancer, and their families and friends, better cope with the disease.

Dollinger, Malin, et al. *Everyone's Guide to Cancer Therapy.* 4th ed. Kansas City, Mo.: Andrews McMeel, 2002. A comprehensive review of treatments available, with topics that include cryotherapy, radio frequency treatment, genetic risk assessment, and managed care.

Greaves, M. F. *Cancer: The Evolutionary Legacy.* New York: Oxford University Press, 2002. In this book, cancer researcher Greaves illuminates what is known of cancer's causes and the obstacles to research. His personal, almost chatty style helps the nontechnical reader through some of the complicated immunological and genetic issues, and it also humanizes a topic that can easily overwhelm the reader.

McKinnell, Robert Gilmore, ed. *The Biological Basis of Cancer.* New York: Cambridge University Press, 1998. This text is designed to be used for an undergraduate course on cancer. It covers everything from the molecular to the clinical aspects of the subject, with a lengthy bibliography.

Weinberg, Robert. *The Biology of Cancer.* New York: Garland Science, 2006. History of research into understanding the causes of cancer. The author himself carried out many of the discoveries related to oncogenes described in the book.

Candidiasis

Disease/disorder

Anatomy or system affected: Abdomen, bladder, blood, gastrointestinal system, genitals, immune system, mouth, reproductive system, skin, urinary system

Specialties and related fields: Epidemiology, family medicine, immunology, internal medicine

Definition: An acute or chronic fungal infection of humans and animals that can be superficial or deep-seated, caused by a species of the fungus *Candida.*

Key terms:

acquired immunodeficiency syndrome (AIDS): a severe and usually fatal disease caused by infection with the human immunodeficiency virus (HIV); infection results in progressive impairment of the immune system

antifungal agents: drugs that can result in the inhibition of growth or killing of fungi; these drugs may be topical or systemic in application

cell-mediated immunity: protection mediated by thymus-derived lymphocytes; this type of immunity is particularly important for certain types of pathogenic organisms such as *Candida*

chlamydoconidia (chlamydospores): budding organisms that form directly from vegetative mycelia (molds); they differ from true spores, which are the result of sexual reproduction

culture: the propagation of organisms, such as fungi, on artificial media; *Candida* organisms grow in many kinds of media in both the yeast and mold forms

dimorphism: the ability of a fungus to exist in two forms, yeasts and molds; yeasts are unicellular round, oval, or cylindrical cells, and molds are branching tubular structures called hyphae

germ tube test: an initial laboratory test used to identify unknown yeasts and performed by microscopically examining a colony of yeast inoculated into rabbit or human plasma

histopathology: the study of the appearance and structure of abnormal or diseased tissue under the microscope

phagocytosis: the progress of ingestion and digestion by cells that are part of the immune system; this process is one of the ways that mammals use to defend themselves against infectious invaders, including *Candida* organisms

Causes and Symptoms

Candida is a genus of dimorphic fungi found widely in nature. This fungus may be found in soil, inanimate objects, plants, and most important, as a harmless parasite of humans and other mammals. It can exist in two forms: as a yeast and as a mold. In the yeast phase, this fungus exists as a normal inhabitant in and on human bodies. Nearly all infections are of such endogenous origin, but human-to-human transmission may occasionally occur from mother to newborn or between sexual partners. The yeasts reproduce asexually by budding, and a sexual stage has been recognized only in a few species. Pseudohyphae develop when yeasts and

INFORMATION ON CANDIDIASIS

CAUSES: Fungal infection
SYMPTOMS: Dependent on region; may include white patches on tongue, difficult or painful swallowing, endocarditis, vaginal discharge, intense itching, diaper rash, urinary tract infection
DURATION: Temporary or chronic
TREATMENTS: Antifungal drugs, removal of foreign material or infected tissue

their progeny adhere to one another, forming chains. Hyphae, the branching tubular structures of molds, are formed in tissue invaded by the fungus.

Identification of *Candida* as the causative agent in clinical infections depends largely on the microscopic examination of infected tissue or secretions and on a culture of *Candida* prepared from infected material. Histopathological examination may reveal yeast forms and/or hyphal or pseudohyphal forms. The microscopic appearance of these organisms is similar to those of some other fungi, and a culture is necessary to confirm this fungus as the responsible pathogen. *Candida* will grow on many types of artificial microbiologic media and can usually be grown on the same media used to grow bacteria. With some types of infection, however, the use of special media or techniques may lead to a higher yield from cultures. After an unknown yeast is grown on artificial media, tests must be performed to determine its identity. Most laboratories initially use the germ tube test, in which yeast is introduced into rabbit or human plasma at 35 degrees Celsius for one to two hours. In this test, a structure called a germ tube is observed if the yeast is *Candida albicans*, *Candida stelloidea*, or rare strains of *Candida tropicalis*. If this test is positive (a germ tube is produced), then most laboratories assume that the microorganism is *C. albicans*—it is by far the most common species causing disease—and conduct no further, and usually more expensive, tests. Simple cultural tests may also be used to identify *C. albicans*, including the formation of spiderlike colonies on eosin methylene blue agar or the production of chlamydoconidia on cornmeal agar. The identification of *Candida* antigens in the serum of patients with widespread or disseminated infection is sometimes used to assist in the diagnosis of candidiasis, but this test is neither sensitive nor specific.

The bodies of humans and other mammals possess multiple defense mechanisms against candidiasis. The skin and mucous membranes provide a protective wall, but breaks in the mucocutaneous barrier may occur in many ways, including trauma, surgery, and disease. A balanced microbial flora in the gastrointestinal tract prevents the overgrowth of *Candida* organisms, which can lead to penetration of this fungus into the lining of the gastrointestinal tract and its entrance into the bloodstream. When invasion occurs, phagocytic cells (including monocytes, neutrophils, and eosinophils) further protect the body by ingesting and killing *Candida* organisms. Phagocytosis is assisted by serum proteins called opsonins. Lymphocytes are also important defenders against this fungus and are part of the cell-mediated immune system. Candidiasis may result when cell-mediated immunity is defective, as is the case with the hereditary condition of chronic mucocutaneous candidiasis or with acquired immunodeficiency syndrome (AIDS). Approximately 80 percent of healthy people exhibit delayed hypersensitivity reactions to *Candida* antigens, indicating the presence of a previously induced cell-mediated immunity directed against such an infection.

Candidiasis may be divided into superficial mucocutaneous and deep-seated, tissue-invasive types. There are more than one hundred fifty species of this fungus, but only ten are recognized as human pathogens, and *C. albicans* is the most important. Oral candidiasis, or thrush, is a common infection characterized by white patches on the tongue and oral mucosal surfaces (oropharyngeal infection). Scrapings taken from these patches contain masses of yeasts, pseudohyphae, and hyphae. Culturing is not as useful as clinical appearance and microscopic examination, since *Candida* organisms can be grown from normal mouths. Thrush is particularly common when the immune system is impaired, as in patients with cancer or AIDS or in asthmatics treated with inhaled steroids. Infection of other parts of the gastrointestinal tract, especially the esophagus, may occur in patients with a variety of underlying conditions, including an impaired immune system, gastrointestinal surgery, and antibiotic treatment. Esophageal involvement often results in difficult or painful swallowing. Only about half of patients with esophageal candidiasis will also have the more easily diagnosed oropharyngeal infection. Some patients with gastrointestinal candidiasis will develop systemic or disseminated infection.

Vaginal candidiasis, the most common type of vaginitis, is a common form of the infection associated with an overgrowth of *Candida* organisms in the vagina followed by mucocutaneous invasion. The patient will have a thick, curdlike vaginal discharge and itching of the surrounding skin areas. Antibiotic therapy, pregnancy, birth control pills, diabetes, and AIDS all predispose women to this form of infection. Recurrent or chronic infection can occur and may be associated with tissue invasion or impaired response of lymphocytes to the infection in some patients.

Cutaneous infection is common with candidiasis. This fungus is often the cause of diaper rash in infants; the condition often results from infection of skin under wet diapers by *Candida* organisms from the gastrointestinal tract. Intertrigo is another skin condition produced by candidiasis in the warm, moist area of skin folds, and similar environments result in perianal or scrotal infections that cause intense itching (pruritus). A widespread eruption of infection involving the trunk, thorax, and extremities is occasionally seen in both children and adults. Disseminated candidiasis, usually in association with persistent candidemia (the presence of the fungus in the bloodstream), may be associated with widely distributed, nodular skin lesions. Candidiasis of the skin, mucous membranes, hair, and nails beginning early in life and associated with defective cell-mediated immunity has been called chronic mucocutaneous candidiasis. This disease is often associated with a variety of endocrine diseases, including diabetes mellitus and decreased function of the parathyroid, thyroid, and adrenal glands.

Deep-organ involvement with candidiasis is serious and often life-threatening. The placement in the body of foreign material used for medical therapy may provide the initial breeding ground for the infection. Examples of these devices are vascular catheters, artificial heart valves, artificial vascular grafts, and artificial joints and other orthopedic implants. The environment created by these foreign materials makes it impossible for the normal defense mechanisms of the body to function.

Urinary tract infection with *Candida* organisms is seen in association with urinary catheters, especially when usage is chronic. Colonization of the urine with *Candida* organisms may also occur following a course of antibiotics or in diabetic patients. Infection of the kidney can result if the candidiasis spreads upward from the bladder through the ureter or via the bloodstream. Renal involvement has been reported in up to 80 percent of patients with disseminated candidiasis. In disseminated disease, infection is spread to the kidney through the bloodstream, with the formation of renal abscesses. Primary renal infection occurs when the kidney is invaded directly without concomitant invasion through the blood. Such direct infection may occur in association with urinary catheters or following surgical procedures involving the genital and urinary tracts. A particularly severe form of ascending renal infection, more frequent in diabetic patients, causes necrosis of the renal papillae and renal failure.

Ocular candidiasis (endophthalmitis) may occur when the eye is infected with *Candida* organisms either by direct invasion or through the bloodstream. Virtually any portion or structure of the eye may be involved. Examination of the retina using an ophthalmoscope can reveal white spots, resembling cotton balls, indicating *Candida* organisms in the blood vessels of the eye. This finding may also be a clue to infection elsewhere in the body that has spread through the bloodstream to the eye.

Endocarditis (inflammation of the lining of the heart) occurs when a native or artificial heart valve becomes infected. Candidiasis is an increasingly frequent cause of endocarditis of the native valves of intravenous drug abusers and artificial valves of all varieties. Such endocarditis is presumptively diagnosed when the organism is grown from blood specimens in the presence of a heart murmur. Abnormal growth on the heart valves, called vegetation, can usually be demonstrated using echocardiography. Fragments of vegetation may break off and circulate in the bloodstream, leading to the obstruction of vessels in many organs of the body, including the brain, eyes, lungs, spleen, and kidneys. Without treatment, this disease is uniformly fatal.

Disseminated candidiasis is seen in the most susceptible patients, including those with cancer, prolonged postoperative illness, and extensive burns. In these patients, further risk is associated with the use of central venous or arterial catheters, broad-spectrum antibiotic therapy, artificial feeding, or abdominal surgery. Dysfunction of neutrophils, or neutropenia, may increase the susceptibility of the patient to widespread infection with *Candida* organisms and can also be seen with AIDS. The kidney, brain, heart, and eye are the most common organs to be involved. Despite severe and extensive disease, specific diagnosis of disseminated candidiasis is difficult during life and is often only made at the time of postmortem examination.

Treatment and Therapy

Candidiasis may be prevented by avoiding or ameliorating the underlying predisposing factor or disease state and by decreasing or halting growth of the fungi. Dry or cracked skin can be treated with dermatologic lubricants. Invasive devices used for medical treatment should be placed in the body under the most sterile conditions and only employed when absolutely necessary. Care of these devices, including urinary catheters, intravascular lines, and peritoneal renal dialysis catheters, must be performed by skilled personnel using the most sterile approach possible. If antibacterial therapy is used excessively, fungal overgrowth may occur; *Candida* organisms can grow with ease in the gastrointestinal tract and vagina when bacteria are inhibited or killed by antibiotics, and overgrowth can lead not only to local infection but also to bloodstream invasion and secondary infection elsewhere in the body. Moreover, the treatment of underlying disease states such as diabetes mellitus, neoplasia, and AIDS will lessen the detrimental effects of candidiasis on the immune system.

Growth of *Candida* organisms can be decreased by altering the local conditions that favor their proliferation. For example, changing a baby's diaper frequently and applying a drying powder can avoid the wet and warm conditions that can result in diaper rash. Obese patients can lose weight, which will minimize skin fold infections. Wearing nonocclusive clothing, especially cotton fabrics, is often helpful in discouraging candidiasis.

Antifungal agents are often used to prevent candidiasis. Hospitalized patients recovering from surgery who have received antibacterial agents are given nystatin, an oral, nonabsorbed antifungal, to prevent the overgrowth of *Candida* organisms in the gastrointestinal tract. For cancer patients receiving chemotherapy, systemic antifungal drugs are often employed during the period when the cancer chemotherapy has had the most deleterious effects on the immune system.

Antifungals are employed by the topical, oral, parenteral (through a blood vessel or muscle), or irrigation routes for treatment of candidiasis. Among the many antifungal agents, nystatin, flucytosine, amphotericin B, and a variety of imidazole agents are the most commonly used. Antifungals utilize a number of different mechanisms that impede the metabolic activities of the organism or disrupt the integrity of the cell membrane on the outer surface of the fungus. Amphotericin B and fluconazole are useful in the treatment of systemic or deep-organ disease. Amphotericin B is produced by the fungus *Streptomyces nodosus* and is administered intravenously for systemic and deep-organ disease and by bladder irrigation for lower urinary tract infection (cystitis). When administered intravenously, amphotericin B has serious side effects, including fever, chills, kidney failure, liver abnormalities, and bone marrow suppression. Fluconazole has fewer adverse effects and can be administered by the oral or intravenous routes; for these reasons, it is now commonly used as the initial therapy for candidiasis. Amphotericin B remains the treatment of choice for serious or life-threatening infection or when a *Candida* species isolated from a patient has been demonstrated by laboratory testing to be resistant to other antifungal agents.

In addition to antifungals, removal of foreign material or infected tissue is often necessary to treat severe candidiasis. Catheters, vascular grafts, artificial heart valves, artificial joints, and other devices must be removed and then replaced, if necessary, while the patient is receiving antifungal therapy or after the infection is cured. In some cases, such as with endocarditis, the infected tissue must be surgically removed to ensure a cure.

As with prevention, treatment of the underlying disease state greatly assists other measures directed against candidiasis. Gaining control of hyperglycemia in diabetes mellitus patients, viral infection in AIDS patients, and bone marrow suppression in cancer patients will aid in the treatment of candidiasis when it is present.

Perspective and Prospects

More than two thousand years ago, the Greek physicians Hippocrates and Galen described oral lesions that were probably thrush, but it was not until 1839 that fungi were found in such lesions. Deep-seated infection was first described in 1861, and endocarditis was identified in 1940. Candidiasis was recognized as an indicator disease in the 1987 surveillance definition for AIDS by the Centers for Disease Control in the United States. *Candida* ranks among the most common pathogens in hospital-acquired infections.

Candidiasis is on the increase largely because of increasingly sophisticated medical therapies and the worldwide epidemic of AIDS. Medical devices, immunosuppressive medical therapies, and organ transplantation are all becoming more common, and it is anticipated that candidiasis will increase in a corresponding manner. Likewise, as patients infected with human immunodeficiency virus (HIV) progress to clinical illness, the cases of candidiasis are expected to rise dramatically.

More effective preventive and therapeutic measures will be necessary to combat such an increase in cases of candidiasis. New antifungal agents will need to be developed to treat resistant strains of *Candida*. Laboratory testing to determine whether various antifungal agents can kill or inhibit the growth of *Candida* species isolated from patients will need to be more widely available and more frequently performed if organisms resistant to antifungals are to be identified. Early identification of resistant organisms will benefit patients by providing more effective antifungal therapy early in the course of treatment. Testing procedures will need to employ better methodology that is standardized to enable laboratories in different locations to compare results and determine regional or national trends in antifungal resistance.

—*H. Bradford Hawley, M.D.*

See also Endocarditis; Fungal infections; Rashes; Women's health.

For Further Information:

Betts, Robert F., Stanley W. Chapman, and Robert L. Penn, eds. *Reese and Betts' A Practical Approach to Infectious Diseases*. 5th ed. Philadelphia: Lippincott Williams & Wilkins, 2003. A well-written and very popular text. This clinically oriented, multiauthor book on infectious diseases, including candidiasis, contains carefully chosen, annotated references at the end of each chapter.

Biddle, Wayne. *A Field Guide to Germs*. Rev. ed. New York: Random House, 2002. This comprehensive book is easily accessible to the nonspecialist and includes a discussion of nearly every virus, bacterium, and fungus known to cause human and nonhuman animal disease.

Kwon-Chung, K. J., and John E. Bennett. *Medical Mycology*. Philadelphia: Lea & Febiger, 1992. A fine text concerning fungal diseases. All aspects of these diseases, including their diagnosis and treatment, are covered.

Mandell, Gerald L., John E. Bennett, and Raphael Dolin, eds. *Mandell, Douglas, and Bennett's Principles and Practice of Infectious Diseases*. 6th ed. New York: Elsevier/Churchill Livingstone, 2005. An outstanding textbook in infectious diseases, with chapters on the various diseases caused by *Candida*, illnesses and conditions associated with this fungus, and antifungal agents.

Martin, Jeanne Marie. *Complete Candida Yeast Guidebook: Everything You Need to Know About Prevention, Treatment, and Diet*. Rev. ed. New York: Crown, 2000. Covers a range of relevant information to the disorder and offers suggestions for treatment that involves diet and hygiene.

Parker, James N., and Philip M. Parker, eds. *The Official Patient's Sourcebook on Genital Candidiasis*. San Diego, Calif.: Icon Health, 2002. Draws from public, academic, government, and peer-reviewed research to provide a wide-ranging handbook for patients with *Candida*.

Winn, Washington C., Jr., et al. *Koneman's Color Atlas and Textbook of Diagnostic Microbiology*. 6th ed. Philadelphia: Lippincott Williams & Wilkins, 2006. A practical text with excellent tables, charts, and photographs of microorganisms, including *Candida*. Also contains information on the collection of specimens from patients, the processing of cultures, and the interpretation of laboratory data.

Canker sores

Disease/disorder

Also known as: Aphthous ulcers, ulcerative stomatitis

Anatomy or system affected: Mouth, skin

Specialties and related fields: Dentistry, family medicine

Definition: Small, round ulcers of the mucous membranes that line the mouth.

Causes and Symptoms

Aphthous ulcers are the most common lesions of the mucous membranes that line the mouth. The cause of this easily recognized problem is not known; however, some evidence points to infection with the human herpesvirus 6, one of a family of viruses that cause a variety of diseases, including cold sores, genital herpes, and shingles.

In most cases, a canker sore is a painful, small, round ulcer on a red base with a yellowish center. The redness also surrounds the lesion like a halo. Sores are usually about 1 to 2 millimeters in diameter but may be as large as 1 to 2 centimeters. They may occur as either single or multiple lesions and are found on the mucous membranes lining the mouth and tongue. These lesions tend to recur; the recurrences may be associated with stress or illness. The associated pain usually lasts for a week to ten days, and the ulcers heal completely within three weeks. Major aphthous ulcers, another variety, start out

INFORMATION ON CANKER SORES

CAUSES: Unknown; possibly herpesvirus infection, stress, or illness
SYMPTOMS: Small, round ulcers of mucous membranes in mouth
DURATION: Acute, often recurrent
TREATMENTS: Pain relief (steroid-containing gel or paste, anesthetic spray, mouthwash), oral steroids

as nodules under the mucous membranes, which then break down and form craterlike ulcers that may last more than a month.

Aphthous ulcers may occur on their own, but they may also be associated with some diseases and disorders of the collagen, certain gastrointestinal problems, and Behçet's disease. This last condition is a syndrome that involves painful ulcers of the tongue and oral mucous membranes, in addition to a variety of eye, skin, joint, gastrointestinal, and central nervous system problems.

TREATMENT AND THERAPY

The treatment of canker sores is geared toward relieving the pain rather than curing the lesion. Treatments include a steroid-containing gel or paste applied directly to the ulcer, an anesthetic spray, or a mouthwash that the patient "swishes and spits." In severe cases, oral steroids tapered over one week may provide relief.

PERSPECTIVE AND PROSPECTS

In patients with human immunodeficiency virus (HIV) infection, aphthous ulcers may be extremely painful or extensive. If the ulcers do not respond to conventional treatment, then the drug thalidomide may be useful. However, it must be used with extreme caution, as this drug is known to cause severe birth defects if taken during pregnancy.

—Rebecca Lovell Scott, Ph.D., PA-C

See also Cold sores; Dental diseases; Dentistry; Dentistry, pediatric; Herpes; Shingles; Skin; Skin disorders; Stress; Ulcers; Viral infections.

FOR FURTHER INFORMATION:

Beers, Mark H., et al., eds. *The Merck Manual of Medical Information, Second Home Edition.* Whitehouse Station, N.J.: Merck Research Laboratories, 2003.

Cook, Allan R., ed. *Oral Health Sourcebook: Basic Information About Diseases and Conditions Affecting Oral Health.* Detroit: Omnigraphics, 1998.

Komaroff, Anthony, ed. *Harvard Medical School Family Health Guide.* New York: Free Press, 2005.

National Institutes of Health. National Institute of Dental Research. *Fever Blisters and Canker Sores.* Rev. ed. Bethesda, Md.: Author, 1992.

CARCINOGENS

DISEASE/DISORDER
ANATOMY OR SYSTEM AFFECTED: All
SPECIALTIES AND RELATED FIELDS: All
DEFINITION: A substance or agent that causes or precipitates cancer.

TYPES AND EFFECTS

Carcinogens include chemicals, radiation, or viruses that can alter the deoxyribonucleic acid (DNA) in a normal human cell and eventually transform it into a cancer cell. Some carcinogens change DNA structure directly, while others make DNA more susceptible to damage from other sources or increase the possibility of DNA changes by causing cells to divide faster than normal.

Susceptibility to different carcinogens varies widely from person to person and is highly dependent upon genetic makeup, physiology, exposure time, dose of the carcinogen, and nutrition.

The *Report on Carcinogens* (RoC) released by the U.S. government in January, 2005, lists 246 cancer-causing agents. Of these carcinogens, 58 are known to produce cancer in humans, while 188 may very likely produce human cancer. For the first time, the list includes viral carcinogens, including hepatitis B virus (HBV), hepatitis C virus (HVC), and human papillomaviruses (HPVs). A list of carcinogens is also published by the International Agency for Research on Cancer (IARC).

CLASSIFICATION AND REDUCING RISK

Identification and classification of carcinogens is made from human observation and from laboratory studies that include animal experimentation and cell cultures. The RoC data include information about the ability of each substance to cause cancer, its ability to damage genes, and the biological changes that it can produce in the body. It also reports the potential for human exposure to the listed substances and the federal regulations that are imposed to limit exposure.

A number of important measures can lower the risk of exposure to carcinogens. Avoiding cigarette smoking, excessive alcohol consumption, and abnormal exposure to ultraviolet (UV) radiation from sunlight reduces the risk of many cancers. Being informed about carcinogens that may be present in the workplace or in the home and exercising necessary precautions with them provides protection. It is very important to follow the directions on any chemical containers.

Perspective and Prospects

The identification of carcinogens dates back to the 1930's when dozens of substances, including industrial and tobacco smoke, were classified as carcinogens. U.S. federal law requires that the secretary of Health and Human Services publish the RoC through the National Toxicology Program (NTP) every two years. In addition to listing carcinogens, the IARC report also lists substances that have been studied and determined not to be carcinogens.

Recent RoC and IARC reports indicate that acrylamide, a chemical in french fries and potato chips, is a possible carcinogen, as well as the charred residue on barbecued meats. The Food and Drug Administration (FDA) reported that in a test of 124 cosmetics, over half of them contained the carcinogens triethanolamine (TEA) and diethanolamine (DEA). Not all carcinogens can be absolutely avoided. For example, tamoxifen, used effectively in the treatment of breast cancer, increases the risk of some types of uterine cancer.

—Alvin K. Benson, Ph.D.

See also Asbestos exposure; Cancer; Environmental diseases; Environmental health; Hepatitis; Human papillomaviruses (HPV); Mutation; Smoking.

For Further Information:

Benigni, Romualdo, ed. *Quantitative Structure-Activity Relationship (QSAR) Models of Mutagens and Carcinogens*. Boca Raton, Fla.: CRC Press, 2003.

Milman, Harry A., and Elizabeth K. Weisburger, eds. *Handbook of Carcinogen Testing*. 2d ed. Park Ridge, N.J.: Noyes, 1994.

Pohanish, Richard P., ed. *Sittig's Handbook of Toxic and Hazardous Chemicals and Carcinogens*. Vols. 1 and 2. 4th ed. Norwich, N.Y.: Noyes, 2002.

Carcinoma

Disease/disorder

Anatomy or system affected: All

Specialties and related fields: Cytology, dermatology, histology, immunology, oncology

Definition: A malignant neoplasm or tumor that arises in epithelial cells.

Causes and Symptoms

The term "carcinoma" is often used as a synonym for cancer. A carcinoma is a malignant neoplasm or tumor that arises in the epithelial cells of tissues that line the surface layer of skin or that cover the internal organs. The most common carcinomas develop in the lungs, breasts, colon, small intestine, prostate (in men), and cervix (in women). In contrast, a sarcoma is a malignant neoplasm that affects mesenchymal tissue, the precursor to bone, muscle, and fat. Carcinomas are spread in the body through lymphatic fluid, most frequently to nearby lymph nodes, while sarcomas are spread in the body through the blood.

In general, carcinomas appear to be caused by a disturbance in the delicate balance of cell growth and death regulation. The immune system normally detects and stops dysfunctional cell growth, but an abnormality in this system can cause cell growth regulators to malfunction, leading to an eventual development of cancerous cells. Other potential causes of carcinoma include genetics, certain viruses, radiation, toxins, and environmental and social factors such as tobacco, pollution, sunlight, and diet. It is important to understand, however, that the causes of most cancers are still not completely known. Therefore, the best preventive measure against cancer is the avoidance and cessation of products and actions that are definitely known to be cancer-causing. Tobacco has been clearly linked to lung cancer, and excessive sunlight exposure has been linked to skin cancer. A healthy diet, exercise, and regular medical examinations are some of the preventive steps recommended by the American Cancer Society to lessen the risks of developing most cancers.

Symptoms of carcinoma depend on the type and location of the tumor, or neoplasm. For example, skin cancer may appear as a mole that changes in color and texture in a short period of time or an open sore that does not heal properly, while lung cancer may manifest itself as a serious and painful cough accompanied by hoarseness and chest pain. Though some cancers may not have a specific symptomology, certain symptoms are common to most, including headaches, chills, fe-

> **Information on Carcinoma**
>
> **Causes:** Tumor in epithelial cells of skin or internal organs; related to genetics, certain viruses, radiation, toxins, environmental and social factors (tobacco, pollution, sunlight, diet)
>
> **Symptoms:** Dependent on type and location of tumor (*e.g.*, mole or open sore for skin cancer; painful cough, hoarseness, and chest pain for lung cancer); in general, headaches, chills, fever, fatigue, unusual bleeding, unintentional weight loss, vomiting
>
> **Duration:** Chronic, sometimes recurrent
>
> **Treatments:** Surgery, chemotherapy, radiation

ver, fatigue, unusual bleeding, unintentional weight loss, and vomiting.

Treatment and Therapy

The goal of most cancer treatments is to eliminate the carcinoma. The course of treatment taken depends entirely on the location and type of cancer. Three kinds of cancer treatment are most frequently used: surgery, chemotherapy, and radiation. In cases where the carcinoma is confined to a specific organ or lymphatic nodule, surgery may be the prescribed course of treatment. When the carcinoma has spread throughout the body, radiation and chemotherapy may be the best viable options. Some cancers require a combination of all three modes of treatment.

Prognosis depends entirely on the carcinoma and the stage of the cancer when first diagnosed. Some carcinomas are successfully treated with little chance of recurrence, while others prove to be nonresponsive and eventually lead to death.

—*Nicholas Lanzieri*

See also Bladder cancer; Brain tumors; Breast cancer; Cancer; Cervical, ovarian, and uterine cancers; Chemotherapy; Colon cancer; Epstein-Barr virus; Gallbladder cancer; Hodgkin's disease; Kidney cancer; Leukemia; Liver cancer; Lung cancer; Lymphadenopathy and lymphoma; Malignancy and metastasis; Mouth and throat cancer; National Cancer Institute (NCI); Oncology; Prostate cancer; Radiation therapy; Sarcoma; Screening; Skin cancer; Stomach, intestinal, and pancreatic cancers; Testicular cancer; Tumor removal; Tumors.

For Further Information:

Cooper, Geoffrey M. *Elements of Human Cancer*. Boston: Jones and Bartlett, 1992.

Dollinger, Malin, et al. *Everyone's Guide to Cancer Therapy*. 4th ed. Kansas City, Mo.: Andrew McMeel, 2002.

Holleb, Arthur I., ed. *The American Cancer Society Cancer Book: Prevention, Detection, Diagnosis, Treatment, Rehabilitation, Cure*. Garden City, N.Y.: Doubleday, 1986.

Cardiac arrest

Disease/disorder

Anatomy or system affected: Circulatory system, heart

Specialties and related fields: Cardiology, emergency medicine

Definition: A complete cessation of the mechanical and/or electrical activity of the heart.

Causes and Symptoms

Many conditions, such as drug overdoses, drowning, poisoning, and electrocution, can result in cardiac arrest, but the major cause is insufficient oxygen supply to the heart as a result of a heart attack. When a major coronary artery becomes blocked, blood cannot flow to the heart muscle cells to deliver oxygen. Without sufficient oxygen, the heart is unable to pump blood to the rest of the body. Within seconds, the blood flow to the brain is inadequate and the individual loses consciousness and stops breathing. If blood flow is not resumed within several minutes, permanent brain damage will occur, frequently followed by death.

The major symptoms of cardiac arrest are lack of a pulse and lack of normal breathing. Medical personnel can also use an electrocardiogram (ECG or EKG) to identify specific problems with the heart, including too rapid of a heart rate to pump blood, quivering of the heart muscle, the complete absence of electrical activity, or the absence of contractions with normal electrical activity. Any of these cases is a medical emergency and treatment is required.

Treatment and Therapy

Cardiopulmonary resuscitation (CPR) is the initial treatment for cardiac arrest. The sooner the blood flow to the brain is restored, the better is the prognosis. Breathing into the victim's mouth and externally compressing the chest over the heart can circulate oxygenated blood throughout the body. However, emergency

Information on Cardiac Arrest

Causes: Usually a heart attack; also, drug overdose, drowning, poisoning, electrocution
Symptoms: Lack of pulse, loss of consciousness, and cessation of breathing; if blood flow is not resumed quickly, permanent brain damage and sometimes death
Duration: Acute
Treatments: Cardiopulmonary resuscitation (CPR), defibrillation, medications (atropine, epinephrine, lidocaine), sometimes surgery

medical treatment is generally required to get the heart beating on its own. Cardioversion, the use of an external defibrillator to shock the heart, is administered to restore the heart's normal cardiac rhythm. Additionally, medical personnel will administer specific medications such as atropine, epinephrine, and lidocaine. In some extreme cases, emergency surgery is required.

Perspective and Prospects

One of the best strategies to save the lives of those who suffer cardiac arrest is to decrease the time that it takes to restore blood flow and get the heart beating on its own again.

CPR was first promoted to the general public as a tool to save lives in the 1970's. By teaching many individuals how to respond to this emergency situation, the likelihood of receiving CPR quickly increases. Unfortunately CPR cannot save everyone. In recent years, automated external defibrillators (AEDs) have been placed in public areas and worksites to improve survival. AEDs can be administered by nonmedical personnel who have been trained how to use them, thus greatly decreasing the time that it takes to restart a normal cardiac rhythm.

—*Bradley R. A. Wilson, Ph.D.*

See also Brain damage; Cardiac rehabilitation; Cardiology; Cardiology, pediatric; Cardiopulmonary resuscitation (CPR); Circulation; Drowning; Electrical shock; Electrocardiography (ECG or EKG); Emergency medicine; Emergency medicine, pediatric; Heart; Heart attack; Pacemaker implantation; Palpitations; Poisoning; Resuscitation; Shock; Vascular medicine; Vascular system.

For Further Information:

American Medical Association. *American Medical Association Family Medical Guide*. 4th rev. ed. Hoboken, N.J.: John Wiley & Sons, 2004.
Klag, Michael J., et al., eds. *Johns Hopkins Family Health Book*. New York: HarperCollins, 1999.
Komaroff, Anthony L., ed. *Harvard Medical School Family Health Guide*. New York: Free Press, 2005.

Cardiac rehabilitation

Treatment

Anatomy or system affected: Chest, circulatory system, heart
Specialties and related fields: Cardiology, exercise physiology, nursing, nutrition, occupational health, physical therapy, psychology
Definition: The activities that ensure the physical, mental, and social conditions necessary for returning cardiac patients to good health.

Key terms:

aerobic exercise: exercise that requires oxygen for energy production and that can be sustained for prolonged periods of time; involves large muscle groups, increases the heart rate and breathing rate, and is rhythmic and continuous
atherosclerosis: a buildup of fatty deposits or plaques which effectively reduces the inner diameter of the arteries, thus obstructing the normal flow of blood
cardiovascular disease: any of a group of diseases that affect the heart, including coronary artery disease, hypertension, congestive heart failure, congenital heart defects, and valvular heart disease
coronary artery bypass graft (CABG): a surgical procedure in which a blocked coronary artery is bypassed using a vein or artery; this intervention provides a blood supply to areas beyond the distal attachment of the graft
coronary artery disease (CAD): a disease which results in a narrowing of the coronary arteries and a concomitant reduction of oxygen supply to the heart muscle
electrocardiogram (EKG or ECG): a mechanical representation of the electrical activity generated by the heart and recorded on paper or displayed on a cathode-ray tube
invasive testing: techniques involving the puncture or incision of the skin or the insertion of an instrument or foreign material into the body
MET: a measure of human energy expenditure; 1 MET is equal to the amount of energy expended at rest (ap-

proximately 3.5 milliliters of oxygen per kilogram of body weight per minute)

myocardial infarction: irreversible damage to heart muscle tissue caused by insufficient oxygen supply to that tissue

percutaneous transluminal coronary angioplasty (PTCA): a procedure undertaken to increase the internal diameter of a coronary artery by inflating a small balloonlike device at the site or sites where the artery has narrowed because of plaque buildup

risk factors: those habits or conditions that increase the likelihood of developing a disease or disorder

target heart rate range: a heart rate range that is to be maintained during exercise training

INDICATIONS AND PROCEDURES

Cardiovascular disease (CVD), or heart disease, is the leading cause of death and disability in most of the industrialized nations of the world. For those persons who survive a cardiac event, discharge from a hospital or medical setting without further assistance may lead to financial, physical, and mental incapacity.

Just as interventional procedures and medical care are important for the initial treatment of acute cardiac events, such as a myocardial infarction (heart attack) or angina (chest pain), cardiac rehabilitation influences long-term morbidity and mortality. Such preventive cardiology assists persons with CVD in three main areas: education, behavior modification, and patient and family support. The two primary goals of the rehabilitation program are to help increase the patient's functional capacity (the ability to perform activities of daily living) and to counteract or arrest the patient's disease process using a multidisciplined educational approach.

In order to provide direction in prevention and rehabilitation, research studies have clearly defined several modifiable risk factors for heart disease, which are presented to patients. Among the most significant are smoking, high serum cholesterol, hypertension, and physical inactivity. Assistance with education about and modification of these risk factors, through risk factor counseling and participation in physical activity, is provided in modern cardiac rehabilitation programs.

Methods for providing education on risk factor modification can vary greatly from program to program, but include such means as didactic lecturing, slide presentations, printed material for patients to read, demonstrations (such as cooking and stress reduction techniques), providing loaner books, and one-on-one counseling.

The exercise portion of the cardiac rehabilitation is most often the time-consuming element of the program. It involves controlling and monitoring four major variables: mode (type of activity, such as bicycling, walking, or stair-stepping), duration (length of time the patient exercises), frequency (number of times per week that exercise is performed), and intensity (exertion level of the patient, usually assessed by the heart rate response).

To become involved in the cardiac rehabilitation program, a patient is initially screened by a physician, nurse, or other clinical specialist and directed to the appropriate level (or phase) of intervention.

There are three to four clinical phases involved with cardiac rehabilitation, as various groups categorize them differently. The Exercise and Cardiac Rehabilitation Committee of the American Heart Association outlines three phases; the American Association of Cardiovascular and Pulmonary Rehabilitation (AACVPR) outlines four phases.

Phase 1 occurs while the patient is still in the hospital. It begins when the patient's condition is stabilized, sometimes as soon as forty-eight hours after the coronary event or procedure. This phase can begin in the coronary care unit (CCU) or the intensive care unit (ICU). Phase 1 incorporates several disciplines, including physical therapy, nursing, psychiatry, dietetics, occupational therapy, and exercise science. It is designed to prevent the deleterious physiological effects of bed rest.

The physical components of this phase include maintaining a range of motion and gradually returning to activities of daily living. Patients gradually advance through stages until they are able to walk up to 200 or 400 feet. Before discharge, patients are encouraged to walk up and down one flight of stairs. Stair climbing is done while accompanied by a physical therapist or other clinician who monitors heart rate and blood pressure. The level of exertion during the early portion of this phase is normally 1 to 2 METs. Thus, in phase 1, the mode of exercise focuses on motion (sitting, standing, and finally walking), the frequency is seven days per week, the duration of exercise is usually five to ten minutes at a time, and the intensity of activity should not cause the heart rate to exceed twenty beats above the resting rate while standing.

For coronary artery bypass graft (CABG) patients who have not experienced a myocardial infarction, progress during this phase is usually faster than for heart attack patients. Percutaneous transluminal coronary angioplasty (PTCA) patients may receive only a few days of rehabilitation, as they are usually discharged from the hospital sooner than heart attack or CABG patients.

The mental components of phase 1 include risk factor modification education and an introduction to rehabilitation concepts. Risk factor education at this point provides a good foundation for the basic concepts that will be explained during the education program in phase 2. For those patients who are appropriate candidates for a phase 2 program, information on that phase is then provided.

Phase 2 customarily begins within three weeks of discharge from the hospital and lasts for four to twelve weeks. During phase 2, patients are exposed to a level of exertion commensurate with several criteria: the patient's clinical status (stable or unstable, depending on whether the patient is experiencing problems related to the disease); the patient's functional capacity, or fitness level; orthopedic limitations, such as muscle or joint problems; the goals for functional capacity (what tasks the patient wants to be able to perform); and any other special circumstances or situations.

In a given phase 2 program, there are a variety of patients, all with varying levels of physical fitness. Through variations in the mode, duration, frequency, or intensity of exercise, these differing levels of fitness can be accommodated. A variety of exercise modes are presented in the phase 2 program, including walking, stationary cycling, stationary rowing, simulated stair-climbing, water aerobics, swimming, and upper body ergometry. The exercise frequency for this phase is three to six days per week, the duration consists of twenty to forty-five minutes of continuous aerobic activity, and the intensity should produce a heart rate that is 60 to 85 percent of the symptom-limited maximal heart rate. Exercises are monitored by an exercise specialist (one of a number of clinician titles described by the American College of Sports Medicine) and a cardiovascular fitness nurse. Exercise intensity is determined in most cases by heart rate and may be monitored by electrocardiogram (EKG or ECG) telemetry on a number of patients simultaneously.

One of the interesting psychological components to phase 2 cardiac rehabilitation is that most programs are arranged so that new participants are coming into the

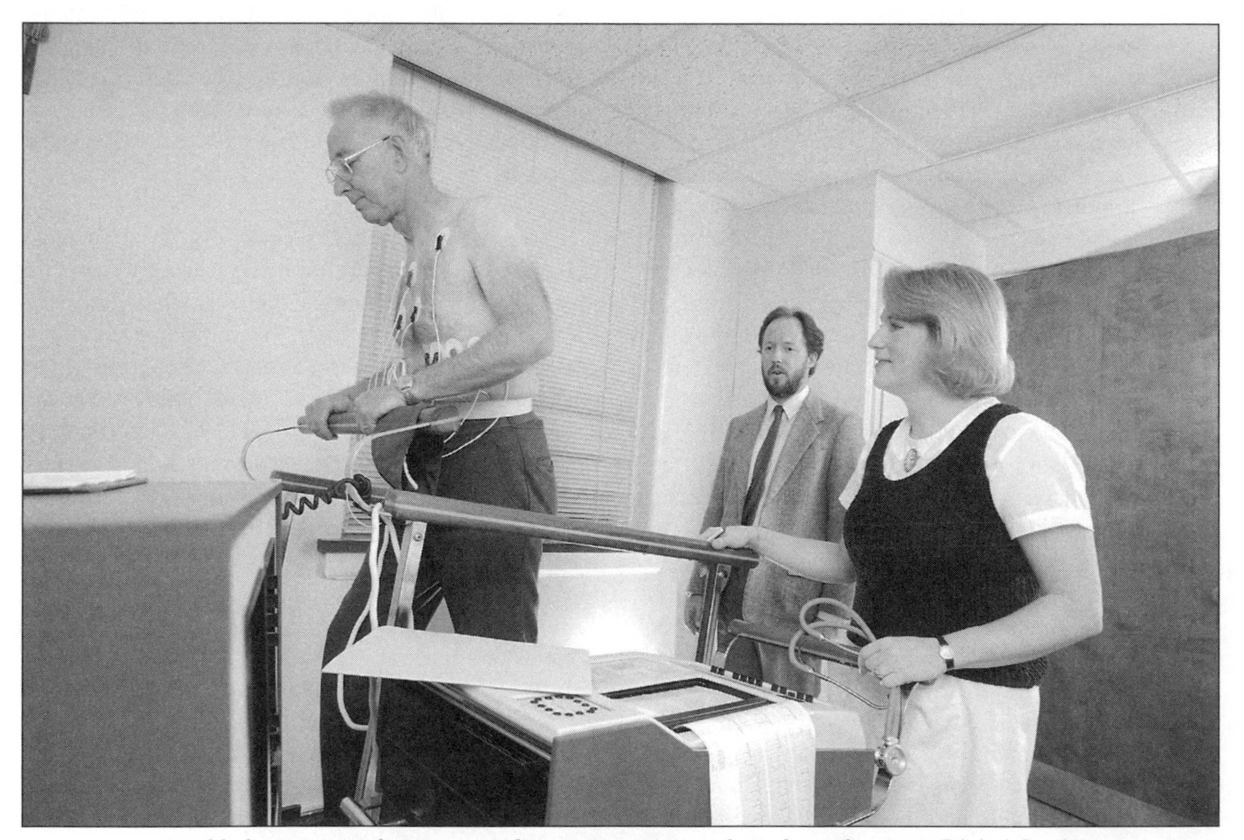

An elderly patient undergoes a cardiac stress test to evaluate heart function. (Digital Stock)

program as participants who have been in the program for several sessions are leaving. Newer participants are able to identify with those already in the program as a result of similarities in cardiac experiences. It has been suggested that this identification decreases the anxiety level of a patient who is just becoming involved in the program.

Patients move into phase 3 of cardiac rehabilitation, a community-based outpatient program, when cardiovascular and physiological responses to exercise have been stabilized and the patient has achieved the goals initially set. Phase 3 is generally considered to be an extended, supervised program which usually lasts from four to six months but which can continue indefinitely.

Participants in phase 3 programs become more involved in and in charge of their own exercises. Typically, these programs do not include EKG monitoring. Individuals are given more responsibility with respect to maintaining their own heart rates in their training heart rate range. Usually, an exercise specialist, nurse, or physician is available to oversee the exercises. The mode, frequency, duration, and intensity of exercise in this phase is similar to that of phase 2.

Phase 4 is a maintenance program. Although many rehabilitation settings label this a phase 3 program, the phase 4 program is considered to be the longest-term, ongoing phase and is of indefinite length. Many phase 2 cardiac rehabilitation program graduates remain in phase 3 or phase 4 programs for years. The mode, frequency, duration, and intensity of the exercise program for phase 4 is also similar to that of phase 2.

USES AND COMPLICATIONS

Traditionally, cardiac rehabilitation has been recommended for individuals convalescing from myocardial infarctions or heart surgery (CABG, PTCA, or valve replacement). More recently, the eligibility for cardiac rehabilitation has been extended to include heart transplant recipients and others with cardiac-related illnesses.

Improvement of work capacity is one of the goals of cardiac rehabilitation. The mechanisms involved in increasing work capacity (aerobic capacity and maximal oxygen consumption) normally include increases in both central (cardiac output, stroke volume, and heart rate) and peripheral (muscle changes, atrioventricular oxygen difference) adaptations. Nevertheless, this does not preclude patients with reduced left ventricular (LV) function from participation in a medically supervised exercise program. For the reduced LV function patient, improvement in exercise tolerance can occur; this improvement may be attributable mainly to peripheral adaptations.

For the low-risk patient, cardiac rehabilitation may seem unnecessary since unsupervised exercise programs have been demonstrated to be safe and effective and to improve exercise capacity. For healthy lifestyle modification to take place, however, the educational component of cardiac rehabilitation may provide the patient with invaluable knowledge. In order to reduce the chance of recurrence or severity of a myocardial infarction in an effective manner, a healthy lifestyle is encouraged. Additional potential benefits of participation include improved self-esteem, positive mental attitude, and decreased anxiety and depression.

Low-risk patients, who account for about one-third to one-half of heart attack patients and about three-quarters of CABG patients, have a first-year mortality of less than 2 percent. Moderate-risk patients have a first-year mortality rate of between 10 percent and 25 percent. High-risk patients' mortality rates are greater than 25 percent. While cardiac rehabilitation is not effective in all circumstances, proper assessment of an individual's clinical situation and competent administration of the program can optimize the outcome for participants.

Increasing numbers of cardiac rehabilitation programs are accepting unconventional patient populations. These patients now include heart transplant recipients, congestive heart failure patients, individuals suffering from ischemic heart disease, and those with arrhythmias and/or pacemakers.

Although most of the prescribed exercise regimens for these patients parallel those for the conventional cardiac patient, there are subtle differences. In the heart transplant population, for example, heart rate response differs from nontransplant patients. The adjustment of heart rate to various workloads lags in acute heart transplant recipients; that is, the heart rate does not increase as rapidly as it does for normal people. To accommodate this difference, researchers have suggested that, in place of heart rate response, clinicians use a "rating of perceived exertion" scale to monitor the patients' responses to exercise.

Even patients who have orthopedic limitations, such as arthritis or chronic injuries, may be accommodated in the exercise portion of the cardiac rehabilitation program. Exercises can be adjusted to allow participants to derive cardiovascular benefits without causing them unnecessary discomfort.

Although cardiac rehabilitation is safe in general, several factors may emerge during graded exercise testing (a screening for entry into a cardiac rehabilitation program) that can identify those patients who may be at increased risk. These factors include a significant depression or elevation of the S-T wave segment from a resting EKG, angina, extensive left ventricular dysfunction and severe myocardial infarction, ventricular dysrhythmias, inappropriate blood pressure response to exercise, achieving a peak heart rate of less than 120 beats per minute (if not taking a negative chronotropic medication, which slows down the heart rate), and a functional exercise capacity of less than 4 to 5 METs. Inclusion in one of these categories does not preclude participation in a cardiac rehabilitation program, but it may warrant specific exercise guidelines and close monitoring.

Among the criteria for exclusion from a cardiac rehabilitation program are unstable angina, acute systemic illness, uncontrolled arrhythmias, tachycardia, diabetes, symptomatic congestive heart failure, a resting systolic blood pressure over 200 millimeters of mercury (mm Hg) or a resting diastolic blood pressure over 110 mm Hg, third-degree heart block without a pacemaker, and moderate to severe aortic stenosis.

For those who meet the criteria for inclusion in a cardiac rehabilitation program, risk stratification (low, moderate, or high) may be employed. This allows an appropriate amount of supervision to be in place based on each patient's goals and condition. Clinical observations and tests allow each patient to be assessed individually. Within each phase, levels of risk may be established. Various proposals have been made for risk stratification prior to entry into a cardiac rehabilitation program, including stratification based on several factors: the degree of left ventricular dysfunction, presence or absence of myocardial ischemia, extent of myocardial injury, and presence of ventricular arrhythmias.

Some of the most widely examined noninvasive assessment tools include the extent of QRS wave abnormalities on a resting EKG and the results of exercise stress testing, twenty-four-hour ambulatory EKG monitoring, radionuclide ventriculography, and echocardiography. A combination of these test results may be used to determine the course of action provided to an individual.

As with any effective therapy, exercise as a form of cardiac rehabilitation is neither without hazard nor always beneficial. If appropriate clinical guidelines are utilized, however, the benefit-risk ratio can be very favorable. In a 1986 study of 51,303 patients from 142 outpatient cardiac rehabilitation programs in the United States (representing 2,351,916 patient-hours of exercise), the incidence rate for fatal and nonfatal cardiac events was 1 in 111,996. This low incidence of cardiac-related events during participation in programs is probably attributable to improved risk stratification, the use of appropriate medical and surgical therapies, and improved exercise guidelines. On the rare occasions when cardiac events occur, reports have indicated that up to 90 percent of all patients with exercise-related cardiac arrest are successfully resuscitated when the patient experiences the event in a properly equipped and supervised program.

Perspective and Prospects

Until the 1940's, patients recovering from acute myocardial infarctions met with restriction of physical activity, bed rest, and psychological apprehension about exertion. Over the next two decades, the deleterious physiological effects of prolonged bed rest began to be described. During this time, a few investigators were beginning to encourage early treatment of the patient who has experienced an acute heart attack, including armchair work and walking within four weeks of the acute event.

In the 1950's, British physician Jeremy Morris and his colleagues conducted research that initiated interest in the relationship between coronary artery disease (CAD) and a sedentary lifestyle. In this study, he found that London bus drivers had twice the risk of developing CAD than their more physically active bus conductor counterparts. In addition, among those drivers and conductors who had experienced a heart attack, the drivers were twice as likely as the conductors to die either during or within two months of their heart attack.

During the 1960's, the beginnings of what are now considered cardiac rehabilitation programs incorporated exercise training on a somewhat limited basis. Restricted exercise regimens began a few weeks after cardiac events and increased in intensity on a very gradual basis. Generally, the patient population considered appropriate for such programs consisted of those individuals who had experienced uncomplicated myocardial infarctions. Some risk factor modification education was initiated, but not on a large scale primarily because data supporting improved patient outcomes were not proven.

Soon afterward, the "On Ward" program, designed to begin on the tenth day following a heart attack, was introduced based on work by William P. Blocker, Jr., and colleagues. In 1971, J. M. Kaufman suggested that rehabilitation of uncomplicated myocardial infarction patients could begin as early as two days after the heart attack. At this time, many hospitals had some form of cardiac rehabilitation program; most of them, however, consisted almost exclusively of exercise training. This approach addressed the physiological changes necessary for improving the functional capacity of the patients but did not address long-term behavior modification and education.

In 1986, Ralph S. Paffenbarger, Jr., published a prominent exercise and heart disease study. In his study using 16,936 Harvard University alumni from thirty-five to seventy-four years of age, he validated the concept that physical inactivity is independently related to CAD. In the next seven years, various research on a total of more than 32,000 people was done confirming that hypothesis.

Also in 1986, another group of physicians and researchers described some of the deleterious effects of bed rest, including decreased physical work capacity, decreased cardiac output, skeletal muscle wasting, orthostatic hypotension (abnormally low blood pressure upon standing), decreased blood volume, loss of muscular strength, and reduced pulmonary function. Exercise was shown to be beneficial in reducing some of these effects.

Based on the information outlined above, a multifactorial approach to cardiac rehabilitation has been undertaken in order to provide patients with the information and skills necessary to alter their lifestyles. This approach includes education, in the form of lectures, handouts, videotapes, and informal discussions; behavior modification, by way of regularly scheduled, supervised aerobic exercise programs and nutritional counseling; and support, by means of cardiac rehabilitation classroom meetings and support groups. With this increased scope of care for the cardiac patient, some institutions are providing cardiac patients with access to a broader base of clinicians. This group may include physicians, nurses, exercise specialists or physiologists, dietitians, physical therapists, social workers, psychologists, and occupational therapists. Even with all these components in place, however, exercise training remains the focal point of most contemporary cardiac rehabilitation programs.

Recent studies using meta-analysis have substantiated the hypothesis that exercise-based cardiac rehabilitation programs that include risk factor/behavior modification significantly decrease mortality. Decreasing the number and/or magnitude of the known risk factors for heart disease has been shown to effect a significant improvement in the cardiovascular risk profile for these patients. Research has demonstrated the fact that, although various degrees of CAD may remain after participation in a cardiac rehabilitation program, patients can achieve a sense of well-being. For some patients, this benefit alone may improve health and reduce the financial burden often associated with postinfarction convalescence.

—*Frank J. Fedel*

See also Angina; Arrhythmias; Bypass surgery; Cardiac arrest; Cardiology; Cardiology, pediatric; Cardiopulmonary resuscitation (CPR); Circulation; Congenital heart disease; Echocardiography; Electrocardiography (ECG or EKG); Exercise physiology; Heart; Heart attack; Heart disease; Heart transplantation; Heart valve replacement; Ischemia; Pacemaker implantation; Physical rehabilitation; Preventive medicine; Stress reduction.

For Further Information:

American Association of Cardiovascular and Pulmonary Rehabilitation. *Guidelines for Cardiac Rehabilitation and Secondary Prevention Programs*. 4th ed. Champaign, Ill.: Human Kinetics, 2004. This short text is laid out well, with many citations of research studies and books on cardiac rehabilitation. A broad-based book that provides information for existing rehabilitation programs and proposes new programs.

Crawford, Michael, ed. *Current Diagnosis and Treatment in Cardiology*. 2d ed. New York: Lange Medical Books/McGraw-Hill, 2003. Discusses advances in cardiac diagnostics, treatments, and prognostic indicators and includes extensive information on prevention techniques.

Eagle, Kim A., and Ragavendra R. Baliga, eds. *Practical Cardiology: Evaluation and Treatment of Common Cardiovascular Disorders*. Philadelphia: Lippincott Williams & Wilkins, 2003. Details advances in cardiac medicine.

Gersh, Bernard J., ed. *The Mayo Clinic Heart Book*. 2d ed. New York: William Morrow, 2000. One of the most respected text for laypeople on heart disease. Covers all aspects of anatomy, physiology, diagnosis, treatment, and prevention.

Gordon, Neil F., and Larry W. Gibbons. *The Cooper Clinic Cardiac Rehabilitation Program*. New York:

Simon & Schuster, 1990. Focused on the philosophy of the Cooper Clinic's founder, Kenneth H. Cooper, this primer provides a wide array of anecdotes for the layperson, as well as a good foundation for the clinician.

Pryor, Jennifer A., and S. Ammani Prasad, eds. *Physiotherapy for Respiratory and Cardiac Problems*. 3d ed. Edinburgh, Scotland: Churchill Livingstone, 2002. This book provides therapists with a great deal of useful information regarding the treatment of individuals with respiratory or cardiac conditions. The appendix offers normal values for vital signs, arterial and venous blood gases, blood chemistry, and pressures in the circulatory and respiratory systems.

CARDIOLOGY

SPECIALTY

ANATOMY OR SYSTEM AFFECTED: Chest, circulatory system, heart

SPECIALTIES AND RELATED FIELDS: Emergency medicine, preventive medicine, vascular medicine

DEFINITION: The branch of medicine concerned with the diagnosis and treatment of diseases of the heart and the coronary arteries, including arteriosclerosis, hypertension, and congenital defects.

KEY TERMS:

acute: referring to the onset of a disease process

chronic: referring to a lingering disease process

coronary arteries: the two arteries that surround the heart and supply the heart muscle with oxygen and nutrients

heart attack: the common term for a myocardial infarction

heart failure: a condition in which the heart pumps inefficiently, allowing fluid to back up into the lungs or body tissue

sudden cardiac death: a situation in which the heart stops beating or beats irregularly, stopping blood flow

SCIENCE AND PROFESSION

Cardiology is the study of the heart and its various diseases: inflammation of the heart muscle, diseases of the heart valves, atherosclerosis and arteriosclerosis (*athero* meaning "deposits of soft material," *arterio* meaning "pertaining to the arteries," and *sclerosis* meaning "hardening"), and congenital defects. This field also concerns related diseases, such as hypertension (high blood pressure) and certain renal, endocrine, and lung disorders.

The heart contains four chambers, the right and left atria on top and the right and left ventricles below. The walls of the heart are three layers of tissue: the outer layer, the epicardium; the middle layer, the myocardium; and an inner layer, the endocardium, which includes the heart valves. The heart is contained in a protective sac, called the pericardium.

The pumping of the heart is a coordinated contraction. The right atrium receives blood from the veins and contracts, pumping blood through the tricuspid valve into the right ventricle. The right ventricle then contracts, pumping blood through the pulmonary valve into the lungs, where it gives up carbon dioxide and receives oxygen. Blood then enters the left atrium, which contracts and sends blood through the mitral valve to the left ventricle. It pumps the blood through the aortic valve into the arterial system, which consists of the aorta and progressively narrower arteries and arterioles. The blood arrives finally in the capillaries, where it delivers nourishment and oxygen to tissues throughout the body and picks up waste products and carbon dioxide. The blood then enters the venous system, first into the venules (tiny veins that lead to larger veins) and finally to one of the two branches of the vena cava: the superior vena cava from the upper part of the body, and the inferior vena cava from the lower. They connect outside the heart and bring blood back into the right atrium.

The heartbeat, the rhythmic contraction of the heart muscle, is controlled by the conduction system. Electrochemical impulses cause muscle fibers to contract, pumping blood through the chambers, and relax, letting the chambers fill again. The contractions are initiated by specialized "pacemaker" tissues in the sinoatrial (S-A) or sinus node, in the junction of the superior vena cava and the right atrium. The pacemaker signal travels to the atrioventricular (A-V) node, near the tricuspid valve. The impulse crosses the A-V node and travels to the bundle of His, specialized fibers that carry it to the ventricles.

Virtually every part of the heart is subject to disease: each layer of the heart muscle, each valve, each chamber, and the coronary arteries. The coronary arteries are quite small and are subject to the accumulation of plaque on their inner walls, a condition known as atherosclerosis. This plaque can be cholesterol, scar tissue, clotted blood, or calcium. As the plaque accumulates, the artery narrows, reducing the flow of blood into the heart muscle. The reduction in blood flow reduces the heart's supply of oxygen, causing myocardial ischemia (lack of blood). There is usually a signal of pain called angina pectoris (*angina* meaning "choking pain" and *pectoris* meaning "of the chest"). Often, the patient feels tightening in the chest with sharp pain behind the sternum. The pain can radiate into either arm or the jaw. It is usually caused by overexertion, exposure to cold, stress, or overeating.

As a rule, an attack of angina pectoris lasts only a few minutes and is relieved by rest, but it can signal the beginning of a heart attack. In addition, coronary arteries contain muscle fibers that can go into spasm and tighten, reducing blood flow into the heart. This condition, too, can cause anginal pain, heart attack, and death. Some patients who have myocardial ischemia do not have anginal pain. This is known as silent ischemia, and it is usually discovered only with an electrocardiogram (ECG) or exercise stress test.

There are four major classes of angina pectoris: stable angina, in which pain begins when the heart's need for oxygen exceeds the amount that it receives; unstable angina, which is significantly more serious than stable angina; variant angina, which is characterized by chest pain at rest and may be caused by spasm of the coronary arteries; and postinfarction angina, unstable angina that appears after acute myocardial infarction.

When atherosclerotic plaque builds up in the coronary arteries, the inner lining of the vessel becomes rough. As a result, a blood clot (thrombus) can form on the plaque, making the vessel even narrower or clogging it completely (coronary thrombosis). When this occurs, blood flow to parts of the heart is stopped, and heart cells die from lack of oxygen. This condition is medically known as myocardial infarction (from *infarct*, meaning "an area of dead cells") and commonly known as a heart attack.

The prognosis for patients who survive a heart attack is variable. In two-thirds of patients, spontaneous thrombolysis (the dissolution of the blood clot) starts to occur within twenty-four hours. About half of heart attack patients, however, will go on to develop postinfarction angina, which usually indicates severe, multivessel coronary artery disease.

Diseases of the conduction system can result in arrhythmias, or disturbances in the regularity of the heartbeat. Arrhythmias can be relatively benign or can severely restrict the patient's physical activity. They can also cause sudden cardiac death. The most common arrhythmias are bradycardia, slowing of the heartbeat, and tachycardia, quickening of the heartbeat.

Normally, the chambers beat in synchronization with each other. In some arrhythmias, the chambers of the heart beat out of synchronization. These arrhythmias include atrial fibrillation, paroxysmal atrial tachycardia, ventricular tachycardia, and ventricular fibrillation. In atrial fibrillation, the atria beat very rapidly (three hundred beats per minute), out of synchronization with the ventricles. When the condition is prolonged, blood clots may form in the atria and may cause a stroke, or the stoppage of blood flow in a blood vessel. With paroxysmal atrial tachycardia, a disturbance in the conduction of the A-V node causes the heart to beat up to two hundred fifty times a minute. The condition is usually not serious, but if it persists, fainting or heart failure could develop. Ventricular tachycardia exists when ectopic, or irregular, beats develop in the ventricular muscle; if they go on, blood pressure falls. In ventricular fibrillation, which is the leading cause of sudden cardiac death, ventricular contractions are weak, ineffective, and uncoordinated. Blood flow stops, and the patient faints. If the condition is not corrected, the patient can die in minutes.

Heart block can be another consequence of conduction disease. If, for various reasons, all the impulses from the sinus node do not pass through the A-V node and the bundle of His, the result is one of three degrees of heart block. First-degree heart block, which is not apparent to the patient, appears on the ECG as a delay in the impulse from the atria to the ventricles. Second-degree heart block occurs when some of the impulses from the atria fail to reach the ventricles. Often, the result is an irregular pulse. This condition can be attributable to a certain heart drug and may disappear when the drug is discontinued. In third-degree heart block, impulses from the pacemaker tissues fail to reach the ventricles. A lower pacemaker assumes the function of stimulating contractions of the ventricles in an "escape rhythm." When this occurs in third-degree heart block, the heart rate often slows down so precipitously that blood flow to the brain and other organs is severely restricted. Dizziness and loss of consciousness may follow. Heart failure can also be the result of a congenital defect, inflammation, myocardial infarction, or other causes.

Disorders in the valves of the heart are most often caused by congenital defects or the effects of rheumatic fever. Rheumatic fever is caused by streptococcal bacteria and usually begins with a throat infection. If this "strep throat" is not treated, rheumatic fever may develop. Acute rheumatic fever is associated with mitral or aortic valve insufficiency (leakage). Chronic rheumatic heart disease can include mitral or aortic stenosis (narrowing). Valves are scarred with fibrous tissue and/or calcific (calcium-containing) deposits that cause the valve openings to become narrower.

Mitral stenosis usually develops slowly. Ten to twenty years after rheumatic fever, the valve narrows so much that blood flow from the atrium into the ventricle is impeded. As blood accumulates in the left atrium, pressure within the atrium increases, and the chamber becomes enlarged. Blood is forced back into the lungs, resulting in pulmonary edema (fluid in the lungs). Blood vessels in the lungs become engorged; the increased pressure forces fluid into the air sacs. Symptoms of mitral stenosis include shortness of breath, fatigue, feelings of suffocation, wheezing, agitation, and anxiety. In severe cases, fluid may also accumulate in the lower extremities. Mitral stenosis can also cause atrial fibrillation, which in turn can generate potentially lethal blood clots.

Mitral "regurgitation," another mitral valve disorder, can also be caused by rheumatic fever. The valve fails to close completely during left ventricle contraction. Blood leaks back into the left atrium, and blood flow into the aorta is reduced. The heart has to work harder to pump blood into the body. Mitral regurgitation may lead to enlargement of the left atrium and left ventricle. Pulmonary edema, shortness of breath, fatigue, and palpitations are late symptoms of severe disease.

Still another disorder is mitral valve prolapse, or mitral insufficiency. The mitral valve consists of two leaflets of tissue that fall apart to open and come together to close. Prolapse occurs when either or both of these leaflets bulge into the left atrium. Some patients experience palpitations and chest pain. In rare cases, significant valve leakage occurs, requiring surgery.

The aortic valve consists of three leaflets or "cusps" that can become fused, calcified, or otherwise compromised because of rheumatic fever or a congenital heart defect. The opening narrows, and blood flow into the aorta is reduced. Pressure increases inside the left ventricle, causing it to pump harder. The wall of the left ventricle thickens, a condition called ventricular hypertrophy. Aortic stenosis may not be evident until it is quite advanced. Symptoms include heart murmur, weakness, fatigue, anginal pain, breathlessness, and fainting.

Tricuspid stenosis and regurgitation occur but are rare, as is pulmonary regurgitation. Pulmonary or pulmonic valve stenosis, however, is a common congenital heart defect. There is a characteristic heart murmur produced by turbulence of blood through the narrow pulmonary valve. Pressure increases in the right ventricle. Fainting and heart failure are possible in severe cases.

In congestive heart failure, the heart pumps inefficiently, failing to deliver blood to the body and allowing blood to back up into the veins. It may occur on the left or the right side, or both. If the left side of the heart is pumping inefficiently, blood flows back into the lungs, causing pulmonary edema. If the right side of the heart is inefficient, blood seeps back into the legs, resulting in edema of the extremities. Blood can also back up into the liver and the kidneys, resulting in engorgement and reduced arterial flow that prevent these organs from getting the nutrition and oxygen they need to function.

Cardiomyopathy refers to diseases of the myocardium. There are many possible causes, including "end-stage" coronary artery disease; infectious agents such as fungi, viruses, and parasites; overconsumption of alcohol; or genetic defects. The three main classes of cardiomyopathy are dilated congestive cardiomyopathy, hypertrophic cardiomyopathy, and restrictive cardiomyopathy. In dilated congestive cardiomyopathy, either all the heart chambers are involved (diffuse), or some but not all chambers are involved (nondiffuse). The cause of this class of cardiomyopathy is usually a viral infection (in which case it is called myocarditis), but drugs, alcohol, and nonviral diseases may be responsible. The heart pumps inefficiently, causing fatigue, breathlessness, and edema in the lower extremities. The heart chambers may enlarge, and blood clots may form. With hypertrophic cardiomyopathy, the myocardium thickens and reduces the cavity of the left ventricle so that blood flow into the aorta is reduced. The condition is usually chronic, with fainting, fatigue, and breathlessness as symptoms. Restrictive cardiomyopathy is rare. With this condition, the heart muscle loses elasticity and cannot expand to fill with blood between contractions. Symptoms include edema, breathlessness, and atrial and ventricular arrhythmias.

The endocardium and the pericardium can become inflamed because of infection or injury, resulting in endocarditis or pericarditis. Bacterial endocarditis usually affects abnormal valves and heart structures that have been damaged by rheumatic fever or congenital defects. Fulminant (sudden and severe) infections can destroy normal heart valves, especially with intravenous drug abuse. The symptoms of bacterial endocarditis are fever, weight loss, malaise, night sweats, fatigue, and heart murmurs. The condition can be fatal if the invading organism is not eradicated. Nonbacterial thrombotic endocarditis or noninfective endocarditis arises from the formation of thrombi on cardiac valves and endocardium caused by trauma, immune complexes, or vascular disease. Pericarditis often occurs concomitantly with, or as a result of, viral respiratory infection. The inflamed pericardium rubs against the epicardium, causing acute pain. Large amounts of fluid may develop and press on the heart in "cardiac tamponade." This condition can impede heart action and blood flow and can be life-threatening. In constrictive pericarditis, the pericardium becomes thicker and contracts. This action prevents the heart chambers from filling, decreasing the amount of blood drawn into the heart and pumped out to the body.

Primary cardiac tumors, those originating in the heart, are rare. While usually benign, they can have fatal complications. Malignant tumors also occur, and metastasis (movement of cancer cells throughout the body) may bring malignancies to the heart.

Congenital heart defects occur in about 0.8 percent of births. Ventricular septal defect, a hole in the wall between the ventricles, is the most common. It is detected by a loud murmur. Atrial septal defect is common but rarely leads to symptoms until the third decade of life.

Diagnostic and Treatment Techniques

The stethoscope, ECGs, and the X ray are basic tools that the cardiologist uses for the diagnosis of heart conditions. By listening to heart sounds through the stethoscope, the physician can learn much about the status of heart function, particularly heart rhythm, congenital defects, and valve dysfunction.

ECG patterns of electrical impulses help the physician discover chamber enlargement and other cardiac abnormalities. In a stress test, the ECG is attached to a patient who is running on a treadmill or riding a bicycle-like apparatus. The test assesses the exercise tolerance of patients with coronary artery disease and other conditions.

The chest X ray provides a picture of the size and configuration of the heart, the aorta, the pulmonary arteries, and related structures. It can detect enlarged chambers and vessels and other disorders. In some cases, radioactive isotopes are injected into the patient, and the patterns that they form in the heart and surrounding arteries are "read" by a scanner to help the physician make a diagnosis. The echocardiogram uses ultrasound to outline heart chambers and detect abnormalities within them and in the myocardium. It is also used to analyze patterns of blood flow.

Newer, more sophisticated instruments the cardiologist uses include fast-computed tomography, called cine-CT because it gives the physician a visualization of heart activity. Magnetic resonance imaging (MRI), MR spectroscopy, and positron emission tomography (PET) scanning help the cardiologist investigate heart function and anatomy.

These techniques and procedures are conducted outside the body. Sometimes it is necessary, however, to go into the body. One such technique is diagnostic catheterization with angiography. A thin flexible tube (catheter) is inserted into a blood vessel in the groin or arm and threaded into a coronary artery or the heart. Pressures and blood oxygen are measured in the heart chambers. A radio-opaque dye is then injected through the catheter. The inside of the artery or the heart becomes visible to the X ray and is recorded on film (a process sometimes called cineangiography). Angiography can also be used with radioactive isotopes. The radiation detected by a scanner can help the physician discover abnormalities in the coronary arteries and the heart.

Diagnosis of angina pectoris is usually based upon the patient's complaint of chest pain. An ECG can help confirm the diagnosis. Yet many patients with coronary artery disease have normal ECGs at rest, so stress testing with the ECG is considered more reliable. Patients may be given pharmacologic stress tests if they are unable to do physical exercise.

Drug therapy for coronary artery disease and angina pectoris is directed at keeping the coronary arteries open and avoiding myocardial ischemia. Primary among the drugs used is nitroglycerin, taken under the tongue or in a transdermal (through-the-skin) patch—or, in emergencies, intravenously. There are many nitrate compounds that fulfill similar functions. Beta-adrenergic blocking agents, or beta-blockers, decrease heart rate and blood pressure, reducing the heart's oxygen requirement and workload, thus reducing the incidence of angina. Some serious arrhythmias are also suppressed. Calcium-channel blockers dilate coronary arteries and maintain coronary blood flow while decreasing blood pressure, reducing heart work, and stabilizing heart rhythm.

If coronary artery disease progresses to the point where there is risk of myocardial infarction, various catheter and surgical procedures may be considered. Coronary angioplasty is used to open a clogged artery mechanically. The cardiologist threads a catheter with a tiny balloon into the clogged artery and inflates the balloon at the site of the blockage. This procedure is repeated until the vessel is open. Another procedure used when coronary arteries are blocked is coronary artery bypass surgery. The surgeon takes sections of vein or artery from another part of the body and implants them between the aorta and the heart, creating new coronary arteries and bypassing those that are clogged.

When clogged coronary arteries cause a myocardial infarction, the patient should be treated in a special medical facility, preferably in a coronary care unit (CCU). Heart attacks rarely begin in the hospital, however, so the medical team must keep the patient alive on the way to the CCU. Primary ventricular fibrillation is the greatest danger, and it must be corrected immediately by medication or electrical defibrillation. Sometimes heart block and profound bradycardia occur, which could cause a drop in blood pressure that could in turn cause cardiac arrest.

The aims of emergency myocardial infarction treatment are to ease discomfort, minimize the mass of infarcted myocardial tissue, reduce heart work, stabilize heart rhythm, and maintain oxygen perfusion throughout the body by regulating blood pressure. Treatment and medications used in the CCU include continuous ECG monitoring (both during and after the heart attack), oxygen, nitroglycerin, antiarrhythmia agents, analgesics for pain, thrombolytic agents to dissolve clots, diuretics, agents to treat shock, and sedatives. Beta-blockers, calcium-channel blockers, anticoagulants, and antianxiety drugs may also be used.

About 60 percent of patients who have suffered from myocardial infarction develop congestive heart failure. In treating congestive heart failure from heart attacks or other causes, the cardiologist uses both dietary instruction and medication. Salt restriction is recommended to reduce edema. The three most commonly prescribed drugs are diuretics to reduce edema, digitalis (digoxin or digitoxin) to increase the force of the heart's contraction, and vasodilators to reduce the resistance of blood vessel walls, to facilitate blood flow, and to reduce heart work. Intractable congestive heart failure may be a reason for a heart transplant.

The main goals of therapy for cardiac arrhythmias are to improve heart function and to prevent sudden cardiac death. Drug therapy must be individualized to correct the particular arrhythmia. Digitalis, quinidine, procainamide, tocainamide, and atropine are often used. Beta-blockers and calcium-channel blockers are also helpful in stabilizing heart rhythm. If heart block becomes severe, an artificial pacemaker is implanted in the chest to regulate the heartbeat.

Disorders of the heart valves are not usually treated with drugs. While awaiting surgery, it may be necessary to treat heart failure, or the effects of valve disease in other parts of the body. For example, diuretics may be required to reduce edema, an antiarrhythmia agent may be needed to control atrial fibrillation, or anticoagulants may be used to prevent blood clots. Some stenotic valves can be opened using a modification of the balloon catheter technique, or surgical reconstruction may be possible. Often, it is necessary to replace the valve with a new one made of human or porcine tissue, or with a mechanical valve.

Pulmonary edema is a severe form of heart failure and is life-threatening. In emergencies, oxygen is given, in severe cases by inserting a breathing tube into the patient's trachea. Medications are given to relieve pulmonary congestion, and if the pumping action of the heart is compromised, digitalis or another medication can strengthen the contractility of the heart.

In treating dilated cardiomyopathy, the cardiologist uses appropriate medications that may include diuretics, vasodilators, antiarrhythmia agents, and digitalis. Alcohol restriction is required.

If bacteria or other microorganisms are involved, appropriate antibiotic therapy must be instituted to eradicate the cause. Patients with congenital or valvular heart disease are high risks for cardiac and valve infection. They are given preventive antibiotic therapy before undergoing surgical or dental procedures.

In acute pericarditis, if excessive fluid builds up, a procedure called pericardiocentesis may be performed to drain the fluid between the pericardium and the heart wall. In cardiac tamponade, pericardiocentesis may be lifesaving. In chronic constrictive pericarditis, an operation may be necessary to remove tissue that has stiffened and strangled the heart.

PERSPECTIVE AND PROSPECTS

Cardiology is a major medical specialty in the United States because heart disease is the major killer of Americans. Today's cardiologist turns increasingly to preventive medicine as a means of reducing morbidity (the relative incidence of a disease) and mortality. These measures include programs against smoking and programs advocating cholesterol reduction, stress reduction, exercise, and other measures that have been found useful in preventing heart disease.

There is much more to be learned about heart disease. It appears to be a consequence of highly industrialized societies, but there are questions that have to be answered, such as why heart disease is so prevalent in the United States but significantly less frequent in other, equally industrial societies.

Ongoing studies continue to accumulate data on increasingly large populations in more and more countries. Links between behavior, habits, nutrition, and ecology may be found that will give a clearer picture of why heart disease became a major killer in the twentieth century. Increased knowledge will improve diagnosis and treatment, improving patient care and the quality of life for sufferers of heart disease.

—C. Richard Falcon

See also Aneurysmectomy; Aneurysms; Angina; Angiography; Angioplasty; Arrhythmias; Arteriosclerosis; Biofeedback; Blue baby syndrome; Bypass surgery; Cardiac arrest; Cardiac rehabilitation; Cardiology, pediatric; Cardiopulmonary resuscitation (CPR); Chest; Cholesterol; Circulation; Congenital heart disease; Cyanosis; Echocardiography; Electrocardiography (ECG or EKG); Endocarditis; Exercise physiology; Heart; Heart attack; Heart disease; Heart failure; Heart transplantation; Heart valve replacement; Hypercholesterolemia; Hypertension; Ischemia; Kawasaki disease; Mitral valve prolapse; Pacemaker implantation; Palpitations; Rheumatic fever; Sports medicine; Thoracic surgery; Thrombolytic therapy and TPA; Thrombosis and thrombus; Transplantation; Vascular medicine; Vascular system.

For Further Information:

Baum, Seth J. *The Total Guide to a Healthy Heart: Integrative Strategies for Preventing and Reversing Heart Disease*. New York: Kensington, 2000. Cardiologist Baum integrates alternative and traditional medicine in the treatment of heart disease. Here he explains in detail the causes, symptoms, and treatments of coronary disease.

Crawford, Michael, ed. *Current Diagnosis and Treatment in Cardiology*. 2d ed. New York: Lange Medical Books/McGraw-Hill, 2003. Discusses advances in cardiac diagnostics, treatments, and prognostic indicators and includes extensive information on prevention techniques.

Eagle, Kim A., and Ragavendra R. Baliga, eds. *Practical Cardiology: Evaluation and Treatment of Common Cardiovascular Disorders*. Philadelphia: Lippincott Williams & Wilkins, 2003. Details advances in cardiac medicine.

Litin, Scott C., ed. *Mayo Clinic Family Health Book*. 3d ed. New York: HarperResource, 2003. Perhaps the best general medical text for the layperson, this book covers the entire medical field. While the information is derived from a wide variety of highly technical sources, the articles are written to be easily understood by a general audience.

Piscatella, Joseph, and Barry Franklin. *Take a Load Off Your Heart: 109 Things You Can Do to Prevent or Reverse Heart Disease*. New York: Workman, 2002. Easy-to-follow guide that details such preventive measures as managing stress, improving diet, and exercising and offers more than one hundred practical tips for preventing, stabilizing, and reversing heart disease.

Swanton, R. H. *Cardiology*. 5th ed. Malden, Mass.: Blackwell Science, 2002. User-friendly reference text designed for those working in the field of cardiology.

Zaret, Barry L., Marvin Moser, and Lawrence S. Cohen, eds. *Yale University School of Medicine Heart Book*. New York: William Morrow, 1992. This book is devoted entirely to the heart. Of particular interest are techniques for prevention and control of heart disease.

Cardiology, pediatric

Specialty

Anatomy or system affected: Chest, circulatory system, heart

Specialties and related fields: Emergency medicine, neonatology, pediatrics, vascular medicine

Definition: The medical field concerned with the diagnosis and treatment of heart diseases in newborns, infants, and children.

Key terms:

echocardiograph: an instrument that uses ultrasound to record activities within the heart and great arteries

electrocardiograph: an instrument for recording heart function

inpatient: one who is treated while held in a medical facility (versus an outpatient, who comes to the facility for treatment as needed)

noninvasive: referring to a procedure that does not require entering the body

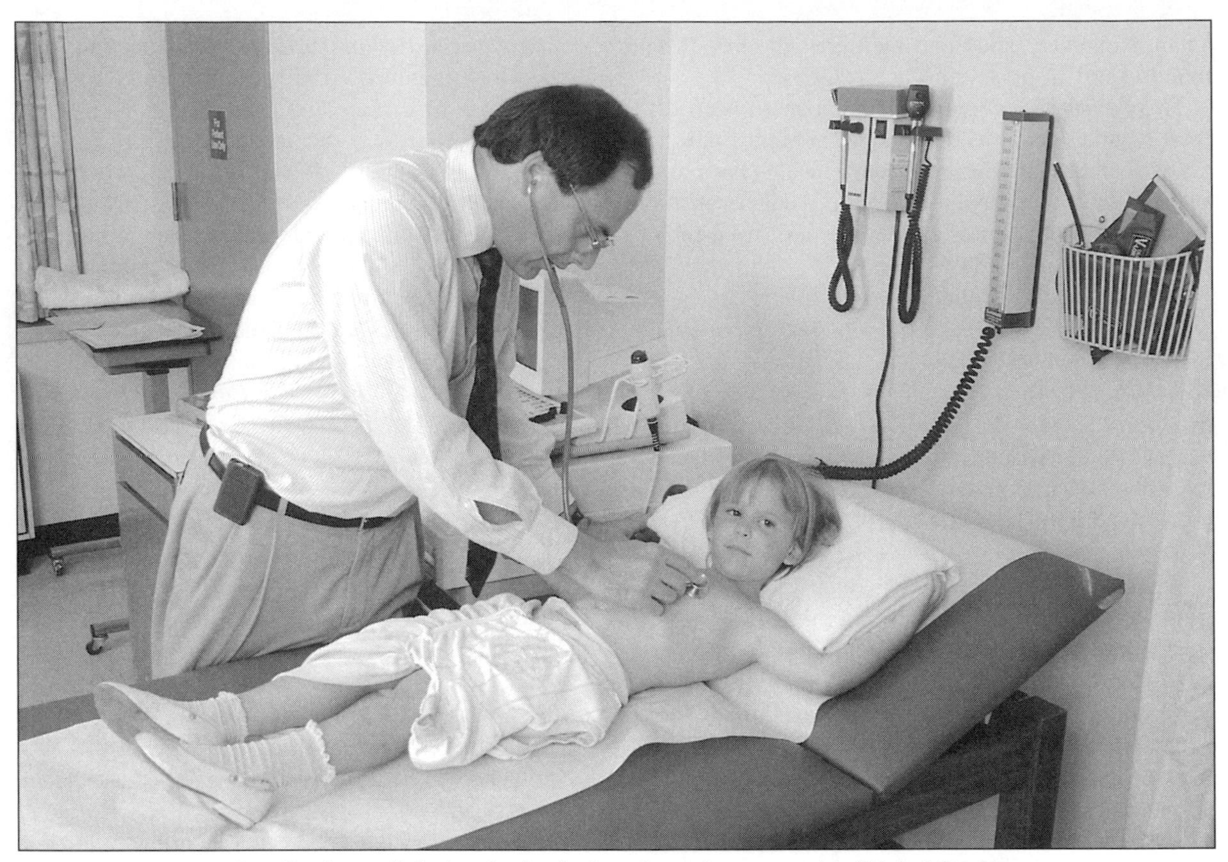

A pediatric cardiologist checks the heartbeat of a young girl. (Digital Stock)

stethoscope: an instrument for listening to sounds in the body, such as the heartbeat

valves: structures that close periodically to allow the passage of blood, such as those that connect heart chambers to each other and to the great arteries

SCIENCE AND PROFESSION

It is imperative that pediatric cardiologists be connected to large, extensive medical facilities in order to have available all the special facilities, instruments, and personnel that are required to treat heart diseases in children. The medical center should have full nursery facilities, including a neonatology section for the care of newborns and premature babies. It should have a surgical facility competent to deal with the special heart problems of children: Most children with heart disease will be treated surgically. It should have a wide range of specialized instruments and skilled personnel for diagnosis and treatment.

Heart disease in adults usually involves the coronary arteries and defects in heart rhythms. It may surface in late youth, middle age, or old age, and is often attributable to or associated with lifestyle (a high-cholesterol diet, smoking, and/or stress) and disease (diabetes mellitus or high blood pressure). In children, however, the most common heart diseases are congenital (present at birth) or caused by infections such as rheumatic fever or Kawasaki disease. About 0.8 percent of newborns have some form of congenital heart defect. Such defects may become manifest in the womb, at birth, in infancy or childhood, or later in life.

In the hospital, the pediatric cardiologist has three major patient groups: inpatient neonates and infants; older inpatient children, who are usually in the hospital for surgery; and outpatient infants and children whose disease conditions are being monitored.

DIAGNOSTIC AND TREATMENT TECHNIQUES

Proper diagnosis of the child's condition is paramount to successful treatment. The cardiac examination begins with the physician's first glance at the patient, during which he or she looks for signs of respiratory difficulty or cyanosis (a bluish tinge to the lips or fingertips). The physician will also measure the child's heart rate and rhythm, blood pressure, and growth pattern.

The pediatric cardiologist has an array of diagnostic tools, including electrocardiography, echocardiography, and stress testing. The main instrument, however, is the stethoscope because many pediatric heart problems are most readily detectable through auscultation, listening to sounds of the body. The pediatric cardiologist must develop extraordinary expertise in detecting and analyzing heart sounds. He or she must learn to differentiate between abnormalities in heart sounds that are functional and benign and those that indicate a disease condition. Through the stethoscope, the physician will hear the heartbeat, murmurs, clicks, and other sounds. Differences in loudness, pitch, variability, and timing are among the factors that must be considered in the diagnosis.

The electrocardiogram, echocardiogram, and other instruments will confirm the diagnosis and help the pediatric cardiologist determine the best course of therapy for the child. Many surgical procedures are used to correct defects in the child's heart: Valves can be repaired or replaced, tissue can be repaired, narrow passages can be opened, and gross abnormalities can be corrected. The success rate of these procedures is excellent, but any heart operation is a major surgery with significant risks. The child who undergoes heart surgery must face a wide range of additional perils. Children with severe heart disease who are cured or significantly helped through surgery must be carefully monitored because there are sometimes postoperative residua (conditions that are partially or wholly uncorrected) or postoperative sequelae (conditions that develop as a result of surgery) and other complications of surgery.

This surveillance by the pediatric cardiologist and other members of the medical team must continue for years. Often, long after the operation, the patient may develop significant arrhythmias and other anomalies. Some of these patients will require implanted pacemakers to avoid sudden death. Some will develop new valvular problems, and some patients who were given prosthetic (artificial) valves may develop infections, blood clots, or obstructions at the site.

PERSPECTIVE AND PROSPECTS

Pediatric heart diseases have existed perhaps since the dawn of the human era. Many children lived as well as they could with their infirmities—some more or less normally, some with moderate or severe restriction on their activities, and some dying in their youth.

Pediatric cardiology has made great strides in maintaining life and improving the physical status of these children. As medical specialists, pediatric cardiologists are relative newcomers, the specialty being less than half a century old. Nevertheless, through their efforts and accomplishments, hundreds of thousands of men, women, and children are alive and well, who might be dead, impaired, or debilitated.

There is still a long way to go. Pediatric heart disease, involving as it often does the physical structure of the heart, would appear comparatively mechanical and straightforward. In fact, these conditions are enormously challenging because of the wide range of anatomic, hemodynamic, and electrophysical problems that they may entail.

Also challenging are the new avenues that have opened for the pediatric cardiologist. Infant heart transplantation, unheard-of a generation ago, is now possible, if not yet commonplace. The dramatic increase in the number of premature babies who are being kept alive involves the pediatric cardiologist as a vital part of the neonatal team. There are also constant, persistent efforts to improve the quality of care both for children requiring surgery and for those who can be helped by other means.

—C. Richard Falcon

See also Aneurysmectomy; Aneurysms; Angina; Angiography; Arrhythmias; Biofeedback; Blue baby syndrome; Bypass surgery; Cardiac arrest; Cardiac rehabilitation; Cardiology; Cardiopulmonary resuscitation (CPR); Chest; Circulation; Congenital heart disease; Cyanosis; Echocardiography; Electrocardiography (ECG or EKG); Endocarditis; Exercise physiology; Genetic counseling; Genetics and inheritance; Heart; Heart attack; Heart disease; Heart failure; Heart transplantation; Heart valve replacement; Ischemia; Kawasaki disease; Mitral valve prolapse; Pacemaker implantation; Palpitations; Pediatrics; Rheumatic fever; Sports medicine; Thoracic surgery; Thrombolytic therapy and TPA; Thrombosis and thrombus; Transplantation; Vascular medicine; Vascular system.

FOR FURTHER INFORMATION:

Anderson, Robert H., et al., eds. *Paediatric Cardiology*. 2 vols. 2d ed. New York: Churchill Livingstone, 2002. A comprehensive text on pediatric and congenital cardiology covering such topics as embryology, morphology, pathophysiology, specific clinical conditions, treatments, and the psychosocial aspects of caring for patients with heart disease.

Garson, Arthur, Jr., et al., eds. *The Science and Practice of Pediatric Cardiology*. 2d ed. Baltimore: Williams & Wilkins, 1998. A text for senior residents, cardiology fellows, teachers, and practitioners. The 146 contributors review all preferred methods of management and their scientific foundations, including basic science topics, such as molecular biology, embryology, anatomy, metabolism, regulation and cardiac pump function, blood flow, and molecular oxygen consumption.

Koenig, Peter, Ziyad M. Hijazi, and Frank Zimmerman, eds. *Essential Pediatric Cardiology*. New York: McGraw-Hill, 2004. A concise guide for the nonspecialist to assist in assessing suspected cardiac disorders in the neonate, child, and adolescent.

Litin, Scott C., ed. *Mayo Clinic Family Health Book*. 3d ed. New York: HarperResource, 2003. Perhaps the best general medical text for the layperson, this book covers the entire medical field. While the information is derived from a wide variety of highly technical sources, the articles are written to be easily understood by a general audience.

Park, Myung K. *The Pediatric Cardiology Handbook*. 3d ed. St. Louis: Mosby, 2003. Handbook that reflects advances in medical management, surgical techniques, and pacemakers in children and covers information on diagnosis and management.

Zaret, Barry L., Marvin Moser, and Lawrence S. Cohen, eds. *Yale University School of Medicine Heart Book*. New York: William Morrow, 1992. A detailed medical text written to educate patients and medical students about the heart, cerebral, and peripheral vascular systems. This text is well written and easy to understand.

Cardiopulmonary resuscitation (CPR)

Procedure

Anatomy or system affected: Circulatory system, heart, lungs, respiratory system

Specialties and related fields: Cardiology, emergency medicine

Definition: A procedure that combines chest compressions and artificial breathing for a person whose breathing and heart contractions have stopped.

Key terms:

automated external defibrillator: a computerized unit that can be used to defibrillate the heart by trained nonmedical personnel

chest compression: pressure applied to the bottom half of the breastbone to pump blood from a heart in cardiac arrest

defibrillation: the sending of an electric shock through the chest to enable the heart to resume normal contractions

mouth-to-mouth breathing: the expiration of air from a rescuer's mouth into a victim's mouth to send oxygen into the victim's lungs

sudden cardiac arrest: the cessation of heart contractions or insufficient contractions to pump blood to the brain and other vital organs

Indications and Procedures

Cardiopulmonary resuscitation (CPR) is generally performed on a person who is in cardiac arrest. In the United States, someone dies from sudden cardiac arrest (SCA) every two minutes. Cardiac arrest occurs when a person has no heartbeats or insufficient heartbeats to pump blood to the brain and other vital organs. Without sufficient blood flow, these organs do not receive enough oxygen to function normally; after about four minutes, they begin to die. This life-threatening situation requires immediate attention to keep the person alive. If medical personnel are not immediately available, then emergency medical services (EMS) should be called and CPR should be initiated.

Cardiac arrest can have many causes. The most common is a severe heart attack. Many heart attacks do not require CPR, but if a person is unconscious with no pulse, then CPR should begin as soon as possible. Other causes of cardiac arrest that may require CPR are drowning, suffocation, drug overdose, electrocution, stroke, and other types of brain damage. In each of these situations, the heart is not contracting and pumping blood.

CPR includes two distinct operations, breathing air into the person's lungs and compressing the chest. In mouth-to-mouth breathing, sometimes called artificial respiration, the rescuer breathes air into the person's lungs, causing the chest to rise and fall with each breath. The rescuer's expired air is 16 percent oxygen, as compared with 21 percent oxygen in room air. This expired air has enough oxygen to maintain life. It is recommended that an individual providing mouth-to-mouth breathing use a protective device, such as a CPR mask or shield, to avoid transmission of potentially infectious body fluids. The mask or shield devices can be purchased for a small cost online or from uniform stores or university medical bookstores.

Chest compressions involve the application of pressure to the lower half of the breastbone. The external pressure increases the pressure in the chest, pushing blood to the brain and the rest of the body. Although this procedure circulates only 25 to 33 percent of normal blood flow, it is sufficient to keep the person alive when used in conjunction with mouth-to-mouth breathing.

In an emergency situation, CPR can be administered by one or two people. One person can alternate mouth-to-mouth breathing and chest compressions. Performing CPR for several minutes, however, can be exhausting. If two certified rescuers are present, one can do the mouth-to-mouth breathing while the other performs chest compressions. Two people can do the procedure more efficiently and for longer periods of time.

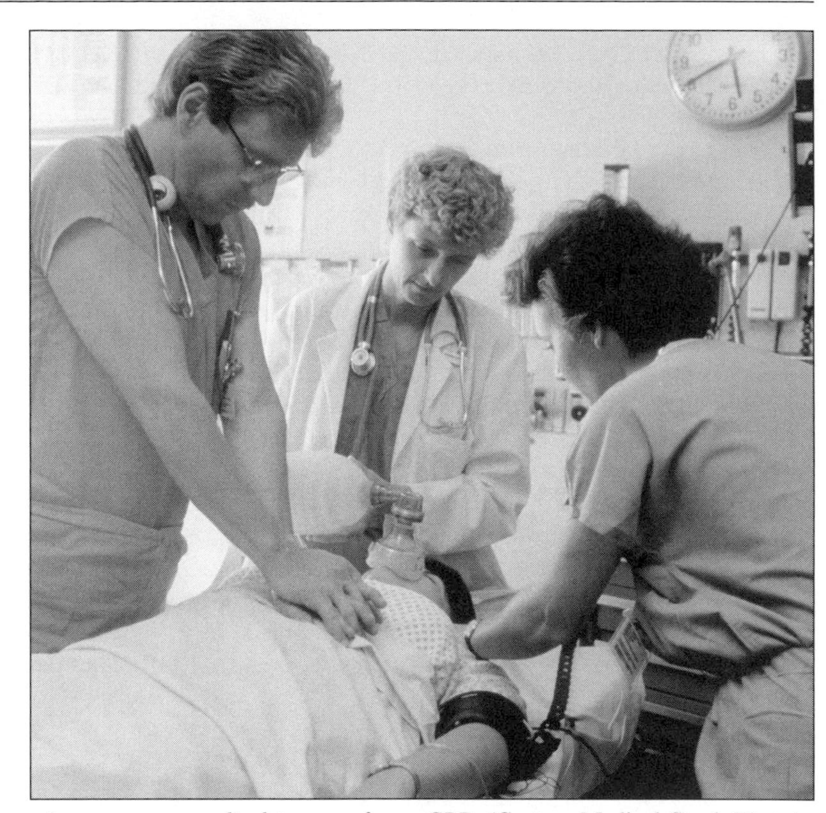

An emergency medical team performs CPR. (Custom Medical Stock Photo)

USES AND COMPLICATIONS

Cardiopulmonary resuscitation should be used only if a person is suffering from cardiac arrest. There are no other applications. Even when CPR is correctly performed by experienced, certified medical personnel, injury can occur to the individual receiving CPR. These injuries may include broken ribs, bruising of the heart, and tearing of the liver and/or the spleen. However, these injuries should not deter an individual from performing CPR. Cardiopulmonary resuscitation is only performed when a person is clinically dead, without a pulse or respiration. Individuals should take a course and become certified to learn the most effective and safest techniques.

Effective CPR sends oxygen to the vital organs to prevent permanent tissue death, but it cannot alter abnormal electrical energy that may be occurring in the heart muscle. This abnormal electrical energy does not allow the heart to pump blood adequately throughout the body. Medical attention is generally needed to restart the heart contractions, and CPR must be continued until EMS personnel arrive. Emergency medical personnel will defibrillate the heart by sending an electric shock through the chest in an attempt to correct the abnormal electrical energy in the heart so that it can resume normal contractions.

Almost anyone can become certified in CPR. The American Heart Association and the American Red Cross offer classes with certification. These organizations are also involved in campaigns to have as many people certified as possible because CPR doubles a victim's chances of sudden cardiac arrest survival. Therefore, the more people that are certified, the more likely it is that someone can perform CPR in an emergency and the more likely it is the victim will survive.

Another program to reduce deaths from sudden cardiac arrest includes the use of automated external defibrillators (AEDs). These units are computerized and allow a person with minimal training to defibrillate a heart. An AED unit has simple steps to follow with voice and print instructions. The machine has built-in safety features to prevent a person from receiving defibrillation that is not needed. AED units have been placed in worksites, stadiums, airports, and other places where large numbers of people are found. Designated people in these areas are trained to use the AEDs. If the first defibrillation shock is administered within six minutes, then the victim has an approximately 45 percent chance of survival.

Perspective and Prospects

Mouth-to-mouth breathing dates to biblical times, when it was used by midwives to resuscitate newborns. However, it fell out of practice until the 1950's, when it was rediscovered by Dr. James Elam and Dr. Peter Safer. In 1960, other physicians found that chest compressions could attain sufficient circulation, and these compressions were combined with mouth-to-mouth breathing to create a CPR procedure similar to what is used today.

—*Bradley R. A. Wilson, Ph.D.; updated by Amy Webb Bull, D.S.N., A.P.N.*

See also Arrhythmias; Cardiac arrest; Cardiac rehabilitation; Cardiology; Cardiology, pediatric; Circulation; Echocardiography; Electrocardiography (ECG or EKG); Emergency medicine; Emergency medicine, pediatric; Heart; Heart attack; Pacemaker implantation; Paramedics; Respiration; Resuscitation.

For Further Information:

Alspach, Grif. "2005 AHA Guidelines for CPR and ECG: New, but Improved?" *Critical Care Nurse* 26, no. 1 (February, 2006): 8-12.

American Heart Association. "Highlights of the 2005 AHA Guidelines for Cardiopulmonary Resuscitation and Emergency Cardiac Care." *Currents* 16, no. 4 (Winter, 2005/2006): 1-28. Also at http://www.americanheart.org/downloadable/heart/1132621842912Winter2005.pdf.

_______. "2005 American Heart Association Guidelines for Cardiopulmonary Resuscitation and Emergency Cardiovascular Care." *Circulation* 112, no. 24, supp. I (December 13, 2005): IV-1-IV-203. Also at http://www.americanheart.org/presenter.jhtml?identifier=3035517.

American Red Cross First Aid: Responding to Emergencies. 4th ed. Yardley, Pa.: StayWell, 2005.

Bergeron, David J., et al. *First Responder*. 7th ed. Upper Saddle River, N.J.: Pearson/Prentice Hall, 2005.

"CPR: Are We Doing It Wrong?" *Harvard Health Letter* 30, no. 7 (May, 2005): 1-3. Overview of CPR and the use of AEDs.

Finucane, Brendan T., and Albert H. Santora. *Principles of Airway Management*. 3d ed. New York: Springer-Verlag, 2003.

Thygerson, Alton, Benjamin Gulli, and Jon R. Krohmer. *First Aid, CPR, and AED*. 5th ed. Sudbury, Mass.: Jones and Bartlett, 2007.

Carpal tunnel syndrome

Disease/disorder

Anatomy or system affected: Arms, hands, joints, nerves, tendons

Specialties and related fields: Neurology, occupational health

Definition: A common disorder that causes discomfort and decreased hand dexterity via excessive pressure on the median nerve at the wrist, often caused by repetitive wrist and hand movements.

Key terms:

carpal tunnel: a narrow tunnel formed by a U-shaped cluster of eight bones called carpals at the base of the palm and the inelastic transverse carpal ligament that lies across the arch

median nerve: a nerve running through the carpal tunnel that carries sensory impulses from the thumb, index and middle fingers, and half of the ring finger to the central nervous system; it has a motor branch that supplies the thenar muscles on the thumb side of the hand

Causes and Symptoms

The carpal tunnel is a narrow passage of ligament and bones that contains the median nerve and tendons. Carpal tunnel syndrome, also known as median nerve palsy, is caused by the transverse carpal ligament compressing the median nerve. This nerve passes through the carpal tunnel alongside nine tendons attached to the muscles that enable the hand to close and the wrist to flex. The tendons have a lubricating lining called the synovium, which normally allows the tendons to glide back and forth smoothly through the tunnel during wrist and hand movements. The median nerve is the softest component within the tunnel and becomes com-

Information on Carpal Tunnel Syndrome

Causes: Repetitive movement of hands and wrists

Symptoms: Discomfort, decreased hand dexterity, numbness, tingling, shooting or burning pain, changes in touch or temperature sensation, clumsiness in the hands

Duration: Temporary or chronic

Treatments: Splinting of wrist, changes in hand movement and problem-causing activity, anti-inflammatory drugs, surgery

pressed when the tendons are stressed and become swollen. Median nerve compression most often results when the synovium becomes thick and sticky as a result of the wear and tear of aging or repeatedly performing stressful motions with the hands while holding them in the same position for extended periods. The carpal tunnel is smaller in some people than in others, predisposing them to carpal tunnel syndrome. Entrapment of the median nerve is less commonly caused by rheumatoid arthritis, diabetes mellitus, poor thyroid gland or pituitary function, excessive fluid retention during pregnancy or menopause, medications, vitamin B_6 or B_{12} deficiency, or bone protruding in the tunnel from previous dislocations or fractures of the wrist.

Initial symptoms of carpal tunnel syndrome include tingling and numbness in the hands, often beginning in the thumb and index and middle fingers, that causes the hand to feel as though it were asleep and shooting pain from the thenar region radiating as far up as the neck. Later symptoms include burning pain from the wrist to the fingers, changes in touch or temperature sensation, clumsiness in the hands, and muscle weakness creating an inability to grasp, pinch, and perform other thumb functions. Swelling of the hands and forearms and changes in sweat gland functioning in the hands may also be noted. Symptoms can be intermittent or constant and often progress to the point of regularly awakening the patient at night. Temporary relief is sometimes available by elevating, massaging, and shaking the hand. Although very treatable if diagnosed early, carpal tunnel syndrome can escalate into persistent pain, which can become so crippling that workplace duties and such simple tasks as holding a cup, writing, and buttoning a shirt are compromised. Carpal tunnel syndrome usually occurs in adults and is more common in women than in men.

A clinical examination for confirmation of median nerve impingement includes wrist examination, an X ray for previous injury and arthritis, and assessment of swelling and sensitivity to touch or pinpricks. Tapping of the median nerve (Tinel's test) will cause tingling or shocklike sensations in the fingers. Holding the wrist in a flexed position for several minutes with the heel of the hands touching for several minutes (Phalen's test) will result in tingling or numbness in the hands. Nerve conduction tests, which measure nerve transmission speed by electrodes placed on the skin, and electromyogram evaluation, which notes muscle function abnormalities, may also assist in a diagnosis. Ultrasound identifies whether motion of the median nerve is impeded.

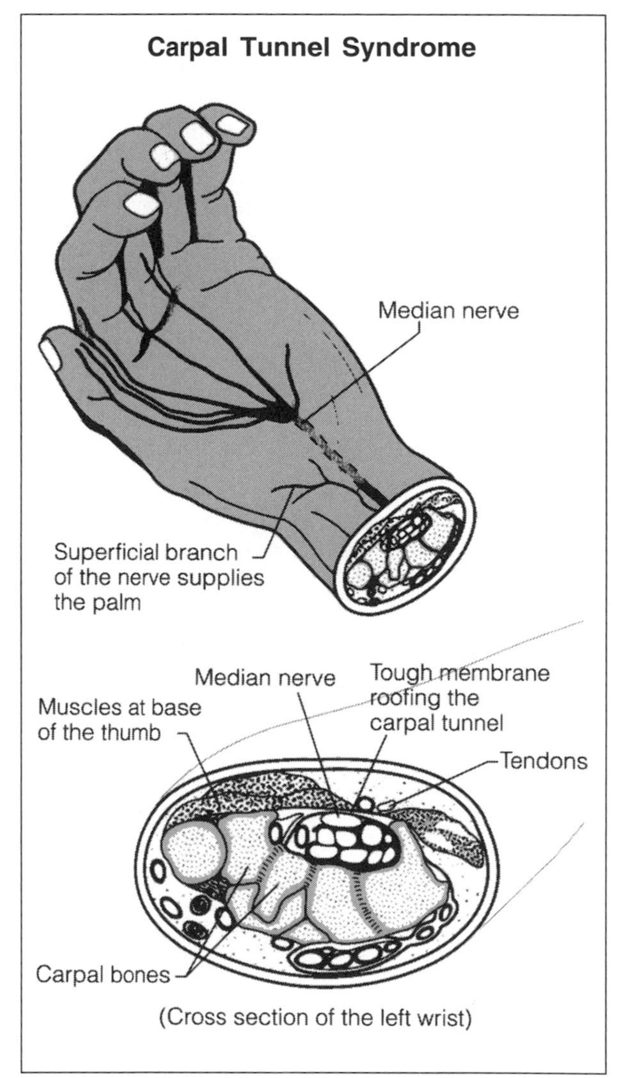

Repetitive wrist motion such as typing may put excessive pressure on the median nerves and cause numbness and tingling in the hands, a condition known as carpal tunnel syndrome. If rest, wrist splints, and painkillers do not alleviate the problem, surgery may be needed to relieve the pressure.

TREATMENT AND THERAPY

Early diagnosis and the taking of appropriate preventive measures, such as ergonomic modifications in the way that upper extremity movements are performed, often reduce the risk of developing advanced carpal tunnel syndrome. The need to compensate for weak muscles with an inappropriate wrist position can be reduced by maintaining a neutral (straight) wrist position instead of a flexed, extended, or twisted wrist position; utilizing the entire hand and all the fingers to grasp and lift objects, instead of gripping solely with the thumb and index finger; minimizing repetitive movements; allowing the upper extremities regular rest periods; using power tools, instead of hand tools; alternating work activities; switching hands; reducing movement speed; and stretching and using strengthening exercises for the hand, wrist, and arm. Keeping the hands warm to maintain good blood circulation and avoiding smoke-filled environments, which reduce peripheral blood flow, are also recommended.

Treatment generally begins with splinting of the wrist and medication, but surgery may be required if symptoms do not subside within three months. Both nocturnal splints and job-specific occupational splints can effectively keep the wrist in a neutral position, thus avoiding the extreme wrist flexion or extension that narrows the carpal tunnel. Wrist supports lying on the desk in front of a computer keyboard are often helpful, but the benefit of strapping on wrist splints while typing is controversial because disuse atrophy may result, potentially creating a muscle imbalance. Aspirin and other oral nonsteroidal anti-inflammatory drugs (NSAIDs) may reduce swelling and inflammation, relieving some nerve pressure. Corticosteroids and cortisone-like medications injected directly into the carpal tunnel can help confirm diagnosis if the symptoms are relieved. Diuretics and vitamin supplementation may also be beneficial. Vitamin B_6 has shown promise in reducing the symptoms of carpal tunnel syndrome. Exercises can be performed, under the guidance of a physical or occupational therapist, to stretch and strengthen the wrists. Acupuncture and chiropractic may benefit some who suffer from carpal tunnel syndrome; however, their effectiveness has not been supported. Pain reduction and improved grip strength has been documented among patients who practice yoga.

If initial symptoms do not subside, pain increases, or the risk of permanent nerve and muscle damage exists, then surgery may be necessary, with subsequent rehabilitation and ergonomic counseling with a physical or occupational therapist. Carpal tunnel release is one of the most common surgical procedures in the United States. It is often recommended for individuals who experience carpal tunnel symptoms for more than six months. This outpatient surgical procedure involves dividing the transverse ligament to open the carpal tunnel to relieve pressure and remove thickened synovial tissue. Endoscopic surgery using a fiber-optic camera allows the surgeon to visualize and cut the carpal ligament. This procedure results in faster recovery and minimizes postoperative discomfort and scarring. Though most patients who have carpal tunnel surgery recover completely, recovery can take months.

Perspective and Prospects

The historic roots of carpal tunnel syndrome can be traced back to the 1860's, when meatpackers complained of pain and loss of hand function, which physicians initially attributed to reduced circulation. Modern occupations that require repetitive motions for extended periods—such as typing on a computer keyboard, construction and assembly-line work, and jack-

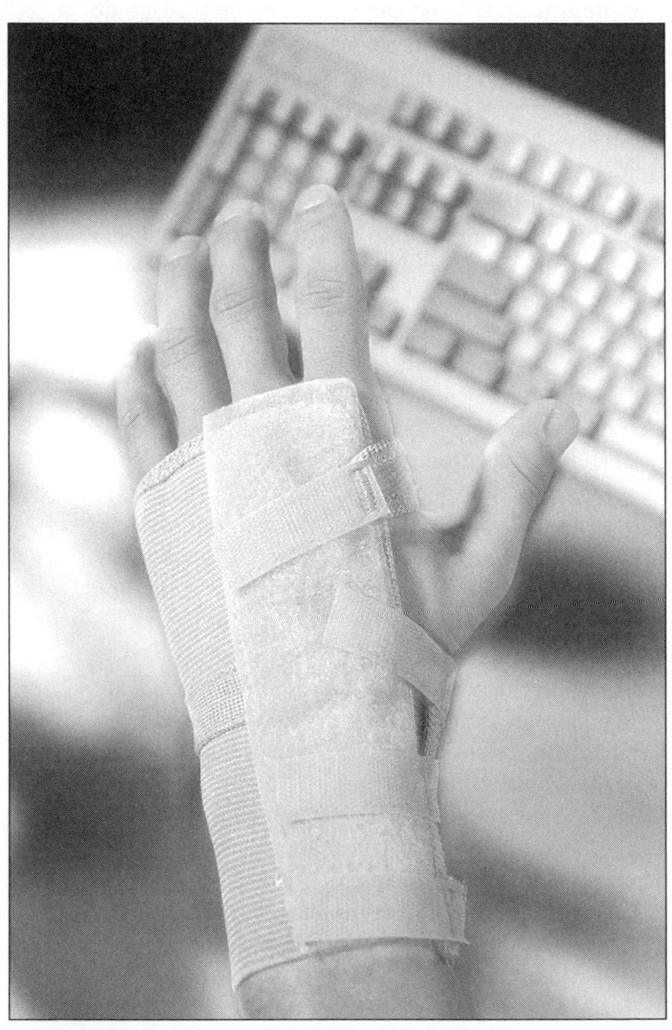

Patients with carpal tunnel syndrome may find that wearing a brace relieves pressure on the nerve in the wrist. (Adobe)

hammer operation—have caused a dramatic rise in cumulative trauma disorders such as carpal tunnel syndrome, while other workplace injuries have leveled off.

—Daniel G. Graetzer, Ph.D.; updated by Sharon W. Stark, R.N., A.P.R.N., D.N.Sc.

See also Nervous system; Neuralgia, neuritis, and neuropathy; Neurology; Neurosurgery; Occupational health; Pain management; Upper extremities.

FOR FURTHER INFORMATION:

Carpal Tunnel Syndrome Place. http://www.ctsplace.com/. Web site offers information about the disorder, ergonomic products for sale, message boards, and myriad research links.

Familydoctor.org. *Carpal Tunnel Syndrome: Pain in Your Hands and Wrists*. http://familydoctor.org/023.xml. Web site from the American Academy of Family Physicians. Provides a diagram of the carpal tunnel ligament and a discussion of the syndrome. Addresses symptoms, diagnosis, helpful and unhelpful treatments, and prevention.

Johansson, Philip. *Carpal Tunnel Syndrome and Other Repetitive Strain Injuries*. Berkeley Heights, N.J.: Enslow, 1999. This text, designed for students in grades eight and above, examines the causes, symptoms, diagnosis, treatment, and prevention of some of the most common repetitive strain injuries, such as carpal tunnel syndrome and tennis elbow. Helpful appendices are included.

McCabe, Steven J. *101 Questions and Answers About Carpal Tunnel Syndrome: What It Is, How to Prevent It, and Where to Turn for Treatment*. New York: McGraw-Hill, 2002. Provides accurate and updated research on the disorder in a user-friendly format.

National Institute of Neurological Disorders and Stroke (NINDS). *Carpal Tunnel Syndrome Fact Sheet*. http://www.ninds.nih.gov/disorders/carpal_tunnel/detail_carpal_tunnel.htm. Web site provides an overview of the syndrome, including symptoms, diagnosis, treatment, and prevention.

Rosenbaum, Richard B., and José L. Ochoa. *Carpal Tunnel Syndrome and Other Disorders of the Median Nerve*. 2d ed. Boston: Butterworth-Heinemann, 2002. This text covers anatomy, clinical presentation, differential diagnosis, relation to other medical conditions, electrodiagnostic methods of evaluation, quantitative sensory testing, thermography, imaging, and acute and chronic mechanical nerve injury.

CAT SCANS. *See* COMPUTED TOMOGRAPHY (CT) SCANNING.

CATARACT SURGERY

PROCEDURE

ANATOMY OR SYSTEM AFFECTED: Eyes

SPECIALTIES AND RELATED FIELDS: Ophthalmology, optometry

DEFINITION: The surgical management of cataracts.

KEY TERMS:

cornea: the transparent, curved front surface of the eye

phacoemulsification: the insertion of an ultrasound device through a small incision in the eye to break a cataract into small fragments, which are then aspirated with the same device

retina: a thin membrane at the back of the eyeball where light is converted into nerve impulses that travel to the brain

ultrasound: high-frequency sound waves

INDICATIONS AND PROCEDURES

Cataract surgery refers to the surgical removal of the lens from the eye, generally because of a decrease in vision or other visual complaints, such as difficulty with night vision, glare, or loss of contrast. The decision to undergo cataract surgery, however, depends most often on the individual's subjective threshold for what constitutes unacceptable vision.

Every eye contains a lens that allows images to be focused on the retina, much like a camera focuses light on film. Over time, most people develop some degree of opacity in their lens, which can only be remedied by surgically removing the lens and replacing it with an artificial one. The artificial lens can be made from a variety of materials, such as silicone, acrylic, or other biocompatible synthetic substances.

Because of the refinement in instrumentation and technique, general anesthesia is rarely indicated in cataract surgery, and the procedure is often performed on an outpatient basis. Anesthesia is generally obtained by injection of the anesthetic solution around the eye or by placing anesthetic drops on the eye. The surgical approach to lens extraction depends to some extent on the nature of the cataract and the surgeon's preference. The majority of surgeons in developed countries use an ultrasound device to break the cataract into small fragments, which are then aspirated with the same device (phacoemulsification). This procedure is often performed through a very small incision, which may be left to close by itself or is closed with one small suture.

The Removal of Cataracts

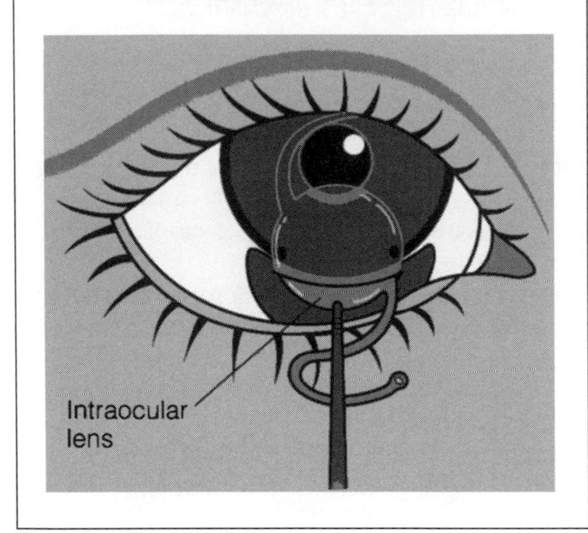

The presence of a cataract, cloudiness of the eye lens that obscures vision, often requires the removal of the entire lens and its replacement with an artificial lens (shown here), which is held in place with loops.

Under certain circumstances, the ophthalmologist may elect to remove the entire lens in a single piece, in which case a larger opening is needed into the eye to gain access to the cataract.

Once the cataract is removed, a clear artificial lens is often placed in its position to allow the eye to continue to focus light properly. This artificial lens may be single-focus (focusing at only one distance) or multifocal (focusing at both near and far distances). In general, cataract surgery is performed on one eye at a time, since a resulting infection in both eyes, albeit rare, can be quite devastating. The length of the procedure is often significantly less than one hour, provided there are no complications or special needs.

In most cases, the patient returns home the same day and may wear a patch over the eye until the next, postoperative day, when he or she is seen on follow-up. The patient is then asked to start using a combination of antibiotic and anti-inflammatory agents to prevent infection and reduce inflammation. Alternatively, some surgeons recommend starting drops immediately following surgery in order to hasten recovery. Some ophthalmologists also suggest using these drops prior to surgery in order to minimize the risk of infection and inflammation even further. Visual recovery varies greatly among individuals and may be as short as a day or as long as several months.

Uses and Complications

Although cataracts are mostly a condition affecting the elderly, they can occur at any age and even in newborns. Cataracts may have various causes, although the most common is related to simple aging and does not necessarily reflect a significant disease of the eye or the body. The presence of cataracts in young children or young adults is never normal, however, and must be promptly addressed, especially in newborns. Potentially more serious conditions may mask themselves as cataracts in the young child. Therefore, unlike the adult cataract, the progression of which can be carefully followed over time, the cataract in the newborn must be quickly referred to an ophthalmologist for surgical care.

With the many refinements in technique and technology, the overall morbidity of this procedure has significantly diminished, and the majority of patients who undergo cataract surgery find it to be a positive life-altering experience. As with most surgical procedures, infection and bleeding can occur during cataract surgery. Although rare (less than 1 in 10,000), a resulting eye infection, known as endophthalmitis, can have devastating consequences and must be addressed immediately. The signs and symptoms of endophthalmitis include decreased vision, pain, and redness. A more common complication of surgery is swelling of the retina (macular edema). This condition may lead to suboptimal vision following surgery but can generally be treated with anti-inflammatory drops. Finally, one or more fragments of the lens may become dislodged in the eye as a result of a rupture of the capsule surrounding the cataract. If the surgeon deems it unsafe to proceed further, then the eye may be closed and approached at a later time with the help of a retinal surgeon, who can then safely remove any remaining fragments from the eye. Other rare but potential complications include the loss of the clarity of the cornea, retinal detachment, glaucoma, or long-standing inflammation.

Perspective and Prospects

The word "cataract" is derived from a Greek and Latin word meaning "waterfall," referring to the visible veil that forms in the pupil. Cataracts constitute the most common cause of preventive blindness throughout the world. In 2003, close to sixteen million people were blind as a result of cataracts. No medical treatments are currently available for cataracts. There is some evidence that a healthy lifestyle with proper precaution against ultraviolet (UV) light can slow the formation or progression of cataracts.

Future trends in the management of cataracts point to less invasive surgical approaches, with smaller incisions and devices that produce less collateral heat. Laser devices for cataract surgery continue to improve and may one day equal or surpass ultrasound devices in their ability to address most cataracts safely.

Significant progress continues to be made in the realm of artificial lenses. Many artificial intraocular lenses (IOLs) can now be folded or injected into the eye through very small incisions. Some progress has been made to manufacture lenses that provide true accommodation, much like a young individual's eyes, thus obviating the need for reading glasses. Finally, with the advent of better antibiotic solutions, the potential risk of infection is significantly reduced.

—Ebrahim Elahi, M.D.

See also Aging; Aging: Extended care; Astigmatism; Blindness; Blurred vision; Cataracts; Corneal transplantation; Eye infections and disorders; Eye surgery; Eyes; Glaucoma; Laser use in surgery; Macular degeneration; Microscopy, slitlamp; Ophthalmology; Optometry; Optometry, pediatric; Vision disorders.

FOR FURTHER INFORMATION:

Albert, Daniel M. *Ophthalmic Surgery: Principles and Techniques*. 2 vols. Malden, Mass.: Blackwell Science, 1999.

Eden, John. *The Physician's Guide to Cataracts, Glaucoma, and Other Eye Problems*. Yonkers, N.Y.: Consumer Reports Books, 1992.

Gottsch, John D., Walter J. Stark, and Morton F. Goldberg, eds. *Ophthalmic Surgery*. 5th ed. New York: Oxford University Press, 1999.

Shulman, Julius. *Cataracts—from Diagnosis to Recovery: The Complete Guide for Patients and Families*. Rev. ed. New York: St. Martin's Griffin, 1995.

Spaeth, George L., ed. *Ophthalmic Surgery: Principles and Practice*. 3d ed. Philadelphia: W. B. Saunders, 2003.

CATARACTS

DISEASE/DISORDER

ANATOMY OR SYSTEM AFFECTED: Eyes

SPECIALTIES AND RELATED FIELDS: Geriatrics and gerontology, ophthalmology, optometry

DEFINITION: Dark regions in the lens of the eye that cause gradual loss of vision.

KEY TERMS:

artificial lens implant: a plastic lens inserted permanently into the eye to replace a defective natural lens that has been removed

cornea: the transparent front surface of the eye; its curvature produces about 60 percent of the focusing power needed to produce an image on the retina

extracapsular cataract extraction: a procedure in which the lens is emulsified (broken up) with an ultrasonic probe and the pieces are suctioned out

intracapsular cataract extraction: a procedure in which the faulty lens is removed in one piece while still inside its capsule

iris: the colored portion of the eye that regulates the amount of light entering the pupil at its center

laser: an intense light beam, used in eye surgery to reattach a detached retina or to open a secondary cataract

microsurgery: surgery performed with the aid of a microscope

retina: the dark membrane on the inside rear surface of the eye, where light is converted into nerve signals sent to the brain

CAUSES AND SYMPTOMS

Cataracts are imperfections in the clarity of the eye lens that reduce its ability to transmit light. They are a very common medical problem. In the United States, cataract removal is the most frequently performed surgery and the largest line-item cost in the Medicare budget. There are many misconceptions about cataracts. Cataracts are not an infection, a growth, a disease, or a film on the surface of the lens. They do not cause pain, redness, teardrops, or other discomforts of the eye. The initial symptom is a gradual deterioration of vision, usually in one eye at a time. There is no known treatment other than to remove the lens surgically. After surgery, neither the lens nor the cataracts can grow back. The formation of cataracts is a normal part of aging, like gray hair or hardening of the arteries. All people would develop cataracts eventually if they lived long enough.

In a discussion of cataracts, it is helpful to review the structure of the human eye. The eye is often compared to a camera, with its lens and film. The camera lens, however, can be moved back and forth slightly to focus on objects at different distances, whereas the eye lens is squeezed into a thicker shape by muscular action to change its focus. Both camera and eye have a variable-size diaphragm to regulate the amount of light that is admitted.

When light enters the eye, it first encounters a trans-

INFORMATION ON CATARACTS

CAUSES: Aging, diabetes, injury, exposure to X rays or nuclear radiation, congenital defect
SYMPTOMS: Loss of clear vision, typically one eye at a time
DURATION: Chronic
TREATMENTS: Surgery

parent, tough outer skin called the cornea. There are no blood vessels in the cornea, but many nerve cells make it sensitive to touch or other irritation. Immediately behind the cornea is the clear aqueous fluid that carries oxygen and nutrients for cell metabolism. Next comes the colored portion, the iris of the eye, with a variable-size opening at its center called the pupil. The pupil has no color, but looks black, like the opening of a cave. A person looking at his or her own eye in a mirror and then shining a flashlight on it can see the black pupil quickly shrink in size.

Next comes the lens of the eye, surrounded by an elastic membrane called the capsule. The lens is suspended by short strands, or ligaments, which are attached to a sphincter muscle. When the muscle contracts, the lens becomes thicker in the middle, thus increasing its focusing strength. The transparent lens has no blood vessels, so its metabolism is provided by the aqueous fluid. Behind the lens is the vitreous fluid, which fills about two-thirds of the eyeball and maintains its oval shape. At the back of the eye is the retina, where special visual cells convert light into electrical signals that travel to the brain via nerve fibers.

The lens of the eye is not simply a homogeneous fluid, but has a unique, internal structure and growth pattern. It continues to grow larger throughout the life of the individual. New cells originate at the front surface of the lens, just inside the capsule enclosure. These cells divide and grow into fibers that migrate toward the middle, or nucleus, of the lens. The whole structure has been compared to the layers of an onion, with the oldest cells at the center. The protein molecules in the nucleus are less soluble and more rigid than those in the outer part of the lens. By the age of forty, in most people the firm nucleus has enlarged until the lens has lost much of its elasticity. Even with considerable muscular strain, the curvature of the lens surface will no longer bulge enough to focus on nearby objects. The eye loses its power of accommodation, and reading glasses will be needed.

The mechanism by which cataracts form in the lens is not yet clearly understood. Like the loss of accommodation, however, it is a normal part of the aging process. One proposed biochemical explanation is the Maillard reaction, in which glucose and protein molecules combine when heated to form a brown product. The Maillard reaction is responsible for the browning of bread or cookies during baking. The same process is thought to occur even at body temperature, but very slowly over a period of years. Some scientists have theorized that wrinkled skin, hardening of the arteries, and other normal features of aging may be caused by this reaction. The biochemistry of aging is an active area of research, in which the deterioration of the eye lens is only one example.

The most common symptom of cataracts is a loss of clear vision that cannot be corrected with eyeglasses. Brighter lighting can partially help to overcome the blockage of light transmission. There is one paradoxical situation reported by some patients, however, whose vision becomes worse in bright light. The explanation for this problem is that brightness causes the pupil to become smaller. If the cataract is centered right in the middle of the lens, it will block a larger fraction of the incoming light. In dimmer light, the pupil opening is larger, so light can pass through the clear periphery of the lens.

By far the most common cataracts are those attributable to normal aging, called senile cataracts. (This has nothing to do with the common use of the term "senility" to describe declining mental ability.) So-called secondary cataracts can also develop in special circumstances. For example, exposure to X rays or nuclear radiation will increase the probability of cataracts, and the eye lens seems to be particularly sensitive to the effects of ionizing radiation. Certain medications such as cortisone, which is used in arthritis treatment, increase the risk of cataracts. A diet deficient in protein, especially in developing countries, has been associated with cataract formation. A blow to the eye from a sports injury or an accident can lead to a cataract. Diabetics are more likely to develop cataracts than the general public. Some studies have suggested that electric shock, ultraviolet rays, or certain environmental pollutants may be other causes.

Some babies are born with cataracts. These are called congenital and are frequently associated with the mother having had German measles (rubella) during the first three months of pregnancy. Surgery on the infant's eye must be done with little delay. Otherwise, the nerve connections between eye and brain will not develop, and permanent blindness can result.

Cataracts are much more prevalent in Israel and India than in Western Europe. It is not clear yet whether race or different diets and life habits are the determining factors. Some ophthalmologists believe that cataracts run in families, suggesting a genetic influence. The evidence is not conclusive, and further studies are needed. What causes cataracts is much less understood than how to treat them surgically.

TREATMENT AND THERAPY

When cataracts begin to form in the eye lens, no medication can remove them and they will not get better on their own. The patient's vision will continue to deteriorate as the cataracts mature, although the process may be quite slow. Fortunately, modern techniques of surgery for cataract removal have a success rate of better than 95 percent.

Consider a typical middle-aged man who believes that his vision is getting worse. When he goes to an optometrist, he is informed that his eye examination has revealed the onset of senile cataracts (as a result of aging). He is referred to an ophthalmologist, who finds no need for surgery at this time, but recommends more frequent, semiannual checkups. The patient is told that reading or other eye-straining activities will not accelerate cataract growth, but that brighter lighting will help him to see more clearly. During the next several years, the cataracts slowly darken and increase in size. Eventually, distant vision in one eye (even with glasses) may deteriorate to 20/160, which means that what he is able to see at 20 feet can be seen by a normal person at 160 feet. The ability of the patient to drive a car is seriously impaired, and surgery is indicated. It is not a medical emergency, but operating on one eye while the other one is still fairly clear is recommended.

Once the decision has been made to go ahead with surgery, it is necessary for the patient to have a thorough physical examination. The doctor checks for possible health problems that could complicate cataract surgery. Among these are diabetes, high blood pressure, kidney disease, anemia, and glaucoma (excess pressure in the eye). Normally, extracting the cata-

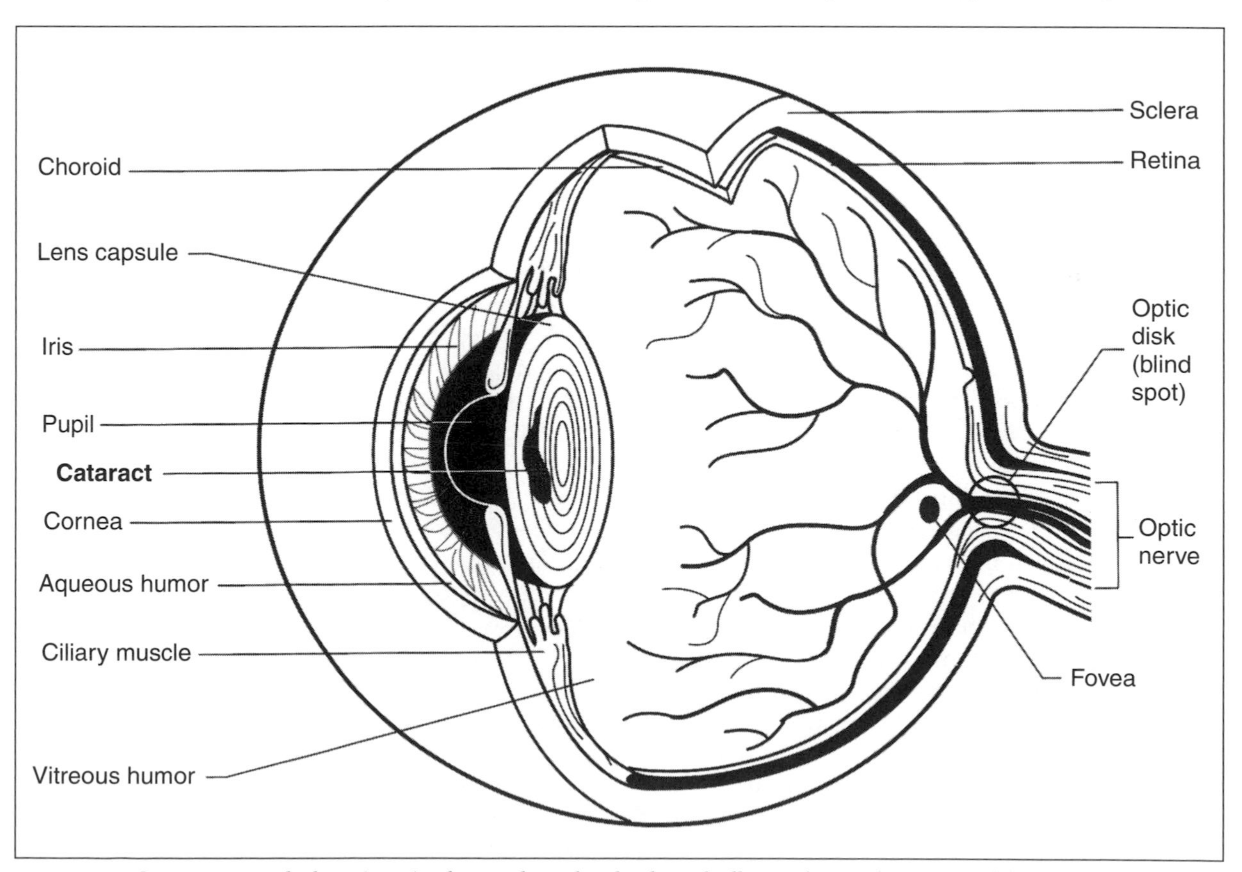

Cataracts are dark regions in the eye lens that lead gradually to obscured vision and blindness.

ractous lens and implanting an artificial, plastic one are done at the same time. Before proceeding with surgery, the ophthalmologist must determine what the proper strength of the implant lens should be, so that light will focus properly on the retina. An accurate measurement is made by reflecting a beam of high-frequency sound waves (ultrasound) from the back of the eye. Measuring the time for an echo to return gives the needed data for calculating the strength of the implant lens.

On the day of the surgery, the patient is given an injection to make him drowsy and eyedrops to dilate the pupil. Gradually, more eyedrops are administered to produce a large dilation, so that access to the lens is easier. In the operating room, local anesthetic is injected to keep the eyelids from closing and to deaden the normally very sensitive surface of the cornea. To prepare for surgery, a microscope is moved into place above the eye. Making an incision in the cornea, removing the defective lens, inserting and fastening the artificial lens, and finally closing the incision with a very fine needle and thread are all performed by the surgeon while looking through the microscope. Its magnification and focus controls are operated using foot pedals, so that both of the surgeon's hands are free.

There are three basic types of cataract extraction. Each method has its advantages and disadvantages. The first method is called intracapsular extraction. The capsule is the membrane that surrounds the lens. Intracapsular means that the lens and capsule are removed together, that is, with the lens still inside its capsule. The advantage of this method is that no part of the lens is left behind to cause possible problems with infection or swelling later. The disadvantage is that the incision at the edge of the cornea must be fairly large to allow the lens and capsule to be pulled out together. Five to ten stitches are needed to close the incision. The patient must avoid strenuous activity for about a month to permit thorough healing. Before 1962, forceps were used to bring the lens and capsule out of the eye. Then Charles D. Kelman introduced the cryoprobe, which uses a freezing process. When the rather slippery lens is touched by the cold probe, it freezes to the probe and can be pulled out in one piece. Most eye surgeons have adopted the cryoprobe for intracapsular extraction.

A second method of cataract surgery is called extracapsular extraction, in which the lens is removed while the capsule is left in the eye. The advantage is that the unbroken back surface of the capsule can prevent leakage of fluid from the rear of the eye and therefore can decrease the chances for damage to the retina. A disadvantage is that small fragments of the lens may remain behind, causing infection or irritation. The size of the incision and the recuperation period are about the same as for the intracapsular method.

The third method of cataract surgery is an improvement of extracapsular extraction, first developed by Kelman in 1967. An ultrasonic probe is used to emulsify, or break up, the lens. The small pieces are then suctioned out of the capsule while fluid is washed into the opening. The main advantage of emulsification is that the incision can be very small, because the lens is brought out in fragments, not as a whole. The incision may be only 3 millimeters long, and a single suture to close it would heal rapidly. This method requires very specialized training, however, because surgeons must learn to operate the microscope, the ultrasonic generator, and the suction apparatus with their feet while manipulating the probe with their hands.

After the eye lens has been extracted, an artificial lens is inserted in its place. The implant is made of clear plastic, about the size of an aspirin tablet. Two spring loops embedded in the plastic are used to center the implant and to keep it there permanently. A variety of different spring loop attachments have been designed by ophthalmologists. In the United States, if a particular design is prone to failure, the Food and Drug Administration (FDA) has the authority to ban its use.

To complete the surgery, the incision in the cornea is closed. During the recuperation period, the patient is instructed to avoid strenuous exercise and to protect the eye from any hard contact. Normally there is little pain, although some eye irritation should be expected during the healing process. A plastic implant lens has a fixed focal length, with no power of accommodation for different distances. It is like a box camera that gives a good picture at a set distance, while near and far objects are somewhat blurry. After the eye has healed thoroughly, the patient is fitted with prescription glasses for reading and for distant vision, respectively.

A number of minor complications can develop after cataract surgery. About one-third of the patients develop a so-called secondary cataract, which is a clouding of the capsule membrane just behind the implant. This condition is easily corrected with a laser beam to open the membrane, requiring no surgery. Another potential complication is astigmatism. The eye is squeezed and flattened slightly, and the curvature of the surface will differ between the flattened and the more rounded regions. During surgery, the symmetry of the corneal surface can be distorted if some sutures are tighter than others. Astigmatism is relatively easy to correct with prescription glasses.

All operations have some risks, and a small percentage of cataract surgeries can lead to serious complications. Among these are a detached retina, glaucoma caused by scar tissue, and hemorrhage into the vitreous fluid in front of the retina. Fortunately, such problems are rare, and the percentage of successful eye surgeries continues to improve.

Perspective and Prospects

In the history of medicine, surgery for cataracts has been traced back to Roman times. The method was called "couching." The physician would insert a needle through the white of the eye into the lens and he would try to push the lens down out of the line of vision, leaving it in the eyeball. The procedure must have been painful, with a high chance for infection. The complete extraction of a lens from the eye was done for the first time in 1745. A French ophthalmologist named Jacques Daviel was performing a couching operation, but was unable to push the lens out of the line of sight. On the spur of the moment, he decided to make a small cut in the cornea, through which he was able to extract the lens. The operation was successful. During the following ten years, he repeated his procedure more than four hundred times with only fifty failures, a much better result than with couching.

A major advance in eye surgery was the discovery of local anesthesia by Carl Koller in 1884. Together with the famous psychiatrist Sigmund Freud, Koller had been investigating the psychological effects of cocaine. He noticed that his tongue became numb from the drug and wondered if a drop of cocaine solution locally applied to the eyes might work as an anesthetic. He tried it first on a frog's eye and then on himself, and the cocaine made his eye numb. He published a short article, and the news spread to other physicians. Synthetic substitutes such as novocaine were developed and came into common use, thereafter making eye surgery virtually painless.

When the lens of the eye is surgically removed, it becomes impossible to focus light on the retina. A strong replacement lens is needed. For example, the French painter Claude Monet had cataract surgery in the 1920's, and photographs show him with the typical thick cataract glasses of that time. Today, contact lenses or artificial lens implants are much better alternatives to restore good vision.

The recovery period after cataract surgery used to be several weeks of bed rest, with the head kept absolutely still, because the cut in the cornea had to heal itself without any stitches. The development of microsurgery made it possible for the surgeon to see the extremely fine thread and needle that can be used for closing the cut. With stitches in place, the patient can usually carry on normal activities within a day after surgery.

In the 1960's, the cryoprobe and the ultrasound probe were developed to replace forceps for removing an eye lens. The size of the required incision was smaller and the healing time correspondingly shorter. In the 1980's, reliable lens implants became available, making near-normal vision possible again. In the future, perhaps drugs can be found that will prevent or delay the onset of cataracts, so that surgery will not be necessary. Further research is needed to obtain a better understanding of biochemical changes in the eye lens that occur with aging.

—Hans G. Graetzer, Ph.D.

See also Aging; Blindness; Cataract surgery; Eye infections and disorders; Eye surgery; Eyes; Ophthalmology; Optometry; Vision disorders.

For Further Information:

Buettner, Helmut, ed. *Mayo Clinic on Vision and Eye Health: Practical Answers on Glaucoma, Cataracts, Macular Degeneration, and Other Conditions*. Rochester, Minn.: Mayo Foundation for Medical Education and Research, 2002. A helpful handbook on all the medical, social, and emotional facets of vision impairment.

Cataracts in America. http://www.cataractsinamerica.com/. A research-oriented site offering comprehensive information on cataracts, new products and treatment technology, bulletin boards, and physician referrals.

Eden, John. *The Physician's Guide to Cataracts, Glaucoma, and Other Eye Problems*. Yonkers, N.Y.: Consumer Reports Books, 1992. The author, an ophthalmologist, describes the medical history of a typical cataract patient in her sixties: the original diagnosis, gradually deteriorating vision, surgery with the insertion of an artificial lens implant, postoperative care, and the fitting of prescription glasses.

Houseman, William. "The Day the Light Returned." *New Choices for Retirement Living* 32 (April, 1992): 54-58. A personal account of a patient who had successful cataract surgery. Under local anesthetic, his faulty eye lens was removed and a plastic lens was inserted. The whole procedure took only half a day.

The initial eye examination and follow-up care after surgery are described.

Parker, James N., and Philip M. Parker, eds. *The Official Patient's Sourcebook on Cataracts*. San Diego, Calif.: Icon Health, 2002. Draws from public, academic, government, and peer-reviewed research to provide a wide-ranging handbook for patients with cataracts.

Sardegna, Jill, et al. *Encyclopedia of Blindness and Vision Impairment*. 2d ed. New York: Facts On File, 2002. All aspects of vision impairment are covered in five hundred entries, including health and social issues, surgery and medications, adaptive aids, education, and helpful organizations. Twelve appendixes provide myriad resources for research, support, and services.

Shulman, Julius. *Cataracts—from Diagnosis to Recovery: The Complete Guide for Patients and Families*. Rev. ed. New York: St. Martin's Griffin, 1995. A well-written book by an ophthalmologist to educate patients who may need cataract surgery. Using nontechnical language and helpful diagrams, Shulman explains several methods for extracting the eye lens.

Taylor, Allen, ed. *Nutritional and Environmental Influences on the Eye*. Boca Raton, Fla.: CRC Press, 1999. This resource contains methodological chapters on grading cataract and macular degeneration and evaluating epidemiological research, chapters on the biology of the eye relevant to nutrition and environmental risk factors, and overviews of epidemiological research on the effects of diet and nutrition, light, and smoking.

Catheterization

Procedure

Anatomy or system affected: Bladder, blood vessels, circulatory system, genitals, heart, reproductive system, throat, urinary system

Specialties and related fields: Anesthesiology, cardiology, critical care, emergency medicine, general surgery, pulmonary medicine, radiology, urology

Definition: The insertion of a tube into a cavity of the body to withdraw fluids from or introduce fluids into that cavity.

Key terms:

bladder: the organ that stores urine until it is discharged from the body

urethra: the tube that transfers urine from the bladder to the outside of the body

Indications and Procedures

Many different types of catheters exist, and they can be used for many different purposes. What they all have in common is the placement of a tube (catheter) into a body cavity. The tube is used to draw a gas or liquid from the cavity or to inject a gas or liquid into the cavity. The most common uses of catheterization are the opening of an airway for breathing, the withdrawal of urine from the bladder, and the injection of dye or other substances such as an intravenous (IV) drip into blood vessels.

Catheterization can be used to assist in the breathing process. This procedure may be necessary when the patient's airway is blocked, the patient is unconscious and unable to breathe, or the patient needs help to breathe. The tube or catheter is placed into the mouth, nose, throat, or lungs. Oxygen passes through the tube and into the lungs, where it can be absorbed by the blood. Catheters can also be used to remove secretions from these same areas to open the airway and improve breathing. They are also necessary in many emergency situations to open and maintain breathing. At times, a catheter must be introduced directly into the lungs through an incision in the neck, near the Adam's apple; this procedure is known as a tracheostomy. A catheter may also be introduced into the patient's nose to transport oxygen into the lungs. Catheterization is important for maintaining breathing during surgery under general anesthesia, when the body's breathing mechanisms are shut down.

Another common catheterization procedure involves the introduction of a urethral catheter. This type of catheter is inserted into the urethra to drain urine from the bladder. Such a procedure may be necessary to empty the bladder when the urethra is blocked, or it may be used to collect urine when the person is unable to control his or her own bladder.

An area where catheters are being used more frequently is heart diagnosis and surgery. In cardiac catheterization, a catheter is inserted into a large blood vessel (a vein or artery) in the upper arm or groin area. The physician then maneuvers the catheter into the heart and uses it to inject a dye directly into the organ. An X ray can show the distribution of the dye within the heart, allowing the physician to see if and where any coronary arteries are blocked. In addition, cardiac catheters can be used to determine blood pressures within the heart, the amount of oxygen in the blood in the heart, and how the valves are functioning. More recently, cardiac catheters have been developed to perform some types of surgery. A good example is balloon angioplasty. Using similar procedures to insert the catheter, the cardiologist guides a specialized catheter into the coronary artery to the area of the blockage. A small balloon on the end of the catheter is inflated, pushing the fatty material blocking the artery against the blood vessel wall and opening the artery to allow for the normal flow of blood.

USES AND COMPLICATIONS

Catheterization has been used safely and successfully for many years. When a person is unable to breathe on his or her own, airway catheters have been instrumental in saving lives and making such patients more comfortable. Such procedures have been widely used on a daily basis, with few complications.

Likewise, urethral catheters are routinely employed to control the flow of urine from the bladder. This type of catheterization can be seen in many clinical settings. Although caution must be used to prevent the introduction of bacteria into the bladder and subsequent infection, this procedure is considered to be safe and effective.

The overall success rate of cardiac catheterization has been good, with few deaths resulting from the procedure. It is a valuable tool for the diagnosis of heart diseases and disorders because a major incision in the chest is avoided. This procedure is performed many times each day in all cardiac care units. Angioplasty has also been successful, but it is useful for only some types of blockages. A major risk of angioplasty is rupture of the artery if the balloon is inflated too much. When this happens, open heart surgery is necessary to prevent death. The death rate from angioplasty is less than 1 percent, however, and the success rate exceeds 90 percent. Another problem with balloon angioplasty is that in 33 percent of the cases, the blockages reform within six months. Nevertheless, this procedure offers a good alternative to coronary artery bypass surgery.

PERSPECTIVE AND PROSPECTS

The use of catheterization for airway management was first tried in 1871 by Friedrich Trendelenburg. Through the years, such procedures have been improved. Catheters will continue to be instrumental for airway management.

The cardiac catheterization of a living human being was done by Werner Forssmann in the 1920's: He performed the procedure on himself. His techniques were further developed by André Frédéric Cournand in the 1940's, for which he won the Nobel Prize in Physiology or Medicine in 1956. Continued advances in the procedure and improved technology have increased the applications of cardiac catheterization. New and better procedures, which will continue to replace some types of open heart surgery, are expected in the future.

—Bradley R. A. Wilson, Ph.D.

See also Amniocentesis; Anesthesia; Anesthesiology; Angiography; Angioplasty; Biopsy; Blood testing; Cardiology; Circulation; Heart; Lumbar puncture; Pharmacology; Phlebotomy; Radiopharmaceuticals; Respiration; Resuscitation; Surgical procedures; Tracheostomy; Transfusion; Urinary system; Urology; Vascular medicine; Vascular system.

FOR FURTHER INFORMATION:

Finucane, Brendan T., and Albert H. Santora. *Principles of Airway Management*. 3d ed. New York: Springer-Verlag, 2003. Third edition of a practical manual on the anatomy, principles, equipment, and techniques of airway management during surgery. Includes complications, pediatric aspects, and mechanical ventilation.

Karch, Amy Morrison. *Cardiac Care: A Guide for Patient Education*. New York: Appleton-Century-Crofts, 1981. Designed to educate the patient diagnosed with heart disease, this resource assesses some of the popular works on the subject. Includes an index.

Kern, Morton J., ed. *Cardiac Catheterization Handbook*. 4th ed. Philadelphia: Mosby, 2003. A handbook designed for medical personnel. Details procedures for patient care, the handling of intravascular equipment, and the collection and evaluation of angiographic, electrocardiographic, and hemodynamic data.

Nordlicht, Scott M., Alan N. Weiss, and Philip A. Ludbrook. *Why Me? Approaching Coronary Heart Disease, Cardiac Catheterization, and Treatment Options from a Position of Strength*. St. Louis: Northern Lights, 1999. Weiss and Ludbrook lead sufferers step-by-step through the basics of the heart and heart disease. Discusses potential treatments, including cardiac catheterization, drug therapy, balloon angioplasty, stents, atherectomy, and bypass surgery.

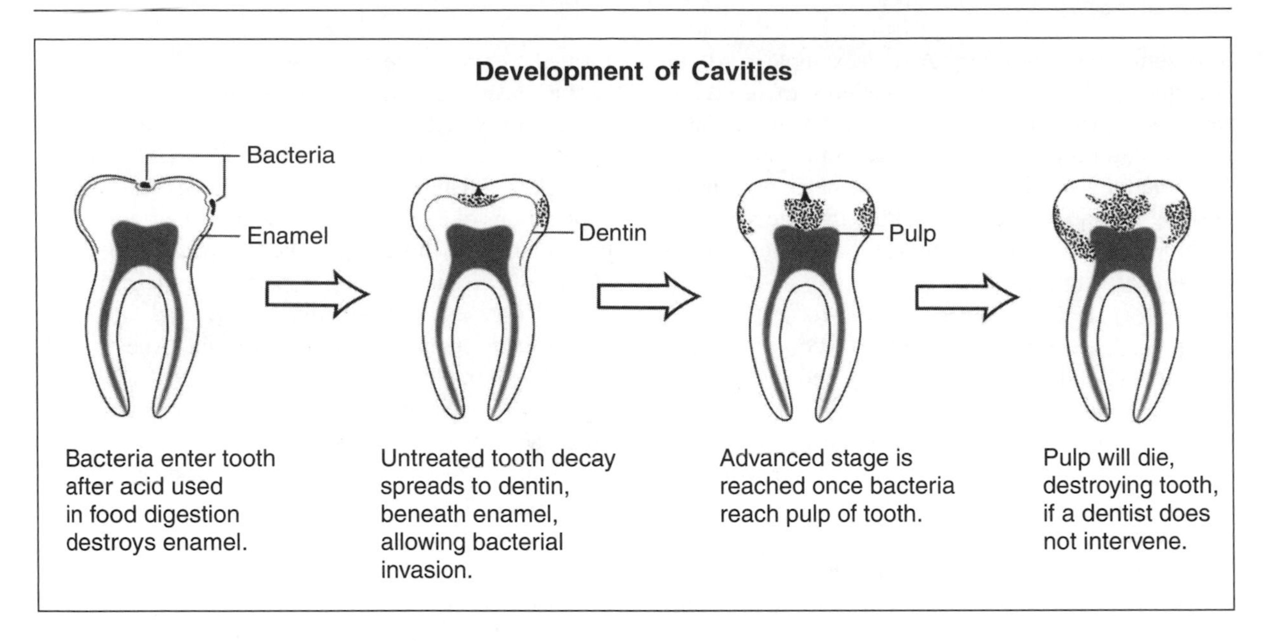

Cavities

Disease/disorder

Also known as: Dental caries

Anatomy or system affected: Gums, teeth

Specialties and related fields: Dentistry

Definition: Cavities are erosions of the surface of teeth that can excavate the tooth surface and damage tooth structure.

Causes and Symptoms

The oral cavity is filled with a variety of bacteria, some of which can ferment foods, especially complex and simple sugars, into organic acids. A mixture of oral bacteria, organic acids, food debris, and saliva combine to form a sticky, creamy-colored substance called plaque. Plaque forms on all teeth, but some are more susceptible to plaque buildup than others. A failure to remove plaque causes it to mineralize into tartar. The combination of plaque and tartar irritates the gums, which results in gingivitis and can ultimately cause an infection of the ligaments and bones that support the teeth (periodontitis). The acids in plaque also dissolve the enamel surface of the tooth, generating a hole that is known as a cavity. Untreated, tooth decay can hollow out a tooth and destroy the nerves and blood vessels inside, resulting in a tooth abscess.

The earliest sign of a cavity is a chalky, white spot on the surface of a tooth, which indicates demineralization of the tooth enamel. At this point, the process is reversible, but the white spot can turn brown and develop into a breach in the enamel. Once the cavity forms, the affected tooth structure cannot be regenerated. Large cavities can cause toothache, particularly after consuming cold, hot, or sweet foods or drinks, but most cavities are typically painless until they grow large enough to affect the nerves. Dental X rays can detect cavities even before they are visible to the naked eye, and cavities usually cause soft spots that are sticky when the tooth is pressed with a probe.

Treatment and Therapy

Treatment of dental cavities requires drilling the tooth to remove the enamel and dentin eroded by the invasion of acid-producing bacteria. Once the affected hard tissues have been removed, a dental filling made from dental amalgam, composite resin, porcelain, or gold is placed into the tooth to restore its structural integrity.

Information on Cavities

Causes: Bacteria, diet (refined sugars or starches), dental plaque, amount and acidity of saliva, quality of tooth enamel, and shape of tooth, leading to destruction of tooth crown; may begin as stains, discolorations, rough spots, or white opaque areas of enamel

Symptoms: Tooth sensitivity to heat or cold, deep aching

Duration: Chronic

Treatments: Fillings made of amalgam, resins, or plastics; artificial crowns

For large cavities that have eroded so much of the tooth structure that restorative material cannot be placed within it, a cap called a crown, made of gold, porcelain, or porcelain fused to metal, is fitted over what remains of the tooth. In some cases, a root canal (endodontic therapy) is necessary if the nervous tissue within the tooth has died as a result of infection. An endodontic file hollows out the tooth, which is then filled with a rubberlike substance called gutta percha. If the level of tooth decay prevents any attempt at restoration, then the tooth is extracted.

Conscientious personal dental hygiene that consists of daily brushing and flossing, regular dental examinations at least twice a year, and diet modification that reduces the intake of simple sugars can reduce the risk of cavities and keep teeth and gums healthy.

—Michael A. Buratovich, Ph.D.

See also Dental diseases; Dentistry; Dentistry, pediatric; Endodontic disease; Gingivitis; Gum disease; Periodontal surgery; Periodontitis; Root canal treatment; Teeth; Tooth extraction; Toothache.

For Further Information:

Frost, Helen, *Food for Healthy Teeth*. Mankato, Minn.: Capstone Press, 2006.

Sutton, Amy, *Dental Care and Oral Health Sourcebook*. Detroit: Omnigraphics, 2003.

Taintor, Jerry F., and Mary Jane Taintor, *The Complete Guide to Better Dental Care*. New York: Checkmark books, 1999.

Celiac sprue

Disease/disorder

Also known as: Nontropical sprue, gluten-sensitive enteropathy

Anatomy or system affected: Intestines, joints

Specialties and related fields: Gastroenterology, internal medicine, nutrition, pediatrics

Definition: Inflammation of the small intestine resulting from an abnormal response to gluten in the diet.

Causes and Symptoms

The most common symptoms of celiac sprue are diarrhea and weight loss. Patients develop an inflammatory reaction to gluten, a protein found in wheat, rye, oats, and barley. This inflammation causes flattening of the fingerlike projections in the small intestine known as villi, thereby decreasing the surface area available for nutrient and fluid absorption. Thus, patients often have anemia (from malabsorption of iron and folic acid) and bone disease (from malabsorption of calcium and vitamin D). Other symptoms of celiac sprue can include muscle weakness, infertility, epilepsy, and psychiatric illnesses, although the mechanisms underlying these manifestations are less clear. Some patients develop a blistering, itching rash on the skin known as dermatitis herpetiformis. Most patients come to medical attention at two years of age, after wheat is introduced into the diet. A small number of people develop the disease as adults. Research suggests that stress can trigger celiac sprue reactions, including extreme emotional stress, pregnancy, surgery, and infections.

Information on Celiac Sprue

Causes: Inflammation of small intestine from gluten in diet

Symptoms: Diarrhea, weight loss, anemia, bone disease

Duration: Chronic, with acute episodes lasting two weeks

Treatments: Elimination of gluten from diet, folic acid supplementation

Treatment and Therapy

The mainstay of therapy is elimination of gluten from the diet, which calms the inflammation and eventually allows the flattened villi to grow back. Symptoms usually improve within two weeks. Lack of improvement is most often the result of incomplete elimination of gluten. Alternative diagnoses must also be considered, including infection, food allergies, inflammatory bowel disease, and lymphoma of the intestines.

The avoidance of gluten sounds straightforward, but it often requires significant dietary changes that must be rigorously followed throughout life. Most breads, pastas, and pastries must be avoided. Patients often benefit from counseling with a nutritionist, since many processed foods contain gluten. Patients may also need to be screened for vitamin and mineral deficiencies. Folic acid supplementation is especially important for women of childbearing age. An X ray to determine bone mineral density is sometimes helpful in patients with suspected vitamin D deficiency.

Perspective and Prospects

Celiac sprue is a genetic disease. It is known to be caused by a mutation on chromosome 6, and attempts to identify the specific gene further are ongoing. Testing to determine whether one has celiac sprue includes blood tests for antibodies against gliadin, the offensive component of gluten. A large scale study done in 2003 found that the incidence rate of celiac sprue is much higher than previously thought, estimated to be about 1 out of every 150 people, or 1.5 million Americans. People at higher risk for celiac sprue are those suffering from diabetes mellitus, Down syndrome, or anemia and those with a family member who has celiac sprue.

—Ahmad Kamal, M.D.; updated by LeAnna DeAngelo, Ph.D.

See also Allergies; Anemia; Diarrhea and dysentery; Gastroenterology; Gastroenterology, pediatric; Gastrointestinal system; Intestinal disorders; Intestines; Malabsorption; Malnutrition; Nutrition; Vitamins and minerals; Weight loss and gain.

For Further Information:

Green, Peter, and Rory Jones. *Celiac Disease: A Hidden Epidemic*. New York: HarperCollins, 2006.

Korn, Danna. *Kids with Celiac Disease: A Family Guide to Raising Happy, Healthy, Gluten-Free Children*. Bethesda, Md.: Woodbine House, 2001.

Parker, James N., and Philip M. Parker, eds. *The Official Patient's Sourcebook on Celiac Disease*. San Diego, Calif.: Icon Health, 2002.

Tessmer, Kimberly A. *Gluten-Free for a Healthy Life: Nutritional Advice and Recipes for Those Suffering from Celiac Disease and Other Gluten-Related Disorders*. Franklin Lakes, N.J.: New Page Books, 2003.

Cells

Biology

Anatomy or system affected: Bones, immune system, musculoskeletal system, nerves, nervous system, skin

Specialties and related fields: Bacteriology, cytology, histology

Definition: The fundamental structural and functional units of all living organisms.

Key terms:

chromosome: one DNA molecule of the cell nucleus, held in combination with chromosomal proteins

cytoskeleton: a network of filaments (including microtubules, microfilaments, and intermediate filaments) that supports the cytoplasm and extensions of the cell surface

endoplasmic reticulum: a system of cytoplasmic membrane-bound sacs that, with attached ribosomes, synthesize proteins destined to enter membranes or to be stored or secreted

gene: a segment of DNA encoding a protein; RNA molecules such as messenger and ribosomal RNA

Golgi complex: a system of membrane sacs in which proteins are chemically modified, sorted, and routed to various cellular destinations

membrane: a thin layer of lipid and protein molecules that controls transport of molecules and ions between the cell and its exterior and between membrane-bound compartments within the cell

mitochondrion: a membrane-bound cytoplasmic organelle that constitutes the primary location of oxidative reactions providing energy for cellular activities

nucleolus: a nuclear structure formed through the activity of chromosome segments in the production of ribosomal RNA and the assembly of ribosomal subunits

peroxisome: a membrane-bound organelle that contains reaction systems linking biochemical pathways taking place elsewhere in the cell; also called a microbody

ribosome: a cytoplasmic particle assembled from ribosomal RNA and ribosomal proteins that uses messenger RNA molecules as directions for synthesizing proteins

Structure and Functions

Cells contain complex biochemical systems that can use energy sources to power cellular activities such as growth, movement, and reaction to environmental changes. The information required to assemble the enzymatic and structural molecules involved in these activities is stored in cells and is duplicated and passed on in cell division.

Cells are divided into two major internal regions, nucleus and cytoplasm, which reflect a fundamental division of labor. In the nucleus are the deoxyribonucleic acid (DNA) molecules that store the hereditary information required for cell growth and reproduction. The nuclear region also contains enzymes that copy the hereditary information into ribonucleic acid (RNA), which is used as instructions for making proteins in the cytoplasm. Enzymes within the nucleus also duplicate the DNA in preparation for cell division. The cytoplasm makes proteins according to the directions copied in the nucleus and also synthesizes most other mol-

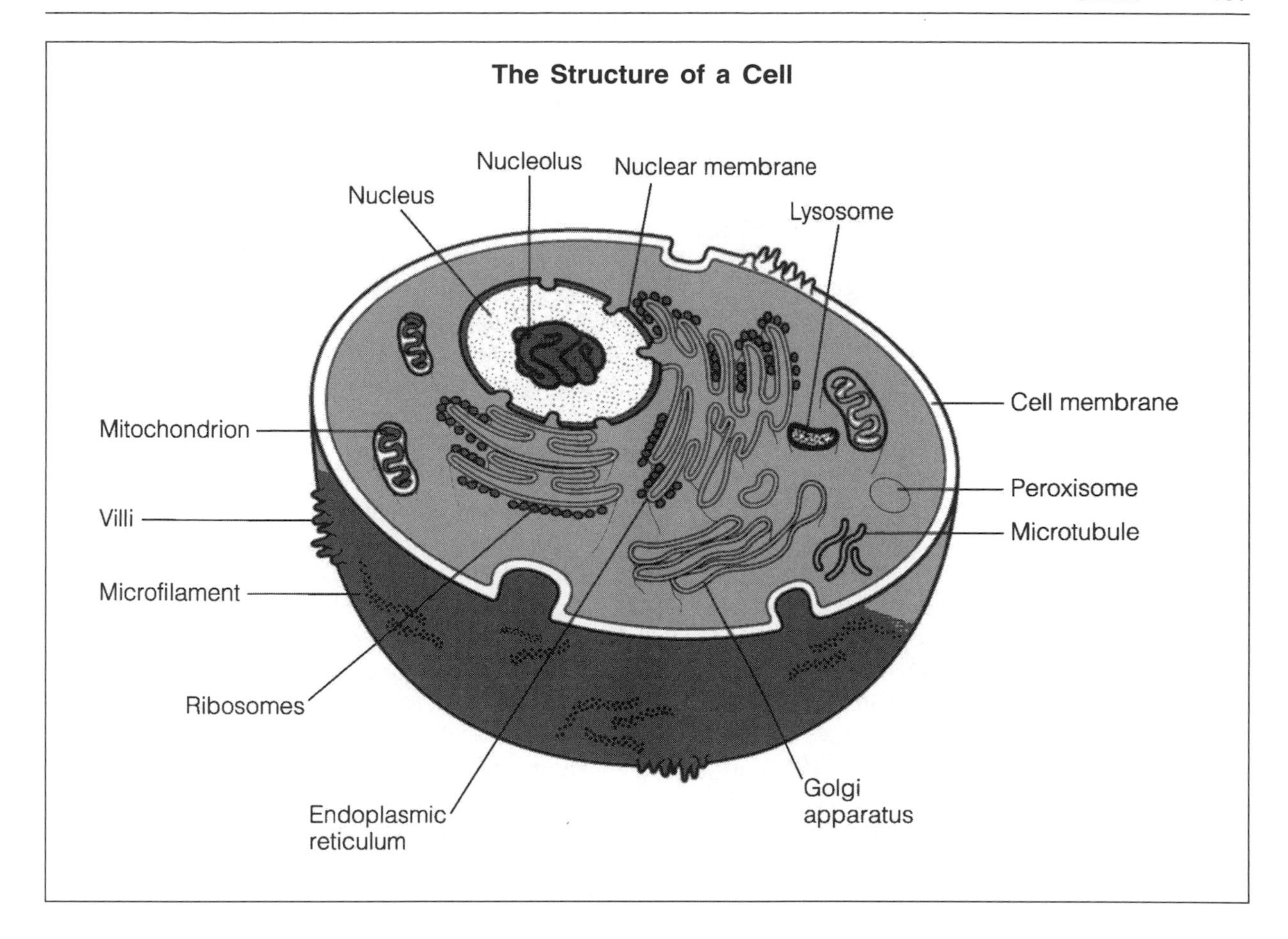

ecules required for cellular activities. The cytoplasm carries out several additional vital functions, including motility and the conversion of fuel substances into usable forms of chemical energy.

Cells are organized by membranes. These layers of lipid and protein molecules, not much more than 7 to 8 nanometers thick, form an outer boundary, the plasma membrane, which separates the cell contents from the exterior. Several internal membrane systems divide the cell interior into specialized compartments called organelles. The lipid part of membranes consists of a double layer of molecules called a bilayer. The lipid bilayer provides the structural framework of membranes and acts as a barrier to the passage of water-soluble substances. Membrane proteins, which are suspended in the lipid bilayer or attached to its surfaces, carry out the specialized functions of membranes.

The plasma membrane forming the outer cell boundary has a variety of functions. The most significant is the transport of substances between the cytoplasm and the cell's exterior, which is carried out by proteins forming channels in the membrane. These channels pass specific water-soluble molecules or ions. The plasma membrane also contains proteins functioning as receptors, which recognize and bind to specific molecules from the surrounding medium. On binding to their target molecules, which include peptide hormones, many receptors trigger internal cellular responses that coordinate the activities of cells in tissues and organs. Other plasma membrane proteins recognize and adhere to molecules on the surfaces of other cells or to extracellular structures such as collagen. These adhesive functions are critical to the development and maintenance of tissues and organs. Other plasma membrane proteins identify cells as part of the individual or as foreign.

The nucleus is separated from the cytoplasm by two concentric membranes, one layered just inside the other, forming a system known as the nuclear envelope. At closely spaced intervals, the envelope is perforated by pores, about 70 to 90 nanometers in diameter, which form channels between the nuclear interior and the surrounding cytoplasm. The pores are filled by a ringlike mass of proteins that controls the movement of large molecules, such as proteins and RNA, through the nuclear envelope.

Within the nucleus are chromatin fibers containing the nuclear DNA, held in association with two major types of proteins, the histone and nonhistone chromosomal proteins. The histones are primarily structural molecules that pack DNA into chromatin fibers. The nonhistones include proteins that regulate gene activity. The hereditary information of the human nucleus is subdivided among forty-six linear DNA molecules. Each individual DNA molecule, with its associated histone and nonhistone proteins, is a chromosome of the nucleus.

Each segment of a chromosome containing the information used to make an RNA copy constitutes a gene. One type of gene encodes messenger RNA (mRNA) molecules, which contain information required to make proteins. Another type of gene encodes ribosomal RNA (rRNA) molecules. Ribosomal RNA forms part of ribosomes, complex RNA-protein particles in the cytoplasm that assemble proteins according to the directions carried in mRNA molecules. The regions of the chromosomes active in making rRNA are collected into structures called nucleoli. Within nucleoli, rRNAs are assembled with proteins into subunits of ribosomes.

The cytoplasm surrounding the nucleus is packed with ribosomes and a variety of organelles. The boundary membranes of the organelles set them off as distinct chemical and molecular environments, specialized to carry out different functions. Ribosomes may be either freely suspended in the cytoplasm or attached to the surfaces of a system of flattened, membranous sacs called the endoplasmic reticulum. Freely suspended ribosomes make proteins that enter the cytoplasmic solution as enzymes, structural supports, or motile elements. Ribosomes attached to the endoplasmic reticulum assemble proteins that become part of membranes or eventually enter small, membrane-bound sacs for storage or release to the cell exterior.

Proteins made in the rough endoplasmic reticulum—those sacs with ribosomes—are modified chemically in another system of membranous sacs, the Golgi complex or apparatus. This system usually appears as a cup-shaped stack of flattened, ribosome-free sacs. The modifications carried out in the Golgi complex may include the addition of chemical groups such as sugars, and the clipping of surplus segments from proteins. Following modification, proteins are sorted into small, membrane-bound sacs that pinch off from the Golgi membranes. These sacs may be stored in the cytoplasm or may release their contents to the cell exterior.

One type of membrane-bound sac containing stored proteins, the lysosome, is particularly important to cell function. Lysosomes contain a group of enzymes collectively capable of breaking down all major molecules of the cell. Many substances taken into cells are delivered to lysosomes, where they are digested by the lysosomal enzymes. Lysosomes may also release their enzymes into the cytoplasm or to the cell exterior. Release within the cell causes cell death, which may be part of pathological conditions or may occur as part of normal development.

Most of the chemical energy required for cellular activities is produced by reactions taking place in another cytoplasmic organelle, the mitochondrion. Mitochondria are surrounded by two separate membranes, one enclosed within the other. Within mitochondria occur most of the oxidative reactions that release energy for cellular activities. Fuel for these reactions is provided by breakdown products of all major cellular molecules, including carbohydrates, fats, proteins, and nucleic acids.

The oxidative functions of mitochondria are supplemented by the activities of peroxisomes (also called microbodies). These structures, which consist simply of a boundary membrane surrounding a solution of enzymes, carry out reactions that link major oxidative pathways occurring elsewhere in the cytoplasm. Microbodies are particularly important to the oxidation of fatty acids.

Almost all cell movements are generated by either of two cytoplasmic structures, microtubules or microfilaments. Microtubules form the motile elements of sperm tails; microfilaments are responsible for the movements of skeletal, cardiac, and smooth muscle. Microtubules are fine, hollow cylinders about 25 nanometers in diameter, assembled from subunits of a protein known as tubulin. Microfilaments are thin, solid fibers 5 to 7 nanometers in diameter, assembled from subunits of a different protein, actin. Both structures produce motion through protein crossbridges that work as transducers converting chemical energy to mechanical energy. One end of a crossbridge attaches to the surface of a microtubule or microfilament; the opposite, reactive end attaches to another microtubule or microfilament or to other cell structures. The crossbridge produces motion by making an attachment at its reactive end, forcefully swiveling a short distance, and then releasing. Distinct proteins form the swiveling crossbridges for the two motile elements.

In addition to their functions in cell motility, both microtubules and microfilaments form supportive networks inside cells collectively called the cytoskeleton. Another group of supportive fibers with diameters averaging about 100 nanometers, the intermediate filaments, also forms parts of the cytoskeleton. Intermediate filaments assemble from a large family of related proteins that is distinct from the tubulins and actins forming microtubules and microfilaments.

Disorders and Diseases

Because cell structure and function underlie the totality of bodily functions, all aspects of health and disease reflect normal and abnormal cellular activities. Perhaps the most critical and important of these activities to contemporary medical science is the conversion of normal to abnormal activity responsible for cancer. In cancer, cells grow and divide uncontrollably, break free from their normal cell contacts, and migrate to other regions of the body.

The cell transformations occurring in the development of cancer involve changes at several levels. Most of these changes reflect an alteration of one or more genes in the cell nucleus from normal to aberrant forms called oncogenes. Most oncogenes prove to encode proteins involved in a relatively small number of activities. These include nonhistone proteins regulating gene activity, growth hormones, receptors in the plasma membrane for peptide hormones, and proteins taking part in internal cellular response systems triggered by receptors. Directly or indirectly, the altered proteins encoded in oncogenes induce internal changes that lead to uncontrolled cell division and loss of normal adhesions to neighboring cells.

For example, the oncogene *src* encodes a protein that adds phosphate groups to other proteins as a cellular control measure. In many types of cancer cells, the *src* gene or its product is hyperactive. One of the targets of the enzyme encoded in the gene is a receptor protein of the plasma membrane. In some cancer cells, uncontrolled addition of phosphate groups to the receptor causes it to lose its attachment to extracellular structures that hold the cells in place. This loss contributes to the tendency of the tumor cells to break loose and migrate to other parts of the body.

In some cases, movement of DNA segments from one chromosome to another is involved in the transformation of cells from normal to cancerous types, including several types of leukemia. For example, in many leukemias, breaks occur in chromosomes 8 and 14 of the human set in cell lines producing leukocytes, and segments are exchanged between the chromosomes. The exchange moves the gene *myc* from its normal location in chromosome 8 to a region of chromosome 14 that encodes a major segment of antibody proteins. In its normal location, the *myc* gene encodes a chromosomal regulatory protein that controls genes involved in cell division. When translocated to chromosome 14, *myc* comes under the influence of DNA sequences that promote the high activity of the antibody gene. As a result, *myc* becomes hyperactive in triggering cell division and contributes to the uncontrolled division of white blood cells characteristic of leukemias.

Alterations in cytoplasmic organelles are also directly responsible for some human diseases. The enzymes contained in lysosomes are abnormally secreted in many human diseases. The degenerative changes of arthritis, for example, are suspected to be caused in part by the abnormal release of enzymes from the lysosomes of bone or lymph cells into the fluids that lubricate joints. Some of the damage to lung tissues caused by inhalation of silica fibers in silicosis is also related to lysosomal function. Microscopic silica fibers are taken in by macrophages and other cells in the lungs; these fibers are delivered to lysosomes for breakdown, as are many other substances. The fibers accumulate in the lysosomes, causing lysosomal enlargement and eventually breakage, with destructive release of lysosomal enzymes into the cytoplasm. Some human diseases related to lysosomes are caused by inherited mutations destroying the activity of lysosomal enzymes. For example, an inherited deficiency in one lysosomal enzyme, hexosaminidase, interferes with reactions clipping carbohydrate segments from molecules removed from the cell surface. As a result, the subparts of these molecules accumulate in lysosomes and cannot be recycled. Their concentration on cell surfaces is diminished; loss of these molecules from nerve cells, particularly a group called gangliosides, can lead to seizures, blindness, loss of intellect, and early death.

Human disease has also been linked to inherited changes in mitochondria. The mutations interfere with the oxidative reactions inside the organelle or have detrimental effects on the transport of substances through the mitochondrial membranes. The mutations cause the most severe problems in locations where the energy supplied by mitochondria is highly critical, particularly in the central nervous system and skeletal and cardiac muscle. Mitochondrial deficiencies in these locations are typically responsible for symptoms such as muscular weakness, irregularities in the heartbeat, and epilepsy.

Deficiencies in motile systems based on microtubules and microfilaments are also associated with human disease. For example, a group of inherited defects known as the immotile cilia or Kartagener's syndrome is characterized by acute bronchitis, sinusitis, chronic headache, male sterility, and reversal of the position of the heart from the left to the right side of the body. In individuals with the disease, the cyclic crossbridges driving microtubule-based motion are missing. Male sterility results from loss of motility by sperm tails; other deficiencies result from the immotility of cilia on cells lining the respiratory system and the cavities of the brain. (Cilia are microtubule-based cellular appendages that beat like sperm tails to maintain the flow of fluids over cell surfaces.) In the respiratory system, loss of ciliary beating stops the flow of mucus that normally removes irritating and infectious matter from the lungs and respiratory tract. This deficiency explains the sinusitis and bronchitis. Presumably, an insufficient flow of fluids in the ventricles of the brain, normally maintained by ciliated cells lining these cavities, produces the headaches. The reversed position taken by the heart remains unexplained.

Even the cytoskeleton has been associated with human disease. For example, deficiencies in intermediate filaments of the cytoskeleton have been implicated in the hereditary disease epidermolysis bullosa. In this disease, skin cells are fragile, and slight abrasions that would cause little or no problem in normal individuals lead to severe blistering, ulceration, and scarring.

PERSPECTIVE AND PROSPECTS

Knowledge of cell structure and function developed gradually from the first morphological descriptions of cells in the seventeenth century. By the 1830's, enough information had accumulated for Theodor Schwann and Matthias Schleiden to propose that all living organisms are composed of one or more cells and that cells are the minimum functional units of living organisms. Their conclusions were supplemented in 1855 by a third postulate by Rudolf Virchow: that all cells arise only from preexisting cells by a process of division. Further work established that the cell nucleus contains hereditary information and that the essential feature of cell division is transmission of this information from parent to daughter cells.

The study of cell chemistry and physiology began in the late eighteenth and early nineteenth centuries. By the end of the nineteenth century, investigators had isolated, identified, and synthesized many organic substances found in cells and worked out the structural components of proteins and nucleic acids. This chemical work was complemented by biochemical studies leading to the discovery of enzymes. The gradual integration of cell structure, physiology, and biochemistry continued; by the 1930's, the field had shifted from morphological observations to biochemical and molecular studies of cell function. Crucial to this shift was the research of George Beadle and Edward Tatum, who concluded from their studies that mutant genes encode a faulty form of an enzyme necessary to produce a substance needed for normal growth. On this basis, they proposed that each gene codes for a single enzyme—the famous "one gene-one enzyme" hypothesis.

Further biochemical work revealed the oxidative reactions providing chemical energy for cell activities. This research was integrated with structural studies of cytoplasmic organelles by Albert Claude, who developed a technique for isolating and purifying cell parts by cell fractionation and centrifugation. Claude and his associates successfully isolated ribosomes, endoplasmic reticulum, Golgi complexes, lysosomes, microbodies, and mitochondria by these methods, which allowed biochemical analysis of the fractions. This work was facilitated by development of the electron microscope, allowing elucidation of the ultrastructure of many of the organelles studied biochemically in cell fractions.

Experiments in the 1940's implicating DNA as the hereditary molecule sparked an intensive effort to work out the three-dimensional structure of this molecule, culminating in the discovery of DNA structure in 1953 by James D. Watson and Francis Crick. Their discovery led to an effort to determine the molecular structure of genes and their modes of action, which was greatly facilitated by the development of rapid methods for nucleic acid sequencing. Using these methods, many genes have been completely sequenced; the sequences, in turn, allowed deduction of the amino acid sequences of many proteins. The comparisons of gene and protein sequences and structure in normal and mutant forms made possible by these developments provided fundamental insights into the mechanisms controlling and regulating genes and the molecular functions of proteins, revolutionizing biology and medicine.

—Stephen L. Wolfe, Ph.D.

See also Amniocentesis; Antibiotics; Bacteriology; Biopsy; Cancer; Cholesterol; Chorionic villus sampling; Cloning; Cytology; Cytopathology; DNA and RNA; Enzymes; Gene therapy; Genetic engineering; Genetics and inheritance; Glycolysis; Gram staining; Immunology; Immunopathology; Karyotyping; Laboratory tests; Microbiology; Microscopy; Mutation; Oncology; Pathology; Proteomics; Stem cell research.

For Further Information:

Alberts, Bruce, et al. *Molecular Biology of the Cell*. 4th ed. New York: Garland, 2002. Describes the evolution of cells and introduces cell structure and function. The text is clearly written at the college level and is illustrated by numerous diagrams and photographs.

Campbell, Neil A., et al. *Biology: Concepts and Connections*. 5th ed. San Francisco: Pearson/Benjamin Cummings, 2006. This classic introductory textbook provides an excellent discussion of essential biological structures and mechanisms. Of particular interest are the five chapters making up the unit titled "The Cell."

Kindt, Thomas J., Richard A. Goldsby, and Barbara A. Osborne. *Kuby Immunology*. 6th ed. New York: W. H. Freeman, 2007. Presents research advances in the field and gives a good overview of the cells and organs involved in the immune system.

Lewin, Benjamin. *Genes IX*. 9th rev. ed. Sudbury, Mass.: Jones & Bartlett, 2007. A college textbook that discusses the entire field of molecular biology and genetics, with many references to the structure and activity of the cell nucleus. Although written at the college level, it is readable and accessible to a general audience.

Lodish, Harvey, et al. *Molecular Cell Biology*. 5th ed. New York: W. H. Freeman, 2004. Outlines the evolution of cells and basic cell structure and function and describes technical approaches used in the study of cells.

Rasmussen, Nicolas. *Picture Control: The Microscope and the Transformation of Biology in America, 1940-1960*. Stanford, Calif.: Stanford University Press, 1997. Rasmussen explores the impact of one of the most productive of the new technologies, electron microscopy, on the biological sciences. This study covers the history of the discipline, beginning in the late 1930's.

Wolfe, Stephen L. *Molecular and Cellular Biology*. Belmont, Calif.: Wadsworth, 1993. Chapter 1, "Introduction to Cell and Molecular Biology," presents cell structure and function and outlines the history of developments in cell biology, biochemistry, and molecular biology.

Centers for Disease Control and Prevention (CDC)

Organization

Definition: One of the divisions of the Department of Health and Human Services in the United States; the CDC is the highest level of governmental health organization in the country.

Key terms:

Department of Health and Human Services: a federal organization, headed by a member of the U.S. president's cabinet, concerned with the health of the nation's citizens

health organizations: organizations that help to shape people's ability to respond effectively to health-related issues by protecting and promoting good health

Role in the United States

The Centers for Disease Control and Prevention (CDC) is located in Atlanta, Georgia. The mission of the CDC is to promote health and quality of life by preventing and controlling disease, injury, and disability. The organization is charged with protecting the public health of the United States by providing leadership and direction in the prevention and control of disease and other preventable conditions and responding to public health emergencies. The CDC claims to hold three core values. The first is accountability. As diligent stewards of public trust and public funds, the CDC acts decisively and compassionately in service of the people's health. The CDC ensures that its research and services are based on sound science and meet real public needs to achieve public health goals. The second is respect. The CDC respects and understands the interdependence of all people both inside the agency and throughout the world. It values their contributions and individual and cultural diversities. The CDC is committed to achieving a diverse workforce at all levels of the organization. The third is integrity. The CDC is honest and ethical in all it does. The CDC prizes scientific integrity and professional excellence.

The CDC is responsible for maintaining, recording, and analyzing disease trends of all types of diseases, including communicable diseases and diseases resulting from lifestyle, occupational, and environmental causes. The CDC also publishes reports on all these diseases, including the *Morbidity and Mortality Weekly*

Report (MMWR), which reports the most current incidence and prevalence statistics for forty-nine reportable diseases. The MMWR also provides a means of disseminating and describing new regularity changes or health information pertinent to public health and safety for local communities. As a federal government health agency, the CDC supports state and local health departments and cooperates with similar national health organizations of other nations. The CDC also provides guidelines for disease prevention. The structure of the CDC is formed by centers, institutes, and officers, which carry out the diverse functions of disease prevention and control. Its divisions are responsible for specific aspects of public health.

The mission of the National Center for Environmental Health (NCEH) is to provide national leadership through science, which promotes health and quality of life by preventing or controlling disease, birth defects, disabilities, or deaths that result from interactions between people and their environment. NCEH especially is committed to safeguarding the health of populations that are particularly vulnerable to certain environmental hazards, including children, the elderly, and people with disabilities.

NCEH conducts research in the laboratory and in the field to investigate the effects of the environment on health. NCEH tracks and evaluates environment-related health problems through surveillance systems. NCEH also helps domestic and international agencies and organizations prepare for and respond to natural, technologic, humanitarian, and terrorism-related environmental emergencies. The scope of NCEH work also includes educating various audiences about environmental health, developing new standards and guidelines in this field, helping formulate public policy, and providing training and technical assistance for officials of state and local health agencies in preventing and responding to public health challenges.

The National Center for Health Statistics (NCHS) is the U.S. government's principal vital and health statistics agency. The mission of NCHS is to provide statistical information that will guide policies to improve the health of the American people. Since 1960, when the National Office of Vital Statistics and the National Health Survey merged to form NCHS, the agency has provided a wide variety of data to monitor national health. NCHS data systems include data on vital events, such as birth and death, as well as information on health status, lifestyle, and exposure to unhealthy influences, the onset and diagnosis of illness and disability, and the uses of health care. These data are used by governmental policymakers, by medical researchers, and by others in the health community.

The National Vital Statistics System in NCHS includes birth data, mortality data, fetal death data, and linked births/infant deaths. Some of the important NCHS health data systems include National Health Interview Survey, National Health Interview Survey on Disability, National Health and Nutrition Examination Survey, National Health Care Survey, Ambulatory Health Care Data, Hospital Discharge and Ambulatory Surgery Data, National Home and Hospice Care Survey, National Nursing Home Survey, National Employer Health Insurance Survey, National Survey of Family Growth, National Maternal and Infant Health Survey, and National Immunization Survey.

Prevention and Health Promotion

The mission of the National Center for Chronic Disease Prevention and Health Promotion is to prevent death and disability from chronic diseases; to promote maternal, infant, and adolescent health; to promote healthy personal behaviors; and to accomplish these goals in partnership with health and education agencies, major voluntary associations, the private sector, and other federal agencies.

Chronic diseases are health conditions that last longer than three months. In the United States, the leading causes of death are chronic diseases, such as heart disease, cancer, stroke, and diabetes, which are often the result of an unhealthy lifestyle. Within the center, there are divisions of cancer prevention and control, diabetes, arthritis, epilepsy, genomics, smoking and health, nutrition and physical activity, reproductive health, oral health, adolescent and school health, and adult and community health.

Within this center there are three divisions: the Division of HIV/AIDS Prevention, the Division of Sexually Transmitted Diseases Prevention, and the Division of Tuberculosis Elimination. As the name implies, the mission of the Division of HIV/AIDS Prevention is to prevent HIV infection and reduce illness and death related to HIV/AIDS. In collaboration with community, state, national, and international partners, the Division of HIV/AIDS Prevention conducts research on behavioral intervention, program evaluation, and epidemiology of HIV/AIDS. It also provides community assistance, technical information, training, and prevention services related to HIV/AIDS.

The Division of Sexually Transmitted Diseases Prevention provides national leadership through research, policy development, and support of effective services to prevent sexually transmitted diseases (STDs) and their complications, such as infertility, adverse outcomes of pregnancy, and reproductive tract cancer. The Division of STD Prevention assists health departments, health care providers, and nongovernmental organizations through the development of goals and policies; synthesis, translation, and dissemination of timely science-based information; and the development and support of science-based programs that meet the needs of communities. The Division of STD Prevention also conducts surveillance; epidemiological, behavioral, and operational research; and program evaluation related to STDs, including syphilis, gonorrhea, chlamydia, human papillomavirus, genital herpes, and hepatitis B.

The Division of Tuberculosis Elimination works to provide leadership in preventing, controlling, and eventually eliminating tuberculosis (TB) from the United States. The activities that are carried out in the Division of Tuberculosis Elimination include developing and advocating effective and appropriate TB prevention and control policies; supporting a nationwide framework for monitoring TB morbidity and mortality; detecting and investigating TB outbreaks; conducting clinical, epidemiological, behavioral, and operational research to enhance TB prevention and control efforts; evaluating prevention effectiveness; providing funding and technical assistance to state and local health departments; and providing training, education, and technical services to state and local health departments.

The mission of the National Center for Infectious Diseases (NCID) is to prevent illness, disability, and death caused by infectious disease in the United States and around the world. Infectious diseases are diseases that are caused by bacteria, viruses, or other microorganisms and can be transmitted from one person to another. With universal immunization and effective antibiotics, infectious diseases are no longer a public health threat in industrialized countries. However, infectious diseases are the leading cause of death worldwide. Deaths from infectious disease in the United States have been increasing recently because new diseases emerge, old diseases rebound, and inappropriate use of antibiotics results in drug-resistant germs. To meet this challenge, NCID conducts surveillance, epidemic investigations, epidemiological and laboratory research, training, and public education programs. NCID also develops, evaluates, and promotes prevention and control strategies for infectious diseases.

As the lead federal agency for injury prevention, the National Center for Injury Prevention and Control (NCIPC) works closely with other federal agencies; national, state, and local organizations; state and local health departments; and research institutes to prevent and reduce injury, disability, death, and costs associated with injuries outside the workplace. Injury is the leading cause of death and disability among children and young adults. Injury is a serious public health problem because of its impact on the health of the United States, including premature death, disability, and the burden on the health care system. Common unintentional injuries are falls, fires, drownings, poisonings, motor vehicle crashes, recreational activities accidents, and playground and day care accidents. Intentional injuries are related to suicide, youth violence, family and intimate partner violence, and homicide. Injury prevention strategies focus primarily on environmental design, such as road construction that permits optimum visibility, product design, human behavior, education, and legislative and regulatory requirements that support environmental and behavioral change.

Vaccination and Immunization

The National Vaccine Program Office is designated to provide leadership and coordination among federal agencies and to oversee that they work together to carry out the goals of the National Vaccine Plan. The National Vaccine Plan provides a framework, including goals, objectives, and strategies, for pursuing the prevention of infectious diseases through immunizations. This office develops and implements strategies for achieving the highest possible level of prevention of human diseases through immunization and the highest possible level of prevention of adverse reactions to vaccines.

The National Immunization Program (NIP) is a disease prevention program that provides leadership for the planning, coordination, and conduct of immunization activities nationwide. NIP provides consultation, training, and statistical, educational, epidemiological, and technical services to assist health departments in planning, developing, and implementing immunization programs. NIP assists health departments in developing vaccine information management systems to facilitate identification of children who need vaccinations, to help parents and providers to ensure that all children are immunized at the appropriate age, to assess vaccination levels in state and local areas, and to monitor the safety and efficiency of vaccines by linking vaccine administration information to adverse event reporting and disease outbreak patterns. NIP also administers research and operational programs for the prevention and control of vaccine-preventable diseases.

OTHER AGENCIES AND OFFICES

As a federal agency, the National Institute for Occupational Safety and Health (NIOSH) is responsible for conducting research into the full scope of occupational disease and injury and making recommendations for the prevention of work-related disease, injury, and disability. The occupational diseases range from lung disease in miners to carpal tunnel syndrome in computer users. Each day, an average of 9,000 U.S. workers sustain disabling injuries on the job, 17 workers die from an injury sustained at work, and 137 workers die from work-related diseases. The economic burden of occupational health problems is high. NIOSH is a diverse organization made up of professionals representing a wide range of disciplines including industrial hygiene, nursing, epidemiology, engineering, medicine, and statistics. NIOSH investigates potentially hazardous working conditions when requested by employers or employees and provides training to occupational safety and health professionals.

The overall health of the United States depends on the health status of its minority population. The major minority groups in the United States include African Americans, Asian and Pacific Islander Americans, Native Americans, and Hispanic Americans, who may be of any race. Compared to the United States as a whole, minority populations, particularly African Americans, suffer higher rates of morbidity and mortality. Native Americans and Hispanics also have worse health outcomes than the total population. Although Asian American and Pacific Islanders overall have reasonably good health indicators, some subgroups have very poor health status. By providing health promotion and communication strategies, policy recommendations, research, and program development, the Office of the Associate Director for Minority Health is committed to developing cooperative and interagency agreements among various federal, state, local, and private agencies and organizations concerned with minority health.

Because of the globalization of the world economy, health problems associated with global movements of people and commerce are increasing. One country's health problems today can become another country's health problems tomorrow. Diseases are losing their boundaries, and global health efforts are necessary. The mission of the Office of Global Health is to improve health worldwide by providing leadership, coordination, and support for the CDC's global health activities in collaboration with the CDC's global health partners. This office provides leadership in the development of cross-cutting policy, plans, and programs related to the CDC's global health interests; assists the CDC's divisions, other federal agencies, or nongovernmental agencies in the implementation of appropriate policy, plans, and programs for which they have responsibilities; and enhances global health partnerships by serving as the entry point for external organizations with an interest in the CDC's global health activities.

Advances in human genetics have demonstrated the potential public health impact of effectively applying genetics to disease prevention. Several CDC programs have been heavily involved with genetics for many years. The Office of Genetics and Disease Prevention works to integrate advances in human genetics into public health research, policy, and program development and evaluation and to provide a coordinated focus for the CDC's genetics efforts with particular emphasis on communication and training.

PERSPECTIVE AND PROSPECTS

The CDC had its origin in the U.S. antimalaria program of World War II and was recognized as the Communicable Disease Center in 1946, when the main health problems were infectious diseases. It became the Center for Disease Control in 1970, then the Centers for Disease Control in 1980, and the words "and Prevention" were added in 1992, though Congress requested that the CDC remain the agency's initials. Currently, the CDC conducts research into the origin and occurrence of communicable diseases as well as noncommunicable diseases and develops methods for their control and prevention. The CDC is a powerful leader in the public health of the United States.

—Kimberly Y. Z. Forrest, Ph.D.

See also Accidents; Acquired immunodeficiency syndrome (AIDS); Bacterial infections; Bacteriology; Childhood infectious diseases; Ebola virus; Environmental diseases; Environmental health; Epidemiology; Immunization and vaccination; Microbiology; National Institutes of Health (NIH); Occupational health; Preventive medicine; Safety issues for children; Safety issues for the elderly; Tuberculosis; Viral infections; World Health Organization.

FOR FURTHER INFORMATION:

Etheridge, Elizabeth W. *Sentinel for Health: A History of the Centers for Disease Control*. Berkeley: University of California Press, 1992. A history of the Centers for Disease Control from its inception during World War II through the mid-1980's, written by a professor of history.

Giesecke, Johan. *Modern Infectious Disease Epidemiology*. 2d ed. New York: Oxford University Press, 2002. Divided into two sections, the first covers the tools and principles of epidemiology from an infectious disease perspective. The second covers the role of contact pattern from an assessment angle, exploring such topics as infectivity, incubation periods, seroepidemiology, and immunity.

McCormick, Joseph B., Susan Fisher-Hoch, and Leslie Alan Horvitz. *Level 4: Virus Hunters of the CDC*. Rev ed. New York: Barnes and Noble Books, 1999. A popular account of the role of the CDC in identifying, tracking, and containing viruses.

Mintzer, Richard. *The National Institutes of Health*. Philadelphia: Chelsea House, 2002. An excellent book for teens which traces the history of infectious disease epidemics in the United States, as well as the history of the National Institutes of Health, the structure and role of that institution, and current major health concerns that are its focus.

Regis, Edward. *Virus Ground Zero: Stalking the Killer Viruses with the Centers for Disease Control*. New York: Pocket Books, 1996. Relates the CDC's role in the containment of an outbreak of the Ebola virus in Kikwit, Zaire, in 1995.

Rom, Mark Carl. *Fatal Extraction: Kimberly Bergalis, the Centers for Disease Control, Health Care Workers, and HIV*. San Francisco: Jossey-Bass, 1997. Written by the principal investigator for the Government Accounting Office's investigation into the CDC's handling of the case of Bergalis, who allegedly contracted AIDS from her dentist.

CEREBRAL PALSY

DISEASE/DISORDER

ALSO KNOWN AS: Little's disease

ANATOMY OR SYSTEM AFFECTED: Brain

SPECIALTIES AND RELATED FIELDS: Dentistry, epidemiology, family medicine, neurology, obstetrics, orthopedics, pediatrics, physical therapy, podiatry, preventive medicine, psychology, public health, speech pathology

DEFINITION: A motor disability evident early in life (often by one year of age and certainly by age two) that is caused by a brain abnormality present by the end of the newborn period (one month of age) and unchanged after that time.

KEY TERMS:

athetosis: involuntary movements that are slow and writhing

chorea: rapid involuntary movements

in utero: occurring in the womb

intraventricular: within the brain spaces called the lateral ventricles

Moro reflex: an involuntary movement in which both arms go outward and upward

motor disability: difficulty in carrying out voluntary movements

posterior rhizotomy: a surgical procedure done on the lower back in which some of the sensory (posterior) nerve roots to the leg muscles are cut

premature infant: an infant born before thirty-seven weeks of pregnancy

prevalence: the number of persons with a disorder divided by the number of persons in the population

primitive reflexes: reflexes present in infants but gone by one year of age

term infant: an infant born after thirty-seven weeks of pregnancy

white matter: the brain fibers that connect neurons

CAUSES AND SYMPTOMS

Cerebral palsy is not a single disorder. Rather, it is a group of disorders that affect the brain at some time before a child is one month old, resulting in a lack of normal control of movements. While problems with making normal movements may be apparent at birth, this symptom is often not noticeable until the child is nine or ten months of age; on occasion, it may not be apparent before eighteen or twenty-four months of age because the areas of the brain that control movement are immature and not very effective early in life. Until the child reaches an age at which these areas are functional, a lack of function may go unrecognized. For example, problems using the legs may not be evident until the child is old enough to try to walk. Sometimes, a child is so severely affected that the motor problems—noticeable as either decreased or increased motor tone, or tension on the tendons—may be apparent in the first days or months of life.

Abnormal motor function can have both negative and positive symptoms. Negative symptoms can in-

Information on Cerebral Palsy

Causes: Unknown; likely a brain abnormality that develops in utero
Symptoms: Lack of normal control of movements, unusual arm or leg postures, weak muscle tone, facial distortion, labored speech
Duration: Chronic
Treatments: None

clude the inability to do normal motor activities such as reach for a toy, pick up a raisin with the fingers, or walk. Positive symptoms can consist of abnormal movements such as the involuntary flexion of the foot when trying to walk, resulting in toe walking, or the persistence of primitive reflexes (such as the Moro reflex), which impede voluntary movements. These positive manifestations can result in unusual arm or leg postures that make some of these children easily recognizable. On the other hand, many children with cerebral palsy do not have these symptoms and are normal in appearance. Others have motor problems so mild that they are never diagnosed but are simply considered clumsy or maladroit.

By definition, any brain abnormality that causes cerebral palsy is not progressive, which means that the brain does not deteriorate. Actually, most of these children show improved motor coordination as they become older. A child with mild cerebral palsy at one year of age may be able to move normally by the second grade. Children correctly diagnosed with cerebral palsy early in life may no longer suffer from the disorder later in life. Therefore, the number of children with cerebral palsy decreases with age. The rate in developed countries is approximately two per one thousand school-age children. The vast majority of children with cerebral palsy reach adulthood, with most having a full life span. As a group, those who are never able to walk are more likely to die younger.

There is no single cause of cerebral palsy. Any abnormality of the brain that can develop either in utero or before the infant is one month old can cause cerebral palsy. Cerebral palsy is more common among children born prematurely; they account for approximately one-third of all children with cerebral palsy. One theory holds that these children develop a brain abnormality while in the womb which causes the child both to be born prematurely and to have cerebral palsy. Alternatively, especially among very low birth weight infants, their difficult first weeks of life may cause intraventricular hemorrhage and brain injury, most commonly of the white matter adjacent to the lateral ventricles. The pattern referred to as diplegia, in which the legs are more severely affected than the arms, is characteristic in premature infants with cerebral palsy.

Approximately 78 percent of term infants who develop cerebral palsy are healthy at birth. Only later, when they reach the appropriate developmental stage, does their condition become apparent. It is widely believed that these children have a brain abnormality that occurred while the brain was developing in the womb. The underlying cause of such abnormalities is unclear. Among the other 12 percent of term infants with cerebral palsy is a group of babies who are unwell at birth. These children have had various physiological insults—including stroke, infection, or lack of oxygen—either in the womb or at the time of birth. Children who suffer a lack of oxygen or hypotension (low blood pressure) during the birth process account for only about 10 percent of infants who develop cerebral palsy. Sometimes, maternal hemorrhage or placental abnormalities deprive the infant of oxygen. Errors committed by the delivering doctor or midwife are an uncommon cause of cerebral palsy. Enhanced fetal monitoring during labor and delivery using electronic devices or delivery by cesarean section has not lowered the rate of cerebral palsy.

Since cerebral palsy is a motor disorder, it is classified by motor patterns. Children with cerebral palsy are generally divided into two major groups: those with increased tone (also called spasticity) and those with decreased tone. This is a somewhat artificial distinction since some children have decreased tone in infancy and increased tone later in life while others may have decreased tone when lying down but increased tone when sitting or standing. A major advantage of this division is the recognition that persistent and severe decrease in motor tone makes walking more difficult while increased tone makes the development of contractures (shortened tendons) more likely. In addition, children are classified by pattern of limb involvement. The common pattern in children born prematurely is diplegia, in which the legs are more severely affected than the arms. About 50 percent of children affected with diplegia are able to walk. Another common pattern is hemiplegia, in which the arm and leg on one side are affected and the other side is normal. The arm is more severely involved than the leg, and the prognosis for walking is good, with almost all these children able to walk if they do not have any other motor problem. When all four limbs are involved, the condition is called quadriplegia (or double hemiparesis or tetraplegia). These youngsters have the least likelihood of being able to walk and are most likely to have associated problems such as mental retardation. The pattern wherein the limbs produce markedly abnormal movements whenever the child attempts voluntary movements is uncommon. These abnormal movements can be sharp and sudden in nature (called chorea) or slower and more writhing (called athetosis), although often the movements are a combination of the two patterns and thus not easily classified. In the past, this motor pattern was caused by severe hyperbilirubinemia (a very high accumulation of bilirubin) shortly after birth. Today, modern therapies such as exchange transfusion and light therapy usually prevent the bilirubin level from rising to dangerous levels.

The motor impairment can affect more than the child's limbs. Speech, chewing, drinking, and swallowing can be abnormal when the motor disability affects the face, tongue, and lips. This is most commonly seen in children with quadriplegia. It is widely noted that many of these children have weak face muscles and tend to keep their mouths open and to drool. When speech is affected, the patient often speaks slowly, has a nasal quality to the voice, and has poor enunciation. When this disability is severe, patients may find it impossible to speak any intelligible words even when their understanding of speech is not affected. Children with this type of motor problem may have difficulty with the fine lip and tongue movements necessary for chewing and may be able to eat only soft foods. Some of these children also have difficulty handling liquids such as water and may choke on clear liquids; they may prefer thickened soft foods. The motor disability can be severe enough that the swallowing movements of the esophagus and stomach are disturbed. Normally, there is a well-organized progression of such movements that propel food down the esophagus and through the stomach into the intestines. When this normal motor progression does not occur, children may regurgitate their food, since the food is inadvertently propelled up and out instead of down and into the intestines. This is referred to as reflux. When present to a minor degree, reflux can be merely a cosmetic problem, and the child may need to wear a bib much of the day. When present to a more severe degree, reflux can interfere with normal nutrition. Having food returning into the mouth in a child who has difficulty coordinating swallowing can lead to aspiration, the inadvertent passage of food down the windpipe and into the lungs, which can cause frequent bouts of pneumonia.

The brain abnormalities that cause cerebral palsy can produce other brain-related disabilities. In a survey of children with cerebral palsy in Atlanta, 75 percent had another disability, 65 percent had mental retardation, 46 percent had epilepsy, and 15 percent had sensory loss. Many of the children had more than one additional disability. Children with quadriplegia are the most likely to have other disabilities.

Treatment and Therapy

Only in unusual circumstances is there any direct treatment available for the brain abnormality that causes the motor disability of cerebral palsy. On the other hand, a variety of resources are available for helping the child cope with motor problems. Physical aids such as wheelchairs, walkers, and crutches have long been available. Modern ones are extremely adjustable and made of lightweight and durable materials. Lightweight plastic can be custom molded and fitted to supplement or replace the more traditional leg braces. Physical therapy helps interfere with involuntary and primitive reflex patterns that hinder voluntary movements. Therapy can also facilitate normal patterns of arm and leg use. Occupational therapy focuses on developing fine motor skills and improving the ability to dress, eat, write, and perform other daily activities. To be successful, all these therapies must be done every day. As a practical matter, this means performing the activities at home with parental assistance under the periodic supervision of a therapist. Orthopedic surgery when used judiciously can improve muscle balance, release contractures, and correct scoliosis. The surgeon must consider carefully how the child's growth in height and weight in the years following the surgery might affect the outcome either favorably or adversely.

Abnormal tone is difficult to alter. No medicines exist that can increase tone, while several medications such as diazepam, dantrolene, and baclofen can sometimes decrease tone for children who have spasticity. Side effects such as sleepiness greatly limit the use of such medications. In addition, many children have both weakness and increased tone. The tone often helps them do activities such as standing, since the tone stiffens their legs. The loss of tone can actually make the child less able to stand. A surgical procedure called posterior rhizotomy can decrease the tone for children with diplegia who have mild gait abnormalities. These youngsters can walk with minimal assistance, usually walking up on their toes, and they have no problem with truncal balance. In this surgical procedure performed on the lower back, some of the sensory (posterior) innervating nerves to the leg muscles are severed. The procedure can produce some postoperative sensory loss, which usually disappears. Long-term adverse effects include weakness and scoliosis. It is generally believed that to be effective, the procedure should be accompanied by an aggressive program of physical therapy.

School programs have become increasingly sophisticated in assisting pupils with motor disabilities. Techniques include the use of computers for written work as well as computers with voice simulators for youngsters who cannot speak adequately to participate in the classroom. All schools in the United States are required to be physically accessible to motor-disabled students and to structure gym and recess programs so that all students can participate.

Perspective and Prospects

The brightest hope lies in research to understand better the abnormalities of fetal development that lead to cerebral palsy, in the expectation of finding preventive measures. In addition, since premature infants are disproportionately represented among those with cerebral palsy, the prevention of prematurity and improvements in the management of children born prematurely also provide hope for decreasing the occurrence of the disorder. Newer medicines such as gabapentin that hold the potential for decreasing the adverse effects of increased tone with fewer side effects are also appearing. Finally, the potential of computers and computer-assisted physical devices to help motor-impaired persons is being actively explored.

—Robert J. Baumann, M.D.

See also Birth defects; Motor skill development; Muscle sprains, spasms, and disorders; Muscles; Nervous system; Neurology; Neurology, pediatric; Palsy; Reflexes, primitive; Seizures.

For Further Information:

Geralis, Elaine, ed. *Children with Cerebral Palsy: A Parent's Guide*. 2d ed. Bethesda, Md.: Woodbine House, 1998. This extensive overview of cerebral palsy and its associated conditions details the characteristics, possible causes, and associated disabilities. Discusses the types of services families may need and provides information to help families when choosing or accessing services.

Grether, Judith K., and Karin B. Nelson. "Maternal Infection and Cerebral Palsy in Infants of Normal Birth Weight." *Journal of the American Medical Association* 278, no. 3 (July 16, 1997): 207-211. A study which suggests that many people with cerebral palsy who were born at term were exposed to an infection before birth.

Hutton, J. L., T. Cooke, and P. O. Pharoah. "Life Expectancy in Children with Cerebral Palsy." *British Medical Journal* 309, no. 6952 (August 13, 1994): 431-435. A modern examination of the life span of children with cerebral palsy which shows that most of them do well.

Kramer, Laura Shapiro. *Uncommon Voyage: Parenting a Special Needs Child*. 2d ed. Berkeley, Calif.: North Atlantic Books, 2001. A personal account of a mother who explored a range of alternative therapies and medicines after her son was diagnosed with cerebral palsy. The therapies greatly diminished his symptoms. Includes a resource guide to medical, therapeutic, and counseling organizations, as well as to experts in various alternative therapies.

Pimm, Paul. *Living with Cerebral Palsy*. Austin, Tex.: Raintree Steck-Vaughn, 1999. Designed for grades three through five, this book discusses cerebral palsy through the stories of children experiencing the disease. The four children highlighted here range in age from nine to eighteen and are affected to varying degrees by the disease.

Stanton, Marion. *The Cerebral Palsy Handbook*. London: Random House U.K., 2002. A guide to caregivers of cerebral palsy patients. Covers the early stages, routine care, types of treatment available, support networks, school and legal rights, and benefits.

Swaiman, Kenneth F., Stephen Ashwal, Donna M. Ferriero, eds. *Pediatric Neurology: Principles and Practice*. 4th ed. Philadelphia: Mosby Elsevier, 2006. Contains a detailed and authoritative review of cerebral palsy written for specialists in the field.

United Cerebral Palsy. http://www.ucp.org/. A comprehensive site with information about the disease and sections dedicated to such topics as education, transportation, sports and leisure, and employment.

CERVICAL, OVARIAN, AND UTERINE CANCERS

DISEASE/DISORDER

ANATOMY OR SYSTEM AFFECTED: Genitals, lymphatic system, reproductive system, uterus

SPECIALTIES AND RELATED FIELDS: Gynecology, immunology, obstetrics, oncology

DEFINITION: The primary cancers of the female reproductive system.

KEY TERMS:

benign: referring to a tumor made of a mass of cells which do not leave the site where they develop

cancer: one of a group of diseases in which cells divide uncontrollably; cancerous tissues do not contribute to the function of the body

cervix: the narrowest part of the uterus, which opens into the vagina

endometrium: the inner lining of the uterus, which normally thickens and then is sloughed off during each menstrual cycle; estrogens cause its growth and development, and progesterone prepares it for possible pregnancy

malignant: referring to a tumor which is capable of losing cells, which can travel via blood or lymph fluid to other sites

metastasis: the process by which malignant tumors invade other tissues either locally or distally

neoplasm: the new and abnormal formation of a tumor

ovary: the female gonad located in the pelvic cavity, where egg production occurs; the principal organ that produces the hormones estrogen and progesterone

tumor: a mass of cells characterized by uncontrolled growth; it can be either benign or malignant

uterus: the female organ in which the embryo develops; it is located in the pelvic cavity and is connected to the ovaries by the uterine tubes

CAUSES AND SYMPTOMS

Although people commonly talk about cancer as a single disease, it actually includes more than one hundred different diseases. These diseases do appear to have a common element to them. All cancer cells divide without obeying the normal control mechanisms. These abnormal cells have altered deoxyribonucleic acid (DNA) that causes them to divide and form other abnormal cells, which again divide and eventually form a neoplasm, or tumor.

If the neoplasm has the potential to leave its original site and invade other tissues, it is called malignant. If the tumor stays in one place, it is benign. One major difference between these tumors is that malignant cells seem to have lost the cellular glue that holds them to one another. Therefore, they can metastasize, leaving the tumor and infiltrating nearby tissues. Metastatic cells can also travel to distant sites via the blood or lymph systems.

Medical scientists do not know exactly what causes a cell to become cancerous. In fact, it is likely that several different factors in some combination cause cancer. Genetic, viral, hormonal, immunological, toxic, and physical factors may all play a role. Whatever the cause, cancer is a common disease, resulting in one out of five deaths in the United States. Tumors of the reproductive tract occur in relatively high rates in women. Cervical cancer accounts for 6 percent, ovarian cancer 5 percent, and cancer of the lining of the uterus (endometrial cancer) 7 percent of all cancers in women.

Cervical cancer is most frequently found in women who are between forty and forty-nine years of age, but the incidence has been steadily increasing in younger women. Several factors appear to be involved in initiating this cancer: young age at first intercourse, number of sexual partners (as well as the number of the partner's partners), infection with sexually transmitted diseases such as herpes simplex type 2 and human papillomavirus, and cigarette smoking. Since most patients do not experience symptoms, regular checkups are necessary. The Pap (Papanicolaou) smear performed in a physician's office will detect the presence of cervical cancer. In this procedure, the physician obtains a sample of the cervix by swabbing the area and placing the cells on a microscope slide for examination.

Ovarian cancer accounts for more deaths than any other cancer of the female reproductive system. While

INFORMATION ON CERVICAL, OVARIAN, AND UTERINE CANCERS

CAUSES: Genetic, viral, hormonal, immunological, toxic, and/or physical factors

SYMPTOMS: Abdominal pain and swelling, gastrointestinal disorders (changes in bowel habits), bloating, abnormal vaginal bleeding

DURATION: Chronic, possibly recurrent

TREATMENTS: Surgical removal of affected organ, hormonal therapy, chemotherapy, radiation

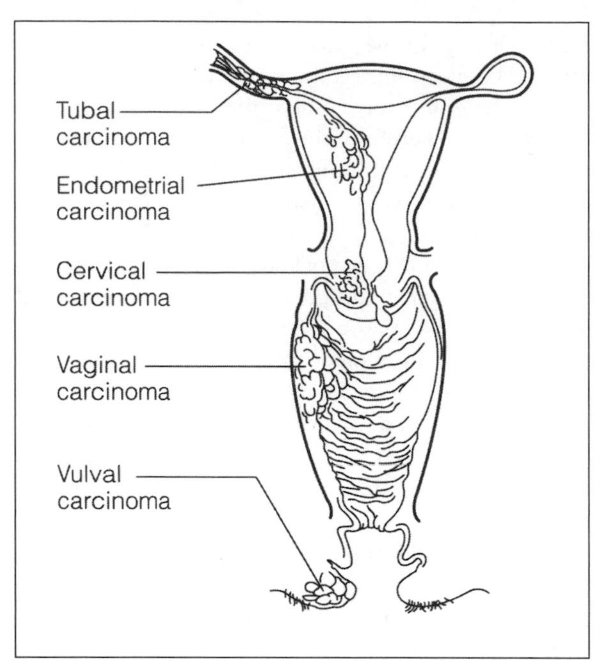

Common sites of cancer in the female reproductive system.

the cause of ovarian cancer is unknown, the risk is greatest for women who have not had children. Researchers recently discovered that the genes BRCA1 and BRCA2, usually associated with hereditary forms of breast cancer, are also connected to an increased rate of ovarian cancer. About 5 to 10 percent of ovarian cancers appear to have a strong hereditary association, particularly in patients who develop the cancer at a young age. Its incidence is slightly decreased in women who use oral contraceptives for many years. Ovarian tumors generally affect women over fifty years of age.

There are two major types of ovarian cancer: epithelial and germ cell neoplasms. About 90 percent of ovarian cancers are epithelial and develop on the surface of the ovary. These tumors often are bulky and involve both ovaries. Germ cell tumors are derived from the eggs within the ovary and, if malignant, tend to be highly aggressive. Malignant germ cell neoplasms tend to occur in women under the age of thirty.

Ovarian cancer is generally considered a silent disease, as the signs and symptoms are vague and often ignored. Abdominal pain is the most obvious symptom, followed by abdominal swelling. Some patients also report gastrointestinal disorders such as changes in bowel habits. Abnormal vaginal bleeding may occur but like the other symptoms is not specific for the disease. Diagnosis is made using imaging techniques such as ultrasound, computed tomography (CT) scanning, and magnetic resonance imaging (MRI). The presence and identification of the BRCA1 and BRCA2 genes also allows a woman to aggressively monitor her health, even though her predisposition for ovarian cancer cannot be changed.

Uterine cancer, also known as endometrial cancer, most frequently affects women between the ages of fifty and sixty-five. Like most cancers, the cause of endometrial cancer is not clear. Nevertheless, relatively high levels of estrogens have been identified as a risk factor. For example, obese women, women who have an early onset of their first period (menarche), and women who never became pregnant tend to have high estrogen levels for longer durations than those without these conditions. Medical scientists believe not only that it is estrogens that are important but also that the other ovarian hormone, progesterone, must be lower than normal for the cancer to develop. Therefore, progesterone appears to have a protective effect in endometrial cancer. Detection of endometrial cancer is accomplished by having a physician take a small tissue sample (biopsy) from the lining of the uterus. The sample can be examined under the microscope to determine if the cells are cancerous.

Treatment and Therapy

A variety of treatments are available for patients with cancers of the reproductive tract: surgical removal of the organ, hormonal therapy, chemotherapy, or radiation therapy.

The treatment of cervical cancer depends on the size and location of the tumor and whether the cells are benign or malignant. If the patient is no longer capable of or interested in childbearing, then she may choose to have her uterus, including the cervix, removed in the procedure known as hysterectomy. The physician may also use a laser, cryotherapy (use of a cold instrument), or electrocautery (use of a hot instrument) to destroy the tumor without removing the uterus. Malignant tumors may require a total hysterectomy and removal of associated lymph nodes, which can trap metastatic cells. This surgery may be followed by radiation or chemotherapy if there is a possibility that all cancer cells have not been removed.

Cervical cancer diagnosed in a pregnant patient can complicate the treatment. Fortunately, only about 1 percent of cervical cancers are found in pregnant women. If the cancer is restricted to the cervix (that is, it has not metastasized), treatment is usually delayed until after childbirth. It is interesting to note that a normal vaginal

IN THE NEWS: CERVICAL CANCER VACCINE; FOUR-PROTEIN TEST FOR OVARIAN CANCER; CHEMOTHERAPY PUMPED INTO ABDOMEN

In June, 2006, the U.S. Food and Drug Administration (FDA) approved the first vaccine for cervical cancer and made it available for females between the ages of nine and twenty-six. Manufactured by Merck and known as Gardasil, it protects against the two main strains of human papillomavirus (HPV) that cause nearly 70 percent of all cervical cancer cases. Although it does not protect against existing HPV infections nor against the other ten or so HPV types that can produce cervical cancer, the vaccine will protect an individual against future infections of the two main viruses that cause cervical cancer. No serious side effects were reported from the vaccine, which is administered as a series of three shots over a period of six months. Eventually, Pap smear tests may not be needed.

In May, 2005, medical researchers at Yale University, George Washington University, and the Nevada Cancer Institute reported a test that measures the levels of four cancer-related proteins in the blood that proved successful in the early detection of ovarian cancer with an accuracy of 95 percent. Starting with measurements of 169 cancer-related protein markers in the blood of ovarian cancer patients and healthy women, the studies were narrowed down to four proteins that were relatively simple to detect: leptin, prolactin, osteopontin, and insulin-like growth factor II. For widespread implementation, the test needs to be improved to achieve more than 99 percent accuracy. This level may be reached by including a few additional protein markers. Previously, the blood test used to detect ovarian cancer measured the concentration of the CA-125 protein. It only identified about 10 percent of females experiencing early ovarian cancer.

Medical research results published in early 2006 report that pumping chemotherapy drugs into a patient's abdomen, known as intraperitoneal therapy, can extend the lives of ovarian cancer victims by an additional year or more. The downside is serious side effects that include stomach pain, numbness to the extremities, and possible infection, resulting in a lower quality of life for these patients compared to those taking only an intravenous (IV) regimen. One year after termination of treatment, patients who received IV or intraperitoneal therapy experienced the same quality of life. In January, 2006, the National Cancer Institute recommended an individualized combination of IV and intraperitoneal therapy for ovarian cancer patients.

—*Alvin K. Benson, Ph.D.*

delivery may occur without harming the mother or the infant. Malignant cervical cancer must be treated in a similar way as in nonpregnant women. If the cancer is found in the first trimester, a hysterectomy or radiation therapy or both is used to help eradicate the malignancy. Obviously, these approaches terminate the pregnancy. During the second trimester, the uterus must be emptied of the fetus and placenta, followed by radiation therapy or removal of the affected reproductive organs. In the third trimester, the physician will typically try to delay treatment until he or she believes that the fetus has developed sufficiently to stay alive when delivered by cesarean section. A vaginal delivery is not recommended, as it has been shown to lower the cure rate of malignant cervical cancer. Treatment after delivery consists of surgery, radiation therapy, and chemotherapy.

The prognosis in patients who have elected surgical removal of the tumor is a five-year survival rate of up to 90 percent. Cure rates for patients undergoing radiation therapy are between 75 and 90 percent. Chemotherapeutic agents have not had as much effect, as they significantly reduce only 25 percent of tumors. It is important to note that the best outcomes are achieved with early diagnosis.

Ovarian cancers are treated with a similar approach. Surgery may involve the removal of the ovaries, uterine tubes, and uterus, as well as associated lymph nodes depending upon the extent of malignancy. Radiation and chemotherapy are usually employed but oftentimes are not effective. The drug taxol is a relatively new agent which shows some promise in treating ovarian cancers. This drug was isolated from the bark of the yew tree and shows some specificity for ovarian tumors. Taxol prevents cell division in ovarian tumors, slowing the progression of the disease.

The outcome for ovarian cancer is usually not as good as for cervical and endometrial cancers, since the disease is usually in an advanced stage by the time that it is diagnosed. The overall survival rate without evidence of recurrence in patients with epithelial ovarian cancers is between 15 and 45 percent. The more uncommon germ cell ovarian cancers have a much more variable prognosis. With early diagnosis, aggressive surgery, and the use of newer chemotherapeutic agents, the long-term survival rate for all ovarian cancer patients approaches 70 percent.

Surgery is often the treatment of choice for endometrial cancer. As with cervical cancer, however, treatment depends upon the extent of the disease and the patient's wishes relative to reproductive capabilities and family planning. A hysterectomy—removal of the uterine tubes, ovaries, and surrounding lymph nodes—is usually indicated. Chemotherapy and radiation therapy are occasionally utilized as adjunctive therapy, as is progesterone. Progesterone (medroxyprogesterone or hydroxyprogesterone) may benefit patients with advanced disease, as it seems to cause a decrease in tumor size and regression of metastases. In fact, progesterone therapy in patients with advanced or recurrent endometrial cancer leads to regression in about 40 percent of cases. Progesterone therapy also has produced regression in tumors that have metastasized to the lungs, vagina, and chest cavity.

The outcome of endometrial cancer is influenced by the aggressiveness of the tumor, the age of the woman (older women tend to have a poorer prognosis), and the stage at which the cancer was detected. Almost two-thirds of all patients live without evidence of disease for five or more years after treatment. Unfortunately, 28 percent die within five years. For cancer identified and treated early, almost 90 percent of patients are alive five years after treatment.

Perspective and Prospects

Even though medical science has advanced the ability to detect and treat cancers much earlier, many lives are still lost to cancer each year. Therefore, as with most diseases, prevention may be a significant way to reduce one's chances of getting cancer, as well as of reducing the effects of cancer itself.

The National Institutes of Health and the American Cancer Society have made several suggestions which can be followed to reduce the risk of cancer. The dietary guidelines include reducing fat intake to less than 30 percent of total calories, eating more high-fiber foods such as whole-grain breads and cereals, and eating more fruits and vegetables in general and in particular those high in vitamins A, C, and E.

Scheduling regular checkups with a health care provider may increase the likelihood of detecting cervical, ovarian, and uterine cancers early, even if no symptoms are present. Pelvic examinations should be performed every three years for women under the age of forty and yearly thereafter. Pap smear tests for cervical cancer should be undertaken yearly from the time that a woman becomes sexually active. Some physicians will take an endometrial tissue biopsy from women at high risk and at the time of the menopause.

Some data suggest that modifying lifestyle may help reduce the incidence of cervical cancer. The cervix is exposed to a variety of factors during intercourse, including infections and physical trauma. Multiple sexual partners increases the risk of sexually transmitted diseases which may predispose the cervix to cancer. This factor is compounded by the fact that infectious agents and other carcinogens can be transmitted from one individual to another. Therefore, theoretically the cervix can be exposed to carcinogens from a partner's sexual partners. Regular intercourse begun in the early teens also predisposes one to cervical cancer, as the tissue of the cervix may be more vulnerable at puberty. Barrier methods of contraception, mainly the condom, reduce the risk of developing cervical cancer by reducing the exposure of the cervix to potential carcinogens. Smoking also increases the risk of cervical cancer, perhaps because carcinogens in tobacco enter the blood which in turn has access to the cervix. Thus, such lifestyle changes as safer sexual practices, quitting smoking, and dietary changes would be beneficial to someone wanting to reduce the chance of having cervical cancer.

Women who are twenty or more pounds over ideal body weight are twice as likely to develop endometrial cancer, and the risk increases with increased body fat. Some estrogens are produced in fat tissue, and this additional estrogen may play a role in the development of endometrial cancer. Therefore, reduction of excess body fat through diet and exercise would be important for a woman who wished to reduce her chances of developing uterine cancer.

—Matthew Berria, Ph.D.

See also Biopsy; Cancer; Cervical procedures; Chemotherapy; Cryosurgery; Endometrial biopsy; Genital disorders, female; Gynecology; Human papillomavirus (HPV); Hysterectomy; Malignancy and metastasis; National Cancer Institute (NCI); Pap smears; Radiation therapy; Reproductive system; Screening; Women's health.

For Further Information:

American Cancer Society (ACS). http://www.cancer.org/docroot/home/index.asp. Web site is divided into sections for patients, family, and friends; survivors; health information seekers; ACS supporters; and professionals. Information on all cancers is wide ranging.

Eyre, Harmon J., Dianne Partie Lange, and Lois B. Morris. *Informed Decisions: The Complete Book of Cancer Diagnosis, Treatment, and Recovery*. 2d ed. Atlanta: American Cancer Society, 2002. This text is intended for the layperson. It is exemplary in its discussion of cancer.

Leikin, Jerrold B., and Martin S. Lipsky, eds. *American Medical Association Complete Medical Encyclopedia*. New York: Random House Reference, 2003. This encyclopedia lists in alphabetical order medical terms, diseases, and medical procedures. It does an excellent job of explaining the different types of cancers and their treatments.

McGinn, Kerry Anne, and Pamela J. Haylock. *Women's Cancers: How to Prevent Them, How to Treat Them, How to Beat Them*. Alameda, Calif.: Hunter House, 2003. A thorough guide that addresses breast, cervical, ovarian, uterine, and vaginal cancers, discussing prevention, diagnosis, and traditional as well as alternative therapies.

National Cervical Cancer Coalition. http://www.nccc-online.org/. Site describes this grassroots advocacy coalition for issues concerning cervical cancer screening and the traditional Pap smear.

Santoso, Joseph T., and Robert L. Coleman. *Handbook of GYN Oncology*. New York: McGraw-Hill, 2001. Myriad information related to cancers of the female reproductive system, including types of gynecologic cancers, complications, management, surgical procedures, peri-operative care, chemotherapy, radiation oncology, and surgical nutrition.

Stewart, Susan Cobb, and the American Medical Women's Association. *The Women's Complete Healthbook*. New York: Dell Books, 1996. This book by the oldest organization of female physicians in the United States is an invaluable guide for the layperson on female-specific diseases.

Sutton, Amy L., ed. *Cancer Sourcebook for Women: Basic Consumer Health Information About Leading Causes of Cancer in Women*. 3d ed. Detroit: Omnigraphics, 2006. An excellent overview of female cancers, with topics such as risk factors, screening methods for early detection, symptoms, diagnostic tests, treatment options, pregnancy during cancer, and fertility after cancer treatment. A directory of resources for cancer patients is also included.

Cervical procedures

Procedure

Anatomy or system affected: Genitals, reproductive system, uterus

Specialties and related fields: Gynecology

Definition: Such procedures as biopsy, conization, cryosurgery, and electrocauterization, which are performed to analyze cervical tissue for abnormal cell development and/or to remove abnormal or cancerous tissue from the cervix.

Indications and Procedures

Surgical procedures performed on the cervix (the opening of the uterus into the vagina) such as biopsy, conization, cryosurgery, and electrocauterization are used to diagnose and treat cervical abnormalities. The first indication of a potential problem is usually a routine gynecological examination that reveals inflammation of the cervix or an abnormal Pap smear. In the Pap smear, a cell sample is scraped from the surface of the cervix and analyzed microscopically. Abnormal results range from slightly abnormal cell growth (dysplasia) to invasive cancer. If the Pap smear results indicate a condition more serious than dysplasia, further tests are conducted.

The first step in the diagnosis of a cervical abnormality is colposcopy and cervical biopsy. The colposcope is a lighted magnifying instrument similar to a pair of binoculars. When placed at the vaginal opening, it permits detailed viewing of the cervix. Abnormal areas are visualized, and a tissue sample of cervical cell layers is punched out for further analysis. Cervical biopsy is performed in a doctor's office and does not require anesthesia because there are no nerve cells in the cervix.

In cases of severe dysplasia or cancer localized to the cervix, a cone biopsy may be performed. Conization is conducted in a hospital under general anesthesia. A circular incision is made around the cervical opening with a knife or laser and is extended up at an angle to obtain a cone of tissue, including some from the cervical canal. The edges of the incision are sutured or cauterized. Examination of the cone can determine the severity and extent of cancer. In some cases, excision of the cone may have eliminated all the cancerous cells from the cervix.

Cryosurgery, also known as cryotherapy, freezes and destroys abnormal tissue with liquid nitrogen. This procedure can be done in a doctor's office and takes only a few minutes to perform. It can be used successfully to treat dysplasia, localized cancer cells, and reddened areas that sometime develop around the cervical opening, called cervical erosions.

Dysplasia, cancer, and cervical erosions are also treated with electrocauterization in which an electrically heated instrument is used to destroy abnormal cells. This procedure is performed in a doctor's office, without anesthesia, just after a woman's menstrual period. A speculum is used to open the vagina, and the tip of the electrocautery device is applied to the abnormal tissue. A scab forms and allows new healthy tissue to grow. Healing is complete in seven to eight weeks.

Pregnant women who have a history of miscarriage during the second trimester of pregnancy due to cervical incompetence may undergo a cervical cerclage, a procedure used to temporarily stitch the cervix closed. A cervical cerclage will help keep the cervix closed as the baby grows. The stitches are generally removed at the thirty-seventh week of pregnancy, allowing for a normal delivery. The procedure successfully prevents miscarriage or premature delivery due to cervical incompetence in 85 to 90 percent of cases.

USES AND COMPLICATIONS

Mild dysplasias typically revert to a normal state spontaneously and are merely monitored for possible slow progression to a more serious state. When Pap smears and/or punch biopsies indicate more serious development of abnormal cells, cryotherapy or electrocauterization is used to destroy the suspicious tissue. While colposcopy is nearly painless, a punch biopsy may cause some cramping. Side effects of electrocauterization include cervical swelling, discharge for up to three weeks, and, rarely, infection or infertility caused by the removal of too many cervical mucous glands. Scarring may occur, making future Pap smears difficult to interpret. Cryotherapy causes much less damage to the cervical opening than electrocauterization, but it may produce a temporary watery discharge and changes in cervical mucus.

If repeated colposcopies or Pap smears confirm severe dysplasia or localized cancer, and if the abnormal tissue extends into the cervical canal, a cone biopsy is performed. If analysis of the cone reveals that the abnormal tissue extends beyond the borders of the biopsied tissue, a second, larger conization may be performed. Conization is major surgery performed under general anesthesia, and bleeding and infection are common complications. Removal of too many cervical mucous glands may lead to infertility. Removal of cervical muscle may lead to an incompetent cervix, an inability of the cervix to maintain a pregnancy to term. There are surgical interventions, however, that can eliminate this problem.

If tests indicate that the cancer has become invasive and has spread beyond the borders of the cervix, a hysterectomy and possible removal of the lymph nodes is performed. This serious surgery renders the woman infertile and carries the same risks as any major surgery.

PERSPECTIVE AND PROSPECTS

In the 1940's, George Papanicolaou discovered that premalignant as well as malignant changes caused the cervix to shed cells that could be analyzed microscopically. Simultaneously, the colposcope was developed. Together Pap smears and colposcopies caused a revolution in the early detection and prevention of cervical cancer.

Cervical cancer has become a more preventable and easily monitored disorder. Advances in the classification of abnormalities from mild to severe and the discovery that exposure to genital herpes virus, multiple sexual partners or mates with a history of multiple partners, smoking, and environmental toxins all contribute to the development of cervical malignancies. Public education may lead to a decrease in the incidence of this disease.

New surgical techniques have improved the efficiency of abnormal tissue destruction, with fewer side effects. The loop electrosurgical excision procedure (LEEP) uses a low-voltage, high-frequency radio wave which runs through a thin wire loop to scoop out abnormal tissue from the cervix in a matter of seconds. Carbon dioxide laser treatment uses a laser beam to destroy cells in a small area, without damaging healthy tissue. Little bleeding occurs, and healing is rapid. Future advances in deoxyribonucleic acid (DNA) analysis may help to identify those who may be at risk for developing cervical cancer so that they may take preventive action and be closely monitored for early, successful treatment.

—*Karen E. Kalumuck, Ph.D.*

See also Biopsy; Cervical, ovarian, and uterine cancers; Cryosurgery; Electrocauterization; Gynecology; Hysterectomy; Infertility, female; Oncology; Pap smear; Women's health.

For Further Information:

Boston Women's Health Collective. *Our Bodies, Ourselves: A New Edition for a New Era*. 35th anniversary ed. New York: Simon & Schuster, 2005. Discusses a broad range of topics concerning women's health. An excellent reference book for all women. A listing of local, national, and international resources is included.

Carlson, Karen J., Stephanie A. Eisenstat, and Terra Ziporyn. *The New Harvard Guide to Women's Health*. Cambridge, Mass.: Harvard University Press, 2004. This popular text addresses issues in women's health and hygiene.

Gray, Mary Jane, et al., eds. *The Woman's Guide to Good Health*. Yonkers, N.Y.: Consumer Reports Books, 1991. A helpful guide to women's health and hygiene. Includes bibliographical references and an index.

McGinn, Kerry Anne, and Pamela J. Haylock. *Women's Cancers: How to Prevent Them, How to Treat Them, How to Beat Them*. Alameda, Calif.: Hunter House, 2003. A thorough guide that addresses breast, cervical, ovarian, uterine, and vaginal cancers, discussing prevention, diagnosis, and traditional as well as alternative therapies.

Rushing, Lynda, and Nancy Joste. *Abnormal Pap Smears: What Every Woman Needs to Know*. Amherst, N.Y.: Prometheus Books, 2001. Explains the causes of cervical neoplasia and the treatment procedures used. Numerous diagrams show the stages of cervical disease.

Stewart, Susan Cobb, and the American Medical Women's Association. *The Women's Complete Healthbook*. New York: Dell Books, 1996. This book by the oldest organization of female physicians in the United States is an invaluable guide for the layperson on female-specific diseases.

Cesarean section

Procedure

Anatomy or system affected: Abdomen, reproductive system, uterus

Specialties and related fields: Anesthesiology, emergency medicine, general surgery, gynecology, neonatology, obstetrics, perinatology

Definition: The surgical procedure used to remove a fetus by incisions into the mother's abdominal and uterine walls.

Key terms:

amniotic fluid: the liquid that surrounds the fetus to protect it from injury and to help maintain a stable temperature

breech: a commonly encountered abnormal fetal presentation in which any part other than the head presents first

cervix: the lower part of the uterus, which is continuous with the vaginal canal; it must enlarge significantly prior to vaginal delivery

incision: a cut made with a scalpel during a surgical procedure

labor: the physiological process by which the fetus and placenta are expelled from the uterus; labor involves strong uterine contractions

placenta: the spongy organ containing blood vessels that provides the fetus with nutrients and oxygen from the mother via the umbilicus

umbilicus: the cord that contains the blood vessels connecting the fetus to the placenta

Indications and Procedures

Cesarean section is performed when it is impossible or dangerous to deliver a baby vaginally. For example, the operation is necessary if the baby is unable to fit through the mother's pelvis or if it shows signs of fetal distress. Fetal distress is detected by abnormal changes in the fetal heart rate, which may indicate that the baby is not receiving adequate oxygen from the placenta. Other reasons for the procedure include a placenta that is lying over the cervix, which blocks the opening to the birth canal (placenta previa); scarring of the uterus from other surgical procedures (or previous cesarean section), which reduces the ability of the uterus to contract; unsuccessful induction of labor with oxytocin (Pitocin); breech presentation, in which any part other than the head presents first; and postmaturity, in which gestation and fetal development indicate that labor should have begun yet is delayed.

A cesarean section allows the delivery of a baby through a horizontal or vertical incision through the mother's abdominal and uterine walls. Prior to surgery, an anesthesiologist gives the mother an epidural or spinal anesthetic so that she can remain conscious but free of pain during the procedure. Occasionally, under certain emergency conditions such as severe fetal distress, a general anesthetic is given. The use of epidural anesthesia, however, is preferred in the majority of deliveries. The anesthesiologist administers epidural anesthesia by injecting a locally acting anesthetic into the space that surrounds the spinal cord. This space is known as the epidural space, and when it is filled with

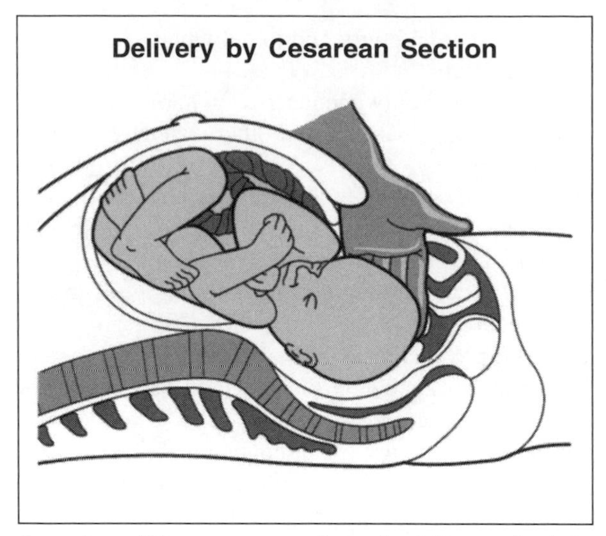

Several conditions may necessitate the delivery of a baby through an incision in the lower abdomen instead of through the birth canal, including fetal distress or the inability of the baby's head to fit through the mother's pelvis.

anesthetic agents, the nerves to the abdominal and pelvic cavities are blocked.

A catheter is inserted into the urinary bladder to empty it prior to making an incision into the abdomen. Typically, a horizontal incision is made just above the pubic bone, as this type of cut heals more readily and is more cosmetically acceptable. Once the pregnant uterus is exposed, a second transverse incision is made in the lower region of the uterus. The amniotic fluid is drained off by suction, and the baby is delivered. Once the infant's head is exposed, its mouth and nose are cleared of any fluid that may hinder respiration. After completely removing the baby from the uterine cavity, the physician clamps the umbilical cord, cuts and ties it, and hands the baby to the parents or a member of the surgical team. Vertical incisions are more likely to be made in emergency situations, since they allow for quicker delivery; however, they result in poorer healing of the uterine muscle. After the placenta is delivered, the physician sutures the uterine and abdominal walls and provides postoperative care to the patient. A drug known as ergonovine can be used after delivery of the infant to stimulate uterine contractions and to aid in preventing postpartum bleeding. A patient in pain or discomfort may be given analgesics such as meperidine or morphine as needed. The medical staff closely monitors the patient's vital signs, such as her heart rate, blood pressure, and urine flow, as well as the status of the uterus, including abnormal bleeding.

Uses and Complications

The major adverse effects to women undergoing cesarean section have been complications caused by anesthesia, infection, hemorrhaging, and blood-clotting disorders, such as thromboembolic episodes in which a blood clot breaks loose from a vessel and causes a stroke, heart attack, or pulmonary embolism. One of the most frequent complications from cesarean section is postoperative fever. Physicians can reduce the incidence of fever, however, by administering antibiotics prophylactically. Some women also experience damage to internal organs during the surgery, especially the bowel and bladder. Risks to the fetus include entrapment of a fetal head or limb in the uterine incision, which may result in injury to the head or spine and in limb fractures, and wounding of the fetus when the incision is made in the uterine wall.

Patients and their health care providers must weigh these potential adverse effects against the benefits of cesarean sections. Very rarely is a cesarean section performed when a normal vaginal delivery is possible. When an obstetrician recommends a cesarean section, he or she believes the benefits outweigh the potential complications. For most patients who are failing to progress in labor or whose baby is in the breech position or in distress, a cesarean section is indicated. It is not always necessary, however, for a cesarean section to be performed on a patient who has had a previous cesarean section. Attempted vaginal births after cesarean (AVBACs) do occur but are decreasing in frequency because of the likelihood of complications.

Perspective and Prospects

Cesarean section was first performed in ancient Rome when the law required physicians to examine the fetus in the event of a mother's death. Some medical historians have proposed that Julius Caesar was delivered in this way; the term for the procedure is derived from his name. Whether this story is truth or legend, however, is still a matter of debate. In the eighteenth century, many women attempted to perform the procedure as a method of abortion. These self-surgeries usually resulted in the mother's death.

Today, cesarean sections are safe for both the mother and the child when they are performed in a medical facility. The rate for delivery by cesarean section has increased in the United States since the 1960's. In 1965, 4.5 percent of babies were born via cesarean section. By 2002, more than one-fourth of all children born in the United States were delivered by cesarean; the total cesarean delivery rate of 26.1 percent was the highest level ever reported in the United States. The cesarean delivery rate declined during the late 1980's through the mid-1990s but has been on the rise since 1996. Since fetal monitoring during labor is much more sophisticated than it was in the past, problems with the fetus are more easily detected, leading to an increased number of cesarean sections but fewer major problems resulting from the labor or delivery process.

—Matthew Berria, Ph.D., and Douglas Reinhart, M.D.; updated by Robin Kamienny Montvilo, Ph.D.

See also Childbirth; Childbirth complications; Emergency medicine; Obstetrics; Reproductive system; Women's health.

FOR FURTHER INFORMATION:

Crombleholme, William R. "Obstetrics." In *Current Medical Diagnosis and Treatment 2006*, edited by Lawrence M. Tierney, Jr., Stephen J. McPhee, and Maxine A. Papadakis. New York: Lange Medical Books/McGraw-Hill, 2006. A chapter in an annual text that is a point of reference for physicians and other health care practitioners. It incorporates the previous year's biomedical research discoveries that have immediate, relevant, and applicable use for the patient.

Cunningham, F. Gary, et al., eds. *Williams Obstetrics*. 22d ed. New York: McGraw-Hill, 2005. This standard textbook in obstetrics would complement a similar text in gynecology. Provides wide coverage of events related to pregnancy and childbirth. A well-written text for the serious reader who wants in-depth information.

Greene, R. A., C. Fitzpatrick, and M. J. Turner. "What Are the Maternal Implications of a Classical Caesarian Section?" *Journal of Obstetrics and Gynaecology* 18, no. 4 (July, 1998): 345-347. This article consists of a detailed chart review of sixty-two cases of cesarean section involving a vertical upper uterine segment incision performed at the Coombe Women's Hospital between January, 1983, and December, 1995.

Menacker, F., E. Declercq, and M. F. Macdorman. "Cesarean Delivery: Background, Trends, and Epidemiology." *Seminars in Perinatology* 30, no. 5 (2006): 235-241. A review of the history of cesarean deliveries with an emphasis on recent trends.

Moore, Michele, and Caroline de Costa. *Cesarean Section: Understanding and Celebrating Your Baby's Birth*. Baltimore: Johns Hopkins University Press, 2003. Offers support and practical information for mothers facing cesarean sections. Discusses the issues behind the decision to perform the procedure, anesthesia, surgery, and recovery.

Tower, Clare L., B. K. Strachan, and P. N. Baker. "Long-Term Implications of Caesarean Section." *Journal of Obstetrics and Gynaecology* 20, no. 4 (July, 2000): 365. Tower, Strachan, and Baker investigated long-term effects of primary cesarean section on subsequent fertility and pregnancies for a group of women delivering in a teaching hospital in the 1990s and correlated these effects to the indication for the initial delivery.

CHAGAS' DISEASE

DISEASE/DISORDER

ANATOMY OR SYSTEM AFFECTED: Immune system, nervous system, skin

SPECIALTIES AND RELATED FIELDS: Family medicine, public health

DEFINITION: An acute disease that is most common in children and caused by the protozoan *Trypanosoma cruzi*.

CAUSES AND SYMPTOMS

Chagas' disease is a parasitic disease that affects millions of persons in both North and South America. More than 15 million persons are infected—most from Mexico south throughout South America—and about 50,000 die from the disease each year. More than 100 million are at risk of contracting the disease.

The protozoan *Trypanosoma cruzi* that causes Chagas' disease is transmitted by the conenose bug (order Hemiptera, family Reduviidae, subfamily Triatominae), also known as the reduviid, assassin, or kissing bug. The feces of the bugs contain the parasites, which enter a human host through broken skin or mucous membranes. Entry of the parasites into cells in the subcutaneous tissue triggers an acute local inflammatory reaction. Within one to two weeks of infection, the trypanosomes spread to the regional lymph nodes and begin to multiply in the cells that phagocytose (digest) them. Chagas' disease can also be transmitted via transfusions of blood from infected individuals.

Chagas' disease is manifested in acute and chronic phases. Symptoms of the acute phase (most common in children) include anemia, loss of strength, nervous disorders, chills, muscle and bone pain, and varying de-

Information on Chagas' Disease

Causes: Protozoan transmitted by conenose bug (also called reduviid, assassin, or kissing bug) through bite or feces
Symptoms: Acute phase includes anemia, loss of strength, nervous disorders, chills, muscle and bone pain, heart failure, sometimes death; chronic phase also includes central and peripheral nervous system dysfunction eventually leading to heart failure
Duration: Acute and chronic
Treatments: Nifurtimox and benznidazole for acute infections

grees of heart failure. Death may ensue three to four weeks after infection. Symptoms of the chronic phase (most common in adults) include those of the acute phase, plus central and peripheral nervous dysfunction, which may last for many years and eventually lead to heart failure.

Treatment and Therapy

Unlike many other trypanosomes of humans, *T. cruzi* does not respond well to chemotherapy. The most effective drugs kill only the extracellular protozoa, but the intracellular forms defy the best efforts at eradication. The reproductive stages, which occur inside living host cells, seem to be shielded from the drugs. Nifurtimox and benznidazole have been shown to be somewhat effective in curing acute infections, but they require long treatment durations and have significant side effects.

Perspective and Prospects

In 1910, Carlos Chagas dissected a number of assassin bugs and found their hindguts swarming with trypanosomes some twenty years before they were known to cause disease. A century later, progress in controlling this harmful disease has been slow.

The 2005 report of the Scientific Working Group on Chagas' Disease calls for, among other things, pediatric formulations of the two main drugs used to treat the disease, better diagnostic tools, better ways to screen donated blood to prevent transmission by transfusion, and improvements in control of the insects involved in transmission of the disease.

—Jason A. Hubbart, M.S.; updated by David M. Lawrence

See also Bites and stings; Insect-borne diseases; Leishmaniasis; Parasitic diseases; Protozoan diseases; Sleeping sickness; Tropical medicine; Zoonoses.

For Further Information:

Perleth, Matthias. *Historical Aspects of American Trypanosomiasis (Chagas' Disease)*. Frankfurt am Main, Germany: Peter Lang, 1997.

Tarleton, Rick L. "Pathology of American Trypanosomiasis." In *Immunology and Molecular Biology of Parasitic Infections*, edited by Kenneth S. Warren. 3d ed. Boston: Blackwell Scientific, 1993.

World Health Organization. *Control of Chagas Disease: Second Report of the WHO Expert Committee on Chagas Disease*. Geneva, Switzerland: Author, 2002.

Chemotherapy

Treatment

Anatomy or system affected: All

Specialties and related fields: Alternative medicine, genetics, microbiology, nuclear medicine, oncology, pharmacology, preventive medicine, toxicology

Definition: The use of chemical compounds to treat diseases, especially infectious diseases and cancer.

Key terms:

adjuvant chemotherapy: the use of combinations of drugs or treatments in addressing metastatic cancer

antibiotics: substances produced by groups of microorganisms that are cytotoxic to other groups of microorganisms

cancer stem cells: the small proportion of cells in cancers that have the potential for long-term replication and metastasis

cytotoxic: referring to the cell-killing properties of a drug

selective toxicity: the properties of a drug that make it selectively destructive to an infectious agent or diseased cell, without harming normal cells of the body

Indications and Procedures

Chemotherapy refers to the concept of using chemicals in a therapeutic manner. Although chemotherapy is commonly associated with cancer, its concept and history actually encompass the use of medicinal approaches to treat many different types of human disease, such as bacterial and viral infections. In the early part of the twentieth century, Paul Ehrlich coined the term "chemotherapy" and defined it descriptively as a "chemical knife," in effect a "magic bullet." The work of Ehrlich established the principle that chemical substances could be used effectively in the treatment of human diseases. The success of chemotherapy is based on the simple principle of selective toxicity, which can be defined as the capacity of a drug to recognize and destroy an infectious agent or diseased cell without seriously harming the human body. The chemical knife envisioned by Ehrlich must be a selective one, or both the host and the pathogen will die.

In antibiotics, this targeting is achieved largely because of the vast structural differences between bacterial cells and human cells. For example, penicillin, discovered by British scientist Alexander Fleming as a product of the mold *Penicillium notatum*, targets a unique compound found only in bacterial cells. When antibiotics such as penicillin target the bacterial cell wall, the bacterial cell lyses, or falls apart and dies. Human cells lack cell walls and peptidoglycan; therefore, the cells of the body are not affected by the antibiotic. Most antibiotics follow this principle of selective cytotoxicity by targeting bacterial structures or metabolic processes unique to bacterial cells, thereby permitting the human host, which is designed differently, to survive the attack.

Many of the same principles have been applied to the development of chemical approaches to cancer treatment; however, the target in cancer therapy is significantly different from that of bacterial antibiotics. One of the most challenging and intractable problems in the treatment of cancer involves the fact that cancer cells are derived from host cells within the body and share many similarities to the cells and tissues of origin, thereby complicating treatment approaches. Unlike bacteria, which differ profoundly from human cells in both form and function, cancer cells evolve within the host and share many if not most cytologic and immunologic properties.

How, then, can the principle of selective cytotoxicity be utilized in the treatment of cancer? Traditional approaches have targeted the abnormal functions of tumor cells, which are largely associated with abnormalities of cell proliferation. For this reason, chemicals that interfere with processes associated with cell reproduction were the major therapeutic approach in the treatment of cancer in the second half of the twentieth century. This theoretical approach targets quantitative differences, such as the rates of deoxyribonucleic acid (DNA) synthesis and/or cell division, rather than qualitative differences, such as structural or biochemical differences, as the basis or rationale for selective targeting treatment approaches. These treatment approaches have largely involved the use of drugs that target DNA synthesis or that block mitosis (cell division), since these are the principal pathways that are quantitatively dysregulated in malignant tumor cells.

This mode of selective toxicity, however, is less precise than the chemical knife of antibiotic therapies, which are based on qualitative rather than quantitative differences between the target and host. This lack of precision is attributable to the fact that the processes of DNA synthesis and mitosis are not restricted only to cancer cells but occur in many other tissues of the body. Many of the side effects of chemotherapy—including anemia, immunosuppression, nausea and vomiting, mouth ulcers, and hair loss—are the result of the effects of these chemicals on normally dividing cells of the body. These side effects are largely temporary, and normal tissue functions are restored once chemotherapy treatments are completed. Chemotherapy may also produce cumulative and long-term effects on organ systems of the body such as the heart, kidneys, and nervous system, depending on the drug regimen, the time course, and the total accumulated dose received by the patient.

Thus, the similarities between cancer cells and normally dividing cells of the body make it much more difficult to design chemotherapy in a way that selectively targets the tumor while sparing the normally dividing cells of the body. Any selective targeting that is achieved depends on the increased rate of cell division in the tumor cells as compared to normal cells. The observed selective toxicity of a chemotherapeutic drug for a tumor is referred to as its therapeutic index, which refers to the ratio between its cytotoxicity for the tumor cells versus normally dividing cells of the body. The higher the therapeutic index, the more selective and presumably effective is the chemotherapeutic drug for a given tumor type. The intrinsic similarities between cancer cells and their normal tissue counterparts, however, ultimately limits the maximum tolerable doses of chemotherapeutic drugs and their clinical effectiveness.

An important concept related to therapeutic index is that of growth fraction, which is defined as the percentage of cells in a normal tissue or tumor that is actively proliferating. Since most chemotherapeutic drugs target cells that are engaged in DNA synthesis or mitosis, malignancies with a higher growth fraction (such as leukemias) will be more sensitive to these drugs than are tumors with a low growth fraction (such as many solid tumors). Most standard chemotherapeutic drugs affect cycling cells, that is, cells that are in the active cell division cycle. These drugs are classified as phase-specific since they are active against tumor cells only in certain phases of the cell cycle. Because they are phase-specific, they are much more cytotoxic to rapidly dividing cells than to nondividing cells.

Another important principle of chemotherapy involves the observation that most conventional chemotherapeutic drugs kill cancer cells with first-order kinetics, which means that the drug induces death in a constant percentage of cells over time rather than a constant number of cells. Therefore, even if the drug is 99.9 percent effective, 0.1 percent of the total number of cancer cells will remain even after drug treatment is completed. This small remaining base of tumor cells may eventually produce tumor recurrence. This problem of tumor recurrence as a result of the mechanism of cell destruction may be countered in part by a combined chemotherapy approach, utilizing multiple drugs, in which each targets a different abnormal component of the cancer cell.

Combined therapy is also designed to address the problem of drug resistance, which has shadowed oncologists and their patients since the earliest treatments for leukemia were developed in the 1950's. In fact, the early therapy protocols involving the use of 6-mercaptopurine and methotrexate in the treatment of childhood acute lymphoblastic leukemia (ALL) immediately exposed some of the fundamental difficulties associated with the use of chemotherapy. Initially, many children with ALL died immediately after treatment, since it was not realized that the therapeutic index of these drugs was so low that overdoses readily occurred. When the dosing regimen was finally adjusted, many children treated with these new drugs recovered rapidly, displaying dramatic drops in white cell counts and restored health. Sadly, some of these children subsequently suffered relapses of disease that no longer responded to chemotherapy. From these early clinical studies, the problem of drug resistance was first identified, and it remains one of the main reasons that chemotherapy treatments may ultimately fail.

More than half a century has passed since the early clinical trials with 6-mercaptopurine in childhood ALL, and oncologists still do not completely understand the phenomenon of drug resistance, although many studies have suggested that it is linked to abnormal gene function and the genetic instability of tumor cells. Most important, more recent research studies have provided significant evidence that, regardless of the mechanism of action, chemotherapeutic drugs ultimately trigger cell death "suicide" pathways that are regulated by the damaged cell. Activation of these internally regulated cell death pathways involves a complex process called apoptosis. A key finding that has emerged from these studies is that, as a result of defects in genes such as the tumor suppressor p53, cancer cells may be less able to enter the death pathway and commit "suicide" in response to chemotherapy than are normal cells whose death pathways are intact.

Uses and Complications

Conventional chemotherapeutic drugs are divided into separate groups depending on their chemical properties and mechanism of cell destruction. Most clinical treatment protocols involve combination chemotherapy using several drugs with different cell targets. This approach is designed to employ multifaceted targeting as a way of achieving maximum cell destruction in a single round of treatment and, in conjunction with high-dose or "dose dense" approaches, is thought to produce maximum effects with the least likelihood of triggering the new growth of drug-resistant tumors. All treatment protocols are designed and implemented only after rigorous preclinical trials are conducted to ascertain their effectiveness against a particular type of cancer. The important classes of standard anticancer drugs are summarized below.

Alkylating agents block the synthesis of DNA by chemically modifying its structure. The nitrogen mustards were the first chemical drugs to be used in the treatment of cancer. Today, cyclophosphamide is commonly used in combined treatment approaches in patients with leukemia and lymphoma. The nitrosoureas, a second group of alkylating agents, interact with DNA by forming chemical cross-links that result in DNA strand breakage. They can enter the cerebrospinal fluid and are therefore used to treat brain tumors. Examples include carmustine and busulfan.

The antimetabolites share structural similarities to DNA precursor components. There are three general groups of antimetabolites: folate antagonists (methotrexate), purine analogues (6-mercaptopurine), and pyrimidine analogues (5-flurouracil). Each of these antimetabolites blocks a normal pathway required for DNA synthesis in the tumor cell, thereby blocking its reproduction.

The anticancer antibiotics are the natural products of

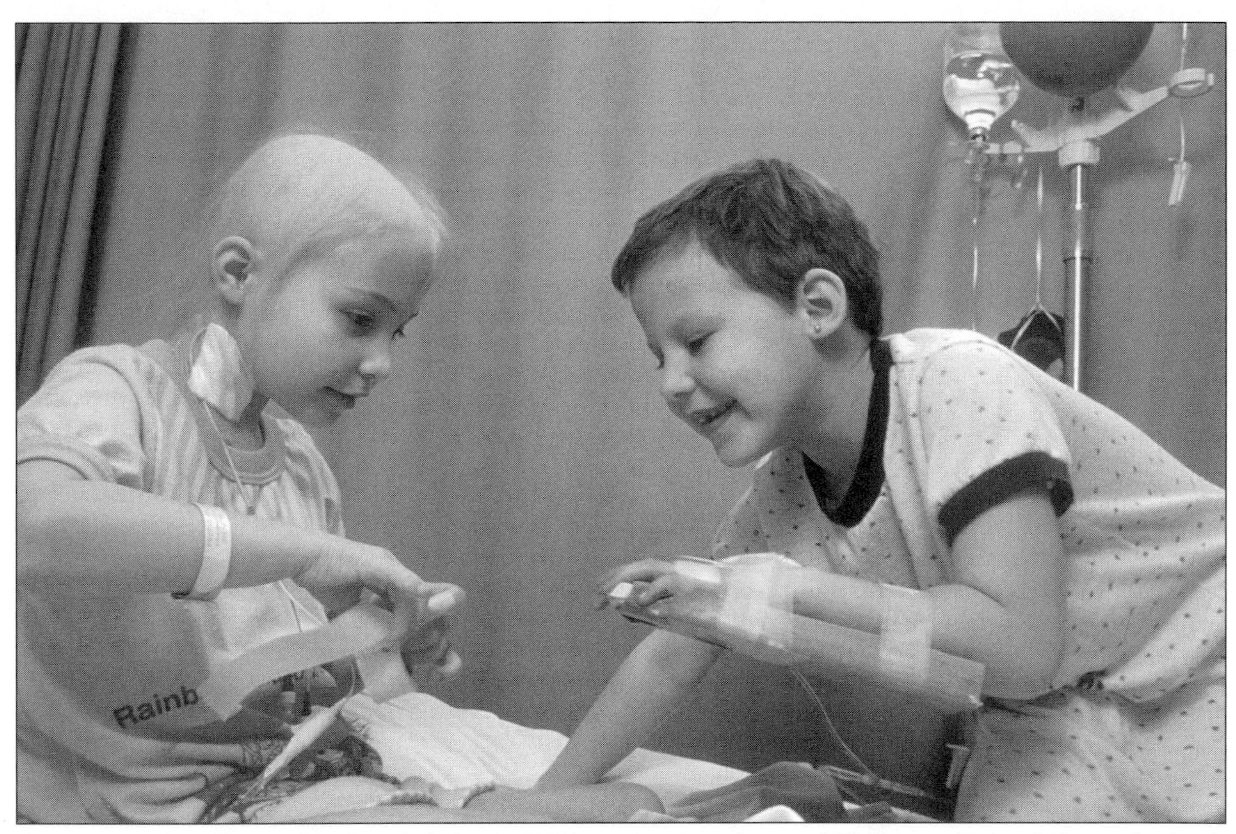

Two young girls with acute lymphocytic leukemia (ALL) receive chemotherapy. (Bill Branson/National Cancer Institute)

microorganisms that display toxic effects toward cancer cells. In general, they interfere with the processes of DNA synthesis or messenger ribonucleic acid (RNA) production. Doxorubicin (Adriamycin) inserts itself between the base pairs of DNA in a process called intercalation, which greatly disrupts DNA structure and function. This drug is effective for many types of cancer; however, its use is limited by its cumulative cytotoxic effects on the heart, which restrict the maximum lifetime dosage that a patient can receive.

Hormonal therapy may be effective against cancers arising in tissues whose growth is hormonally sensitive, such as cancers of the breast and prostate gland. Tamoxifen is a competitive estrogen receptor (ER) antagonist, which means that it binds to estrogen receptors in competition with estrogen. Tamoxifen use has significantly decreased the recurrence of breast cancer in patients with estrogen-sensitive tumors, by 60 percent. Studies with a different class of antiestrogens called aromatase inhibitors, which block estrogen synthesis directly, have also shown very promising results.

A number of naturally occurring products have been found to display anticancer properties. Important members of this group are the vinca alkaloids, which are the natural products of periwinkle plants. Vincristine and vinblastine, the best-known chemical agents of this group, both work by blocking the process of mitosis. These drugs are commonly used in combined therapies with other chemotherapeutic drugs to treat leukemias and lymphomas. Another naturally occurring product is etoposide, a toxic plant alkaloid found in the mandrake (mayapple) plant. It induces a cell cycle arrest that blocks cell proliferation and is used to treat several types of cancer.

A recently discovered drug is paclitaxel, better known as Taxol. This drug, originally isolated from the bark of the rare Pacific yew tree, was found to disrupt the process of mitosis by binding to the filaments called microtubules that pull the chromosomes apart during the process of cell division. Taxol freezes these structures, thereby paralyzing the cell division machinery. In synthetic form, it is used to treat ovarian and breast cancer.

Most recently, there has been a renewed interest in some of the naturally occurring components of herbal medicines and plants that have been used for centuries in the treatment of myriad ailments and diseases. One of the most dramatic examples is the traditional Chinese medicine used to treat patients in rural China with a rare form of leukemia called acute promyelocytic leukemia (APL). The results convinced a team of European and American oncologists to visit rural China and study the properties of this curative herbal extract. After the many components of this complex herbal medicine were purified, it was found that the active anticancer component was arsenic. Indeed, further studies showed that very low dose arsenic by itself was capable of eliciting complete remission in patients with formerly incurable APL. Many other plants and flowers produce anti-inflammatory substances with documented anticancer properties. Perhaps the best known is aspirin. Its chemical name is acetylsalicylic acid, and it occurs naturally in the bark of the willow tree. For centuries, it was used as an anti-inflammatory agent, and over the past few years it has been shown to have chemopreventive effects against colon cancer. The chemically synthesized cyclo-oxygenase-2 (COX-2) inhibitors may also have anticancer effects, further strengthening the suggested link between abnormal inflammatory pathway activities within the cell and responses to chemotherapy.

Beginning in the late twentieth century, the understanding of the molecular basis of cancer has increased dramatically, and oncologists have been extremely eager to apply this knowledge to the development of newer targeted treatment approaches that would selectively destroy cancer cells and spare the normal cells of the body. One of the greatest successes in this area of research to date has been in the treatment of a form of leukemia called chronic myeloid leukemia (CML) with a drug called Gleevec, produced by Novartis Pharmaceutical Company, that selectively targets the primary gene product that is abnormal in this type of leukemia. CML patient responses to Gleevec were so dramatic that the drug was quickly approved by the U.S. Food and Drug Administration (FDA). Because of its greater selective toxicity as a result of a gene-targeted mechanism of action, Gleevec causes few side effects, unlike traditional chemotherapeutic drugs.

Perspective and Prospects

The idea of chemotherapy is not a new one; it dates back to the days of antiquity. Approximately 2,500 years ago, ancient Egyptian writings about cancer first appeared, along with treatment recommendations such as the use of barley, castor beans, and pig ears to treat cancers of the stomach and uterus. After the ancient Egyptians, among the earliest recorded chemotherapies involved the use of mercury to treat outbreaks of syphilis in Europe in the late 1400's. In North America, early American Indians chewed the bark of the cinchona tree to ward off malaria, and by 1630 it was recognized by Europeans that this medicinal bark contained an antimalarial substance called quinine, which eventually became a widely used treatment for malarial infections.

One of the most significant advances in the development of modern chemotherapy was the pioneering work of Paul Ehrlich in the early part of the twentieth century. His efforts to find a "magic bullet" to selectively destroy infectious disease agents culminated in the isolation of a synthetic arsenic compound called salvarsan, which was used in the treatment of syphilis.

In 1929, Alexander Fleming made the monumental discovery that penicillin, an extract from a common mold, could kill infectious bacterial pathogens. He made this astonishing finding upon examining a set of moldy, contaminated culture dishes that he was preparing to discard when he noticed that no bacterial colonies grew in the vicinity of the mold. Thus the modern age of antibiotics was born. In 1935, Gerhard Domagk, a scientist at Bayer Pharmaceutical Company, isolated a chemical substance whose active component, sulfanilamide, was capable of killing several types of infectious bacteria and was later used to save his own daughter from a near-fatal streptococcal infection. This was the first sulfonamide, and it led to the chemical synthesis of a class of related drugs with antimicrobial activity called sulfa drugs. Selman Waksman, another pioneer of this time, isolated the antibiotic streptomycin from the soil microbe *Streptomyces griseus*. It was Waksman who first proposed the term "antibiotic" to define a chemical substance made by one microorganism that kills other microorganisms at low concentrations. Since those early days of drug discovery, many antibiotics and synthetic drugs have been developed. These discoveries transformed the world of medicine and have saved countless lives worldwide.

During the second half of the twentieth century, the term "chemotherapy" became increasingly associated with the treatment of cancer. Several important discoveries of this time were largely responsible for this transition in modern thinking. The earliest discovery occurred in the 1930's as scientists were studying the aftermath of World War I and the effects of sulfur mustard on soldiers exposed to this toxic gas. These findings and later studies on nitrogen mustard showed that among the side effects of exposure to these poisonous gases were decreases in white blood cell (lymphocyte) production by the bone marrow. Ultimately, this led to the notion that low doses of these toxic chemicals might be used as a medicinal approach in the treatment of leukemias and lymphomas resulting from the abnormal production of lymphocytes in the bone marrow. Nitrogen mustard was used for the first time to treat lymphoma in the 1940's. Early promising results quickly established the principle that toxic chemicals could be used to destroy cancer cells within the body. In 1951, landmark research by Gertrude Elion and George Hitchings led to the synthesis of a chemical called 6-mercaptopurine, which was found to block DNA synthesis in rapidly dividing leukemia cells. 6-mercaptopurine was used successfully to treat the most common form of childhood leukemia, ALL. Before this treatment was developed, the average survival time for children diagnosed with ALL was only three to four months. Upon introduction of this new chemotherapeutic treatment, approximately 80 percent of children diagnosed with ALL improved or recovered from this disease.

Since those early days of cancer chemotherapy, more than fifty chemotherapeutic drugs have been used successfully in the treatment of cancer. The greatest successes have been observed for childhood leukemia, Hodgkin's disease, some adult leukemias and lymphomas, and some other rare childhood tumors. The mixed results and lower success rates obtained for many adult epithelial carcinomas have prompted continued research into the development of novel therapeutic approaches to the treatment of cancer.

The twenty-first century promises to be the beginning of a new era in the history of chemotherapy. As the molecular basis of disease is increasingly well understood, the scope of potential targets for therapy and prevention steadily increases. Some of these developments have resulted from the discovery that some cancers express unusual proteins on their surface, unique to the tumor, which may serve as targets for new forms of treatments. For example, certain types of cancers, including breast cancer and some leukemias, may develop from what have been called cancer stem cells. These represent the small minority of cells that are capable of growing or metastasizing; most of the other cells which constitute the cancer do not metastasize and have limited tumorigenic potential. It was found these stem cells often have unique markers on their surface, markers which differentiate themselves from either normal cells or other cancer cells which have limited survival potential. The development of methods of chemotherapy which target only these stem cells may provide another mechanism to target certain cells.

Another form of treatment has been called adjuvant chemotherapy, the use of combination of drugs. By using these drugs sequentially, it is sometimes possible to reduce their concentrations, thereby reducing the extent of side effects while at the same time providing effective therapy. Adjuvant chemotherapy has shown some evidence of success in treating metastatic cancers such as those associated with breast or lung cancer.

—Sarah Crawford, Ph.D.;
updated by Richard Adler, Ph.D.

See also Antibiotics; Bacterial infections; Bacteriology; Cancer; Carcinoma; Cells; Drug resistance; Immune system; Immunology; Leukemia; Lymphadenopathy and lymphoma; Malignancy and metastasis; Microbiology; Oncology; Pharmacology; Radiation therapy; Sarcoma; Tumor removal; Tumors.

For Further Information:

Bruning, Nancy. *Coping with Chemotherapy*. Rev. ed. New York: Ballantine Books, 1993. Takes a practical approach to dealing with the difficulties and side effects of cancer chemotherapy.

Brunton, Laurence L., et al., eds. *Goodman and Gilman's The Pharmacological Basis of Therapeutics*. 11th ed. New York: McGraw-Hill, 2006. This reference book provides a detailed explanation of the principles of cancer drug treatments. Offers comprehensive coverage at a somewhat advanced level.

Clarke, Michael, et al. "Stem Cells: The Real Culprit in Cancer?" *Scientific American* 295, no. 1 (July, 2006): 52-59. Discusses the possible significance of cancer stem cells and their potential as a target for chemotherapy.

Fischer, David S. *The Cancer Chemotherapy Handbook*. 6th ed. St. Louis: Mosby, 2003. Presents a broad-based approach to cancer chemotherapy, nutritional supplements, and basic treatment approaches.

Quillin, Patrick. *Beating Cancer with Nutrition*. Rev. ed. Sarasota, Fla.: Bookworld Services, 2001. Describes nutritional approaches as a way of enhancing cancer therapies and their effectiveness.

Chest

Anatomy

Anatomy or system affected: Circulatory system, lungs, muscles, musculoskeletal system, respiratory system

Specialties and related fields: Cardiology, pulmonary medicine

Definition: The region of the body from the diaphragm to the neck, both within the rib cage (heart and lungs) and in front of it (breasts and muscles).

Key terms:

breast: the mammary gland, along with the nipple in front of it and the surrounding fatty tissue

diaphragm: a curved muscular sheet that separates the chest cavity from the abdominal cavity

heart: a muscular pump that propels the blood through the circulatory system

lungs: the air sacs that are the principal respiratory organs; located in the chest

ribs: the bones that support the chest and define its outline

thoracic: pertaining to the chest

thorax: another name for the chest region

Structure and Functions

The chest, or thorax, consists of those parts of the body lying between the diaphragm and the neck. Included here are the rib cage, diaphragm, heart, lungs, chest muscles, and breasts.

The skeletal support of the chest consists of the thoracic vertebrae and rib cage. In humans, there are usually twelve pairs of ribs and twelve thoracic vertebrae. Each thoracic vertebra consists of a cylindrical portion, the centrum or body, and a neural arch attached to the dorsal side of the centrum. The neural arch surrounds and protects the spinal column. A spinous process extends dorsally from the neural arch of each thoracic vertebra and serves as a site for muscle attachment. Near the base of each neural arch are two pairs of articular processes (zygapophyses). The superior pair of one vertebra face toward each other and articulate with the inferior articular processes of the adjacent vertebrae.

Attached to each thoracic vertebra is a rib. There are usually twelve pairs of ribs, but this number occasionally varies. Each rib consists of a bony portion and a cartilaginous extension, the costal cartilage. At its vertebral end, each rib has two articulating processes, the head (capitulum) and the tubercle (tuberculum). The costal cartilages of the first seven ribs (the number occasionally varies) extend all the way to the sternum. The next two or three ribs have costal cartilages that attach to the costal cartilage above them. The remaining ribs have costal cartilages that are "floating" and have no attachments. Together, the ribs make up a cagelike structure called the rib cage, which shapes the chest and protects the heart and lungs from injury.

The sternum, or breastbone, runs along the front of the chest in the midline of the body. It consists of a flattened top portion called the manubrium, a long, extended body (corpus), and an extension called the xiphoid process, which is made mostly of cartilage. The manubrium has notches for the attachment of the clavicle and the first rib on either side. The attachment for the second rib lies between the manubrium and corpus and is shared by both bones. The corpus of the sternum is formed by the fusion of five individual parts called sternebrae. The costal cartilages of the second through seventh ribs articulate with the corpus of the sternum and mark the boundaries between the individual sternebrae. Beyond the notch for the attachment of the seventh costal cartilage, the xiphoid process extends downward along the midline.

A muscular diaphragm marks the boundary between the chest cavity and the abdominal cavity. Although it is located at the lower end of the chest cavity, it originates in the neck region and derives its nerve supply, the phrenic nerve, from within the neck. The diaphragm is the principal muscle used in breathing. Normally dome-shaped and bowed upward, the diaphragm flattens when its muscles contract, expanding the chest cavity and resulting in the inhalation of air. Relaxation of the diaphragm returns the curvature of the dome upward, compressing the chest cavity and resulting in the exhalation of air. The diaphragm has openings for the passage of the esophagus and the major blood vessels, especially the descending aorta and inferior vena cava.

The heart and major blood vessels lie within the chest cavity and are protected by the rib cage. The heart is a muscular pump that has four chambers (two atria and two ventricles) in all adult mammals. The right atrium receives oxygen-poor blood from the body's organs via the superior vena cava (from the head and upper extremities) and the inferior vena cava (from the abdominal region, pelvic region, and lower extremities). Blood from the right atrium passes through the tricuspid valve to the right ventricle, from which it is pumped into the pulmonary artery. The pulmonary artery then divides in two branches that run separately to each lung. Oxygen-rich blood from the lungs returns to the heart by means of the pulmonary veins, which empty into the left atrium. Blood from the left atrium passes through the bicuspid valve and empties into the left ventricle, which has an extremely thick, muscular wall. Contraction of the left ventricle propels the blood out of the aorta and through the body via the arteries.

Contractions of the heart originate in a location known as the sinoatrial node, located on the surface of the right atrium. From this point, contractions spread to the atrioventricular node, located at the point where all four chambers meet. The wave of contraction then spreads rapidly down the septum between the two ventricles and up the side walls of each ventricle. A specialized bundle called the bundle of His, composed of modified muscle fibers (Purkinje fibers), is responsible for this rapid conduction.

Except for the pulmonary arteries, the arteries of the chest region are all branches of the aorta, the major artery that flows out from the left ventricle of the heart in an upward direction. The aorta can be subdivided into an initial portion (the ascending aorta), an aortic arch, and a longer descending aorta which extends from the thoracic region into the pelvis. The coronary arteries are small but important branches that arise from the ascending aorta as it leaves the heart. These arteries supply blood to the muscular wall of the heart itself. From the arch of the aorta, the most common pattern of branching is that of a brachiocephalic trunk, which then splits into a right common carotid and right subclavian artery, followed by a left common carotid artery and then a left subclavian artery. There is considerable variation, however, in this pattern of branchings. The carotid arteries run up the sides of the neck to supply blood to the head and neck.

The subclavian arteries of either side run first upward and then laterally through the chest cavity, continuing toward the upper extremity as the axillary artery. Along its course, each subclavian artery gives off the following branches: vertebral artery, thyrocervical trunk, internal thoracic artery, costocervical artery, and descending scapular artery. The vertebral artery, the largest branch, supplies blood to the vertebrae of the neck region and ultimately to the base of the brain. The short thyrocervical trunk divides almost immediately into three branches: an inferior thyroid artery to the lar-

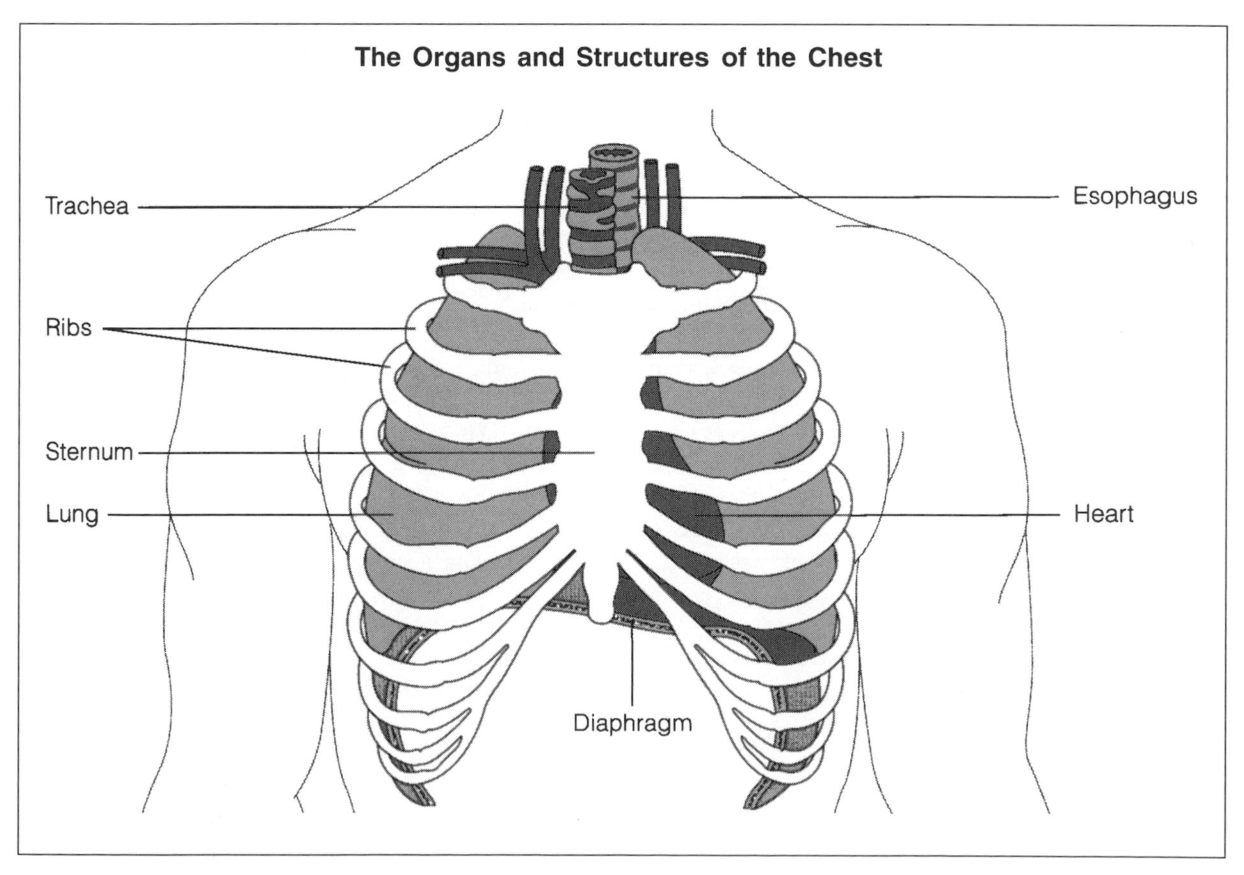

ynx, trachea, esophagus, and surrounding muscles; a suprascapular artery to the subclavius and sternocleidomastoid muscles and to the overlying skin; and a transverse cervical artery to the muscles of the shoulder region.

The right and left internal thoracic arteries (also called internal mammary arteries) run along the ventral side of the chest, just beneath the costal cartilages and just to either side of the sternum. Each internal thoracic artery gives off branches to the diaphragm, the pleura, the pericardium, the thymus, the transverse thoracic muscle, the ribs and intercostal muscles, the pectoral muscles, and the mammary glands. Beyond the sixth rib, each internal thoracic artery divides into a musculophrenic branch to the last six ribs and the diaphragm and a superior epigastric artery, which descends along the abdominal surface, supplying the muscles of this region before meeting the inferior epigastric artery that ascends from the pelvic region.

The veins of the chest region include the external and internal jugular veins, draining the head and neck, and the subclavian veins, draining the upper extremities. These veins come together to form the right and left brachiocephalic veins, which then drain into the superior vena cava. The superior vena cava also receives several smaller tributaries, including the azygos vein, the paired internal thoracic and inferior thyroid veins, the highest intercostal vein, and several smaller veins of the vertebral column. The azygos vein (on the right) and the hemizygous vein (on the left) run parallel to each other on either side of the vertebral column along the dorsal or rear wall of the chest cavity, draining blood from the muscles of the back, the bronchi, the ribs, and the mediastinum. The right and left internal thoracic veins receive tributaries from the ribs and intercostal muscles as well as the diaphragm, pericardium, and mediastinum. The highest intercostal veins drain the first two or three intercostal spaces on either side, also receiving smaller tributaries from the bronchi and the upper portion of the diaphragm. The inferior thyroid veins drain the thyroid gland, esophagus, trachea, and larynx. In addition to the above, the veins of the heart muscle all drain into a coronary sinus, which runs between the left atrium and ventricle, then drains directly into the right atrium near the inferior vena cava.

The lungs, the principal organs of respiration, consist of several lobes. The right lung has superior, medial, and inferior lobes; the left lung has superior and inferior lobes only. Inhalation of air, or inspiration, is brought about by the lowering (contraction) of the diaphragm and by the raising and outward expansion of the rib cage. Exhalation of air, or expiration, is brought about by the raising (relaxation) of the diaphragm and by the relaxation of the intercostal muscles, lowering and contracting the rib cage. Under most conditions, inspiration is an active process requiring muscular contraction, while expiration takes place passively as the muscles relax.

Together, the heart, the lungs, and the thoracic portion of the esophagus occupy the thoracic cavity, or chest cavity. Each of these organs is surrounded by a thin membrane, the visceral pleura. This membrane is continuous with the parietal pleura, another thin membrane that lines the outer walls of the chest cavity. The right and left visceral pleura come together to form a septum called the mediastinum, which separates the bulk of the thoracic cavity into right and left pleural cavities, each containing one of the lungs. The pericardial cavity, containing the heart, is inserted between the layers of the mediastinum. Also occupying part of the thoracic cavity is a large mass of lymphoid tissue, the thymus body. The thymus is irregular in shape and occupies the highest portion of the thoracic cavity above the heart.

Muscles of the chest region may be divided into those associated developmentally with the upper extremity and those that are associated instead with the trunk of the body. One muscle, the trapezius, is a modified gill muscle that belongs developmentally to neither group. Fibers of the trapezius muscle originate from the cervical and thoracic vertebrae, including the adjoining ligaments and the adjacent part of the skull. These fibers converge onto the spine and acromion of the scapula and onto the clavicle. The muscles associated with the trunk of the body are called axial muscles. Of those in the chest or thoracic region, four are responsible primarily for movements of the shoulder blade (scapula), twelve for movements of the rib cage, and another eleven for movements of the vertebral column.

The levator scapula runs from the transverse processes of the first four cervical vertebrae to the vertebral border of the scapula; by contracting, it raises and rotates the scapula. The two rhomboid muscles run from the vertebral column to the vertebral border of the scapula. The rhomboideus minor originates from the spinous processes of the seventh cervical and the first thoracic vertebra and from the nuchal ligament that runs from these spinous processes to the skull. The rhomboideus major originates from the spinous processes of the second through fifth thoracic vertebrae. Both rhomboideus muscles run diagonally from the vertebral column to the vertebral border of the scapula, including the base of the scapular spine. The serratus anterior, also called serratus ventralis, is a sheetlike muscle that lies between the scapula and the rib cage. Its fibers originate from the ribs as a series of strips that converge slightly; they all insert onto the vertebral border of the scapula. The attachments of this muscle to the ribs resemble a series of angular saw-teeth (serrations) that give the muscle its name. The four preceding muscles all share a common embryological origin, and all have a common nerve supply from the dorsal scapular nerve.

The axial muscles associated with movements of the rib cage include the scalenus anterior, scalenus medius, scalenus posterior, intercostals, subcostals, levatores costarum, transversus thoracis, serratus posterior superior, serratus posterior inferior, rectus abdominis, and diaphragm. The three scalene muscles, as their name implies, are all shaped like elongated scalene triangles (with three sides of different lengths). The scalenus anterior arises from the transverse processes of the third through sixth cervical vertebrae and inserts (attaches) onto the first rib. The largest of the scalene muscles is the scalenus medius, which runs from the transverse processes of the last six cervical vertebrae to an insertion on the first rib. The scalenus posterior arises from the transverse processes of the last two or three cervical vertebrae and inserts onto the second rib.

The intercostal muscles run between the ribs in two sets of fibers. The external intercostals run from each rib to the next in a diagonal direction; the upper end of each fiber is situated closer to the vertebral column than is the lower end. The internal intercostals also run diagonally from each rib to the next, but deep to the fibers of the external intercostals and perpendicular to them, so that the lower end of each fiber is closer to the vertebral end of each rib than is the upper end. Both sets of intercostals are broad, extending nearly along the entire extent of each rib, but the fibers are in each case short, extending only from one rib to the next. The subcostals are similar in position and orientation to the internal intercostals, except they are usually confined to the last few ribs and they span two or three intercostal spaces at a time. The levatores costarum are a continuation of the external intercostals onto the transverse processes of the vertebrae, from the last cervical vertebra to the eleventh thoracic vertebra. Each levator costarum is a triangular slip located in the angle between one of the ribs and the vertebra in front of it, running from the transverse process of the vertebra onto the rib.

The transversus thoracis is a flat muscle which covers part of the inside of the rib cage. Its fibers originate from the corpus and xiphoid process of the sternum; these fibers radiate both horizontally and diagonally upward to insert on the deep surfaces of the second through sixth ribs. The serratus posterior superior arises from the spinous processes of the first few thoracic vertebrae and the seventh cervical vertebra, as well as from the ligaments connecting these spinous processes with one another and with the skull. The fibers converge only slightly and are inserted in four separate slips onto the superior margins of the second through fifth ribs. The serratus posterior inferior is a similar but broader muscle located further down the spine. It arises from the spinous processes of the last two thoracic and first few lumbar vertebrae, runs diagonally upward, and divides into four separate slips that insert onto the inferior margins of the last four ribs. The rectus abdominis, obliquus externus, obliquus internus, and transversus abdominis are abdominal muscles that pull down on the chest and particularly on the rib cage. The rectus abdominis consists of a strip of muscle fibers running vertically along the ventral midline. The other abdominal muscles are sheetlike and cover the majority of the abdominal surface. Contractions of these muscles generally pull downward on the ribs and oppose the expansion of the rib cage.

The diaphragm is also an axial muscle of the chest cavity. Its muscle fibers originate from the inside of the xiphoid process of the sternum (the sternal portion), from the inner surfaces of the last six ribs and their costal cartilages (the costal portion), and from two muscular arches and two tendinous crura that make up the lumbar portion. The medial lumbocostal arch forms a passage for the greater psoas muscle, while the lateral lumbocostal arch forms a passage for the lumbar quadrate muscle. The right and left crura arise from the ventral surfaces of the first few lumbar vertebrae. Together, the sternal, costal, and lumbar portions of the diaphragm converge upon a sheetlike central tendon, which is divided into large left and right leaflets and a small middle leaflet.

The axial muscles concerned with movements of the thoracic vertebrae include the longus and splenius muscles and the muscles of the erector spinae complex. The longus colli arises from the centra of the last few cervical and first few thoracic vertebrae along their ventral surfaces; it runs upward to insert onto the bodies of the first four cervical vertebrae and the transverse processes of the fifth and sixth cervical vertebrae. The splenius capitis originates from the spinous processes of the last cervical and the first three or four thoracic vertebrae and from the ligaments connecting these processes to one another and to the back of the skull. The muscle inserts onto the occipital and temporal bones on the back of the skull, including the mastoid process. The splenius cervicis arises from the spinous processes of the third through sixth thoracic vertebrae and runs to an insertion on the transverse processes of the first few cervical vertebrae. The muscles of the erector spinae complex include the iliocostalis, longissimus, spinalis, semispinalis, multifidius, rotatores, and intertransversarii. Collectively, these muscles are responsible for dorsal movements (extension) of the vertebral column throughout the lumbar, thoracic, and cervical regions.

The muscles associated developmentally with the extremities are called appendicular muscles. Appendicular muscles of the chest region include the pectoralis, latissimus dorsi, and subclavius. The pectoralis major is triangular in shape; it originates from the sternum, costal cartilages, and a portion of the clavicle, from which its fibers converge toward an insertion onto the greater tuberosity of the humerus. The pectoralis minor originates from the third through fifth ribs and inserts onto the coracoid process of the scapula. The latissimus dorsi is a broad, flat muscle that originates from the lower half of the vertebral column (and part of the ilium) by way of a tough tendinous sheet (the lumbar aponeurosis); it inserts high on the humerus. The subclavius muscle runs from the bottom surface of the clavicle diagonally onto the first rib. Upon contraction, this muscle helps pull the shoulder inward and the rib cage upward.

Each of the paired breasts consists of a mammary gland, nipple (papilla), areola, and surrounding fat tissue. The breasts are small in children and remain small in most adult men, but they become larger during puberty in women and enlarge even more during late pregnancy and throughout lactation. Toward the end of pregnancy, the gland begins to secrete milk, a white, nutritive fluid containing lactose (milk sugar), proteins, and some fats (more sugar and less fat than in cow's milk). The secretion of milk is known as lactation. During lactation, the mammary gland continues to secrete milk as long as the baby continues nursing. When the child is weaned, the mammary gland undergoes a process of involution (shrinkage). The smaller ducts of the mammary gland collect into larger ducts, each draining a wedge-shaped section of the breast. These larger ducts converge toward a raised nipple (papilla) from which the milk exudes. The nipple is surrounded by a circular area, the areola, characterized by thin skin which is a bit more heavily pigmented (usually redder) than the remainder of the breast.

DISORDERS AND DISEASES

A wide variety of medical problems can occur in the chest region, including a number of diseases and traumatic injuries. Because of the presence of the heart and lungs, injuries and diseases of the chest region are often life-threatening and may be fatal. These include diseases of the heart and major vessels, diseases of the lungs and bronchi, and cancer of the breast. Common heart disorders include myocardial infarction, coronary artery disease, and chest pain (angina pectoralis); less common disorders include arrhythmias and heart murmurs. Disorders of the lungs and bronchi include lung cancer, pulmonary emphysema, and such infectious diseases as tuberculosis, lobar pneumonia, and bronchial pneumonia.

Thoracic specialists include heart specialists (cardiologists), respiratory specialists (pulmonologists), cancer specialists (oncologists), neuromuscular specialists, and neurologists. Thoracic surgeons specialize in the surgery of the chest. Thoracotomy is a cutting into the thoracic cavity, usually for the repair of the heart, the lungs, or both. Thoracotomy is the first step in open heart surgery, coronary bypass surgery, pacemaker implantation, and heart or lung transplants.

Disorders of the breast are so distinctive that many different specialists are involved. The most feared and most fatal of these diseases is breast cancer, often treated by surgical removal of the tumor or of the entire breast. Other breast disorders include mastitis, an inflammation of the breast in women. Rare conditions include the presence of extra (supernumerary) breasts in either sex. Also rare are the hormonal or reproductive disorders that result in the premature enlargement of the female breast or in its failure to develop during adolescence. Enlargement of the breast in males is a condition known as gynecomastia; it often results from abnormal levels of steroid hormones associated with marijuana abuse, but it may arise from other causes. Usually only the fat tissue enlarges in this condition (and never as much as in women); the mammary gland, nipple, and areola remain underdeveloped. Much less common is a condition called Klinefelter syndrome, in which a tall, thin male develops breasts comparable in size to those of a thirteen-year-old girl. This condition is controlled by a chromosomal defect (XXY). The opposite chromosomal defect (XO) results in Turner syndrome, in which a short, web-necked female has breasts that enlarge only slightly and that never develop fully. Both Klinefelter and Turner syndromes result in a degree of mental retardation and in sterility.

Breast surgery may be performed by several types of surgeons, including general surgeons, thoracic surgeons, cancer surgeons, and plastic surgeons. Common surgical operations include the removal of a breast tumor (lumpectomy) or of the entire affected breast (mastectomy) in cases of breast cancer. In addition, plastic surgeons may perform such cosmetic operations as breast augmentation (using implants) or breast reduction.

PERSPECTIVE AND PROSPECTS

The heart, lungs, breasts, and major muscles and bones of the chest region were studied by the ancients. The Latin names that are used today are derived in large measure from the writings of Galen, or Caius Galenus, physician to the Roman army in the second century. Renaissance artists such as Leonardo da Vinci (1452-1519) and Michelangelo (1475-1564) dissected human corpses illegally in order to gain further knowledge of the anatomical structures visible on the body's surface. These studies were followed by the well-illustrated anatomical texts of Andreas Vesalius (1514-1564), who corrected many of Galen's errors.

Good medical understanding of the circulatory system began with the studies of the Renaissance physician William Harvey (1578-1657), who examined the veins in the arms of many patients. It was Harvey who discovered the valves in the veins and who proved that the blood circulates outward from the heart and then back. Anatomists who have described the finer details of the structure of the heart include Jan Evangelista Purkinje (1787-1869) and Wilhelm His, Jr. (1863-1934).

—Eli C. Minkoff, Ph.D.

See also Anatomy; Aspergillosis; Asthma; Avian influenza; Bones and the skeleton; Breasts, female; Bronchitis; Bypass surgery; Cardiac rehabilitation; Cardiology; Cardiology, pediatric; Choking; Chronic obstructive pulmonary disease (COPD); Common cold; Congenital heart disease; Coughing; Croup; Cystic fibrosis; Electrocardiography (ECG or EKG); Embolism; Emphysema; Heart; Heart transplantation; Heart valve replacement; Heartburn; Hyperbaric oxygen therapy; Interstitial pulmonary fibrosis (IPF); Legionnaires' disease; Lung cancer; Lungs; Pacemaker implantation; Pleurisy; Pneumonia; Pulmonary diseases; Pulmonary medicine; Pulmonary medicine, pediatric; Respiration; Respiratory distress syndrome; Resuscitation; Thoracic surgery; Tuberculosis; Wheezing; Whooping cough.

FOR FURTHER INFORMATION:

Agur, Anne M. R., and Arthur F. Dalley. *Grant's Atlas of Anatomy*. 11th ed. Philadelphia: Lippincott Williams & Wilkins, 2005. Contains many excellent, detailed illustrations.

Crouch, James E. *Functional Human Anatomy*. 4th ed. Philadelphia: Lea & Febiger, 1985. A very readable book with good explanations; a very good beginning reference.

Marieb, Elaine N. *Essentials of Human Anatomy and Physiology*. 8th ed. San Francisco: Pearson/Benjamin Cummings, 2006. Nonscientists at the advanced high school level or above will be able to understand this fine textbook that emphasizes the interrelationships of body organ systems, homeostasis, and the complementarity of structure and function.

Rosse, Cornelius, and Penelope Gaddum-Rosse. *Hollinshead's Textbook of Anatomy*. 5th ed. Philadelphia: Lippincott-Raven, 1997. A very thorough, modern, detailed reference with good descriptions and illustrations.

Standring, Susan, et al., eds. *Gray's Anatomy*. 39th ed. New York: Elsevier Churchill Livingstone, 2005. A classic work with the most thorough descriptions. Most of the excellent color illustrations offer realistic detail, and the rest emphasize well-selected highlights.

CHEST PAIN. *See* ANGINA; HEART ATTACK; PAIN.

CHICKENPOX

DISEASE/DISORDER

ALSO KNOWN AS: Varicella

ANATOMY OR SYSTEM AFFECTED: Mouth, nose, skin

SPECIALTIES AND RELATED FIELDS: Dermatology, epidemiology, family medicine, immunology, pediatrics, public health, virology

DEFINITION: A highly infectious viral disease occurring primarily in children. Chickenpox is characterized by weakness, fever, and a generalized body rash.

KEY TERMS:

antihistamine: a medicine used to treat allergic reactions

encephalitis: inflammation of the brain

malaise: a feeling of weakness or discomfort

pruritus: itching

vesicles: small, fluid-filled bumps

CAUSES AND SYMPTOMS

Chickenpox is an acute, highly infectious viral disease occurring primarily, but not exclusively, in children. Each year, between three and four million cases are reported, with the highest incidence occurring during the late winter and early spring. About two out of every thousand of those affected fall so ill as to require hospitalization.

The varicella-zoster virus is responsible for chickenpox infection. Physical contact with an infected individual is not required, as the virus is transmitted from person to person via an airborne route.

Symptoms begin to appear about eleven to fifteen days after exposure. At first, they may resemble those of the common cold: sore throat, runny nose, malaise, and fever. Soon, red spots appear on the body, usually beginning on the trunk and scalp and spreading outward. Occasionally, the mucous membranes are affected as well, with spots appearing in the mouth and nasal passages. The spots develop into vesicles—raised bumps with clear, "teardrop" blisters that turn rapidly to crusty lesions within six to eight hours. The rash occurs in waves, with new spots developing as old ones heal and disappear. By the fifth or sixth day, no new lesions will develop, and the crusts will be gone in less than twenty days.

Chickenpox causes intense itchiness. The impulse to scratch can be overwhelming and can lead to one of the most common complications: bacterial skin infections. Scratching the lesions can also lead to ugly pox scarring. Other possible complications of chickenpox include viral pneumonia and viral encephalitis.

INFORMATION ON CHICKENPOX

CAUSES: Infection with varicella-zoster virus

SYMPTOMS: Generalized body rash, intense itching, malaise, weakness, fever, sore throat, runny nose

DURATION: Two to three weeks

TREATMENTS: None; alleviation of symptoms

The diagnosis of chickenpox is almost always done on the basis of its symptoms, most notably its characteristic rash accompanied by fever. In the event that confirmation of the disease is necessary, the fluid in the lesions can be cultured, although by the time results are obtained (five to ten days), the disease is usually on its way to resolution.

TREATMENT AND THERAPY

In children, chickenpox, uncomfortable although it may be, is not considered a serious illness. The vast majority of cases are uncomplicated and resolve themselves within two to three weeks. Treatment is therefore primarily symptomatic, with an emphasis on controlling itching and reducing fever.

Oral antihistamines such as Benadryl (diphenhydramine) or Atarax (hydroxyzine) are effective in managing pruritus. Topical treatments, such as calamine lotion, may offer almost immediate relief. Fever is treated with either acetaminophen or ibuprofen. Aspirin is not an option because of its link to Reye's syndrome, a potentially fatal condition characterized by vomiting, disorientation, and eventually coma.

Some parents trim short the fingernails of infected children to keep them from scratching away the crusts of chickenpox lesions. This is one way of reducing the risk of secondary bacterial infections. Frequent bathing is also helpful in preventing this complication.

Although there is no cure for chickenpox, the oral antiviral drug acyclovir has been shown to be effective in decreasing the intensity of itching, hastening the healing of skin lesions, and generally shortening the duration of the disease. In order to be effective, treatment must begin within twenty-four hours of the appearance of the rash.

The use of acyclovir is not recommended in children under thirteen because of the relatively benign nature of the disease in this age group. In adolescents older than thirteen and in adults, however, chickenpox may have severe complications, and this increased risk may be lessened with acyclovir therapy.

PERSPECTIVE AND PROSPECTS

Chickenpox has been around for so long that there are conflicting accounts about how it got its name. One theory has it that when chickenpox was first described, it was noted that its lesions looked as if they were placed upon the skin rather than arising from the skin itself. They were compared to chickpeas—hence the name. Another idea is that the name "chickenpox" was intended to distinguish this weaker pox illness from the more life-threatening smallpox—"chicken" being used, as in "chickenhearted," to mean weak or timid.

Chickenpox was not considered a distinct rash disease until 1553, when the Italian physician Filippo Ingrassia differentiated it from scarlet fever. In 1785, the English physician William Heberden gave the earliest clear description of varicella, having distinguished it from smallpox in 1768. In 1924, T. M. Rivers and W. S. Tillett reported the isolation of the chickenpox virus.

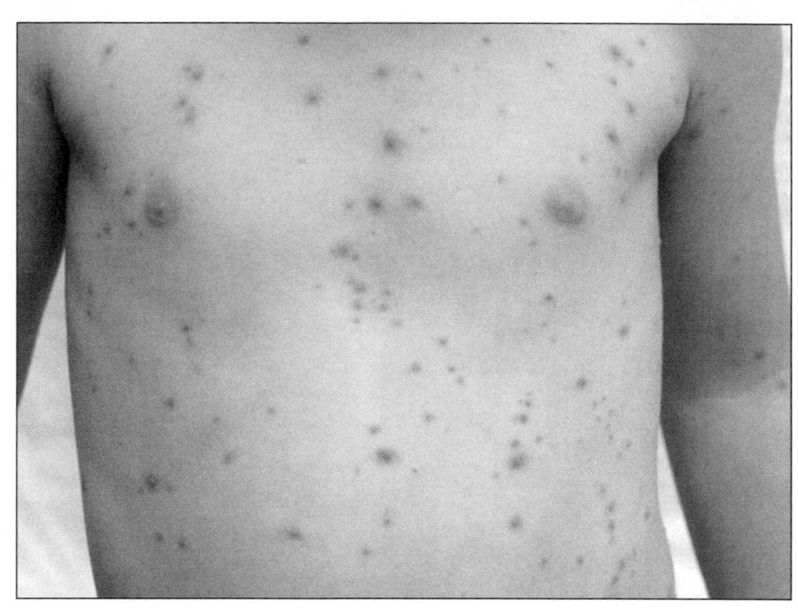

A chickenpox rash. (Custom Medical Stock Photo)

Throughout history, the treatment of chickenpox has been symptomatic. In the 1970's, however, a vaccine became available for persons in high-risk categories. In 1995, a vaccine called Varivax was approved for use in children over the age of one. Varivax is 70 to 90 percent effective in preventing chickenpox over the short term. Vaccinated individuals who still develop chickenpox get a milder form of the disease. Immunity from the vaccine may wane over time, so booster shots may be needed. Because of the vaccine's recent introduction, its ability to provide long-term protection from chickenpox is still unknown.

—Robert T. Klose, Ph.D.

See also Childhood infectious diseases; Herpes; Immunization and vaccination; Infertility, male; Itching; Rashes; Shingles; Skin disorders; Viral infections.

FOR FURTHER INFORMATION:

Behrman, Richard E., Robert M. Kliegman, and Hal B. Jenson, eds. *Nelson Textbook of Pediatrics*. 17th ed. Philadelphia: Saunders, 2004. This standard pediatrics textbook contains complete discussions of all common (and uncommon) causes of infectious disease in children. Many chapters are well written and easily understood by the nonspecialist.

Carpi, John. "A Pox on the Pox." *Scientific American* 273, no. 4 (October, 1995): 32-33. The new vaccine against chickenpox has raised both hopes and doubts. Many pediatricians are skeptical because chickenpox is so mild and complications from the disease are so infrequent and rare.

Kiple, Kenneth F., ed. *The Cambridge World History of Human Disease*. New York: Cambridge University Press, 1993. In addition to being an encyclopedia describing human diseases, this book provides an epidemiological history of disease and discusses possible origins and treatments. The authors target a general population.

Kump, Theresa. "Chicken-Pox Survival Guide." *Parents* 69, no. 5 (May, 1994): 29-31. Sooner or later, almost everyone develops chickenpox, and 90 percent of those suffering from the rash are children under age fifteen. Tips for coping with chickenpox are presented.

Marquis, Julie. "Chickenpox Vaccine Is Swaying Skeptics." *Los Angeles Times*, June 21, 2000, p. 1. The United States' first community-wide study of the chickenpox vaccine, conducted in the Antelope Valley of California, suggests that inoculations led to an 80 percent reduction in cases over five years and could end the disease's long run as a painful, itchy, and occasionally dangerous rite of childhood.

Rees, Alan M. *Consumer Health USA: Essential Information from the Federal Health Network*. Phoenix, Ariz.: Oryx Press, 1995. Provides information on the prevention, diagnosis, and treatment of diseases and disorders such as AIDS and other sexually transmitted diseases, cancer, blood diseases, diabetes, genetic diseases, mental and emotional health, neurological disorders, and women's health.

Sadovsky, Richard. "Safety and Effectiveness of Varicella Vaccine." *American Family Physician* 61, no. 7 (April 1, 2000): 2209. This article reviews a report on the safety and efficacy of the varicella vaccine compiled by the Northern California Kaiser Permanente Medical Care Program, which instituted varicella vaccination into its preventive care program in April, 1995.

Ward, Mark A. "Varicella." In *Conn's Current Therapy*, edited by Robert E. Rakel. 49th ed. Philadelphia: W. B. Saunders, 1997. This chapter in a standard reference work provides an overview of the topic and offers guidelines for disease management.

Woolf, Alan D., et al., eds. *The Children's Hospital Guide to Your Child's Health and Development*. Cambridge, Mass.: Perseus, 2002. An authoritative and comprehensive guide to children's health, providing a guide to every common illness or condition that affects children and a carefully designed emergency section.

Child abuse. *See* Domestic violence.

Childbirth

Biology

Anatomy or system affected: Reproductive system, uterus

Specialties and related fields: Gynecology, neonatology, obstetrics, perinatology

Definition: The process whereby a fetus moves from the uterus to outside the mother's body—a natural event that normally requires no, or minimal, medical intervention.

Key terms:

birth canal: the passageway from the uterus to the outside of the mother's body formed by the fully opened cervix in continuity with the vagina

cervix: a ring of tissue at the lowest and narrowest part of the uterus forming a canal that opens into the vagina

contraction: a squeezing action of the uterus that results in birth

dilation: the opening of the cervix to allow passage of the fetus through the birth canal

hormone: a chemical carried in the blood that acts as a messenger between two or more body parts

labor: the period in the birth process in which forceful and rhythmic uterine contractions are present

parturition: the process or action of giving birth

placenta: a structure located inside the uterus during pregnancy that provides oxygen to the fetus, removes fetal wastes, and produces hormones; also known as the afterbirth

prostaglandins: chemical messengers that are not carried in the blood and that function only locally

uterus: the organ in the female pelvis that supports the fetus during pregnancy and expels it during birth; also known as the womb

vagina: the stretchy tubular structure that leads from the uterus to the outside of the mother's body; part of the birth canal

Process and Effects

In humans, pregnancy lasts an average of forty weeks, counting from the first day of the woman's last menstrual cycle. Actually, ovulation, and therefore conception and the start of pregnancy, does not normally occur until about two weeks after the beginning of the last menstrual period, but because there is no good external indicator of the time of ovulation, obstetricians typically count the weeks of pregnancy using the easily observed last period of menstrual bleeding as a reference point. Because of the uncertainty about the actual time of ovulation and conception, the calculated due date for an infant's birth may be inaccurate by as much as two weeks in either direction.

There is incomplete understanding of the processes that determine the timing and initiation of childbirth. Near the end of pregnancy, the uterus undergoes changes that prepare it for the birth process: The cervix softens and becomes stretchy, the cells in the uterus acquire characteristics that enable them to contract in a coordinated fashion, and the uterus becomes more responsive to hormones that cause contractions.

A number of substances are involved in the preparation of the uterus for birth, including the hormones estrogen and progesterone (produced within the placenta), the hormone relaxin (from the maternal ovary and/or uterus), and prostaglandins (produced within the uterus). The fetus participates in this preparation, since it provides precursors necessary for the uterine synthesis of estrogens. In addition, the amnion and chorion (the placenta and umbilical cord), two membranes surrounding the fetus, are capable of producing prostaglandins that assist in the preparation of the uterus.

Once labor begins, the hormone oxytocin (from the maternal pituitary gland) and uterine prostaglandins cause uterine contractions. It is not known what triggers the onset of labor or how the preparatory hormones and prostaglandins work together.

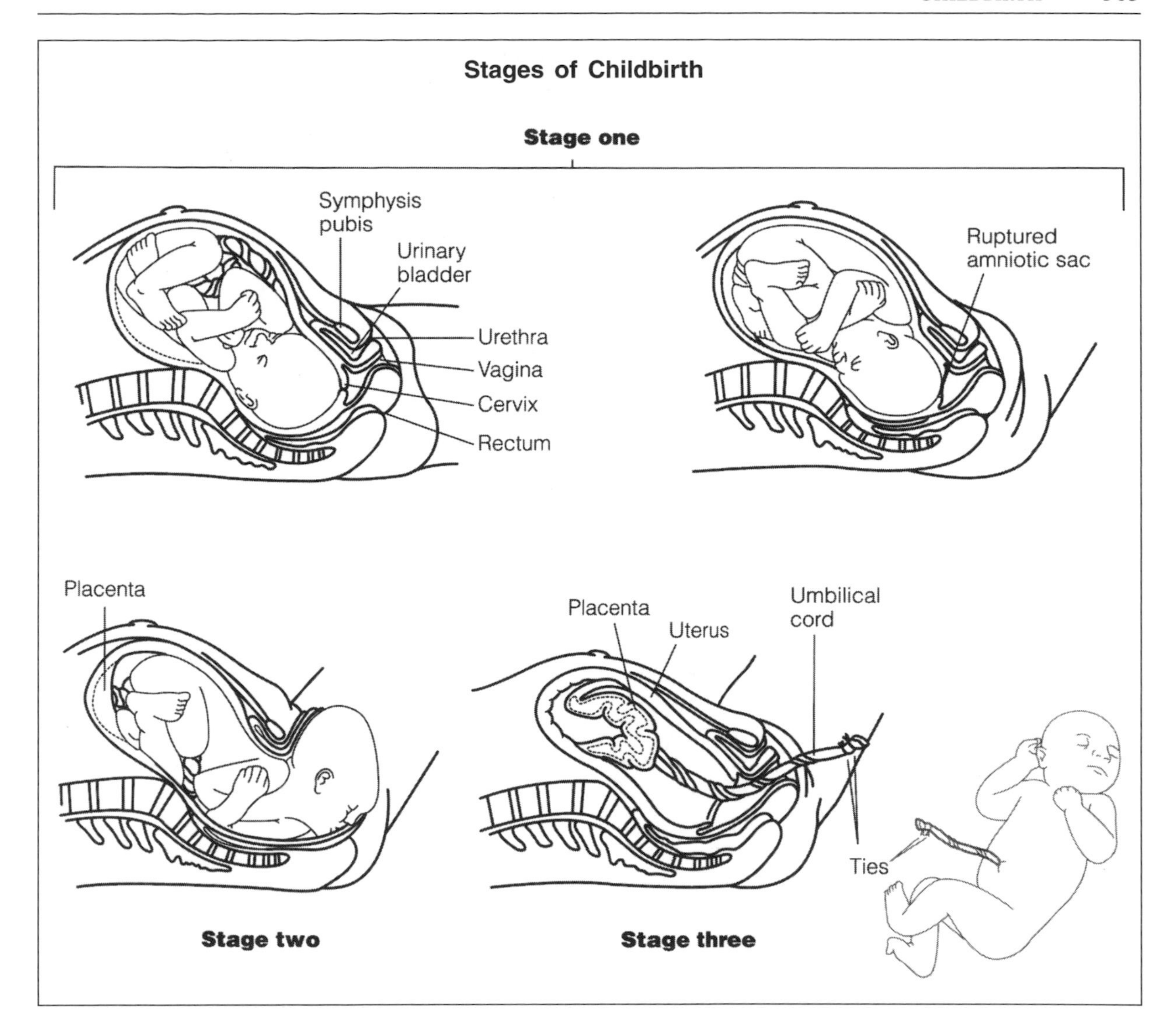

In humans, the onset of labor is indicated by one or more of three signs: the beginning of regular, rhythmic uterine contractions; the rupture of the amniotic membrane, a painless event that is usually accompanied by the leakage of clear fluid from the vagina; and the expulsion of a slightly bloody mucus plug from the cervix, which is an indication that the cervix is beginning to dilate. These signs may appear in any order, or occasionally one sign may be absent or unnoticed. For example, the amniotic membrane may fail to rupture spontaneously; in this case, the attendant will usually pierce the membrane in order to facilitate the birth.

Uterine contractions are the most prominent indication of labor, which is divided into three stages. In the first stage of labor, the contractions have the effect of dilating the cervix from its initial size of only a few millimeters to full dilation of 10 centimeters, large enough to permit the passage of the fetus. When the first stage of labor starts, the contractions may be up to twenty minutes apart, with each contraction of relatively short duration. As the first stage progresses, the contractions become longer and closer together, so that by the end of the first stage there may be only a minute between contractions. There is no downward movement of the fetus during the first stage of labor, but the contractions do force the fetus against the cervix, and this force is important in causing cervical dilation. This first stage lasts for an average of eleven hours in women giving birth for the first time, but up to twenty hours is considered normal. The average length of the first stage of labor in women who have previously delivered is reduced to seven hours, with a norm of up to fourteen hours.

In the second stage of labor, the fetus moves downward through the fully dilated cervix and then into the vagina as a result of the force exerted by the continuing uterine contractions. Voluntary contractions of the abdominal muscles by the mother can help shorten this stage of labor by applying additional force, but in the absence of voluntary contractions (as with an anesthetized mother), the uterine contractions are usually sufficient to cause delivery. In 96 percent of human births, the fetus is situated so that the head is downward and thus is first to pass through the birth canal. Because the vagina does not lie in the same line as the cervix and uterus, the head of the fetus must flex and rotate as the fetus progresses downward past the mother's pelvic bones. The final barrier to the birth of the fetus is the soft tissue surrounding the vaginal opening; once the head of the fetus passes through and stretches this opening, the rest of the body usually slips out readily. The average duration of this second stage of labor in women delivering for the first time is slightly more than one hour; the average duration is shortened to twenty-four minutes in women who have previously delivered. Most women agree that the actual birth of the child during the second stage is less uncomfortable than the strong uterine contractions that occur at the very end of the first stage of labor, when the cervix is dilating the last centimeter or so.

Most infants begin to take regular, deep breaths immediately upon delivery. These breaths serve to inflate the lungs with air for the first time. The infant now becomes dependent on breathing to supply oxygen to the blood, whereas oxygen had been supplied to the fetal blood by circulation through the placenta.

Following delivery of the infant, the mother enters the third stage of labor, during which continued uterine contractions serve to reduce the size of the uterus and expel the placenta. The placenta usually separates from the uterus and is expelled five to fifteen minutes after the birth of the infant.

Uterine contractions do not end with the delivery of the placenta; they continue, with decreasing frequency and intensity, for as long as six weeks following childbirth. These later contractions, known as afterpains, serve to reduce bleeding from the site of placental attachment and to return the uterus and cervix to their prepregnancy condition.

Another significant process that occurs in the mother's body following delivery is the onset of milk production. During pregnancy, the breasts are prepared for later milk production by a number of hormones, but actual milk production does not begin until about the second day after delivery. It appears that the decrease in progesterone levels caused by the removal of the placenta at birth allows milk production to commence.

Most obstetrical attendants agree that the ideal childbirth situation is a labor and delivery with a minimum of medical intervention. If all goes well, the role of the attendant will be primarily that of a support person. Most women are admitted to a hospital or birthing center during the first stage of labor. The mother's blood pressure and temperature will be frequently checked. In addition, the strength and timing of contractions will be assessed either by a hand placed lightly on the abdomen or by an electronic monitor that detects uterine activity through a sensor belt placed around the abdomen. The fetal heart rate will be measured with a stethoscope or by this same electronic tocomonitor placed on the mother's abdomen. Fetal well-being may also be monitored by an electrode placed on the scalp of the fetus through the cervix. This scalp pH probe indicates whether the fetus is tolerating labor well or is in distress. Cervical dilation can be assessed by a vaginal examination: The attendant will insert one or more fingers into the cervix to determine its state of dilation. It is also important that the attendant provide emotional support and reassurance to the mother throughout the delivery.

During the second stage of labor, the attendant will monitor the progress of the fetus through the birth canal. By inserting a hand into the vagina and feeling for the fetal skull bones, the attendant can determine the exact placement of the fetus within the birth canal. As the infant's head appears at the vaginal opening, an incision called an episiotomy is usually performed to prevent accidental tearing of these tissues. Many physicians believe that episiotomy should be done to prevent possible vaginal tearing, since a planned incision is easier to repair than an accidental tear. Another advantage of episiotomy is that it tends to speed the expulsion of the infant, which may be an advantage to both the mother and the child at this stage. The episiotomy incision is made after the injection of a local anesthetic to numb the area, and the incision is stitched closed following the delivery of the placenta.

Once the infant's head has emerged from the vagina, the attendant uses a suction device to clear the infant's nose and mouth of fluid. As the rest of the infant emerges, the attendant supports the body; a quick examination is conducted at this time to determine whether the infant has any major health problems. The umbilical cord that joins the infant to the placenta is usually cut within a few minutes after birth. When the placenta is delivered, the attendant will examine it for completeness and then will perform a thorough examination of the mother and child to ensure that all is well.

Complications and Disorders

If the labor and delivery do not progress normally, the attendant has available a number of medical interventions that will promote the safety of both the mother and the baby. For example, labor may be induced by administration of oxytocin through an intravenous catheter. Such induction is performed if the amniotic membrane ruptures without the spontaneous onset of uterine contractions or if the pregnancy progresses well beyond the due date or for maternal indicators such as hypertension. The induction of labor has been found to be safe, but careful monitoring of the progress of labor is required.

Another fairly common procedure is the use of forceps to assist delivery. These tonglike instruments have two large loops that are placed on the sides of the fetal head when the head is in the birth canal. Forceps are not used to pull the fetus from the birth canal; instead, they are used to guide the fetus through the birth canal and to assist in the downward movement of the fetus during contractions. The use of forceps can help to speed the second stage of labor, and injury to the fetus or the mother is minimal when the forceps are not applied until the fetal head is well within the birth canal, as is the convention. Some type of anesthesia is always used with a forceps delivery. In some areas, vacuum extraction of the fetus is preferred. As the name implies, vacuum extraction makes use of a suction cup on the end of a vacuum hose; the suction cup is affixed to the fetal scalp.

Many women require some type of pain relief during labor, although this need can be reduced by thorough education and preparedness during the pregnancy. A wide range of pain-reducing drugs (analgesics), sedatives, and tranquilizers is available for use during the first stage of labor. These are typically administered by injection; they work at the level of the brain to alter the perception of pain and to promote relaxation. The goal is to use the minimum drug dose that allows the woman to be comfortable. The main danger is that these drugs reach the fetus through the placental circulation; side effects in the infant, which can persist for many hours after delivery, may include depressed respiration, irregular heart rhythm or rate, and sleepiness accompanied by poor suckling response.

Anesthetics that numb pain-carrying nerves in the mother may also be used during the first and second stages of labor. Two routes of delivery are in common use: epidural and spinal, both of which involve the injection of anesthetic drugs into or near the membranes around the mother's spinal cord. The epidural route of injection places the anesthetic in a space that lies outside the spinal cord membranes; with spinal anesthesia, the injection is made slightly deeper into the membranous layers. An advantage of both methods is that the mother remains awake during the delivery and can assist by pushing during the second stage.

Although the disadvantages of both anesthetics, and especially of epidurals, have been downplayed, these procedures do impose restrictions on the mother. Once an epidural has been given, for example, a woman must stay in bed because it will be difficult for her to move her legs; some hospitals do offer "mobile epidurals," which use a type of drug that blocks the pain while still allowing the woman to walk around, but these are the exception, not the rule. Because walking helps to stimulate labor, the use of epidurals can be counterproductive. The use of epidurals is also associated with a prolongation of the second stage of labor and with increased need for forceps to assist delivery. Headaches, backaches, low blood pressure, nausea, and other side effects may result in the mother following the use of anesthetics. Moreover, contrary to past evidence, recent studies have suggested that the drugs in epidurals cross the placenta to the baby, causing health risks.

General anesthesia refers to the use of drugs that induce sleep; they may be administered by inhalation or by injection. Because of profound side effects in both the mother and child, most physicians use general anesthesia only in an emergency situation requiring an immediate cesarean section.

Cesarean section refers to the delivery of the fetus through an incision made in the mother's abdominal and uterine walls. (The name derives from an unsubstantiated legend that Julius Caesar was delivered in this way.) Cesarean deliveries may be planned in advance, as when a physician notes that the fetus is in a difficult-to-deliver position, such as breech (buttocks downward) or transverse (sideways). Multiple fetuses may also be delivered by cesarean section in order to spare the mother and her infants excessive stress. Alternatively, cesarean delivery may be performed as an emergency measure, perhaps after labor has started. As fetal monitoring techniques have improved, problems are noted more quickly and with greater frequency, leading to a larger number of cesarean sections. One indication of the need for emergency cesarean delivery is fetal distress, a condition characterized by an abnormal fetal heart rate and rhythm. Fetal distress is thought to be an indication of reduced blood flow to the placenta, which may be life-threatening to the fetus. Cesarean section may be performed using spinal or epidural anesthesia, as well as general anesthesia. A woman who delivers one child by cesarean section does not necessarily require a cesarean for later deliveries; each pregnancy is evaluated separately. Attempted vaginal births after cesareans (AVBACs) are still being done but are decreasing in frequency due to increased likelihood of problems.

Perspective and Prospects

Prior to 1800 in the United States, most women were attended during childbirth by female midwives. In some areas, a midwife was provided a salary by the town or region; her contract might stipulate that she provide services to all women regardless of financial or social status. In other areas, midwives worked for fees paid by the clients. Midwives of this time had little, if any, formal training and learned about birth practices from other women. Because birth was considered a natural event requiring little intervention on the part of the attendant, the midwife's medical role was limited and the few doctors available were consulted only in difficult cases. Although birth statistics were not kept at the time, anecdotal accounts from the diaries of midwives and doctors suggest that the births were most often successful, with rare cases of maternal or infant deaths.

The nineteenth century saw a gradual shift away from the use of midwives to a preference for formally trained male doctors. This shift was made possible by the establishment of medical schools that provided scientific training in obstetrics. Because these schools were generally closed to women, only men received this training and had access to the instruments and anesthesia that were coming into use.

Maternity hospitals came into being during the 1800's but were at first used primarily by poor or unmarried women. Women of higher social status still preferred to deliver their children in the privacy of their homes. Indeed, home birth was safer than hospital birth, since the building of hospitals had outpaced the knowledge of how to sanitize them. Rates of infection and maternal and infant death were higher in hospitals than in homes.

By the 1930's, the situation had reversed: Hospital births had become safer than home births, because sanitation and surgical procedures had improved. There followed an increasing trend for women to enter hospitals for delivery, so that the percentage of women giving birth in hospitals increased from about 25 percent in 1930 to almost 100 percent by 1960. In the same period, maternal and infant mortality showed a dramatic reduction. The shift to hospital birth had coincided with an interventionist philosophy: Most women were anesthetized during delivery, and forceps deliveries and episiotomy became more common.

By the 1960's, the older idea of "natural" childbirth—that is, a birth which encourages active labor and the use of drug-free types of pain relief with as little medical intervention as possible—had regained popularity. This change in attitude was brought about in part by recognition that analgesic and anesthetic drugs often had profound effects on the infant and often prevented strong mother-infant bonding in the immediate hours after delivery.

It was also brought about by the Lamaze method of childbirth, conceived by French doctor Fernand Lamaze and introduced to the United States with Marjorie Karmel's book *Thank You, Dr. Lamaze* (1959). In this method, women learn controlled breathing techniques to relax and to cope with contractions during labor. A labor coach, who is often the baby's father, helps to initiate and facilitate these techniques. Because natural childbirth must be learned, usually through childbirth classes offered in hospitals during the last trimester of pregnancy, it is also called prepared childbirth. As an extension of natural childbirth, the LeBoyer method has been proposed, allowing for delivery to take place underwater, so that the fetus is expelled from the fluid-filled amniotic sac into a warm, peaceful, fluid-filled environment, allowing for an easier transition to extrauterine life.

By the latter part of the twentieth century, a compromise between the more radical approaches of the past seemed to have been reached, with common practice in obstetrics being to allow the birth to proceed naturally when possible, but with the advantage of having refined drugs, diagnostics, and surgical techniques available if needed. The midwife had been reinstated as a specially trained nurse who could supervise normal births and provide educated assistance at difficult ones.

—Marcia Watson-Whitmyre, Ph.D.;
Cassandra Kircher, Ph.D.;
updated by Robin Kamienny Montvilo, Ph.D.

See also Amniocentesis; Assisted reproductive technologies; Birth defects; Breast-feeding; Cesarean section; Childbirth complications; Chorionic villus sampling; Conception; Ectopic pregnancy; Embryology; Episiotomy; Fetal alcohol syndrome; Gynecology; In vitro fertilization; Miscarriage; Multiple births; Neonatology; Obstetrics; Perinatology; Placenta; Postpartum depression; Pregnancy and gestation; Premature birth; Reproductive system; Stillbirth; Ultrasonography; Umbilical cord; Women's health.

FOR FURTHER INFORMATION:

Ammer, Christine. *The New A to Z of Women's Health: A Concise Encyclopedia*. 5th ed. New York: Checkmark Books/Facts On File, 2005. A respected classic that covers the full spectrum of women's health issues, including the reproductive system and childbearing.

Childbirth.org. http://www.childbirth.org/. A site that helps users learn about childbirth options and how to find the best possible care during pregnancy. Includes many links of educational, informational, and personal nature.

Creasy, Robert K., and Robert Resnik, eds. *Maternal-Fetal Medicine: Principles and Practice*. 5th ed. Philadelphia: Saunders, 2004. This complete text covers all aspects of pregnancy and delivery, from conception to medical care of the newborn. Chapters cover normal physiology as well as problems and their treatment.

Cunningham, F. Gary, et al., eds. *Williams Obstetrics*. 22d ed. New York: McGraw-Hill, 2005. This standard medical school text is still named in honor of its first author, J. Whitridge Williams, who was a professor of obstetrics at The Johns Hopkins Medical School at the beginning of the twentieth century. Although written for the medical specialist, this work is fairly easy to read.

Klaus, Marshall H. John H. Kennell, and Phyllis H. Klaus. *Doula Book: How a Trained Labor Companion Can Help You Have a Shorter, Easier, and Healthier Birth*. 2d ed. Reading, Mass.: Perseus, 2002. Explores the growing trend of doulas in the labor room, giving advice on finding and working with a doula and detailing the way in which doulas statistically reduce the need for cesarean section, shorten the length of labor, decrease the pain medication required, and enhance bonding and breast-feeding.

Klein, M. C., et al. "Why Do Women Go Along with This Stuff? *Birth* 33, no. 3 (September, 2006): 245-250. A review of the use of monitoring techniques during pregnancy and labor, as well as discussion of induction, anesthesia, and surgical delivery.

Lees, Christoph, Karina Reynolds, and Grainne McCarten. *Pregnancy and Birth: Your Questions Answered*. Rev. ed. New York: DK, 2007. Written by two obstetricians and a midwife, this easy-to-read question-and-answer book covering pregnancy and childbirth is illustrated with numerous photographs, drawings, and charts.

Nabukera, S., et al. "First-Time Births Among Women Thirty Years and Older in the United States: Patterns and Risk of Adverse Outcomes." *Journal of Reproductive Medicine* 51, no. 9 (September, 2006): 676-682. Discusses the trend in the United States of women waiting longer to have their first baby and the increase in adverse outcomes in those who do.

Quilligan, Edward J., and Frederick P. Zuspan, eds. *Current Therapy in Obstetrics and Gynecology*. 5th ed. Philadelphia: Saunders, 2000. This compact book contains a wealth of information, such as charts showing fetal weight at different points in pregnancy, the responsibilities of various members of the obstetrical team, and the criteria used in determining specific treatments.

Simkin, Penny, Janet Whalley, and Ann Keppler. *Pregnancy, Childbirth, and the Newborn: The Complete Guide*. 3d ed. Minnetonka, Minn.: Meadowbrook Press, 2003. This comprehensive guide is written in easy-to-understand language and is medically accurate and up to date. Contains many excellent illustrations and charts. The authors are associated with the Childbirth Education Association of Seattle.

CHILDBIRTH COMPLICATIONS

DISEASE/DISORDER

ANATOMY OR SYSTEM AFFECTED: Reproductive system, uterus

SPECIALTIES AND RELATED FIELDS: Gynecology, neonatology, obstetrics

DEFINITION: The difficulties that can occur during childbirth, either for the mother or for the baby.

With medical monitoring and diagnostic tests, about 5 to 10 percent of pregnant women can be diagnosed as high-risk pregnancies, and appropriate precautions and preparations for possible complications can be made prior to labor. Yet up to 60 percent of complications of labor, childbirth, and the postpartum period (immediately after birth) occur in women with no prior indications of possible complications. Difficulties in childbirth can be placed into two general categories—problems with labor and problems with the child—and encompass a wide range of causes and possible treatments.

Complications of labor. Cesarean birth (also called cesarean section, C-section, or a section) is the surgical removal of the baby from the mother. About one in ten infants is delivered by cesarean birth. In this procedure, one incision is made through the mother's abdomen and a second through her uterus. The baby is physically removed from the mother's uterus, and the incisions are closed. This type of surgery is very safe but carries with it the general risks of any major surgery and requires approximately five days of hospitalization. In some cases, diagnosed preexisting conditions suggest that a cesarean birth is necessary and can be planned; in the majority of cases, unexpected difficulties during labor dictate that an emergency cesarean section be performed.

Some conditions leave no question about the necessity of a cesarean section. These absolute indications include a variety of physical abnormalities. Placenta previa is a condition in which the placenta has implanted in the lower part of the uterus instead of the normal upper portion, thereby totally or partially blocking the cervix. The baby could not pass down the birth canal without dislodging or tearing the placenta, thereby interrupting its blood and oxygen supply. Placenta previa is frequently the cause of bleeding after the twentieth week of pregnancy, and it can be definitively diagnosed by ultrasound. For women with this condition, bed rest is prescribed, and the baby will be delivered by cesarean birth at the thirty-seventh week of pregnancy.

Placental separation, also known as placenta abruptio, is the result of the placenta partially or completely separating from the uterus prior to the normal separation time after birth. This condition results in bleeding, with either mild or extreme blood loss depending on the severity of the separation. If severe, up to four pints of blood may be lost, and the mother is given a blood transfusion. If the pregnancy is near term, an emergency cesarean section is indicated to deliver the child.

Occasionally, as the baby begins traveling down the birth canal, the umbilical cord slips and lies ahead of the baby. This condition, called prolapsed cord, is very serious because the pressure of the baby against the cord during a vaginal delivery would compress the cord to the extent that the baby's blood and oxygen supply would be cut off. This condition necessitates an emergency cesarean section.

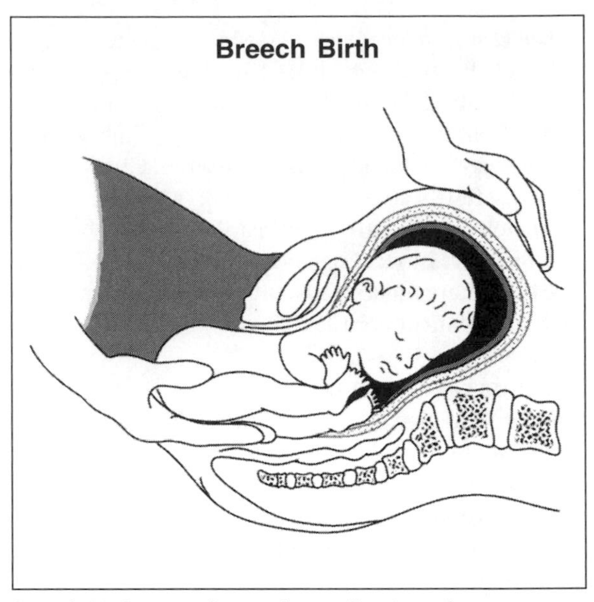

Breech birth, one of several complications that may occur during childbirth, is the emergence of the infant buttocks-first rather than head-first; such a birth is risky for the child, and often birth is accomplished by cesarean section, a surgical procedure to eliminate that risk.

Some conditions that occur during labor are judged for their potential for causing harm to either the mother or the baby. The physician's decision to proceed with vaginal delivery will be based on the severity of the complication and consideration of the best option for the mother and baby. A few of the more common indicators for possible cesarean section which occur during labor include a fetal head size that is too large for the mother's birth canal; fetal distress, evidenced by insufficient oxygen supply reaching the baby; rupturing of the membranes without labor commencing or prolonged labor after membranes burst (usually twenty-four hours); and inelasticity of the pelvis in first-time mothers over forty years of age.

Other maternal conditions are diagnosed prior to the onset of labor, and the physician may or may not recommend a cesarean birth based on the severity of the complication. These include postmaturity, in which the onset of labor is at least two weeks overdue and degeneration of the placenta may compromise the health of the baby; maternal diseases, such as diabetes mellitus and toxemia, in which the stress of labor would be highly risky to the mother; and previous cesarean section.

Complications with the baby. Premature labor can occur between twenty and thirty-six weeks gestation, and a premature infant is considered to be any infant whose birth weight is less than 5.5 pounds. Certain maternal illnesses or abnormalities of the placenta can lead to premature birth, but in 60 percent of the cases there is no identifiable cause. If labor begins six weeks or more prior to the due date, the best chance of infant survival is to be delivered and cared for at a hospital with a perinatal center and specialized intensive care for premature infants. Prior to twenty-four weeks development, a premature infant will not survive as a result of inadequate lung development. The survival rate of premature infants increases with age, weight, and body system maturity.

In about 4 percent of births, the baby is in the breech position—buttocks first or other body part preceding the head—rather than in the normal head-down position. Delivery in this position is complicated because the cervix will not dilate properly and the head may not be able to pass through the cervix. Other complications of breech position are prolapse or compression of the umbilical cord and trauma to the baby if delivered vaginally. Manual techniques may be used to rotate the baby into the correct position. Vaginal delivery may be attempted, frequently aided by gentle forceps removal of the baby. Breech babies are frequently born by cesarean section.

Cephalopelvic disproportion is a condition in which the baby's head is larger than the pelvic opening of the mother. This can be determined only after labor has begun, because the mother's muscles and joints expand to accommodate the baby's head. If at some point during labor the doctor determines that the baby will not fit through the mother's pelvic opening, a cesarean section will be performed.

—*Karen E. Kalumuck, Ph.D.*

See also Birth defects; Cesarean section; Childbirth; Diabetes mellitus; Episiotomy; Gestational diabetes; Multiple births; Obstetrics; Placenta; Postpartum depression; Preeclampsia and eclampsia; Pregnancy and gestation; Premature birth; Reproductive system; Stillbirth; Toxemia; Umbilical cord; Women's health.

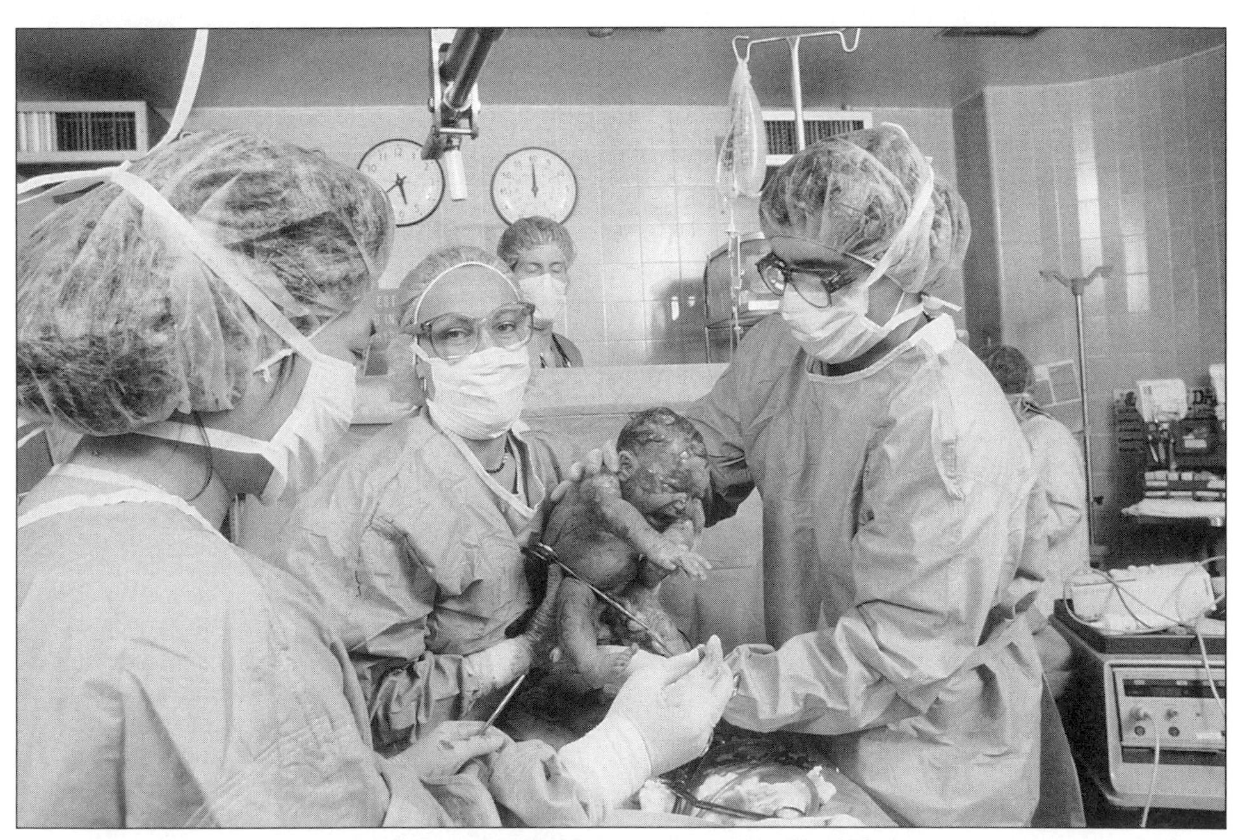

A newborn is delivered by cesarean section. (PhotoDisc)

For Further Information:

Campos, Bonnie C., and Jennifer Brown. *Protect Your Pregnancy*. New York: McGraw-Hill, 2003. A pregnancy guide with a special focus on at-risk pregnancies. Reviews how to recognize signs and symptoms of pregnancy complications and explores preexisting and developing medical conditions that can lead to premature delivery, among other topics.

Carlson, Karen J., Stephanie A. Eisenstat, and Terra Ziporyn. *The New Harvard Guide to Women's Health*. Cambridge, Mass.: Harvard University Press, 2004. This popular text addresses issues in women's health and hygiene.

Gonik, Bernard, and Renee A. Bobrowski. *Medical Complications in Labor and Delivery*. Cambridge, Mass.: Blackwell Scientific, 1996. Organized by system, covering cardiovascular, renal, neurological, and other potentially life-threatening diseases, this new pocket guide provides management protocols needed to stabilize the mother and ensure the safe delivery of the baby.

Hotchner, Tracie. *Pregnancy and Childbirth*. Rev. ed. New York: Avon Books, 1997. This very readable book addresses a wide range of topics: the physical and psychological changes to mother and fetus; complications; prenatal testing; choosing an obstetrician, midwife, and hospital; labor and delivery; and new baby care.

Mishell, Daniel R., et al. *Management of Common Problems in Obstetrics and Gynecology*. 4th ed. Boston: Blackwell, 2002. More than one hundred chapters focus on obstetrics, gynecology, gynecological urology, gynecological oncology, reproductive endocrinology, infertility, and family planning. One chapter devoted to complications during pregnancy.

Moore, Keith L., and T. V. N. Persaud. *The Developing Human*. 7th ed. Philadelphia: W. B. Saunders, 2003. An outstanding textbook on human embryonic development, with specific information about the causes of congenital malformations and common defects occurring in each of the body's systems.

Sears, William, and Martha Sears. *The Birth Book: Everything You Need to Know to Have a Safe and Satisfying Birth*. Boston: Little, Brown, 1994. This helpful resource guide is divided into three parts: "Preparing for Birth," "Easing Pain in Labor," and "Experiencing Birth." You'll find details about vaginal births, cesareans, VBACs, water births, home births, best birthing positions, drugs, pain, how to design your own birth plan, and pages and pages of birth stories.

Stoppard, Miriam. *Conception, Pregnancy, and Birth*. Rev. ed. New York: DK, 2000. Revised edition of a complete guide to having a baby. Advice includes current information on the ideal diet and exercise, the impact of pregnancy and birth on fathers, and ways to prepare older children for a new sibling.

Childhood infectious diseases

Disease/disorder

Anatomy or system affected: Gastrointestinal system, immune system, lungs, muscles, musculoskeletal system, nose, respiratory system

Specialties and related fields: Bacteriology, epidemiology, family medicine, immunology, internal medicine, pediatrics, public health, virology

Definition: A group of diseases including diphtheria, tetanus, measles, polio, rubella (German measles), mumps, varicella (chickenpox), hepatitis, and pertussis (whooping cough).

Key terms:

anorexia: diminished appetite or aversion to food

conjunctivitis: inflammation of the conjunctiva, which lines the back of the eyelid, extends into the space between the lid and the globe of the eye, and goes over the globe to the transparent tissue covering the pupil

erythematous: related to or marked by reddening

malaise: a general feeling of discomfort, of being "out of sorts"

nuchal rigidity: stiffening of the back of the neck

oophoritis: inflammation of the ovary

orchitis: inflammation of the testis

photophobia: dread or avoidance of light

prodrome: a forewarning symptom of a disease

rhinitis: inflammation of the nasal mucous membrane

salivary glands: the glands that produce saliva

Causes and Symptoms

Acute communicable diseases occur primarily in childhood because most adults have become immune to such diseases, either by having acquired them as children or by having been inoculated against them. For example, prior to the use of vaccine for measles—a highly contagious disease found in most of the world—the peak incidence of the disease was in five- to ten-year-olds. Most adults were immune. Before a vaccine was developed and used against measles, epidemics occurred at two- to four-year intervals in large cities. Today, most cases are found in nonimmunized preschool children or in teenagers or young adults who have received only one dose of the vaccine.

A person infected with red measles (also known as rubeola) becomes contagious about ten days after exposure to the disease virus, at which time the prodromal stage begins. Typically, the infected person experiences three days of slight to moderate fever, a runny nose, increasing cough, and conjunctivitis. During the prodromal stage, Koplik's spots appear inside the cheeks opposite the lower molars. These lesions—grayish white dots about the size of sand particles with a slightly reddish halo surrounding them that are occasionally hemorrhagic—are important in the diagnosis of measles.

After the prodrome, a rash appears, usually accompanied by an abrupt increase in temperature (sometimes as high as 104 or 105 degrees Fahrenheit). It begins in the form of small, faintly red spots and progresses to large, dusky red confluent areas, often slightly hemorrhagic. The rash frequently begins behind the ears but spreads rapidly over the entire face, neck, upper arms, and upper part of the chest within the first twenty-four hours. During the next twenty-four hours, it spreads over the back, abdomen, entire arms, and thighs. When it finally reaches the feet after the second or third day of the rash, it is already fading from the face. At this point, the fever is usually disappearing as well.

The chief complications of measles are middle-ear infections, pneumonia, and encephalitis (a severe infection of the brain). There is no correlation between the severity of the case of measles and the development of encephalitis, but the incidence of the infection of the brain runs to only one or two per every thousand cases. Measles can also exacerbate tuberculosis.

The incubation period for rubella (German measles) lasts between fourteen and twenty-one days, and the disease occurs primarily in children between the ages of two and ten. Like the initial rash of measles, the initial rash of rubella usually starts behind the ears, but children with rubella normally have no symptoms save for the rash and a low-grade fever for one day. Adolescents may have a three-day prodromal period of malaise, runny nose, and mild conjunctivitis; adolescent girls may have arthritis in several joints that lasts for weeks. The red spots begin behind the ears and then spread to the face, neck, trunk, and extremities. This rash may coalesce and last up to five days. Temperature may be normal or slightly elevated. Complications from rubella are relatively uncommon, but if pregnant women are not immune to the disease and are exposed to the rubella virus during early pregnancy, severe congenital anomalies may result. Because similar symptoms and rashes develop in many viral diseases, rubella is difficult to diagnose clinically. Except in known epidemics, laboratory confirmation is often necessary.

The patient with mumps is likely to have fever, malaise, headache, and anorexia—all usually mild—but "neck swelling," a painful enlargement of the parotid gland near the ear, is the sign that often brings the child to a doctor. Maximum swelling peaks after one to three days and begins in one or both parotid glands, but it may involve other salivary glands. The swelling pushes the earlobe upward and outward and obscures the angle of the mandible. Drinking sour liquids such as lemon juice may increase the pain. The opening of the duct inside the cheek from the affected parotid gland may appear red and swollen.

The painful swelling usually dissipates by seven days. Abdominal pain may be caused by pancreatitis, a common complication but one that is usually mild. The most feared complication, sterility, is not as common as most believe. Orchitis rarely occurs in prepubertal boys and occurs in only 20 to 30 percent of older males. In 35 percent of patients with orchitis, both testes are involved, and a similar percentage of affected testes will atrophy. Surprisingly, impairment of fertility in males is only about 13 percent; absolute infertility is rare. Ovary involvement in women, with pelvic pain and tenderness, occurs in only about 7 percent of postpubertal women and with no evidence of impaired fertility. Mumps during early pregnancy may cause miscarriage, but this is a rare complication for females who have been immunized.

Measles, rubella, and mumps are all viral illnesses, but *Hemophilus influenzae* type B is the most common cause of serious bacterial infection in the young child. It is the leading cause of bacterial meningitis in children between the ages of one month and four years, and it is the cause of many other serious, life-threatening bacterial infections in the young child. Bacterial meningitis, especially from *Hemophilus influenzae* and pneumococcus, is the major cause of acquired hearing impairment in childhood.

Poliomyelitis (polio), an acute viral infection, has a wide range of manifestations. The minor illness pattern accounts for 80 to 90 percent of clinical infections in children. Symptoms, usually mild in this form, include slight fever, malaise, headache, sore throat, and vomiting but do not involve the central nervous system. Major illness occurs primarily in older children and adults. It may begin with fever, severe headache, stiff neck and back, deep muscle pain, and abnormal sensations, such as of burning, prickling, tickling, or tingling. These symptoms of aseptic meningitis may go no further or may progress to the loss of tendon reflexes and asymmetric weakness or paralysis of muscle groups. Fewer than 25 percent of paralytic polio patients suffer permanent disability. Most return in muscle function occurs within six months, but improvement may continue for two years. Twenty-five percent of paralytic patients have mild residual symptoms, and 50 percent recover completely. A long-term study of adults who suffered the disease has documented slowly progressive muscle weakness, especially in patients who experienced severe disabilities initially.

Tetanus is a bacterial disease which, once established in a wound of a patient without significant immunity, will build a substance that acts at the neuromuscular junction, the spinal cord, and the brain. Clinically, the patient experiences "lockjaw," a tetanic spasm causing the spine and extremities to bend with convexity forward; spasms of the facial muscles cause the famous "sardonic smile." Minimal stimulation of any muscle group may cause painful spasms.

Diphtheria is another bacterial disease that produces a virulent substance, but this one attacks heart muscle and nervous tissue. There is a severe mucopurulent discharge from the nose and an exudative pharyngitis (a sore throat accompanied by phlegm) with the formation of a pseudomembrane. Swelling just below the back of the throat may lead to stridor (noisy, high-pitched breathing) and to the dark bluish or purplish coloration of the skin and mucous membranes because of decreased oxygenation of the blood. The result may be heart failure and damaged nerves; respiratory insufficiency may be caused by diaphragmatic paralysis.

Clinically, pertussis (whooping cough) can be divided into three stages, each lasting about two weeks. Initial symptoms resembling the common cold are followed by the characteristic paroxysmal cough and then convalescence. In the middle stage, multiple, rapid coughs, which may last more than a minute, will be followed by a sudden inspiration of air and a characteristic "whoop." In the final stage, vomiting commonly follows coughing attacks. Almost any stimulus precipitates an attack. Seizures may occur as a result of hypoxia (inadequate oxygen supply) or brain damage. Pneumonia can develop, and even death may occur when the illness is severe.

Varicella (chickenpox) produces a generalized itchy, blisterlike rash with low-grade fever and few other symptoms. Minor complications, such as ear infections, occasionally occur, as does pneumonia, but serious complications such as infection in the brain are rare. It is a very inconvenient disease, however, requiring the infected person to be quarantined for about nine days or until the skin lesions have dried up completely. Varicella, a herpes family virus, may lie dormant in nerve linings for years and suddenly emerge in the linear-grouped skin lesions identified as herpes zoster. These painful skin lesions follow the distribution of the affected nerve. Herpes zoster is commonly known as shingles.

Hepatitis type B is much more common in adults than in children, except in certain immigrant populations in which hepatitis B viral infections are endemic. High carrier rates appear in certain Asian and Pacific Islander groups and among some Inuits in Alaska, in whom perinatal transmission is the most common means of perpetuating the disease. Having this disease in childhood can cause problems later in life. An estimated five thousand deaths in the United States per year from cirrhosis or liver cancer occur as a result of hepatitis B. Carrier rates of between 5 and 10 percent result from disease acquired after the age of five, but between 80 and 90 percent will be carriers if they are infected at birth. The serious problems of hepatitis B occur most often in chronic carriers. For example, approximately, 15 to 40 percent of carriers will ultimately develop liver cancer. The virus is fifty to one hundred times more infectious than human immunodeficiency virus (HIV), the virus that causes acquired immunodeficiency syndrome (AIDS). Health care workers are at high risk of contracting hepatitis B, but virtually everyone is at risk for contracting this disease because it is so contagious.

Hepatitis type A is a virus that causes jaundice, fatigue, abdominal pain, nausea, diarrhea, and fever. Approximately 15 percent of those who have the disease will have relapsing symptoms for six to nine months. Hepatitis A is usually spread through fecal contamination, and during epidemic years over 35,000 cases are diagnosed in the United States.

Treatment and Therapy

The Centers for Disease Control and Prevention (CDC) and the U.S. Department of Health and Human Services recommend immunizing all infants soon after birth and again at age one to two months, with a final dose after the age of twenty-four weeks. The Committee on Infectious Diseases of the American Academy of Pediatrics recommends extending hepatitis B immunization to all adolescents, if possible. Based on field trials, the hepatitis B vaccine appears to be between 80 and 90 percent effective. The plasma-derived vaccine is protective against chronic hepatitis B infection for at least nine years. Newer, yeast-derived vaccines appear to be safe for administration to all, including pregnant women and infants: Both the vaccine and a placebo evoke the same incidence of reactions. These yeast-derived vaccines will be monitored to see if a booster dose is needed.

The incidence of infection with hepatitis B increases rapidly in adolescence, but teenagers are less likely to comply with immunization than are infants. Asking adolescents to participate in a three-dose immunization program over a six-month period is likely to result in high dropout rates. Therefore, the American Academy of Pediatrics' committee has recommended combining vaccination at birth with vaccination of teenagers. Two states, Alaska and Hawaii, have implemented universal immunization of infants with hepatitis B vaccine, and so have twenty nations. Thirty-four states require vaccination for students before entry to middle school. Hepatitis A vaccine is recommended by the CDC for all children between twelve and twenty-three months of age. Two doses of the vaccine should be given at least six months apart.

Primary vaccination with DTaP (diphtheria, tetanus, and acellular pertussis) vaccine is recommended at two months, four months, and six months of age, followed by boosters at fifteen to eighteen months and upon entry into school (at four to six years of age).

Once a child reaches fifteen months of age, only one dose of the *Hemophilus influenzae* type B vaccine is necessary, but vaccination should begin at two months of age. Three vaccines are licensed for use in infants. Depending upon which vaccine is used, shots are given at ages two, four, and six months, with a booster between twelve and fifteen months. These vaccines are safe and at least 90 percent effective in preventing serious illness, such as sepsis and meningitis, from influenza B.

At two and four months of age, infants should receive an inactivated poliovirus vaccination, with boosters between six and eighteen months and upon entry into school (four to six years of age).

MMR (measles, mumps, rubella) vaccination should take place at twelve and fifteen months and at four to six years of age. If the infant lives in a high-risk area, the first dose should occur at twelve months of age. While women who are pregnant or plan to become pregnant in the next three months should not receive MMR vaccination, children may receive the vaccine even if the mother is pregnant, since the viruses are not shed by immunized individuals.

Children who have not received the second dose should be vaccinated at eleven to twelve years. In the 1990's, researchers announced that they had developed a vaccine to prevent chickenpox. Preliminary trials show the vaccine to be safe and effective even in immunocompromised patients. Varicella vaccine should be given at or after twelve months of age to those children who have not had chickenpox.

Other available vaccines to prevent serious infections in children are recommended only in special circumstances. These include vaccines to prevent classic viral flu and pneumococcal disease. (The viral flu is to be distinguished from the bacterial vaccine to prevent influenza B.) Vaccination with the viral influenza vaccine is recommended especially for elderly and high-risk persons, their household contacts, and health care personnel who may come in contact with such patients. Any child who has a heart disease, lung disease, diabetes, or other serious chronic disease should receive the vaccine. This includes the child who is immunocompromised, even if he or she is HIV-positive.

Pneumococcal vaccine is now routinely given to children aged two to twenty-three months and to certain children aged twenty-four to fifty-nine months who are at risk of overwhelming pneumococcal infections. For example, children without spleens and children with sickle cell disease should be considered for vaccination against pneumococcal disease.

Some parents refuse to have their children vaccinated against pertussis because of concerns about the vaccine's safety. Media focus on the safety of pertussis vaccines, as well as legal suits, has frightened many physicians as well, the result being that they may be overly cautious in interpreting vaccine contraindications. Yet primary care physicians have also been sued for failing to give timely immunizations, which may result in complications from preventable disease. The Tennessee Medicaid Pertussis Vaccine Data should reassure them of the vaccine's safety. Other pertussis vaccine safety information is also available, including reports from the American Academy of Pediatrics' Task Force on Pertussis and Pertussis Immunization. Some parents fear that there is a link between vaccinations and neurological disorders such as autism; this is an area of ongoing research.

The means exist to prevent many serious illnesses from infectious diseases in childhood, but both parents and health care professionals must make the effort to vaccinate all children at the appropriate times in their lives.

Perspective and Prospects

Some vaccines are more protective than others; effectiveness may hinge on a number of factors. In 1989, for example, 40 percent of people who developed measles had been vaccinated correctly under the old guidelines of one dose. Recommendations were therefore revised to include a booster dose. In the case of the hepatitis B vaccine, initial recommendations for administration of the vaccine established no injection site (only intramuscular), but studies revealed that there were fewer vaccine failures in recipients who were vaccinated in the deltoid region of the arm as opposed to the buttocks. The recommendation for injection site was therefore revised.

In the United States, vaccine coverage increased by the last 1990's after having been woefully inadequate during the 1980's: One state's department of health, in a 1987 study, discovered that only 64 percent of children who were two years old were adequately vaccinated with DTaP, oral polio, and MMR vaccines. However, by 2000, percentages were closer to 80 percent. Undoubtedly, multiple and interacting factors have inhibited full vaccine coverage for all American children, including physicians' attitudes and practice behaviors. For parents, the cost of vaccination, lack of health insurance, and other barriers to health care frustrate their efforts to get their children immunized. Some parents, for ideological or other reasons, may even be disinterested in or opposed to vaccination. In today's highly mobile society, however, all persons should keep a standard personal immunization record to facilitate immunization coverage.

—Wayne R. McKinny, M.D.;
updated by Lenela Glass-Godwin, M.WS.

See also Bacterial infections; Bacteriology; Bronchiolitis; Chickenpox; Common cold; Epidemiology; Epiglottitis; Family medicine; Fifth disease; Giardiasis; Hand-foot-and-mouth disease; Hemolytic uremic syndrome; Hepatitis; Herpes; Immunization and vaccination; Impetigo; Infection; Influenza; Kawasaki disease; Measles; Microbiology; Mononucleosis; Mumps; Noroviruses; Parasitic diseases; Pediatrics; Pinworms; Poliomyelitis; Rabies; Rheumatic fever; Roseola; Rotavirus; Roundworms; Rubella; Scarlet fever; Smallpox; Strep throat; Tapeworms; Tetanus; Tonsillitis; Tuberculosis; Viral infections; Whooping cough; Worms.

For Further Information:

Beers, Mark H., et al. *The Merck Manual of Diagnosis and Therapy*. 18th ed. Whitehouse Station, N.J.: Merck Research Laboratories, 2006. Published since 1899, this classic work is well indexed and easy to use. Discussions of the various infectious diseases of childhood are usually brief but thorough.

Behrman, Richard E., Robert M. Kliegman, and Hal B. Jenson, eds. *Nelson Textbook of Pediatrics*. 17th ed. Philadelphia: Saunders, 2004. This standard pediatrics textbook contains complete discussions of all common (and uncommon) causes of infectious disease in children. Many chapters are well written and easily understood by the nonspecialist.

Biddle, Wayne. *A Field Guide to Germs*. 2d ed. New York: Anchor Books, 2002. This comprehensive book is easily accessible to the nonspecialist and includes a discussion of nearly every virus, bacterium, and fungus known to cause human and nonhuman animal disease. The history of the microbe and the treatment of diseases are included.

Burg, Fredric D., et al., eds. *Treatment of Infants, Children, and Adolescents*. Philadelphia: W. B. Saunders, 1990. One can quickly find specific information about vaccine dosages and other valuable information in this text.

Kimball, Chad T. *Childhood Diseases and Disorders Sourcebook: Basic Consumer Health Information About Medical Problems Often Encountered in Preadolescent Children*. Detroit: Omnigraphics, 2003. Offers basic facts about common illnesses, serious diseases, and chronic conditions in children. Discusses frequently used diagnostic tests, surgeries, and medications. Long-term care for seriously ill children is also presented.

Kumar, Vinay, Abul K. Abbas, and Nelson Fausto, eds. *Robbins and Cotran Pathologic Basis of Disease*. 7th ed. Philadelphia: Elsevier Saunders, 2005. An excellent textbook that combines the clinical and the pathological beautifully.

Woolf, Alan D., et al., eds. *The Children's Hospital Guide to Your Child's Health and Development*. Cambridge, Mass.: Perseus, 2002. An authoritative and comprehensive guide to children's health, providing a guide to every common illness or condition that affects children and a carefully designed emergency section.

CHIROPRACTIC

SPECIALTY

ANATOMY OR SYSTEM AFFECTED: Back, bones, hips, musculoskeletal system, nervous system, spine

SPECIALTIES AND RELATED FIELDS: Neurology, orthopedics, preventive medicine

DEFINITION: The art and science of adjusting the spine and other bony articulations of the body in order to restore and maintain normal structure and function in the nervous system.

KEY TERMS:

adjustment: a thrust delivered into the spine or its articulations with the purpose of reestablishing normal joint and nerve function

nerve interference/pressure: chiropractic term that refers to a disturbance of normal nerve impulse transmission, usually via compression, stretch, or chronic irritation

neuromusculoskeletal: pertaining to the interrelationship between the nerves, muscles, and skeletal aspects of the body

palpation: the act of feeling with the hand; the application of the fingers with light pressure to the surface of the body for the purpose of determining the consistence of the parts beneath for physical diagnosis

subluxation: an incomplete or partial dislocation of a joint, which creates abnormal neurological and physiological symptoms in neuromusculoskeletal structures and/or other body systems via interference with nerve impulse transmission

SCIENCE AND PROFESSION

In the United States, chiropractic has the second largest patient base in the health care system. Licensed in every state, chiropractors are acknowledged as physicians along with medical doctors and osteopathic doctors, dentists, podiatrists, optometrists, and psychologists. Patients can consult with chiropractic physicians without referral. The scope of chiropractic practice varies from state to state, and reference must be made to specific state laws for exact information. The major premise of this field states that vertebrae of the spine can, and frequently do, become misaligned, causing interference in normal conduction of nerve impulses from the brain to the organs and tissues of the body. Although most spinal misalignments are corrected naturally through normal body movement, some become fixated. As a result, normal nerve transmission is impaired for long periods, and health suffers.

What distinguishes doctors of chiropractic from other health care professions is that they work primarily to identify, analyze, and adjust the vertebrae and pelvis back to their correct positions. Treatment is directed at restoring and maintaining normal structure and mechanical function of the spine to reduce irritation of the spinal cord and spinal nerves. These irritations lead to pain and distress of the muscles and joints of the body. Less acknowledged and still in want of corroborating research is the relationship between the subluxation, the neuromusculoskeletal system, and internal organ dysfunction. Contrary to popular belief, the scope of chiropractic is recognized for its ability to promote the total health and integration of the body from the inside out. In addition to spinal adjusting, chiropractors encourage those whom they treat to take personal responsibility for their lives by teaching ways to preserve health rather than wait until symptoms of disease appear.

Doctors of chiropractic may examine, diagnose, analyze, and use X rays for diagnostic purposes according to generally recognized procedures taught in accredited chiropractic colleges. Clinical practice generally encompasses consultation and taking a history of the patient; physical, neurological, orthopedic, and chiropractic examinations; X-ray analysis of the spine and articulating structures; the administration of adjustments; physiotherapy; nutritional support; and the use of orthopedic supports. In most states, chiropractic practice does not include the prescription or administration of medicine or drugs, performance of surgery, practice of obstetrics, administration of radiation therapy, treatment of infectious or sexually transmitted diseases, performance of internal exams, reduction of fractures, or administration of anesthetics. Historically, chiropractic physicians practice either solo or in a group setting with other chiropractors and do not have hospital privileges. This is changing as some chiropractic physicians are entering into group practice settings with other health care specialists and gaining admittance to hospitals in a limited capacity.

Chiropractic history dates back to 1895 when D. D. Palmer experimented with a spinal adjustment on Harvey Lillard. Lillard, a janitor, had experienced a "popping sensation" in his upper spine caused by heavy lifting and subsequently had a loss of hearing. After treatment, Lillard's hearing improved and Palmer for-

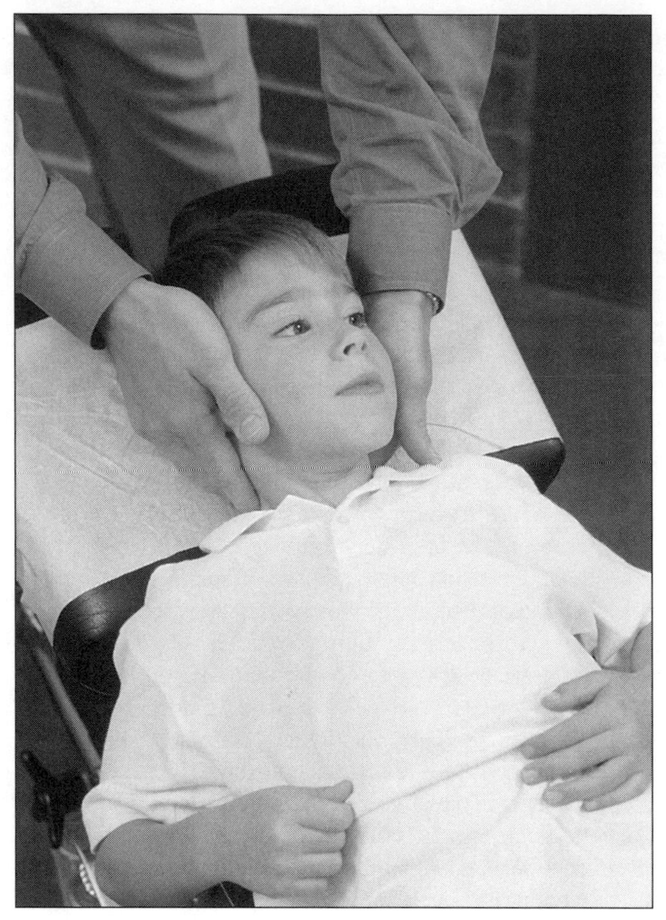

A chiropractor performs a manipulation on the neck of a young patient. (PhotoDisc)

mulated early chiropractic scientific premise and philosophy: that illness is essentially functional in nature and becomes organic only as an end process. His son, B. J. Palmer, is credited with refining and promoting the work of his father. Chiropractic lays claim to a colorful and compelling history into its first century. From its humble beginnings, it has survived as a viable alternative health care system in America and has emerged as the second largest health care entity in the industry. The early educational program organized by D. D. Palmer was admittedly crude, abbreviated, and inadequate. As the profession grew and matured, however, so did the educational standards to the current level, which is beyond reproach.

Chiropractic colleges are sanctioned as degree-granting institutions by the same regional accrediting agencies that regulate all other colleges and universities. Chiropractic colleges are accredited by the Council on Chiropractic Education, which is in turn approved by the United States Office of Education. Programs of study in chiropractic colleges parallel those in medical colleges except that chiropractic theory and practice replace surgery and medical theory. The medical curriculum is designed to prepare the medical student to diagnose and combat systemic diseases, with great emphasis on the use of drugs and surgery. The chiropractic curriculum, on the other hand, is designed to prepare the chiropractic student to evaluate and manage conservatively conditions from a holistic point of view, in which the various factors that affect a person's health are taken into consideration, including diet, nutritional supplementation, exercise, stress, and lifestyle.

Chiropractors have a full medical curriculum enabling them to make diagnoses. The education of a chiropractor begins with two years of preprofessional college study, with concentration in the human sciences. Although this prerequisite of two years is all that is required, the majority of students entering chiropractic college possess at least a bachelor's degree. The student then begins the Doctor of Chiropractic (D.C.) course of study at an accredited chiropractic college. The D.C. program is composed of four academic years of study most often divided into semesters or trimesters. The initial phase of study is much like any curriculum in the medical, dental, or veterinary schools, consisting of courses in the basic sciences: organic chemistry, biochemistry, anatomy of the musculoskeletal system (including limbs, trunk, and head), anatomy of the internal structures of the body (including all the organs, blood vessels, and internal systems), neuroanatomy (the anatomy of the brain, spinal cord, and entire nervous system), physiology (the study of how these systems function), neurophysiology, pathology (the study of disease), bacteriology, histology (the microscopic study of body tissues), and microbiology. The remainder of the courses are concentrated on the clinical sciences: X-ray physics, positioning, and interpretation; laboratory diagnosis (blood and urine studies); physical examination and diagnosis; neurology; orthopedics; cardiology; obstetrics and gynecology; pediatrics; geriatrics; dermatology; gastrointestinal and genitourinary systems; physical therapy nutrition; and chiropractic adjustment techniques.

During the later part of the student chiropractor's matriculation, he or she will see patients in a college-affiliated clinic as an "extern," which prepares the future doctor for patient care and management. In addition to the basic chiropractic curriculum, there are residencies available in both radiology and orthopedics. A chiropractic graduate may apply to study an additional three years in order to become either a chiropractic radiologist or a chiropractic orthopedist. The training received in these programs is highly specialized, and both of these chiropractic specialists are the equal of their medical counterparts in terms of diagnostic abilities. In addition, comprehensive 360-hour programs of study in orthopedics, neurology, radiology, and sports medicine exist; doctors completing such programs are eligible to sit for an examination to be awarded Diplomate status by chiropractic boards in the corresponding specialties. Postgraduate education for the practicing chiropractor includes seminars and workshops in soft tissue injuries, disk syndromes, low back pain, and other common and difficult conditions. Interdisciplinary seminars and conferences in nutrition, fitness, biochemical imbalances, and numerous other areas of common interest allow physicians from every discipline the opportunity to exchange views and perspectives.

The licensing procedure for the graduate chiropractic doctor varies from state to state. During the formal educational process, chiropractic students are exposed to thorough written examinations in all basic science and clinical subjects, which are administered by the National Board of Chiropractic Examiners. Successful completion of these written tests is a prerequisite to licensure in many states. Otherwise, completion of a written and practical examination administered by the respective state board is required, and in some states completion of the National Board Examinations and a state-administered written board are both required. The majority of states require doctors to attend certified educational seminars for continued licensure. The chiropractic profession is generally organized on a state basis through professional state associations and on a national basis through national organizations.

Diagnostic and Treatment Techniques

To understand fully how chiropractic health care works, it is necessary to understand the spine and the role that it plays in overall body function. The nervous system—consisting of the brain, cranial nerves (nerves that originate in the head), the spinal cord, and thirty-one pairs of spinal nerves that branch out much as the limbs of a tree do—generates and regulates all activities in the body. While no one knows exactly how the nervous system functions, it is known that signals, or impulses, travel along the nerve fibers conveying information between the brain and the rest of the body. Since every tissue and organ of the body is connected to and controlled by nerves from the spinal cord and brain, removal or nerve interference can bring dramatic results. Interference with the transmission of these impulses results in alteration of normal body function. The cranium (skull) and spinal column, composed of twenty-four bones called vertebrae, house the brain and spinal cord. In addition to protecting the spinal cord, the spine is the core of the skeletal framework that supports upright posture, provides for organ and muscle attachment, and allows for the dynamics of human movement. Given this monumental job, the spine and its connecting framework are subject to much activity and abuse.

In order for the mechanics of body motion to occur properly, there must be full, free, and harmonious movement in every one of the spinal joints. The working unit of the spine is referred to as the motor unit. The motor unit is composed of two vertebrae joined by cartilage cushions called disks and four posterior joints called facet joints, two located to attach the superior vertebra and two to attach the inferior vertebra. The disks separate the vertebrae while allowing flexibility and shock absorption for the spine. They also maintain openings between the vertebrae that are necessary for the passage of the spinal nerves. The facet joints provide additional movement and are limited in their range of motion by ligaments. Restriction in any of them can be compensated for only by the other joints and adjoining structures (such as ribs, muscles, or tendons), thus producing strain in the compensating structures.

It is at the location of the facet joints of the spine where subluxation occurs—an alteration of the alignment and proper movement of the spinal joint resulting in irritation of the exiting spinal nerve via compression, stretch, or chronic (constant) irritation—and leads to alteration of normal body functions. Subluxations can result from various factors, including trauma, toxic irritation, muscular imbalance caused by disuse and/or repetitive tasks, ligamental weakening, organic dysfunction, and stress. The altered nerve impulse transmission, left uncorrected, results in accumulative dysfunction in the tissue cells of the body.

Spinal biomechanics, the basis of the chiropractor's evaluation, refers to the manner in which the spine works in movement. Restoration of spinal motion is the primary treatment on which chiropractors depend to alleviate patients' symptoms. The single most unique element of chiropractic procedures is the spinal adjustment. This chiropractic adjustment is a technique of physically moving the spine by hand or by instrument with the objective of mobilizing a fixated joint. It is a gentle but dynamic thrust applied to a specific joint in a way that generates joint movement in a specific direction. Basically, it is a way to "coax" a restricted joint into moving. Applied repeatedly over a period of time, spinal adjustments are capable of restoring mobility to even the most chronic spinal subluxations. Deep-rooted subluxations that have existed for several years typically require months of care. Fixations of lesser duration and severity respond in less time, often the mildest in one treatment. The procedure works because the restoration of the proper mechanics of spinal motion via the spinal adjustment improves joint function, corrects specific joint problems, and helps prevent injury through increased spinal strength brought about by spinal joints that function properly.

Chiropractic health care can be useful for the detection and correction of existing health problems and/or for preventive purposes. In lieu of concentrating on bacterial or viral infections or treating the end-symptoms of disease processes, chiropractors look for the reason that a patient's symptom developed, including such contributing factors as environmental conditions, lifestyle, systemic stress, and malfunction. For example, instead of giving medication to stop the pain of headache, the chiropractor analyzes possible irritating factors, including subluxation, that may be causing the headache and addresses that factor first. Thus, in many cases, the prescription of medication can be avoided.

Perspective and Prospects

Chiropractic originated in the second half of the nineteenth century during a time when many theories of healing were being promulgated. Chiropractic and osteopathy shared their early beginnings amid the emergence of several alternatives to the regular school of healing (medicine), including the Thomsonian system (the use of botanicals), the Hygienic movement (the use of fresh fruits and vegetables, fresh air, exercise, and better food preparation), and homeopathy. Daniel David Palmer, born in 1845 in Canada, was involved in making and losing several small mercantile fortunes when he made his way to Iowa in 1886 to become a magnetic healer. Over the next decade, he would attract patients from throughout the Midwest until one day in September, 1895, a janitor named Harvey Lillard came into his office, received an "adjustment," and regained his lost hearing. Soon afterward, the term "chiropractic" (Greek meaning "done by hand") was coined by Samuel Weed, a Palmer patient. D. D. Palmer began giving instruction at Dr. Palmer's School and Cure, later becoming Palmer Institute and Chiropractic Infirmary and finally Palmer Chiropractic College.

Brian Inglis, a distinguished British historian, commentator, and author of the two-volume work *The History of Medicine* (1965), has declared: "The rise of chiropractic . . . has been one of the most remarkable social phenomena in American history . . . yet it has gone virtually unexplored." In spite of its humble origins and formulative years, chiropractic has had a decided impact on the evolution of health care attitudes in the United States and to some degree in other parts of the Western world. For more than three-quarters of a century, it fought for its very survival, overcoming a strong medical lobby in 1977 when the American Medical Association (AMA) reversed its long-standing policy against professional interrelationships between medical doctors and chiropractors. In March, 1977, the AMA's Judicial Council announced:

> A physician may refer a patient for diagnostic or therapeutic services to another physician, a limited practitioner, or any other provider of health care services permitted by law to furnish such services, whenever he believes that this may benefit the patient. As in the case of referrals to physician-specialists, referrals to limited practitioners should be based on their individual competence and ability to perform the services needed by the patient.

Despite the AMA's policy change toward chiropractic, however, complete acceptance by the medical profession has not occurred. This reluctance has not been attributable solely to the attitudes of the medical profession. Rather, it is the result of a combination of the continued opposition of the medical profession and the resistance of chiropractors to subordinate themselves to medical prescription, as with physical therapists who practice under medical supervision. Chiropractors have been independent practitioners for too long, functioning at a high level in the diagnosis and treatment of illness, for them to be willing to regress in status.

It is likely that the chiropractic profession will continue on its present course of becoming a health profession with parallels to medicine. Emphasizing the uniqueness of chiropractic treatment and the contrasting philosophical approaches of health maintenance and therapy, chiropractic has not only survived but also flourished. Whether used as a preventive means to ensure good health or as a way to help the body cure itself of disease, chiropractic has sometimes succeeded where other health care measures have failed.

—*Cindy Nesci, D.C.*

See also Alternative medicine; Anxiety; Bone disorders; Bones and the skeleton; Massage; Muscle sprains, spasms, and disorders; Muscles; Pain; Pain management; Physical rehabilitation; Spinal cord disorders; Spine, vertebrae, and disks; Stress; Stress reduction.

FOR FURTHER INFORMATION:

Altman, Nathaniel. *Everybody's Guide to Chiropractic Health Care*. New York: St. Martin's Press, 1990. A consumer's handbook written to inform the layperson who is searching for an alternative to traditional, medical health care.

Coulter, Ian Douglass. *Chiropractic: A Philosophy for Alternative Health Care*. Boston: Butterworth-Heinemann, 1999. Explores how chiropractic differs from orthodox medicine in its approach to health care and patient problems.

Haldeman, Scott, ed. *Principles and Practice of Chiropractic*. 3d ed. New York: McGraw-Hill, 2005. A collection of articles by leading authorities in the fields of history, sociology, neurophysiology, spinal biomechanics, and clinical chiropractic. Written with the purpose of presenting an accurate overview of the latest developments in the field.

Lenarz, Michael, and Victoria St. George. *The Chiropractic Way*. New York: Bantam, 2003. Explores the healing qualities of a rapidly growing alternative health field. Basic principles of spinal health, chiropractic techniques, and complementary diet, exercise, and stress-relief programs are covered.

Peterson, David H., and Thomas F. Bergmann. *Chiropractic Technique: Principles and Procedures*. 2d ed. St. Louis: Mosby, 2002. Traces the historical and scientific roots of chiropractic care and gives hands-on guidance to techniques.

Tousley, Dirk, and David M. Lees. *The Chiropractic Handbook for Patients*. 3d ed. Independence, Mo.: White Dove, 1985. This popular work on chiropractic is written with the general reader in mind. Contains information that will help patients understand their treatment.

CHLAMYDIA

DISEASE/DISORDER

ANATOMY OR SYSTEM AFFECTED: Eyes, genitals, lungs, lymphatic system, reproductive system, urinary system

SPECIALTIES AND RELATED FIELDS: Gynecology, microbiology

DEFINITION: The most common sexually transmitted disease in the United States, which primarily infects the reproductive tract and is caused by the bacterium *Chlamydia trachomatis*.

KEY TERMS:

contact tracing: also known as partner referral; a process that consists of identifying sexual partners of infected patients, informing the partners of their exposure to disease, and offering resources for counseling and treatment

screening procedures: tests that are carried out in populations which are usually asymptomatic and at high risk for a disease in order to identify those in need of treatment

sexually transmitted disease: an infection caused by organisms transferred through sexual contact (genital-genital, orogenital, or anogenital); transmission of infection occurs through exposure to lesions or secretions which contain the organisms

CAUSES AND SYMPTOMS

Chlamydia is the most common sexually transmitted disease (STD) in the United States, with a prevalence of about 10 percent in sexually active men and women. Chlamydia is caused by a bacterium called *Chlamydia trachomatis* that infects cells on mucosal surfaces, such as the genital tract, urinary tract, anorectal tract, eyes, and throat. These infections cause inflammation of the cervix, urethra, prostate, or epididymis. In women, symptoms may include urinary discomfort, lower abdominal pain, and abnormal vaginal discharge. In men, symptoms may involve urinary discomfort and unusual discharge from the urethra.

Most cases of chlamydia are asymptomatic, and many patients are diagnosed based on screening procedures. Nevertheless, asymptomatic patients are able to infect others and can suffer serious consequences of chlamydia infection, such as pelvic inflammatory disease (PID) and infertility. PID occurs when chlamydia infection ascends the female reproductive tract to involve the uterus, Fallopian tubes, and pelvic cavity. This infection of the upper reproductive tract can lead to scarring of these organs and puts the

Information on Chlamydia

Causes: Bacterial infection of mucosa (genital tract, urinary tract, anorectal tract, eyes, throat) through sexual transmission or childbirth
Symptoms: Often none, but may include urinary discomfort, lower abdominal pain, abnormal discharge from vagina or urethra, complications such as pelvic inflammatory disease (PID) and infertility; in infants, eye infection, visual impairment, blindness, respiratory tract infection
Duration: Chronic until treated
Treatments: Antibiotics (doxycycline, azithromycin, erythromycin, ofloxacin)

patient at increased risk of infertility and ectopic pregnancy.

In rare cases, chlamydia can travel to regional lymph nodes and cause abscesses, a condition termed lymphogranuloma venereum. This condition is commonly accompanied by systemic symptoms such as fever, chills, and muscle and joint aches.

An infant may contract chlamydia as it passes through the birth canal of an infected mother. The disease can lead to eye infection that results in visual impairment and blindness, as well as infection of the respiratory tract.

Treatment and Therapy

A patient receives antibiotic therapy if laboratory tests indicate infection with *C. trachomatis*. Uncomplicated chlamydia infection can be treated effectively with antibiotics such as doxycycline, azithromycin, erythromycin, or ofloxacin. A patient with risk factors for STDs or symptoms of the disease is treated presumptively with antibiotic therapy, even before the results of laboratory tests for chlamydia return.

Because chlamydia is associated with other STDs, such as gonorrhea, human immunodeficiency virus (HIV), syphilis, and hepatitis B and C, the patient undergoes testing for these diseases as well. Up to 50 percent of patients with chlamydia also have gonorrhea, so an antibiotic against gonorrhea is given along with an antibiotic for chlamydia, unless laboratory tests have declared the patient free of gonorrhea. If chlamydia and gonorrhea are treated early, complications such as PID or infertility can be avoided.

In addition to antibiotics, a key component of chlamydia treatment involves counseling in the prevention of STDs. To minimize future exposure to chlamydia and other STDs, patients are encouraged to use barrier methods such as condoms during intercourse and to avoid high-risk sexual behaviors.

Another key component to the treatment of chlamydia and other STDs is contact tracing, which occurs once the infection is confirmed with laboratory testing. With the cooperation of the patient, all sexual partners of the patient are notified regarding their exposure to disease. Partners are encouraged to seek medical attention, even if they have no symptoms themselves, in order to prevent reinfection of the patient during subsequent sexual encounters or further spread of the disease to other sexual partners.

In the United States, erythromycin eyedrops are given prophylactically to all newborns to prevent eye infections with chlamydia that could lead to visual impairment.

Perspective and Prospects

Diseases caused by *C. trachomatis* have been described as early as ancient Egyptian times. It was not until 1907, however, that the bacterium was actually identified. In the 1960's, a clinically useful diagnostic test was developed that allowed screening of a large number of bacterial specimens within a few days. The development of a relatively easy test for chlamydia enabled physicians to screen a large number of asymptomatic but at-risk patients (such as those under age twenty-five or those with multiple sexual partners).

A promising area of research is the search for a vaccine to *C. trachomatis*. This research focuses on identifying antigens on the bacterium that are important for its function, such as proteins responsible for bacterial attachment to or uptake into cells. The premise is to use these proteins to generate an immune response in patients so that when patients are exposed to chlamydia, their immune systems are prepared to respond against it.

—Anne Lynn S. Chang, M.D.

See also Acquired immunodeficiency syndrome (AIDS); Antibiotics; Bacterial infections; Blindness; Conjunctivitis; Epidemiology; Genital disorders, female; Genital disorders, male; Gonorrhea; Gynecology; Hepatitis; Herpes; Human immunodeficiency virus (HIV); Infertility, female; Men's health; Pelvic inflammatory disease (PID); Reproductive system; Screening; Sexually transmitted diseases (STDs); Syphilis; Trachoma; Women's health.

For Further Information:

Centers for Disease Control. "1998 Guidelines for the Treatment of Sexually Transmitted Diseases." *Morbidity and Mortality Weekly Report* 47, no. RR-1 (January, 1997): 1-115.

Holmes, King K., et al., eds. *Sexually Transmitted Diseases*. 3d ed. New York: McGraw-Hill, 1999.

Kasper, Dennis L., et al., eds. *Harrison's Principles of Internal Medicine*. 16th ed. New York: McGraw-Hill, 2005.

Ryan, Kenneth J., and C. George Ray, eds. *Sherris Medical Microbiology: An Introduction to Infectious Diseases*. 4th ed. New York: McGraw-Hill, 2004.

Choking

Disease/disorder

Anatomy or system affected: Chest, lungs, neck, respiratory system, throat

Specialties and related fields: Emergency medicine

Definition: A condition in which the breathing passage (windpipe) is obstructed.

Information on Choking

Causes: Blockage of airway, injury
Symptoms: Coughing, red face, grabbing at throat
Duration: Acute
Treatments: Heimlich maneuver, emergency care

Causes and Symptoms

A person who is choking may cough, turn red in the face, clutch his or her throat, or any combination of the above. If the choking person is coughing, it is probably best to do nothing; the coughing should naturally clear the airway. The true choking emergency occurs when a bit of food or other foreign object completely obstructs the breathing passage. In this case, there is little or no coughing—the person cannot make much sound. This silent choking calls for immediate action.

Treatment and Therapy

An individual witnessing a choking emergency should first call for emergency help and then perform the Heimlich maneuver. The choking person should never be slapped on the back. The Heimlich maneuver is best performed while the choking victim is standing or seated. If possible, the person performing the Heimlich maneuver should ask the victim to nod if he or she wishes the Heimlich maneuver to be performed. If the airway is totally blocked, the victim will not be able to speak and may even be unconscious.

The individual performing the Heimlich maneuver positions himself or herself behind the choking victim and places his or her arms around the victim's waist. Making a fist with one hand and grasping that fist with the other hand, the rescuer positions the thumb side of the fist toward the stomach of the victim—just above the navel and below the ribs. The person performing the maneuver pulls his or her fist upward into the abdomen of the victim with several quick thrusts. This action should expel the foreign object from the victim's throat, and he or she should begin coughing or return to normal breathing.

The Heimlich maneuver is not effective in dislodging fish bones and certain other obstructions. If the airway is still blocked after several Heimlich thrusts, a finger sweep should be tried to remove the obstruction. First the mouth of the victim must be opened: The chin is grasped, and the mouth is pulled open with one hand. With the index finger of the other hand, the rescuer sweeps through the victim's throat, pulling out any foreign material. One sweep should be made from left to right, and a second sweep from right to left. The Heimlich maneuver may then be repeated if necessary.

—Steven A. Schonefeld, Ph.D.

See also Asphyxiation; Coughing; Cyanosis; Heimlich maneuver; Hyperventilation; Respiration; Resuscitation; Unconsciousness.

For Further Information:

American College of Emergency Physicians. *Pocket First Aid*. London: DK, 2003. An excellent reference guide illustrated with photographs and written in a clear, step-by-step format. Covers many first aid methods, from resuscitation of conscious and unconscious choking victims, to how to deal with bleeding, shock, spinal injuries, poisoning, seizures, fractures, and bandages.

Castleman, Michael. "Life Saving Moves from EMS Experts." *Family Circle* 107, no. 4 (March 15, 1994): 37. Tips are presented for care of nine medical emergencies, including bleeding and shock. First aid help should be given with care, because certain injuries can be made worse with improper treatment.

Mosby's Medical Dictionary. 7th ed. St. Louis: Mosby/

Elsevier, 2006. Offers a basic presentation of medical terms and concepts.
Stern, Loraine. "Mom, I Can't Breathe!" *Woman's Day* 57, no. 6 (March 15, 1994): 18. The various ailments that can cause breathing problems in children are described. The signs that could signal serious illness include inability to swallow, difficulty speaking or finishing a sentence, and breathing difficulties that rapidly become more severe.

Cholecystectomy

Procedure

Anatomy or system affected: Abdomen, gallbladder, gastrointestinal system

Specialties and related fields: General surgery

Definition: The surgical removal of a diseased gallbladder.

Indications and Procedures

Cholecystectomy is indicated when the patient exhibits nausea, vomiting, and abdominal pain and examination reveals gallstones. Gallstones, which consist mostly of crystallized cholesterol and bile, form in the gallbladder and may lodge in the bile duct. The stones can be dissolved with medication or broken up with ultrasound and passed from the body. They can (and often do) form again, however, with renewed symptoms. Removal of the gallbladder is the method of choice to prevent the recurrence of symptoms. Surgery is performed under general anesthesia.

In open surgery, the abdomen is cleaned and a 7.5- to 15-centimeter (3- to 6-inch) incision made with a scalpel through the skin and abdominal tissues. The gallbladder is isolated from the liver. A duct and artery are tied off with surgical staples or sutures, and they are cut in order to free the gallbladder. The organ is removed, and the tissues are closed with sutures or staples.

In laparoscopic surgery, the surface is cleaned and the surgeon makes four small holes. A 1.3-centimeter (0.5-inch) cut is made at or near the navel and another just below the breastbone, as well as two small punctures to the right of the incisions. The laparoscope, with a video camera and light, is inserted into the navel incision. Long, thin dissecting instruments are passed through the three punctures, and the gallbladder is cut free as in open surgery. The organ is removed through the navel incision, which is then closed with sutures or staples. The punctures are closed with small adhesive bandages.

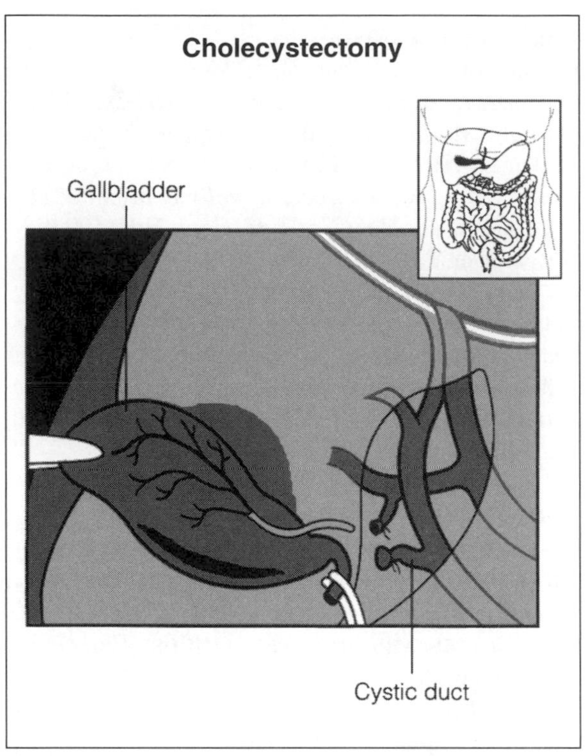

The removal of the gallbladder may be indicated with severe infection of the organs or with repeated attacks of biliary colic caused by the presence of gallstones; the inset shows the location of the gallbladder.

Uses and Complications

Open surgery for cholecystectomy requires a hospital stay of five to eight days and a recovery time of four to six weeks. Complications occur in 1.0 to 9.4 percent of the surgeries and range from postoperative bleeding and diarrhea to intestinal obstruction. The mortality rate is low: 0.2 to 0.6 percent.

Laparoscopic surgery usually requires an overnight stay and a recovery period of five to seven days. Complications occur in 5.1 percent of the surgeries and are similar to those in open surgery, but they may also include severing the common bile duct that connects the liver and small intestine and puncturing major blood vessels, including the largest one, the aorta. Laparoscopy is relatively new, and the preliminary mortality rate is 0.1 percent.

—*Albert C. Jensen, M.S.*

See also Cholecystitis; Gallbladder cancer; Gallbladder diseases; Gastroenterology; Gastrointestinal system; Laparoscopy; Stone removal; Stones.

For Further Information:

Büchler, M. W., et al., eds. *Five Years of Laparoscopic Cholecystectomy: A Reappraisal.* Farmington, Conn.: S. Karger A. G., 1996.

Chellappa, M. *Laparoscopic Cholecystectomy.* Teaneck, N.J.: World Scientific, 1994.

Dunn, David C., and Christopher J. E. Watson. *Laparoscopic Cholecystectomy: Problems and Solutions.* Cambridge, Mass.: Blackwell Science, 1992.

Jakimowicz, J. J., and T. J. Ruers, eds. *Laparoscopic Cholecystectomy: State of the Art.* Farmington, Conn.: S. Karger A. G., 1991.

Parker, James N., and Philip M. Parker, eds. *The Official Patient's Sourcebook on Gallstones.* San Diego, Calif.: Icon Health, 2002.

Cholecystitis

Disease/disorder

Anatomy or system affected: Abdomen, gallbladder, gastrointestinal system, liver, pancreas

Specialties and related fields: Emergency medicine, family medicine, gastroenterology, internal medicine, pathology

Definition: An inflammation of the gallbladder.

Causes and Symptoms

There are basically two types of cholecystitis, calculous and acalculous, both of which could present as acute or chronic inflammation of the gallbladder. The calculous type is seen in 90 percent of cases and is caused by an obstruction of the neck of the gallbladder by gallstones, which are usually composed of cholesterol. The cholesterol stones may block the gallbladder neck and cause an acute attack of cholecystitis, or they may act as chemical irritants and result in chronic inflammation. About 10 percent of cases of cholecystitis are not the result of gallstones and are hence called acalculous. A variety of factors may precipitate an acute attack, such as sepsis, severe trauma, severe burns, and even the postpartum state. Approximately 75 percent of patients with acute cholecystitis are female.

Information on Cholecystitis

Causes: Usually obstruction of gallbladder by gallstones; sometimes sepsis, severe trauma, severe burns

Symptoms: Severe, progressive upper-right abdominal pain, with nausea, vomiting, fever, sometimes jaundice

Duration: Often chronic, with acute episodes lasting one to three days

Treatments: None (spontaneous resolution), sometimes gallbladder removal

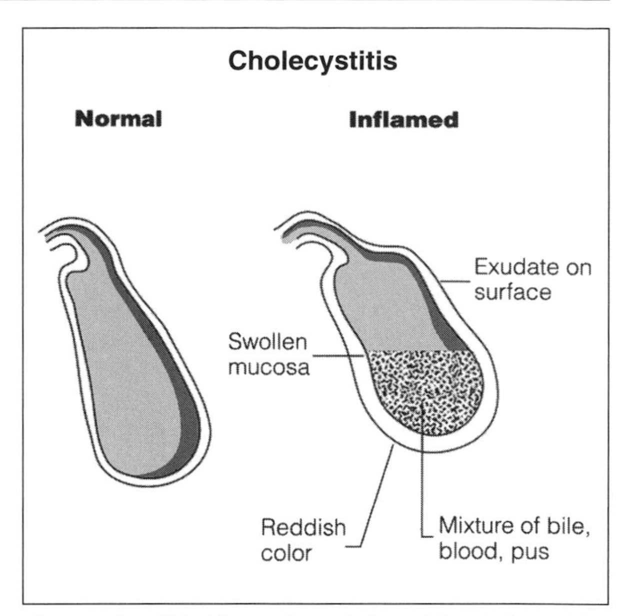

A normal gallbladder and one inflamed by cholecystitis.

Acute cholecystitis may first come to a medical attention in the emergency room, with the patient complaining of severe progressive right upper abdominal pain, which may be associated with nausea, vomiting, and fever. The pain could radiate to the back, in which case it is known as biliary colic. Jaundice (yellowish skin) may or may not be present, depending on the degree of obstruction of the gallbladder neck. The attack usually follows a large fatty meal and can last one to three days. Chronic cholecystitis is usually more insidious in onset and may arise following multiple attacks of acute cholecystitis. The presentation could vary, manifesting as mild upper-right abdominal distress or longstanding pain.

Diagnosis is usually made with an ultrasound of the abdomen that demonstrates calcified gallstones. Obstruction of the gallbladder neck cannot be visualized, however, and thus requires another imaging test called a hepatobiliary iminodiacetic acid (HIDA) scan. An elevated white blood cell count is also seen in most cases.

Treatment and Therapy

Most acute attacks of cholecystitis may resolve spontaneously, but they should always be considered for surgery, as removal of the gallbladder (cholecystectomy) is the only definitive therapy for the disease. The gallbladder is usually removed using laparoscopic surgery, wherein small incisions are made in the abdomen through which instruments and a fiber-optic camera are passed. In acute attacks, it may also be necessary to maintain adequate nutrition and fluid replacement. A low-fat diet is usually recommended for these patients.

In those patients who decide against surgery, there is a risk of perforation of the gallbladder, which has a 25 percent mortality rate.

—*Rashmi Ramasubbaiah, M.D., and Venkat Raghavan Tirumala, M.D., M.H.A.*

See also Cholecystectomy; Gallbladder diseases; Gastroenterology; Internal medicine; Stone removal; Stones.

For Further Information:

American Medical Association. *American Medical Association Family Medical Guide*. 4th rev. ed. Hoboken, N.J.: John Wiley & Sons, 2004.

Frazier, Margeret Schell, and Jeanette Wist Drzymkowski. *Essentials of Human Diseases and Conditions*. 3d ed. St. Louis: Saunders, 2004.

Kasper, Dennis L., et al., eds. *Harrison's Principles of Internal Medicine*. 16th ed. New York: McGraw-Hill, 2005.

Rakel, Robert E., ed. *Textbook of Family Practice*. 6th ed. Philadelphia: W. B. Saunders, 2002.

Tapley, Donald F., et al., eds. *The Columbia University College of Physicians and Surgeons Complete Home Medical Guide*. 3d rev. ed. New York: Crown, 1995.

Cholera

Disease/disorder

Anatomy or system affected: Circulatory system, gastrointestinal system, intestines, kidneys

Specialties and related fields: Environmental health, epidemiology, gastroenterology, internal medicine, microbiology, public health

Definition: An acute bacterial disease transmitted by polluted water and contaminated food.

Key terms:

epidemic: an acute disease prevalent and spreading rapidly in a community

pandemic: a worldwide epidemic

pathogen: a disease-causing organism

rice-water stools: extremely dilute feces comprising a whitish liquid containing rice-shaped flecks of solid mucus material; a characteristic symptom of cholera

Causes and Symptoms

The comma-shaped bacterium *Vibrio cholerae* causes the life-threatening disease cholera. The organism is spread when people ingest water or raw food contaminated with fecal matter. Studies have shown that the bacterium can live in both oceanic salt water and freshwater. In the ocean, it adheres to a type of zooplankton called copepods, which are eaten by certain types of shellfish. Therefore, people who consume shellfish grown in contaminated water can ingest the cholera organism. Also, people eating crops fertilized with human feces can ingest the organism.

Cholera affects particularly underdeveloped nations with poor sewage disposal and sanitation practices. It is endemic in Africa, Southeast Asia, the Indian subcontinent, and Central and South America. Even in developed nations, however, cholera may emerge after major disasters, such as hurricanes and earthquakes. Fewer than 250 cases were reported in the United States from 1996 to 2006, primarily around the Gulf Coast. Most of those cases were caused by the ingestion of contaminated raw shellfish.

After a person ingests contaminated food or water, between twenty-four and seventy-two hours elapse before the symptoms of cholera develop. Normally, between ten million to a billion *V. cholerae* bacteria must be present to cause infection, due to the large number that die in stomach acid. If an individual has taken antacids to neutralize stomach acid, however, then only about one thousand organisms are necessary to cause infection. Fewer organisms are also required if they enter the body via food, because the food protects some of the bacteria from the stomach acid.

The organisms that survive travel to the small intestine, attach to the epithelial cells there, and produce a toxin that causes a tremendous loss of water and electrolytes though extreme diarrhea and sometimes vomiting. Patients can lose more than twenty quarts of fluid per day. The extremely dilute feces are primarily a whitish liquid containing flecks of solid mucus material resembling rice grains, and hence are commonly called rice-water stools. The tremendous loss of fluids and electrolytes can lead to hypotension (low blood pressure), an increase in both pulse and respiratory rates, cardiac arrhythmia, kidney failure, and the appearance of sunken eyes and cheeks. Shock, resulting from changes in blood acidity and extremely low blood volume, can lead to death within a few hours, especially in children.

Information on Cholera

Causes: Bacterial infection via contaminated food or water
Symptoms: Diarrhea, vomiting
Duration: Several days
Treatments: Fluid and electrolyte replacement, antibiotics

Some strains of *V. cholerae* may produce almost no symptoms or only mild diarrhea in some individuals, but the majority of infected people experience very severe disease. Left untreated, approximately 60 percent of patients die; however, immediate rehydration therapy normally saves all but about 1 percent of patients. Nonfatal cases spontaneously resolve themselves after a few days, since both the organisms and the toxin that they produce are ejected from the patient's body in the diarrhea.

Treatment and Therapy

The best method for controlling cholera is prevention. Societies with adequate sanitation and sewage treatment are normally protected, except for contaminated seafood. Underdeveloped nations should be encouraged to improve their sanitation and sewage treatment practices and to cease using human feces as crop fertilizer. Also, especially in infected areas, raw foods and unpurified water should be avoided.

Although different vaccines have been developed, the immunity that they produce appears to be short-lived and not effective against all strains. Prophylactic antibiotic treatment for travelers entering affected areas has not been shown to be effective. Given the large number of bacteria needed for the disease to occur, however, proper hygienic practices alone should provide sufficient protection.

Treatment for cholera patients is primarily supportive, with rehydration and restoration of the electrolyte balance being paramount. Secondary treatment with antibiotics may reduce the presence of organisms and their production of toxin, thus ameliorating the symptoms. Because of the high volume of watery diarrhea, the antibiotic tends to be released from the body very rapidly. Doxycycline is usually the preferred drug, but trimethoprim-sulfamethoxazole or tetracycline have also been used. Unfortunately, certain strains of *V. cholerae* have been discovered to be resistant to the latter two antibiotics. Using antibiotics to more effectively eliminate the organism may be important, since it has been estimated that up to 20 percent of patients continue to carry *V. cholerae* asymptomatically for a time after recovery from the disease.

Perspective and Prospects

Historically, cholera has been a very important epidemic pathogen credited with causing seven different pandemics. These pandemics have affected various areas, including Asia, the Middle East, and Africa. Between 1832 and 1836, two pandemics (the second and fourth) affected the North American continent, resulting in 200,000 American deaths. While studying and trying to limit the effects of the 1854 cholera epidemic in London, physician John Snow founded the science of epidemiology and introduced techniques that are still in use today. The seventh pandemic occurred in 1961, starting in Indonesia and spreading to South Asia, the Middle East, and portions of both Europe and Africa.

In 1991, Peru suddenly reported new cases after being free of cholera for more than a century. Contaminated bilge water discharged from a freighter into the Peru harbor has been hypothesized as being responsible for the disease's reappearance. The water supply in the capital city of Lima was not chlorinated, and the organism rapidly multiplied and infected the inhabitants. In two years, more than 700,000 cases and 6,323 deaths were recorded in South and Central America, and spread of this cholera strain continues today.

The 1961 pandemic strain has caused over five million cases of cholera and more than 250,000 deaths. In 1992, a genetic variant of this strain appeared in Bangladesh, causing an epidemic. Whether this cholera strain will eventually initiate an eighth pandemic remains to be seen.

—*Steven A. Kuhl, Ph.D.*

See also Bacterial infections; Bacteriology; Diarrhea and dysentery; Environmental health

For Further Information:

Ezzell, Carol. "It Came from the Deep." *Scientific American* 280 (June, 1999): 22-24.

Pennisi, Elizabeth. "Infectious Disease: Cholera Strengthened by Trip Through Gut." *Science* 296 (June, 2002): 1783-1784.

Reidl, Joachim, et al. "*Vibrio cholerae* and Cholera: Out of the Water and into the Host." *FEMS Microbiological Reviews* 26 (June, 2002): 125-139.

Wachsmuth, Kaye, et al. *"Vibrio cholerae" and Chol-*

era: Molecular to Global Perspectives. Washington, D.C.: American Society for Microbiology. 1994.

Zimmer, Carl. "Infectious Diseases: Taming Pathogens—An Elegant Idea, but Does It Work?" *Science* 300 (May, 2003): 1362-1364.

Cholesterol

Biology

Anatomy or system affected: Blood vessels, cells, circulatory system, gastrointestinal system

Specialties and related fields: Biochemistry, cytology, family medicine, internal medicine, nutrition, preventive medicine, vascular medicine

Definition: A lipid substance that is a structural component of cell membranes and which makes up the surface of lipoproteins.

Key terms:

cholesterol: a lipid substance that is a component of cell membranes and the surface of circulating lipoproteins

cholesteryl ester: cholesterol linked to a fatty acid; it is stored in lipid droplets in the cytoplasm of cells and circulates in the core of lipoproteins

lipids: substances that are poorly soluble in water; in animal tissues, the principal lipids are triglycerides (fat), phospholipids, cholesterol, and cholesteryl esters

lipoproteins: lipid aggregates that transport fat and cholesteryl esters in the circulation; associated apolipoproteins determine how rapidly they are taken up by the liver or other tissues

sterols: a class of chemically related lipids; cholesterol is the principal sterol in vertebrates, but in plants its functions are served by related substances

Structure and Functions

Living cells are bounded by a cell membrane composed of a double layer of phospholipid, associated with and traversed by proteins that have catalytic, transportation, and signaling functions. Variable amounts of sterol are interspersed among the molecules of phospholipid in each membrane layer. Sterols are essential components in the membranes of fungal, plant, and animal cells (but not in bacteria). In vertebrates, the predominant sterol is cholesterol. There is little or no cholesterol in plant cell membranes; its place is taken by chemically related substances, chiefly sitosterol. This fact is of nutritional significance; only animal products add cholesterol to the diet.

In mammals, cholesterol is the precursor of steroid hormones, which are essential for mineral balance, adjustment of the body to stress, and normal reproductive function. It is also the precursor of bile acids, which are required for the absorption of dietary lipids. Bile acids play a role in cholesterol balance, since their formation and secretion by the liver, along with some free cholesterol, is the only significant pathway for removal of cholesterol from the body.

Cholesterol itself is required for normal functioning of the mammalian cell membrane. Cholesterol alters the membrane's fluidity—the ease with which proteins embedded in the membrane can move about and interact with one another—and also affects the activity of enzymes and transport proteins embedded in the membrane. Cultured cells that are prevented from making their own cholesterol will not grow unless it is provided in the medium.

Free cholesterol is confined to cellular membranes. Cholesterol content is highest (about one molecule of cholesterol for every one or two molecules of phospholipid) in the outer cell membrane that forms the boundary between a cell and its environment. It is much lower in intracellular membranes. Although cholesterol synthesis is completed within the endoplasmic reticulum, the ratio of cholesterol to phospholipid in this membrane is less than one to twenty. In a typical cell, it is estimated that between 80 and 90 percent of the total free cholesterol is located in the outer cell membrane.

Cholesterol in excess of normal proportions is coupled (esterified) to long-chain fatty acids. The resulting cholesteryl ester accumulates, along with triglyceride, in lipid droplets in the cytoplasm. The activity of the enzyme catalyzing this esterification is increased when cholesterol is imported into the cell in excess of its needs. The ability to esterify and sequester cholesterol defends the cell against excessive membrane concentration of the free sterol.

Free cholesterol and cholesteryl ester are carried in plasma in lipoproteins. Lipoproteins are aggregates of several thousand molecules of lipid and one or more molecules of specific proteins (apolipoproteins). Each lipoprotein particle consists of a core of triglyceride and cholesteryl ester surrounded by a single layer of phospholipid and free cholesterol. The apolipoproteins are embedded in the surface of the particle. Lipoproteins differ in size and relative lipid composition. In humans, about two-thirds of circulating cholesterol is contained in low-density lipoprotein (LDL), a core of cholesteryl ester with a single molecule of apolipoprotein B on the surface. LDL transports cholesterol from the liver to peripheral tissues. Most of the remaining circulating cholesterol is carried in high-density lipoprotein (HDL), which transports cholesterol from peripheral tissues back to the liver for disposal. Under normal conditions, LDL is the principal source of exogenous cholesterol available to a cell.

Uptake of LDL is mediated by a specific protein on the cell's surface, the LDL receptor, which is concentrated in pockets in the cell membrane termed coated pits. LDL receptors bind apolipoprotein B and particles such as LDL that contain this protein. Coated pits continually pinch off to form sealed vesicles (endosomes) inside the cell. At the same time, new coated pits form on the cell surface. When a coated pit pinches off, it carries with it LDL receptors and associated LDL. The fluid within the endosome is acidified, which causes LDL to dissociate from its receptor and float free. The LDL is transferred to lysosomes, where cholesteryl ester is cleaved to liberate cholesterol; along with the free cholesterol that formed part of the LDL surface, this liberated cholesterol is now available for use within the cell. The LDL receptor is returned to the cell surface, where it can again become associated with a coated pit and participate in a new round of LDL uptake.

The rate at which LDL is removed from the circulation depends on the concentration of LDL receptors in cells of the liver and other tissues. (Although there are other mechanisms for removing LDL, these are less efficient than uptake via the LDL receptor.) This process is subject to feedback regulation. When a cell contains an adequate supply of cholesterol, the synthesis of new LDL receptors is inhibited. This inhibition occurs at the transcriptional level: The rate at which the gene for the LDL receptor is copied into messenger ribonucleic acid (mRNA) is reduced. With less mRNA for this protein reaching the cytoplasm, the rate at which new copies of the protein are made also falls. Following normal turnover of existing receptors, the concentration of LDL receptors at the cell surface declines and the uptake of cholesterol is accordingly reduced.

The gene for the LDL receptor contains short stretches of deoxyribonucleic acid (DNA), termed sterol response elements (SREs), that make transcription sensitive to cholesterol-induced "down-regulation." These can be spliced out and inserted into another gene that codes for a bacterial protein. The foreign gene can be inserted into a mammalian cell, which will then begin to produce the corresponding protein. If the foreign gene does not contain an SRE, the rate of synthesis of the coded protein is unaffected by the cholesterol content of the recipient cell. When an SRE has been inserted into the gene in an appropriate location, however, excess cholesterol down-regulates transcription of the foreign gene just as it does that for the LDL receptor.

The signal that causes down-regulation of the cholesterol receptor has not been clearly identified. It is possible that an internal "regulatory" pool of cholesterol—such as the cholesterol content of certain internal membranes or the concentration of individual cholesterol molecules bound to some cytoplasmic protein carrier—is responsible. Some evidence, however, points to oxysterol analogues of cholesterol, rather than to cholesterol itself, as mediators of down-regulation. These analogues arise as minor metabolites of cholesterol and as intermediates and by-products of cholesterol synthesis. They are much more potent than cholesterol itself in inhibiting the synthesis of LDL receptors. A cytoplasmic oxysterol-binding protein has been identified whose affinity for different oxysterols parallels their relative potency in down-regulating the transcription of LDL receptor genes.

Mammalian cells also have the capacity to synthesize their own cholesterol. The enzymes catalyzing the successive reactions along this pathway are located in the cytoplasm and in the membranes of the endoplasmic reticulum. The starting material from which cholesterol is made is acetic acid in the form of acetyl coenzyme A (acetyl CoA). This material is generated in mitochondria as an intermediate in the oxidation of glucose and of fatty acids. To be utilized for synthesis of cholesterol, it must first be transported from the mitochondria to the cytoplasm; a specific shuttle exists for this purpose. The synthesis of fatty acids from acetyl CoA also takes place in the cytoplasm, and more of the translocated precursor is used for this purpose than to make cholesterol.

An early step on the pathway to cholesterol is the reduction of hydroxymethylglutaryl coenzyme A (HMG CoA) to mevalonic acid, catalyzed by HMG CoA reductase. The enzymatic capacity to catalyze this reaction is substantially lower than that for other steps on the pathway, so that the overall rate of cholesterol synthesis is largely determined by the activity of this enzyme. Both amount and activity are regulated to match the rates of cholesterol synthesis to the needs of the cell. When the cell has adequate supplies of cholesterol, HMG CoA reductase activity is low and, simultaneously, uptake via the LDL receptor is reduced. Conversely, when more cholesterol is needed, HMG CoA reductase activity and overall cholesterol synthesis are increased, as are expression of the LDL receptor and the uptake of cholesterol.

HMG CoA reductase activity is regulated at several points, including transcription of the gene, efficiency with which its mRNA is translated into protein, turnover of the enzyme protein, and inactivation by chemical modification. Regulation of the transcription of the HMG CoA reductase gene and regulation of the LDL receptor gene appear to have the same fundamental mechanism. The gene for HMG CoA reductase contains an SRE similar in sequence to those in the gene for the LDL receptor. Oxysterols that repress transcription of the LDL receptor exert the same effect on transcription of the gene for HMG CoA reductase, and with the same relative potency. Mutant cells that have lost the capacity to respond to oxysterols by repressing the synthesis of LDL receptors also fail to respond by repressing the synthesis of HMG CoA reductase.

Excess cholesterol also increases the rate at which HMG CoA reductase is broken down. This might be a response to changes in cholesterol concentration in the internal membranes in which HMG CoA reductase is embedded. When the gene for HMG CoA reductase is altered to remove the sequences that anchor it to the membrane and the altered gene is inserted into a recipient cell, the mutant protein is located unattached in the cytoplasm. In contrast to the native enzyme, the rate of turnover of the altered gene product is not affected by the cholesterol content of the recipient cell.

Phosphorylation (attachment of a phosphate to specific amino acid residues) of HMG CoA reductase is a third mechanism by which the synthesis of cholesterol is altered. This is best documented in the liver (which is also the principal site within the body for the synthesis of cholesterol). Liver cells contain an enzyme that phosphorylates and inactivates HMG CoA reductase; the same enzyme also phosphorylates and inactivates the enzyme catalyzing the rate-determining step in the synthesis of fatty acids, acetyl CoA carboxylase. The phosphorylation of both enzymes is promoted, and the synthesis of fatty acids and cholesterol is correspondingly inhibited, under fasting conditions. In the fed state, the reverse is true. These changes appear to be a response to circulating levels of the hormone insulin.

Most of the mevalonic acid that is produced by HMG CoA reductase activity is converted to cholesterol. Since its formation is the rate-determining step on the pathway, the addition of mevalonic acid itself to the cell results in much higher rates of cholesterol synthesis than can be achieved with acetyl CoA as starting material. Moreover, the synthesis of cholesterol from mevalonic acid is not controlled by feedback inhibition. Under these circumstances, expression of HMG CoA reductase and expression of the LDL receptor are maximally repressed.

Mevalonic acid is also the precursor of other substances needed by the cell. These include dolichol (a coenzyme needed for the addition of carbohydrate residues to proteins), ubiquinone (a participant in electron transport reactions in mitochondria), and isoprenyl side chains that are attached to specific proteins. Although their synthesis consumes only a minor portion of the mevalonic acid produced by HMG CoA reductase, these substances are essential to normal cell function. When HMG CoA reductase is inhibited by lovastatin, a drug that competes with the substrate HMG CoA for binding to the enzyme, cell growth is inhibited even when supplies of cholesterol in the medium are adequate. Resumption of cell growth requires the addition of small amounts of mevalonic acid as well as cholesterol. Mutant cell lines have been obtained that, even without lovastatin, are unable to grow unless mevalonic acid is present. The requirements of these cells can be met with a large amount of mevalonic acid in the medium or with a small amount of mevalonic acid plus a large amount of cholesterol.

The multiple roles of mevalonic acid are also reflected in the way that HMG CoA reductase activity is regulated. Although transcription of the HMG CoA reductase gene is reduced when cholesterol levels in the cell are high, some transcription continues to allow enough mevalonic acid to be produced to meet other needs of the cell. Adding small amounts of mevalonic acid further decreases the synthesis of HMG CoA reductase by decreasing the rate at which its mRNA is translated into protein. In contrast, expression of the LDL receptor is not under dual regulation; maximal suppression can be obtained with cholesterol alone.

DISORDERS AND DISEASES

Excessive levels of LDL cholesterol are associated with an increased risk of coronary heart disease and stroke. Efforts to reduce LDL cholesterol through changes in diet or through drugs take advantage of what is known about cholesterol balance in individual cells and in the body as a whole. The latter is determined by three factors: the dietary intake of cholesterol, the rate of cholesterol synthesis within the body (principally by the liver), and the rate of cholesterol disposal (also principally by the liver, through secretion of free sterol into the bile and by the conversion of cholesterol to bile acids). Accordingly, levels of LDL cholesterol can be diminished by limiting the intake and synthesis of new cholesterol, reducing cholesterol secretion by the liver (in the form of an LDL precursor particle), promoting LDL uptake by the liver (mediated by the LDL receptor), and increasing the formation and secretion of bile acids and free cholesterol.

The body can meet its need for cholesterol through synthesis; there is no dietary requirement. Cholesterol deficiency does not arise in humans even on a purely vegetarian (cholesterol-free) diet. The average Western diet, rich in meat and dairy products, contains between 250 and 500 milligrams of cholesterol per day. Small amounts of cholesterol in the diet are fairly well absorbed, but efficiency declines with larger quantities; on average, about half of the cholesterol consumed per day is assimilated. Absorption of cholesterol and other lipids in the small intestine requires the presence of bile acids. These mix with cholesterol and partially degraded dietary triglyceride to form small droplets that facilitate the absorption of lipids by the cells lining the small intestine. In the process, most of the bile acid (as well as cholesterol secreted in the bile) is reabsorbed and returned to the liver. The absorbed cholesterol is esterified and secreted into the lymph, along with triglyceride, in the core of chylomicrons. These large lipoproteins are reduced in size by removal of triglyceride in capillary beds, and the remnants, containing all the original cholesteryl ester, are taken up by the liver. Thus, the cholesterol absorbed in the intestine passes initially to the liver.

The liver is the most important site for cholesterol synthesis within the body. As explained above, hepatic synthesis of cholesterol is under feedback control. HMG CoA reductase activity and cholesterol synthesis are suppressed when large amounts of dietary cholesterol reach the liver and are augmented when the diet is cholesterol-free. Drugs such as lovastatin that inhibit HMG CoA reductase are useful in reducing cholesterol levels in the circulation, since they limit the ability of the liver to respond by making more cholesterol when the dietary intake is reduced.

Cholesterol within the liver may be incorporated into very low-density lipoprotein (VLDL) and secreted into the circulation. VLDL is secreted primarily to transport triglyceride to other tissues for use as a metabolic fuel or for storage. After serving this function, most of the VLDL remnants return to the liver. Those that escape hepatic reabsorption are transformed in the circulation into LDL. LDL is also taken up by the liver (and elsewhere), but at a much slower rate than VLDL remnant particles, so that this lipoprotein accumulates in the circulation. It is deposition of LDL in the lining of blood vessels that initiates the formation of atherosclerotic plaques—the beginning of atherosclerotic disease. Since cholesterol is required for the secretion of VLDL, HMG CoA reductase inhibitors that cause a partial depletion of cholesterol in liver cells reduce the rate at which it enters the bloodstream. By the same means, they also increase expression of LDL receptors in liver cells, which results in a more rapid removal of LDL from the circulation. Both mechanisms reduce circulating levels of LDL cholesterol.

Cholesterol in the liver may also be converted to bile acids and secreted in the bile. Although most of the secreted bile acid comes back to the liver, some escapes reabsorption in the small intestine. The bile acid that is lost must be replaced by the metabolization of more cholesterol. Bile acid sequestrants such as cholestyramine are also used to reduce circulating cholesterol. They act by forming complexes with bile acids in the small intestine and interfere with their reabsorption. A larger fraction of the secreted bile acid is thus lost by excretion, and the rate of conversion of cholesterol to bile acid in the liver is correspondingly increased.

The liver secretes a large amount of free cholesterol into the bile. Most of this biliary cholesterol is reabsorbed and returned to the liver. Since bile acids are required for the intestinal uptake of cholesterol, a second beneficial action of bile acid sequestrants is to increase the fraction of biliary cholesterol that escapes reabsorption and is excreted. The combination of bile acid sequestrant and HMG CoA reductase inhibitor is especially effective in lowering blood levels of LDL cholesterol by limiting the uptake of cholesterol from the diet, limiting the synthesis of cholesterol in the liver, increasing the clearance of cholesterol from the blood by the liver, and increasing the conversion of hepatic cholesterol to bile acids.

Other drugs used to reduce circulating LDL cholesterol levels include nicotinic acid, fibiric acid derivatives, and probucol. Nicotinic acid (niacin) is also a vitamin, but the amounts required to affect plasma cholesterol levels are far in excess of the daily requirement for this compound as an essential nutrient. At these pharmacologic doses, side effects such as itching, facial flushing, and gastric distress are common. Nicotinic acid decreases the formation of VLDL triglyceride in the liver and therefore reduces the formation of LDL; it also promotes the uptake of LDL through LDL receptors and increases the concentration of HDL cholesterol (cholesterol being returned to the liver for disposal). The underlying mechanisms for these actions have not been determined. Fibric acid derivatives, such as gemfibrazole, also reduce VLDL secretion and promote LDL uptake by the liver; again the mechanism of drug action is uncertain. Probucol acts primarily to prevent chemical modification of LDL in the circulation that makes it more likely to be deposited in the walls of blood vessels.

Although high circulating levels of LDL cholesterol call for drug intervention, the risk of atherosclerotic disease can be reduced in most adults by attention to the dietary factors that affect cholesterol balance. Dietary studies have had a controversial history because of frequently contradictory findings. A few principles are, however, well supported by the data. First, eliminating cholesterol from the diet, with no other intervention, produces a significant drop in the levels of cholesterol in circulating LDL. Second, intake of calories beyond actual energy needs raises serum cholesterol. Excess fuel is stored as triglycerides, which to a large extent are formed in the liver and exported in VLDL. Since VLDL contains cholesterol, and since it is the precursor of LDL, high rates of triglyceride formation in the liver promote the accumulation of cholesterol in plasma LDL—which is especially likely to occur if the calories are ingested in the form of triglyceride. Not only does this increase the requirement for the liver to secrete VLDL, but the fatty acids derived from triglyceride also stimulate cholesterol synthesis. Third, saturated fatty acids have the strongest tendency to elevate plasma cholesterol levels. This is the case even when these fatty acids are consumed as vegetable oils (such as palm oil and coconut oil) unaccompanied by cholesterol. The basis for this effect is not well understood but appears to result from decreased expression of LDL receptors in the liver. The American Heart Association recommends that not more than 200 milligrams per day of cholesterol be consumed in a diet which is matched to caloric need and in which not more than 30 percent of calories are consumed as fat (and not more than 10 percent as saturated fat).

PERSPECTIVE AND PROSPECTS

The average adult body contains about 150 grams of cholesterol. Less than 5 percent of this cholesterol is in circulating lipoproteins or trapped in atherosclerotic lesions. The remainder performs essential functions as a structural component of membranes and as the precursor of other vital substances. Although researchers have learned much about the subcellular distribution, the pathway for biosynthesis, and the mechanisms for transport of cholesterol, important questions remain. It is not known how cholesterol is transported within the cell or what determines its relative distribution among different cellular membranes. It is not known what signals suppress the synthesis of HMG CoA reductase and LDL receptors or how the message is transmitted to the nucleus to diminish transcription of these genes. Some product of mevalonic acid metabolism other than cholesterol also regulates the expression of HMG CoA reductase, but this factor has not yet been identified. It is not known why cholesterol is an absolute requirement for functioning of mammalian cell membranes. It is not known what determines the fraction of dietary cholesterol that is absorbed across the intestinal lining. Finally, there is much to learn about factors that regulate the secretion and reuptake of lipoproteins by the liver and that control the return to the liver of cholesterol in HDL.

These questions are of practical as well as academic interest. Coronary heart disease and other complications of atherosclerosis are the leading causes of death in the United States. Controlling and reversing this process is a serious medical challenge. While other factors such as hypertension, smoking, and diabetes mellitus contribute to the risk of atherosclerosis, reducing the level of cholesterol that circulates as a component of LDL and increasing the level transported in HDL have been shown to provide significant protection. Knowledge of how cholesterol is normally produced and assimilated has contributed to the design of drugs that reduce circulating levels by interfering with the absorption and synthesis of cholesterol and promoting its metabolism and excretion. This field of investigation continues to be a major concern of both basic and pharmaceutical scientists.

—Lauren M. Cagen, Ph.D.

See also Arteriosclerosis; Blood and blood disorders; Blood testing; Cells; Digestion; Food biochemistry; Heart disease; Hypercholesterolemia; Hyperlipidemia; Metabolism; Nutrition; Preventive medicine; Strokes.

FOR FURTHER INFORMATION:

Dietschy, John M. "Physiology in Medicine: LDL Cholesterol: Its Regulation and Manipulation." *Hos-*

pital Practice 25 (June 15, 1990): 67-78. An excellent nontechnical introduction to the subject of cholesterol balance and its regulation by a major contributor to the field. The article discusses the effect of diet and drug interventions.

Grundy, Scott M. *Cholesterol and Atherosclerosis.* Philadelphia: J. P. Lippincott, 1990. The author provides a general overview of cholesterol balance, elevated plasma cholesterol, and its management by diet and drugs. Although intended for physicians, the book is written in a simple and direct style and is profusely illustrated.

HeartInfo.org. http://www.heartinfo.org/. Site provides information on lowering cholesterol levels, cholesterol and the heart, and the opportunity to join a cholesterol discussion group.

Hirsch, Anita. *Good Cholesterol, Bad Cholesterol: An Indispensable Guide to the Facts About Cholesterol.* New York: Avalon, 2002. In an easy-to-browse format, medical facts about cholesterol, lifestyle guidance to managing cholesterol levels, and recipes for low cholesterol meals are included.

Leaf, David A. *Cholesterol Treatment: A Guide to Lipid Disorder Management.* Reprint. Durant, Okla.: EMIS, 2000. The primary purpose of this book is to provide in a convenient reference much of the information that the practicing physician and supportive health care clinicians need to manage patients with lipid disorders.

McGowan, Mary P., et al. *Fifty Ways to Lower Cholesterol.* New York: McGraw-Hill, 2002. Advocates a multifaceted approach to lowering cholesterol levels, including diet, weight management, exercise, and medical intervention.

Nesto, N. W., and Lisa Christenson. *Cholesterol-Lowering Drugs: Everything You and Your Family Need to Know.* New York: William Morrow, 2000. Includes profiles of commonly used cholesterol-lowering prescription drugs (Questran, Lescol, Pravachol, Zocor, Lopid, nicotinic acid) and a discussion of side effects, interactions, and warnings. Includes special information for women, children, and seniors. Addresses the causes and dangers of high cholesterol; the effect of diet, exercise, and smoking; and age, gender, and genetic factors.

Rinzler, Carol Ann, and Martin Graf. *Controlling Cholesterol for Dummies.* New York: Wiley, 2002. Part of a popular series of books, this one offers advice on managing cholesterol intake through exercise and diet, explains the differences between "good" and "bad" cholesterol, and provides a test to rate your risk of heart disease.

Yeagle, Philip L. *Understanding Your Cholesterol.* San Diego, Calif.: Academic Press, 1991. This popular work explains cholesterol and the risk factors that can lead to atherosclerosis. Includes a bibliography.

Chorionic villus sampling

Procedure

Anatomy or system affected: Reproductive system, uterus

Specialties and related fields: Embryology, genetics, obstetrics, perinatology

Definition: The collection of a small sample of chorionic villi tissue from the fingerlike projections of the placenta at the point of attachment to the uterine wall. These cells are examined for genetic and chromosomal abnormalities by means of karyotyping.

Indications and Procedures

Chorionic villus sampling can be performed between the tenth and twelfth weeks of pregnancy to detect genetic and chromosomal abnormalities. The procedure is recommended when there is increased risk of genetic disorders in the fetus such as Down syndrome, sickle cell disease, and muscular dystrophy.

Chorionic villus sampling involves collecting a small sample of the chorionic villi, the fingerlike projections on the developing placenta, which delivers food and oxygen to the fetus. A sample of chorionic villi can be obtained either by inserting a needle through the abdomen or by entering the cervix with a small flexible catheter through the vagina. The choice of approach depends on the position of the placenta. Ultrasound is used to locate the fetus and the placenta and its villi.

A 10- to 25-milligram sample is collected using a syringe, which is then purified and sometimes cultured. Since the chorionic villi originate from the same cell as the fetus, they normally have the same genetics. Results are available within days.

Uses and Complications

Along with exposing genetic and chromosomal disorders, chorionic villus sampling can be used to determine the sex of the embryo but should never be used for this purpose alone because of the risks involved. Testing can be done early in the pregnancy. Therefore, if the woman should choose to terminate her pregnancy, an easier first-trimester abortion can be per-

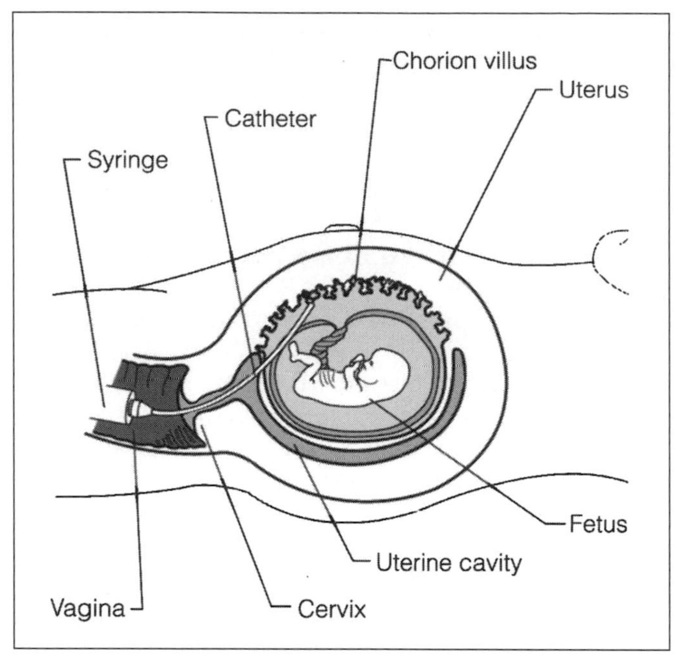

Chorionic villus sampling is one method of obtaining embryonic cells from a pregnant woman; examination of these cells helps physicians determine fetal irregularities or defects, which allows time to assess the problem and make recommendations for treatment.

formed. If the results from the test are favorable, the parents have an early peace of mind.

Possible complications from chorionic villus sampling include vaginal bleeding and cramping. More serious risks involve spontaneous abortion and even possible fetal injury. The rate of miscarriage is about 1 percent higher with chorionic villus sampling than with amniocentesis, performed after sixteen weeks and yielding the same information.

Some studies suggest that chorionic villus sampling itself may cause some birth defects; others do not. Also, the procedure can be inaccurate. Abnormalities may occur in some placental cells but not in the fetus. This might lead to aborting a healthy fetus. With the guidance of a physician, the risks and benefits should be compared with other available procedures.

—Paul R. Boehlke, Ph.D., and Pavel Svilenov; updated by Robin Kamienny Montvilo, Ph.D.

See also Abortion; Amniocentesis; Birth defects; Down syndrome; Embryology; Fetal surgery; Genetic counseling; Genetic diseases; Karyotyping; Miscarriage; Muscular dystrophy; Obstetrics; Perinatology; Pregnancy and gestation; Reproductive system; Sickle cell disease; Ultrasonography; Women's health.

For Further Information:

Caughey, Aaron B., Linda M. Hopkins, and Mary E. Norton. "Chorionic Villus Sampling Compared with Amniocentesis and the Difference in the Rate of Pregnancy Loss." *Obstetrics and Gynecology* 108, no. 3 (September, 2006): 612-616.

Ettorre, Elizabeth, ed. *Before Birth: Understanding Prenatal Screening*. Burlington, Vt.: Ashgate, 2001.

Filkins, Karen, and Joseph F. Russo, eds. *Human Prenatal Diagnosis*. 2d rev. ed. New York: Marcel Dekker, 1990.

Harper, Peter S. *Practical Genetic Counselling*. 6th ed. New York: Oxford University Press, 2004.

Lichtman, Ronnie, Lynn Louise Simpson, and Allan Rosenfield. *Dr. Guttmacher's Pregnancy, Birth, and Family Planning*. Rev. ed. New York: New American Library, 2003.

Moore, Keith L., and T. V. N. Persaud. *The Developing Human*. 7th ed. Philadelphia: W. B. Saunders, 2003.

Pierce, Benjamin A. *The Family Genetic Sourcebook*. New York: John Wiley & Sons, 1990.

Chromosomal abnormalities. *See* Birth defects; Genetic diseases.

Chronic fatigue syndrome

Disease/disorder

Anatomy or system affected: Immune system, muscles, musculoskeletal system, psychic-emotional system

Specialties and related fields: Family medicine, hematology, immunology, internal medicine, psychiatry

Definition: Chronic fatigue syndrome is a multifaceted disease state characterized by debilitating fatigue.

Key terms:

adenopathy: the enlargement of any gland (often the lymph gland)

cell-mediated immune response: an immune response that involves cells rather than antibodies, particularly T lymphocytes rather than B lymphocytes

cytokines: proteins secreted by immune cells which contribute to immune responses and inflammation

fibromyalgia: a condition of generalized pain that is similar to chronic fatigue syndrome

infectious mononucleosis: acute self-limiting infection of lymphocytes by the Epstein-Barr virus

interleukin-2: a protein messenger that regulates T cell activity and differentiation during the immune response

lymphocytes: agranular leukocytes that differentiate into B lymphocytes and T lymphocytes and play a fundamental role in the immune response

polymerase chain reaction: a laboratory method used to increase the amount of DNA found in small quantities

suppressor T cell: a type of T lymphocyte that is believed to modulate the immune response

CAUSES AND SYMPTOMS

Chronic fatigue syndrome is a heterogenous disease state that has been difficult to define, diagnose, and treat because of poorly understood cause-and-effect relationships. The disease can be best described in terms of long-lasting and debilitating fatigue, the etiology of which has been linked to such external factors as microbial agents, stress, and lifestyle as well as such internal factors as genetic makeup and the body's immune response. The fact that it is a physical disease with psychological components has also caused confusion in the medical community.

Among the many names that have been used for the disease, the three that demonstrate the many factors that contribute to chronic fatigue syndrome are chronic Epstein-Barr virus syndrome, chronic fatigue immune dysfunction syndrome, and "Yuppie flu." Because of the marked immunological aspects of the disease and the fact that different viruses have been found in patients with chronic fatigue, the disease is referred to as chronic fatigue immune dysfunction syndrome by many involved in the study. The Centers for Disease Control and Prevention (CDC) continues to refer to it as chronic fatigue syndrome (CFS).

Although the disease is not specific by race, sex, or age group, there is demographic evidence that young white females make up two-thirds of the known cases. It is estimated by the CDC that between 1 and 10 of every 10,000 people in the United States have CFS. The disease has also been identified as a problem in Europe and Australia.

CFS can manifest itself in acute and chronic phases, although some patients do not remember an acute phase presentation. Acute phase symptoms are general and flulike, with a low-grade fever, sore throat, headache, muscle pain, painful lymph nodes, and overall fatigue. Unlike with a bout of influenza, the symptoms do not subside with time, instead intensifying into a chronic phase. The fatigue can become disabling, with severe muscle and joint pain, swollen and painful lymph nodes, and the inability to develop proper sleep patterns. The similarity of CFS to fibromyalgia, diffuse muscular pain throughout the body, has resulted in cross diagnosis by many physicians of the two syndromes. Some researchers blame psychological and emotional stress, with a viral infection having triggered the initial acute phase. Although the psychological description does not fit all cases, problems of concentration, attention, and depression have been implicated to the point that researchers recognize both psychological and physical components. The working definition from both a research and a clinical perspective requires that the fatigue cause at least 50 percent incapacitation and last at least six months. The ineffectiveness of treatment, compounded by the inability to provide a concrete diagnosis, further complicates the psychological aspects of the disease for the patient.

Although the environment provides an array of agents that could trigger the physical condition of CFS, the hypothesis for a viral cause is supported by the flulike symptoms, occasional clustering of cases, and presence of antiviral antibodies in the patient's serum. The involvement of the Epstein-Barr virus in some forms of CFS seems likely because of its role as the etiological agent of mononucleosis and Burkitt's lymphoma, which are similar diseases. In both of these diseases, the Epstein-Barr virus has a unique and harmful effect on the immune system because it directly invades B lymphocytes, the antibody-producing cells of the body, using them to grow new virus particles while disrupting the proper functioning of the immune system. Like CFS, mononucleosis is characterized by

INFORMATION ON CHRONIC FATIGUE SYNDROME

CAUSES: Unknown; possibly microbial agents, stress, lifestyle factors, genetic makeup, immunological factors

SYMPTOMS: Debilitating fatigue, low-grade fever, sore throat, headache, muscle pain, painful lymph nodes, disturbed sleep patterns

DURATION: Chronic

TREATMENTS: None; alleviation of symptoms

flulike symptoms and fatigue, but the disease is self-limiting and the patient eventually recovers.

Despite this seeming difference in outcome, the Epstein-Barr virus can cause a chronic condition. The viruses that infect humans can become dormant within the cells that they infect. The nucleic acid of a virus can become incorporated into the DNA of its host cell, and the body no longer shows physical signs of their presence. A virus can become active at times of physical or emotional stress and can once again trigger the physical symptoms of disease. For example, herpes simplex virus 1 remains dormant in its host cell but periodically, in response to environmental factors, causes a cold sore lesion.

Immunological dysfunction has been observed in CFS patients because they demonstrate increased allergic sensitivity to skin tests when compared to normal individuals. Cells and cellular chemicals directly involved with protective immunity and the regulation of the immune response have been found in these patients in abnormal concentrations. For example, they have abnormal numbers of the natural killer cells and suppressor T cells that are essential to cell-mediated immunity. A variety of cytokines, such as gamma interferon, and various interleukins which regulate the activities of the cells in the cell-mediated and humoral immune responses are seen in abnormal concentrations in some CFS patients. Some of these cytokines are already known to mediate the immune response to viral infections. Infectious agents such as bacteria, viruses, yeast, intracellular parasites, and even cancer cells are eliminated from the body when humoral and cell-mediated immune systems are operating properly. The presence of abnormally high concentrations of these cytokines may contribute to inflammatory processes sometimes found in patients with CFS. When the immune system is not working properly, however, not only is the body more susceptible to a variety of infectious agents but the immune system can begin to damage or destroy normal tissues as well. Such disease states are referred to as autoimmune diseases. Inflammation and allergic reactions are other examples of uncontrolled immune responses.

The psychological and emotional aspects of CFS are also in question. Some studies indicate that the brain is physically affected by inflammation and hormonal changes. Other studies demonstrate that some of the known viral infective agents can have neurological effects. Psychiatric studies give ample evidence that depression, memory loss, and concentration are significant problems for some CFS patients. The extent to which stress is a factor in the disease is unknown.

Treatment and Therapy

Defining and treating chronic fatigue syndrome has been difficult because it manifests itself as a systemic disease with confusing cause-and-effect relationships involving external factors such as infectious viruses, internal factors such as the immune response, and a psychological component that is difficult to assess in the light of the biological changes occurring in the body. The symptoms, provided by patient histories, physical examinations, and laboratory findings, involve neuromuscular, psychoneurological, and immunological changes that vary between patients. The variety of factors to consider has caused difficulty in establishing diagnostic criteria for primary care in a clinical setting or further definition of the disease and treatments in a research setting.

In 1988, the CDC established diagnostic criteria that are divided into two major criteria, eleven minor symptom criteria, and three minor physical criteria. The first major criterion defines chronic fatigue as lasting at least six months and causing debilitation to 50 percent of the patient's normal activity. The second major criterion requires that all other disease conditions that could fit the patient history, physical examination, and appropriate laboratory tests be ruled out. The categories of disease that might be similar to CFS are cancers, chronic degenerative disease, autoimmune disorders, microbial and parasitic disease, and chronic psychiatric disease. Combinations of some minor criteria that would fit a general flulike condition must be demonstrated.

In 1993, a meeting at the CDC attempted to evaluate what had been learned over the previous five-year period and to make recommendations regarding a case definition. It was suggested that the case definition format involve inclusion and exclusion criteria that would increase the number and range of cases being studied because of the heterogeneous nature of the disease. The cases should also be subcategorized to provide a homogeneity that would allow for subgroup identification and comparison. The inclusion evidence should be simple, with a descriptive interpretation of the fatigue being essential and having objective criteria to define a 50 percent reduction of physical activity. Symptoms that are specific to unexplained fatigue should be used, while the physical exam information should not be included. It was also suggested that exclusion of any cases should involve an in-depth history (both medical and psychiatric), a physical examination, and standardized testing that would involve medical, laboratory, and psychiatric information.

Because it appears that CFS overlaps with many other medical and psychiatric conditions that can be identified and treated, there is debate as to how to interpret CFS as it relates to patient care and research. Some believe that an in-depth history is fundamental to the understanding of CFS and that CFS could be the final pathway that occurs from a variety of biological and psychosocial insults to the body.

The minor criteria used to define CFS involve both symptom and physical criteria that have not been proved adequate to validate or define the condition. In fact, the conflicting data have only served to emphasize further the clinical heterogeneity of the disease and suggest a heterogeneity of cause. Suggestions have been made to drop the concept of minor criteria, use symptoms that are specific for the unexplained fatigue, and drop all physical examination criteria. The argument for eliminating physical criteria is that more specific criteria exist for a case definition. Because physical symptoms are inconsistent or periodic, it is believed that a documented patient history would provide more case-specific information.

Although symptom criteria have widespread support in the case definition of CFS, symptoms with the greatest sensitivity and specificity are also being debated. Night sweats, cough, gastrointestinal problems, and new and worsening allergies are not presently considered and are believed by some to be more specific than fever or chills and sore throat. Others have proposed that symptoms should be reduced to chills and fever, sore throat, neck or axilla adenopathy, and sudden onset of a main symptom complex. The most prevalent symptoms are believed to be muscle weakness and pain, problems in concentration, and sleep disturbance.

The importance of the psychiatric component in CFS continues to be a problem in case definition. Some believe that the neurological component is a major criterion in case definition and that behavior symptoms, including stress and psychiatric illness, must be emphasized in clinical diagnosis as well as in therapy. It has been recommended that objective neuropsychological testing be used to determine cognitive dysfunction and depression. There is agreement that CFS patients have impaired concentration and attention, but forgetfulness and memory problems are questioned. There is also evidence that the duration and severity of myalgia are closely associated with psychological distress and that psychotherapy improves physical symptoms. Finally, it has been argued that the psychiatric component of the case definition is essential because there is evidence that the disease directly affects the brain and that CFS can cause both isolation and limitation of the patient's normal lifestyle.

Whatever the case definition, the second major criterion will be expressed in some form. Proper patient care necessitates extensive evaluation in order to identify the biological or psychological reasons for the problem. Proper CFS patient care demands the elimination of other serious disease possibilities that may appear superficially similar. Primary care physicians may find it difficult to make a diagnosis without a team of specialists in the areas of hematology, immunology, and psychiatry. Numerous laboratory tests must be made available. Although there are no specific recommended tests, those that must be performed should be tailored to specific patients and used by the team of specialists for their care.

The possibility of infectious disease, either as part of CFS (as in the case of certain viral agents) or as an autonomous infection having no relation to CFS, requires a variety of antibody tests to detect such viruses as Epstein-Barr or HIV. Skin tests such as the purified protein derivative (PPD) test for tuberculosis are used. Polymerase chain reaction and tissue culture for cytopathic effects have been developed to detect certain retroviruses for ultimate use in diagnosis at the clinical level.

The immune system is so intimately interactive with the entire body that most disease conditions are affected by or affect its function. The measure of its components provides a clue to the identity of the disease that is operating because they indicate whether normal protection activity or immune dysfunction (or a combination) is occurring in the patient.

The components of the immune system can be measured in numerous ways, from methodologies used in standard clinical laboratory procedures to research protocols used to study immune function and disease treatment. Tests are available that can measure total antibody concentration and the various subgroups IgG, IgM, IgA, IgE, and IgD; cytokines such as interleukin-2 and gamma interferon; cellular components such as T cells and their subtypes (such as suppressor T cells and natural killer cells); and B cells.

Autoimmune diseases and allergies are immune dysfunction diseases in their own right. Because there is an immune dysfunction component to CFS, tests for these conditions are important considerations. An antinuclear antibody (ANA) test determines the presence of antibodies that attack the tissues of the patient, as in systemic lupus erythematosus. The type and extent of allergic reactions can be measured using the radioimmunosorbent (RIST) tests for total IgE concentration and radioallergosorbent (RAST) tests for IgE concentration for particular antigens.

Systemic disease states, including CFS, often involve generalized inflammation that is considered part of the body's protective response. While inflammation is important to the elimination of various infective agents, it is also involved in neurological and muscle tissue damage. C-reactive protein (CRP) and the erythrocyte sedimentation rate (ESR) tests measure the intensity of the inflammatory response. A variety of other tests provide information that indicates the extent of muscle, liver, thyroid, and other vital organ damage.

Although a diagnosis can be made for CFS, there is no standard treatment. Clinical treatment essentially takes the form of alleviating the symptoms. Antidepressants such as doxepin (Sinequan) are useful in the treatment of depression and are also used to control muscle pain, lethargy, and sleeping problems. Nonsteroidal anti-inflammatory drugs (NSAIDs) provide relief for headache and muscle pain. Two drugs that have demonstrated antiviral activities are acyclovir and ampligen; ampligen can also modulate the immune response.

An example of research to develop therapies that might alleviate other symptoms of CFS involves the treatment of a number of patients with dialyzable leukocyte extract and psychologic treatment in the form of cognitive-behavioral therapy. The patients' cell-mediated immune response after therapy was evaluated by peripheral blood T cell subset analysis and delayed hypersensitivity skin testing. Psychologic analysis was performed using numerous cognitive tests. Both therapies proved to be inconclusive.

Because of the systemic nature of the disease, including its psychoneurological component, consideration must be given to holistic medical treatment. Any treatment protocol must be able to address the interactive factors of CFS that are still being defined in terms of cause and effect. Some researchers believe that therapeutic treatment should comprise diet, exercise, vitamins, and homeopathic medicine. They further believe that psychoemotional treatment should allow patients to be responsible for their own recovery and help them to develop a personal lifestyle that provides general good health.

Perspective and Prospects

The vague, often "flulike" symptoms used to define chronic fatigue syndrome have historically been associated with numerous infectious agents, such as *Brucella* (brucellosis), *Coxsiella*, Epstein-Barr virus infections (infectious mononucleosis), and other chronic viral diseases. In most cases, a specific etiological agent was discovered. Association with a specific agent allowed for treatment in many cases, or at the least a means to define the illness.

Since being linked with the Epstein-Barr virus, CFS has been the subject of many studies that support its definition as a heterogenous illness, including a category of postinfective fatigue syndromes that follow viral infections. The case definition provided by the CDC in 1988 has allowed the disease to be diagnosed and treated at the clinical level and to be identified and compared at the research level. The disease state has proven to be elusive, however, and the case definition too complex and open to interpretation. It is believed that the refinement of the case definition proposed by the CDC in 1993 will promote greater understanding of the problem at both clinical and research levels, particularly because more objective criteria to validate and define CFS have not emerged.

As indicated by its very definition, CFS has presented the health care system with a challenge whereby the primary care physician receives information provided by a team of specialists. Continued technological advances and research into both the immune system and the nature of viral infection will provide new insights into more traditional treatment protocols, including the role played by immune responses to the triggering agent. The neuropsychological components of the disease, as well as evidence demonstrating intimate ties between these components and the immune system, require a personal, active approach by the patient to achieving a healthy state. CFS provides a challenge to the patient to adapt to a personal lifestyle that will create a healthy mind and body.

CFS must also be considered in terms of the society in which it is manifest as a serious and genuine illness. Medical treatment and diagnostic testing can be costly as well as useless, particularly as the health care community continues to refine its understanding of the condition. Patients must remain vigilant regarding phony or trendy treatments that have no correlation to acceptable research findings; such treatments not only can be expensive but also could lead to deteriorating health. Furthermore, the definition and diagnosis of CFS have legal ramifications that have an impact on insurance and other forms of medical care compensation.

—Patrick J. DeLuca, Ph.D.; updated by Richard Adler, Ph.D.

See also Fatigue; Fibromyalgia; Immune system; Immunology; Mononucleosis; Multiple chemical sensitivity syndrome; Stress.

FOR FURTHER INFORMATION:

Afari, Niloofar, and Dedra Buchwald. "Chronic Fatigue Syndrome: A Review." *American Journal of Psychiatry* 160 (February, 2003): 221-236. Summary of the current state of knowledge addressing possible causes and treatment of CFS. The authors acknowledge that diagnosis is based upon symptoms rather than any specific pathology.

Berne, Katrina. *Chronic Fatigue Syndrome, Fibromyalgia, and Other Invisible Illnesses: The Comprehensive Guide*. 3d ed. Alameda, Calif.: Hunter House, 2002. Explores the interactions among the brain, emotions, and the immune system and reviews the current state of research.

Bested, Alison, and Alan Logan. *Chronic Fatigue Syndrome and Fibromyalgia*. Nashville: Cumberland House, 2006. Review of possible causes and treatments for chronic pain and fatigue. Addressed primarily to the lay audience.

CFIDS Association of America. http://www.cfids.org/. A group dedicated to conquering chronic fatigue and immune dysfunction syndrome (CFIDS). Focuses on increasing the pace of CFIDS research, achieving public policy victories for people with CFIDS, and directing mainstream attention to the disease.

Englebienne, Patrick, and Kenny DeMeirleir, eds. *Chronic Fatigue Syndrome: A Biological Approach*. Boca Raton, Fla.: CRC Press, 2002. Reviews research advances in understanding the disease from the perspective of various fields of the biomedical sciences, such as protein biochemistry, virology, and pharmacology.

Friedberg, Fred. *Fibromyalgia and Chronic Fatigue Syndrome: Seven Proven Steps to Less Pain and More Energy*. Oakland, Calif.: New Harbinger, 2006. A layperson's directive on living with the clinical features of the illness as well as behaviors which may reduce any symptoms.

Patarca-Montero, Roberto. *Chronic Fatigue Syndrome and the Body's Immune Defense System*. New York: Haworth Medical Press, 2002. Patarca-Montero, a leading immunologist, examines the connections between the disease and immunology; reviews how therapeutic tools such as herbal medicine, vaccines, and cell therapy are being used in CFS research; and discusses the connection between CFS and fibromyalgia, Gulf War syndrome, sick building syndrome, and multiple chemical sensitivity.

Sticherling, Michael, and Enno Christophers, eds. *Treatment of Automimmune Disorders*. New York: Springer, 2003. Explores the basic mechanisms of autoimmune disorders; neurological, gastrointestinal, ophthalmological, and skin diseases; and current and future therapeutic options.

Wessely, Simon, Matthew Hotopf, and Michael Sharpe. *Chronic Fatigue and Its Syndromes*. New York: Oxford University Press, 1998. The authors consider chronic fatigue to be similar to any other illness in that its onset and course are influenced by physical, psychological, and social factors. Chapters review these topics as well as the history of chronic fatigue and neurasthenia and the influence of social circumstances.

CHRONIC OBSTRUCTIVE PULMONARY DISEASE (COPD)

DISEASE/DISORDER

ANATOMY OR SYSTEM AFFECTED: Lungs, respiratory system

SPECIALTIES AND RELATED FIELDS: Geriatrics and gerontology, public health, pulmonary medicine

DEFINITION: A progressive, irreversible disease of the lungs that causes expiratory airflow obstruction. The most common form of COPD is a combination of chronic bronchitis and emphysema.

KEY TERMS:

alpha 1 antitrypsin: a protein that protects the lungs

alveoli: air sacs in the lungs that exchange oxygen and carbon dioxide

barrel chest: a rounded chest in which the anterior and posterior diameter is increased

bronchial tubes: branches in the airways in the lungs that allow for the exchange of oxygen and carbon dioxide

chronic bronchitis: a condition involving the inflammation and eventual scarring of the lining of the bronchial tubes and the production of excess mucus in the lungs

emphysema: airway disease involving permanent distension of distal airspaces and damage to alveolar walls of the lungs
exacerbation: worsening or intensifying
expiratory phase: exhalation, or breathing out
hypoxic: having low oxygen levels
pursed lip breathing: slow expirations from the abdomen against pursed lips
tachypnea: rapid breathing greater than twenty breaths per minute

Causes and Symptoms

Patients suffering from chronic obstructive pulmonary disease (COPD), a combination of chronic bronchitis and emphysema, have a chronic cough and shortness of breath that progressively limits their tolerance for physical activity. A physical examination may appear normal in the early stages of COPD, but as the disease progresses, tachypnea and wheezing occur. Over time, the occasional cough becomes more frequent and greater effort is exerted to breathe. In later stages of COPD, the heart may be affected because the lungs can no longer supply an adequate amount of oxygen to the body. Other signs of COPD are a barrel chest, pursed lip breathing, and a prolonged expiratory phase of respirations. Coughing produces phlegm that becomes increasingly difficult to expel as it thickens. Persons with advanced COPD cannot lie flat to sleep and eventually may sit in an semiupright position in order to breathe.

The major risk factor for COPD is smoking. Other risk factors are air pollution (including exposure to mining), textile manufacturing (such as steel and cement), a history of childhood respiratory infections, and low socioeconomic status. In chronic bronchitis, the lining of the bronchial tubes become irritated, inflamed, and filled with mucus that blocks the airways, making it difficult to breathe. In emphysema, the alveoli become irritated, stiffen, and cannot transfer oxygen and carbon dioxide in the blood. Thus far, a deficiency of the enzyme alpha 1 antitrypsin is the only identified genetic cause of COPD.

COPD is an insidious disease that presents few symptoms until it is well developed in the lungs. It is usually not identified until the patient is fifty to sixty years old, although COPD caused by a deficiency of alpha 1 antitrypsin may be identified by thirty to forty years of age.

Confirmation of the diagnosis of COPD is made by pulmonary function tests (PFTs). PFTs are helpful in diagnosing COPD in its early stages and may be helpful in convincing patients to stop smoking, if necessary, so as to slow the progression of COPD. Spirometry measures the amount of air exhaled in one second, or forced expiratory volume (FEV1). The total amount of air exhaled, or forced vital capacity (FVC), is compared to the FEV1 to determine the extent of airway obstruction. A peak flow meter can show the severity of breathing impairment; after a deep breath, the patient blows into the instrument as forcefully and for as long as possible. Arterial blood gas tests measure the level of oxygen in and carbon dioxide in the blood. Serum alpha-1-antitrypsin levels are measured by blood samples. Finally, chest X rays, pulmonary ventilation-perfusion scans, and chest magnetic resonance imaging (MRI) scans may all help to identify the degree of lung damage caused by COPD.

Information on Chronic Obstructive Pulmonary Disease (COPD)

Causes: Unknown; risk factors include smoking, air pollution, textile manufacturing, childhood respiratory infections
Symptoms: Chronic cough, shortness of breath, wheezing, limited physical activity
Duration: Chronic and progressive
Treatments: None; alleviation of symptoms (bronchodilators, antibiotics, steroids, oxygen therapy, vaccination against pneumonia and influenza, smoking cessation, pulmonary rehabilitation)

Treatment and Therapy

Since no cure exists for COPD, treatment focuses on decreasing symptoms and reducing complications. Bronchodilator medications, antibiotics, steroids, oxygen, and vaccination against pneumonia and influenza are used to treat or prevent symptoms, slow the progression of the disease, and manage any complications. Smoking cessation is vitally important for slowing the progress of COPD. Nicotine replacement therapy, antidepressant therapy, and counseling are some of the methods used to assist in smoking cessation.

Patients with COPD who are hypoxic require long-term oxygen therapy to improve their functional status and rate of survival. The purpose of oxygen therapy is to maintain adequate oxygen levels to prevent respiratory difficulties.

Pulmonary rehabilitation can help reduce hospitalizations and improve the quality of life for those with COPD, improving their overall functional status. Pulmonary rehabilitation includes therapies to enhance breathing, physical training to improve muscle strength and stamina, and the pacing of activities to avoid overexertion. Pursed lip breathing helps to relieve abnormal breathing (dyspnea) and to slow respirations.

Lung transplantation and lung reduction surgery may be options for people who suffer from severe emphysema. Lung reduction surgery, which is still in the experimental stages, is the partial removal of the most damaged areas of the lungs in order to allow for better lung expansion of the normal areas of the lung. Gene therapy and alpha-1-antitrypsin replacement therapy are presently under evaluation as treatments for alpha-1-antitrypsin deficiency, but the long-term effects of these treatments are unknown.

Perspective and Prospects

COPD costs in the United States exceed $32 billion annually. Between 80 and 90 percent of all cases are caused by smoking. COPD is the fourth leading cause of death in the United States. The incidence of this disease is increasing every year. Those with COPD are prone to recurrent respiratory infections, and their quality of life gradually declines as the disease worsens. Smoking cessation is the single most important prevention method.

—*Sharon W. Stark, R.N., A.P.R.N., D.N.Sc.*

See also Asbestos exposure; Aspergillosis; Bronchitis; Chest; Cyanosis; Emphysema; Environmental diseases; Environmental health; Geriatrics and gerontology; Influenza; Lungs; Nicotine; Occupational health; Oxygen therapy; Pneumonia; Pulmonary diseases; Pulmonary medicine; Respiration; Smoking; Wheezing.

For Further Information:

Barnett, Margaret. *Chronic Obstructive Pulmonary Disease in Primary Care*. New York: Wiley, 2006. Provides health professionals with practical advice and coping strategies for patients living with COPD.

Calverley, Peter M. A., et al., eds. *Chronic Obstructive Pulmonary Disease*. 2d ed. New York: Oxford University Press, 2003. Discusses the improvements in patient care and the development of new treatment methods.

Haas, François, and Sheila Sperber Haas. *The Chronic Bronchitis and Emphysema Handbook*. Rev. ed. New York: John Wiley & Sons, 2000. Provides an overview of the respiratory system; COPD symptoms and progression; smoking cessation; oxygen, drug, and alternative therapies; and surgical interventions for treating COPD.

Jenkins, Mark. *Chronic Obstructive Pulmonary Disease: Practical, Medical, and Spiritual Guidelines for Daily Living with Emphysema, Chronic Bronchitis, and Combination Diagnosis*. Center City, Minn.: Hazelden Information Education, 1999. Provides management techniques and references to resources for maintaining optimal physical and mental health during the course of COPD.

Parker, James N., and Philip M. Parker, eds. *The 2002 Official Patient's Sourcebook on Chronic Obstructive Pulmonary Disease*. San Diego, Calif.: Icon Health, 2002. Provides information for investigating a variety of topics related to COPD from multiple perspectives.

Chronic wasting disease (CWD)

Disease/disorder

Anatomy or system affected: Brain, nervous system

Specialties and related fields: Neurology

Definition: A neurological disease of deer and elk caused by an infectious protein particle called a prion.

Causes and Symptoms

Chronic wasting disease (CWD) is an invariably fatal neurological disease that affects deer, elk, and moose in North America. The disease was first described in the late 1960's in captive animals in Colorado. As of 2006, CWD-infected animals—from either wild or captive populations—have been found in Colorado, Illinois, Kansas, Montana, Nebraska, New Mexico, New York, Oklahoma, South Dakota, Utah, West Virginia, Wisconsin, Wyoming, and New Mexico in the United States and in the provinces of Alberta and Saskatchewan in Canada. In the late stages of the disease, infected animals show progressive weight loss, listlessness, increased salivation and urination, increased water consumption, depression, and death.

The brains of dead animals show characteristic vacuoles, or holes, that give the brain the appearance of a sponge. This pathology is characteristic of all the transmissible spongiform encephalopathies (TSEs), including bovine spongiform encephalopathy (BSE) of cows

Information on Chronic Wasting Disease (CWD)

Causes: Prion disease in deer and elk
Symptoms: In animals, progressive weight loss, listlessness, increased salivation and urination, increased water consumption, depression, death; possible transmission to humans through infected game
Duration: Chronic and progressive
Treatments: None

(so-called mad cow disease), scrapie of sheep, and Creutzfeldt-Jakob disease (CJD) of humans. Although CWD is similar to these other diseases, it is not identical to them. These diseases appear to be caused by the misfolding of a small protein (prion) normally located in the membranes of neurons and other cells. The normal function of this protein is unknown, but when misfolded, it accumulates in the brain, resulting in the death of neurons. The misfolded, pathogenic prion appears to be able to direct the misfolding of any normal prion present in a cell, thus replicating its aberrant structure.

Prion diseases can be either inherited or transmitted. Humans can inherit CJD or contract it from contaminated blood or brain tissue. Evidence suggests that variant CJD in humans can result from consuming beef contaminated with the BSE prion. There is concern about whether the CWD prion in deer and elk can also "jump" the species barrier to humans in a manner similar to BSE.

CWD is believed to be transmitted from animal to animal through contact with body fluids or feces. Research published in 2006 indicated that the disease is most easily transmitted via saliva and blood, although other modes of transmission have not been ruled out. Two recent studies found no strong clinical or epidemiological evidence that the disease can be transmitted to humans via the consumption of contaminated meat. Laboratory studies indicate that such transmission is possible, however. Because of the long incubation period for the disease, however, it is difficult to prove or disprove transmission from deer, elk, or moose to humans.

Perspective and Prospects

Many states where CWD is prevalent have banned the baiting of deer and are thinning the deer population. Deer and elk in crowded populations, particularly captive herds, appear to be more susceptible to CWD.

Research efforts are focused on developing a sensitive field diagnostic test. Definitive diagnosis is made by autopsy, but tests based on tonsil biopsy and antibodies to detect prions in body fluids are also being developed. Transgenic mouse models of each of the known TSEs are also being created in order to learn more about transmission and pathology.

—Michele Arduengo, Ph.D.;
updated by David M. Lawrence

See also Brain; Brain disorders; Creutzfeldt-Jakob disease (CJD); Food poisoning; Nervous system; Neurology; Prion diseases.

For Further Information:

Brown, David R., ed. *Neurodegeneration and Prion Disease.* New York: Springer, 2005.

Harris, David A., ed. *Prions: Molecular and Cellular Biology.* Portland, Oreg.: Horizon Scientific Press, 1999.

Prusiner, Stanley B., ed. *Prion Biology and Diseases.* 2d ed. Cold Spring Harbor, N.Y.: Cold Spring Harbor Laboratory Press, 2004.

U.S. Geological Survey. "Chronic Wasting Disease." http://www.nwhc.usgs.gov/disease_information/chronic_wasting_disease/index.jsp.

Chronobiology

Specialty

Anatomy or system affected: All

Specialties and related fields: Alternative medicine, endocrinology, neurology, preventive medicine

Definition: The study of the biological cycles in the functioning of organisms; in humans, knowledge of such cycles as circadian rhythms may aid in the diagnosis and treatment of diseases.

Key terms:

circadian rhythm: a cyclical variation in a biological process or behavior that has a duration of slightly greater than twenty-four hours

jet lag: the malaise, headache, fatigue, gastrointestinal disorders, and other symptoms that may result from traveling across several time zones within a few hours

melatonin: a hormone produced by the pineal gland within the epithalamus of the forebrain; it is usually released into the blood during the night phase of the light-dark cycle

period: the length of one complete cycle of a rhythm; ultradian rhythms are about twenty-four hours (twenty to twenty-eight hours), and infradian rhythms are longer than twenty-eight hours

seasonal affective disorder (SAD): a manic depression which undergoes a seasonal fluctuation as a result of various factors, both unknown and known

suprachiasmatic nuclei (SCN): two clusters of nerve cell bodies located in the hypothalamus of the forebrain; these structures display circadian rhythms and seem to be the source of rhythmicity for many of the body's other cycles

SCIENCE AND PROFESSION

Chronobiology refers to the study of various cycles or rhythms that are fundamental to living organisms, including human beings. Many of the early observations were made on plants and nonhuman animals, but the basic concepts also apply to human biology and medicine. In the twentieth century, early findings about cyclical changes in symptoms, body weight, pulse rate, and body temperature were substantiated and broadly expanded to include numerous aspects of human biology and medicine. Well-informed physicians now expect rhythms in their patients' behavior, physiology, and response to therapy. The extensive research on biological rhythms in diverse organisms makes up the specialized field called chronobiology. The presence of circadian, menstrual, weekly, seasonal (circannual), and other rhythms in humans necessitates a consideration of these cycles in any comprehensive approach to medical practice.

Despite their importance, the exact nature of these rhythms has not been resolved. Living organisms behave as though they have internal oscillators or biological clocks that time their activities. Some research provides evidence that many of the body's cells each have such internal timers. Until the exact causes for the various biological rhythms have been identified, there will be some limitations to the benefits derived from knowledge of their characteristics. An unsettled dispute concerns whether the actual timing information for circadian and other rhythms comes from within the organism (endogenous) or from the environment (exogenous). It is expected that travel to space beyond the moon may ultimately answer this question. Astronauts may have sufficient internal timing information to survive, or it may be necessary to create a rhythmic environment of change in light-dark cycles and perhaps magnetic field variations to provide vital timing information. In the meantime, there is much that is known in chronobiology.

In mammals, an important circadian timing mechanism resides in a cluster of cells called the suprachiasmatic nuclei, or SCN, which are located in the hypothalamus of the forebrain. From studies on laboratory mammals, it has been learned that removal of the SCN abolishes many of the body's circadian rhythms. In humans, chance tumors in this area are often found to disrupt the circadian rhythms of the patient. In laboratory mammals, it has been shown that there is a separate pathway from the eyes to the SCN that allows information about changes in the light-dark schedule to reach this part of the brain. Therefore, there is intense interest in learning more about the SCN and how they regulate circadian rhythms.

Additionally, the pineal gland, a small gland attached to the epithalamus of the forebrain, receives information from the SCN about the light-dark schedule. A hormone produced by the pineal gland called melatonin is released into the bloodstream at night and suppressed during daylight. Melatonin plays a significant role in the timing of body rhythms and sleep cycles. When melatonin levels rise, the brain interprets this as bedtime, a factor that has led to its increasing use as a treatment for jet lag.

The general physiology of the other tissues of the body is organized according to rhythmic processes. The exact question of whether such rhythms are dependent on the SCN is still a point of controversy. Nevertheless, the greater application of chronobiology to medicine does not have to await the solution of such theoretical questions. Even now, a wide variety of examples can be cited of the utility of chronobiologic principles in medicine.

DIAGNOSTIC AND TREATMENT TECHNIQUES

Four medical applications of chronobiology will be discussed. One area from psychiatry is the treatment of seasonal affective disorder. Three from other areas of medicine are the chronobiological treatment of asthma, cancer, and jet lag.

Seasonal affective disorder, or SAD, is characterized by depression beginning each year as daylight shortens and fully remitting when days start to lengthen, sometimes switching to mania. The condition is related to where people live and the corresponding hours of sunlight; the condition remits in a few days when sufferers travel to sunnier climes and worsens as they travel to areas where the days are shorter. As many as one in four persons in the northern latitudes may suffer from SAD, and female sufferers outnumber male ones. Although the disorder has been recognized only recently, for years writers and poets have noted seasonal depression in themselves and others.

Some patients take a mid-winter vacation to a sunny climate to alleviate the condition. For those who cannot travel, the use of artificial lights has been introduced. Glow lights are placed in the homes of SAD patients and used early in the morning as well as after sunset to lengthen daylight hours. Morning lights appear to bring particularly prompt relief. Relapses have been reported when light is withdrawn. Research is currently under way to determine when during the day light is most effective, how much light is needed, and the mechanisms by which light works to fight SAD.

Some details are emerging about this process. The human forebrain contains a small organ about the size of a pea that produces the hormone melatonin according to a circadian schedule. Melatonin is usually released into the bloodstream during the night. The use of bright light therapy seems to inhibit the release of melatonin and thereby to cause other changes in the brain chemistry. In some mammals, this mechanism may be important in regulating their seasonal behavior. In humans, the situation is more complex, and an adequate theory for the neurochemical basis of SAD and other mental disorders has yet to be advanced.

Asthma sufferers have long known that their symptoms worsen at night. This increase in coughing, wheezing, and breathlessness at night has been only recently identified with circadian rhythms rather than environmental factors. At first, some researchers thought that asthma was worse at night because the patients were lying down. It has been shown, however, that the symptoms show their circadian periodicity whether the person is lying down or not. The normal nightly decrease in airway passage diameter in the lungs of normal persons is exaggerated in the asthmatic. The most dangerous hours for the asthmatic are the very early morning hours, a time when there are more deaths among asthmatics. Interestingly, asthmatics who become adapted to a nighttime work schedule shift their most severe asthma symptoms to the daytime sleep period.

Experts in the field such as Michael H. Smolensky of the University of Texas contend that much more research needs to be done on the role of circadian rhythms in asthma and its treatment. For example, adrenocortical hormones, which are powerful anti-inflammatory agents, have been used successfully to treat asthmatics. It was discovered that the time of day when the hormones were given was of great importance. If the hormones are given in the evening, the patient's own adrenal gland is inhibited. Therefore, the best time to give such hormones is in the early morning, near the time when they are normally released in the body.

Theophylline is a drug that has been very successful in ameliorating the symptoms of asthmatics. It has been found that certain types of sustained-release theophylline are effective in reducing the early morning symptoms if the drug is taken the night before. In the study of asthma, the benefit of considering chronobiology has become obvious, and any new products to treat asthma need to be evaluated chronobiologically before they are made available to the general public.

Cancer diagnosis and treatment are aspects of medicine that are receiving increased consideration by chronobiologists. The normal growth of tissues occurs by cell division, or mitosis, a rhythmic process that is normally precisely regulated. Cancer is essentially unregulated mitosis, resulting in the growth of a tumor that is no longer subject to the control mechanisms of the body. Yet even this breakdown in regulation has its seasons. In human males, some types of testicular cancer are more often diagnosed in the winter, and in females some types of cervical cancer have a peak occurrence in the summer.

The treatment of cancer involves the use of surgery, radiation, or chemotherapy in an attempt to remove or kill the cancerous cells without substantial damage to the normal tissues. Early studies in animal models demonstrated that there are often specific times of the day that these types of cancer treatment can be most effective. In a few cases, the tumor may have a rhythm of mitosis that is no longer synchronized to the rhythm of the surrounding tissue. In these cases, it may be possible to administer drugs or radiation that inhibits mitosis according to a schedule that will affect the cancer cells but will not harm the host tissue. More often, there will be a mixed effect of the timed treatment, so that some suppression of mitosis occurs along with some side effects.

The application of chronobiology to the treatment of breast cancer has raised hopes that there can be a marked improvement for survival rates of women who undergo breast surgery. William J. M. Hrushesky of Albany Medical College found that women who had breast surgery near to the time of menses had a more than fourfold higher risk of recurrence and death than those patients who had surgery near the middle of the menstrual cycle. These findings are under review, and the final conclusions await the evaluation of more cases. It has also been observed that the diagnosis of breast cancer in the United States has a two-peaked seasonal rhythm in the spring and the fall. There is also evidence that the body temperature of the breast in normal women has a circadian rhythm along with perhaps an additional seven-day periodicity, whereas breasts with tumors have abnormal temperature rhythms of about twenty hours. This information may help in the early diagnosis of breast cancer if suitable automatic monitoring devices are used to measure breast temperature.

Jet lag may appear to be more of an inconvenience than a serious medical problem until one considers the disastrous consequences of a plane crash caused by pilot error or a poorly made decision by a diplomat in an international crisis. Wiley Post and Harold Gatty, on their 1931 plane trip around the world, were the first persons to suffer from this disorder. Essentially, the body is subjected to a shift in the day-night schedule, with sleep and meal times shifted earlier or later depending on the number of time zones crossed and the direction of the flight. The symptoms are general malaise, headaches, fatigue, disruptions of the sleep-wake cycle, and gastrointestinal disorders. There are individual differences in the time required to overcome jet lag. In general, younger and healthier people are better able to cope with such change.

A shift of six hours, such as a flight between New York and Paris, requires a substantial reorganization of one's circadian rhythms. It can take from two days to two weeks to resynchronize. Adaptation is slowest when one stays indoors and continues on a "home-time" schedule. Eastward flights are less easily tolerated than westward flights; the delays in resynchronization can take almost twice as long. The reason for the difference is that when one flies east, the sun comes up earlier relative to "home-time." It is easier for most people to "advance" than to shift "backward"—that is, to go from day to night than to go backward from night to day. For this reason, it is suggested that travelers fly early in the day when flying east and later in the day when flying west.

Unfortunately, little consideration has been given to chronobiology in scheduling work time and time off. Pilots, diplomats, businesspersons, and other time zone travelers often perform poorly when their body rhythms are disturbed by jet lag. Similarly, people who must change their work shift every few weeks often find their performance level dropping. The rate at which work shifts should be rotated forward to increase worker effectiveness is now coming under considerable study.

It should be realized that the living body has myriad hormones, enzymes, and other important constituents that have rhythms of several different periods. Maintaining the correct time relationship between the rhythms can be critical for normal health. In the diagnosis of disease, chronobiology has to be taken into account. Erhard Haus of the St. Paul-Ramsey Medical Center has spent many years detailing the circadian and other rhythms that must be considered. What is normal for the morning hours may be pathological for the evening hours. These rhythmic values are yet to be determined for many important diagnostic measurements.

In 2005, a research study by the Feinberg School of Medicine and Northwestern University confirmed previous findings that school start times for adolescents are too early. In adolescents, melatonin, the hormone that helps induce sleep, increases later in the evening, causing melatonin levels to stay at high levels until approximately 8:00 A.M. There is no known way to change melatonin levels; for example, going to bed earlier does not cause melatonin to decrease earlier. The researchers encouraged parents and school districts to start later, as research consistently shows that adolescents have their poorest academic performance in the morning and have consistently better cognitive functioning later in the day. The researchers noted that school start times are easily modified. Many previous studies have shown the same effect, and some school districts have instituted later start times, with many schools reporting improved cognitive functioning and mood among students.

Perspective and Prospects

One of the earliest written observations of a biological cycle was by Androsthenes, a soldier marching with Alexander the Great in the fourth century B.C.E., who recorded that the tamarind tree opens its leaves during the day and closes them at night. In experiments on similar leaf movements in other plants, the astronomer Jean Jacques d'Ortous de Mairan in 1729 found that plants held in the dark continued to open and close their leaves on a roughly twenty-four-hour schedule. Thus, circadian rhythms were shown not to be simple responses to the rising and setting of the sun but rather internal oscillations.

Early observers more interested in humans also identified rhythms. In the fifth century B.C.E., Hippocrates reported that his patients had twenty-four-hour fluctuations as well as longer-term rhythms in their symptoms. Herophilus of Alexandria in the third century B.C.E. observed a daily change in the human pulse rate. The Italian scientist Sanctorius in 1711 made repeated measurements of his own body weight and the turbidity of his urine, both of which he found to vary during the month. Later, he went to the extreme measure of constructing a giant scale and living on its huge pan so that a frequent record could be made of his changing weight. The French scientists A. Seguin and A. L. Lavoisier in 1790 did research that revealed circadian rhythms in the body weight of men. These researchers suggested that men who did not show such circadian rhythms in body weight should be suspected of being ill. The British scientist J. Davy in 1845 reported that he had found both circadian and circannual (yearlong) rhythms in his own body temperature.

Yet the historical citations of persons taking an interest in chronobiology in past centuries were only of passing concern and did not, in most cases, help to establish this field. Chronobiology as a discipline has received attention from the medical community only since about the 1970's, and many of its contributions to improving health are yet to be realized. The foremost student of chronobiology as applied to medicine has been Franz Halberg of the University of Minnesota. He has repeatedly called the attention of the medical community to the importance of biological rhythms in maintaining health and in the diagnosis and treatment of disease. Halberg has promoted the use of "autorhythmometry," or the self-measurement of one's physiological variables to monitor one's changing health. It has been shown that this method can be used effectively even by groups of schoolchildren.

The phase or the timing of the peaks and troughs of circadian rhythms is germane in both diagnosis and treatment. The advent of portable automatic recording devices that store physiological data on computer chips is opening up a means of documenting a patient's circadian rhythms around the clock for weeks at a time. Eventually, when patients visit physicians there will then be a complete record of body temperature, blood pressure, and other physiological variables. This database will provide a much better basis for decisions than the limited data normally taken during infrequent medical visits.

The diagnosis of diabetes mellitus has been shown to depend to an extent on the time of day that the various tests, such as the glucose tolerance test, are administered. Some diabetics are "matinal" diabetics and do not have trouble regulating their blood glucose levels until the afternoon. These persons need to have glucose tolerance tests administered in the afternoon in order to reveal their diabetes. Many additional examples of the importance of chronobiology in diagnosis and treatment exist. As more physicians and health professionals become familiar with the concepts and application of chronobiology, the effectiveness of health care will be enhanced.

—John T. Burns, Ph.D.;
Miriam Ehrenberg, Ph.D.;
updated by LeAnna DeAngelo, Ph.D.

See also Asthma; Cancer; Chemotherapy; Depression; Hormones; Light therapy; Melatonin; Metabolism; Physiology; Psychiatry; Seasonal affective disorder (SAD); Sleep disorders; Stress; Stress reduction.

FOR FURTHER INFORMATION:

Coleman, Richard M. *Wide Awake at 3:00 A.M.: By Choice or by Chance?* New York: W. H. Freeman, 1990. A popular presentation of the essentials of human chronobiology. Coleman is a former director of the Stanford University Sleep Disorders Clinic, and his coverage of this subspecialty is noteworthy. Shift work and jet lag are also discussed.

Columbus, Frank, ed. *Frontiers in Chronobiology Research*. New York: Nova Science, 2006. Covers topics from cell biology, developmental biology, ecology, endocrinology, genetics, molecular biology, neurobiology, and pharmacology. Focuses on circadian, tidal, seasonal, and annual rhythms.

Dunlap, Jay, Jennifer Loros, and Patricia Decourse, eds. *Chronobiology: Biological Timekeeping*. Sunderland, Mass.: Sinauer Associates, 2003. Provides a general introduction. Compares the anatomy, physiology, genetics, and molecular biology of organisms with circadian clocks.

Endres, Klaus-Peter, and Wolfgang Schad. *Moon Rhythms in Nature: How Lunar Cycles Affect Living Organisms*. Translated by Christian von Arnim. Edinburgh, Scotland: Floris Books, 2002. A nonscientific introduction to the lunar influences on Earth's biosphere.

Palmer, John D. *The Living Clock: The Orchestrator of Biological Rhythms*. New York: Oxford University Press, 2002. An engaging exploration of a range of mammalian behavior affected by internal biological clocks.

Rosenthal, Norman E. *Winter Blues: Everything You Need to Know to Beat Seasonal Affective Disorder*. New York: Guilford Press, 2006. Written at the popular level, this book gives the layperson an overview of the symptoms and treatment of seasonal affective disorder.

Sehgal, Amita. *Molecular Biology of Circadian Rhythms*. Hoboken, N.J.: Wiley-Liss, 2004. Reviews research advances in understanding biological rhythms and discusses the linkages to the understanding of cell and body biochemistry, health, and aging, and the molecular control of behavior.

Waterhouse, J. M., et al. *Keeping in Time with Your Body Clock*. New York: Oxford University Press, 2003. Explains how the body clock works, how it can malfunction, and ways to optimize health and well-being.

Circulation

Biology

Anatomy or system affected: Blood, blood vessels, circulatory system, liver

Specialties and related fields: Cardiology, hematology, vascular medicine

Definition: The flow of blood throughout the body; the circulatory system consists of the heart, lungs, arteries, and veins.

Key terms:

aneurysm: a localized enlargement of a vessel, usually an artery

atherosclerosis: accumulation of plaque within the arteries

calcification: the deposit of lime salts in organic tissue, leading to calcium in the arterial wall

capillaries: hairlike vessels that connect the ends of the smallest arteries to the beginnings of the smallest veins

claudication: muscle cramps that occur when arterial blood flow does not meet the muscles' demand for oxygen

diastole: the period of relaxation in the cardiac cycle

hypertension: a blood pressure higher than what is considered to be normal

lumen: the space within an artery, vein, or other tube

stenosis: the constriction or narrowing of a passage

systole: the period of contraction in the cardiac cycle

thrombus: a blood clot that, commonly, obstructs a vein but may also occur in an artery or the heart

vasoconstriction: a decrease in the diameter of a blood vessel

vasodilation: an increase in the diameter of a blood vessel

Structure and Functions

The cardiovascular system is made up of the heart, arteries, veins, and lungs. The heart serves as a pump to deliver blood to the arteries for distribution throughout the body. The veins bring the blood back to the heart, and the lungs oxygenate the blood before returning it to the arterial system.

Contraction of the heart muscle forces blood out of the heart. This period of contraction is known as systole. The heart muscle relaxes after each contraction, which allows blood flow into the heart. This period of relaxation is known as diastole. A typical blood pressure taken at the upper arm provides a pressure reading during two phases of the cardiac cycle. The first number is known as the systolic pressure and represents the pressure of the heart during peak contraction. The second number is known as the diastolic pressure and represents the pressure while the heart is at rest. A typical pressure reading for a young adult would be 120/80. When blood pressure is abnormally elevated, it is commonly referred to as high blood pressure, or hypertension.

The heart is separated into two halves by a wall of muscle known as the septum. The two halves are known as the left and right heart. The left side of the heart is responsible for high-pressure arterial distribution and is larger and stronger than the right side. The right side of the heart is responsible for accepting low-pressure venous return and redirecting it to the lungs.

Because of these pressure differences from one side of the heart to the other, the vessel wall constructions of the arteries and the veins differ. Strong construction of the arterial wall allows tolerance of significant pressure elevations from the left heart. The arterial wall is made up of three major tissue layers, known as tunics. Secondary layers of tissue that provide strength and elasticity to the artery are known as elastic and connective tissues. As with the artery, the wall of the vein is made up of three distinct tissue layers. Compared to that of an artery, the wall of a vein is thinner and less elastic, which allows the wall to be easily compressed by surrounding muscle during contraction.

While the heart is at rest, between contractions, newly oxygenated arterial blood passes from the lungs and enters the left heart. Each time the heart contracts, blood is forced from the left heart into a major artery known as the aorta. From the aorta, blood is distributed throughout the body. Once depleted of nutrients and oxygen, arterial blood passes through an extensive array of minute vessels known as capillaries. A significant pressure drop occurs as blood is dispersed throughout the immense network of capillaries. The capillaries empty into the venous system, which carries the blood back to the heart.

The primary responsibility of the venous system is to return deoxygenated blood to the lungs and heart. Much more energy is required from the body to move venous flow compared to arterial flow. Unlike the artery, the vein does not depend on the heart or gravity for energy to move blood. The venous system has a unique means of blood transportation known as the "venous pump," which moves blood toward the heart.

The components making up the venous pump include muscle contraction against the venous wall, intra-abdominal pressure changes, and one-way venous valves. Compression against the walls of a vein induces movement of blood. Muscle contraction against a vein wall occurs throughout the body during periods of activity. Activity includes every movement, from breathing to running. Variations in respiration cause fluctuations in the pressure within the abdomen, which produces a siphonlike effect on the veins, pulling venous blood upward. Valves are located within the veins of the extremities and pelvis. A venous valve has two leaflets, which protrude inward from opposite sides of the vein wall and meet one another in the center. Valves are necessary to prevent blood from flowing backward, away from the heart.

The venous system is divided into two groups known as the deep and superficial veins. The deep veins are located parallel to the arteries, while the superficial veins are located just beneath the skin surface and are often visible through the skin.

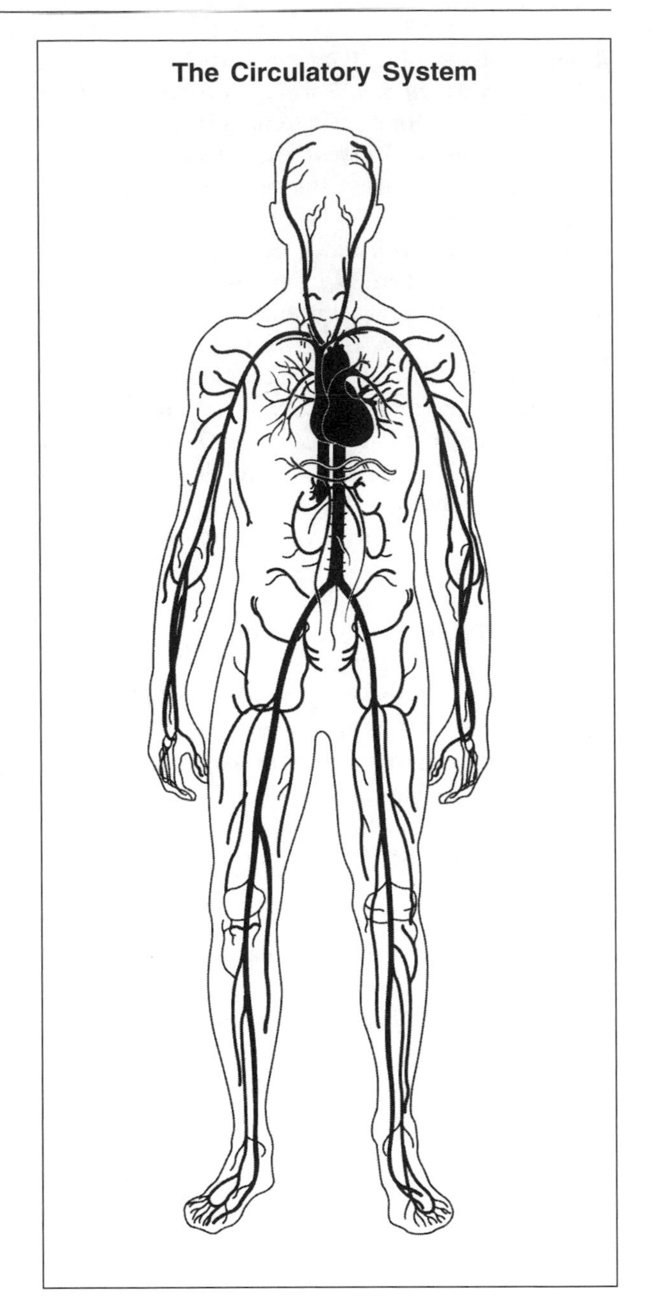

DISORDERS AND DISEASES

Numerous variables may affect the flow of blood. The autonomic nervous system is connected to muscle within the wall of the artery by way of neurological pathways known as sympathetic branches. Various drugs and/or conditions can trigger responses in the sympathetic branches and produce constriction of the smooth muscle in the arterial wall (vasoconstriction) or relaxation of the arterial wall (vasodilation). Alcohol consumption and a hot bath are examples of conditions that produce vasodilation. Exposure to cold and cigarette smoking are examples of conditions that produce vasoconstriction. Various drugs used in the medical environment are capable of producing similar effects. The diameter of the lumen of an artery influences the pressure and the flow of blood through it.

Another condition that alters the arterial diameter is atherosclerosis, a disease primarily of the large arteries, which allows the formation of fat (lipid) deposits to build on the inner layer of the artery. Lipid deposits are more commonly known as atherosclerotic plaque. Plaque accumulation reduces the diameter of the arterial lumen, causing various degrees of flow restriction.

Plaque is similar to rust accumulation within a pipe which restricts the flow of water. A restriction of flow is referred to as a stenosis. The majority of stenotic lesions occur at the places where arteries divide into branches, also known as bifurcations. In advanced stages of plaque development, plaque may become calcified. Calcified plaque is hard and may become irregular, ulcerate, or hemorrhage, providing an environment for new clot formation and/or release of small pieces of plaque debris downstream.

An arterial wall may become very hard and rigid, a condition commonly known as "hardening of the arteries." Hardened arteries may eventually become twisted, kinked, or dilated as a result of the hardening process of the arterial wall. A hardened artery which has become dilated is known as an aneurysm.

Normal arterial flow is undisturbed. When blood cells travel freely, they move together at a similar speed with very little variance. This is known as laminar flow. Nonlaminar (turbulent) flow is seen when irregular plaque or kinks in the arterial wall disrupt the smooth flow of cells. Plaque with an irregular surface may produce mild turbulence, while a narrow stenosis produces significant turbulence immediately downstream from the stenosis.

Many moderate or severe stenoses can be heard with the use of a standard stethoscope over the vessel of interest. A high-pitched sound can be heard consequent to the increased velocity of the blood cells moving through a narrow space. (A similar effect is produced when a standard garden hose is kinked to create a spray and a hissing sound is heard.) Medically, this sound is often referred to as a bruit. *Bruit* (pronounced "broo-ee") is a French word meaning noise.

Patients with significant lower extremity arterial disease will consistently experience calf pain and occasionally experience thigh discomfort with exercise. The discomfort is relieved when the patient stands still for a few moments. This is known as vascular claudication and occurs from a pressure drop as a consequence of a severely stenotic (reduced in diameter by greater than 75 percent) or occluded artery. If the muscle cannot get enough oxygen as a result of reduced blood flow, it will cramp, forcing the patient to stop and rest until blood supply has caught up to muscle demand. Alternate pathways around an obstruction prevent pain at rest, when muscle demand is low. Alternate pathways are also referred to as collateral pathways. Small, otherwise insignificant branches from a main artery become important vessels when the body uses them as collateral pathways around an obstruction. Time and exercise help to collateralize arterial branches into larger, more prominent arterial pathways. If collateral pathways do not provide enough flow to prevent the patient from experiencing painful muscle cramps while performing a daily exercise routine or to heal a wound on the foot, it may be necessary to perform either a surgical bypass around the obstruction or another interventional procedure such as angioplasty, atherectomy, or laser surgery.

Claudication may also occur in the heart. The main coronary arteries lie on the surface of the heart and distribute blood to the heart muscle. Patients suffering from coronary artery disease (CAD) may experience tightness, heaviness, or pain in the chest subsequent to flow restriction to the heart muscle as a result of atherosclerotic plaque within the coronary arteries. These symptoms are known as angina pectoris, or simply angina, usually occurring with exercise and relieved by rest. Intensity of the symptoms is relative to the extent of disease. A myocardial infarction (heart attack) is the result of a coronary artery occlusion.

Unlike the arteries, the venous system is not affected by atherosclerosis. The primary diseases of the veins include blood clot formation and varicose veins. A varicose vein is an enlarged and meandering vein with poorly functioning valves. A varicosity typically involves the veins near the skin surface, the superficial veins, and is often visualized as an irregular and/or raised segment through the skin surface. Varicosities are most common in the lower legs.

Valve leaflets are common sites for development of a thrombus. Thrombosis is the formation of a clot within a vein, which occurs when blood flow is delayed or obstructed for many hours. Several conditions that may induce venous clotting include prolonged bed rest (postoperative patients), prolonged sitting (long airplane or automobile rides), and use of oral contraceptives. Cancer patients are at high risk of clot formation secondary to a metabolic disorder which affects the natural blood-thinning process.

Because numerous tributaries are connected to the superficial system, it is easy for the body to compensate for a clot in this system by rerouting blood through other branches. The deep venous system, however, has fewer branches, which promotes the progression of a thrombus toward the heart. A thrombus in the deep venous system is more serious because the risk of pulmonary emboli, commonly known as blood clots in the lungs, is much higher than superficial vein thrombosis.

The further a thrombus propagates, the higher the risk to the patient.

Lower extremity venous return must take an alternate route via the superficial venous system when the deep system is obstructed by a thrombus. This is known as compensatory flow around an obstruction.

PERSPECTIVE AND PROSPECTS

Historically, the vasculature of the human body was evaluated by placing one's fingers on the skin, palpating for the presence or absence of a pulse, and making note of the patient's symptoms. Prior to the 1960's, treatment of the circulatory system was very limited or nonexistent, resulting in a high death rate and large numbers of amputations, strokes, and heart attacks. The development of arteriography (the angiogram), a procedure in which dye is injected into the vessels while X rays are obtained, revealed more about the vasculature and the nature of disease involving it. In conjunction with arteriography came corrective bypass surgery.

This period of development was followed by vast improvements in diagnostics, treatment, and knowledge of preventive maintenance. Today, synthetic bypass grafts are commonplace and are used to reroute flow around an obstruction. In many cases, procedures such as atherectomy and angioplasty, in which plaque or a thrombus is removed through a catheter inserted into the vessel, are often performed as outpatient procedures.

Diagnostic imaging of the cardiovascular system and the study of hemodynamics with the use of ultrasound have been useful for patient screening, the monitoring of disease progression, and the postoperative evaluation of surgical/interventional procedures. Ultrasound is a particularly valuable diagnostic tool because, compared to X rays or arteriography, it is less expensive; it is also quick, painless, and noninvasive (no radiation, needle, or dye is required).

In addition to technological advances, new medications have been made available to reduce the risk of graft rejection, hypertension, and clotting and to lower blood cholesterol. Preventive measures, however, constitute the most effective approach to good health. Much new information has been made available to improve the knowledge of the general public regarding diet, exercise, and the avoidance of unhealthy habits as the way to create and maintain a healthier cardiovascular system.

—*Bonnie L. Wolff*

See also Aneurysmectomy; Aneurysms; Angina; Angiography; Angioplasty; Arteriosclerosis; Biofeedback; Bleeding; Blood and blood disorders; Blood testing; Bypass surgery; Cardiopulmonary resuscitation (CPR); Catheterization; Chest; Cholesterol; Claudication; Cyanosis; Diabetes mellitus; Dialysis; Disseminated intravascular coagulation (DIC); Echocardiography; Edema; Embolism; Endarterectomy; Exercise physiology; Heart; Heart disease; Heat exhaustion and heat stroke; Hematology; Hematology, pediatric; Hemorrhoid banding and removal; Hemorrhoids; Hormones; Hypercholesterolemia; Hypertension; Ischemia; Kidneys; Lymphatic system; Phlebitis; Phlebotomy; Preeclampsia and eclampsia; Pulmonary hypertension; Shock; Shunts; Stents; Strokes; Systems and organs; Thrombolytic therapy and TPA; Thrombosis and thrombus; Transfusion; Transient ischemic attacks (TIAs); Varicose vein removal; Varicose veins; Vascular medicine; Vascular system; Venous insufficiency.

FOR FURTHER INFORMATION:

Bick, Rodger L.. ed. *Disorders of Thrombosis and Hemostasis: Clinical and Laboratory Practice*. 3d ed. Philadelphia: Lippincott Williams & Wilkins, 2002. An excellent introduction to the diagnosis and management of clotting and bleeding disorders.

Guyton, Arthur C., and John E. Hall. *Human Physiology and Mechanisms of Disease*. 6th ed. Philadelphia: W. B. Saunders, 1997. A well-written text for medical students interested in learning the physiological effects of disease. Parts 3 and 4 pertain to the heart and circulation.

Marieb, Elaine N., and Katja Hoehn. *Human Anatomy and Physiology*. 7th ed. San Francisco: Pearson Benjamin Cummings, 2007. Nonscientists at the advanced high school level or above will be able to understand this fine textbook. It includes a complete glossary, index, pronunciation guide, and other helpful features.

Saltin, Bengt, et al., eds. *Exercise and Circulation in Health and Disease*. Champaign, Ill.: Human Kinetics, 2000. This book is a compilation of integrated topics in cardiovascular regulatory physiology from more than forty authors.

Strandness, D. Eugene, Jr. *Duplex Scanning in Vascular Disorders*. 3d ed. New York: Raven Press, 2002. This book is written for medical vascular specialists and is somewhat technical in nature; however, it is well written. The beginning of each chapter defines the importance of that particular subject and the clinical presentation, treatment, and typical course of the vascular disease involved.

CIRCUMCISION, FEMALE, AND GENITAL MUTILATION

PROCEDURE

ANATOMY OR SYSTEM AFFECTED: Genitals, reproductive system

SPECIALTIES AND RELATED FIELDS: General surgery, gynecology, plastic surgery, psychiatry

DEFINITION: The partial or complete surgical removal of the clitoris, labia minora, and labia majora for cultural reasons.

KEY TERMS:

clitoridectomy: the removal of the entire clitoris, the prepuce, and adjacent labia

deinfibulation: an anterior episiotomy

episiotomy: the incision of the labia

infibulation: a clitoridectomy followed by the sewing up of the vulva

pharaonic circumcision: another term for infibulation

prepuce: the covering of the clitoris

sunna circumcision: the removal of the tip of the clitoris and/or the prepuce

INDICATIONS AND PROCEDURES

The various forms of female circumcision, although not universal to all cultures, have been practiced in numerous societies of the world for nearly two thousand years. Recorded evidence cites that female circumcision predates the advent of both Christianity and Islam and that early Christians, Muslims, and the Jewish group Falashas practiced circumcision on young girls. Historically, during the nineteenth century and until the 1940's, clitoridectomies were performed in Europe and America as a procedure to "cure" female masturbation, nervousness, and other specific types of perceived psychological dysfunction.

The 1989-1990 Demographic Health Survey of Circumcision stated that circumcision is still performed annually on an estimated 80 to 114 million women; 85 percent of these procedures involve clitoridectomy, while approximately 15 percent involve infibulation. Certain contemporary cultures of Africa, the Middle East, and parts of Yemen, India, and Malaysia continue these practices. Contemporary Middle Eastern countries practicing female circumcision and genital mutilation are Jordan, Iraq, the two Yemens, Syria, and southern Algeria. In Africa, it is practiced in the majority of the countries, including Egypt, Ivory Coast, Kenya, Mali, Mozambique, Sudan, and Upper Volta. It has been estimated that 99 percent of northern Sudanese women aged fifteen to forty-nine are circumcised. In and around Alexandria, Egypt, 99 percent of rural and lower-income urban women are circumcised.

Cross-culturally, there are essentially four types of female genital circumcision and female genital mutilation. Circumcision or sunna circumcision is removal of the prepuce or hood of the clitoris, with the body of the clitoris remaining intact. Sunna means "tradition" in Arabic. Excision circumcision or clitoridectomy is the removal of the entire clitoris (both prepuce and glans) and all or part of the adjacent labia majora and the labia minora.

Intermediate circumcision is the removal of the clitoris, all or part of the labia minora, and sometimes part of the labia majora.

Infibulation or pharaonic circumcision is the removal of the clitoris, the labia minora, and much of the labia majora; on occasion, the remaining sides of the vulva are stitched together to close up the vagina, except for a small opening maintained for the passage of blood and urine.

All types of female genital mutilation frequently create severe, long-term effects, such as pelvic infections that usually lead to infertility, chronic recurrent urinary tract infections, painful intercourse, obstetrical complications, and, in some cases, surgically induced scars that can cause tearing of the tissue, and even hemorrhaging, during childbirth. In fact, it is not unusual for women who have been infibulated to require surgical enlargement of the vagina on their wedding night or when delivering children. Unfortunately, babies born to infibulated women frequently suffer brain damage because of oxygen deprivation (hypoxia) caused by a prolonged and obstructed delivery. The baby may die during the painful birthing process because of a damaged birth canal. Other physical and psychological difficulties for the circumcised woman may be sexual dysfunction, delayed menarche, and genital malformation.

From a cultural perspective, there are numerous reasons for these surgical procedures. It is a rite of passage and proof of adulthood. It raises a woman's status in her community, because of both the added purity that circumcision brings and the bravery that initiates are called upon to demonstrate. It is also thought to confer maturity and inculcate positive character traits, such as the ability to endure pain and to be submissive. In some cultures, the circumcision ritual is a positive one in which the girl is the center of attention and receives presents and moral instruction from her elders. It creates a bond between the generations, as all women in the society must undergo the procedure and thus have shared an important experience.

It is thought that a girl who has been circumcised will not have her conscience troubled by lustful thoughts or sensations or by physical temptations such as masturbation. Therefore, there is less risk of premarital relationships that can end in the stigma and social difficulties of illegitimate birth. The bond between husband and wife may be closer because one or both of them will never have had sex with anyone else. The relationship may be motivated by love rather than lust because there will be no physical drive for the wife, only an emotional one. There is little incentive for extramarital sex for the wife; hence, the marriage may be more secure. Children may be better cared for because the husband can be more confident that they are his. Generally, a girl who is not circumcised is considered "unclean" by local villagers and therefore unmarriageable. In some societies, a girl who is not circumcised is believed to be dangerous, even deadly, if her clitoris touches a man's penis.

Unfortunately, female genital circumcision and female genital mutilation surgeries are invariably conducted in unsanitary conditions in which a midwife or close female relative uses unsterile sharp instruments, such as pieces of glass, razor blades, kitchen knives, or scissors. The induction of tetanus, septicemia, hemorrhaging, and even shock are not uncommon. Human immunodeficiency virus (HIV) can be transmitted. No anesthesia is used. These procedures usually are experienced by the child at approximately three years of age, although the actual age depends upon the customs of the particular society or village. In order to minimize the risk of the transmission of viruses, countries such as Egypt have made it illegal for female genital mutilation to be practiced by anyone other than trained doctors and nurses in hospitals.

Treatment and Therapy

There is no information regarding the surgical restoration of severed or damaged genitals. Because of severe cultural sanctions by the participating groups, which continue to hold tenaciously to such practices, female genital circumcision is seldom discussed with outsiders. Those who follow these customs do not report their occurrence. Consequently, there are few data concerning the frequency of female genital circumcision and female genital mutilation within the United States, despite the knowledge that some immigrant groups from Africa, the Middle East, and Asia continue to practice these surgeries. Health care workers estimate that, within the United States, approximately ten thousand girls undergo these surgical procedures each year. Usually, the procedure is conducted in the home. Those who can pay physicians to perform the surgery may do so; in these cases, local anesthesia is used and the risk of infection is less.

Perspective and Prospects

Because of the high number of female genital mutilations and the deaths that this procedure has caused, it is now prohibited in Great Britain, France, Sweden, Switzerland, and some countries of Africa, such as Egypt, Kenya, and Senegal. The National Organization of Circumcision Information Resource Centers (NOCIRC) is opposed to the procedures, as well as to male circumcision. The United Nations Children's Fund (UNICEF) and the World Health Organization (WHO) consider female genital mutilation to be a violation of human rights, recommending its eradication. In the United States, former Congresswoman Patricia Schroeder introduced a bill that would outlaw female genital mutilation. The bill, called the Federal Prohibition of Female Genital Mutilation Act of 1995, was passed in 1996. The Canadian Criminal Code was enacted to protect children who are ordinarily residents in Canada from being removed from the country and subjected to female genital mutilation.

Both female genital circumcision and female genital mutilation perpetuate customs that seek to control female bodies and sexuality. It is hoped that with increasing legislation and attitude changes regarding bioethical issues, fewer girls and young women will undergo these mutilating surgical procedures. One problem in this campaign is the conflict between cultural self-determination and basic human rights. Feminists, physicians, and ethicists must work respectfully with, and not independently of, local resources for cultural self-examination and change.

—John Alan Ross, Ph.D.

See also Bleeding; Childbirth; Childbirth complications; Circumcision, male; Episiotomy; Ethics; Genital disorders, female; Gynecology; Infertility, female; Menstruation; Psychiatry; Reproductive system; Septicemia; Sexual dysfunction; Sexuality; Stillbirth; Women's health.

FOR FURTHER INFORMATION:

Benedek, Wolfgang, et al., eds. *The Human Rights of Women: International Instruments and African Experiences*. London: Zed, 2002. Examines a range of issues as they affect women around the globe. Genital mutilation is discussed specifically.

"Female Genital and Sexual Mutiliation." *WIN News* 26, no. 2 (Spring, 2000): 51-59. A look at the problem of female genital and sexual mutilation around the world. More than 149 million girls have been mutilated in Africa alone.

Gruenbaum, Ellen. *The Female Circumcision Controversy: An Anthropological Perspective*. Baltimore: Johns Hopkins University Press, 2000. Argues that Western outrage over female circumcision often fails to appreciate the diversity of cultural contexts, the complex meanings, and the conflicting responses to change among citizens of developing nations, thus resulting in a strong backlash against Western intervention.

James, Stanlie M., and Claire C. Robertson, eds. *Genital Cutting and Transnational Sisterhood: Disputing U.S. Polemics*. Urbana: University of Illinois Press, 2002. In five essays, authors use a historical approach, feminist perspectives, and cultural relativism to argue that Western outrage over female circumcision is arrogant and ethnocentric.

Larsen, Ulla, and Sharon Yan. "Does Female Circumcision Affect Infertility and Fertility? A Study of the Central African Republic, Cote d'Ivoire, and Tanzania." *Demography* 37, no. 3 (August, 2000): 313-321. In Cote d'Ivoire and Tanzania, circumcised women had lower childlessness, lower infertility by age, and higher total fertility rates than women who were not circumcised; the reverse pattern prevailed in the Central African Republic.

Walker, Alice, and Pratibha Parmar. *Warrior Marks: Female Genital Mutilation and the Sexual Blinding of Women*. New York: Harcourt Brace, 1993. Describes Walker's journey around the world to interview a group of women trying to eliminate the traditional practice of female circumcision, a practice forced on women by the men of diverse societies, in a study that includes a new introduction offering an update on the issue.

Williams, Deanna Perez, William Acosta, and Herbert A. McPherson, Jr. "Female Genital Mutilation in the United States: Implications for Women's Health." *American Journal of Health Studies* 15, no. 1 (1999): 47-52. Female genital mutilation has become a public health concern in the United States because of an influx of immigrants from countries that practice it. The Centers for Disease Control estimates that 168,000 females in the United States are at risk for this procedure.

CIRCUMCISION, MALE

PROCEDURE

ANATOMY OR SYSTEM AFFECTED: Genitals, reproductive system

SPECIALTIES AND RELATED FIELDS: General surgery, pediatrics, urology

DEFINITION: The removal of the foreskin (prepuce) covering the head of the penis.

KEY TERMS:

chordee: the downward curvature of the penis, most apparent on erection, caused by the shortness of the skin on the downward side of the penile shaft

glans or *glans penis:* the head of the penis

necrosis: the death of one or more cells or a portion of a tissue or organ resulting from irreversible damage

phimosis: the narrowing of the opening of the skin covering the head of the penis sufficient to prevent retraction of the skin back over the glans

sepsis: an infection in the circulating blood

smegma: a pasty accumulation of shed skin cells and secretions of the sweat glands which collects in the moist areas of the foreskin-covered base of the glans

urinary tract infections: infections of the bladder, the kidneys, the urethra (which connects the bladder to the opening at the end of the penis), and the ureters (which connect the bladder to the kidneys); infection may be limited to one area of these organs or spread throughout the urinary tract

INDICATIONS AND PROCEDURES

Routine circumcision of the newborn male—in which the foreskin of the penis is stretched, clamped, and cut—is becoming an increasingly controversial procedure. Famed pediatrician Benjamin Spock once contended that circumcision is a good idea, especially if most of the boys in the neighborhood are circumcised; then a boy feels "regular." Yet, many wonder if that is justification for circumcision. Allowing routine circumcision of newborns as a religious and cultural rite still leaves the debate over medical necessity. The United States is the only country in the world that circumcises a majority of newborn males without a religious reason. In fact, circumcision has been termed a "cultural surgery."

True medical indications for the surgery are seldom present at birth. Such conditions as infections of the head and/or shaft of the penis may be indications for circumcision; an inability to retract the foreskin in the newborn (phimosis) is not an indication. Some argue that circumcision should be delayed until the foreskin has become retractable, making an imprecise surgical procedure presumably less traumatic. In 96 percent of infant boys, however, the foreskin is not fully retractable; it is normally so tight and adherent that it cannot be pulled back and the penis cleaned. By age three, that percentage decreases to 10 percent.

There are other definite contraindications to newborn circumcision. Circumcising infants with abnormalities of the penal head or shaft makes treatment more difficult because the foreskin may later be needed for use in reconstruction. Prematurity, instability, or a bleeding problem also preclude early circumcision. The foreskin is a natural protective membrane, representing 50 to 80 percent of the skin system of the penis, having 240 feet of nerve fibers, more than 1,000 nerve endings, and 3 feet of veins, arteries, and capillaries. It keeps the sensitive head protected, facilitating intercourse, and prevents the surface of the glans from thickening and becoming desensitized. Also, within the inner surface of the foreskin are a series of tiny ridged bands that contribute significantly to stimulating the glans.

The two most persistent arguments for the operation, however, are the risks of infection and cancer in the uncircumcised. Without circumcision, smegma accumulates beneath the base of the covered head of the penis. This cheeselike material of dead skin cells and secretions of the sweat glands is thought to be a cause of cancer of the penis and prostate gland in uncircumcised men and cancer of the cervix in their female partners. Doctors who argue against circumcision, however, say that the presence of smegma in the uncircumcised is simply a sign of poor hygiene and that poor sexual hygiene, inadequate hygienic facilities, and sexually transmitted diseases cause an increased incidence of cancer in ethnic groups or populations that do not practice circumcision. Doctors who argue against circumcision also point out that complete circumcision is found as often in male partners of women without cancer of the cervix as in male partners of women who have cervical cancer. In Sweden, moreover—where newborn circumcision is not routinely practiced but where good hygiene is practiced—the rates of these cancers are essentially the same as those found in Israel, where ritualistic circumcision is practiced.

The increased incidence of urinary tract infections and sexually transmitted diseases (STDs) in uncircumcised males sufficiently argues for circumcision, say its proponents. They warn that the intact foreskin invites bacterial colonization, which leads to urethral infection ascending to the bladder that ultimately may spread upward to the kidneys and sometimes cause permanent kidney damage. On the other hand, no proof exists that uncircumcised male infants who sustain urinary tract infections will have future urologic problems. Furthermore, the operation is not a simple procedure and is not without peril. Penile amputation, life-threatening infections, and even death have been well documented.

Slightly increased rates of infection with sexually transmitted diseases in the uncircumcised argue the case for some proponents, but it is acquired immunodeficiency syndrome (AIDS) that they most fear. In Africa, where circumcision is seldom practiced, the acquisition of AIDS by heterosexual men from infected women during vaginal intercourse is the most common mode of transmission.

Proponents say that infection with human immunodeficiency virus (HIV), the virus that leads to AIDS, depends on a break or an abrasion of the skin to gain entry. The intact foreskin provides a site for transfer of infected cervical secretions. In Africa, doctors at the University of Nairobi noted a relationship of HIV infection to genital ulcers and lack of circumcision. Uncircumcised men had a history of genital ulcers more often than did the circumcised, and they were more often HIV-positive. They were also more frequently HIV-positive even if they did not have a history of genital ulcer disease.

Every evaluation of circumcision, pro or con, should reflect the confounding genetic and environmental variables, as well as the actual increased risks and benefits. All the pros and cons should be explained to parents before informed consent is obtained.

USES AND COMPLICATIONS

In 1989, the American Academy of Pediatrics' Task Force on Circumcision concluded that "newborn circumcision has potential medical benefits and advantages as well as disadvantages and risks. When circumcision is being considered, the benefits and risks should be explained to the parents and informed consent obtained." This neutral statement does not lessen the anxiety of parents who are trying to weigh the pros and cons of routine newborn circumcision, but examination of the evidence does allow parents to weigh the individual benefits and risks and see if the scale tips in either direction.

Worldwide studies of predominantly uncircumcised populations have shown a higher incidence of urinary tract infection in boys during the first few months of life, which is the reverse of what is found in older infants and children, where girls predominate. In 1986, Brooke Army Medical Center in Fort Sam Houston, Texas, took a closer look. The doctors found the incidence of urinary tract infection in circumcised infant males to be 0.11 percent but 1.12 percent in the uncircumcised. Even without proof that the uncircumcised male infants who get urinary tract infections will have future urologic problems, the proponents for the surgical procedure claim about a 1 percent advantage.

The evidence for an increase in sexually transmitted diseases (such as genital herpes, gonorrhea, and syphilis) among the uncircumcised is conflicting. Furthermore, apparent correlations between circumcision status and these diseases do not reflect confounding genetic and environmental variables. It is also difficult to factor in the risk from HIV infections. The studies from Africa do not look at any variables in the transmission of HIV except circumcision status and previous history of genital ulcers. The nutritional and economic status of the men was not examined, even though it is known that malnourishment suppresses the immune systems. Moreover, if everyone practiced "safe sex," the argument for circumcision would be moot.

Almost all the surgical complications of circumcision can be avoided if doctors performing the procedure adhere to strict asepsis, are properly trained and experienced in the procedure, remove the appropriate and correct amount of tissue, and provide adequate hemostasis. The variety of circumstances, populations, and physicians affects the incidence of complications. In the larger, teaching hospitals, often the newest physicians with the least experience or supervision perform the operation. As a result, complications may arise. Excessive bleeding is the most frequent complication. The incidence of bleeding after circumcision ranges from 0.1 percent to as high as 35 percent in some reports. Most of the episodes are minor and can be controlled by simple measures, such as compression and suturing, but some of these efforts can lead to diminished blood supply to the head and shaft of the penis with necrosis of the affected part. Chordee can result if improper technique or bad luck intervenes, and such penile deformity begets the risk of emotional distress. The urethral opening on the end of the penis can become infected or ulcerated when the glans is no longer protected by foreskin; such infection rarely occurs in the uncircumcised. Finally, any surgical procedure runs the risk of infection. These localized infections rarely spread to the blood, but death from sepsis and its sequelae has been documented.

Overall, the surgical complication rate after circumcision runs around 0.19 percent, which could be lowered with strict protocols, meticulous technique, strict asepsis, and well-trained, experienced physicians. Strict protocols, it is hoped, would ensure that absolute contraindications to the procedure—such as anomalies of the penis, prematurity, instability, or a bleeding disorder—were honored.

Another human factor must be considered. Many insurance companies do not provide payment for newborn care, since it is considered preventive medicine. In 1997, a physician's fee for performing a circumcision ranged to approximately $400, with a nationwide average of $137. Interestingly, a growing number of circumcised men are undergoing expensive foreskin restoration procedures.

In part because of an additional cost that arises with anesthesia, the vast majority of infant circumcisions are performed without pain control. The surgery is painful, yet some physicians claim that the minute that the operation ends, the circumcised baby no longer cries and frequently falls asleep. Continuing pain, therefore, is probably not present.

Another perspective to examine is the experience of adult males, who are circumcised by their own choice. Many complain of at least a week's discomfort after the operation. The most compelling argument against adult circumcision, however, comes from their answer to "Would you do it again?" In one study of several hundred men who were circumcised as adults, they were asked five years later if they would do it again. All said no.

PERSPECTIVE AND PROSPECTS

Routine newborn circumcision originated in the United States in the 1860's, ostensibly as prophylaxis against disease. Some medical historians, however, believe that nonreligious circumcision was a deliberate surgical procedure to desensitize and debilitate the penis to prevent masturbation. During this era, and for nearly a hundred years afterward, most American physicians viewed masturbation as an inevitable cause of blindness, weak character, insanity, nervousness, tuberculosis, venereal disease, and even death. One physician maintained that a painful circumcision would have a salutary effect upon the newborn's mind, so that pain would be associated with masturbation. As late as 1928, the *American Medical Journal* published an editorial that justified male circumcision as an effective means of preventing the dire effects of masturbation. During World Wars I and II, soldiers were forcibly circumcised under threat of court martial, being told that the surgery was for reasons of hygiene and the prevention of epilepsy and other diseases.

Eventually, a general change in attitude occurred, notably in Great Britain and New Zealand, which virtually have abandoned routine circumcision. Rates of circumcision have also fallen dramatically in Canada, Australia, and even the United States. As recently as the mid-1970's, approximately 90 percent of U.S. male babies were circumcised. Not until 1971 did the American Academy of Pediatrics determine that circumcision is not medically valid. By 2001, the incidence of newborn circumcision had declined to 55 percent.

In 1971, the American Academy of Pediatrics' Committee on the Fetus and Newborn issued an advisory that said, "There are no valid medical indications for routine circumcision in the neonatal period." In 1978, when the American College of Obstetricians and Gynecologists affirmed this statement, the circumcision rate had already declined to an estimated 70 percent of newborn males, compared to previous rates of between 80 and 90 percent.

Undoubtedly, the future will bring improved surgical techniques. More emphasis will be placed on avoiding surgical complications by more rigid monitoring of the operation and who performs the procedure. It is unlikely that circumcision will disappear completely.

Organizations such as Doctors Opposing Circumcision and the National Organization to Halt the Abuse and Routine Mutilation of Males, however, are actively proposing an end to routine neonatal circumcision. Some nursing groups and concerned mothers have formed local groups to oppose circumcision in male neonates. They argue that subjecting a baby to this procedure may impair mother-infant bonding. Another question posed by some physicians and parents is the ethics involved in the unnecessary removal of a functioning body organ, particularly without the patient's consent. Others claim that the baby's rights are being violated, noting that it is the child who must live with the outcome of the decision to perform a circumcision. As a result of these efforts, the rates of circumcision will probably continue to fall.

—Wayne R. McKinny, M.D.; updated by John Alan Ross, Ph.D.

See also Circumcision, female, and genital mutilation; Ethics; Genital disorders, male; Men's health; Neonatology; Pediatrics; Reproductive system; Urology, pediatric.

FOR FURTHER INFORMATION:

Apuzzio, Joseph J., Anthony M. Vintzileos, and Leslie Iffy, eds. *Operative Obstetrics*. 3d ed. New York: Taylor & Francis, 2006. Examines obstetric surgical procedures, including the methods used in circumcision.

Behrman, Richard E., Robert M. Kliegman, and Hal B. Jenson, eds. *Nelson Textbook of Pediatrics*. 17th ed. Philadelphia: Saunders, 2004. This standard pediatric textbook briefly covers the medical risks and benefits of routine newborn circumcision fairly and without bias or excessive medical jargon. Draws no conclusions.

Bigelow, Jim. *The Joy of Uncircumcising! Exploring Circumcision—History, Myths, Psychology, Restoration, Sexual Pleasure, and Human Rights*. Rev. ed. Aptos, Calif.: Hourglass, 1998. This book provides an alternative view of this controversial procedure.

Gollaher, David L. *Circumcision: A History of the World's Most Controversial Surgery*. New York: Basic Books, 2000. Gollaher sets out to make "the strange familiar," but also "the familiar strange," in this book about the persistent practice of circumcision, which has been found in a variety of different cultures around the world.

King, Lowell R., ed. *Urologic Surgery in Neonates and Young Infants*. Philadelphia: W. B. Saunders, 1998. J. W. Duckett's contribution, "The Neonatal Circumcision Debate," is an excellent review of the controversies surrounding this operation. Although written for doctors, it will present minimal difficulty for laypersons.

Snyder, Howard M. "To Circumcise or Not." *Hospital Practice* 26 (January 15, 1991): 201-207. This widely available medical journal article examines in detail the medical evidence for and against circumcision. With a minimum of medical jargon, the author also states his own personal bias against the routine use of the procedure.

CIRRHOSIS

DISEASE/DISORDER

ANATOMY OR SYSTEM AFFECTED: Liver

SPECIALTIES AND RELATED FIELDS: Family medicine, internal medicine, psychology

DEFINITION: The formation of scar tissue in the liver, which interferes with its normal function.

CAUSES AND SYMPTOMS

The liver is a large, spongy organ that lies in the upper-right abdomen. Regarded as primarily part of the digestive system because it manufactures bile, the liver has many other functions, including the synthesis of blood-clotting factors and the detoxification of such harmful substances as alcohol.

Cirrhosis describes the fibrous scar tissue (or nodules) that replaces the normally soft liver after repeated long-term injury by toxins such as alcohol or viruses. The liver may form small nodules (micronodular cirrhosis), large nodules (macronodular cirrhosis), or a combination of the two types (mixed nodular cirrhosis). Cirrhosis is a frequent cause of death among middle-aged men, and increasingly among women. While alcoholism is the most common cause, chronic hepatitis and other rarer diseases can also produce the irreversible liver damage that characterizes cirrhosis. The resulting organ is shrunken and hard, unable to perform its varied duties. Because of its altered structure, the cirrhotic liver causes serious problems for surrounding organs, as blood flow becomes difficult. The barrier to normal circulation leads to two serious complications: portal hypertension (the buildup of pressure in the internal veins) and ascites (fluid leakage from blood vessels into the abdominal cavity).

TREATMENT AND THERAPY

Diagnosis is usually made from a history of alcoholism; a physical examination revealing a small, firm liver; a fluid-filled abdomen (ascites); and laboratory studies that show low concentrations of the blood products that the liver manufactures. A definitive diagnosis can be made only by biopsy, although radiographic methods such as computed tomography (CT) scanning and magnetic resonance imaging (MRI) can be quite conclusive.

The mortality rate is very high, as the damage is irreversible. Deaths from internal vein rupture and hemorrhage (the results of portal hypertension) and from kidney failure are most common. Repeated hospitalizations attempt to control the variety of complications that arise with agents that stop bleeding, bypass tubes that relieve pressure, the removal of the ascitic fluid, and nutritional support for malnutrition. Eventually, kidney failure ensues or one of these control measures

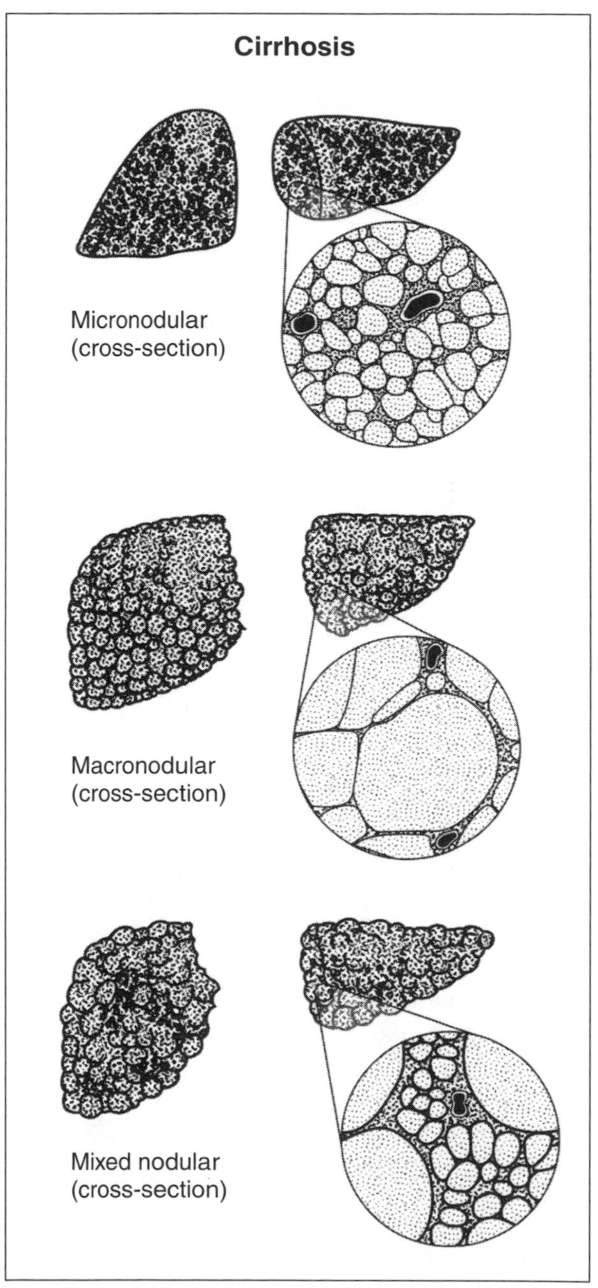

Cirrhosis appears in three forms, detectable under the microscope, each depending primarily on the cause of the liver damage. All are characterized by the replacement of normally soft, spongy tissue with hard, fibrous scarring. Alcohol-related cirrhosis usually produces the micronodular form.

Information on Cirrhosis

Causes: Buildup of scar tissue in liver from toxins (alcohol, viruses)
Symptoms: May include jaundice, fatigue, weakness, appetite loss, easy bruising
Duration: Chronic
Treatments: None

fails, and death rapidly follows. Cases of mild cirrhosis, where sufficient normal tissue remains, have a clearly better course.

—*Connie Rizzo, M.D., Ph.D.*

See also Alcoholism; Hepatitis; Jaundice; Liver; Liver cancer; Liver disorders; Liver transplantation; Nonalcoholic steatohepatitis (NASH).

For Further Information:

Fishman, Mark, et al., eds. *Medicine*. 5th ed. Philadelphia: Lippincott Williams & Wilkins, 2004. A standard reference source which focuses on internal medicine. Includes bibliographical references and an index.

Goldman, Lee, and Dennis Ausiello, eds. *Cecil Textbook of Medicine*. 22d ed. Philadelphia: W. B. Saunders, 2004. This is a standard textbook of medicine. Although it is somewhat difficult, it is complete, beginning with normal conditions and progressing through disease process, diagnosis, and treatment.

Mulvihill, Mary Lou, et al. *Human Diseases: A Systemic Approach*. 6th ed. Upper Saddle River, N.J.: Pearson Prentice Hall, 2006. This well-written and interesting book uses a case-oriented approach to explore the essential concepts of physiology and health. Numerous examples of pathologies relating to steroids or steroid hormones are illustrated.

Parker, James N., and Philip M. Parker, eds. *The Official Patient's Sourcebook on Primary Biliary Cirrhosis*. San Diego, Calif.: Icon Health, 2002.

_______. *The 2002 Official Patient's Sourcebook on Cirrhosis of the Liver*. San Diego, Calif.: Icon Health, 2002. Provides comprehensive information drawn from public, academic, government, and peer-reviewed research.

Claudication

Disease/disorder

Anatomy or system affected: Blood vessels, circulatory system, legs

Specialties and related fields: Vascular medicine

Definition: Pain in the calf or thigh muscle brought on by walking and relieved by rest.

Causes and Symptoms

Claudication is pain that develops in the calf or thigh muscle during walking. The pain increases if the patient continues walking and is relieved within a few minutes after walking is terminated. The medical term for this condition is intermittent claudication. The pain is caused by a narrowing in the arteries that supply the leg with blood. This narrowing is commonly caused by atherosclerosis, in which fatty material that builds up on the inside wall of the artery. At first, as the fatty material accumulates in the artery, it creates no symptoms. Only after more than 50 percent of the artery is narrowed do symptoms occur. The first symptom is mild cramping or heaviness that develops during a long walk. Over time, the narrowing increases and the distance that the individual is able to walk decreases. If not treated, the narrowing of the artery may increase further and the pain will be present all the time, signaling a more serious condition called rest pain that may lead to limb loss.

Factors that may lead to this condition include smoking, high blood pressure, heart disease, high cholesterol, and advanced age. Elderly people are more likely to develop intermittent claudication, but younger individuals with multiple risk factors for vascular disease may develop this problem at any age. Sometimes a

Information on Claudication

Causes: Narrowing in leg arteries from atherosclerosis; risk factors include smoking, high blood pressure, heart disease, high cholesterol, advanced age
Symptoms: Mild cramping or heaviness during long walks, progressing to leg pain at rest and sometimes amputation
Duration: Chronic, progressive without treatment
Treatments: Smoking cessation, lowering of cholesterol levels, program of long-distance walking, medications (pentoxifylline, cilostazol), surgery (angioplasty, bypass surgery, stents)

thrombus may obstruct an artery, causing claudication symptoms to occur suddenly instead of slowly as with atherosclerosis.

The diagnosis of claudication is fairly simple. Clinically, true intermittent claudication can be differentiated from a similar but unrelated condition by noting if the symptoms happen every time that the patient walks a similar distance. True claudication will develop every time, while pain from other conditions will occur at some times but not others.

To be more precise in diagnosing this condition, a Doppler study can be performed on an outpatient basis in a hospital or a doctor's office. The examination, called an ankle-brachial index (ABI), is simple and painless. Blood pressures are taken at the ankles and in the arms before and after exercise. If the pressure at the ankles drops with exercise and goes back to normal a few minutes later, then the diagnosis of intermittent claudication can be made. Ultrasound imaging or angiogram studies may be done to identify the exact location of the narrowing.

Treatment and Therapy

Treatment depends on the severity of the symptoms. Stopping smoking, lowering cholesterol levels, and beginning a program of long-distance walking may provide enough relief to allow some patients to return to near-normal routines. Medications such as pentoxifylline (Trental or Pentoxil) or cilostazol (Pletal) may provide limited relief from symptoms. More severe cases may require angioplasty, surgery to bypass the narrowed artery, or stenting of the diseased artery.

Perspective and Prospects

Claudication has become more common in the United States as the population ages and sedentary lifestyles become more popular. Although some treatments are effective, it is a difficult problem to manage. Education programs are available to help those at risk for this condition make necessary lifestyle changes that may lessen their chances of developing this ailment. Those changes may include getting plenty of exercise (brisk walking being the best), not smoking, lowering cholesterol, and keeping diabetes under control.

—Steven R. Talbot, R.V.T.

See also Arteriosclerosis; Bypass surgery; Cholesterol; Circulation; Exercise physiology; Hypercholesterolemia; Lower extremities; Pain management; Stents; Thrombosis and thrombus; Vascular medicine; Vascular system.

For Further Information:

Hershey, Falls B., Robert W. Barnes, and David S. Sumner, eds. *Noninvasive Diagnosis of Vascular Disease.* Pasadena, Calif.: Appleton Davies, 1984.

Rutherford, Robert B., ed. *Vascular Surgery.* 6th ed. Philadelphia: W. B. Saunders, 2005.

Zwiebel, William J., and John S. Pellerito, eds. *Introduction to Vascular Ultrasonography.* 5th ed. Philadelphia: Saunders, 2005.

Cleft lip and palate

Disease/disorder

Anatomy or system affected: Bones, musculoskeletal system

Specialties and related fields: Neonatology, otorhinolaryngology, pediatrics, plastic surgery, speech pathology

Definition: A fissure in the midline of the palate so that the two sides fail to fuse during embryonic development; in some cases, the fissure may extend through both hard and soft palates into the nasal cavities.

Key terms:

alveolus: the bony ridge where teeth grow

ectrodactyly: a congenital anomaly characterized by the absence of part or all of one or more of the fingers or toes

hard palate: the bony portion of the roof of the mouth, contiguous with the soft palate

Logan's bow: a metal bar placed, for protection and tension removal, on the early postoperative cleft lip

obturator: a sheet of plastic shaped like a flattened dome which fits into the cleft and closes it well enough to permit nursing

soft palate: a structure of mucous membrane, muscle fibers, and mucous glands suspended from the posterior border of the hard palate

syndactyly: a congenital anomaly characterized by the fusion of the fingers or toes

uvula: the small, cone-shaped projection of tissue suspended in the mouth from the posterior of the soft palate

Causes and Symptoms

Cleft palate is a congenital defect characterized by a fissure along the midline of the palate. It occurs when the two sides fail to fuse during embryonic development. The gap may be complete, extending through the hard and soft palates into the nasal cavities, or may be partial or incomplete. It is often associated with cleft lip

Information on Cleft Lip and Palate

Causes: Congenital defect
Symptoms: Craniofacial abnormalities, greater susceptibility to colds, poor muscle reactivity, dental problems
Duration: Correctable, usually at between seven and twelve months of age
Treatments: Surgery

or "harelip." About one child in eight hundred live births is affected with some degree of clefting, and clefting is the most common of the craniofacial abnormalities.

Cleft palate is not generally a genetic disorder; rather, it is a result of defective cell migration. Embryonically, in the first month, the mouth and nose form one cavity destined to be separated by the hard and soft palates. In addition, there is no upper lip. Most of the upper jaw is lacking; only the part near the ears is present. In the next weeks, the upper lip and jaw are formed from structures growing in from the sides, fusing at the midline with a third portion growing downward from the nasal region. The palates develop in much the same way. The fusion of all these structures begins with the lip and moves posteriorly toward, then includes, the soft palate. The two cavities are separated by the palates by the end of the third month of gestation.

If, as embryonic development occurs, the cells that should grow together to form the lips and palate fail to move in the correct direction, the job is left unfinished. Clefting of the palate generally occurs between the thirty-fifth and thirty-seventh days of gestation. Fortunately, it is an isolated defect not usually associated with other disabilities or with mental retardation.

If the interference in normal growth and fusion begins early and lasts throughout the fusion period, the cleft that results will affect one or both sides of the top lip and may continue back through the upper jaw, the upper gum ridge, and both palates. If the disturbance lasts only part of the time that development is occurring, only the lip may be cleft, and the palate may be unaffected. If the problem begins a little into the fusion process, the lip is normally formed, but the palate is cleft. The cleft may divide only the soft palate or both the soft and the hard palate. Even the uvula may be affected; it can be split, unusually short, or even absent.

About 80 percent of cases of cleft lip are unilateral; of these, 70 percent occur on the left side. Of cleft palate cases, 25 percent are bilateral. The mildest manifestations of congenital cleft are mild scarring and/or notching of the upper lip. Beyond this, clefting is described by degrees. The first degree is incomplete, which is a small cleft in the uvula. The second degree is also incomplete, through the soft palate and into the hard palate. Another type of "second-degree incomplete" is a horseshoe type, in which there is a bilateral cleft proceeding almost to the front. Third-degree bilateral is a cleft through both palates but bilaterally through the gums; it results in a separate area of the alveolus where the teeth will erupt, and the teeth will show up in a very small segment. When the teeth appear, they may not be normally aligned. In addition to the lip, gum, and palate deviations, abnormalities of the nose may also occur.

Cleft palate may be inherited, probably as a result of the interaction of several genes. In addition, the effects of some environmental factors that affect embryonic development may be linked to this condition. They might include mechanical disturbances such as an enlarged tongue, which prevents the fusion of the palate and lip. Other disturbances may be caused by toxins introduced by the mother (drugs such as cortisone or alcohol) and defective blood. Other associated factors include deficiencies of vitamins or minerals in the mother's diet, radiation from X rays, and infectious diseases such as German measles. No definite cause has been identified, nor does it appear that one cause alone can be implicated. It is likely that there is an interplay between mutant genes, chromosomal abnormalities, and environmental factors.

There are at least 150 syndromes involving oral and facial clefts. Four examples of cleft syndromes that illustrate these syndromes are EEC (ectrodactyly, ectodermal dysplasia, cleft lip/palate), popliteal pterygium syndrome, van der Woude's syndrome, and trisomy 13 syndrome. EEC and trisomy 13 both result in mental retardation as well as oral clefts, plus numerous other disabilities more serious than clefting. Popliteal pterygium has as its most common feature skin webbing (pterygium), along with clefts and skeletal abnormalities. Van der Woude's syndrome usually shows syndactyly as well as clefting and lower-lip pitting.

Problems begin at birth for the infant born with a cleft palate. The most immediate problem is feeding the baby. If the cleft is small and the lip unaffected, nursing may proceed fairly easily. If the cleft is too large, however, the baby cannot build up enough suction to nurse efficiently. To remedy this, the hole in the nipple of the bottle can be enlarged, or a plastic obturator can be fitted to the bottle.

Babies with cleft palate apparently are more susceptible to colds than other children. Since there is an open connection between the nose and mouth, an infection that starts in either location will easily and quickly spread to the other. Frequently, the infection will spread to the middle ear via the Eustachian tube. One end of a muscle is affixed to the Eustachian tube opening, and the other end is attached to the middle of the roof of the mouth (palate). Normal contraction opens the tube so that air can travel through the tube and equalize air pressure on both sides of the eardrum. As long as the eardrum has flexibility of movement, the basics for good hearing are in place. Children with cleft palates, however, do not have good muscle reactions; therefore, air cannot travel through the tube. If the tube remains closed after swallowing, the air that is trapped is absorbed into the middle-ear tissue, resulting in a vacuum. This pulls the eardrum inward and decreases its flexibility, and hearing loss ensues. The cavity of the middle ear then fills with fluid, which often breeds bacteria, causing infection. The infection may or may not be painful; if there is no pain, the infection may go unnoticed and untreated. The accumulated fluid can cause erosion of the tiny bones, which would decrease sound transmission to the auditory nerve. This conductive hearing loss is permanent. Persistent and prolonged fluid buildup can also cause accumulation of dead matter, forming a tumorlike growth called a cholesteotoma.

Other problems associated with cleft palate are those related to dentition. In some children there may be extra teeth, while in others the cleft may prevent the formation of tooth buds so that teeth are missing. Teeth that are present may be malformed; those malformations include injury during development, fusion of teeth to form one large tooth, teeth lacking enamel, and teeth that have too little calcium in the enamel. If later in development and growth the teeth are misaligned, orthodontia may be undertaken. Another possible problem met by patients with a cleft palate is maxillary (upper jaw) arch collapse; this condition is also remedied with orthodontic treatment.

TREATMENT AND THERAPY

One of the first questions a parent of a child with a cleft palate will pose regards surgical repair. The purpose of surgically closing the cleft is not simply to close the hole—although that goal is important. The major purpose is to achieve a functional palate. Whether this can be accomplished depends on the size and shape of the cleft, the thickness of the available tissue, and other factors.

Cleft lip surgery is performed when the healthy baby weighs at least seven pounds; it is done under a general anesthetic. If the cleft is unilateral, one operation can

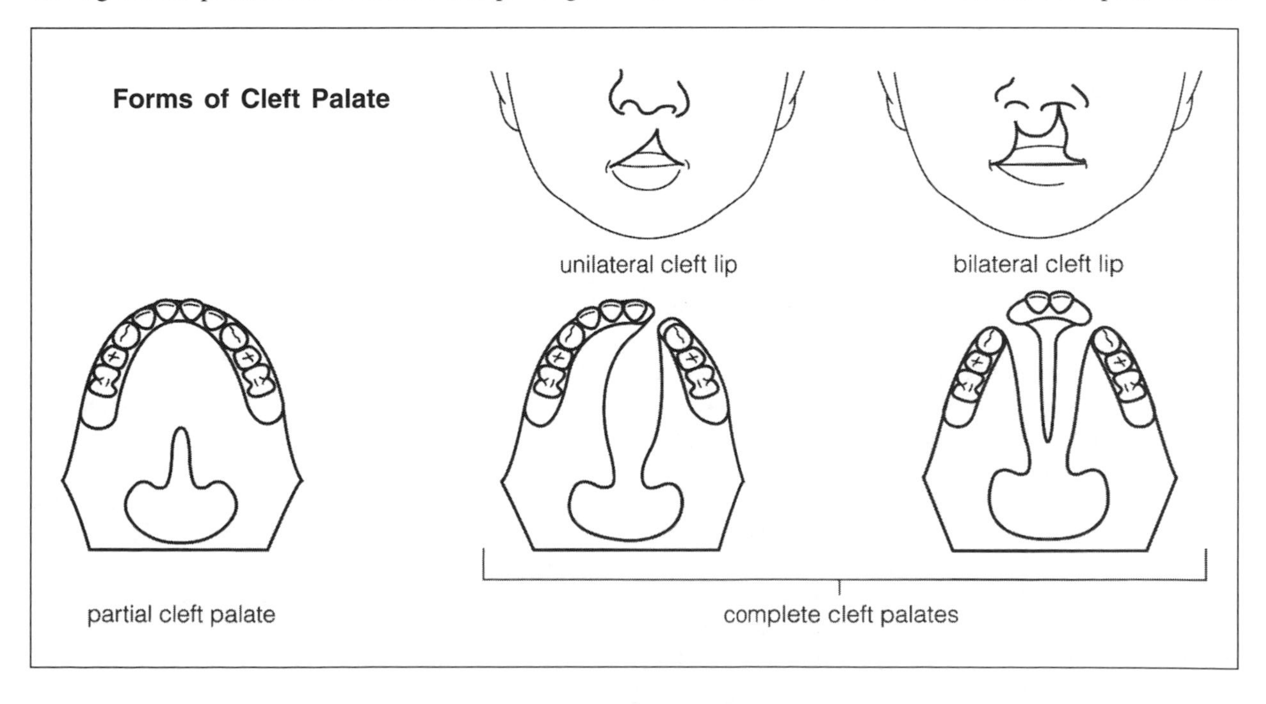

accomplish the closure, but a bilateral cleft lip is often repaired in two steps at least a month apart. When the lip is repaired, normal lip pressure is restored, which may help in closing the cleft in the gum ridge. It may also reduce the gap in the hard palate, if one is present. Successive operations may be suggested when, even years after surgery, scars develop on the lip.

Surgery to close clefts of the hard and soft palate is typically done when the baby is at least nine months of age, unless there is a medical reason not to do so. Different surgeons prefer different times for this surgery. The surgeon attempts to accomplish three goals in the repair procedure. The surgeon will first try to ensure that the palate is long enough so that function and movement will result (this is essential for proper speech patterns). Second, the musculature around the Eustachian tube should work properly in order to cut down the incidence of ear infections. Finally, the surgery should promote the development of the facial bones and, as much as possible, normal teeth. This goal aids in eating and appearance. All of this may be accomplished in one operation, if the cleft is not too severe. For a cleft that requires more procedures, the surgeries are usually spaced at least six months apart so that complete healing can occur. This schedule decreases the potential for severe scarring.

At one time, it was thought that if surgery were performed before the child began talking, speech problems would be avoided. In reality, not only did the surgery not remedy that problem, but the early closure often resulted in a narrowing of the upper jaw and interference with facial growth as well. Thus, the trend to put off the surgery until the child was four or five years of age developed; by this age, more than 80 percent of the lateral growth of the upper jaw has occurred. Most surgeons can perform the corrective surgery when the child is between one and two years of age without affecting facial growth.

Successful repair greatly improves speech and appearance, and the physiology of the oral and nasal cavities is also improved. Additional surgery may be necessary to improve appearance, breathing, and the function of the palate. Sometimes the palate may partially reopen, and surgery is needed to reclose it.

When the baby leaves the operating room, there are stitches in the repaired area. Sometimes a special device called a Logan's bow is taped to the baby's cheeks; this device not only protects the stitches but also relieves some of the tension on them. In addition, the baby's arms may be restrained in order to keep the baby's hands away from the affected area. (The child has been fitted for elbow restraints before surgery; the elbows are encased in tubes which prevent them from bending.) A parent of a child that has just undergone cleft palate repair should not panic at the sight of bleeding from the mouth. To curb it, gauze may be packed into the repaired area and remain about five days after surgery. As mucus and other body fluids accumulate in the area, they may be suctioned out.

During the initial recovery, the child is kept in a moist, oxygen-rich environment (an oxygen tent) until respiration is normal. The patient will be observed for signs of airway obstruction or excessive bleeding. Feeding is done by syringe, eyedropper, or special nipples. Clear liquids and juices only are allowed. The child sits in a high chair to drink, when possible. After feeding, the mouth should be rinsed well with water to help keep the stitches clean and uncrusted. Peroxide mixed with the water may help, as well as ointment. Intake and output of fluids are measured. Hospitalization may last for about a week, or however long is dictated by speed of healing. At the end of this week, stitches are removed and the suture line covered and protected by a strip of paper tape.

An alternative to surgery is the use of an artificial palate known as an obturator. It is specially constructed by a dentist to fit into the child's mouth. The appliance, or prosthesis, is carefully constructed to fit precisely and snugly, but it must be easily removable. There must be enough space at the back so the child can breathe through the nose. While speaking, the muscles move back over this opening so that speech is relatively unaffected.

Speech problems are the most likely residual problems in the cleft palate patient. The speech of the untreated, and sometimes the treated, cleft palate patient is very nasal. If the soft palate is too short, the closure of the palate may leave a space between the nose and the throat, allowing air to escape through the nose. There is little penetrating quality to the patient's voice, and it does not carry well. Some cleft palate speakers are difficult to understand because there are several faults in articulation. Certainly not all cleft lip or palate patients, however, will develop communication problems; modern surgical procedures help ensure that most children will develop acceptable speech and language without necessitating the help of a speech therapist.

Genetic counseling may help answer some of the family's questions about why the cleft palate occurred, whether it will happen with future children, and whether there is any way to prevent it. There are no universal answers to these questions. The answers depend on the degree and type of cleft, the sex of the child, the presence of other problems, the family history, and the history of the pregnancy. Genetic counseling obtained at a hospital or medical clinic can determine whether the condition was heritable or a chance error and can establish the risk level for future pregnancies.

PERSPECTIVE AND PROSPECTS

Oral clefts, as well as other facial clefts, have been a part of historical records for thousands of years. Perhaps the earliest recorded incidence is a Neolithic shrine with a two-headed figurine dated about 6500 B.C.E. The origination and causative agent of such clefts remain mysterious today.

Expectant parents are rarely alerted prior to birth that their child will be born with a cleft, so it is usually in the hospital, just after birth, that parents first learn of the birth defect. Even if it is suspected that a woman is at risk for producing a child with a cleft palate, there is no way to determine if the defect is indeed present, as neither amniocentesis nor chromosomal analysis reveals the condition. When the baby is delivered, the presence of the cleft can evoke a feeling of crisis in the delivery room. Shocklike reactions may be caused by the unexpectedness of the event or can occur because the doctors and medical personnel in the room have had little exposure to the defect. The parents may feel personal failure.

The problems accompanying clefting may alter family morale and climate, increasing the complexity of the problem. A team of specialists usually works together to help the patient and the family cope with these problems. This team may include a pediatrician, a speech pathologist, a plastic surgeon, an orthodontist, a psychiatrist, a social worker, an otologist, an audiologist, and perhaps others.

The cooperating team should monitor these situations: feeding problems, family and friends' reactions to the baby's appearance, how parents encourage the child to talk or how they respond to poor speech, and whether the parents are realistic about the long-term outcome for their child. The grief, guilt, and shock that the parents often feel can be positively altered by how the professional team tackles the problem and by communication with the parents. Usually the team does not begin functioning in the baby's life until he or she is about a month old. Some parents have confronted their feelings, while others are still struggling with the negative feeling that the birth brought to bear. Therefore, the first visit that the parents have with the team is important, because it establishes the foundation of a support system which should last for years.

If the cleft were only a structural defect, the solution would simply be to close the hole. Yet, problems concerning feeding and health, facial appearance, communication, speech, dental functioning, and hearing loss, as well as the potential for psychosocial difficulties, may necessitate additional surgical, orthodontic, speech, and otolaryngological interventions. In other words, after the closure has been made, attention is focused on aesthetic, functional, and other structural deficits.

—*Iona C. Baldridge*

See also Birth defects; Cleft lip and palate repair; DiGeorge syndrome; Speech disorders.

FOR FURTHER INFORMATION:

Berkowitz, Samuel, ed. *Cleft Lip and Palate: Diagnosis and Management*. 2d ed. New York: Springer, 2006. A review of treatment approaches. Offers facial and palatal growth studies.

Cleft Palate Foundation. http://www.cleftline.org/. Web site is divided into two sections, one for patients and families and one for professionals. The group offers publications, Cleftline (a toll-free phone number for information and support), and annual research grants.

Clifford, Edward. *The Cleft Palate Experience*. Springfield, Ill.: Charles C Thomas, 1987. This author writes from the perspective of a cleft palate team participant and incorporates the value of the team in his chapters. Much space is given to the child's development of a positive self-image and the parents' role, from birth, in forming this image.

Gruman-Trinker, Carrie T. *Your Cleft-Affected Child: The Complete Book of Information, Resources, and Hope*. Alameda, Calif.: Hunter House, 2001. An excellent guide to cleft disorders, including topics such as surgical procedures, financial assistance, emotional impact, and forming support groups.

Lorente, Christine, et al. "Tobacco and Alcohol Use During Pregnancy and Risk of Oral Clefts." *American Journal of Public Health* 90, no. 3 (March, 2000): 415-419. This study examines the relationship between maternal tobacco and alcohol consumption during the first trimester of pregnancy and oral clefts. Multivariate analyses showed an increased risk of cleft lip with or without cleft palate associated with smoking and an increased risk of cleft palate associated with alcohol consumption.

Stengelhofen, Jackie, ed. *Cleft Palate*. New York: Churchill Livingstone, 1989. Explores the various communication problems met by those with a cleft palate. An appeal to the entire team of professionals treating the patient and their partnership with parents. Case histories are discussed.

Wyszynski, Diego F., ed. *Cleft Lip and Palate: From Origin to Treatment*. New York: Oxford University Press, 2002. An excellent reference covering all aspects of cleft lip and palate formation, etiology, treatment, and prevention.

CLEFT LIP AND PALATE REPAIR

PROCEDURE

ANATOMY OR SYSTEM AFFECTED: Bones, gums, mouth, musculoskeletal system, skin

SPECIALTIES AND RELATED FIELDS: General surgery, neonatology, otorhinolaryngology, pediatrics, plastic surgery

DEFINITION: The surgical closure of cleft lip and cleft palate, deformities of the mouth that are often described as either the failure of tissue migration to allow fusion or the failure of tissue ingrowth (filling in).

INDICATIONS AND PROCEDURES

Cleft lip is more common in males than in females. Additionally, males tend to have more severe cleft deformities than females. Cleft lip repair is classically performed according to the rule of tens: The infant should be ten weeks old, weigh at least ten pounds, and have a white blood cell count under ten thousand (no infections) and a hemoglobin count of ten grams (not anemic). Today, many surgeons prefer to perform repairs earlier in healthy, full-term newborns ranging in age from one day to fourteen days. Cleft lip repairs typically involve making flaps around the lip area and merging the gaping sides. The muscular layer around the mouth must be sealed into a functional unit, as must the skin.

Cleft palate is more prevalent in females than males by a 2:1 ratio. A cleft palate may involve only the soft palate, or it may involve both the hard and the soft palates. Suckling can be a greater challenge with a cleft palate than with cleft lip. Moreover, middle-ear disease and infections are a greater problem for an infant with a cleft palate, because the reflux of fluids or solids into the nasal or middle-ear regions can occur. Surgical closure of a cleft palate usually is performed on infants between nine months and one year of age; delays can permanently retard speech and phonation development, while premature closure can stunt facial bone growth and contribute to dentition problems. Typically, if both the hard and the soft palates are open, they will be surgically closed at the same time. Closure of the soft palate occurs in a three-layer manner, while closure of the hard palate is done in a two-layer approach.

Cleft lip coupled with cleft palate is more common in males and tends to be left-sided more often than right-sided. Combined cleft lip and palate repair follows the same plans as described above, but there is greater concern about the well-being of an infant with the combined deformity.

—Mary C. Fields, M.D.

The Repair of Cleft Lip

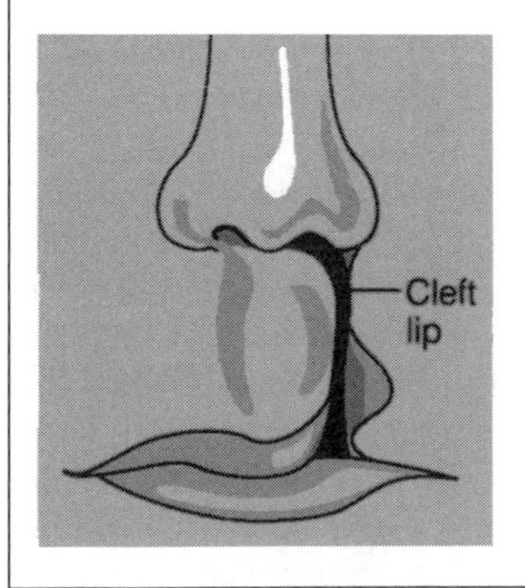

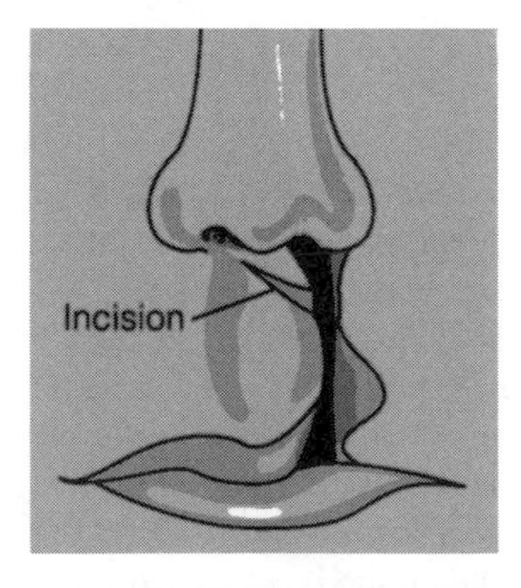

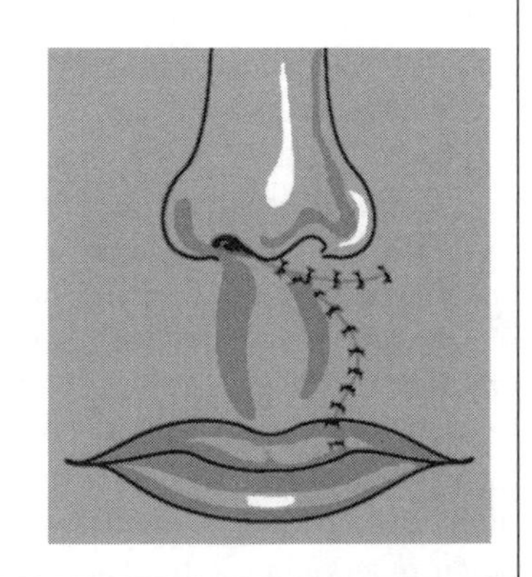

A cleft lip, a congenital deformity in which the tissues between the lip and nostril have failed to fuse, can be corrected surgically through realignment and suturing.

See also Birth defects; Bones and the skeleton; Cleft lip and palate; Pediatrics; Plastic surgery; Surgery, pediatric.

For Further Information:

Berkowitz, Samuel, ed. *Cleft Lip and Palate: Diagnosis and Management*. 2d ed. New York: Springer, 2006.

Clifford, Edward. *The Cleft Palate Experience*. Springfield, Ill.: Charles C Thomas, 1987.

Dronamraju, Krishna R. *Cleft Lip and Palate*. Springfield, Ill.: Charles C Thomas, 1986.

Gruman-Trinker, Carrie T. *Your Cleft-Affected Child: The Complete Book of Information, Resources, and Hope*. Alameda, Calif.: Hunter House, 2001.

Watson, A. C. H. *Management of Cleft Lip and Palate*. Philadelphia: Whurr, 2001.

Wynn, Sidney K., and Alfred L. Miller. *A Practical Guide to Cleft Lip and Palate Birth Defects*. Springfield, Ill.: Charles C Thomas, 1984.

Wyszynski, Diego. *Cleft Lip and Palate: From Origin to Treatment*. New York: Oxford University Press, 2002.

Clinical trials

Procedure

Anatomy or system affected: All

Specialties and related fields: All

Definition: Research studies that test new drugs or treatments on human subjects to determine whether and at what dosage they are safe, effective, and better than similar products already in use.

Key terms:

blinded or *single-blind:* a study in which the patients are not told whether they are in an experimental or control group

control group: a group of patients receiving either a standard treatment or a placebo, allowing comparison with the experimental treatment

double-blind: referring to a study in which neither the patients nor the research staff knows which patients are receiving which treatment

informed consent: consent for treatment by a patient who has been educated fully about the purpose, benefits, and risks of a clinical trial

Institutional Review Board (IRB): a committee that oversees informed consent, reviews the progress of clinical trials, and safeguards participants' rights

placebo: an inactive substance resembling the experimental drug that might be given to a control group, especially when no standard treatment exists

protocol: a lengthy, technical document outlining the rules for inclusion in, scientific rationale of, and procedures for a clinical trial

randomization: assigning, by chance, patients with similar characteristics to either the experimental or the control group in a clinical trial

Indications and Procedures

Clinical trials offer the most reliable process for bringing new drugs and medical treatments into public use. The process has features that can protect human participants, avoid biases, ensure that patient improvements are due to the experimental treatment and not to other factors, and allow accurate comparison of the experimental treatment with others on the market. Clinical trials are usually initiated and managed by academic institutions (often with grant funding), pharmaceutical companies, or government research agencies, such as the National Cancer Institute.

In 1998, it was estimated that the cost of developing a new drug was, on average, $500 million, and the process could take twelve to fifteen years—from discovery and laboratory testing, through clinical trials, to U.S. Food and Drug Administration (FDA) approval, and finally getting the drug to market. By the late 1990's, a new drug might go through sixty-eight clinical trials. The average number of patients enrolled in a trial was 3,800.

Clinical trials fit into one of four types. Phase I trials, which usually involve only twenty to one hundred seriously ill patients, try to determine how to administer a new drug, the maximally tolerated dose (MTD), how the human body processes the drug, and any significant side effects. Phase II trials, which are usually randomized, treat up to several hundred patients who all have measurable rates of disease. These trials study the effectiveness of the drug. Phase III trials, which are usually randomized and blinded and which treat hundreds or thousands of patients, have more relaxed criteria for inclusion and are usually multicenter (held simultaneously at more than one site). These trials try to determine whether the new drug is better than current, standard ones. Phase IV trials, conducted once a drug is on the market, are often informal. Pharmaceutical companies may simply ask physicians to submit reports on how their patients are responding to the drug.

Uses and Complications

The 1979 Belmont Report detailed three ethical principles to guide clinical trials. They include respect for persons (abiding by their opinions and choices as autonomous agents), beneficence (do no harm and maximize the possible benefits while minimizing possible harm), and justice (distributing the benefits and burdens of research fairly).

Two standard features of clinical trials help ensure that ethical principles are being followed. First, all clinical trials in the United States must be approved and monitored by an Institutional Review Board (IRB), which includes both scientists and laypersons. Multicenter trials must also have a data safety and monitoring board composed of independent experts. This group monitors data from the trial regarding the treatment's effectiveness and any adverse reactions. Second, the detailed informed consent document that patients must carefully consider and sign gives a number of categories of information. Most important, anticipated physical risks and discomforts are explained, as are financial risks.

Perspective and Prospects

In October, 1948, *The British Medical Journal* published an article reporting on what was probably the first study using all the methodological features of the randomized clinical trial. Since then, the randomized clinical trial has come to be regarded as perhaps the most important medical achievement of the twentieth century. It transformed biomedical research and allowed physicians to make treatment choices based on scientific evidence rather than personal opinion and experience.

The National Cancer Institute (NCI) and other sources reported a small participation rate in clinical trials—ranging in the late 1990's from 3 to 20 percent of patients. One of many causes was that insurance companies and managed care providers frequently refused payment for experimental treatments. Their concerns were that they might be liable for adverse reactions or additional care after the trial ends and that clinical trials are more costly than conventional treatments. Because so many insurers would not cover the costs of clinical trials, researchers had trouble finding patients willing to participate, thus slowing the development of more effective drugs and treatments. Insurers gradually realized that more widespread coverage of the costs of trials might speed the development of better drugs, which could ultimately save them money. In 1998, states began to pass laws requiring insurers to cover the routine medical costs (such as tests and office visits) of treatment in clinical trials of drugs for life-threatening diseases.

Criticism has been leveled at clinical trials for insufficient inclusion of women, children, people of color, and the aged. When these groups are underrepresented, there is no certainty that a drug will be effective or without side effects for them.

In June, 2000, the FDA added a regulation that would place a clinical hold on a phase I trial of a drug or treatment for a life-threatening disease affecting both women and men if either gender was excluded because of risk to their reproductive potential. That same month, President Bill Clinton signed an executive memorandum directing Medicare to reimburse senior citizens for routine medical costs incurred in clinical trials. A major impetus for this change came from reports that only 33 percent of cancer clinical trial participants were over sixty-five, while 63 percent of all cancer patients are over sixty-five.

—Glenn Ellen Starr Stilling, M.A., M.L.S.

See also Animal rights vs. research; Cancer; Death and dying; Disease; Ethics; Food and Drug Administration (FDA); Iatrogenic disorders; Invasive tests; National Cancer Institute (NCI); Noninvasive tests; Over-the-counter medications; Pharmacology; Pharmacy; Screening; Terminally ill: Extended care.

For Further Information:

CenterWatch Clinical Trials Listing Service. http://www.centerwatch.com/.

ClinicalTrials.gov. http://www.clinicaltrials.gov/.

Finn, Robert. *Cancer Clinical Trials: Experimental Treatments and How They Can Help You.* Sebastopol, Calif.: O'Reilly, 1999.

Green, Stephanie, Jacqueline Benedetti, and John Crowley. *Clinical Trials in Oncology.* 2d ed. Boca Raton, Fla.: Chapman & Hall, 2003.

Harrington, David P. "The Randomized Clinical Trial." *Journal of the American Statistical Association* 95, no. 449 (March, 2000): 312-315.

Malay, Marilyn. *Making the Decision: A Cancer Patient's Guide to Clinical Trials.* Sudbury, Mass.: Jones and Bartlett, 2002.

Quinn, Susan. *Human Trials: Scientists, Investors, and Patients in the Quest for a Cure.* Cambridge, Mass.: Perseus, 2002.

CLONING

PROCEDURE

ALSO KNOWN AS: Nuclear transplantation

ANATOMY OR SYSTEM AFFECTED: Cells

SPECIALTIES AND RELATED FIELDS: Biotechnology, embryology, ethics, genetics

DEFINITION: From a scientific perspective, the term "clone" signifies an exact genetic copy of a segment of deoxyribonucleic acid (DNA), cell, or organism. Cloning is a procedure conducted by teams of molecular biologists, geneticists, and embryologists to introduce the genetic information from one cell into another for the purpose of producing a clone.

KEY TERMS:

blastocyst: the stage during early embryonic development, just prior to implantation in the uterus, in which the cells form a large hollow ball; at this point, the cells are undifferentiated

complementary DNA (cDNA): DNA that is made from messenger ribonucleic acid (mRNA) and thus represents the genes actively being expressed in a cell at a given time

eukaryotic: referring to a type of cell that contains a nucleus and membrane-bound organelles; all animal cells are eukaryotic, as are those of plants and fungi

parthenogenesis: the development of an adult from an unfertilized egg

pluripotent: a description for stem cells that have begun differentiation and are capable of forming limited cell types

totipotent: an undifferentiated cell that still retains the ability to form any other cell type of the adult organism; cells of this type are commonly referred to as stem cells

transduction: the incorporation of a piece of DNA into the genome of a bacterium using a virus as a vector

transformation: the incorporation into a cell of cell-free DNA from the environment

transgenic: referring to an organism that contains genetic material from two or more species

transformation: the incorporation into a cell of cell-free DNA from the environment

vector: a system that is used to carry a fragment of DNA for molecular cloning

USES AND COMPLICATIONS

Scientists use the word "cloning" to indicate an experimental process by which an exact genetic duplicate is made of a molecule, cell, or organism. It is frequently divided into two general categories. Molecular cloning involves copying genes, short segments of DNA, or cells (sometimes also called cellular cloning) for the purpose of producing multiple copies of a molecule or cell for further scientific study. The cloning of DNA is commonly called recombinant DNA technology or genetic engineering. Cloning at the organismal level, also called nuclear transplantation, has been used to create genetically identical organisms and has the potential to produce genetically identical tissues and organs from a donor.

The procedure for molecular cloning involves choosing a vector for the study of the target DNA. The choice of the vector depends on the size of the genetic information being studied and whether it is genomic DNA or complementary DNA (cDNA). Common vectors include plasmids (small circular pieces of bacterial DNA), viruses, and artificial chromosomes. For example, if the length of the DNA being studied is small, then the researcher may choose to insert it into a plasmid. By the process of transformation, the selected plasmid is moved into the bacteria (usually *E. coli*), and as the bacteria divide, cells are produced that are clones for the DNA in the plasmid vector. If the researcher is unsure what area contains the gene to be cloned, then the genome is first fragmented and individual fragments are placed into viruses, or bacteriophages. This creates a library of genetic information. Each bacteriophage vector then infects a bacterium by a process called transduction. The infected bacterium is allowed to divide, producing a colony of bacteria that are clones for the information contained within the bacteriophage vector. These colonies may then be screened using molecular techniques to isolate a colony that contains the desired section of DNA.

If the DNA fragment is larger, as is frequently the case with studies of genomic DNA, then the researcher may decide to create an artificial chromosome. The purpose is to create a small pseudo-chromosome that is replicated by the host cell prior to cell division. Bacterial artificial chromosomes (BACs) and yeast artificial chromosomes (YACs) are commonly used, but the formation of human artificial chromosomes (HACs) has recently been announced. In all cases, the purpose is to create cells that are genetically identical, or cloned, for a specific stretch of DNA. While this is a useful technique, molecular cloning is not able to produce an entire organism that is genetically identical to the original.

In eukaryotic organisms, the result of sexual reproduction is to produce offspring that contain new combinations of the parents' genomes. While this provides variability to the species, it complicates medical research since it effectively shuffles the genome every generation. Identical, or monozygtic, twins are the closest thing to clones in humans, but between even their cells small genetic differences exist. For scientific studies of development and cell biology, large numbers of cloned cells are needed.

The process of nuclear transplantation, or cloning as it is commonly called, has the ability to create large numbers of genetically identical cells. In theory, cloning is not a difficult process: Simply remove the DNA from the host cell, replace it with the DNA from the donor cell, and encourage the new cell to divide. Procedures such as this have been performed on amphibians since the 1950's, but nuclear transplantation in mammals is slightly more complicated. For example, mammalian egg cells, called oocytes, are vastly smaller than those of amphibians.

Technological advances in microscopy and embryology helped to remedy this problem. In mammalian nuclear transplantation, a researcher, frequently an embryologist, uses a microscope equipped with a micropipette. The micropipette is effectively a microscopic needle that is controlled remotely by the researcher. During the procedure, the egg is held in place by a second pipette to allow for greater control. The researcher then inserts the needle from the first pipette into the oocyte through the zona pellucida (outer covering of the oocyte) and gently removes the genetic material from the cell. At this stage, the oocyte contains only the zona pellucida, cytoplasm, and the internal organelles of the cell, such as the mitochondria. The researcher then inserts a donor cell, complete with DNA, into the area between the oocyte and the zona pellucida. At this point, there are effectively two cells alongside each other—one containing nothing but cytoplasm, the other containing the donor DNA. In order to form a single cell, the plasma membranes of the two cells must be fused. This is done using a process called electrofusion, in which a small current is applied to the cells, temporarily disrupting the membranes and allowing the cytoplasm of the two cells (and the donor DNA) to mix. The end result is an egg cell than contains the DNA of a second cell.

However, this is not yet technically a clone. In order to produce a group of cells that are identical to the original donor cell, the oocyte must be persuaded to divide. In some systems, the first cell divisions occur naturally in response to electrofusion, but this is not always the case. Frequently, growth factors or other chemical signals need to be applied to make the cell divide. As the cells divide, they form a blastocyst, in which all cells are clones of one another and the DNA in the original donor cell.

The development of improved technologies in nuclear transplantation has enabled scientists to create organisms that are genetically the same. In the media, the use of the term "clone" usually signifies an organism produced by this procedure. To create a cloned organism, the researcher must insert the blastocyst into the uterus of a surrogate mother, who will carry the organism to term. To do this, scientists have adapted the techniques of in vitro fertilization. During in vitro fertilization, eggs are fertilized by sperm cells in the laboratory and then transferred into the uterus of the female. Cloning does not require the fertilization step, since the blastocyst contains the ball of cloned cells. Theoretically, once implanted, the cloned blastocyst should develop in the same manner as an embryo from a natural fertilization event.

An additional form of cloning is gathering significant attention from the scientific community, therapeutic cloning. The purpose of therapeutic cloning is to generate a large number of stem cells that have been cloned from a donor's DNA for the purpose of treating a disease. The idea is that since embryonic stem cells are totipotent, or have the ability to produce all cell types, then if they are reintroduced into the donor the stem cell theoretically has the ability to take the place of damaged or diseased cells. Only embryonic stem cells are totipotent, however, so the key is to introduce a donor's DNA into an oocyte by nuclear transplantation, allowing it to divide and form a blastocyst. Within the blastocyst forms a group of cells called the inner cell mass (ICM) that contains totipotent stem cells. These cells can then be harvested and grown under laboratory conditions that persuade the cells to develop into new tissues, such as nerves or skin cells.

Recently, researchers have proposed a new technique to generate these stem cells involving parthenogenesis, or the development of an unfertilized egg. Parthenogenesis is common in amphibians and insects, but it does not occur naturally in humans. If a female egg cell could be chemically persuaded to form blastocysts without having to go through the process of nuclear transplantation, then the resulting stem cells could be used to generate new organs or tissues for the female. The process could not be done the same way in males, since sperm cells lack the cytoplasmic components found in egg cells.

Indications and Procedures

By definition, the purpose of cloning is to produce genetically identical cells or individuals for scientific studies. Yet even identical, or monozygotic, twins, whose cells are derived from the same fertilized egg, are not truly identical. For example, monozygotic twins do not have the same fingerprint pattern, even though they possess the same genes for ridges on the fingers. The reason for this difference is environmental. For twins, the genes establish a general pattern, but it is the touch of the fingers on the inner wall of the uterus that establishes the final pattern of fingerprints. Environment plays a significant role in the development of the embryo, and this fact has presented a challenge for scientists who wish to produce identical genetic clones.

Dolly, a cloned ewe, was not an exact copy of her donor, even though she possessed the same genetic information as the donor ewe. The reason is that Dolly was raised in the uterus of a surrogate mother and thus was exposed to the minor, but important, environmental variations specific to the surrogate mother. It is known that, by a process called genomic imprinting, the mother can override certain traits in the embryo and impose her own traits, regardless of the genes present in the embryo. The mother also provides all the nutrients needed for the developing embryo, and thus any metabolic problems with the surrogate mother may inhibit proper development in the cloned embryo.

Another problem with nuclear transplantation is that not all the DNA in the cell is located within the nucleus. Mitochondria, the energy factories of a cell, contain small circular pieces of DNA. The genes on this DNA are inherited along with the mother's cytoplasm, so that individuals receive all mitochondrial DNA from the maternal line. During nuclear transplantation, mitochondria are not removed from the host cell, so once transplantation is complete the new cell contains donor DNA but both host cell and donor cell mitochondria. Because mitochondrial genetic disorders exist, it is known that the genes in the mitochondria contribute to the characteristics of the organism.

Cells age and have a finite life span. This appears to be at least partially controlled by the length of the chromosome, specifically the ends of the chromosome called the telomeres. After each cell division, the telomeres shorten like a genetic fuse, until the cell is no longer able to divide. A prime concern among those involved with cloning is whether the cloned cells inherit the telomere length (and thus age) of the donor cell or whether the telomere length is reset in the blastocyst. Claims have been made that support both ideas, and research is ongoing in this area. What is important, however, is the fact that the cloned cell, although totipotent, may not be perfect and may bring with it the genetic flaws of the donor cell.

One of the greatest challenges facing the process of cloning is ethical, which involves the opinion of the general public regarding the cloning of mammals and, potentially, humans. Some consider the cloning of organisms to be an unnatural event, while others question the source of embryonic stem cells. The greatest concern among the general public is the debate on the cloning of humans and the moral right of people to create life by artificial processes. Many of these same debates occurred when in vitro fertilization was introduced. The arguments both for and against human cloning appear to be endless and will continue into the foreseeable future. What should be noted is that the majority of scientists involved in cloning research are interested in either the therapeutic benefits of cell cloning or the study of embryonic development and cell differentiation, not the creation of a cloned human.

Perspective and Prospects

While for many people the history of cloning may appear to have begun in 1996, when Ian Wilmut of the Roslin Institute in Scotland introduced the world to Dolly the cloned ewe, the reality is that the cloning of organisms had been going on for some time. The making of cloned plants had been occurring for decades and now represents a common occurrence in agriculture. If one restricts the discussion to animals, then Dolly does not really even represent the first cloned mammal, but rather the first adult animal cloned from the cells of another adult animal.

The cloning of animals by nuclear transplantation has its roots in the late nineteenth century, when early embryologists were studying cell division in the eggs of invertebrate animals. The first experiments that transferred a nucleus from one cell to another in a vertebrate animal were conducted in the early 1950's by Robert Briggs and Thomas King. Briggs and King worked with nuclear transplantation in amphibians. These researchers were not interested in the creation of a cloned frog but rather the question of nuclear programming, or whether the cells isolated from the blastocyst had the genetic ability to form a new adult frog. These experiments examined the use of embryonic cells to produce a functionally adult organism.

In later experiments, researchers, including Briggs

and King, set out to determine at what age of embryonic development cells differentiate to the point where they cannot be used to produce a functioning adult. In essence, they were studying the potency of the cells and beginning to distinguish between totipotent cells and pluripotent cells. For the next several decades, scientists perfected methods of nuclear transplantation in a variety of organisms, including mammals such as mice and rabbits.

In 1996, the researchers at the Roslin Institute used tissue from the mammary gland of an adult ewe in a nuclear transplantation experiment. The result was Dolly, the first mammal to be cloned from an adult cell. Although this experiment was widely reported as producing the first cloned mammal, its real importance was the demonstration that the genes of an adult cell could be expressed in an embryo to produce a living organism. For decades, scientists had debated whether adult cells were capable of being used in cloning. Adult cells are highly specialized, and many of their developmental genes are inactivated. The experiments with Dolly demonstrated that, under the right conditions, the environment within the blastocyst allows DNA from adult cells to be used. In other words, the DNA from differentiated tissue can be used to create undifferentiated stem cells. This remains a major advance in the understanding of cellular processes.

The question may then be asked as to why scientists pursue experiments involving the cloning of organisms. Since public opinion is against the cloning of humans and no immediate need exists to clone an individual, then research in this area would appear to be at an impasse. The reality, however, is that the process of nuclear transplantation and organism cloning gives scientists the ability to answer some important questions about cellular differentiation, especially during embryonic development, and the patterns of expression of genes within cells during development.

Furthermore, while the cloning of humans may not be morally acceptable, cloning can serve society in many other ways, such as in studies using transgenic organisms and in tissue and organ transplantation. Scientific research frequently involves the use of transgenic organisms for study. In the study of human genetics and biochemistry, mice are frequently used as a model system. The ability to study the effects of a particular gene in a transgenic organism is dependent on that organism being genetically pure (homozygous) for that trait. In animals, it can take up to fifteen generations of inbreeding to develop a pure line. For organisms with long gestation periods or a small number of offspring per generation, this becomes both cost- and time-prohibitive. The cloning of new organisms, which are at least genetically the same as the donor, can facilitate research with transgenics.

Organ transplantation in humans is a difficult process. Recipients of organ transplants must be carefully matched with donors for a variety of biochemical factors to ensure that the new organ is not rejected by the recipient's immune system. Even when a match is close, the use of immunosuppressant drugs increases the chances of infection in the recipient. The process of nuclear transplantation may alleviate some of these problems. Rather than being matched with a donor, a patient would contribute genetic material for nuclear transplantation. Stem cells could then be harvested and chemically induced to form the required tissue, or someday even the entire organ. Experiments are currently under way to manufacture skin for burn victims using this type of procedure. The applications of nuclear transplantation are almost endless, and developments in this area of research have the potential to influence directly the lives of the majority of people alive today.

—Michael Windelspecht, Ph.D.;
updated by Jeffrey A. Knight, Ph.D.

See also Assisted reproductive technologies; Cells; Conception; Embryology; Ethics; Fetal tissue transplantation; Gene therapy; Genetic diseases; Genetic engineering; Genetics and inheritance; Genomics; In vitro fertilization; Law and medicine; Multiple births; Pregnancy and gestation; Transplantation.

FOR FURTHER INFORMATION:

Cibelli, Jose, Robert Lanza, Michael West, and Carol Ezzell. "The First Human Cloned Embryo." *Scientific American* 286 (January, 2002): 44-51. Discusses the process by which clones are generated for therapeutic purposes, as well as a new strategy for producing cloned cells using only unfertilized eggs. Illustrations of cloning procedure are included.

McKinnell, Robert, and Marie Di Berardino. "The Biology of Cloning: History and Rationale." *Bioscience* 49 (November, 1999): 875-885. Reviews the history of cloning from the nineteenth century onward, including the scientific experiments that led to the cloning of amphibians and the advances in mammalian cloning.

National Institutes of Health. Department of Health and Human Services. *Regenerative Medicine 2006.*

Bethesda, Md.: NIH Press, 2006. A collection of articles describing advances in stem cell and cloning technologies since this resource was first published in 2001.

Nussbaum, Martha, and Cass Sunstein, eds. *Clones and Clones: Facts and Fantasies About Human Cloning*. New York: W. W. Norton, 1998. A series of contributed essays on all aspects of human cloning, including science, ethics, and legal issues.

Pasternak, Jack J. *An Introduction to Human Molecular Genetics*. 2d ed. Hoboken, N.J.: Wiley-Liss, 2005. An excellent primer on many technologies as applied to humans, including genetic engineering, stem cell research, cloning, and gene therapy.

Wilmut, Ian, Keith Campbell, and Colin Tudge. *The Second Creation: Dolly and the Age of Biological Control*. New York: Farrar, Straus and Giroux, 2000. Coauthored by one of the creators of Dolly, this book examines the process of cloning and the steps that led to the cloning of the first mammal. It also provides insight into the reason that Dolly was cloned.

Club drugs

Disease/disorder

Also known as: Designer drugs, psychedelics

Anatomy or system affected: All

Specialties and related fields: Alternative medicine, critical care, emergency medicine, pharmacology, preventive medicine, psychiatry, psychology, public health, toxicology

Definition: A slang term for a variety of substances of abuse that generally are used in social situations, have hallucinogenic properties, and may either excite or sedate the user.

Key terms:

amnesia: a diverse condition where there is complete or partial loss of memory for specific periods of time, for specific types of information, or both

blackout: memory loss, usually as a result of taking substances known to disrupt memory, in which the affected person may function as if aware of what is happening, despite having no memory of activities

psychedelic drugs: substances that cause alterations in perception and thinking, such as changes in awareness or sense of self and hallucinations

raves: social gatherings that are distinguished by long periods of music, dancing, and often a percentage of individuals using psychedelic drugs and other substances of abuse

synergistic effects: the combined effects of drugs interacting with one another, such that the effects of the drugs together have a compounded effect, greater than that of any one alone

Causes and Symptoms

Less expensive, easily accessible, intoxicating drugs can often be attractive to persons wanting a momentary high or psychedelic experience, when they are at a rave, dance party, or bar with friends. This desire, combined with a belief that club drugs seem safe, leads people to trying club drugs and sometimes using them regularly. Club drugs are often first used in dance clubs or with friends. The belief that such drugs are natural forms of prescription drugs or are not necessarily always illegal fuels a misconception of their safety. Because the drugs are psychedelic, the reactions that individual users have can vary quite significantly depending on the user's emotional state, concurrent use of other substances, underlying psychiatric conditions, personality, and past experience with the drug. Additionally, as they are street drugs, usually subject to some variability in their contents (such as being mixed with less expensive drugs), their quality may vary substantially. Finally, the individual situations where the substances are used can pose a variety of dangers of varying levels.

Club drugs go by many different names. They include substances such as gamma-hydroxybutyrate (GHB, Georgia Home Boy, Liquid X), ketamine hydrochloride (ketamine, special K), lysergic acid diethylamid (LSD, acid, blotter), methylenedioxymethamphetamine (MDMA, Adam, ecstasy, X), and rohypnol (roofies, roach, roche). They also include herbal ecstasy (herbal X, cloud nine, herbal bliss), which is a drug made from ephedrine or pseudoephedrine and caffeine. These substances vary in their effects but as a group cause a variety of positive reactions, including euphoria, feelings of well-being, emotional clarity, a decreased sense of personal boundaries, and feelings of empathy and closeness to others. They also can cause, however, significant negative reactions, including panic, impaired judgment, amnesia, impaired motor control, insomnia, paranoia, irrational behavior, flashbacks, hallucinations, rapid heartbeat, high blood pressure, chills, sweating, tremors, respiratory distress, convulsions, and violence. It is not uncommon for individuals to mix these drugs with alcohol, prescription drugs, and illegal drugs. Taken in combination, these substances can make these very dangerous reactions even worse.

Treatment and Therapy

The effects of club drugs vary somewhat by substance; as such, treatment also varies by substance. In general, though, club drugs may tend to be seen more in emergency care settings than in primary health care settings. This is due to the fact that some of the problems that they cause, as a group, are often of an emergency nature. For instance, overdose, strokes, allergic shock reactions, blackouts, loss of consciousness, and accidents related to these conditions may require emergency care. Similarly, dehydration and heat exhaustion can result from prolonged periods of dancing or other physical exertion, as can occur in rave situations, and result in a need for emergency care. Finally, because date rapes have been known to occur with these drugs, particularly rohypnol, injuries due to sexual assault also may need attention.

Certainly the long-term impact of problems like those described above may require some type of psychotherapy. In addition, problems related to the abuse of or dependence upon club drugs would be addressed in much the same manner as for other substances of abuse. General addiction treatment would be advised. A special area of treatment may also include exploration of what it is like to deal with blackouts, amnesia, and flashbacks, as these are features that are commonly reported with psychedelic drugs.

Perspective and Prospects

Club drugs emphasize that there is a continuing need for the social awareness of the dangers of substances that may otherwise seem harmless. Just because a substance is not listed as an illegal drug does not mean that it cannot be dangerous. Any drug, whether sold over the counter, by prescription, or any other place, can be misused and can be dangerous. Where drugs are used, how much is used, with whom they are used, and with what they are used can all make a difference.

Club drugs are also a reminder that in efforts to find ways of joining with each other, finding community, and discovering themselves and their relationships, people will sometimes resort to experimenting with substances. While the experimental use of psychedelic substances for psychotherapeutic work continues and may prove beneficial to certain groups of patients, such work is balanced by investigations into neurology, physiology, psychopharmacology, and psychology to ensure that the benefits do not outweigh the risks. Continued exploration of the neuronal, developmental, social, and other health effects of using club drugs is likely, as they pose a significant danger to public health, particularly that of younger populations.

—*Nancy A. Piotrowski, Ph.D.*

See also Addiction; Amnesia; Emergency medicine; Hallucinations; Herbal medicine; Intoxication; Marijuana; Panic attacks; Paranoia; Pharmacology; Seizures; Trembling and shaking.

For Further Information:

Holland, Julie. *Ecstasy: The Complete Guide—A Comprehensive Look at the Risks and Benefits of MDMA.* Rochester, Vt.: Inner Traditions International, 2001.

Jansen, Karl. *Ketamine: Dreams and Realities.* Ben Lomond, Calif.: Multidisciplinary Association for Psychedelic Studies (MAPS), 2004.

Kuhn, Cynthia, et al. *Buzzed: The Straight Facts About the Most Used and Abused Drugs from Alcohol to Ecstasy.* 2d ed. New York: W. W. Norton, 2003.

O'Neill, John, and Pat O'Neill. *Concerned Intervention: When Your Loved One Won't Quit Alcohol or Drugs.* Oakland, Calif.: New Harbinger, 1992.

Stafford, Peter. *Psychedelics.* Berkeley, Calif.: Ronin, 2003.

Cluster headaches

Disease/disorder

Anatomy or system affected: Blood vessels, brain, head, nerves, nervous system

Specialties and related fields: Neurology

Definition: The most severe headache syndrome, characterized by paroxysmal onset of one side of the head, short duration, and episodic occurrence. Cluster headaches are often confused with migraine headaches, which are a similar syndrome but with different causes, patterns, and treatments.

Key terms:

alarm clock headaches: an earlier term for cluster headaches, emphasizing the characteristic awakening of sufferers during the night

circadian rhythm: the biological clockwise regularity associated with many body processes; most sufferers of cluster headaches have attacks at the same time of day during the same season of the year

cluster period: a time period, from two weeks to four months, during which cluster headaches occur; they usually disappear, or "enter remission," after the cluster period ends

paroxysmal: having a sudden, spasmlike, and painful onset

trigeminal-autonomic reflex pathway: the nerve pathway at the base of the brain activated during cluster attacks; the trigeminal nerve, the most important facial nerve for sensations such as temperature and pain, causes the "hot-poker-in-the-eye" pain typical of cluster headaches

unilateral: occurring only on one side (for example, on one side of the head or behind one eye)

Causes and Symptoms

Cluster headache is a well-defined, rare, but often misdiagnosed syndrome characterized by excruciatingly severe unilateral headaches that last from a half hour to three hours, with an average duration of forty-five minutes. Its features include paroxysmal onset of one side of the head, a short duration, and episodic occurrence. The pain often wakes sufferers one to two hours after they fall asleep. "Cluster" refers to the original perception that the headaches emerged in groups over a period of time (called the cluster period) lasting weeks to months, followed by periods that are free of pain and attacks (called remission or interim periods). The International Headache Society divides cluster headaches into episodic cluster and chronic cluster, with chronic further subclassified into primary and secondary variants. Chronic cluster headaches do not have a cessation, or interim, period but recur for years.

The precise cause of cluster headaches is unknown, although the season of the year is the most common trigger. Because they usually begin with spring or autumn, cluster headaches are often misattributed to seasonal allergies (such as hay fever) or seasonal-related stress (such as the beginning of school, final examinations, or the height of business cycles).

Positron emission tomography (PET) scanning has revealed that in cluster headaches the hypothalamus activates the trigeminal nerve, which is responsible for most of the severe pain. Located deep in the brain, the hypothalamus is also responsible for the internal biological clock that regulates the approximately twenty-four-hour sleep-wake cycle. The production and activity of the neurotransmitter serotonin, which is important in the self-regulation of these circadian rhythms, is also altered during attacks. Cluster headache is not related to the development of tumors or lesions.

Cluster headaches are rare. No more than .03 percent of the population ever experiences them. Men suffer them more than women do, although with improvements in epidemiological techniques the known ratio has been changed from 7:1 to 2:1. The age of onset is usually in the late twenties. As with migraine headaches, cluster headaches tend to run in families, with a fourteenfold increase in the chances of having them if a first-degree relative (mother, father, son, daughter, brother, or sister) suffers from the syndrome. In addition, a statistically significant incidence of migraine headaches exists in families with a cluster headache sufferer.

Cluster headache attacks, which are excruciatingly severe, debilitating, and dramatic, are almost always unilateral and occur from one to six times a day. They are most intense in, around, or behind one eye. Because the pain, commonly described as "boring" or "stabbing," often spreads into the upper teeth, jaw, neck, or temple, the headaches can be misdiagnosed as coming from dental or sinus problems. The attacks are rapid, peaking in five to ten minutes, and are occasionally, but not frequently, preceded by a visual aura. Attacks are much more likely to occur if tobacco and/or alcohol have been recently used, and they even more frequently will awaken sufferers during their first hour of napping or sleeping.

While migraine headache sufferers seek quiet, darkened places and try to remain still, cluster headache sufferers feel more pain if they try to lie down or recline in a chair. Typically, cluster headache sufferers are restless, pacing back and forth, or want to sit upright, holding their heads with their hands. A sufferer may even bang his or her head against a wall to obtain relief.

Information on Cluster Headaches

Causes: Unknown; may be seasonal

Symptoms: Sudden headache on one side of head, with intense pain behind one eye often spreading to teeth, jaw, neck, or temple; occasionally preceded by visual aura

Duration: Recurrent, with acute episodes occurring one to six times a day and lasting a half hour to three hours each during cluster periods

Treatments: For symptom alleviation, oxygen therapy, injections of sumatriptan or dihydroergotamine, zolmitriptan tablets, intranasal lidocane, ergotamine; for prevention, verapamil, ergotamine, lithium, methysergide, prednisone, valproic acid, divalproex

Treatment and Therapy

Treatments are oriented either toward abortive therapies or prophylactic therapies. Abortive approaches attempt to shorten the duration and/or intensity of an individual attack. Prophylactic approaches attempt to shorten or prevent the cluster periods themselves. While a fortunate characteristic of the attacks is their brevity, this feature also limits the range of abortive measures that can be undertaken; by the time that some agents are metabolized, the attack is over.

Although not always practical, a successful and safe abortive treatment is simply breathing 100 percent oxygen for ten to twenty minutes through a nonrebreathing mask. Also not always practical but effective are subcutaneous injections of sumatriptan (Imitrex) or intravenous, intramuscular, or subcutaneous injections of dihydroergotamine (Migranal). Other effective first-line therapies for acute intervention include zolmitriptan (Zomig) tablets, intranasal lidocane, or ergotamine (Cafergot).

Prophylactic, or preventive, treatments prevent attacks or at least lessen their intensity. All cluster headache sufferers should be on a prophylactic regimen (unless their cluster periods are less than two weeks, which is rarely the case). Verapamil (marketed as Calan, Covera, Isoptin, Tarka, and Verelan) is the most commonly prescribed medication because its mechanism as a calcium-channel blocker is well understood and it is usually effective. Occasionally, higher-than-typical doses must be employed. For those who do not respond well or receive sufficient relief on verapamil alone, a second medication such as ergotamine, lithium, methysergide (Sansert), or prednisone is often added. Sometimes, these second medications are effectively used alone, as are valproic acid and divalproex (Depakote).

In the event that pharmacology proves ineffective, several surgical or radiation techniques can block the trigeminal-autonomic reflex pathway. The benefits of these, or any, invasive treatments must be weighed against potential harm. For example, corneal anesthesia, needed to carry out these procedures, can put the eye at risk.

Perspective and Prospects

People have suffered from cluster headaches as long as people have suffered from headaches, although the rarity, seasonal occurrence, and symptoms of cluster headaches have made their recognition as a distinct syndrome difficult. Through PET scanning, neurovascular research has identified three areas of the brain particularly affected by cluster headaches. Because two of these areas are affected every time any sort of pain is felt, research is being concentrated on the third area, hypothalamic gray matter. Researchers expect that probes here will resolve their biggest debate: Is the vasodilation associated with cluster headache the primary problem or the result of activation of the trigeminal vascular system? Researchers do agree that cluster headaches, while distinct, belong to a family of related conditions, the cranial neuralgias.

—Paul Moglia, Ph.D.

See also Brain; Brain disorders; Head and neck disorders; Headaches; Migraine headaches; Pain management; Stress.

For Further Information:

Dalessio, Donald J. "Relief of Cluster Headache and Cranial Neuralgias." *Postgraduate Medicine* 109, no. 1 (January, 2001): 69-78.

Kudrow, L. "Cluster Headache: Diagnosis and Management." *Headache* 19 (1979): 141-148.

Newman, Lawrence C., Peter Goadsby, and Richard B. Lipton. "Cluster and Related Headaches." In *Headache*, edited by Ninan T. Mathew. Philadelphia: W. B. Saunders, 2001.

Cognitive development

Development

Anatomy or system affected: Brain, nervous system, psychic-emotional system

Specialties and related fields: Environmental health, genetics, pediatrics, psychology

Definition: The growth and age-related changes that occur over time in children's mental processes and in activities related to the faculties of attending, learning, perceiving, problem solving, thinking, and remembering.

Key terms:

adaptation: change or adjustment made to create a balance between existing thought structures and the environment

assimilation: the process of attempting to explain a new experience in terms of existing schemes

cognition: the activity of knowing and the processes through which knowledge is acquired and used

cognitive equilibrium: a term used by psychologist Jean Piaget to describe the balanced relationship between an individual's mental processes and the environment *conservation:* understanding that an object's properties remain unchanged when its appearance is altered

egocentrism: seeing the world only from one's own point of view; being unable to acknowledge or recognize different perspectives

equilibration: the process of adapting or adjusting one's existing knowledge or mental structures to the new situation, thus constructing more complex and sophisticated structures

miseducation: the tendency to hurry and pressure children to perform activities and tasks for which they are not cognitively or physically ready

reflexive: referring to an automatic response to external stimuli

reversibility: the ability to negate an action by mentally reversing it or imagining its opposite

scheme: a pattern of thought constructed by the child to organize experience in a meaningful way

PHYSICAL AND PSYCHOLOGICAL FACTORS

The mental capabilities and skills of humans develop gradually over a period of time during childhood and adolescence. The quality of the processes by which an individual responds to and adapts thinking to particular situations and evaluates, plans, and solves problems also changes over time.

In childhood, the brain develops very rapidly. At birth, the human brain already weighs about 25 percent of its adult weight. By six months of age, this figure is 50 percent. By the age of five, the child's brain has achieved 90 percent of its eventual weight. While the basic structure of the brain is genetically and biologically determined, environment and experience play a significant role in the growth of cognition. Children's biological constitutions may affect the way in which they interact with and respond to their environment.

According to the Swiss psychologist Jean Piaget, the cognitive growth of all children follows a universal or holistic pattern of development through infancy, childhood, and adolescence. The thought processes of young children are less mature and complex than those of older children, and as children grow and experience life, their cognitive structures become more sophisticated, as well as qualitatively different from those of children in earlier or later stages of development. Cognitive structures, or "schemes" as Piaget called them, are thought patterns that children construct to explain, understand, or interpret their experiences. When children's schemes or thought processes are in harmony with their environment, they experience cognitive equilibrium. When children encounter new and puzzling events or objects, they are in a state of imbalance or disequilibrium and must achieve equilibrium through a process called equilibration. This process consists of adapting or adjusting one's existing knowledge or mental structures to the new situation, thus constructing more complex and sophisticated structures. Adaptation takes place through the processes of assimilation and accommodation.

Assimilation refers to the process of attempting to explain a new experience in terms of existing schemes. For example, a child who sees a pony for the first time may call it a "kitty" because a cat is the existing model of that child for four-legged animals. Noticing that there are differences between the scheme of a cat and the reality of the pony, however, the child soon attempts to modify existing mental structures to fit the new experience. This process of modification is accommodation. Through assimilation and accommodation, children organize their knowledge into schemes which better explain their world.

Piaget's theory of cognitive development, with its emphasis on continuous and active organization and adaptation involving assimilation and accommodation, implies that children actively construct their own knowledge. This construction is based on the child's current stage of cognitive development: Piaget proposed that all children in a specific, universal cognitive stage construct similar interpretations of similar experiences.

According to Piaget, cognitive development can be divided into four major stages. The order in which these stages occur is universal, and all individuals must experience each stage. No stage can be skipped, although the rates at which children go through a stage may vary. The basis for Piaget's insistence on the unvarying sequence of cognitive stages is a concept known as epigenesis, which he used to explain the gradual development of thinking processes. Each new structure or cognitive skill is based on and develops from an earlier one. Hence, each stage, and each structure within each stage, is necessary for the development of new, more advanced structures. Piaget called this feature of development "hierarchization."

The four stages of cognitive development identified by Piaget are the sensorimotor stage (up to age two), the preoperational stage (two to seven years of age), the concrete operations stage (seven to eleven years of age), and the formal operations stage (age eleven and up).

During the sensorimotor stage, children act upon their environment and acquire knowledge of it through their senses and motor activities. In the first two years, cognition progresses from reflexive actions, such as sucking and grasping, to primitive symbolic functions or representation, such as language use and symbolic play. The sensorimotor stage can be further divided into six substages. Substage 1 lasts from birth to one month and centers on exercising basic reflexes, including eye movements, sound orientation, and vocalization, and assimilating and accommodating objects into reflexive schemes. Substage 2, from one to four months, consists of simple repetitive actions, such as thumb sucking, which are discovered by chance and acquired through repeated trials. Piaget called these actions primary circular reactions. Substage 3 appears between four and eight months of age. Piaget named this period secondary circular reactions. Infants notice stimulating events in the environment beyond their bodies—such as a noise made by squeezing a toy or a movement caused by touching an object—and attempt to re-create the events.

Between eight and twelve months of age, infants experience substage 4, or the coordination of secondary schemes. This means that infants can use two already acquired schemes to reach a simple goal. For example, they are able to remove an object to grasp a hidden toy. These early coordinations reflect intentional behavior and simple problem solving. Tertiary circular reactions are characteristic of substage 5, appearing between the ages of twelve and eighteen months. Infants display curiosity, experiment actively, and find new ways of solving problems. Their behaviors are goal-directed but are carried out through trial and error. Substage 6, from eighteen to twenty-four months, reflects inner experimentation or new mental combinations. The infant now displays symbolic functioning through language, imagery, and symbolic play. Children also begin to acquire a sense of cause and effect.

During the sensorimotor stage, children develop the ability to imitate. Piaget believed that novel actions could be imitated by infants around eight to twelve months of age and needed much practice. The ability to imitate absent models, called deferred imitation, appears between twelve and twenty-four months of age.

Another important milestone of the sensorimotor stage is the development of a sense of object permanence. Before the age of four months, objects are of interest to infants only if they can be experienced by the senses. They lose interest in objects that are hidden; such objects no longer exist for them. Between four and eight months of age, they may retain interest in partially hidden objects, and by twelve to eighteen months of age, the concept of objects is stronger. The idea that objects have permanence even when not seen appears around the age of eighteen months, when children can represent objects mentally.

The preoperational stage, the second of Piaget's stages of cognitive development, occurs between the ages of two and seven. During this stage, children increase their use of words and images to represent objects and experiences. Piaget called this stage "preoperational" because he believed that children had not yet achieved "operations," or cognitive schemes to think logically. The preoperational stage can further be divided into a preconceptual period (two to four years of age) and an intuitive period (four to seven years of age).

Characteristics of the preconceptual period include growth of symbolic representation, expressed through developing language and pretend play. Children in this stage demonstrate animism; that is, they attribute life to nonliving things. They are egocentric, seeing the world as revolving around themselves and having difficulty in seeing other points of view.

Although still egocentric during the intuitive period, children are less so than before. Piaget argued that they also display centered thinking, or the capacity to classify objects according to one feature or attribute even though several may be evident. Children in this stage find it hard to conserve, or understand that a substance or object's properties can remain unaltered even when its appearance changes. They cannot reverse actions mentally, such as realizing that water poured from a tall glass into a flat dish is the same amount of water and would look as high as before if poured back into the glass.

In the concrete operations stage, between the ages of seven and eleven, children's cognitive structures develop to include operations that help them think more competently and logically about objects and events experienced. Children are less egocentric; are able to classify, sequence, and quantify more efficiently; and display skills of conservation and reversibility. Piaget believed, however, that children are still unable to hypothesize or think about abstract concepts during this stage.

From eleven years onward, children enter the formal operations stage. They can hypothesize and reason inductively about abstract concepts such as religion, goodness, or beauty. According to Piaget, this transition from concrete to formal operations is very gradual. He also suggested that many adults reason at the formal operations level only if a problem is important or interesting to them.

Another approach to cognitive development compares individuals as information-processing systems to computers. The hardware in this system consists of physical components such as the brain, the sensory receptors, and the nervous system. The software consists of the mental processes and strategies used to store, interpret, access, and analyze information. The information-processing mechanisms of young children are elementary and immature. As children grow, as their nervous systems and brains develop, their information-processing strategies improve and become more sophisticated, like modern computers.

Humor and the appreciation of humor have also been associated with an individual's level of cognitive development. A child whose mental structures and language acquisition have developed enough to enable the child to notice incongruities or deviations from the usual and expected can perceive humor in incongruous situations. To a two-year-old, calling a bird a cat may seem hilarious or making barking sounds and pretending to be a dog may provoke much laughter. A picture of a fish in a tree will amuse a three-year-old. Seven-year-olds who can understand the double meanings inherent in language will laugh at puns and "knock-knock" jokes and can create riddles. As children's understanding of language ambiguities matures and becomes more sophisticated, they are able to appreciate more complex humor.

Sociocultural Factors

The Russian psychologist Lev Vygotsky believed that cognition is sociocultural, that it is influenced by values and beliefs of cultures as well as by the specific tools that each culture uses for adaptation and problem solving. Children are born with simple mental processes like attention, memory, perception, and sensation. These processes develop into what Vygotsky called higher mental functions, or more competent ways of using intellectual capabilities. The strategies and tools for thinking are taught to children by their culture and develop as young children interact and collaborate with capable adults or peers, who guide and model problem-solving techniques that encourage cognitive development. Vygotsky called the difference between children's level of achievement when working independently and their potential development when guided by a competent adult the zone of proximal development.

For Vygotsky, language plays an important role in cognitive growth. Adults use language to transmit the culture's ways of thinking to the child. The child uses language to plan and regulate activities and behavior and to solve problems. Language helps children organize thought and reach objectives. Younger children verbalize phrases and words aloud during this process, but older children and adults internalize speech that, although no longer uttered aloud, still organizes and guides thinking and action.

Disorders and Effects

The importance of experience on the cognitive development of children implies that when children live in intellectually impoverished environments, their cognitive development may be stunted or fail to reach its potential. Studies show the children whose parents play and interact in a variety of ways with them and provide stimulating materials to engage their interest and attention do better in school than children who lack this cognitive stimulation. Verbal interactions between parents and children, collaborative activities with competent peers, and guided activities with adults have been found to help children improve their thinking and planning abilities. Mary Ainsworth's research on mother-infant attachment showed that mothers who interacted with their infants had securely attached children who, in turn, felt confident enough to explore their environment more independently than less securely attached infants. In this way, cognitive growth was affected by social functioning. Some longitudinal studies have found that securely attached children demonstrated more cognitive competence through childhood and adolescence than children who did not have secure attachments. Parental support and responsiveness encouraged cognitive growth over time.

The effects of the curriculum within programs and schools for children can maximize or discourage cognitive development. The Cognitively Oriented Curriculum, developed at the High/Scope Institute by David Weikart and his associates, focused on active learning. It was based on Piagetian principles and involved children in planning and other cognitively oriented activities. The games that children play can also affect their thinking and can be utilized in the curriculum. Research by Constance Kamii and Rheta DeVries has shown how the use of games and play-oriented activities can help children develop numerical thinking, language competency, and other cognitive abilities, while promoting autonomy or the ability to think independently and enhancing cooperative and social skills.

As an understanding of the negative effects of poverty and lack of enriching experiences increased during the 1950's and 1960's, initiatives such as Head Start and various other compensatory early childhood programs were established in the United States to reverse the effects of early cognitive deprivation. Initial studies on the effects of such programs were extremely encouraging, and gains in intelligence quotient (IQ) scores and cognitive performance were found to be significant. It was later discovered, however, that such gains could be lost if intellectual stimulation was not maintained. The need to continue to provide stimulating educational experiences was recognized. It was found that positive attitudes toward schooling and a sense of self-esteem also occur when compensatory education and enrichment programs are provided.

The increasing evidence of brain research concerning the importance to the developmental process of stimulating experiences during the first few years of life, as well as knowledge about the growth and weight of the brain in infancy, suggests the need to provide such experiences from a very early age. Prenatal experiences and their impact on cognitive and other areas of development are also being studied.

The concept of cognitive development as a highly active process that occurs in a series of stages has certain implications for the education and well-being of children. One implication is that children in a particular stage of development should not be hurried but should be allowed to develop and mature at their own pace. Hurrying children beyond their developmental capacity can cause mental and emotional damage. David Elkind uses the term "miseducation" to refer to the tendency to hurry and pressure children to perform activities and tasks for which they are not cognitively or physically ready. He believes that miseducation is an increasingly common problem in the United States.

Another implication of the active nature of cognitive development is that children should be given numerous opportunities to explore materials and the environment, and thus acquire knowledge for themselves. Materials, equipment, and knowledge to be discovered should be appropriate to the stage of the child and should be based on the child's existing structures and schemes.

Perspective and Prospects

The cognitive and intellectual development of children was not studied seriously or scientifically until the late nineteenth century in Europe and America. G. Stanley Hall was the first person to develop an instrument—the questionnaire—to study the minds of children. The twentieth century saw the emergence of developmental theories such as the psychoanalytic theory of Sigmund Freud and the psychosocial theory of Erik Erikson. Behaviorism, which viewed children's learning and development as passive and therefore controllable, dominated much of the earlier part of the century. John Watson proposed that children were like blank tablets on which anything could be written. In other words, children's development was shaped by their environment and by the people around them. This view had been held in the seventeenth century by the philosopher John Locke. Watson's theory was extended by B. F. Skinner, who evolved a learning theory based on the use of reinforcement and external stimuli to influence and control behavior. Albert Bandura's theory of social cognition departed from the earlier passive learning theories of Watson and Skinner. He believed that individuals actively process information. Bandura also emphasized the role of observational learning, or learning by observing others and thinking about outcomes, in the process of children's development.

During the 1950's, a cognitive revolution occurred as the theory and research of Jean Piaget became known. Piaget was interested in how children think, in their "wrong" answers as indicators of their stage of cognitive development, and in their active construction of knowledge. He observed his own children's early interactions and explorations. He also utilized the clinical method, in which he interviewed children of different ages to understand the nature of their hypotheses and problem-solving strategies. The questions in this method were flexible and depended on the responses given by the child.

Piaget's theories were later criticized and were seen to underestimate children's abilities. His assumption of the heterogeneity or universality of cognitive stages was also questioned. Critics charged that Piaget did not give enough credit to the role of cultural and social factors in cognitive development. The impact of culture and social interaction on the child's thinking and use of strategies as culturally transmitted tools of thought was studied by Lev Vygotsky. In the last decades of the twentieth century, Vygotsky's ideas aroused much interest. The difference in learning styles was also studied, and it was recognized that learning styles vary across cultures as well as from individual to individual.

Many neo-Piagetian theories attempted to integrate some Piagetian assumptions with information-processing approaches. These approaches examined cognitive processes such as memory and attention and demonstrated their influence on children's cognitive development.

The influence of the environment and various activities cannot be overemphasized in its importance to cognitive development. As technologies continue to develop for use by children, ranging from toys to educational tools, it will be crucial to consider all aspects of development carefully. One example is recent research evaluating the impact on brain development of frequent videogame and computer use by children. The research suggested that activities which encourage vision and movement skills, to the exclusion of other skills important to development, may be problematic. The concern is that some capacities may become overused, while others may not receive enough stimulation to encourage adequate development. More research is certainly needed to examine the potential impact of new technologies and exposure to diverse stimuli. Important lessons can be learned from history in an effort to guard against anything that impoverishes a child's learning environment.

—Nillofur Zobairi, Ph.D.; updated by Nancy A. Piotrowski, Ph.D.

See also Bonding; Developmental stages; Learning disabilities; Mental retardation; Motor skill development; Psychiatric disorders; Psychiatry, child and adolescent; Reflexes, primitive.

For Further Information:

Berk, Laura E. *Child Development*. 7th ed. Boston: Pearson/Allyn and Bacon, 2006. A text that reviews theory and research in child development, cognitive and language development, personality and social development, and the foundations and contexts of development.

Berk, Laura E., and Adam Winsler. *Scaffolding Children's Learning: Vygotsky and Early Childhood Education*. Washington, D.C.: National Association for the Education of Young Children, 1995. The authors examine Lev Vygotsky's life and the key concepts of his developmental approach, which stresses the strong links between a child's social, cognitive, and psychological existence, in a clear and understandable way. Implications for early childhood education are discussed.

Bjorklund, David F. *Children's Thinking: Developmental Function and Individual Differences*. 4th ed. Belmont, Calif.: Thomson/Wadsworth, 2005. The book provides a detailed description of theory and research in the field of cognitive development. It includes discussions on the biological foundations of cognition, individual differences, and the impact of culture and schooling.

Elkind, David. *Miseducation: Preschoolers at Risk*. New York: Alfred A. Knopf, 1987. The author discusses the many pressures on modern children, explaining how their physical and emotional health may be at risk when schools and parents attempt to "miseducate" them before they are developmentally ready. Elkind's examples can be appreciated by both professionals and laypeople.

Nathanson, Laura Walther. *The Portable Pediatrician: A Practicing Pediatrician's Guide to Your Child's Growth, Development, Health, and Behavior from Birth to Age Five*. 2d ed. New York: HarperCollins, 2002. An engaging, easy-to-read guide for parents to assess their child's development, medical symptoms, and behavioral problems.

Shore, Rima. *Rethinking the Brain: New Insights into Early Development*. Rev. ed. New York: Families and Work Institute, 2003. The author summarizes research on the brain and discusses implications for development, especially in the first three years of life. The material is presented in a readable and understandable style.

Cold sores

Disease/disorder

Also known as: Fever blisters

Anatomy or system affected: Mouth, skin

Specialties and related fields: Family medicine

Definition: An infectious disease characterized by thin-walled vesicles around the mouth.

Causes and Symptoms

Cold sores are an infectious disease caused by the herpes simplex virus. Cold sores and fever blisters are two terms used for sores that develop around the mouth. They are among the most common disorders around the mouth area, causing pain and annoyance to millions of Americans. An estimated 45 to 80 percent of adults and children in the United States have had at least one cold

Information on Cold Sores

Causes: Infection by herpes simplex virus
Symptoms: Sores around mouth that dry to form scabs; preceded by tingling, burning, or itching sensation
Duration: Chronic, with acute outbreaks lasting from three to ten days
Treatments: Keeping area clean and dry, avoidance of sore irritation or stress; prevention through antiviral compounds (acyclovir, valacyclovir, foscarnet)

sore. There are two types of herpes simplex. Type 1 usually causes oral herpes, or fever blisters, while type 2 usually causes genital herpes. About 95 percent of the fever blisters located on the mouth are caused by herpes simplex type 1.

Fever blisters are highly contagious, more so in the first day or two of an eruption. Once the blister has formed a dry scab, transmission is low and the herpes simplex virus usually cannot be recovered from the site. The virus can spread to others through touch; frequently, infection spreads through kissing. The chance of infection is higher if the body's defenses are weakened by stress, illness, or injury.

Once a person is infected with oral herpes, the virus remains in the nerve located near the fever blister. It may stay dormant at this site for years. People who have had fever blisters in the past can sometimes predict when an outbreak is going to occur. The appearance of cold sores may be preceded by a few hours of a tingling, burning, or itching sensation, a phenomenon called a prodrome. Typically, the sores erupt in a small cluster, with each blister about the size of a large pimple. The blisters quickly dry to form a scab. Generally, no scarring or loss in sensation occurs. Outbreaks usually last from three to ten days.

Treatment and Therapy

Treatment includes keeping the area clean and dry to prevent bacterial infection. The patient should avoid irritating the sores, as touching them may spread the virus. For example, if a person rubs the sore and then rubs an eyelid, a new sore may appear on the eyelid in a few days. When the fever blister is contagious, kissing should be avoided. People whose cold sores appear in response to stress should try to avoid stressful situations. Some investigators have suggested that adding L-lysine to the diet or eliminating certain foods (such as nuts, chocolate, and seeds) may help, although no research studies have validated these suggestions. Even sunlight has been linked as a trigger for fever blisters. The National Institute of Dental and Craniofacial Research recommends the use of sunscreen on the lips to prevent sun-induced recurrences of herpes.

Because no cure exists for herpes, treatments are directed toward controlling outbreaks. Currently available antiviral compounds include nucleoside analogues, which selectively interfere with viral deoxyribonucleic acid (DNA) replication. Oral acyclovir (Avirax or Zovirax) and valacyclovir (Valtrex), antiviral drugs that keep the virus from multiplying, can be taken to prevent recurrence. Acyclovir applied locally has also been found effective, and foscarnet (Foscavir) is useful in treating acyclovir-resistant infections. Two topical preparations, Zovirax and penciclovir (Vectavir), have been shown to influence the eruption and duration of cold sores when applied during the prodromal stage. Antibiotics may be used in treating secondary infections. An ophthalmologist should treat any eye lesions.

Some cold sore treatments that have been successful in selected people are solvents such as ether, alcohol, povidone iodine, and antiseptic mouthwash. Other patients have applied ice or toothpaste to the sores. While none of these treatments has scientific backing, eating an ice pop or applying an ice cube to the blister may relieve the discomfort.

Perspective and Prospects

Future research is aimed at determining the precise form and location of the inactive herpesvirus in nerve cells. This information might allow scientists to design antiviral drugs that can attack the virus while it lies dormant in nerves. Researchers are also trying to learn more about how sunlight, injury, and stress act as triggers so that the cycle of recurrences can be stopped. An experimental new herpes treatment derived from an herb known as *Prunella vulgaris* may one day help prevent and treat both types of herpes.

—*Janet Mahoney, R.N., Ph.D., A.P.R.N.*

See also Blisters; Canker sores; Herpes; Skin; Skin disorders; Stress; Stress reduction; Ulcers; Viral infections.

For Further Information:

Ignatavicius, Donna D., and M. Linda Workman, eds. *Medical-Surgical Nursing: Critical Thinking for*

Collaborative Care. 5th ed. Philadelphia: Saunders, 2006.

Lewis, Sharon Mantik, et al., eds. *Medical-Surgical Nursing: Assessment and Management of Clinical Problems*. 6th ed. 2 vols. St. Louis: Mosby, 2004.

National Institutes of Health. National Institute of Dental Research. *Fever Blisters and Canker Sores*. Rev. ed. Bethesda, Md.: Author, 1992.

Smeltzer, Suzanne C., and Brenda G. Bare, eds. *Brunner and Suddarth's Textbook of Medical-Surgical Nursing*. 10th ed. Philadelphia: Lippincott Williams & Wilkins, 2004.

Colic

Disease/disorder

Anatomy or system affected: Gastrointestinal system, intestines, psychic-emotional system

Specialties and related fields: Gastroenterology, pediatrics

Definition: As a general term, a paroxysm of acute abdominal pain caused by spasm, obstruction, or twisting of a hollow abdominal organ. As a specific entity, infantile colic is a group of behaviors displayed by young infants including crying, facial grimacing, drawing-up of the legs over the abdomen, and clenching of the fists.

Key terms:

flatulence: the presence of excessive gas in the stomach and intestines, which is expelled from the body

irritability: a state of general overreaction to external stimuli

spasm: an involuntary muscle contraction; a painful spasm is called a cramp

Causes and Symptoms

As a general term, colic can arise from any site in the abdomen. For example, cramplike pain caused by a stone obstructing the bile ducts or a stone obstructing the urinary tract are known as biliary colic or renal colic, respectively. More specifically, the term "colic," when unmodified, generally refers to infantile colic.

The crying of colicky infants tends to be more prominent in the evening, although they cry more than other infants at other times of day. The "rule of threes" of infantile colic holds that infants with colic cry for more than three hours per day for more than three days per week for more than three weeks. The associated gestures suggest to some that the infant is experiencing abdominal pain and is responsible for the use of the term "colic" to describe the condition.

Several causes of infantile colic have been postulated, but conclusive evidence is lacking for any of them. This combination of behaviors has been interpreted as abdominal pain, leading to the idea that cramping somewhere in the intestine is the cause. Neurobehavioral explanations have been offered. The most common is that colic represents a state of agitation that may not require a noxious stimulus for agitation and crying to continue. Rarely is colic the result of organic disease, and the prevailing opinion is that it is a variant of normal infant behavior. It appears to be unrelated to caregiving style or intensity. Other proposed mechanisms include difficult temperament, sleep disturbance, diarrhea, child abuse, and irritable bowel syndrome (IBS). Some theories ascribe colic to hypersensitivity to dietary protein—usually proteins derived from cow's milk, which can be secreted in breast milk—thus explaining the occurrence of colic in breast-fed infants. Intestinal gas, either from air swallowed during feeding or from fermentation of incompletely absorbed carbohydrates in the colon, has also been implicated. Parents of colicky infants frequently describe flatulence as an associated symptom.

Treatment and Therapy

The medical treatment of the infant with colic begins with a thorough medical history and a careful physical examination. While the likelihood of finding a cause of the infant's symptoms are slight, the thoroughness of this approach provides an effective basis for reassurance and demonstrates that the parents' complaint is taken seriously.

Infantile colic virtually always resolves spontaneously, leaving the infant healthy and thriving. The essentials of therapy are demystification, reassurance, and support for the haggard and anxious parents. Demystification is the explanation of the source of the infant's distress, which alleviates the anxiety attendant on diagnostic hypotheses that occur to or are suggested to the parents. It is important for pediatricians to deal with the anxiety aroused by the infant's symptoms with reassurance, pointing out that the baby will be fine; the only risk of lasting damage is to the parents.

Quick, superficial attempts to solve the problem with formula changes or medications, particularly when not accompanied by patient demystification and reassurance, reinforce the parents' suspicion that there is something wrong with the child, ultimately increasing parental perception of the child's vulnerability. The results of studies in the medical literature investigating

Information on Colic

Causes: Unknown; abdominal pain suspected
Symptoms: Crying for long periods of time, facial grimacing, drawing of legs over abdomen, clenching of fists
Duration: Typically one to three months
Treatments: Switching formulas, swaddling, mimicking of in utero motion, medications

the usefulness of switching formulas and using agents such as simethicone to deal with intestinal gas are mixed. Dicyclomine, an anticholinergic medication used in the past, should not be given to infants under six months of age because of the possibility that it will interfere with the baby's breathing.

More frequent, smaller feedings may help, as may increased carrying (called "walking the floor") and rocking. One theory holds that mimicking the environment in the womb is reassuring—closeness to a warm person with a detectable heartbeat, swaddling (wrapping the baby in a blanket to restrict movement of the extremities), and rhythmic stimulation provided by background music and car or stroller rides. One commonly used method involves placing the baby in an infant seat on top of a running washer or dryer, thus exposing the infant to constant vibration. Care must be taken to stay with the baby or to secure the infant seat to prevent injury resulting from a fall off the appliance. Most colicky infants have excessive gas, and "gas pains" have long been suspected as responsible for colic. Since virtually all the gas in the intestine is swallowed air, minimizing air swallowing and maximizing burping after feedings are important measures in reducing colic. The use of cereal to ease the infant's hunger and decrease the vigor with which he or she sucks on the nipple results in less air being swallowed. Unfortunately, many parents are advised to put the cereal in the bottle; this increases the negative pressure required to suck the slurry of milk and cereal and increases the amount of air swallowed.

Perspective and Prospects

One theory holds that infantile colic is related to a familial prevalence of irritable bowel syndrome, also called irritable colon or spastic colon. IBS is viewed in this context as a familial abnormality in the regulation of intestinal motility that produces different symptoms at different ages. According to this theory, if one is born into an "irritable colon" family, one proceeds through distinct, age-related symptom complexes, the first of which is infantile colic. Between six months and three years of age, irritable colon syndrome of infancy (also called chronic nonspecific diarrhea or toddler diarrhea) is prominent, manifest as recurrent, watery diarrhea with no other symptoms and no repercussions on growth and development. Recurrent, periumbilical abdominal pain, frequently exacerbated by meals in schoolchildren between five and twelve years of age, is the third of these symptom complexes. It is followed by the development of similar symptoms in adulthood, usually accompanied by alternating diarrhea and constipation. In fact, infants with irritable bowel syndrome of infancy have a higher-than-normal incidence of having had prolonged or severe infantile colic, and several studies show that children with symptoms of irritable colon have a higher-than-normal prevalence of other family members with symptoms of irritable colon. It is useful to identify other members of the family with such symptoms to aid in demystifying the illness.

—Wallace A. Gleason, Jr., M.D.

See also Bonding; Diarrhea and dysentery; Gastroenterology, pediatric; Gastrointestinal system; Lactose intolerance; Neonatology; Pediatrics.

For Further Information:

Barr, Ronald G. "Changing Our Understanding of Infant Colic." *Archives of Pediatrics and Adolescent Medicine* 156, no. 12 (December, 2002): 1172-1175. Argues that many of the symptoms of colic, including a pattern of repeated crying, are now understood to be behaviors likely universal to normal infant development.

Brazelton, T. Berry. *Calming Your Fussy Baby: The Brazelton Way.* Cambridge, Mass.: Perseus, 2002. Brazelton, a well-known pediatrician, offers advice for calming infants and covers colic and effective ways of addressing it.

Lampe, John B. "Infantile Colic: Follow-up at Four Years of Age." *Clinical Pediatrics* 29, no. 10 (October, 2000): 620. A now four-year-old group of formerly colicky infants and controls was reexamined with respect to possible persistent differences in behavior, temperament, eating and sleeping habits, psychosomatic complaints, growth, and family atmosphere.

McCormick, David P. "The Challenge of Colic." *Clinical Pediatrics* 39, no. 7 (July, 2000): 401-402. McCormick offers his reaction to a study on colic by

Susan Levitzky, a pediatrician, and Robyn Cooper, a psychologist, published in the same issue.

Thompson, June. "Infantile Colic: What Is It and Are There Effective Treatments?" *Community Practitioner* 73, no. 9 (September, 2000): 767. Infantile colic, also called three month colic and evening colic, has been studied extensively, and many possible causes and factors have been suggested. Thompson reviews some of the research on the etiology and effectiveness of treatments for this phenomenon.

_______. "Low Birth Weight and Colic 'Linked.'" *Community Practitioner* 73, no. 8 (August, 2000): 727. It has been hypothesized that depletion of nutrition during critical stages of organ development influences organ function, and impaired fetal growth has been associated with a large number of diseases. This study aimed to describe how fetal growth and gestational age affect infantile colic while considering other potential risk factors.

Walling, Anne D. "Diagnosing Biliary Colic and Acute Cholecystitis." *American Family Physician* 62, no. 6 (September 15, 2000): 1386. Approximately 500,000 cholecystectomies are performed annually in the United States. Symptomatic gallstones are the most common indication for cholecystectomy.

Waltman, Alicia Brooks. "The Crying Game." *Parenting* 14, no. 3 (April, 2000): 128-132. Waltman offers information about the latest research on colic and the best ways to soothe a crying baby. For many babies, a surefire soother is a breast or a bottle.

White, Barbara Prudhomme, et al. "Behavioral and Physiological Responsivity, Sleep, and Patterns of Daily Cortisol Production in Infants with and Without Colic." *Child Development* 71, no. 4 (July/August, 2000): 862-877. To describe the behavioral and physiological responses associated with colic, the responses of twenty two-month-old infants with and twenty without colic were studied during a physical examination.

Colitis

Disease/disorder

Anatomy or system affected: Abdomen, gastrointestinal system, intestines, stomach

Specialties and related fields: Gastroenterology, internal medicine

Definition: A potentially fatal but manageable disease of the colon that inflames and ulcerates the bowel lining, occurring in both acute and chronic forms.

Key terms:

diarrhea: persistent liquid or mushy, shapeless stool

dysentery: bloody diarrhea caused by infectious agents affecting the colon

ileum: the last section of the small bowel, which passes food wastes to the colon through the ileocecal valve

inflammation: swelling caused by the accumulation of fluids and chemical agents

mucosa: the membrane of cells that lines the bowel; admits fluids and nutrients but also serves as the first-line protection against infectious agents and other materials foreign to the body

procedure: any medical treatment that entails physical manipulation or invasion of the body

stoma: an opening, formed by surgery, from the bowel to the exterior surface of the body

stool: the food wastes mixed with fluid, bacteria, mucus, and dead cells that exit the body upon defecation

ulcer: an area of the mucosa that has been abraded or dissolved by infection or chemicals, creating an open sore

Causes and Symptoms

The colon is the section of the lower bowel, or intestines, extending from the ileocecal valve to the rectum. It is wider in diameter than the small bowel, although shorter in length at about one meter. From behind the pelvis, the colon rises along the right side of the body (ascending colon), turns left to cross the upper abdominal cavity (transverse colon), and then turns down along the left side of the body (descending colon) until it joins the sigmoid (S-shaped) colon. The sigmoid colon empties into the rectum, a pouch that stores the waste products of digestion that are excreted through the anus. The colon absorbs most of the fluid passed to it from the small bowel, so that wastes solidify; meanwhile, bacteria in the colon break down undigested proteins and carbohydrates, creating hydrogen, carbon dioxide, and methane gases in the process.

A key structure in colonic activity is its mucosa. This thin sheet of cells lining the bowel wall permits passage of fluids and certain nutrients into the bloodstream but resists bacteria and toxins (poisonous chemical compounds). When the mucosa is torn or worn away, bacteria and toxins enter, infecting the bowel wall. The body responds to infection by rushing fluids and powerful chemicals to the endangered area to confine and kill the infecting agents. In the process, the tissues of the bowel wall swell with the fluids; this is known as inflammation. The medical suffix denoting this response is *-itis*; when it occurs in the colon, physicians call it colitis.

A variety of agents can cause colitis, which is divided into two major types depending on the duration of the disease: acute colitis and chronic ulcerative colitis. Acute colitis is a relatively brief, single episode of inflammation. It is often caused by bacteria or parasites. For example, *Giardia lamblia*, a bacterium in many American streams, is a common infectious agent in colitis, and the amoebas in polluted water supplies are responsible for the type of colitis known as amebic dysentery. Some medicines, however, especially antibiotics, can also induce colitis. Acute colitis either disappears on its own or can be cured with drugs. Untreated, however, it may be fatal.

Chronic ulcerative colitis and Crohn's disease constitute a category of serious afflictions called inflammatory bowel disease (IBD) whose primary physical effects include swelling of the bowel lining, ulcers, and bloody diarrhea. Although some medical researchers think that these afflictions may be two aspects of the same disease, ulcerative colitis affects only the colon, whereas Crohn's disease can involve the small bowel as well as the colon. Moreover, colitis chiefly involves the colonic mucosa, but Crohn's disease delves into the full thickness of the bowel wall.

Chronic ulcerative colitis is a permanent disease that manifests itself either in recurring bouts of inflammation or in continuous inflammation that cannot be cleared up with drugs. It is commonly called ulcerative colitis because ulcers, open sores in the mucosa, spread throughout the colon and rectum, where the disease usually starts. Researchers have not yet discovered the causes of chronic ulcerative colitis, although there are many theories, of which three are prominent. The first is bacterial or viral infection, and many agents have been proposed as the culprit. Because such a multitude of organisms commonly reside in or pass through the colon, researchers have enormous difficulty separating out a specific kind in order to show that it is always present during colitis attacks. Second is autoimmune reaction. Research in other diseases has shown that sometimes the body's police system, enforced by white blood cells, mistakes native, healthy tissue for a foreign agent and attacks that tissue in an attempt to destroy it. Yet no testing in chronic ulcerative colitis has yet proven the theory. Third is a combination of foreign infection and autoimmune response; it is as if the immune system overreacts to an infectious agent and continues its attack even after the agent has been neutralized. Many researchers have suspected that the disease is inherited, because certain families have higher rates of the disease than others. This genetic theory is not universally accepted, however, because it is just as likely that family members share infection rather than having passed on a genetic predisposition for the disease. Other theories propose food allergies as the cause; even toothpaste has been considered.

Regardless of the cause, there is no doubt that colitis is a painful, disabling, bewildering disease. When the bowel inflames, the tissues heat up and fever results. Cramps are common, and sufferers feel an urgent, frequently uncontrollable urge to defecate. When they reach the toilet (if they do so in time), they have soft, loose stool or diarrhea, which can seem to explode from the anus. They may have as many as ten to twenty bowel movements a day. Because ulcers often erode blood vessels, blood can appear in the stool, as well as mucus and pus from the bowel wall. Severe weight loss, anemia, lack of energy, dehydration, and anorexia often develop as the colitis persists. The symptoms may clear up on their own only to recur months or years later; attacks may come with increasing frequency thereafter. The first attack, if it worsens rapidly, is fatal in about 5 to 10 percent of patients, although the death rate can rise to 25 percent among first-time sufferers who are more than sixty years old.

Complications from colitis can be life-threatening. These include perforation of the bowel wall, strictures, hemorrhaging, and toxic megacolon (hyperinflation of the colon, an emergency medical condition). Furthermore, studies show that patients who have had ulcerative colitis for more than ten years have about a 20 percent chance of developing cancer in the colon or rectum.

Information on Colitis

Causes: Unknown; possibly bacterial or viral infection, genetic factors, exposure to antibiotics, autoimmune reaction

Symptoms: Swelling of bowel lining, ulcers, bloody diarrhea, pain, fever, severe weight loss, anemia, lack of energy, dehydration, uncontrollable urge to defecate

Duration: Chronic, with acute episodes

Treatments: Medications (anti-inflammatory agents), surgery, dietary restrictions

Because colitis is a relapsing, embarrassing disease, patients often suffer psychological turmoil. In *Colitis* (1992), Michael P. Kelly reports the results of his study of forty-five British colitis patients. According to Kelly, they typically denied that early symptoms were the signs of serious illness, passing them off as the result of overeating or influenza. The denial continued until the continual, desperate urge to defecate made them despair of controlling their bowels without help. Often, they suffered embarrassment because they had to flee family gatherings or work in order to find a toilet or because they passed stool inadvertently in public. Many feared being beyond easy access to a toilet, shunned public places, and felt humiliated. Only then did some visit a physician, and even after chronic ulcerative colitis was diagnosed, a portion hoped they could still cope on their own. When they could not, they grew depressed, insomniac, angry at their fate, or antisocial. Even with treatment, the strain of enduring the disease can be debilitating.

Treatment and Therapy

Fortunately, medical science has several well-tested methods of controlling or curing colitis. In the case of acute colitis, patients usually resume normal bowel functions on their own and emerge as healthy as they were before the onset of symptoms. For chronic ulcerative colitis patients, however, the body is rarely the same again, and they must adjust to the effects of medication, surgery, or both—an adjustment that some authors claim is essentially a redefinition of the self.

After interviewing a patient and assessing the reported symptoms, the physician suspecting colitis orders a stool sample to check for blood, bacteria, parasites, and pus. If any of these are present, the physician directly examines the rectum and colon by inserting a fiberoptic endoscope into the rectum and up the colon. Early in the disease, the mucosa looks granular with scattered hemorrhages and tiny bleeding points. As the disease progresses, the mucosa turns spongy and has many ulcers that ooze blood and pus. An X ray often helps determine the extent of inflammation, and tissue samples taken by endoscopic biopsy can establish if it is ulcerative colitis or infection, and not Crohn's disease, that is present.

There is no easy treatment for chronic ulcerative colitis. Dietary restrictions—especially the elimination of fibrous foods such as raw fruits and vegetables or of milk products—may reduce the irritation to the inflamed colon, and symptoms then may improve if the disease is mild. Antidiarrheal drugs can firm the stool and reduce the patient's urgency to defecate, although such drugs must be used very cautiously to avoid dangerous dilation of the bowels.

Such nonspecific measures are seldom more than delaying tactics, and drugs are needed to counteract the colon's inflammation. Two types are most common. The first, sulfasalazine, is a sulfa drug developed in the 1940's. It is an anti-inflammatory agent that is most effective in mild to moderate ulcerative colitis and helps prevent recurrence of inflammation. Corticosteroids, the second type, behave like the hormones produced by the adrenal gland that suppress inflammation. The drug works well in relieving the symptoms of moderate to moderately severe attacks. Both types of drugs have serious side effects, so physicians must carefully tailor dosages for each patient and check repeatedly for reactions. In some patients, sulfasalazine induces nausea, vomiting, joint pain, headaches, rashes, dizziness, and hepatitis (liver inflammation). The effects of corticosteroids include sleeplessness, mood swings, acne, high blood pressure, diabetes, cataracts, thinning of the bones (especially the spine), and fluid retention and swelling of the face, hands, abdomen, and ankles. Women may grow facial hair, and adolescents may have delayed sexual maturation. In most cases, the side effects clear up when patients stop taking the drugs.

With medication, people who suffer mild or moderate chronic ulcerative colitis can control it for years, often for the rest of their lives. Severe colitis requires surgery, and sometimes patients with milder forms choose to have surgery rather than live with the disease's unpredictable recurrence or the ever-present side effects of drugs. In any case, surgery is the one known cure for chronic ulcerative colitis, although fewer than one-third of patients undergo surgical procedures. Several types of these surgeries have high success rates.

Because ulcerative colitis eventually spreads throughout the colon, complete removal of the large bowel and rectum is the surest way to eliminate the disease. This "total proctocolectomy" takes place in three steps. The surgeon first cuts through the wall of the abdomen, the incision extending from the mid-transverse colon to the rectum, and removes the colon. Next, the end of the ileum is pulled through a hole in the abdomen to form a stoma (a procedure called an ileostomy). Finally, the rectum is removed and the anus sutured shut. Thereafter the patient defecates through the stoma. Either of two arrangements prevents stool from simply spilling out unchecked. Most patients affix plastic bags around their stomas into which stool flows without their control; when full, the bag is either emptied and reattached or thrown away and replaced. To avoid external bags, some patients prefer a "continent ileostomy," so called because it allows them to control defecation. The surgeon constructs a pouch out of a portion of the ileum and attaches it right behind the stoma, a procedure called a Kock pouch after its inventor, Nils Kock of Sweden. When this pouch is full, the patient empties it with a catheter inserted through the stoma. Some patients can choose to have an ileoanal anastomosis. In this procedure, the surgeon forms the end of the ileum into a pouch, which is attached to the anus and collects wastes in place of the rectum. The patient continues to defecate through the anus rather than through a stoma.

None of these surgical procedures is free of problems, and all require extensive recovery in the hospital and rehabilitation. Moreover, both infections and mechanical failures can occur. If healthy portions of the colon are left intact, they often flare with colitis later, and more operations become necessary. Patients with stomas are vulnerable to bacterial inflammation of the small intestine, resulting in diarrhea, vomiting, and dehydration. Stomas and pouches sometimes leak or close up, and even after successful operations patients lose some capacity to absorb zinc, bile salts, and vitamin B_{12}, although food supplements can make up for these deficiencies.

Any major surgery is an emotional trial. One that leaves a basic function of the body permanently altered, as with proctocolectomy or ileostomy, is difficult to accept afterward, even when the surgery was an emergency measure to save the patient's life. Patients must live with a bag of stool on their abdomen or a pouch that they must empty with a plastic straw—bags and pouches that sometimes leak stool or gas and that, even when functioning smoothly, are not pleasant to handle. They must pay close attention to body functions that they rarely had to think about before the ulcerative colitis began. The changes can severely depress patients, who then may need psychiatric help and antidepressant drugs to recover their spirits. Patients with anastomoses, who continue to defecate through their anus, also find their bowel functions changed, although not so severely. For example, it takes many months before normal stool forms, and diarrhea plagues these patients.

After their operations, patients have access to considerable help in addition to physicians and surgeons. Special nurses train patients to care for their stomas, check regularly for infection or malfunction, and generally ease them into their new lives. Formal support groups and informal networks are common, through which the afflicted can get information and reassurance. In the United States, the National Foundation for Ileitis and Colitis arranges many support groups, as well as sponsoring medical research and education programs.

PERSPECTIVE AND PROSPECTS

Acute forms of colitis, especially amebic dysentery, have long been recognized as among the endemic diseases of polluted water, and until the development of antibiotics, they regularly killed significant portions of local populations, especially the young and elderly. Chronic ulcerative colitis was first described in 1859, but no effective treatment for it existed until the 1940's. At that time, Nana Svartz of Sweden noticed that when rheumatoid arthritis patients were given sulfasalazine, the bowel condition of those who had colitis improved as well. J. Arnold Bargen, an American physician, confirmed Svartz's observation in a formal clinical trial, and sulfasalazine soon was mass-produced for distribution in the United States and later throughout the world. Since the 1940's, medications and surgical techniques for ulcerative colitis have proliferated, although none restores a patient's original state of health.

Because the agents causing ulcerative colitis are unknown, the historical and geographical origin of the disease likewise cannot be determined. Nevertheless, three somewhat odd social facets of the disease are recognized.

Evidence suggests that ulcerative colitis is a disease of urban industrial society. Along with Crohn's disease, colitis appears to be entrenched in Scandinavia, the United States, Western Europe, Israel, and England. It rarely occurs in rural Africa, Asia, or South America, despite the poor nutrition and sanitation in some of these areas. Yet the disease does not appear to vary solely by racial type or nationality, although Jewish people tend to fall ill with it more often than any other group. For example, African Americans, whether from families long-established in the United States or recently immigrated, show an incidence of colitis as high as residents of European descent.

Furthermore, ulcerative colitis strikes the young. It most often begins between the ages of fifteen and thirty; men and women are equally likely to come down with it. This fact, taken with the high rate of inflammatory bowel disease (IBD) sufferers who have family members also with the disease (20 to 25 percent), has led some researchers to believe that a genetic factor creates a susceptibility for IBD.

Finally, IBD patients bear some social stigma, or at least believe they do. Ulcerative colitis involves bowel incontinence and often ends with surgical replacement of the anus with a stoma; in such cases, bowel movements can dominate a patient's life and become obvious to family members, coworkers, and even strangers. Because the subject of stool is taboo to many and the odor offends most people, patients can feel severe embarrassment and come to see themselves as pariahs. Even though the causes of ulcerative colitis remain obscure and the treatment is often distressing, modern medicine saves people who otherwise would die.

—*Roger Smith, Ph.D.*

See also Colon and rectal surgery; Colon cancer; Crohn's disease; Diarrhea and dysentery; Diverticulosis and diverticulitis; Gastroenterology; Gastrointestinal disorders; Gastrointestinal system; Intestinal disorders; Intestines; Irritable bowel syndrome (IBS).

For Further Information:

Beers, Mark H., et al. *The Merck Manual of Diagnosis and Therapy.* 18th ed. Whitehouse Station, N.J.: Merck Research Laboratories, 2006. This is a reference work for physicians, and the nomenclature can be daunting. It is best consulted after more general introductory reading. The sections on colitis describe the physical symptoms, tests, and treatments systematically and thoroughly.

Brandt, Lawrence J., and Penny Steiner-Grossman, eds. *Treating IBD: A Patient's Guide to the Medical and Surgical Management of Inflammatory Bowel Disease.* Reprint. Philadelphia: Lippincott-Raven, 1996. One of the most thorough introductions to ulcerative colitis and Crohn's disease. Illustrations, tables, and very helpful glossaries accompany the text.

Crohn's and Colitis Foundation of America. http://www.ccfa.org/. Provides support groups and a wide range of educational publications and programs on Crohn's and ulcerative colitis.

Kalibjian, Cliff. *Straight from the Gut: Living with Crohn's Disease and Ulcerative Colitis.* Cambridge, Mass.: O'Reilly and Associates, 2003. Shares numerous personal stories from those suffering from colitis and offers advice on all aspects of living with the disease.

Kelly, Michael P. *Colitis.* New York: Routledge, 1992. Kelly begins his book with a description of symptoms and treatments, but his is primarily a sociological study. Based on interviews with forty-five patients, the work discusses typical effects that the disease had on their lives and how they coped with the treatments, especially surgical procedures.

Parker, James N., and Philip M. Parker, eds. *The 2002 Official Patient's Sourcebook on Ulcerative Colitis.* San Diego, Calif.: Icon Health, 2002. Draws from public, academic, government, and peer-reviewed research to provide a wide-ranging reference about the causes, treatments, and risk factors of colitis.

Saibil, Fred. *Crohn's Disease and Ulcerative Colitis: Everything You Need to Know.* Rev. ed. Toronto: Firefly Books, 2003. A leading expert on IBD, Saibil covers topics such as signs and symptoms, how the gastrointestinal system works normally and how IBD affects it, procedures and instruments used to diagnose IBD, effects of diet, children and IBD, and effects on sexual activity and child-bearing.

Sklar, Jill, Manual Sklar, and Annabel Cohen. *The First Year—Crohn's Disease and Ulcerative Colitis: An Essential Guide for the Newly Diagnosed.* New York: Avalon, 2002. A unique guide for patients with specific gastrointestinal disorders, setting expectations and answering questions related to the first week of diagnosis, the first months, and the first year. Topics include treatment options, dietary choices, fertility issues, and holistic alternatives.

Steiner-Grossman, Penny, Peter A. Banks, and Daniel H. Present, eds. *The New People, Not Patients: A Source Book for Living with Inflammatory Bowel Disease.* Rev. ed. Dubuque, Iowa: Kendall/Hunt, 1997. Written to help IBD patients live with the disease, this book combines very practical information—about support groups and patients' rights, for example—with overviews of symptoms and treatments.

Colon and rectal polyp removal

Procedure

Anatomy or system affected: Abdomen, anus, gastrointestinal system, intestines

Specialties and related fields: Gastroenterology, general surgery, proctology

Definition: The surgical removal of overgrowths of the tissue lining the rectum and colon.

Indications and Procedures

Rectal and colon polyps are growths of tissue that occur in the mucous membranes lining the colon and rectum.

They are usually not malignant. Common types of colorectal polyps are juvenile polyps, Peutz-Jeghers polyps (hamartomas), hyperplasias, adenomas, and mixed hyperplastic-adenomatous polyps. Adenomas are both the most dangerous and the most common type of colon polyp.

Rectal or colon polyps are removed when they are found, even if they cause no symptoms, because identifying the kind of polyp helps doctors determine whether cancer is likely to develop. The type of polyp is determined in the laboratory after surgical removal, using microscopic techniques

The presence of polyps does not mean that a patient has cancer, although larger polyps (greater than 1 centimeter) indicate a higher risk for cancer than do smaller ones. Certain types of polyps also are more likely than others to develop into cancer. Hyperplasias are polyps with no potential to develop into cancer. Juvenile polyps and Peutz-Jeghers polyps are associated with inherited disorders that indicate an increased risk for colon cancer, but they do not always develop into malignant tumors. Colorectal adenomas are particularly dangerous when they occur in conjunction with a genetic condition known as familial adenomatous polyposis (FAP). In patients with FAP, untreated colorectal adenomas develop into colon cancer virtually 100 percent of the time. Mixed hyperplastic-adenomatous polyps, although not as risky as pure adenomas, can develop into colon cancer, and patients with a diagnosis of this type of polyp should be closely monitored.

Colon polyps often cause no symptoms. They are usually detected by routine screening for colorectal cancers. The most common symptoms, when they occur, are bleeding from the anus (visible on underwear or toilet paper), constipation or diarrhea lasting more than a week, and blood in the stool, which can appear as red streaks or an overall darkening of fecal matter. The fecal occult blood test will detect blood that is not visible.

When polyps are suspected, the physician will perform a rectal examination or special tests such as barium enema X rays, flexible sigmoidoscopy, or colonoscopy. In a rectal examination, the doctor feels the rectal tissue with his fingers, looking for abnormalities. Barium makes healthy intestinal tissue look white on an X ray, and polyps appear dark against the white background. The sigmoidoscope is a flexible fiberoptic tube that can be inserted through the anus. The tube has a light and small video camera so that the doctor can visualize the lower third of the large intestine. Colonoscopy is similar to sigmoidoscopy, but the colonoscope allows the physician to visualize the entire intestine.

Removal is most commonly accomplished using colonoscopy to visualize the polyps and specialized forceps to detach and remove the growths. Snare forceps can be used to surround a polyp and cut it from the lining of the colon or rectum. Other methods of removal include a laser beam, burning, or ultrasound, depending on the size of the polyp. Bleeding during the procedure can be controlled with electrocautery forceps, which use heat to sever the polyp from the surrounding healthy tissue and seal off blood vessels, or by pressing epinephrine-soaked gauze against the removal site.

Special precautions must be taken during surgery to remove gas from the colon so that the combustion of hydrogen or methane gas does not occur. These gases are normally produced by bacteria that inhabit the colon.

A polyp in the lower portion of the colon may be removed using similar procedures during the sigmoidoscopy. In some cases, the patient may undergo surgery to remove the polyp through the abdomen.

Uses and Complications

Since colonoscopy is somewhat uncomfortable for the patient, sedatives are usually given, but general anesthesia is usually not necessary. Rectal and colon polyp removal is typically done as an outpatient procedure.

Because of the gas that enters the intestine during the procedure, patients may experience bloating, pressure, and intestinal cramps in the twenty-four hours following removal. This discomfort subsides as the gas passes out of the intestine.

Repeat colonoscopy should be performed so that recurrent polyps can be removed and examined for malignancy. Colorectal cancer is the second leading cause of cancer deaths in the United States, and the majority of these cancers arise from colorectal polyps.

—Matthew Berria, Ph.D.,
and Douglas Reinhart, M.D.;
updated by Caroline M. Small

See also Biopsy; Cancer; Colon and rectal surgery; Colon cancer; Colonoscopy and sigmoidoscopy; Electrocauterization; Endoscopy; Enemas; Gastroenterology; Gastrointestinal system; Hemorrhoid banding and removal; Hemorrhoids; Intestinal disorders; Intestines; Oncology; Proctology; Screening.

For Further Information:

American Cancer Society. *American Cancer Society's Complete Guide to Colorectal Cancer.* New York: Author, 2005.

Burke, Carol and James Church, eds. *Hereditary Colorectal Cancer Syndromes.* New York: Blackwell, 2007.

Corman, Marvin L. *Colon and Rectal Surgery.* 5th ed. Philadelphia: Lippincott Williams & Wilkins, 2005.

Longo, Walter E., and John M. A. Northover, eds. *Reoperative Colon and Rectal Surgery.* New York: Martin Dunitz, 2003.

National Institutes of Health. National Cancer Institute. *Cancer of the Colon and Rectum.* Rev. ed. Bethesda, Md.: Author, 1991.

________. *What You Need to Know About Cancer of the Colon and Rectum.* Rev. ed. Bethesda, Md.: Author, 1999.

Zollinger, Robert M., Jr., and Robert M. Zollinger, Sr. *Zollinger's Atlas of Surgical Operations.* 8th ed. New York: McGraw-Hill, 2003.

Colon and rectal surgery

Procedure

Anatomy or system affected: Abdomen, anus, gastrointestinal system, intestines

Specialties and related fields: Gastroenterology, general surgery, proctology

Definition: Surgery that is required to correct pathologies of the colon, rectum, and anus.

Key terms:

abscess: a pocket of infection or inflammation
acute: referring to a short, immediate disease state
chronic: referring to an enduring disease state
ulcer: a lesion that destroys tissue

Indications and Procedures

The large intestine, or colon, is shaped like an inverted *U*. It starts at the lower right side of the pelvis, where the small intestine empties into the cecum. The colon rises from the cecum to the center of the abdomen, crosses to the left, and descends to the S-shaped sigmoid colon, the rectum, and the anus. Common disorders of the colon, rectum, and anus that require surgery are hemorrhoids, Crohn's disease, ulcerative colitis, cancer, diverticulosis, and diverticulitis.

Hemorrhoids are swollen veins in the lower part of the rectum and the anus. They protrude as nodes or lumps that can cause severe pain, itching, and inflammation. Hemorrhoids can be tied off with tiny rubber bands. After a few days, they fall off painlessly. Medications can shrink internal hemorrhoids, or hemorrhoidal tissue can be removed by photocoagulation, a process that uses electromagnetic energy to eradicate affected tissues. Sometimes, a hemorrhoidectomy is required. This procedure involves the extensive excision of hemorrhoidal tissue and can be quite painful.

Crohn's disease and ulcerative colitis are chronic inflammatory bowel diseases (IBDs) that can affect the colon. Crohn's disease usually occurs in the small intestine, although it may be limited to the colon. When Crohn's disease is severe and restricted to the colon, the surgeon may perform an ileostomy. This procedure involves removing the entire lower intestine, rectum, and anus. The anal opening is closed, and a new opening, or stoma, is made in the abdominal wall. The ileum, the lower end of the small intestine, is then attached to the opening. A removable pouch is sealed to the opening to collect fecal matter, which must be emptied manually.

Ulcerative colitis may exist with no symptoms other than an occasional flare-up, or it can be a chronic, serious, or life-threatening disease. It is characterized by a series of ulcers on the inner wall of the colon. Bloody diarrhea, abdominal pain, and painful bowel movements are symptoms. In severe cases, there is danger of perforation of the colon wall or of swelling (toxic megacolon), either of which can be life-threatening. Ulcerative colitis may also be a precursor of colon cancer. In severe cases of ulcerative colitis, surgery is required. Ileostomy is the surgical procedure usually performed, but recently a procedure was developed called ileoanal anastomosis. As in ileostomy, the surgeon removes the entire colon and rectum but leaves the anal sphincter muscles. The ileum is then attached to the anus. This procedure allows the patient to have natural bowel movements and avoids the necessity of the ileostomy pouch.

Cancers of the colon or rectum, called colorectal cancers, are major causes of morbidity and mortality. The possibility of colon cancer is often signaled by the presence of polyps on the lower intestinal wall. Symptoms such as mucus or blood in the stool may alert the physician to look for polyps and determine whether they are likely to become cancerous. Benign polyps are usually removed surgically.

When polyps are likely to become cancerous, and in the presence of actual colorectal cancer, surgery is usually performed to remove diseased tissue. This often requires excising part or all of the colon. Sometimes a colostomy is performed, an operation similar to an ileostomy. In this procedure, the diseased sections of the colon, the rectum, and the anus are removed. The anal opening is sealed, and the remaining colon is brought to an opening in the abdominal wall. This opening, or stoma, is fitted with a removable colostomy bag or pouch to collect fecal matter.

Diverticula are small, saclike pouches that develop in the colon wall, most often in the sigmoid colon. Their presence is known as diverticulosis. These sacs can collect stagnant fecal matter and become inflamed, resulting in diverticulitis. Abscesses and infection may develop. As inflammation progresses or recurs, the wall of the colon thickens, reducing the width of the passage and increasing the possibility of obstruction and distension of the colon. Perforations in the colon wall may develop and cause peritonitis (infection of the membrane that covers the abdomen).

In severe cases, it may be necessary to perform a temporary colostomy. The diseased section of colon is removed, and the rectum and anus are closed. A stoma is made in the abdominal wall and attached to the remaining colon and covered by a pouch to collect fecal matter. After the bowel has healed, the rectum and anus can be reopened and attached to the colon.

Uses and Complications

Patients with permanent ileostomies and colostomies have a hole in their abdomens that is often 5 or more centimeters (2 or more inches) in diameter. Patients are required to wear removable pouches sealed to their stomas to collect fecal matter so that it can be eliminated. The apparatus is cumbersome, and the entire process can be unpleasant enough to cause serious depression in the patient. Patients' spouses and other family members are often involved in changing and emptying the bags, particularly with older, infirm persons. Ileoanal anastomosis solves some of these problems because it allows natural bowel movements, but it is useful only in certain conditions.

Perspective and Prospects

Current surgical procedures are often effective in serious colorectal conditions. The success rate of these surgeries for the treatment of cancer is quite high if the cancer is caught before it spreads to other parts of the body. Nevertheless, patients may have to endure the inconvenience of ostomy bags and paraphernalia for the rest of their lives. Ostomy equipment has been improved: Better sealing adhesives are now in use so that the bags do not slip or leak as they once did. The configuration of belts, bags, and other appliances has been altered to make them more convenient and easier to live with. New surgical procedures that could maintain normal bowel function for more patients, however, would be a major advancement.

—C. Richard Falcon

See also Abdomen; Abdominal disorders; Biopsy; Cancer; Colitis; Colon and rectal polyp removal; Colon cancer; Colonoscopy and sigmoidoscopy; Crohn's disease; Diverticulitis and diverticulosis; Electrocauterization; Endoscopy; Enemas; Fistula repair; Gastroenterology; Gastrointestinal system; Hemorrhoid banding and removal; Hemorrhoids; Hernia repair; Hernias; Ileostomy and colostomy; Intestinal disorders; Intestines; Oncology; Proctology; Tumor removal; Tumors.

For Further Information:

Feldman, Mark, Lawrence S. Friedman, and Lawrence J. Brandt, eds. *Sleisenger and Fordtran's Gastrointestinal and Liver Disease: Pathophysiology, Diagnosis, Management*. 8th ed. 2 vols. Philadelphia: W. B. Saunders, 2006. A comprehensive textbook of gastrointestinal diseases and physiology. Contains excellent chapters on all disorders mentioned in the text, as well as some beautiful endoscopic photographs.

Kapadia, Cyrus R., James M. Crawford, and Caroline Taylor. *An Atlas of Gastroenterology: A Guide to Diagnosis and Differential Diagnosis*. Boca Raton, Fla.: Pantheon, 2003. Provides a fully illustrated, nonspecialist understanding of myriad gastrointestinal diseases, including heartburn, dyspepsia, diarrhea, irritable bowel syndrome, and pancreatitis. Includes bibliographic references and index.

Litin, Scott C., ed. *Mayo Clinic Family Health Book*. 3d ed. New York: HarperResource, 2003. Perhaps the best general medical text for the layperson, this book covers the entire medical field. While the information is derived from a wide variety of highly technical sources, the articles are written to be easily understood by a general audience.

Phillips, Robert H. *Coping with an Ostomy: A Guide to Living with an Ostomy for You and Your Family*. Wayne, N.J.: Avery, 1986. Writing for soon-to-be ostomates, Phillips summarizes types of operations and their typical causes, then concentrates on the emotional and social aspects of living with a stoma.

Zollinger, Robert M., Jr., and Robert M. Zollinger, Sr. *Zollinger's Atlas of Surgical Operations*. 8th ed.

New York: McGraw-Hill, 2003. A comprehensive examination of surgery. Covers basic surgical anatomy and vascular, gynecologic, gastrointestinal, and miscellaneous abdominal procedures.

COLON CANCER

DISEASE/DISORDER

ANATOMY OR SYSTEM AFFECTED: Abdomen, anus, gastrointestinal system, intestines, lymphatic system

SPECIALTIES AND RELATED FIELDS: Gastroenterology, genetics, immunology, oncology, proctology

DEFINITION: Cancer occurring in the large intestine, which is the second deadliest type of this disease.

CAUSES AND SYMPTOMS

With an estimated sixty thousand deaths per year in the United States, cancer of the colon and rectum (also called large bowel or colorectal cancer) is the second most deadly cancer, ranking only behind lung cancer. About 90 percent of colorectal cancers arise from the glandular epithelium lining the inner surface of the large bowel and are termed adenocarcinomas. The cells of this layer are constantly being replaced by new cells. This fairly rapid cell division, along with the relatively hostile environment within the bowel, promotes internal cellular errors that lead to the formation of aberrant cells. These cells can become disordered and produce abnormal growths or tumors. Often, colorectal tumors protrude into the lumen (the spaces within the bowel), forming growths called polyps. Some polyps are benign and do not spread to other parts of the body, but they may still disturb normal bowel functions. Other polyps become malignant by forming more aggressive cell types, which allows them to grow larger and spread to other organs. The cancer can grow through the layers of the colon wall and extend into the body cavity and nearby organs such as the urinary bladder. Cancer cells can also break away from the main tumor and spread (metastasize) through the blood or lymphatic vessels to other organs, such as the lungs or liver. If not controlled, the spreading cancer eventually causes death by impairment of organ and system functions.

The tendency to develop colorectal polyps and cancer can be inherited; this genetic predisposition may be responsible for about 5 to 7 percent of all colorectal cancers. One example is an inherited disorder called familial adenomatous polyposis (FAP), in which multiple polyps develop in the colon; it often leads to colorectal cancer. Some of the defective genes that cause this and other types of colorectal cancers have been identified and are being studied to determine their role. The interplay between the various oncogenes (mutated cell division and growth genes) and tumor suppressor genes (cell division and growth inhibitor genes) has been determined. Whether inherited or caused by carcinogens, damage to these specific genetic regions disrupts the delicate balance that regulates orderly and perfectly timed cell reproduction and development, producing cancer cells. Irritable bowel syndrome (IBS) and exposure to certain occupational carcinogens are also known to increase the risk.

INFORMATION ON COLON CANCER

CAUSES: Hereditary and/or environmental factors, dietary habits, colon polyps, long-standing ulcerative colitis

SYMPTOMS: Fatigue, weakness, shortness of breath, change in bowel habits, narrow stools, diarrhea or constipation, red or dark blood in stool, weight loss, abdominal pain, cramps, bloating

DURATION: Chronic

TREATMENTS: Surgery, chemotherapy, radiation

TREATMENT AND THERAPY

The chances for survival are greatly increased when colorectal cancer is detected and treated at an early stage. Early detection in the general population is possible with the use of three common medical tests: digital rectal examination, in which the physician checks the inner surface of the rectal wall with a gloved finger for abnormal growths; fecal occult blood test, in which a stool sample is tested for hidden blood that may have emanated from a cancerous growth; and sigmoidoscopy, in which the physician examines the rectal and lower colon inner lining with a narrow tubular optical instrument inserted through the anus. In 2002, researchers announced an encouraging step toward early detection of the disease. A new screening test, which looks for a gene that is usually faulty in the earliest stages of colon cancer and is sloughed off into the stool, found cancer in 57 percent of early colon cancer patients. Researchers hope to refine the test within three to five years in order to make the test 70 percent accurate.

Once cancer is suspected, further tests will be done to arrive at a diagnosis. These tests may include a computed tomography (CT) scan, double-

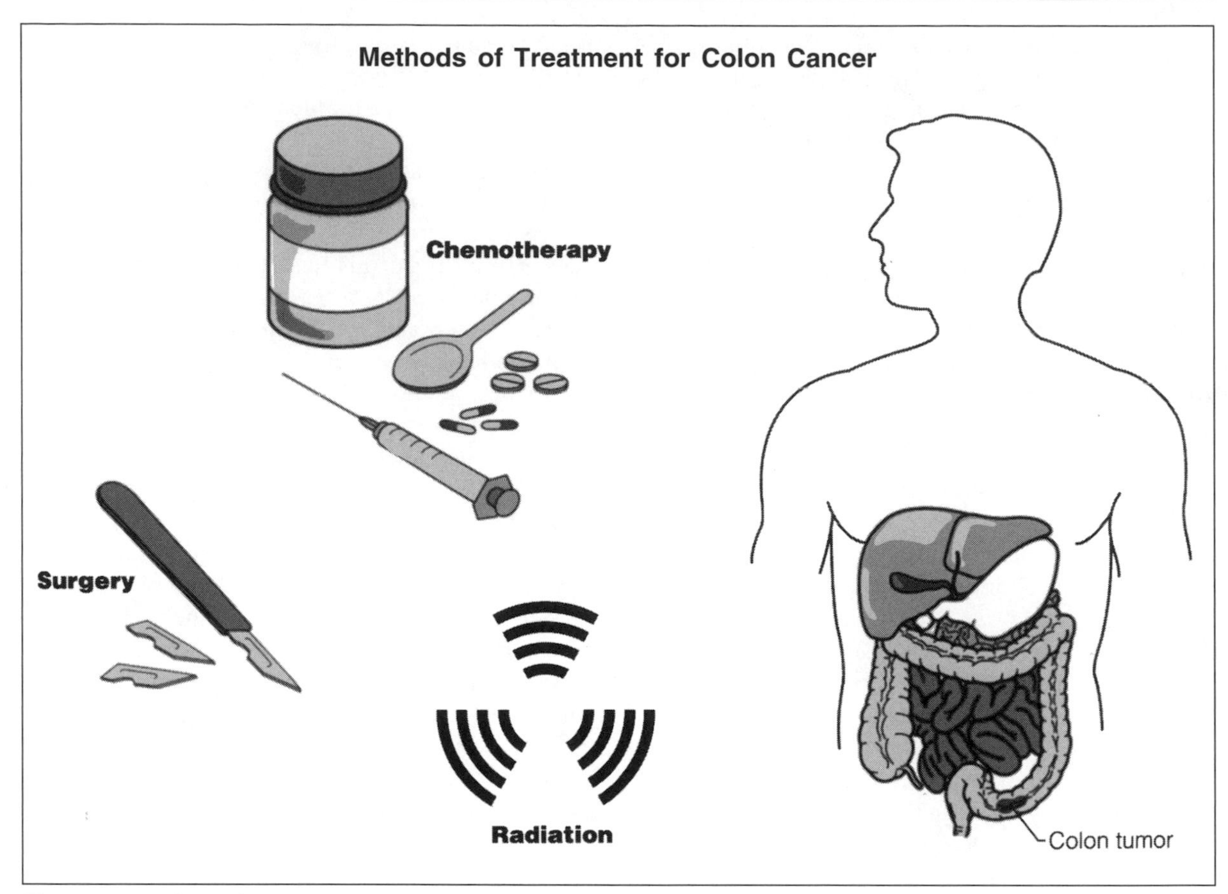

The presence of a malignant tumor in the colon requires some form of treatment or a combination of treatments, usually beginning with its surgical removal and followed by radiation therapy and/or chemotherapy (the use of anticancer drugs).

contrast barium enema X-ray series, and colonoscopy. The CT scan and contrast X rays reveal abnormal growths, and colonoscopy is similar to sigmoidoscopy but uses a longer, flexible tube in order to inspect the entire colon. During sigmoidoscopy and colonoscopy, the physician can remove polyps and obtain tissue samples for biopsy. Microscopic examination of the tissue samples by a pathologist can determine the stage or extent of growth of the cancer. This is important because it helps determine the type of treatment. In one type of staging, the following criteria are used: stage 0 (cancer confined to epithelium lining of the bowel), stage 1 (cancer confined to the bowel wall), stage 2 (cancer penetrating through all layers of the bowel wall and possibly invading adjacent tissues), stage 3 (cancer invading lymph nodes and/or adjacent tissues), and stage 4 (cancer spreading to distant sites, forming metastases).

Surgery is the primary treatment for colorectal cancer. Very small tumors in stage 0 can be removed surgically with the colonoscope. Tumors in more advanced stages require abdominal surgery in which the tumor is removed along with a portion of the bowel and possibly some lymph nodes. For cases in which the bowel cannot be reconnected, an opening is created through the abdominal wall (colostomy). This is usually a temporary procedure, and the hole will be closed when the bowel can be rejoined. Some advanced cancers cannot be cured by surgery alone. Adjuvant therapies—chemotherapy, radiation therapy, and biological therapy—may be used in combination with surgery. Chemotherapy drugs kill spreading cancer cells. The most common is 5-fluorouracil (5-FU), a chemical that interferes with the production of deoxyribonucleic acid (DNA) in dividing cells. 5-FU is more effective when given together with leucovorin (a compound similar to folic acid) and levamisole (an immune system stimulant).

In 2002, the Food and Drug Administration (FDA) approved the use of the Eloxatin injection in combination with 5-FU and leucovorin for the treatment of patients whose cancer has recurred or become worse following initial drug therapy. This approach was shown to shrink tumors in some patients and delay resumed tumor growth. Levamisole and other treatments that reinforce the immune system are forms of biological therapy. Radiation therapy, given either before or after surgery, is helpful in killing undetected cancer cells near the site of the tumor.

Perspective and Prospects

More than 150,000 new cases of colorectal cancer are diagnosed in the United States each year, or roughly 15 percent of all cancers. The incidence of colorectal cancer is lower among females than males and rises dramatically after the age of fifty. Colorectal cancer is more common in developed countries such as the United States and in densely populated, industrialized regions. American mortality rates from colorectal cancer are higher in the Northeast and north-central regions of the country than in the South and Southwest. Populations moving from low-risk parts of the world, such as Asia or Africa, to high-risk areas, such as the United States or Europe, take on the higher risk within a generation or two, and vice versa.

Research is ongoing in discerning the risk factors of and creating treatments for colorectal cancers. Recent epidemiological evidence has supported the use of nonsteroidal anti-inflammatory drugs (NSAIDs) as a means of reducing the risk of cancers of the colon and rectum, as well as the risk of intestinal cancers resulting from exposure to carcinogens. The studies focused only on the daily use of aspirin, but similar results have been reported following long-term use of sulindac and indomethacin. Sulindac has shown an ability to induce regression of colon polyps in patients with familial adenomatous polyposis. Researchers are still working on finding the right balance in dose and frequency since sulindac has potentially severe side effects and aspirin may induce bleeding if high doses are maintained on a daily basis.

—Rodney C. Mowbray, Ph.D.;
updated by Connie Rizzo, M.D., Ph.D.

See also Biopsy; Cancer; Chemotherapy; Colon and rectal polyp removal; Colon and rectal surgery; Colon therapy; Colonoscopy and sigmoidoscopy; Ileostomy and colostomy; Intestinal disorders; Intestines; Malignancy and metastasis; National Cancer Institute (NCI); Oncology; Radiation therapy; Stomach, intestinal, and pancreatic cancers; Tumor removal; Tumors.

For Further Information:

Adrouny, Richard. *Understanding Colon Cancer*. Jackson: University Press of Mississippi, 2002. An excellent lay guide to the disease, offering information on topics such as diagnosis, prognosis, treatment, demographics, high-risk conditions, the sequence from bowel polyps to cancer, the warning signs, the stages of the disease, and theories of how colon cancer spreads.

American Cancer Society (ACS). http://www.cancer.org/docroot/home/index.asp. Web site is divided into sections for patients, family, and friends; survivors; health information seekers; ACS supporters; and professionals. Information on all cancers is wide ranging.

Bub, David S., et al. *One Hundred Questions and Answers About Colorectal Cancer*. Sudbury, Mass.: Jones and Bartlett, 2003. Provides authoritative answers to questions about treatment options, post-treatment quality of life, and sources of support.

De Vita, Vincent T., Jr., Samuel Hellman, and Steven A. Rosenberg, eds. *Cancer: Principles and Practice of Oncology*. 7th ed. Philadelphia: Lippincott Williams & Wilkins, 2005. This thoroughly revised and updated classic reflects the latest breakthroughs in every aspect of oncology, from molecular biology, to multimodality treatment, to new data on cancer prevention by drugs and diet.

Dollinger, Malin, et al. *Everyone's Guide to Cancer Therapy*. 4th rev. ed. Kansas City, Mo.: Andrews & McMeel, 2002. An excellent source of medical information about cancer, written for the general public. Various cancer sites in the body are described and a helpful glossary of medical terminology is provided.

Eyre, Harmon J., Dianne Partie Lange, and Lois B. Morris. *Informed Decisions: The Complete Book of Cancer Diagnosis, Treatment, and Recovery*. 2d ed. Atlanta: American Cancer Society, 2002. The American Cancer Society endorses this excellent book, which provides a complete consumer reference for cancer diagnosis, treatment, and recovery. From assessing different therapy options and coping with stress and depression, this provides an excellent all-around survey of cancer's special decision-making requirements.

Goldman, Lee, and Dennis Ausiello, eds. *Cecil Textbook of Medicine*. 22d ed. Philadelphia: W. B. Saunders, 2004. This is a standard textbook of medicine. Although it is somewhat difficult, it is complete, beginning with normal conditions and progressing through disease process, diagnosis, and treatment.

Levin, Bernard, et al., eds. *American Cancer Society's Complete Guide to Colorectal Cancer.* Atlanta: American Cancer Society, 2006. An accessible guide with a foreward by journalist Katie Couric.

Miskovitz, Paul, and Marian Betancourt. *What to Do If You Get Colon Cancer: A Specialist Helps You Take Charge and Make Informed Choices.* New York: Wiley, 1997. Designed for patients and families of patients with colon cancer, this volume has three sections: discovery, treatment, and recovery. The appendices are useful, containing information on financial aid and insurance considerations.

Parker, James N., and Philip M. Parker, eds. *The Official Patient's Sourcebook on Colon Cancer.* San Diego, Calif.: Icon Health, 2002. Draws from public, academic, government, and peer-reviewed research to provide a wide-ranging reference about the causes, treatments, and risk factors of colon cancer.

Colon therapy

Treatment

Also known as: Colonic irrigation, colon hydrotherapy

Anatomy or system affected: Abdomen, anus, gastrointestinal system, intestines

Specialties and related fields: Alternative medicine

Definition: Irrigation of the colon, or large intestine, with water in order to detoxify it.

Indications and Procedures

Colon therapy involves washing out the entire approximately 5-foot length of the colon with pure water in order to dislodge any impacted fecal material. Some practitioners believe that the colon may not function properly because of poor dietary habits, insufficient fluid intake, and physical or emotional stress or illness. Such malfunction can lead to a buildup of hardened, impacted fecal material, which may stagnate and decay in the colon. Bacterial decomposition of the material may create toxins that are absorbed into the bloodstream. This in turn could cause other body organs to overwork themselves as they attempt to detoxify the waste materials and could lead to a variety of illnesses, from colds to cardiovascular disease.

During this procedure, a flexible tube is inserted into the rectum and water is slowly pumped into the intestine. The pressure is regulated in order to avoid injury. Alternation of warm and cool water leads to contraction and relaxation of the intestinal walls, which helps to remove impacted pieces of dry feces from the walls. Feces, gas, mucus, and bacteria exit through the same tube. A cleaner internal surface of the colon provides more surface area for the absorption of nutrients and water. Approximately 20 gallons of water are used in the procedure, which lasts about one hour.

Uses and Complications

Irrigation of the entire colon came into prominence during the late nineteenth century in Russia. In the United States, Dr. John Harvey Kellogg espoused colonic irrigation along with other health and fitness regimes at his sanatorium in Battle Creek, Michigan, in the early twentieth century. The procedure fell into obscurity during the late 1940's, when medical research indicated no benefit to the procedure. Renewed interest in colonics in the late twentieth century led to the establishment of the International Association for Colon Hydrotherapy, which provides training and certification for practitioners. While colon therapy regained enthusiastic followers, mainstream physicians point out that waste products in the colon cannot "toxify" the body. They also believe that colonics may interfere with the natural balance of helpful bacteria that keep the intestines functioning normally.

After a procedure, some patients report feeling energized and lighter, while others report nausea, headaches, or flulike symptoms. These symptoms generally subside within a few hours. Other side effects may include diarrhea and a loss of necessary intestinal bacteria.

—Karen E. Kalumuck, Ph.D.; updated by LeAnna DeAngelo, Ph.D.

See also Alternative medicine; Gastrointestinal system; Hydrotherapy; Intestines; Preventive medicine.

For Further Information:

Collings, Jillie. *Principles of Colonic Irrigation: The Only Introduction You'll Ever Need.* New York: Thorsons, 1996.

Goldberg, Burton, John Anderson, and Larry Trivieri, eds. *Alternative Medicine: The Definitive Guide.* 2d ed. Berkeley, Calif.: Ten Speed Press, 2002.

Jonas, Wayne, ed. *Mosby's Dictionary of Complementary and Alternative Medicine.* St. Louis: Elsevier Mosby, 2005.

Colonoscopy and sigmoidoscopy

Procedures

Anatomy or system affected: Gastrointestinal system, intestines

Specialties and related fields: Gastroenterology, general surgery

Definition: The insertion of a flexible tube into the rectum to look at the inside surface of the colon.

Key terms:

biopsy: removal of a piece of tissue for examination under a microscope

colitis: inflammation of the inner surface of the colon

lumen: the space inside a tubelike structure such as the colon

mucosa: the layer of tissue that lines the inside of a tubelike structure such as the colon

polyp: a small piece of tissue that extends from the surface of the colon into the lumen

Indications and Procedures

Colonoscopy and sigmoidoscopy are common procedures to evaluate the lower part of the gastrointestinal tract. Colonoscopy refers to examination of the entire large bowel, whereas sigmoidoscopy examines only the part closest to the rectum (known as the sigmoid colon). The advantage of sigmoidoscopy is that it is less time-consuming and can be performed without sedation. Since sigmoidoscopy evaluates only part of the colon, however, full colonoscopy is often preferred. The most common reason for having a colonoscopy is to screen for colon cancer. If sigmoidoscopy is used for this purpose, it must be combined with a barium enema and an X ray to evaluate the upper part of the colon.

Prior to colonoscopy, the bowel must be cleaned of stool to enable the physician to see the underlying mucosa. Patients are often asked to go on a diet of clear liquids (such as chicken broth, gelatin, and juice) for one to three days prior to the procedure. The night before the procedure, patients ingest a purgative to clear out any residual stool. The two most common preparations are polyethylene glycol (GoLytely) and a sodium phosphate mix (Fleet Phospho-Soda). Following ingestion of these solutions, patients should have clear or very light-colored liquid bowel movements. Regular medications that may cause excessive bleeding from biopsy sites, such as aspirin, warfarin, and nonsteroidal anti-inflammatory drugs (NSAIDs), are often discontinued prior to the procedure. Patients should also discontinue iron supplements, since they may create a black coating that makes it difficult for the physician to see the mucosa.

When patients enter the colonoscopy suite, they are given an intravenous (IV) catheter to administer fluids, as well as sedative and analgesic medications. Patients are asked not to eat or drink anything the day of the procedure. Sedative medications sometimes cause nausea, and any food that is present in the stomach may be vomited. Blood pressure, pulse, and oxygen saturation are monitored throughout the procedure. The patient is positioned on his or her left side, and a colonoscope is inserted through the rectum into the colon. The colonoscope is a long, flexible tube with a fiber-optic channel connected to a camera. The image of the inside of the colon is transmitted to a television screen. The colonoscope also has channels to administer air or water, as well as a suction channel. Air is introduced to expand the walls of the colon, enabling better viewing. Water is used to remove residual stool that may obstruct the view of the colon. The colonoscope is advanced to the cecum (the first part of the large bowel) or even the terminal ileum (the last part of the small bowel). The instrument is then slowly withdrawn while any abnormalities in the mucosa are noted. Following the procedure, patients are often observed for a period of time to make sure that no complications occur. If sedative medications were used, patients should not drive or operate machinery for the rest of the day.

Uses and Complications

In addition to screening for colon cancer, colonoscopy and sigmoidoscopy can be used to evaluate blood in the stool, chronic diarrhea or other changes in bowel habits, and unexplained abdominal pain. Common findings include polyps, which may be biopsied. It is common practice to remove a polyp completely, in case it turns out to be the precancerous type (known as an adenomatous polyp). Other findings include diverticula, small outpouchings of the colon which have very thin walls and are prone to spontaneous bleeding. They may also become infected, resulting in a condition known as diverticulitis. Other findings during colonoscopy may be useful in establishing the presence of a particular disease. Yellowish pseudo-membranes line the gut in colitis associated with the bacterium *Clostridium difficile*. A dusky hue is often seen in cases of ischemic colitis caused by diminished blood supply to the colon. Characteristic findings are also seen in inflammatory bowel disease.

Colonoscopy is a very safe procedure. One common aftereffect is abdominal discomfort as a result of the air used to distend the colon. This condition usually resolves over a few hours as the air is passed. The most serious complications of colonoscopy are perforation and bleeding. Perforation refers to a hole in the colon. It is an extremely rare occurrence, but it can be deadly. Patients with perforations often have severe abdominal pain and a rigid abdomen. If it is large and results in free air in the abdomen, a perforation requires emergency surgery. Rarely, very small perforations can be treated with observation and antibiotics. Bleeding is a risk if a biopsy is taken during the procedure. Most of the time, the bleeding stops by itself, but in some cases repeat colonoscopy may be required to control the bleeding. Rarely, bleeding may occur a few hours to several days after colonoscopy, so patients should report these symptoms to their physician. Whenever sedation is used, there is a risk of too much being given, which can lead to respiratory or cardiac arrest. Other possible complications include pain and inflammation at the site of the catheter and allergic reactions to sedative or analgesic medications.

—*Ahmad Kamal, M.D.*

See also Colon and rectal polyp removal; Colon and rectal surgery; Colon cancer; Diverticulitis and diverticulosis; Endoscopy; Enemas; Gastroenterology; Gastrointestinal system; Intestines; Invasive tests; Oncology; Proctology; Screening; Tumor removal; Tumors.

For Further Information:

Church, James M. *Endoscopy of the Colon, Rectum, and Anus*. New York: Igaku-Shoin, 1995.

Drossman, Douglas A., et al., eds. *Handbook of Gastroenterologic Procedures*. 4th ed. Philadelphia: Lippincott Williams & Wilkins, 2005.

Waye, Jerome D., Douglas K. Rex, and Christopher B. Williams, eds. *Colonoscopy: Principles and Practice*. Malden, Mass.: Blackwell, 2003.

Color blindness

Disease/disorder

Anatomy or system affected: Eyes

Specialties and related fields: Brain, optometry

Definition: An inability to distinguish certain colors resulting from an inherited defect in the light receptor cells in the retina of the eye.

Causes and Symptoms

The retina of the eye is a thin, fragile membrane that contains millions of photoreceptor cells. They convert light energy into an electrical signal, which is transmitted to the brain via the optic nerve. On a microscopic scale, the structure of the retina is like a carpet with its many fibers sticking upward. There are two types of photoreceptor cells, called rods and cones because of their distinctive shapes. Only the cones are important for color vision. There are three varieties of cones with peak sensitivities for red, green, and blue, respectively. The shades and tints of all other colors are mixtures of these three.

Color blindness involves a deficiency in these photoreceptor cells. A deficiency of green photoreceptor cells is much more common than a deficiency of red photoreceptors. Some people are totally colorblind, which means that they are completely unable to distinguish among red, orange, yellow, and green. Color blindness is quite rare in females (less than 1 percent of the population) but is more prevalent in males (about 8 percent).

Diagnostic tests are available to determine the extent of color blindness. The Ishihara color test, named after a Japanese ophthalmologist, consists of a mosaic of colored dots containing a letter of the alphabet made up of dots of a different color—for example, yellow dots in a background of green ones. Color-blind individuals would be unable to distinguish the letter because yellow and green look the same to them.

A more precise diagnostic test makes use of the Nagel anomaloscope, which has two colored light sources whose brightness can be adjusted. The patient tries to match a given color by superimposing the two light beams while varying their intensities. For normal eyes, red and green lights of similar intensities can be superimposed to create yellow. However, a patient who requires a considerably larger green component to create yellow evidently has a deficiency of green photoreceptor cells.

Treatment and Therapy

Color blindness is a genetic defect from birth, not a disease. No procedure is known by which it can be corrected. Color-blind people must find ways to counter the effects of their condition. For example, they can obtain driver's licenses because they learn that stoplights are always red on top, yellow in the middle, and green on the bottom. Color-blind individuals may need help, however, with tasks such as clothing selection. Good

> **INFORMATION ON COLOR BLINDNESS**
>
> **CAUSES:** Genetic defect resulting in photoreceptor deficiency
> **SYMPTOMS:** Inability to distinguish between certain colors (red, orange, yellow, green)
> **DURATION:** Lifelong
> **TREATMENTS:** None

color discrimination is required for some occupations, such as interior decorating, graphic design, advertising, or airplane piloting. Fortunately, color blindness is not a deterrent for most jobs.

—*Hans G. Graetzer, Ph.D.*

See also Eye infections and disorders; Eyes; Genetic diseases; Vision disorders.

FOR FURTHER INFORMATION:

Cameron, John R., James G. Skofronick, and Roderick M. Grant. *Medical Physics: Physics of the Body*. Madison, Wis.: Medical Physics, 1992.

Kasper, Dennis L., et al., eds. *Harrison's Principles of Internal Medicine*. 16th ed. New York: McGraw-Hill, 2005.

"Vision." In *Encyclopaedia Brittanica*. 15th ed. Chicago: Encyclopaedia Britannica, 2002.

COMA

DISEASE/DISORDER

ANATOMY OR SYSTEM AFFECTED: Brain, head, nervous system, psychic-emotional system

SPECIALTIES AND RELATED FIELDS: Critical care, emergency medicine

DEFINITION: A loss of consciousness from which a person cannot be aroused; a symptom signifying a variety of causes.

KEY TERMS:

alcoholic coma: coma accompanying severe alcohol intoxication

apoplectic coma: coma induced by cerebral, cerebellar, or brain-stem hemorrhage, as well as by embolism or cerebral thrombosis

brain death: irreversible brain damage so extensive that the organ enjoys no potential for recovery and can no longer maintain the body's internal functions

coma: a loss of consciousness from which the patient cannot be aroused

conscious: having an awareness of one's existence

hepatic coma: coma accompanying cerebral damage caused by the degeneration of liver cells (especially that associated with cirrhosis of the liver)

traumatic coma: coma following a head injury

CAUSES AND SYMPTOMS

Consciousness is defined by the normal wakeful state, with its self-aware cognition of past events and future anticipation. Disease or dysfunction that impairs this state usually causes readily identifiable conditions such as coma. The self-aware, cognitive aspects of consciousness depend largely on the interconnected neural networks of the cerebral hemispheres. Normal conscious behavior depends on the continuous, effective interaction of these systems. Loss of consciousness from medical causes can be brief (a matter of minutes to an hour or so) or it can be sustained for many hours, days, or sometimes even weeks. The longer the duration of the comatose state, the more likely it is to reflect structural damage to the brain rather than a transient alteration in its function.

The word "coma" comes from the Greek *koma*, meaning to put to sleep or to fall asleep. This state of unarousable unresponsiveness results from disturbance or damage to areas of the brain involved in conscious activity or the maintenance of consciousness—particularly parts of the cerebrum (the main mass of the brain), upper parts of the brain stem, and central regions of the brain, especially the limbic system. A wide spectrum of specific conditions can injure the brain and cause coma. The damage to the brain may be the result of a head injury or of an abnormality such as a brain tumor, brain abscess, or intracerebral hemorrhage. Often there has been a buildup of poisonous substances that intoxicates brain tissues. This buildup can occur because of a drug overdose, advanced kidney or liver disease, or acute alcoholic intoxication. Encephalitis (inflammation of the brain) and meningitis (inflammation of the brain coverings) can also cause coma, as can cerebral hypoxia (lack of oxygen in the brain, possibly attributable to the impairment of the blood flow to some areas). Whatever the underlying mechanism, coma indicates brain failure, and the high degree or organization of cerebral biochemical systems has been disrupted. Coma is easily distinguishable from sleep in that the person does not respond to external stimulation (such as shouting or pinching) or to the needs of his or her body (such as a full bladder).

Comas are classified according to the event or condition that caused the comatose state. Some of the most frequently encountered types of comas are traumatic coma, alcoholic coma, apoplectic coma, deanimate coma, diabetic coma, hepatic coma, metabolic coma, vigil coma, pseudo coma, and irreversible coma. Traumatic coma follows a head injury. It enjoys a somewhat more favorable outcome than that of comas associated with medical illness. About 50 percent of patients in a coma from head injuries survive, and the recovery is closely linked to age: The younger the patient, the greater the chance for recovery. Alcoholic coma refers to the coma accompanying severe alcohol intoxication, usually more than 400 milligrams alcohol per 100 milliliters of blood. This coma is marked by rapid, light respiration, usually with tachycardia and hypotension. Apoplectic coma is induced by cerebral, cerebellar, or brain-stem hemorrhage, as well as by embolism or cerebral thrombosis. The term "deanimate coma" refers to a deep coma with loss of all somatic and autonomic reflex activity. The maintenance of life depends wholly upon such supportive measures as assisted respiration, and cardiac arrest will quickly follow if the respirator is stopped; this may be a transient or irreversible state. Diabetic coma is the coma of severe diabetic acidosis. Hepatic coma is the coma accompanying cerebral damage resulting from degeneration of liver cells, especially that associated with cirrhosis of the liver. "Metabolic coma" is the term applied to the coma occurring in any metabolic disorder in the absence of a demonstrable macroscopic physical abnormality of the brain. Vigil coma is defined as a state of stupor in which the patient is mute and shows no verbal or motor responses to stimuli although the eyes are open and give a false impression of alertness. Pseudo coma refers to states resembling acute unconsciousness but with self-awareness preserved. Irreversible coma, or brain death, occurs when irreversible brain damage is so extensive that the organ enjoys no potential for recovery and can no longer maintain the body's internal functions.

Information on Coma

Causes: Head injury, disease, brain tumor, brain abscess, intracerebral hemorrhage, drug overdose, hypoxia, acute alcoholic intoxication

Symptoms: No response to external stimulation (such as shouting or pinching)

Duration: Ranges from minutes to several weeks or months

Treatments: Maintenance of oxygenation and circulation, intravenous administration of glucose or thiamine, control of generalized seizures, restoration of blood acid-base and osmolar balance

Treatment and Therapy

Of the acute problems in clinical medicine, none is more difficult than the prompt diagnosis and effective management of the comatose patient. The difficulty exists partly because the causes of coma are so many and partly because the physician possesses only a limited time in which to make the appropriate diagnostic and therapeutic judgment.

Measurements of variations in the depth of coma are important in its assessment and treatment. Varying depths of coma are recognized. In less severe forms, the person may respond to stimulation by, for example, moving an arm. In severe cases, the person fails to respond to repeated vigorous stimuli. Yet even deeply comatose patients may show some automatic responses, as they may continue to breathe unaided or may cough, yawn, blink, or show roving eye movement. These actions indicate that the lower brain stem, which controls these responses, is still functioning.

Assessment of the patient in coma includes an evaluation of all vital signs, the level of consciousness, neuromuscular responses, and reaction of the pupils to light. In most hospitals, a printed form for neurologic assessment is used to measure and record the patient's responses to stimuli in objective terms. The Glasgow coma scale also provides a standardized tool that aids in assessing a comatose patient and eliminates the use of ambiguous and easily misinterpreted terms such as "unconscious" and "semicomatose." Additional assessment data should include evaluation of the gag and corneal reflexes. Abnormal rigidity and posturing in response to noxious stimuli indicate deep coma.

The definitive treatment of altered states of consciousness requires removing, correcting, or halting the specific process responsible for the state to whatever degree possible. Often, accurate diagnosis and specific therapy require time, and the first priority is to protect the brain from permanent damage.

General treatment measures that apply to all patients include the following: assurance of an adequate airway passage and oxygenation; maintenance of proper circulation; intravenous administration of glucose or thiamine if the patient is undernourished; any measures necessary to stop generalized seizures; the restoration of the blood acid-base and osmolar balance; the treatment of any detected infection; the treatment and control of extreme body temperatures; the administration of specific antidotes for situations such as drug overdoses; control of agitation; and the protection of the corneas.

In the absence of the gag reflex, regurgitation and aspiration are potential problems. Tube feeding, if necessary, must be done slowly and with the head of the bed raised during the feeding and for about half an hour later. Absence of the corneal reflex can inhibit blinking and natural moistening of the eye. The cornea cannot be allowed to dry, since blindness can result; therefore, artificial tears are instilled in the eyes to keep them moist.

Once the cause leading to the comatose state has been determined, the appropriate steps should be taken to minimize or eliminate it whenever possible. For many causes of coma, rapid intervention and treatment can mean recuperation for the patient, such as in the cases of diabetes, removable hematomas, and drug overdose.

Comatose patients are predisposed to all the hazards of immobility, including impairment of skin integrity and the development of ulcers, contractures and joint disabilities, problems related to respiratory and circulatory status, and alterations in fluid and electrolyte balance. All these factors must be taken into consideration when dealing with the comatose patient.

The outcome from severe medical coma depends on its cause and, with the exception of depressant drug poisoning, on the initial severity and extent of neurologic damage. Depressant drug poisoning reflects a state of general anesthesia, and, barring severe complications, almost all patients who survive drug intoxication can recover physically unscathed.

The clinical tests most valuable for estimating the capacity for recovery after medical coma are identical to those used in making the initial diagnosis. Within a few hours or days after the onset of coma, many patients show neurologic signs that can differentiate, with a high probability, the future extremes of either no improvement or the capacity for good recovery. After a period of about six hours (except for patients on drugs), certain neurological findings begin to correlate with the potential for neurologic recovery and can predict the outcome of about one-third of patients who will do badly. By the end of the first day, tests can predict the two-thirds of the patients who will do well. With each successive day, the signs develop greater predictive power. Persistence of coma in an adult for more than four weeks is almost never associated with later complete recovery.

Perspective and Prospects

Attempts to define *coma* must give at least brief consideration to the concepts of consciousness. Consciousness involves not only the reception of stimuli but also the emotional implications of such stimuli, as well as the construction of intricate mental images.

Since the days of the ancient Greeks, people have known that normal conscious behavior depends on intact brain function and that disorders of consciousness are a sign of cerebral insufficiency. The range of awake and intelligent behavior is so rich and variable, however, that clinical abnormalities are difficult to recognize unless there are substantial deviations from the norm. Impaired, reduced, or absent conscious behavior implies the presence of severe brain dysfunction and demands urgent attention if recovery is to be expected. The brain can tolerate only a limited amount of physical or metabolic injury without suffering irreparable harm, and the longer the failure lasts, the narrower the margin between recovery and the development of permanent neurologic invalidism.

Since such researchers as Pierre Mollaret and Maurice Goulon first examined the question in 1959, many others have tried to establish criteria that would accurately and unequivocally determine that the brain is dead, or about to die no matter what therapeutic measures one undertakes. In 1968, the Harvard Medical School Ad Hoc Committee to Examine the Definition of Brain Death established criteria for determining irreversible coma, or brain death. These criteria are often used to complement the traditional criteria for determining death. All other existing guidelines, such as the Swedish, British, and United States Collaborative Study Criteria, include nearly identical clinical points but contain some differences as to the duration of observation necessary to establish the diagnosis as well as the emphasis to be placed on laboratory procedures in diagnosis.

Techniques such as computed tomography (CT) scanning and electroencephalography (EEG) have transformed the process of diagnosis in clinical neurology, with technology sometimes replacing clinical deduction. The art of diagnosis, however, is to comprehend the whole picture—where the lesion is, what it comprises, and above all, what it is doing to the patient.

Advances in resuscitative medicine have made obsolete the traditional clinical definition of death, that is, the cessation of heartbeat. Cardiac resuscitation can salvage patients after periods of asystole lasting up to several minutes. Cardiopulmonary bypass machines permit the patient's heartbeat to cease for several hours with full clinical recovery after resuscitation. While respiratory depression formerly meant death within minutes, modern mechanical ventilators can maintain pulmonary oxygen exchange indefinitely. Such advances have permitted many patients with formerly lethal cardiac, pulmonary, and neuromuscular disease to return to relatively full and useful lives. Abundant clinical evidence, however, demonstrates that severe damage to the brain can completely destroy the organ's vital functions and capacity to recover, even when the other parts of the body still live. The result has been to switch the emphasis in defining death to a cessation of brain function. Brain death occurs when brain damage is so extensive that the organ has no potential for recovery and cannot maintain the body's internal functions. Countries worldwide have adopted the principle that death occurs when either the brain or the heart irreversibly fails in its functions. In the United States, the time of brain death has been accepted as the time of the person's death in legal terms.

The determination of whether a comatose patient is brain-dead or can possibly recuperate is extremely important. Issues such as organ transplant programs that require donation of healthy organs and the economic and emotional expense involved in the treatment and care of a comatose patient make it critical to know when to fight for life and when to diagnose death.

In carrying out the many details of the physical care and assessment of the comatose patient, health care personnel must not lose sight of the fact that the patient is a fellow human being and a member of a family. One cannot always be sure exactly how much the patients are aware of what is being said or done as care is given. Whatever the level of awareness and response, comatose patients should be told what will be done to and for them, as they deserve the same respect afforded alert and aware patients.

—*Maria Pacheco, Ph.D.*

See also Concussion; Death and dying; Ethics; Euthanasia; Unconsciousness.

For Further Information:

Bongard, Frederick, and Darryl Y. Sue, eds. *Current Critical Care Diagnosis and Treatment*. 2d ed. New York: Lange Medical Books/McGraw-Hill, 2002. A medical text that combines medical and surgical perspectives with diagnostic and treatment knowledge. Covers forty topics in critical care basics, medical critical care, and essentials of surgical intensive care and includes information on pregnancy, psychiatric disorders, imaging procedures, and transport, among other topics.

Goldman, Lee, and Dennis Ausiello, eds. *Cecil Textbook of Medicine*. 22d ed. Philadelphia: W. B. Saunders, 2004. Offers in-depth coverage of numerous medical conditions and a comprehensive presentation of the comatose state. The discussion is technical, however, and requires a good science background.

Leikin, Jerrold B., and Martin S. Lipsky, eds. *American Medical Association Complete Medical Encyclopedia*. New York: Random House Reference, 2003. A concise presentation of numerous medical terms and illnesses. A very good general reference.

Miller, Benjamin F., Claire Brackman Keane, and Marie T. O'Toole. *Miller-Keane Encyclopedia and Dictionary of Medicine, Nursing, and Allied Health*. Rev. 7th ed. Philadelphia: W. B. Saunders, 2005. Contains a concise presentation of the topic of coma.

Plum, Fred, and J. B. Posner. *The Diagnosis of Stupor and Coma*. 3d ed. New York: Oxford University Press, 2000. An excellent book dealing in detail with the diagnosis, treatment, and management of the comatose patient. Well organized and easy to read, it also includes an excellent bibliography for individuals who are interested in more specific presentations of the topic.

Ropper, Alan H., et al. *Neurological and Neurosurgical Intensive Care*. 4th ed. Philadelphia: Lippincott Williams & Wilkins, 2004. Covers a range of topics related to neurologic injury, including comas, head injury, myasthenia, electrophysiologic monitoring, and metabolic derangements.

Common cold

Disease/disorder

Anatomy or system affected: Chest, lungs, nose, respiratory system

Specialties and related fields: Family medicine, internal medicine, otorhinolarnygology, public health, virology

Definition: A class of viral respiratory infections that form the world's most prevalent illnesses.

Key terms:

acute: referring to a disease process of sudden onset and short duration

chronic: referring to a disease process of long duration and frequent recurrence
coronavirus: a microorganism causing respiratory illness; one of the most prevalent causes of the common cold
pathogen: any disease-causing microorganism
rhinovirus: a microorganism causing respiratory illness; one of the most prevalent causes of the common cold
virus: an extremely small pathogen that can replicate only within a living cell

Information on Common Cold

Causes: Viral infection
Symptoms: Fatigue, runny or congested nose, muscle aches, sore throat, coughing, fever
Duration: Typically several days
Treatments: Bed rest, limiting physical stress, alleviation of symptoms via medications (antihistamines, decongestants, analgesics, cough medicines, etc.)

Causes and Symptoms

One of the reasons that no cure has ever been found for the common cold is that it is caused by literally hundreds of different viruses. More than two hundred distinct strains from eight genera have been identified, and no doubt more will be discovered. Infection by one of these viruses may confer immunity to it, but there will still be scores of others to which that individual is not immune. The common cold is usually restricted to the nose and surrounding areas— hence its medical name, rhinitis (*rhin-* meaning "nose" and *-itis* meaning "inflammation").

Children get the most colds, averaging six to eight per year until they are six years old. From that age, the number diminishes until, for adults, the rate is three to five colds per year. Colds and related respiratory diseases are the largest single cause of lost workdays and school days. Colds and related respiratory diseases are probably the world's most expensive illnesses. In the United States, about a million and a half person-years are lost from work each year; this figure accounts for one-half of all absences. Worldwide, the costs of lost workdays, medications, physician's visits, and the complications that may require extensive medical care are incalculable.

Among the virus types that cause the common cold are rhinovirus, coronavirus, influenza virus, parainfluenza virus, enterovirus, adenovirus, respiratory syncytial virus, and coxsackie virus. They are not all equally responsible for cold infections. Rhinoviruses and coronaviruses between them are thought to cause 25 to 60 percent of all colds. Rhinoviruses appear to be responsible for colds that occur in the peak cold seasons of late spring and early fall. Coronaviruses appear to be responsible for colds that occur when rhinovirus is less active, such as in the late fall, winter, and early spring.

A respiratory syncytial virus can cause the common cold in adults; in children it causes much more severe diseases, including pneumonia and bronchiolitis (inflammation of the bronchioles, small air passages in the lungs). Similarly, influenza and parainfluenza viruses, adenoviruses, and enteroviruses can be responsible for rhinitis and sore throat, but they are also capable of causing more serious illnesses such as pneumonia and influenza.

Viruses are the smallest of the invading microorganisms that cause disease, so small that they are not visible using ordinary microscopes. They can be seen, however, with an electron microscope, and their presence in the body can be detected through various laboratory tests.

Viruses vary enormously in their size and structure. Some consist of three or four proteins with a core of either deoxyribonucleic acid (DNA) or ribonucleic acid (RNA); some have more than fifty proteins and other substances. Viruses can replicate only within living cells. They invade the body and produce disease conditions in different ways. Some travel through the body to find their target host cells. A good example is the measles virus, which enters through the mucous membranes of the nose, throat, and mouth and then finds its way to target tissues throughout the body. Some, such as the viruses that cause the common cold, enter the body through the nasal passages and settle directly into nearby cells.

Rhinoviruses are members of the Picornaviridae family (*pico-* from "piccolo," meaning "very small"; *rna* from RNA, the genetic material that it contains; and *viridae* denoting a virus family). Coronaviruses are members of the Coronaviridae family, and they also contain RNA. Most viruses that are pathogenic to humans can thrive only at the temperature inside the human body, 37 degrees Celsius (98.6 degrees Fahrenheit). Rhinoviruses prefer the cooler temperatures found in the nasal passages, 33 to 34 degrees Celsius

(91.4 to 93.2 degrees Fahrenheit). More than one hundred different rhinovirus types have been identified.

Exactly how a patient contracts a cold is better understood than it once was. Exposure to a cold environment—for example, getting a chill in winter weather—does not cause a cold unless the individual is exposed to the infecting virus at the same time. Fatigue or lack of sleep does not increase susceptibility to the cold virus, and even the direct exposure of nasal tissue to cold viruses does not guarantee infection.

A group in England, the Medical Research Council's Common Cold Unit, studied the disease from 1945 to 1990 and made many fundamental discoveries—even though the researchers never found a cure, or, for that matter, any effective methods to prevent the spread of the disease. As part of their research, they put drops containing cold virus into the noses of volunteers. Only about one-third of the subjects thus inoculated developed cold symptoms, showing that direct exposure to the infecting agent does not necessarily bring on a cold.

What appears to be essential in the spread of the disease is bodily contact, particularly handshaking or touching. The infected individual wipes his or her nose or coughs into his or her hand, getting nasal secretions on the fingers. These infected secretions are then transferred to the hand of another person who, if susceptible, can become infected by bringing the hand up to the mouth or nose. Sneezing and coughing also spread the disease. Many viral and bacterial diseases are transmissible through nasopharyngeal (nose and throat) secretions; these include measles, mumps, rubella, pneumonia, influenza, and any number of other infections.

One or more individuals in a group become infected and bring the disease to a central place, such as a classroom, office, military base, or day care center. In the case of the common cold, transferring infected particles by touch exposes another person to the infection. In other respiratory diseases, breathing, sneezing, or coughing virus-laden particles into the air will spread the disease. The infected individual then becomes the means by which the disease is brought into the home. By far, the largest number of colds are brought into the family by children who have contracted the infection in classrooms or day care centers.

The pathogenesis of the common cold—that is, what happens when an individual is exposed to the cold virus—is not fully understood. It is believed that the virus enters the nasal passages and attaches itself to receptors on a cell of the nasal mucous membrane and then invades the cell. Viruses traveling freely in the blood or lymphatic system are subject to attack by white blood cells called phagocytes in what is part of the body's nonspecific defense system against invading pathogens.

Once inside the host cell, the virus replicates itself by stealing elements of the protoplasm of the cell and using them to build new viruses under the direction of the RNA component. These new viruses are released by the host cell to infect other cells. This process can injure or kill the host cell, activating the body's specific immune response system and starting the chain of events that will destroy the invading virus and create immunity to further infection from it.

In response to cell death or injury, certain chemicals are released that induce inflammation in the nasal passages. Blood vessels in the nasal area enlarge, increasing blood flow to the tissues and causing swelling. The openings in capillary walls enlarge and deliver lymphocytes, white blood cells that produce antibodies to fight the virus, as well as other specialized white blood cells.

Nasal mucosa swell and secretions increase, a condition medically known as rhinorrhea (*-rrhea* meaning "flowing," denoting the runny nose of the common cold). During the first few days of infection, these secretions are thin and watery. As the disease progresses and white blood cells are drawn to the area, the secre-

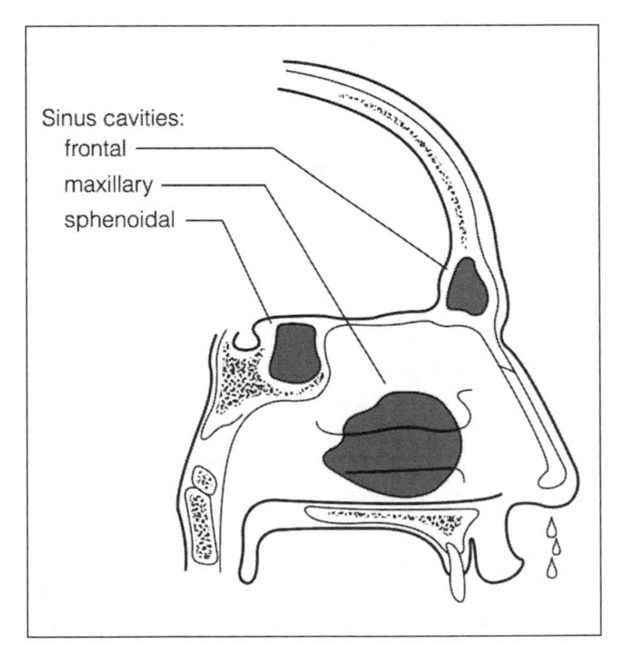

The sinus cavities typically become congested with mucus as the body fights the virus that has caused the cold.

tions become thicker and more purulent, that is, filled with pus. A sore throat is common, as is laryngitis, or inflammation of the larynx or voice box. Fever is not a usual symptom of the common cold, but a cough will often develop as excess mucus or phlegm builds up in the lungs and windpipe.

As mucus accumulates and clogs nasal passages, the body attempts to expel it by sneezing. In this process, impulses from the nose travel to the brain's "sneeze reflex center," where sneezing is triggered to help clear nasal passages. Similarly, as phlegm accumulates in the windpipe and bronchial tree of the lungs, a message is sent to the "cough reflex center" of the brain, where coughing is initiated to expel the phlegm.

The common cold is self-limiting and usually resolves within five to ten days, but there can be complications in some cases. Patients who have asthma or chronic bronchitis frequently develop bronchoconstriction (narrowing of the air passages in the lungs) as a result of a common cold. If severe purulent tracheitis and bronchitis develop, there may be a concomitant bacterial infection. In some patients, the infection may spread to other organs, such as the ears, where an infection called otitis media can develop. Sinusitis, infection of the cavities in the bone of the skull surrounding the nose, is common. If the invading organism spreads to the lungs, bronchitis or pneumonia may develop.

Other possible complications of the common cold depend on the individual virus. Rhinoviruses, usually limited to colds, may infrequently cause pneumonia in children. Coronaviruses, also usually limited to colds, infrequently cause pneumonia and bronchiolitis. A respiratory syncytial virus causes pneumonia and bronchiolitis in children, the common cold in adults, and pneumonia in the elderly. Parainfluenza virus, which causes croup and other respiratory diseases in children, can cause sore throat and the common cold in adults and, rarely, may cause tracheobronchitis in these patients. Influenza B virus, an occasional cause of the common cold, also causes influenza and, infrequently, pneumonia.

Another condition that can closely resemble the common cold, but which is not caused by a virus, is allergic rhinitis. The major form of allergic rhinitis is hay fever. It has many of the same symptoms as the common cold: sneezing, runny nose, nasal congestion, and, sometimes, sore throat. In addition, the hay fever victim may suffer from itching in the eyes, nose, mouth, and throat. Hay fever is an allergic reaction to certain pollens. Because the pollens that cause hay fever are abundant at certain times of the year, it may be prevalent at the same times as some colds. Spring is a peak season for the common cold and also for hay fever, because of the many tree pollens that are carried in the air. In the fall, weed pollens, such as those of ragweed, affect hay fever sufferers during another peak period for colds. Colds occur less frequently in summer, but summer is another peak season for hay fever.

Treatment and Therapy

The nose is the first barrier of defense against the bacteria and viruses that cause upper respiratory infections. The nasal cavity is lined with a thin coating of mucus, a thick liquid that is constantly replenished by the mucous glands. Inner nasal surfaces are filled with tiny hairs, or cilia. Dust, bacteria, and other foreign matter are trapped by the mucus and moved by the cilia toward the nasopharynx to be expectorated or swallowed.

The blood vessels in the nasopharyngeal bed respond automatically to stimulation from the brain. Certain stimuli cause the vessels to constrict, widening air passages and at the same time reducing the flow of mucus. Other stimuli, such as those that are sent in response to a viral infection, allergen, or other irritant, cause blood vessels to dilate and increase the flow of mucus. Nasal passages become swollen, and airways are blocked.

The mucus-covered lining of the nasal passages contains various substances that help ward off infection and irritation by allergens. Lysozyme (*lyso-* meaning "dissolution" and *-zyme* from "enzyme," a catalyst that promotes an activity) attacks the cell walls of certain bacteria, killing them. It also attacks pollen granules. Mucus also contains glycoproteins that temporarily inhibit the activity of viruses. Mucus has small amounts of the antibodies immunoglobulin IgA and IgC that also may inhibit the activity of invading viruses.

Bed rest is usually the first element of treatment. Limiting physical stress may help keep the cold from worsening and may avoid secondary infections. The medications used to treat the common cold are directed at relieving individual symptoms: There is nothing available that will kill the viruses that cause it. Most cases of the common cold are treated at home with over-the-counter cold preparations. Children's colds and the complications that may arise from colds, such as bacterial and viral superinfection, may require the services of a physician.

Many medications for the common cold contain antihistamines. Histamine is a naturally occurring chemical in the body that is released in response to an allergen or an infection. It is a significant cause of the inflammation, swelling, and runny nose of hay fever. When these symptoms are seen with the common cold, however, they are probably caused by the body's inflammatory defense system rather than by histamine.

When antihistamines were first discovered, it was thought that they could inhibit the inflammatory defense against a cold. Patients were advised to take antihistamines at the first sign of a cold, in the hope of avoiding a full infection. Current thinking is that antihistamines have little value in the treatment of the common cold. They may have a minor effect on a runny nose, but there are better agents for this purpose. Antihistamines are usually highly sedative—most over-the-counter sleeping pills are antihistamines—so they may cause drowsiness. Patients taking many antihistamines are cautioned to avoid driving or operating machinery that could be dangerous.

The mainstays of therapy for the common cold are the decongestants that are applied topically (that is, directly to the mucous membranes in the nose) or taken orally. They are also called sympathomimetic agents because they mimic the effects of certain natural body chemicals that regulate many body processes. A group of these, called adrenergic stimulants, regulate vasoconstriction and vasodilation—in other words, they can narrow or widen blood vessels, respectively. Their vasoconstrictive capability is useful in managing the common cold, because it reduces the size of the blood vessels in the nose, reduces swelling and congestion, and inhibits excess secretion.

Topical decongestants are available as nasal sprays or drops. The sprays are squirted up into each nostril. The patient is usually advised to wait three to five minutes and then blow his or her nose to remove the mucus. If there is still congestion, the patient is advised to take another dose, allowing the medication to reach further into the nasal cavity. Nose drops are taken by tilting the head back and squeezing the medication into the nostrils through the nose-dropper supplied with the medication. Clearance of nasal congestion is prompt, and the patient can breathe more easily. Nasal irritation is reduced, so there is less sneezing. Some nasal sprays and drops last longer than others, but none works around-the-clock, so applications must be repeated throughout the day.

Patients who use nasal sprays and drops are advised to follow the manufacturer's directions exactly. Applied too often or in too great a quantity, these preparations can cause unwanted problems, such as rhinitis medicamentosa, or nasal inflammation caused by a medication (also called rebound congestion). As the vasoconstrictive effect of the drugs wears down, the blood vessels dilate, the area becomes swollen, and secretions increase. This reaction may be attributable to the fact that the drug's vasoconstrictive effect has deprived the area of blood, and thus excited an increased inflammatory state, or it may simply be attributable to irritation by the drug. Use of sprays or drops should be limited to three or four days.

Oral decongestants are also effective in reducing swelling and relieving a runny nose, although they do not have as great a vasoconstrictive effect concentrated in the nasal area as sprays or drops. Because they circulate throughout the body, their vasoconstrictive effects may be seen in other vascular beds. There are many patients who are warned not to use oral decongestants unless they are under the care of a physician. These people include patients with high blood pressure, diabetics, heart patients, and patients taking certain drugs such as monoamine oxidase (MAO) inhibitors, guanethidine, bethanidine, or debrisoquin sulfate.

Three kinds of coughs may accompany colds: coughs that produce phlegm or mucus; hyperactive nagging coughs, which result from overstimulation of the cough reflex; and dry, unproductive coughs. If the phlegm or mucus collecting in the lungs is easily removed by occasional coughing, a soothing syrup, cough drop, or lozenge may be all that the patient requires. If the cough reflex center of the brain is overstimulated, there may be hyperactive or uncontrollable coughing and a cough suppressant, such as dextromethorphan, may be needed. Dextromethorphan works in the brain to raise the level of stimulus that is required to trigger the cough reflex. Some antihistamines, such as diphenhydramine hydrochloride, are effective cough suppressants. If coughing is unproductive—that is, if the mucus has thickened and dried and is not easily removed—an expectorant should be taken. Currently, the only expectorant used in over-the-counter drugs is guaifenesin. It helps soften and liquefy mucus deposits, so that coughs become productive. When a cough of a cold is serious enough for a physician to be consulted, prescription drugs may have to be used, such as codeine to stop hyperactive coughing and potassium iodide for unproductive coughs.

For allergic rhinitis or hay fever, avoidance of allergens is recommended but is not always possible. For hay fever outbreaks, antihistamines are the mainstays of therapy, with other agents added to relieve specific symptoms. For example, topical and oral decongestants may be required to relieve a runny nose.

Perspective and Prospects

Viruses are among the most intriguing and baffling challenges to medical science. Great progress has been made in preventing some virus diseases, such as by immunization against smallpox and hepatitis B. There has been only limited success, however, in finding agents to cure viral diseases, and so far nothing has been found to prevent or cure the common cold. Vaccines have been developed against certain rhinoviruses, and no doubt many more could be developed. Yet because the common cold is caused by so many different types of virus—more than two hundred—and vaccines against one virus are not necessarily effective against others, it is questionable whether such vaccines would ever be useful. A helpful vaccine would be one that could immunize against an entire family of viruses such as rhinoviruses or coronaviruses, the two leading causes of the common cold.

The search goes on for agents to cure the common cold. Substances, such as interferons, have been found that are effective against a wide range of viruses. One of the interferons was used by the British Medical Research Council's Common Cold Unit. Those researchers reported that interferon applied as an intranasal spray was highly effective in protecting subjects from cold infection. After some years, however, experimentation with interferon in the common cold was abandoned because the agent had significant side effects, nasal congestion among them.

The science of virology only began in the 1930's, so it is not surprising that viruses continue to hide their mysteries. Nevertheless, many fundamental discoveries have been made and one can predict increasing success. As scientists unravel the intricacies of viral infections, they find clues that help them devise ways of interfering with virus life processes. In some cases, effective drugs have been developed, such as the interferons, acyclovir for herpes simplex, and amantadine for the influenza virus. It is likely that the cure for the common cold will continue to be elusive, unless a broad-spectrum antiviral agent could be developed that works against multiple viral infections in the way that broad-spectrum antibiotics work against multiple bacterial infections.

—C. Richard Falcon

See also Allergies; Antihistamines; Bronchitis; Coughing; Decongestants; Fever; Influenza; Nasopharyngeal disorders; Nausea and vomiting; Noroviruses; Otorhinolarnygology; Pneumonia; Sinusitis; Sore throat; Viral infections.

For Further Information:

American Pharmaceutical Association. *Handbook of Nonprescription Drugs*. 13th ed. Washington, D.C.: Author, 2002. The section on drugs for colds, coughs, and allergies contains a thorough background discussion of these conditions. All major over-the-counter medications are listed.

Biddle, Wayne. *A Field Guide to Germs*. 2d ed. New York: Anchor Books, 2002. This comprehensive book is easily accessible to the nonspecialist and includes a discussion of nearly every virus, bacterium, and fungus known to cause human and nonhuman animal disease. The history of the microbe and the treatment of diseases are included.

Gallo, Robert. *Virus Hunting*. New York: Basic Books, 1991. Gallo gives a good general account of viruses—how they live and how modern medical science is trying to combat them.

Kimball, Chad. *Colds, Flu, and Other Common Ailments*. Detroit: Omnigraphics, 2002. A comprehensive guide for general readers covering treatment issues and controversies surrounding common ailments and injuries. Includes discussions on ailments of the nose, throat, lungs, ears, eyes, and head; common injuries; alternative therapies; choosing a doctor; and buying drugs and finding health information online.

Litin, Scott C., ed. *Mayo Clinic Family Health Book*. 3d ed. New York: HarperResource, 2003. One of the most thorough and accessible medical texts for the layperson.

Woolf, Alan D., et al., eds. *The Children's Hospital Guide to Your Child's Health and Development*. Cambridge, Mass.: Perseus, 2002. An authoritative and comprehensive guide to children's health, providing a guide to every common illness or condition that affects children and a carefully designed emergency section.

Young, Stuart H., Bruce S. Dobozin, and Margaret Miner. *Allergies*. Rev. ed. New York: Plume, 1999. A useful book that covers the treatment of allergic coldlike conditions, such as hay fever, and gives advice on how to manage them.

Computed tomography (CT) scanning

Procedure

Also known as: Computed axial tomography, CAT scan

Anatomy or system affected: Circulatory system, endocrine system, gastrointestinal system, musculoskeletal system, nervous system, reproductive system, respiratory system

Specialties and related fields: Biotechnology, cardiology, emergency medicine, endocrinology, gastroenterology, internal medicine, oncology, preventive medicine, psychiatry, radiology, vascular medicine

Definition: The use of X rays and a computer to produce detailed cross-sectional images of most body regions to aid in diagnosis.

Key terms:

cathode: an electrode that produces electrons

cathode-ray tube (CRT): a vacuum tube whose cathode emits electrons accelerated through a high voltage anode, focused on a fluorescent image screen

slice: a CT cross section of a body part

soft tissue: tissue other than bone

tomogram: the three-dimensional image of a CT slice

X ray: high-energy electromagnetic radiation

Indications and Procedures

Computed tomography (CT) scanning collects X-ray data and uses a computer to produce three-dimensional images, called tomograms, of body cross sections, or slices. The noninvasiveness of CT scanning yields easy and safe body part analysis based on varying tissue opacity to X rays. Bone absorbs X rays well and appears white. Air absorbs them poorly, so the lungs are dark. Fat, blood, and muscle absorb X rays to varying extents, yielding different shades of gray. Tumors and blood clots, for example, appear as areas of abnormal shades in normal tissue.

CT scanning is used to analyze disorders of the brain (brain CT) and most body parts (body CT), yielding tomograms that are hundreds of times more definitive than conventional X rays. For example, conventional abdominal X rays show bones and faintly outline the liver, kidneys, and stomach. Tomograms clearly depict all abdominal organs and large blood vessels.

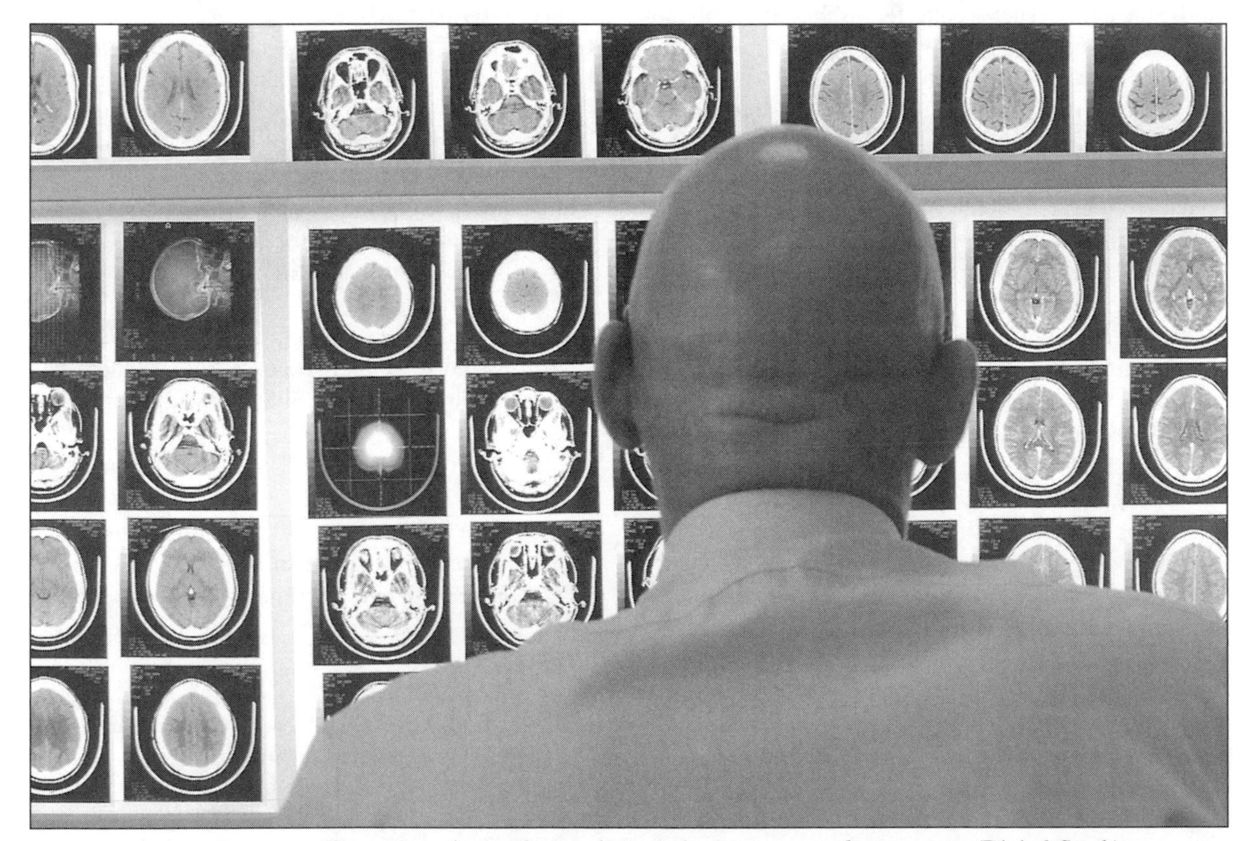

A doctor can use CT scans to detect abnormalities in brain tissue, such as tumors. (Digital Stock)

Physicians call CT scanning the most valuable diagnostic method because, without it, the symptoms that patients describe may not be identified clearly as minor, serious, or life-threatening. For example, a subjective description of repeated headache does not reveal whether the cause is tension, stroke, or brain cancer. Before CT scanning, an accurate diagnosis often required complex or dangerous identification methods.

A CT patient changes into a hospital gown, removes any metal possessions, and lays on a table that can be raised, lowered, or tilted. During a scan, the patient enters a doughnut-shaped scanner that holds an X-ray source, detectors, and computer hookups. In brain CT, the patient's head is in the scanner. Some CT patients have experienced claustrophobia, which can be prevented with faster scanner speeds and less-enclosed scanners. A patient who must stay still for an extended time may be given a sedative. If small anomalies are foreseen, then contrast materials are given before or during the procedure. These materials include barium salts and iodine, X-ray blockers that allow better visualization of specific tissues. Subjects may take the materials orally, by enema, or intravenously.

The CT scanner generates a continuous, narrow X-ray beam while moving 360 degrees around the patient's head or body. The beam is monitored by X-ray detectors sited around the aperture through which the patient passes. Slices are produced as the scanner circles the head or body. Between slices, the table moves through the scanner. Slices become tomograms seen on a CRT and are stored in the computer. The procedure takes twenty to forty minutes in a standard scanner.

In newer spiral CT, a patient is scanned rapidly as the X-ray tube rotates in a spiral. There are no gaps as with slices, and tissue-volume tomograms are produced. A simple spiral scan is completed while the patient holds a breath, aiding the detection of small lesions and decreasing scan artifacts. Spiral CT, twenty times faster than standard CT, is very useful with restless children and critically ill patients. Its slip-ring electrotechnology precludes the need, in standard scanners, to reset after one 360-degree scan before another scan is possible.

USES AND COMPLICATIONS

CT scanning detects organ abnormalities, and a major use is in diagnosing and treating brain disease. Even the earliest scanners could distinguish tumors from clots, aiding in the diagnosis of cancer, stroke, and certain birth defects. Furthermore, brain CT saves lives as physicians avoid risky methods requiring opening of the brain for pretreatment diagnosis. In addition, postsurgical scans can find recurrences or metastases.

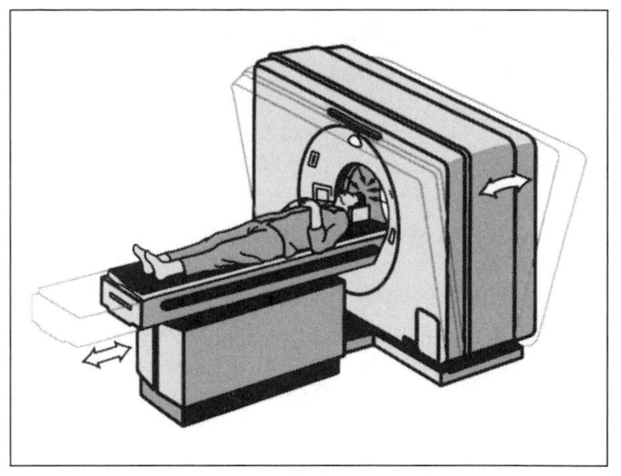

In the imaging technique called computed tomography (CT) scanning (formerly known as a CAT scan), multiple X-ray pictures are taken as the scanner tilts and rotates around the patient. These images are then assembled by a computer to create a three-dimensional view of a body part, such as the head.

Body CT allows for better damage appraisal of broken bones than does conventional X-ray analysis. Another use of body spiral CT is in the diagnosis of pulmonary embolism; it is safer than using pulmonary angiography, which maneuvers a catheter from the heart to the pulmonary artery. CT scans can also guide surgery, biopsy, and abscess drainage and can help fine-tune radiation therapy. Speed and excellent soft tissue elucidation make CT scanning invaluable for trauma detection in emergency rooms.

There are few side effects to CT scanning. Preparation for a scan may be mildly uncomfortable, but it is rarely dangerous. Before body CT, subjects often fast, take enemas to clear the bowels, and receive contrast materials through enemas or IVs. If contrast materials are used, then physicians must be told of allergies, especially to iodine. Contrast materials—enhancers of specific tissue CT—may cause hot flashes. Barium enemas for lower gastrointestinal tract scans cause full feelings and urges to defecate.

PERSPECTIVE AND PROSPECTS

British engineer Godfrey Hounsfeld and American physicist Alan Cormack won the 1979 Nobel Prize in Physiology or Medicine for the theory and development of computed tomography. CT scanning was first used in 1972, after Hounsfeld made a brain scanner holding an X-ray generator, a scanner rotated around a circular chamber, a computer, and a CRT. The patient laid on a gurney, head in the scanner, and emitter detectors rotated 1 degree at a time for 180 degrees. At each position, 160 readings entered the computer, so 28,800 readings were processed.

CT scanning is essential to radiology, which began in 1885 after Wilhelm Conrad Röntgen discovered X rays. The rays soon became medical aids, and for years broad X-ray beams were sent through body parts to exit onto film, yielding conventional X-ray images. Bones absorb X rays well, appearing white, and conventional images can show bone fractures and give some soft tissue data. However, soft tissue evaluation is poor, the tissues superimpose, and estimating their condition is difficult. CT scans allow convenient, noninvasive analysis.

CT scans and stereotaxic neurosurgery, later joined, have improved diagnosis and treatment. For example, the implantation of electrodes in a brain can be monitored using CT, enhancing accuracy. Similar techniques are used in breast biopsy. Current progress in CT scans includes thinner slices, spiral scans, and fast-operating standard scanners. Because complex scans expose patients to more radiation than do conventional X rays, fast scans are preferred to minimize patient risk.

—Sanford S. Singer, Ph.D.

See also Brain; Brain disorders; Headaches; Imaging and radiology; Magnetic resonance imaging (MRI); Neuroimaging; Noninvasive tests; Nuclear medicine; Positron emission tomography (PET) scanning; Strokes; Tumors; Ultrasonography.

For Further Information:

Durham, Deborah L. *Rad Tech's Guide to CT: Imaging Procedures, Patient Care, and Safety*. Malden, Mass.: Blackwell Scientific, 2002. Contains useful information for CT technicians and general readers.

Hsieh, Jiang. *Computed Tomography: Principles, Design, Artifacts, and Recent Advances*. Bellingham, Wash.: SPIE Press, 2003. Illustrated. Covers the title issues and provides an index and a bibliography.

Kalender, Willi A. *Computed Tomography: Fundamentals, System Technology, Image Quality, Applications*. 2d rev. ed. Erlangen, Germany: Publicis, 2005. Covers history and principles, spiral CT, applications, and future prospects. Illustrated and indexed, with a bibliography.

Slone, Richard M., et al., eds. *Body CT: A Practical Approach*. New York: McGraw-Hill, 2000. Covers CT techniques and protocols for many tissues. Illustrated. Contains a bibliography and an index.

Conception

Biology

Anatomy or system affected: Cells, reproductive system, uterus

Specialties and related fields: Embryology, gynecology, obstetrics

Definition: The process of creating new life, encompassing all the events from deposition of sperm into the female to the first cell divisions of the fertilized ovum.

Key terms:

cervix: the lowest part of the uterus in contact with the vagina; contains an opening filled with mucus through which sperm can pass

ejaculation: the reflex activated by sexual stimulation that results in sperm mixed with fluid being expelled from the male's body

fertilization: the union of the sperm and the ovum, which usually occurs in the female's oviduct

menstruation: the process of shedding the lining of the uterus that occurs about once a month

oviduct: the thin tube that leads from near the ovary to the upper part of the uterus; also called the Fallopian tube

ovulation: the process by which the mature ovum is expelled from the ovary

ovum: the round cell produced by the female that carries her genetic material; also called the egg

sperm: the motile cells produced within the male that carry his genetic material

uterus: the organ above the vagina through which the sperm must pass on their way to the ovum; also called the womb

vagina: the stretchy, tube-shaped structure into which the male's penis is inserted during intercourse; the site of sperm deposition

Process and Effects

The process of conception begins with the act of intercourse. When the male's penis is inserted into the female's vagina, the stimulation of the penis by movement within the vagina triggers a reflex resulting in the ejaculation of sperm. During ejaculation, involuntary muscles in many of the male reproductive organs contract, causing semen, a mixture of sperm and fluid, to move from its sites of storage out through the urethra within the penis.

The average volume of semen in a typical human ejaculation is only 3.5 milliliters, but this small volume normally contains 200 million to 400 million sperm. Other constituents of semen include prostaglandins, which cause contractions of involuntary muscles in both the male and the female; the sugar fructose, which provides energy to the sperm; chemicals that adjust the activity of the semen; and a number of enzymes and other chemicals.

In a typical act of intercourse, the semen is deposited high up in the woman's vagina. Within a minute after ejaculation, the semen begins to coagulate, or form a clot, because of the activation of chemicals within the semen. Sperm are not able to leave the vagina until the semen becomes liquid again, which occurs spontaneously fifteen to twenty minutes after ejaculation.

Once the semen liquefies, sperm begin moving through the female system. The path to the ovum (if one is present) lies through the cervix, then through the hollow cavity of the uterus, and up through the oviduct, where fertilization normally occurs. The sperm are propelled through the fluid within these organs by the swimming movements of their tails called flagella, as well as by female organ contractions that are stimulated by the act of intercourse and by prostaglandins contained in the semen. It is not necessary for the woman to experience orgasm, a pleasurable climax, in order for these contractions to occur. The contractions allow sperm to reach the oviduct within five minutes after leaving the vagina, a rate of movement that far exceeds their own swimming abilities.

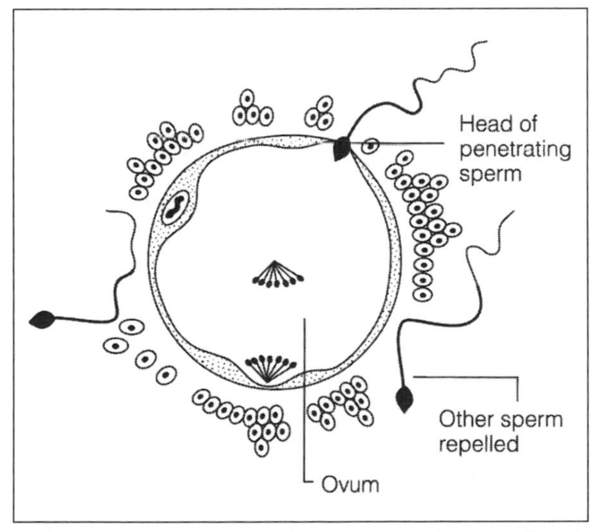

Male sperm cells propel themselves toward the ovum (female egg) by the swimming movements of their tails; fertilization occurs when a sperm cell penetrates the layers surrounding the ovum and fuses its membrane with the membrane of the ovum.

Although some sperm can reach the oviduct quite rapidly, others never enter the oviduct at all. Of the two hundred million to four hundred million sperm deposited in the vagina, it is estimated that only one hundred to one thousand enter the oviducts. Some of the other millions of sperm may be defective, lacking the proper swimming ability. Other apparently normal sperm may become lost within the female's organs, possibly trapped in clefts between cells in the organ linings. The damaged and lost sperm will eventually be destroyed by white blood cells produced by the female.

Sperm movement through the female system is enhanced around the time of ovulation. For example, at the time of ovulation, the hormones associated with ovulation cause changes in the cervical mucus that aid sperm transport. The mucus at that time is extremely liquid and contains fibers that align themselves into channels, which are thought to be used by the sperm to ease their passage through the cervix. The hormones present at the time of ovulation also increase the contractions produced by the uterus and oviduct, and thus sperm transport through the structures is enhanced as well.

During transport through the female, sperm undergo a number of important chemical changes, collectively called capacitation, that enable them to fertilize the ovum successfully. Freshly ejaculated sperm are not capable of penetrating the layers surrounding the ovum, a fact that was uncovered when scientists first began to experiment with in vitro fertilization (the joining of sperm and ovum outside the body). Capacitation apparently occurs during transport of the sperm through the uterus and possibly the oviduct, and it is presumably triggered by some secretion of the female. With in vitro fertilization, capacitation is achieved by adding female blood serum to the dish that contains the sperm and ovum. Capacitation is not instantaneous; it has been estimated that this process requires an hour or more in humans. Even though the first sperm may arrive in the vicinity of the ovum within twenty minutes after ejaculation, fertilization cannot take place until capacitation is completed. In 2003, scientists discovered that sperm has a type of chemical sensor that causes the sperm to swim vigorously toward concentrations of a chemical attractant. While researchers long have known that chemical signals are an important component of conception, the 2003 findings were the first to demonstrate that sperm will respond in a predictable and controllable way, a fact promising for future contraception and infertility research.

The site where ovum and sperm typically come together is within the oviduct. At the time of ovulation, an ovum is released from the surface of the ovary and drawn into the upper end of the oviduct. Once within the oviduct, the ovum is propelled by contractions of the oviduct and possibly by wavelike motions of cilia, hairlike projections that line the inner surface of the oviduct. It takes about three days for the ovum to travel the entire length of the oviduct to the uterus, and since the ovum only remains fertilizable for twelve to twenty-four hours, successful fertilization must occur in the oviduct.

Upon reaching the ovum, the sperm must first penetrate two layers surrounding it. The outermost layer, called the corona radiata, consists of cells that break away from the ovary with the ovum during ovulation; the innermost layer, the zona pellucida, is a clear, jellylike substance that lies just outside the ovum cell membrane. Penetration of these two layers is accomplished by the release of enzymes carried by the sperm. Once through the zona pellucida, the sperm are ready to fertilize the ovum.

Fertilization occurs when a sperm fuses its membrane with the membrane of the ovum. This act triggers a protective change in the zona pellucida that prevents any additional sperm from reaching the ovum and providing it with extra chromosomes. Following fusion of the fertilizing sperm and ovum, the chromosomes of each become mingled and pair up; the resulting one-celled zygote contains a complete set of chromosomes, half contributed by the mother and half by the father.

It is at the moment of fertilization that the sex of the new child is decided. Genetic sex is determined by a pair of chromosomes denoted X and Y. Female body cells contain two X's, and each ovum produced contains only one X. Male body cells contain an X and a Y chromosome, but each sperm contains either an X or a Y chromosome. Men usually produce equal numbers of X- and Y-type sperm. The sex of the new individual is determined by which type of sperm fertilizes the ovum: If it is a Y-bearing sperm, the new individual will be male, and if it is an X-bearing sperm, the new individual will be female. Since entry of more than one sperm is prohibited, the first sperm to reach the ovum is the one that will fertilize it.

Following fertilization, the zygote or early embryo begins a series of cell divisions while it travels down the oviduct. When it arrives at the uterus about three days after ovulation, the zygote will be in the form of a hollow ball of cells called a blastocyte. Initially, this ball of cells floats in the fluid-filled cavity of the uterus, but two or three days after its arrival in the uterus (five to six days after ovulation), it will attach to the uterine lining. Researchers in 2003 made an exciting discovery when they identified how embryos stop and burrow into the lining of a woman's uterus. A protein, called L-selectin, on the surface of the embryo acts like a puzzle piece when it touches and quickly locks to carbohydrate molecules found on the uterine surface. This implantation process must occur in exact synchrony during a very short time in a woman's cycle. (If it occurs outside the uterus, usually in one of the Fallopian tubes, then the result is an ectopic pregnancy, which is often a medical emergency.) Over the next nine months, the body of the embryo will take on a human form and develop the ability to live independently outside the uterus.

Complications and Disorders

Three factors limit the time frame in which conception is possible: the fertilizable lifetime of the ovulated ovum, estimated to be between twelve and twenty-four hours; the fertilizable lifetime of ejaculated sperm in the female tract, usually assumed to be about forty-eight hours; and the time required for sperm capacitation, which is one hour or more. The combination of these factors determines the length of the fertile period, the time during which intercourse must occur if conception is to be achieved. Taking the three factors into account, the fertile period is said to extend from forty-eight hours prior to ovulation until perhaps twenty-four hours after ovulation. For example, if intercourse occurs forty-eight hours before ovulation, the sperm will be capacitated in the first few hours and will still be within their fertilizable lifetime when ovulation occurs. On the other hand, if intercourse occurs twenty-four hours after ovulation, the sperm will still require time for capacitation, but the ovum will be near the end of its viable period. Thus the later limit of the fertile period is equal to the fertilizable lifetime of the ovum, minus the time required for capacitation.

Obviously, a critical factor in conception is the timing of ovulation. In a typical twenty-eight-day menstrual cycle, ovulation occurs about halfway through the cycle, or fourteen days after the first day of menstrual bleeding. In actuality, cycle length varies widely from month to month. It appears that generally the first half of the cycle is more variable in length, with the second half more stable. Thus, no matter how long the entire menstrual cycle is, ovulation usually occurs fourteen days prior to the first day of the next episode of menstrual bleeding. Therefore, it is relatively easy to determine when ovulation occurred by counting backward, but difficult to predict the time of ovulation in advance.

Assessment of ovulation time in women is notoriously difficult. There is no easily observable outward sign of ovulation. Some women do detect slight abdominal pain about the time of ovulation; this is referred to as *Mittelschmerz*, which means, literally, pain in the middle of the cycle. This slight pain may be localized on either side of the abdomen and is thought to be caused by irritation of the abdominal organs by fluid released from the ovary during ovulation. Other signs of ovulation are an increased volume of the cervical mucus and flexibility of the cervix and a characteristic fernlike pattern of the mucus when it is dried on a glass slide. There is also a slight rise in body temperature after ovulation, which again makes it easier to determine the time of ovulation after the fact rather than in advance. It is also possible to measure the amount of luteinizing hormone (LH) in urine or blood; this hormone shows a marked increase about sixteen hours prior to ovulation. Home test kits to detect LH levels are available for urine samples. There are additional signs of the time of ovulation, such as a slight opening of the cervix and a change in the cells lining the vagina, that can be used by physicians to determine the timing and occurrence of ovulation.

Since ovulation time is so difficult to detect in most women on an ongoing basis, most physicians would counsel that, to achieve a pregnancy, couples should plan on having intercourse every two days. This frequency will ensure that sperm capable of fertilization are always present, so that the exact time of ovulation becomes unimportant. A greater frequency of intercourse is not advised, since sperm numbers are reduced when ejaculation occurs often. Approximately 85 to 90 percent of couples will achieve pregnancy within a year when intercourse occurs about three times a week.

Couples often wonder if it is possible to predetermine the sex of their child by some action taken in conjunction with intercourse. Scientists have found no consistent effect of diet, position assumed during intercourse, timing of intercourse within the menstrual cycle, or liquids that are introduced into the vagina to kill one type of sperm selectively. In the laboratory, it is possible to achieve partial separation of sperm in a semen sample by subjecting the semen to an electric current or other procedure due to the physical difference of X- and Y-containing sperm. The separated sperm can then be used for artificial insemination (the introduction of semen through a tube into the uterus). This method is not 100 percent successful in producing offspring of the desired sex and so is available only on an experimental basis.

Some couples have difficulty in conceiving a child, in a few cases as a result of some problem associated with intercourse. For example, the male may have difficulty in achieving erection or ejaculation. The vast majority of these cases are caused by psychological factors such as stress and tension rather than any biological problem. Fortunately, therapists can teach couples how to overcome these psychological problems.

About 15 percent of couples in the United States suffer from some type of biological infertility—that is, infertility that persists when intercourse occurs successfully. In 10 percent of the cases of infertility, doctors are unable to establish a cause. In another 20 percent of couples, both partners are infertile. In the remaining 70 percent of cases, about half the problems are in the male and half in the female.

In men, the most commonly diagnosed cause of infertility is low sperm count. Sometimes low sperm count is caused by a treatable imbalance of hormones. If not treatable, this problem can sometimes be circumvented by the use of pooled semen samples in artificial insemination or through in vitro fertilization. In vitro fertilization may also be a solution for men who produce normal numbers of sperm but whose sperm lack swimming ability. Another cause of male infertility is blockage of the tubes that carry the semen from the body, which may be caused by a previous infection. Surgery is sometimes successful in removing such a blockage.

In women, a common cause of infertility is a hormonal problem that interferes with ovulation. Treatment with one of a number of so-called fertility drugs may be successful in promoting ovulation. Fertility drugs, however, have some disadvantages: They have a tendency to cause ovulation of more than one ovum, thus raising the possibility of multiple pregnancy, which is considered risky; and they may alter the environment of the uterus, making implantation of a resulting embryo less likely.

Another common cause of female infertility is blockage of the oviducts resulting from scar tissue formation in the aftermath of some type of infection. Because surgery is not always successful in opening the oviducts, this condition may require the use of in vitro fertilization or the new technique of surgically introducing ova and sperm directly into the oviduct at a point below the blockage.

Finally, some cases of infertility result from biological incompatibility between the man and the woman. It may be that the sperm are unable to penetrate the cervical mucus, or perhaps that the woman's body treats the sperm cells as foreign, destroying them before they can reach the ovum. Techniques such as artificial insemination and in vitro fertilization offer hope for couples experiencing these problems.

PERSPECTIVE AND PROSPECTS

For most of history, the events surrounding conception were poorly understood. For example, microscopic identification of sperm did not occur until 1677, and the ovum was not identified until 1827 (although the follicle in which the ovum develops was recognized in the 1600's). Prior to these discoveries, people held the belief espoused by early writers such as Aristotle and Galen that conception resulted from the mixing of male and female fluids during intercourse.

There was also confusion about the timing of the fertile period. Some early doctors thought that menstrual blood was involved in conception and therefore believed that the fertile period coincided with menstruation. Others recognized that menstrual bleeding was a sign that pregnancy had not occurred; they assumed that the most likely time for conception to result was immediately after the menstrual flow ceased. It was not until the 1930's that the first scientific studies on the timing of ovulation were completed.

Since there was little scientific understanding of the processes involved in conception, medical practice for most of human history was little different from magic, revolving around the use of rituals and herbal treatments to aid or prevent conception. Gradually, people rejected these practices, often because of religious teachings. By the 1900's, conception had been established as an area of intense privacy, thought by physicians and the general public to be unsuitable for medical intervention.

In the early part of the twentieth century, the role of physicians in aiding conception was mostly limited to educating and advising couples finding difficulty in conceiving. There were few techniques, other than artificial insemination and fertility drug treatment, available to assist in conception at that time.

The situation changed with the first successful in vitro fertilization in 1978. This event ushered in an era of intense medical and public interest in assisting conception. Other methods to aid conception were soon introduced, including embryo transfer, frozen storage of embryos, and surgical placement of ova and sperm directly into the oviduct.

Paralleling the development of these techniques has been demand on the part of society for medicine to apply them. Infertility rates in the United States have been gradually increasing. One reason for increased infertility has been the increasing age at which couples decide to start a family, since the fertility of women appears to undergo a decline past the age of thirty. Another factor affecting fertility rates of both men and women has been an increased incidence of various sexually transmitted diseases, which can result in chronic inflammation of the reproductive organs and infertility caused by scar tissue formation.

People's attitudes toward medical intervention in conception have also changed. The earlier religious taboos against interference in conception have been somewhat relaxed, although some churches still do not approve of certain methods of fertility management. Although there remain ethical issues to be resolved, the general public seems to have accepted the idea that medicine should provide assistance to those who wish to, but cannot, conceive children.

—Marcia Watson-Whitmyre, Ph.D.;
updated by Alexander Sandra, M.D.

See also Assisted reproductive technologies; Childbirth; Cloning; Contraception; Gamete intrafallopian transfer (GIFT); Gynecology; In vitro fertilization; Infertility, female; Infertility, male; Menstruation; Multiple births; Obstetrics; Pregnancy and gestation; Reproductive system; Sperm banks.

FOR FURTHER INFORMATION:

Doherty, C. Maud, and Melanie M. Clark. *Fertility Handbook: A Guide to Getting Pregnant*. Omaha, Nebr.: Addicus Books, 2002. The authors, a reproductive endocrinologist and a former infertility patient, combine their experiences to explore current infertility options and treatments. Addresses the causes, getting diagnoses, choosing a fertility specialist, and utilizing new assisted reproductive technology.

Harkness, Carla. *The Infertility Book: A Comprehensive Medical and Emotional Guide*. Rev 2d ed. Berkeley, Calif.: Celestial Arts, 1992. Presents a comprehensive guide to problems of infertility and combines medical and emotional perspectives. Contains anecdotal accounts in the patients' own words.

Jones, Richard E., and Kristin H. Lopez. *Human Reproductive Biology*. 3d ed. Burlington, Mass.: Elsevier Academic Press, 2006. This college-level textbook provides comprehensive coverage of all biological aspects of human reproduction. There is a separate chapter on fertilization; information on the timing of ovulation, contraception, and infertility treatment is also presented.

Kearney, Brian. *High-Tech Conception: A Comprehensive Handbook for Consumers*. New York: Bantam Books, 1998. An increasing number of specialists are responding to the predicament of childless couples by offering procedures requiring the removal of eggs from the ovaries. Kearney's handbook provides potential high-tech customers with information for critically assessing the potentials and risks of the various techniques.

Weschler, Toni. *Taking Charge of Your Fertility*. Rev. ed. New York: HarperCollins, 2001. An excellent book that encourages women to become responsible for their own reproductive health. Includes discussions of infertility, natural birth control, and achieving pregnancy.

Wisot, Arthur L., and David R. Meldrum. *Conceptions and Misconceptions: The Informed Consumer's Guide Through the Maze of In Vitro Fertilization and Other Assisted Reproduction Techniques*. 2d ed. Point Roberts, Wash.: Hartley & Marks, 2004. Written by two leading fertility experts, this book is an excellent guide. Includes a thorough discussion of the basic physiology of conception and reproduction.

Concussion

Disease/disorder

Anatomy or system affected: Brain, head, nerves, nervous system

Specialties and related fields: Critical care, emergency medicine, neurology, sports medicine

Definition: Mild brain injury that briefly impairs neurological functions.

Key terms:

amnesia: memory loss

disorientation: lack of comprehension of reality

unconsciousness: lack of awareness of one's surroundings

Causes and Symptoms

Annually in the United States, 1.4 million people suffer concussions, with 75 percent of those conditions being considered mild in nature. Concussions can be caused by a variety of traumatic events: motor vehicle accidents, penetrating injuries, sports injuries, and falls. Recent studies indicate that the number of concussions from motor vehicle accidents and falls have decreased, while penetrating injuries (gunshot wounds) and sports-related injuries are on the increase. Concussion is a common athletic injury experienced by approximately 300,000 youths each year. Recent information suggests that children heal more slowly than adults following head trauma. Although concussions are the mildest traumatic brain injuries, they can result in irreversible damage or death if a person suffers another head trauma prior to recovering fully from the initial injury.

People experiencing head trauma that disrupts brain activity and sometimes causes brief unconsciousness, ranging from several seconds to minutes immediately after an impact, are considered to have sustained a concussion. Direct, sudden, powerful blows to the head or an impact to the body that jars the head causes the brain to bounce inside the skull and suffer tissue bruising. Nerve fibers tear, and chemical reactions are altered.

Concussions are described as mild, moderate, or severe, though there is a lack of standardized definitions for each type of concussion. A mild concussion may or may not involve a brief period of unconsciousness; the brain generally recovers quickly and without long-term damage. However, approximately 15 percent of those injured will continue to experience symptoms one year after the initial injury. These symptoms may range from headaches to emotional or behavioral problems. The Centers for Disease Control and Prevention (CDC) and the National Center for Injury Prevention and Control have developed recommendations for standardized terminology, treatment, and prevention of mild traumatic brain injuries. A severe concussion is considered an emergency and requires an extended time for recovery.

Headache, dizziness, nausea, and disorientation immediately following the injury are considered risk factors for long-term complications from the head injury. Each person's brain and injury are unique. Therefore, a wide variety of symptoms may be occur. Patients may experience double vision and suffer hearing problems. People with concussions also report becoming uncoordinated and sensitive to light and noises, and they may

Information on Concussion

Causes: Brain trauma from car accidents, falls, sports injuries, etc.

Symptoms: Unconsciousness, memory loss, headache, dizziness, nausea, disorientation, double vision, hearing problems, lack of coordination, sensitivity to light and noises, sensory changes in smell and taste

Duration: Ranges from several seconds to minutes immediately after impact

Treatments: Dependent on severity; none (mild), rest and alleviation of symptoms (moderate), neck immobilization and hospitalization (severe)

experience sensory changes in smell and taste. Patients may become moody, cognitively impaired, unable to concentrate, and fatigued.

Researchers have determined that the major neuropsychological complications of concussion may occur in the brain's memory, learning, and planning functions. Some concussion patients taking tests, such as the Wechsler Abbreviated Scale of Intelligence, have revealed decreased concentration, reaction, and processing skills in performing intellectual tasks. Their strategies to solve problems are impaired when compared to people who have not suffered concussions.

Medical professionals assess patients with a head injury by physical examination, radiological tests, and a standardized scale that measures level of consciousness called the Glasgow Coma Scale. Computed tomography (CT) and magnetic resonance imaging (MRI) scans may be used. The American Academy of Neurology emphasizes the duration of loss of consciousness to determine the degree of concussions. Evaluations also consider orientation and posttraumatic amnesia. Medical professionals assess patients' responses to stimuli and memory of incidents before their injury, defining the concussion according to the level of confusion, amnesia, and duration of loss of consciousness. Physicians ask patients questions about who and where they are and about the time and date. The duration of amnesia after the brain trauma helps medical professionals determine the extent of the injury and treatments that would be most effective to heal the brain. The Colorado Medical Society developed a popular system, assigning Grades 1 (mild), 2 (moderate), and 3 (severe) to concussions, to guide athletic personnel in examining players who suffer concussions during games and deciding how long they must refrain from participation in order to prevent additional damage.

Brain damage and death can result from serial concussions. Postconcussion complications may include second impact syndrome: If a patient suffers another concussion before healing is complete following the first injury, then the second concussion can be the catalyst for rapid cerebral swelling that causes increased pressure within the rigid structure of the brain. This pressure can cause the brain to press on the brain stem and result in respiratory failure and death. This condition is usually fatal.

More common is postconcussive syndrome (PCS), which consists of such cognitive and physical symptoms as headache, anxiety, vertigo, nausea, and hallucinations. An estimated 30 percent of professional football players suffer from PCS. Researchers have determined that people who experience several concussions, such as athletes and soldiers, are more vulnerable to becoming clinically depressed.

Treatment and Therapy

Research has found that patients who rest for one week following a concussion, with a slow return to previous activities to allow the brain to heal, have fewer long-term complications than do those patients who resume activities more quickly. Specific medications and therapies might be prescribed to alleviate symptoms and assist patients in resuming normal behaviors. Although most patients recover, some experience long-term concussion-related conditions, such as memory loss and neurological impairment.

Severe concussions with increased brain pressure require hospitalization, often in a neurological intensive care unit. The patient's head is maintained in a neutral position. The patient is at risk for stopped breathing due to increased brain pressure. This risk is decreased by placing the patient on a mechanical ventilator. The patient may have suffered internal bleeding in the brain because of the injury, and blood clots can form there. Surgery may be required to remove these clots. Patients with preexisting conditions such as epilepsy and diabetes may develop complications related to those diseases and require longer recovery times.

Physicians recommend wearing helmets to absorb shocks sustained during athletic activities involving the risk of head injury in order to prevent or minimize concussions. The American Academy of Neurology has demanded a ban on boxing because the sport involves knocking out opponents by inflicting concussions. Boxers often suffer permanent brain damage and are at a heightened risk for neurological diseases.

Perspective and Prospects

Muslim physician Rhazes (850-923) was the first person known to describe concussion. He differentiated between a head injury that caused neurological symptoms from those injuries that resulted in lesions and structural damage. In the nineteenth century, medical researchers developed hypotheses, often controversial, regarding the physical and emotional influences of concussion symptoms. Since then, investigators have studied the impact of concussions on neuropsychological functioning and have addressed cognitive impairment and potential and the duration of recovery. Second impact syndrome was first defined in 1984.

The development of sports medicine increased the interest in studying concussions. The understanding of the internal brain damage involved in concussions did not significantly advance, however, until imaging technologies such as CT scanning and magnetic resonance imaging (MRI) were developed in the late twentieth century. In the twenty-first century, medical professionals utilize those techniques to view brain tissues and to observe the physiological reactions to concussion-causing trauma. Positive emission tomography (PET) has been developed to measure chemical changes in the brain. In the case of concussion, the PET scan can be used to evaluate changes that signal areas of injury in the brain.

—Elizabeth D. Schafer, Ph.D.;
updated by Amy Webb Bull, D.S.N., A.P.N.

See also Amnesia; Bleeding; Brain; Brain disorders; Coma; Dizziness and fainting; Head and neck disorders; Nausea and vomiting; Nervous system; Neuroimaging; Neurology; Sports medicine; Unconsciousness.

For Further Information:

Evans, Randolph W., ed. *Neurology and Trauma*. 2d ed. New York: Oxford University Press, 2006.

Kennedy, Jan, Robin Lumpkin, and Joyce Grissom. "A Survey of Mild Traumatic Brain Injury Treatment in the Emergency Room and Primary Care Medical Clinics." *Military Medicine* 171, no. 6 (June, 2006): 516-521.

Kerr, Mary, and Elizabeth Crago. "Acute Intracranial Problems." In *Medical-Surgical Nursing*, edited by Sharon Lewis, Margaret Heitkemper, and Shannon Dirksen. 6th ed. St. Louis: Mosby, 2004.

Metzl, Jordan. "Concussion in the Young Athelete." *Pediatrics* 117, no. 5. (May, 2006): 1813.

National Center for Injury Prevention and Control. *Report to Congress on Mild Traumatic Brain Injury in the United States: Steps to Prevent a Serious Public Health Problem*. Atlanta: Centers for Disease Control and Prevention, 2003. Also at http://www.cdc.gov/ncipc/pub-res/mtbi/mtbireport.pdf.

Shannon, Joyce Brennfleck, ed. *Sports Injuries Sourcebook*. 2d ed. Detroit: Omnigraphics, 2002.

Wrightson, Philip, and Dorothy Gronwall. *Mild Head Injury: A Guide to Management*. New York: Oxford University Press, 1999.

Congenital heart disease

Disease/disorder

Anatomy or system affected: Chest, circulatory system, heart

Specialties and related fields: Cardiology, neonatology, pediatrics, vascular medicine

Definition: Conditions resulting from malformations of the heart that occur during embryonic and fetal development, accounting for about 25 percent of all congenital defects.

Key terms:

atrium: one of two heart chambers that receive blood, the left from the lungs and the right from the body

great arteries and veins: large vessels channeling blood into and out of the heart, including the aorta (to the body), the pulmonary artery (to the lungs), the vena cava (from the body), and the pulmonary veins (from the lungs)

heart failure: the inability of the heart to pump adequate amounts of blood to maintain the organs and tissues of the body; often results in tissue fluid retention and congestion

murmur: a sound made by the heart other than the normal two-step beat; murmurs are caused by the turbulent movement of blood and may indicate a heart defect

septum: a membrane that serves as a wall of separation; in the heart, the interatrial septum divides the two atria and the interventricular septum divides the two ventricles

ventricles: heart chambers that pump blood, the left to the body and the right to the lungs

Causes and Symptoms

Congenital heart disease collectively includes various structural and functional defects of the heart and blood vessels resulting from errors that occur during embryonic development. The defects may cause heart murmurs, high or low blood pressure, congestive heart failure, cyanosis (blue skin), abnormal heart rhythms and rates, and incidences of low oxygen (hypoxia). Congenital heart disease is detected in about 0.7 percent of live births and 2.7 percent of stillbirths. Babies born with congenital heart disease have the most difficulty during the first few weeks of life. Some problems, however, are not easily detected at the time of birth and are discovered at various stages of life. Heart defects may be inherited from parents, induced by environmental agents such as drugs, or caused by an interaction of genetic and environmental factors. Defects are more common in children with genetic disorders such as Down syndrome. With intensive treatment, including surgery, many forms of congenital heart disease can be corrected, allowing those affected to lead normal lives.

Knowledge of normal heart development will help in understanding how congenital heart disease occurs and will provide a means for categorizing these defects. Near the end of the third week of embryonic development, the heart begins to form from two cords of tissue that hollow out and fuse to form a primitive heart tube. This tube undergoes some constrictions and dilations to form the early divisions of the heart, including a receiving chamber, the atrium, and a pumping chamber, the ventricle, which exits into a muscular tube called the truncus arteriosus. At about twenty-two days, the heart begins to contract and pump blood. A day later, it bends or loops upon itself to form an S shape, with the atrium on one side, the truncus arteriosus on the other side, and the ventricle in the middle. If it bends to the left instead of to the right, a rare heart defect called dextrocardia results. The heart will be displaced to the right side of the body and may have some accompanying abnormalities.

During the fourth and fifth week of development, the heart begins to divide into four chambers by first forming a septum (dividing membrane) in the canal between the atrium and the ventricle. This septum is formed by heart tissue called the endocardial cushions. Failure of this septum to form properly causes atrioventricular canal defects. These are often associated with Down syndrome. During the fifth week of development, a spiral septum forms in the truncus arteriosus which divides it into two vessels: the pulmonary artery, which connects to the right ventricle, and the aorta, which connects to the left ventricle. The formation of this septum and the ventricular connections are subject to error and may result in a group of anomalies called conotruncal defects.

As these large arteries are forming, a shunt (bypass) develops between them called the ductus arteriosus. This short vessel allows the blood to be diverted away from the nonfunctional fetal lungs into the aorta and on to the placenta, where it will receive oxygen and nutrients. Persistence of this shunt after birth is responsible for a defect called patent ductus. A septum dividing the atrium into right and left halves also forms during the fourth and fifth weeks of development; however, blood is allowed to pass from the right atrium to the left atrium through a small hole in this septum called the foramen ovale. This hole normally closes after birth but is necessary during fetal life to shunt blood away from the fetal lungs and toward the placenta in a manner similar to that of the ductus arteriosus. At about the same time, a septum forms from the floor of the ventricle and divides it into right and left halves. Failure of the atrial and ventricular septa to form properly and to close at the time of birth results in septal defects.

After the appearance of the four chambers, two pairs of valves form in the heart to prevent the backflow of blood and to ensure greater efficiency in pumping. The semilunar valves (also called the pulmonary and aortic valves) form between the ventricles and their respective outlet arteries (pulmonary artery and aorta), and the atrioventricular valves (bicuspid or mitral on the left and tricuspid on the right) form between the atria and the ventricles. Improperly formed valves can lead to flow defects. During development, the heart also makes connections with veins returning from the general circulation and the lungs. Errors in these connections and other structural errors cause several other less common congenital heart defects.

The most common congenital heart defects are the

Information on Congenital Heart Disease

Causes: Genetic and environmental factors
Symptoms: Shortness of breath, fatigue, sweating while eating, inability to gain weight, lung congestion, altered blood pressure, hypoxia, congestive heart failure
Duration: Ranges from short-term to lifelong
Treatments: Surgery, medications, insertion of balloon catheter

septal defects and patent ductus, which together account for about 37 percent of all heart defects. After birth, because the pressure becomes higher in the left side of the heart, blood moves from left to right through the openings in the heart that come with such defects, causing too much to flow to the lungs and a mixing of systemic and pulmonary blood. The child's lungs will be congested, causing difficulty in breathing and eventually heart failure.

About 29 percent of congenital heart defects are categorized as right-heart and left-heart flow defects. These defects impede the flow of blood from either the right or the left side of the heart to its normal destination. Right-heart flow defects include bicuspid pulmonary valve (a valve with two cusps instead of three), pulmonary valve stenosis (a narrowing of the valve), dysplastic pulmonary valve (a malformed valve), peripheral pulmonary stenosis (a narrowing of the walls of the pulmonary artery), infundibular pulmonary stenosis (a narrowing below the valve), and hypoplastic right ventricle (incomplete formation of the valve). These defects impede blood flow to the lungs, which results in poor oxygenation of the blood (cyanosis). Left-heart flow defects include bicuspid aortic valve, aortic valve stenosis, coarctation of the aorta (narrowing), aortic atresia (a blocked aorta), and hypoplastic left ventricle. These defects impede blood flow to the body and often result in altered blood pressure, hypoxia of body tissues, and congestive heart failure.

The principal conotruncal defects, which account for about 17 percent of heart defects, are tetralogy of Fallot and transposition of the great arteries. Tetralogy of Fallot includes four defects that result in cyanosis: pulmonary stenosis, a ventricular septal defect, an overriding or displaced aorta, and hypertrophy or enlargement of the right ventricle. With transposition of the great arteries, the aorta connects to the right ventricle and the pulmonary artery to the left ventricle, the opposite of the normal formation. The blood is not properly oxygenated, and survival is not possible without medical intervention or a natural shunt such as patent ductus. Other rare conotruncal defects include double outlet right ventricle (the aorta and the pulmonary artery attached to right ventricle), truncus arteriosus (failure of the truncus to separate into the aorta and the pulmonary artery), and aortopulmonary window (an opening between the aorta and the pulmonary artery).

Defects resulting from improper fusion of the endocardial cushions and surrounding tissues cause atrioventricular defects, which affect about 9 percent

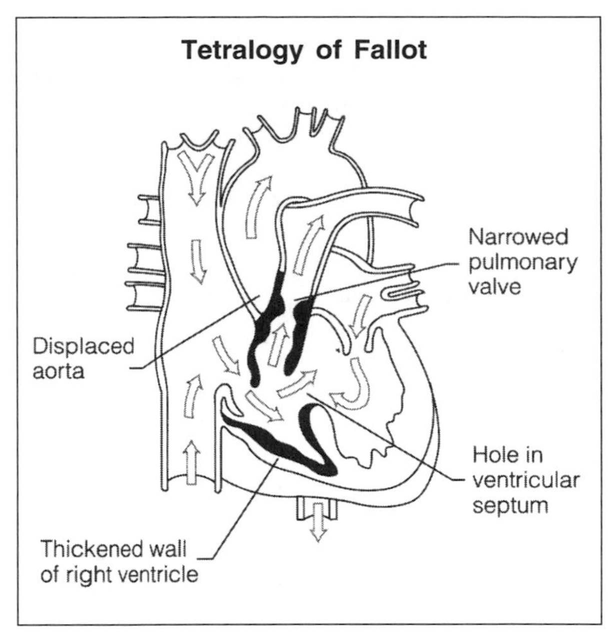

A relatively common congenital heart defect, tetralogy of Fallot comprises four defects: an overriding or displaced aorta, pulmonary stenosis (a narrowed pulmonary valve), a ventricular septal defect (a hole in the ventricular septum), and a thickened, or enlarged, right ventricle. These together result in cyanosis: poor blood oxygenation.

of patients with congenital heart disease. Complete atrioventricular canal defect occurs in about 20 percent of Down syndrome cases, but it is rare outside this group. The defect produces a large open space in the center of the heart, allowing blood to intermix freely between the right and left sides of the heart. The defect is sometimes accompanied by hypoplastic ventricle. If the condition is not treated, the heart will fail. Patent foramen primum or ostium primum is a milder form of atrioventricular canal defect in which the atrial septum fails to fuse with the endocardial cushions, resulting in a problem similar to atrial septal defect. In addition, the mitral valve is usually deformed.

Other less common defects include looping defects such as dextrocardia, in which the apex of the heart points to the right instead of to the left. This change in symmetry normally does not affect heart function, but some looping defects are associated with other problems such as transposition of the great arteries. Another less common defect is anomalous venous return, in which the veins returning blood to the heart from the lungs attach to the right atrium or return to the right atrium by attaching to other large veins rather than to the left atrium. Errors in the coronary artery connections may also occur, causing poor circulation of blood to the heart muscles. Very rarely, the heart may protrude through the chest wall at birth, causing a difficult-to-treat problem called ectopia cordis.

Treatment and Therapy

Congenital heart disease can often be diagnosed shortly after birth, especially if the baby experiences certain symptoms such as cyanosis, shortness of breath, fatigue and sweating while eating, and inability to gain weight. A physical examination by a physician will include checking the heart and breathing rates for abnormalities and listening to the heart for possible murmurs. Heart murmurs are whooshing sounds caused by turbulent movement of blood that may indicate faulty valves, patent ductus, and other heart defects. A cardiologist will make the definitive diagnosis by administering such tests as the electrocardiogram, the Doppler-echocardiogram, and the cardiac catheterization. The electrocardiogram measures the rhythmic electrical signal that passes through the heart with each beat. An abnormal signal will often indicate problems with a particular region of the heart and is especially useful in identifying rhythm disorders. The echocardiogram produces visual images of the heart by sending out ultrasound waves that bounce off and return to a receiving device. Most structural heart defects can be detected with this technique, and many are discovered prenatally with routine fetal ultrasound monitoring. At the same time, a second receiving device (the Doppler) analyzes ultrasound signals from blood moving through the heart and is able to provide information about the speed and direction of blood flow within the heart. This helps detect abnormal functions such as reverse blood flow. The Doppler-echocardiogram has revolutionized congenital heart disease diagnosis and in most cases provides enough information to define the patient's problem accurately.

If the cardiologist believes that it is necessary, further tests can be done. A chest X ray may be taken to determine if there is any lung involvement in the disorder. Cardiac catheterization can add information about the internal heart blood pressures and blood oxygen levels and can help visualize some defects better with the administration of contrast dyes in combination with X-ray analysis. Special monitors can be used to record the electrocardiogram for one or two days to check for intermittent rhythm irregularities, and older children can be monitored while exercising to see how the heart performs under stress. These and other tests allow physicians to assess the seriousness of the problem and to recommend timely and appropriate treatment.

Serious heart malformations need to be treated immediately upon diagnosis. Often these include defects that cause cyanosis, including transposition of the great arteries, left-heart flow defects such as coarctation of the aorta, and defects that cause heart failure, such as truncus arteriosus. Immediate emergency surgery may be needed to save the life of the newborn infant. Additional follow-up surgeries may also be required to correct the defect completely. For example, one way of correcting transposition of the great arteries is by performing an atrial switch operation in which systemic blood returning from the body is diverted to the left side of the heart (so it can be pumped to the lungs) and pulmonary blood from the lungs is diverted to the right side of the heart (so it can be pumped to the body). This is accomplished by first enlarging the foramen ovale with a balloon catheter, a procedure called Rashkind balloon atrial septostomy. A second operation several months later enlarges the opening between the two atria further and installs a flap to enhance the cross flow of blood. This is known as a Mustard or Senning atrial switch operation. A more recently developed procedure for correcting this defect requires only one operation. The misplaced aorta and pulmonary artery are both cut and then reattached to the correct heart chamber; this is called a Jatene arterial switch operation. At the same time, the coronary arteries are moved to the new aorta.

Some defects require no surgery but can be treated with drugs and other less traumatic procedures, such as the balloon catheter. Drugs are also used to help improve heart performance before and after surgery. When fluid accumulates in the lungs or other body tissues, the heart has problems pumping all the blood that returns to it because of the congestion. The overworked heart suffers under this stress, and thus the condition is called congestive heart failure. Diuretics such as Lasix (furosemide) improve the kidneys' ability to remove the excess fluid and relieve the congestion. Another drug, digitalis, can be helpful in treating congestive heart failure by slowing the heart rate and causing the heart to beat more forcefully. An open ductus is beneficial to children born with cyanotic heart defects because it allows a more even distribution of oxygenated blood. Treatment with prostaglandin E1 helps keep the ductus open until corrective surgery can be performed. Indomethacin has the opposite effect and is often used to promote closing of a patent ductus in premature babies. As in adults, drugs such as digitalis, beta-blockers, and calcium channel blockers can be used to treat abnormal heart rhythms (arrhythmia) in children with congenital heart disease. The balloon catheter is used in a nonsurgical technique to enlarge narrow vessels and passages and has been used successfully to treat pulmonary and aortic valve stenosis in a technique called balloon valvuloplasty.

Types of surgery done later in infancy or childhood include closed heart operations such as repair of a patent ductus and partial treatment of some types of cyanosis with a Blalock-Taussig shunt (connecting the subclavian artery to the pulmonary artery to bring more blood to the lungs). Open heart surgery is used to repair defects inside the heart such as septal defects. A heart-lung machine is used to bypass the heart and lungs while the operation is underway, and the body is cooled so that the brain and other tissues require less oxygen. Children with very serious heart defects such as hypoplastic right or left ventricles may require a series of corrective surgical operations, and for some the only hope is a heart transplant. For example, children with hypoplastic right ventricle are given a Blalock-Taussig shunt shortly after birth to improve blood flow to their lungs and then are later given the Fontan operation, which involves closing off the Blalock-Taussig shunt and connecting the pulmonary artery to the right atrium so that blood returning from the body will flow directly to the lungs, completely bypassing the defective right ventricle.

Some heart defects require no treatment. For example, most small septal defects close on their own during the first one or two years of life. Also, mild disorders such as benign valve defects usually require no treatment, and many children with heart murmurs have no detectable problems.

PERSPECTIVE AND PROSPECTS

In the late nineteenth and early twentieth centuries, physicians were beginning to understand that certain congenital heart defects such as patent ductus could be diagnosed by listening to the heart. Treatment, however, was not possible at that time. The *Atlas of Congenital Cardiac Disease* was published in 1936 by Maude Abbot of McGill University. This work greatly assisted other physicians in recognizing and diagnosing congenital heart disease. In 1939, Robert Gross of Boston repaired a patent ductus, and in 1944, Alfred Blalock and Helen Taussig developed and performed their famous shunt operation in order to treat children with tetralogy of Fallot. Open heart surgery had to wait until the mid-1950's, when the heart-lung machine was perfected. Even then, open heart surgery could only be performed on older children. These operations were pioneered by Walton Lillehei of the University of Minnesota and John Kirlin of the Mayo Clinic. Open heart surgery on newborn infants was developed in the 1970's by Brian Barratt-Boyes of New Zealand.

During the period while heart surgery was being developed, cardiac catheterization was also advancing. It was used primarily for diagnosis, but in 1966, William Rashkind of Philadelphia began to use the balloon catheter to enlarge openings in the atrial septum in order to treat transposition of the great arteries. Microsurgical catheters are currently being developed to repair patent ductus and other heart defects without the need for major surgery. The echocardiogram was pioneered by Inge Edler in the 1950's, and the Doppler-echocardiogram came into widespread use as a diagnostic tool in the 1980's. This instrument has greatly reduced the need for other diagnostic tests that were used in the past.

The modern strategy for treatment of congenital heart defects is to perform the corrective surgery as early in infancy as possible. This eliminates the need for numerous hospitalizations and diagnostic tests and reduces the need for extensive drug treatment. Children with multiple defects will still need more than one surgery. Modern treatment also emphasizes the roles of the child, the family, and health care personnel in fostering an understanding of the condition, treatment, and outcome. Even children who have been successfully treated will sometimes have physical limitations. These children need to be encouraged and supported by their families and allowed to pursue their goals to the fullest extent possible. Overcoming congenital heart disease is now possible for the vast majority of those who are afflicted.

—*Rodney C. Mowbray, Ph.D.*

See also Arrhythmias; Birth defects; Blue baby syndrome; Bypass surgery; Cardiology; Cardiology, pediatric; Cyanosis; DiGeorge syndrome; Echocardiography; Genetic diseases; Heart; Heart disease; Heart failure; Heart transplantation; Mitral valve prolapse; Neonatology; Shunts.

FOR FURTHER INFORMATION:

American Heart Association. http://www.americanheart.org/. A group dedicated to reducing disability and death from cardiovascular diseases and stroke. Offers thorough information on a wide range of cardiovascular diseases, referrals to emergency cardiovascular care classes, and research statistics and articles.

Beers, Mark H., et al. *The Merck Manual of Diagnosis and Therapy*. 18th ed. Whitehouse Station, N.J.: Merck Research Laboratories, 2006. Contains complete medical descriptions of the common congenital heart defects and appropriate methods of diagnosis and treatment.

Gersh, Bernard J., ed. *The Mayo Clinic Heart Book*. 2d ed. New York: William Morrow, 2000. One of the most respected texts for laypeople on heart disease. Covers all aspects of anatomy, physiology, diagnosis, treatment, and prevention.

Koenig, Peter, Ziyad M. Hijazi, and Frank Zimmerman, eds. *Essential Pediatric Cardiology*. New York: McGraw-Hill, 2004. An excellent text for the nonspecialist that covers cardiac disorders in the neonate, child, and adolescent.

Kramer, Gerri Freid, and Shari Mauer. *Parent's Guide to Children's Congenital Heart Defects: What They Are, How to Treat Them, How to Cope with Them*. New York: Three Rivers Press, 2001. Experts in pediatric cardiology provide easy-to-understand answers to help parents coping with a child's heart disease. Includes the latest information on diagnosis, treatment options, surgery, aftercare, and growing up with heart defects, as well as stories from parents who have lived through the ordeal.

Moore, Keith L., and T. V. N. Persaud. *The Developing Human*. 7th ed. Philadelphia: W. B. Saunders, 2003. An outstanding textbook on human embryonic development. Includes discussion of the development of the circulatory system. The diagrams and descriptions allow the reader to compare normal and abnormal development and to see exactly how errors in development result in congenital heart defects.

Neill, Catherine A., Edward B. Clark, and Carleen Clark. *The Heart of a Child: What Families Need to Know About Heart Disorders in Children*. 2d ed. Baltimore: Johns Hopkins University Press, 2001. A comprehensive, up-to-date work on heart disease affecting children, written for the layperson by medical professionals. The authors give a thorough description of all congenital heart defects and explain their developmental basis.

Park, Myung K. *The Pediatric Cardiology Handbook*. 3d ed. St. Louis: Mosby, 2003. A text for the medical specialist with discussion of all congenital heart defects, including atrial septal defects, ventricular septal defects, cushion defects, coarctation, and interrupted aortic arch.

Sherwood, Lauralee. *Human Physiology: From Cells to Systems*. 6th ed. Belmont, Calif.: Thomson/Brooks/Cole, 2007. This college textbook contains useful biological information about embryonic development and genetic defects.

Congestive heart failure. *See* Heart failure.

Conjunctivitis

Disease/disorder

Also known as: Pinkeye

Anatomy or system affected: Eyes, immune system

Specialties and related fields: Bacteriology, family medicine, microbiology, ophthalmology, optometry, virology

Definition: An acute inflammatory disease of the eye caused by infection or irritation.

Causes and Symptoms

Conjunctivitis, or pinkeye, is one of the most common eye disorders. The conjunctiva is a thin translucent membrane that overlays the white part of the eye and the inner surface of the eyelids. It protects the eye from foreign objects and infection.

The conjunctiva may become inflamed through infection with a virus or bacterium, allergic reactions, and exposure to certain chemicals. Inflammation of the conjunctiva brings increased blood flow to the eye, producing a red, or bloodshot, appearance. Conjunctivitis causes a feeling of irritation, burning, or mild pain. A discharge often occurs, which may form a crust on the eyelids when it dries. Conjunctivitis does not cause visual loss, fever, or severe pain. It is typically mild and short-lived, lasting from a few days to a few weeks.

Most conjunctivitis is caused by infection and is highly contagious, spreading quickly from one eye to the other and from person to person by touch. Viral conjunctivitis will resolve without treatment, although symptoms may persist as long as a few weeks. Upper-respiratory symptoms often occur simultaneously, since similar viruses cause the common cold. These viruses may live on surfaces for several hours and can be transmitted in poorly chlorinated swimming pools. Bacterial conjunctivitis causes a thicker discharge and more severe crusting. It is caused by various bacteria, and all respond well to topical antibiotics.

Information on Conjunctivitis

Causes: Viral or bacterial infection, allergic reactions, exposure to chemicals or irritants
Symptoms: Red or bloodshot eye, burning sensation, mild pain, discharge forming crust on eyelids
Duration: Ranges from a few days to a few weeks
Treatments: None or topical antibiotics

Allergic conjunctivitis may be stimulated by a reaction to dust, mold, animal dander, or pollen. It causes burning or itching in both eyes and occurs in a seasonal pattern. Chemicals, wind, dust, smoke, and chronic dry eyes can also cause direct irritation of the conjunctiva.

Treatment and Therapy

For viral conjunctivitis, no therapy is required, but the patient may be contagious for as long as two weeks. Common bacterial conjunctivitis resolves quickly with antibiotic eyedrops or ointment. A person remains contagious with bacterial conjunctivitis until after twenty-four hours of antibiotic treatment. The spread of infection can be prevented by washing one's hands frequently, using separate towels, and isolating an infected child from interaction with other children for the first twenty-four hours of treatment. For allergic conjunctivitis, avoiding the offending allergen and using topical antihistamines or artificial tears are effective treatments.

Perspective and Prospects

Conjunctivitis in the United States is generally benign and rarely causes permanent injury. Elsewhere in the world, however, conjunctivitis is a leading cause of blindness. In areas of extreme poverty, repeated infections with trachoma, a bacterial infection spread by flies, lead to permanent scarring of the eyes. Newborns may also contract severe bacterial conjunctivitis from the mother's cervix during birth. For this reason, most developed nations require that all newborns receive antibiotic eyedrops at birth.

—*Christopher D. Sharp, M.D.*

See also Allergies; Bacterial infections; Blindness; Childhood infectious diseases; Eye infections and disorders; Eyes; Keratitis; Trachoma; Viral infections; Vision disorders.

For Further Information:

Johnson, Gordon J., et al., eds. *The Epidemiology of Eye Disease*. 2d ed. New York: Oxford University Press, 2003.

Kasper, Dennis L., et al., eds. *Harrison's Principles of Internal Medicine*. 16th ed. New York: McGraw-Hill, 2005.

Parker, James N., and Philip M. Parker, eds. *The Official Patient's Sourcebook on Conjunctivitis*. San Diego, Calif.: Icon Health, 2002.

Stoffman, Phyllis. *The Family Guide to Preventing and Treating One Hundred Infectious Illnesses.* New York: John Wiley & Sons, 1995.

Turkington, Carol, and Bonnie Lee Ashby. *The Encyclopedia of Infectious Diseases.* 2d ed. New York: Facts On File, 2003.

Constipation

Disease/disorder

Anatomy or system affected: Abdomen, gastrointestinal system, intestines

Specialties and related fields: Family medicine, gastroenterology, internal medicine

Definition: The slow passage of feces through the bowels or the presence of hard feces.

Causes and Symptoms

People of every age group, from infants to the elderly, can experience the unpleasant symptoms of constipation, which is characterized primarily by discomfort. Certain disease states such as diabetes mellitus, paralysis of the legs, colon cancer, and hypothyroidism predispose a person to constipation. Possible causes of constipation are medications, iron supplements, toilet training procedures, pregnancy, lack of adequate fluids, a low-fiber diet, and lack of physical activity.

Treatment and Therapy

Most cases of constipation can be treated by the patient at home. Drinking adequate fluids makes it easier for fecal material to pass through the large intestine. Without adequate hydration, a person may experience small, pelletlike stools. Eight to ten glasses of liquids per day are recommended, including water, milk, cocoa, fruit juice, herbal tea, and soup. Once adequate hydration is achieved, a high-fiber diet can gradually be started. Without enough fluids, a high-fiber diet can worsen the problems of constipation. A high-fiber diet adds bulk to the bowel movement (increasing stool volume, de-

INFORMATION ON CONSTIPATION

CAUSES: Lack of fiber or adequate fluids in diet, certain medications, iron supplements, pregnancy, lack of physical activity, aging
SYMPTOMS: Uncomfortable passage of stools, bloating, abdominal discomfort
DURATION: Ranges from short-term to chronic
TREATMENTS: Adequate hydration, high-fiber diet, exercise, laxatives

creasing pressure within the colon, and decreasing the intestinal transit time of foods) and thus can lead to more regular bowel habits and partial relief of the symptoms. One can increase fiber in the diet by eating prunes, high-fiber breakfast cereals, beans or legumes, raw fruits and vegetables, and whole-grain breads. In order to minimize gastrointestinal discomforts such as increased flatulence (gas), it is recommended to increase one's fiber consumption gradually.

In addition to adequate liquids and a high-fiber diet, exercise is important in treating constipation. Any sort of physical activity, such as walking, running, tennis, or swimming, can help to stimulate the activity of the large intestine.

Laxatives and enemas should not be used until after a discussion with a physician. Mineral oil should also not be used because many essential fat-soluble vitamins (such as vitamins A, D, E, and K) may be excreted as well. Persistent constipation should be evaluated by a physician.

—Martha M. Henze, M.S., R.D.

See also Diarrhea and dysentery; Enemas; Gastroenterology; Gastroenterology, pediatric; Gastrointestinal disorders; Gastrointestinal system; Hemorrhoid banding and removal; Hemorrhoids; Indigestion; Intestinal disorders; Intestines; Obstruction; Over-the-counter medications.

FOR FURTHER INFORMATION:

Berkson, D. Lindsey. *Healthy Digestion the Natural Way*. New York: Wiley, 2000.

Capasso, Francesco. *Laxatives: A Practical Guide*. New York: Springer, 1997.

Gitnick, Gary, and Karen Cooksey. *Freedom from Digestive Distress*. New York: Crown, 2000.

Parker, James N., and Philip M. Parker, eds. *The Official Patient's Sourcebook on Constipation*. San Diego, Calif.: Icon Health, 2002.

Peikin, Steven R. *Gastrointestinal Health*. Rev. ed. New York: HarperCollins, 1999.

Wexner, Steven D., and Graeme S. Duthie, eds. *Constipation: Etiology, Evaluation, and Management*. 2d ed. London: Springer, 2006.

Whorton, James C. *Inner Hygiene: Constipation and the Pursuit of Health in Modern Society*. New York: Oxford University Press, 2000.

CONTRACEPTION

PROCEDURE

ANATOMY OR SYSTEM AFFECTED: Genitals, reproductive system, uterus

SPECIALTIES AND RELATED FIELDS: Gynecology, obstetrics, urology

DEFINITION: The use of techniques to prevent pregnancy, which may interfere with ovulation, sperm transport, or implantation of an embryo.

KEY TERMS:

barrier method: a contraceptive that physically prevents sperm from meeting an egg

cervix: the entrance to the uterus from the vagina

ejaculation: the release of sperm from the male's body during sexual activity

hormone: a chemical signal carried in the blood that allows distant body parts to coordinate their actions

implantation: the process in which the embryo attaches to the uterine lining

ovulation: the monthly release of a mature egg from the ovary

spermicide: a chemical that kills sperm after they are ejaculated

toxic shock syndrome: an infection normally caused by staphylococci that can develop rapidly into severe untreatable shock, which can be fatal

uterus: the organ that supports the embryo during its development

vagina: the tube-shaped cavity of the female into which the male's penis is inserted during intercourse

vas deferens: the tubes in the male reproductive system that carry sperm

METHODS AND EFFECTIVENESS

Contraception is defined as the avoidance of conception by either natural means (abstinence) or artificial means (physical barriers, chemicals, hormones). Pregnancy can be prevented by interfering with the process of conception at any number of sites in the male or female anatomy.

Barrier methods. A male condom, or prophylactic, is

a thin sheath made to fit an erect penis. It can be made of latex (a type of rubber), polyurethane (a type of plastic), or natural products such as lamb's intestines. A condom prevents semen, which contains sperm, from entering a woman's vagina during intercourse. The latex condom is one of the few forms of contraception that can also protect against sexually transmitted diseases (STDs). Men who are not allergic to latex should use latex condoms, as they are the best at preventing pregnancy and STDs. Polyurethane condoms break more easily, and natural condoms are not as effective at preventing STDs.

Male condoms should be used any time a man has intercourse with his partner. If the condom does not have space at the end called a sperm repository, then 0.25 inch of the condom should be left at the tip of the penis to collect semen. To increase the protective birth control value, spermicidal foam or jelly can be used in addition to the condom. According to the American College of Obstetricians and Gynecologists, this combination is 99 percent effective. Vaseline or other types of petroleum jelly, lotion, or oils should not be used as a lubricant with condoms because they weaken the latex rubber. Non-oil-based lubricants or even water can be used with latex condoms. Condoms come in a variety of sizes and can be purchased over the counter at drugstores and pharmacies and in coin machines in many public restrooms. There is no age restriction on buying condoms.

The female condom is a lubricated, thin polyurethane tube that has a flexible ring on each end. The closed end of the tube is inserted into the vagina, and the other end remains outside the vagina, slightly covering the labia. The female condom is 75 percent effective at blocking sperm from entering the vagina. It provides some protection against STDs; however, the male condom provides the best protection against STDs of all contraceptive methods. The female condom should be used only once per intercourse.

A diaphragm is a dome-shaped rubber disk with a flexible rim, which covers the cervix so that sperm are unable to enter the uterus. A diaphragm must be prescribed and sized by a health care professional. It is recommended that a spermicide be applied to the diaphragm to make it more effective. The diaphragm provides birth control protection up to six hours after insertion. A new application of spermicide should be inserted into the vagina with the diaphragm in place for repeated intercourse. In order to be effective, the diaphragm must remain in the vagina six hours after the last intercourse, but never longer than twenty-four hours because of the risk of toxic shock syndrome. The diaphragm is approximately 83 percent effective as a birth control method, but it does not provide any protection against STDs.

The cervical cap is a soft rubber or plastic cup with a round rim, which fits snugly over the cervix. As with a diaphragm, it must be fitted by a health care professional. The cervical cap should be used in combination with a spermicidal cream or jelly for optimal effectiveness. It can provide birth control protection for up to forty-eight hours. The cervical cap should be removed after forty-eight hours because of a low risk of toxic shock syndrome. It does not provide any protection against STDs.

Vaginal spermicides include creams, jellies, films,

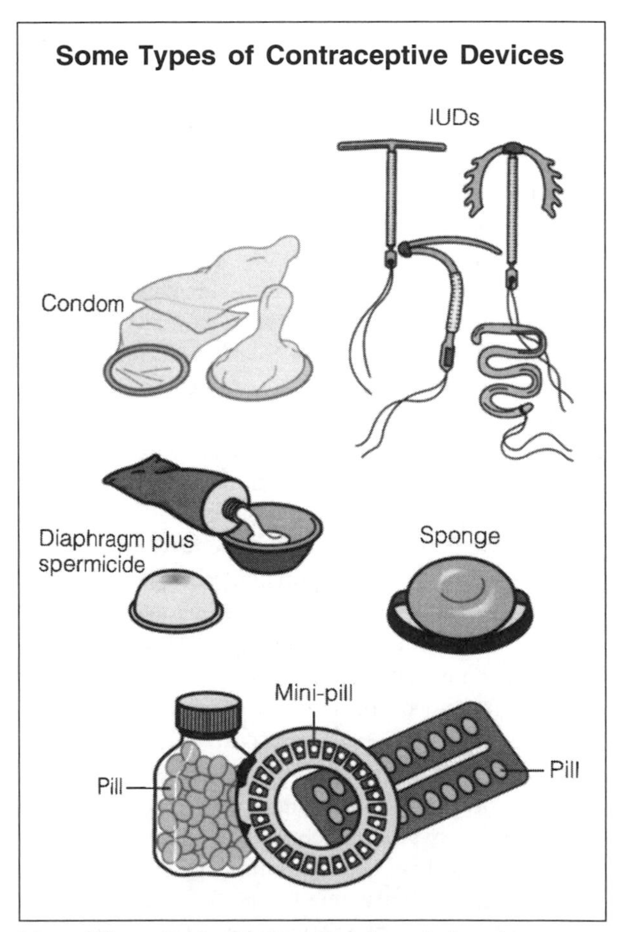

Many different kinds of devices have been designed to prevent pregnancy, from barrier methods such as condoms and diaphragms to hormonal methods such as birth control pills. Each method has its own advantages, disadvantages, and failure rates.

foams, suppositories, and tablets. They contain sperm-killing chemicals and act somewhat as a barrier to sperm entering the uterus. Spermicides used by themselves are up to 79 percent effective for birth control, but when used properly with condoms, they are up to 99 percent effective. They are available without a prescription. In order for spermicides to be effective, they should be inserted into the woman's vagina up to twenty minutes before intercourse and stay in the vagina at least eight hours. A new application of spermicide should be applied for repeated intercourse. Spermicides do not protect against STDs unless they are used in combination with condoms.

Hormonal methods. Oral contraceptives or birth control pills, often simply called "the pill," are the most popular form of reversible birth control in the United States. They contain synthetic hormones that interact with a woman's natural hormones to prevent pregnancy. There are two types of birth control pills, combination estrogen-progestin and progestin alone.

Combination birth control pills stop the ovary from releasing an egg. Available only with a doctor's prescription, they come packaged in twenty-one or twenty-eight pills per month. There are twenty-one active pills in the twenty-one-day pack. The twenty-eight-day pack contains twenty-one active pills and seven sugar pills. With both types, new packs of pills are started every twenty-eight days. Menstruation occurs during the week with no pills or sugar pills. A woman's body needs one to three months to adjust to the pill. Some other form of contraception should be used for the first month in addition to the birth control pill. By the second month, the pill should provide the needed birth control. Pills should be taken at the same time of the day each day. Oral contraceptives are 98 to 99 percent effective in providing birth control, but they provide no protection against STDs. Oral contraceptives can be taken safely by most women, but they are not recommended for women over thirty-five who smoke. A benefit of oral contraceptives is that they can make a woman's menstrual cycle regular and lighter, and they are protective against pelvic inflammatory disease (PID), ovarian cancer, and endometrial cancer.

The second form of oral contraception is the mini-pill. It contains only one hormone, progestin, and works by thickening the cervical mucus so that sperm is unable to reach the egg. Progestin also changes the lining of the uterus so that implantation cannot occur. Mini-pills are 95 percent effective in preventing pregnancy, but they do not offer protection against STDs.

Ortho Evra is a thin patch that releases a combination of estrogen and progestin. It is worn on the upper outer arm, upper torso (excluding the breast), buttocks, or abdomen. Once attached, it delivers hormones through the skin and into the bloodstream. The patch will remain in place during exercise or bathing and in humid conditions. It is worn for three weeks, then removed for one week before a new patch is worn. The patch offers approximately 99 percent birth control protection but no protection from STDs.

Depo-Provera (depo-medroxyprogesterone acetate, or DMPA) contains only the hormone progestin and can be given by a doctor as an injection every three months. Infertility may last up to a year beyond the end of the injections. DMPA works in the same way as the mini-pill. Users of DMPA should be cautious, as both adolescent and adult users have experienced a significant loss of bone density. This bone loss is thought to correct itself when the shots are discontinued. Some studies have implied that DMPA increases a woman's chance of developing cervical or breast cancer. An alternative to DMPA is Lunelle. Lunelle is also an injection, but it contains a combination of progestin and estrogen. Injections are given once a month.

A vaginal ring is a transparent flexible ring that is inserted into the vagina, normally around the cervix. The ring releases estrogen and progestin into the vagina to stop ovulation, thicken cervical mucus, and prevent implantation if fertilization occurs. It is worn for three weeks, followed by a week off during which menstruation occurs. Vaginal rings must be replaced each month. A backup method must be used during the first week after the vaginal ring is inserted for the first time, because it is not effective until seven days after the first emplacement. If the ring slips out of the vagina, you can wash the ring with cold to lukewarm water (avoid hot water) and reinsert it. If more than three hours pass with the ring outside of the vagina, then a woman will have an increased chance of pregnancy, and she should again use a back-up method for another seven days to obtain maximum protection against pregnancy.

Emergency contraceptive pills (ECPs) can be used if sexual assault occurred, if intercourse took place without the use of birth control, or partners found that a condom broke during or after sex or some other method failed. This contraceptive method involves a woman taking simultaneously two oral contraceptives containing both estrogen and progestin within seventy-two hours of unprotected sex. Twelve hours after the initial dose, another two pills must be taken simultaneously. It is often recommended that women also take an antinausea drug, such as dimenhydrinate (Gravol), because the sudden hormone increase in the body can cause nausea and vomiting. A woman should have her menstrual cycle within ten to twenty-one days of taking ECPs, and thereafter her cycle should return to normal. Emergency contraceptive pills prevent conception, rather than cause a miscarriage, by thickening the cervical mucus, thus preventing sperm from fertilizing the egg. In 2003, a Food and Drug Administration (FDA) panel recommended that these so-called morning-after pills by made available over the counter.

Intrauterine devices (IUDs). An IUD is a small device that is inserted by a doctor into a woman's uterus. The shape of the IUD is either a ring or the capital letter *T*; both have a silky or plastic thread attached that comes down into the cervix, allowing for easy removal. The ParaGard T 380A (a *T*-shaped IUD) can be kept in the uterus for ten years. An IUD is thought to prevent pregnancy because it is a foreign object whose presence causes the woman's uterus to function improperly. The IUD interferes with sperm reaching the egg and prevents the egg from implanting in the uterus. IUDs that contain copper are thought to work by the releasing of copper ions into the uterus. The copper in the uterine cavity stops the sperm from making it through the vagina and into the uterus. Copper IUDs should be replaced every ten years. Progestasert is an IUD that releases the hormone progesterone, which results in a thickening of cervical mucus so that sperm cannot reach the egg; it must be replaced every year. Mirena is another progesterone-releasing IUD; it can last up to five years. IUDs are 97 to 99 percent effective in preventing pregnancy but provide no protection from STDs.

Sterilization. Essure is a sterilization device shaped much like a spring. The device is threaded through a thin tube through the vagina and into the Fallopian tubes. Two Essure devices are inserted, one in each Fallopian tube. Once they are in place, a meshlike substance inside the devices irritates the Fallopian tubes, causing scarring of the Fallopian tubes over time. The scarring finally causes permanent closing of the tube. Since this process of blockage in the tubes takes time, women are advised to use another form of birth control for the first three months after the insertion of Essure. The device then provides more than 99 percent effectiveness as birth control. It provides no protection from STDs.

Female sterilization through tubal ligation is one of the most common forms of contraception in the United States. An estimated 700,000 women undergo tubal ligation each year. The procedure involves surgically sealing the Fallopian tubes in order to prevent the egg from being released into the uterus. This surgery also prevents a male's sperm from entering the Fallopian tube, where fertilization normally occurs. The procedure is performed in a hospital or an outpatient surgical clinic under general anesthesia. One or two small incisions are made in a woman's abdomen, and a laparoscope is inserted. Instruments are also inserted and used to burn or seal the passages into the Fallopian tubes. Patients are usually able to return home a few hours after surgery. This procedure is more than 99 percent effective as birth control but provides no protection from STDs.

Male sterilization through vasectomy can be performed in a doctor's office. Local anesthesia is applied and a small incision is made in the upper part of the scrotum. The vas deferens is cut and sealed. This simple operation prevents sperm from traveling out of the testes. There is also a nonsurgical technique in which the doctor locates the vas deferens and holds it in place with a small clamp. A tiny puncture is made in the skin, and the opening is stretched so that the vas deferens can be cut and tied. This procedure requires no stitches because the punctures heal quickly on their own. With either of these methods, a man is able to return home immediately after the procedure and usually needs only a day of rest before resuming his normal activities. It is recommended that another form of birth control be used during the first nine or ten ejaculations to ensure that the seminal fluid no longer contains sperm. This method is 99 to 100 percent effective in preventing pregnancy; however, it provides no protection against STDs.

PERSPECTIVE AND PROSPECTS

Despite the fact that highly effective contraceptive techniques are available both over the counter and through a doctor, almost 60 percent of pregnancies in the United States are not planned and many are unwanted. A direct correlation exists between the correct use of birth control and resulting protection. People who are younger, less educated, or less motivated to prevent pregnancy often fail to use contraception correctly.

Historically, contraception has had the single purpose in society of preventing unwanted pregnancies.

Today, because STDs have become epidemic, contraception has taken on the dual role of both stopping pregnancy and being the primary method of preventing the spread of STDs. Hundreds of millions of people in the United States suffer from some form of STD, while fifteen million more are infected each year. Many of these STDs and unwanted pregnancies could have been prevented if proper contraception techniques had been employed. Both men and women must assume responsibility for protecting themselves and their partners against the life-changing and sometimes life-threatening effects of STDs.

The Contraception and Reproductive Branch of the National Institute of Child Health and Human Development (NICHD), which has as one of its goals to prevent acquired immunodeficiency syndrome (AIDS) and other STDs, is looking into the development of new microcides with spermicidal activity that can provide birth control as well as simultaneous protection against major STDs. One of their top objectives is to link contraceptive technology to AIDS prevention.

—*Toby R. Stewart, Ph.D.*

See also Abortion; Conception; Ethics; Gynecology; Hormones; Hysterectomy; Men's health; Menstruation; Over-the-counter medications; Pregnancy and gestation; Reproductive system; Sterilization; Tubal ligation; Vasectomy; Women's health.

For Further Information:

Beers, Mark H., ed. *The Merck Manual of Medical Information, Second Home Edition*. Whitehouse Station, N.J.: Merck Research Laboratories, 2003. A comprehensive book of medical knowledge, including information on contraception.

Connell, Elizabeth B. *The Contraception Sourcebook*. Chicago: Contemporary Books, 2002. Provides a history and explanation of contraception, from oral contraceptives to male contraception.

Keyzer, Amy Marcaccio. *Family Planning Sourcebook*. Detroit: Omnigraphics, 2001. Contains excellent information on all types of contraception and family planning.

Thornton, Yvonne S. *Woman to Woman: A Leading Gynecologist Tells You All You Need to Know About Your Body and Your Health*. New York: E. P. Dutton, 1998. Divided into six sections covering topics from female physiology to contraception.

Corneal transplantation

Procedure

Anatomy or system affected: Eyes

Specialties and related fields: General surgery, ophthalmology

Definition: A delicate surgical operation involving the removal and replacement of the cornea, the transparent outer covering of the eye.

Key terms:

endothelium: the inner surface of the cornea, which is separated from the rest of the eye by an essential layer of transparent fluid

lamellar keratoplasty: the partial removal or transplantation of a portion of the cornea; usually possible in younger patients or those with less advanced disorders

penetrating keratoplasty: the surgical transplantation of the entire thickness of the cornea, which is made up of four distinct layers of tissue

trephine: a specialized surgical instrument that is used to cut a perfectly vertical incision to remove corneas from both the donor and the recipient

Indications and Procedures

The cornea, which has four distinct layers, is the transparent outer coating of the eye. It serves both to protect the eye and to provide the main refracting surface as light reaches the eye and is transmitted to the lens and retina. Its total thickness is approximately .52 millimeters. The layers of specialized tissue are the epithelium, the stroma, Descemet's membrane, and the endothelium, or inner surface of the cornea.

Several types of corneal disorders may lead to a decision to perform partial or total keratoplasty. Most of these fall under the general term "corneal dystrophy." The most common, or classical, cases of corneal dystrophy involve the deposit of abnormal material in the cornea, resulting in irritation and eventually damage. Frequently, such disorders stem from genetic factors, making it possible to diagnose the dystrophy during the patient's childhood and perform a lamellar keratoplasty. Other dystrophies include granular dystrophy and macular dystrophy. The former involves lesions in the center of the cornea, which may multiply and coalesce. At that stage, they may extend into the deeper layers of the stroma, the second layer of the cornea. Macular dystrophy actually begins in the stroma, causing all layers to become opaque.

Entirely different types of disorders that may call for corneal transplantation are interstitial keratitis (a type of inflammation) and trachoma. The latter condition can reach near epidemic levels in underdeveloped areas of the world, where low levels of hygiene allow the implantation and rapid multiplication of bacteria in the cornea. The effect is a breakdown of tissue accompanied by the discharge of mucus.

Whether the cornea has been affected by disease or injury, the goal of corneal transplantation is to eliminate any opacity that can hamper vision. The graft operation itself may be described in only a few stages, each marked by the need for a high degree of technical skill to increase the likelihood of success. First, the surgeon must calculate the exact size of the graft in question. This is done through the use of a special tool called a trephine, which will make the cuts to remove both the donor and the host eye corneas. Some trephines are equipped with transparent lenses to give the surgeon maximum levels of accuracy. When the two vital incisions are made, great care is taken to obtain a perfectly vertical cut.

Beginning with this initial stage, the surgeon may add a bubble of air through the incision to protect the endothelium and reduce the likelihood of an immune system reaction once the donor cornea has been transplanted. As the transfer occurs, another air bubble is introduced. After suturing, this bubble will be replaced by a balanced salt solution called acetylcholine.

This suturing, which must be very precise, almost always begins with four sutures at the cardinal points to ensure even tension. The last stage of the operation involves checking the wound for leakage of acetylcholine. This step is necessary not only to avoid infection but also to guard against rejection of the cornea by the host organ.

USES AND COMPLICATIONS

Significant differences in the healing process following corneal transplantation occur according to the method of suturing. A choice is made between a continuing or an interrupted series of sutures around the circumference of the cornea. Interrupted sutures may be preferred if there is a chance of uneven healing of the wound, something the physician may judge following examination of the degree of vascularization in particular corneal graft beds. In some cases, surgeons may opt for double suturing.

The chief complication that can follow corneal transplantation is rejection by the immune system. Surgeons try to obviate this risk by close study of the factors that can affect the receptivity of the eye to a new cornea. Earlier literature on corneal transplantation tended to assume that there was a lack of antigenicity—the production of disease-fighting antigens, or antibodies, as a defense system against viruses, bacteria, or foreign tissues—in the cornea. As ophthalmologists developed a fuller understanding of the immunological role of blood vessels and the lymphatic system, however, the need to give considerable attention to the degree of vascularization of the graft bed zone became more obvious. One method that surgeons can use to reduce antigen activity and enhance host acceptance is part of the transplantation operation itself: constant maintenance of a liquid layer between the host tissue and the new cornea tissue being transplanted. In the late 1990's, researchers at the University of Texas Southwestern Medical Center at Dallas announced the creation of an oral vaccine that may prevent rejection. Processed corneal cells in liquid form fed to laboratory mice produced a marked reduction in rejection rates. Current studies focus on the success of the vaccine with humans.

Although the period for healing and suture removal varies from patient to patient, the surgeon looks for the normal development of a gray-tinged scar tissue in the incision area as a sign of success. Failure, if discovered in time, may lead to a second transplantation attempt.

PERSPECTIVE AND PROSPECTS

The first attempts to perform corneal transplantation—all unsuccessful—date from the nineteenth century. In the 1820's, German doctor F. Reisinger experimented with corneal grafts using rabbits and chickens. In the 1830's, Samuel Bigger of Ireland and R. S. Kissam of the United States tried to pioneer surgical grafts on humans, but both made the error of trying to replace human corneas with animal corneas. Success with living tissue (as opposed to the application of a glass product) finally came in 1905 when Moravian doctor Edward Zirm transplanted a child donor's cornea to the eye of a chemical burn victim. Zirm's success was based on cumulative medical knowledge of antiseptics, anesthesia, and technical aids such as the ophthalmoscope and the trephine. After a long period without major changes, in 1935 a Russian scientist named Filatov experimented with two innovations that were copied in other countries: the use of egg membrane to enhance a firm fix and the insertion of a delicate spatula between the cornea and lens to protect the intraocular tissues.

The greatest advances were made soon after antibiotics and steroids were introduced in the 1940's. By the

1950's, the use of extremely delicate surgical needles helped reduce postsurgical rejection rates. Major contributions to the development of delicate surgical instruments were made by the Spanish ophthalmologist Ramón Castroviejo, who performed many operations in the United States. By the 1980's, Castroviejo was urging others to follow the example of Townley Paton, who founded New York's first eye bank some two decades earlier.

By the turn of the twenty-first century, forty thousand people in the United States had received corneal transplants using cells taken from the eyes of donors who had died. However, many patients with severe corneal damage cannot be helped by conventional cornea transplants. Two research teams, onc in Taiwan, at the University of Taoyuan, and one at the University of California at Davis School of Medicine, used stem cells to continually produce new corneal cells within the eye. In Taiwan, stem cells were placed on amniotic membrane, taken from placentas, to grow the tissue. In California, cells were first grown in laboratory dishes and then placed on the amniotic membrane to produce the tissue, which was transplanted to the damaged corneas. The use of this kind of tissue showed improved or restored vision for patients with corneal damage. While these procedures hold great potential for worldwide application, they have been called "investigational" and by no means eliminate the need for cornea donors.

The prospects for increasingly higher success rates in the field of corneal transplantation are linked to technical progress in donor organ conservation and the level of precision that can be achieved in carrying out transplantation operations.

—*Byron D. Cannon, Ph.D.*

See also Eye infections and disorders; Eye surgery; Eyes; Grafts and grafting; Keratitis; Ophthalmology; Trachoma; Transplantation; Vision disorders.

For Further Information:

Brightbill, Frederick S., ed. *Corneal Surgery*. 3d ed. St. Louis: C. V. Mosby, 1999. This rather technical text is divided into sections in which the authors discuss their specific areas of expertise.

Foster, C. Stephen, Dimitri T. Azar, and Claes H. Dohlman, eds. *Smolin and Thoft's The Cornea: Scientific Foundations and Clinical Practice*. 4th ed. Philadelphia: Lippincott Williams & Wilkins, 2005. This covers some cornea-related topics that either are absent from standard texts (for example, congenital anomalies) or reflect recent surgical advances (for example, corneal surgery to make refractive corrections to reduce or remove myopia).

Parker, James N., and Philip M. Parker, eds. *The Official Patient's Sourcebook on Corneal Transplant Surgery*. San Diego, Calif.: Icon Health, 2002. Draws from public, academic, government, and peer-reviewed research to provide a wide-ranging handbook for patients facing corneal transplant surgery.

Spaeth, George L., ed. *Ophthalmic Surgery*. 3d ed. Philadelphia: W. B. Saunders, 2003. The subsections of this text deal with all aspects of eye surgery, including corneal surgery and operations to correct glaucoma, cataracts, and retinal displacement.

Sutton, Amy, ed. *Eye Care Sourcebook: Basic Consumer Health Information About Eye Care and Eye Disorders*. 2d ed. Detroit: Omnigraphics, 2003. A complete guide to eye care that includes such topics as eye anatomy, preventive vision care, refractive disorders and eye diseases, surgical treatment, current research and clinical trials, and a list of organizations.

Cornelia de Lange syndrome

Disease/disorder

Also known as: Amsterdam dwarfism, Brachmann-de Lange syndrome

Anatomy or system affected: Arms, brain, ears, eyes, feet, hair, hands, head, heart, immune system, legs, mouth, nose, teeth

Specialties and related fields: Genetics, neurology, pediatrics, physical therapy

Definition: A disorder with distinctive physical abnormalities and mental retardation usually apparent at birth.

Causes and Symptoms

Cornelia de Lange syndrome occurs at an estimated rate of 1 per 10,000 to 30,000 live births. Sometimes siblings have this syndrome, reinforcing the hypothesis that it is hereditary. Although the precise causation is unknown, researchers are investigating the possibility that a mutated gene on chromosome 3 is responsible.

The physical appearance of children with this syndrome is significantly altered. Patients are smaller in size and weight than average infants, and their growth and motor development are usually delayed. Upper limbs are often deformed, with missing tissues. Although legs attain average size and development appropriate to patients' age, sometimes toes are webbed.

> **Information on Cornelia de Lange Syndrome**
>
> **Causes:** Unknown, possibly genetic
> **Symptoms:** Low size and weight, delayed growth and motor development, deformed upper limbs, webbed toes, small hands, small head, heavy body hair, heart abnormalities, cleft palate, reflux, convulsions, impaired immune system
> **Duration:** Lifelong
> **Treatments:** Incubation to monitor respiration and nutrition, antibiotics, surgical procedures for specific ailments, physical therapy, auditory devices, prosthetics

Hands tend to be tiny. Patients share similar facial characteristics. Heads are abnormally small with upturned nostrils and thin lips and eyebrows. Heavy body hair often grows.

Intellectual development is impeded, particularly affecting vocalization. Hearing and vision sometimes are affected. Patients often suffer heart abnormalities, cleft palate, reflux, and convulsions. They are vulnerable to infections because of impaired immune systems.

Prenatal ultrasounds can reveal if fetuses have physical deficiencies that might be associated with Cornelia de Lange syndrome. Physicians identify the syndrome by observing characteristics evident in infants and toddlers. Genetic professionals confirm diagnoses, especially in patients whose symptoms are less obvious.

Treatment and Therapy

Many newborns with Cornelia de Lange syndrome require incubation to monitor respiration and nutrition. Antibiotics and other medications, as well as surgical procedures, are administered to treat specific ailments affecting these individuals. Physical therapy, auditory devices, and prosthetics can aid children. Some patients have shortened life spans and are unable to live autonomously. Heart conditions cause most of the deaths associated with this syndrome.

Although no known cure or prevention exists, medical awareness and treatment of this syndrome can extend the life span and enhance the quality of life for many patients. Some patients with milder conditions survive to average life expectancies. Adults with this syndrome attain a height from four to five feet and undergo puberty at normal ages. Various therapies can assist patients who exhibit aggressive and self-destructive behaviors and improve communication and social skills.

Perspective and Prospects

In 1916, Dr. Winfried R. Brachmann became the first physician to document this syndrome's characteristics in an infant. Dutch pediatrician Cornelia C. de Lange clinically described two patients in 1933 and discussed her work at neurological conferences. By the early twenty-first century, researchers had established a Cornelia de Lange syndrome database to coordinate information. Geneticists, particularly Dr. Ian Krantz and his colleagues, conducted molecular investigations to determine the genetic causation of this syndrome. A mutation in a gene known as NIPBL is now known to be one cause of this relatively rare disorder. This gene provides direction for the making of a protein, delangin, which is very important in developmental regulation of a number of body parts in the fetus. In the United States, the Cornelia de Lange Syndrome-USA Foundation provides support for affected families.

—Elizabeth D. Schafer, Ph.D.;
updated by Lenela Glass-Godwin, M.WS.

See also Birth defects; Dwarfism; Genetic diseases; Genetics and inheritance; Mental retardation.

For Further Information:

Benson, M. "Cornelia de Lange Syndrome: A Case Study." *Neonatal Network* 21, no. 3 (April, 2002): 7-13.

Berg, J. M., et al. *The De Lange Syndrome*. New York: Pergamon Press, 1970.

Cornelia de Lange Syndrome-USA Foundation. http://www.cdlsusa.org/.

Gardner, R. J. M. "Another Explanation for Familial Cornelia de Lange Syndrome." *American Journal of Medical Genetics* 118A, no. 2 (April 15, 2003): 198.

Gilbert, Patricia. *Dictionary of Syndromes and Inherited Disorders*. 3d ed. Chicago: Fitzroy Dearborn, 2000.

Corns and calluses

Disease/disorder

Anatomy or system affected: Feet, hands, skin
Specialties and related fields: Dermatology, podiatry
Definition: Areas of thickened skin that form as a result of constant pressure or friction over a bony prominence.

Causes and Symptoms

Both corns (clavi) and calluses (tylomas or tyloses) occur when chronic pressure or friction causes hypertrophy of the dermal skin layer and a proliferation of keratin as a protective response. Both corns and calluses usually occur on the feet. Corns develop from pressure on normally thin skin. Calluses develop over areas where the skin is normally thicker. They commonly develop on the plantar (sole) surface of the foot and on the palmar (palm) surface of the hand. Corns are frequently painful, whereas calluses usually are not painful. Corns are small, flat, or slightly elevated lesions with a smooth, hard surface. Calluses cover a larger area than corns and are less well demarcated.

There are two classifications of corns: hard and soft. Hard corns have a conical structure composed of keratin, with the point of the cone directed inward, causing pain when pressed into the soft, underlying tissue. Hard corns have a circumscribed border that demarcates the lesions from the surrounding soft tissue. Hard corns usually develop on the top or sides of the toes, where shoes press on the interphalangeal joints of the toes, or the plantar surface of the foot, where pressure is exerted against bony prominences.

Soft corns develop in areas where a bony prominence causes constant pressure against soft tissue, resulting in a blanched thickening of the skin. Because soft corns commonly develop on interdigital surfaces, such as between the fourth and fifth toe, they are characteristically moist and macerated and can become inflamed.

Calluses develop as a protection against continual pressure. They do not have the central core of keratin and as a result are not sensitive to pressure. Normal skin markings are present over callused areas. Calluses usually develop on weight-bearing areas of the foot under the metatarsal heads and the heel. Calluses on the palm are frequently the result of manual occupations.

Information on Corns and Calluses

Causes: Constant pressure or friction over bony prominence, often from improperly fitting shoes

Symptoms: Pain, inflammation, rough skin

Duration: Typically short-term, occasionally chronic

Treatments: Better-fitting footwear, over-the-counter medications, occasionally surgery

Treatment and Therapy

Treatment of corns and calluses depends on symptoms. Since corns and calluses are caused by chronic pressure, preventive measures include removing the source of friction or pressure. Well-fitting shoes that do not crowd the toes relieve pressure on interdigital areas. Soft, sufficiently wide or open-toed shoes are good choices. Soft insoles and properly fitting stockings also reduce pressure. Wrapping lamb's wool or other padding over pressure points can increase air circulation and reduce pressure and discomfort. Corns and calluses can be treated with over-the-counter keratolytic agents. Salicylic acid plasters are used to soften the tissue, which can then be removed with a pumice stone. When corns, or occasionally calluses, become inflamed or painful, they can be removed by paring or trimming. This should be done by a health care provider, especially in patients with compromised circulation to the feet. In rare circumstances, surgery may be required if a corn or callus becomes infected or if the chronic pressure on particular areas is caused by a structural abnormality of the foot, such as a hammertoe.

—Roberta Tierney, M.S.N., J.D., A.P.N.

See also Bunions; Dermatology; Feet; Foot disorders; Hammertoe correction; Hammertoes; Hypertrophy; Podiatry; Skin; Skin disorders.

For Further Information:

Copeland, D. P. M. Glenn, and Stan Solomon. *The Foot Doctor: Lifetime Relief for Your Aching Feet.* Emmaus, Pa.: Rodale Press, 1986.

Lippert, Frederick G., and Sigvard T. Hansen. *Foot and Ankle Disorders: Tricks of the Trade.* New York: Thieme, 2003.

Lorimer, Donald L., et al., eds. *Neale's Disorders of the Foot.* 7th ed. New York: Elsevier Churchill Livingstone, 2006.

Mackie, Rona M. *Clinical Dermatology.* 5th ed. New York: Oxford University Press, 2003.

MAGILL'S
MEDICAL GUIDE

Entries by Anatomy or System Affected

ABDOMEN

ANUS

ARMS

BACK

BREASTS

CELLS

CHEST

Pacemaker implantation
Pityriasis rosea
Pleurisy
Pneumonia
Pulmonary diseases
Pulmonary medicine
Pulmonary medicine, pediatric
Respiration
Respiratory distress syndrome
Resuscitation
Sneezing
Thoracic surgery
Tuberculosis
Wheezing
Whooping cough

CIRCULATORY SYSTEM

Aneurysmectomy
Aneurysms
Angina
Angiography
Angioplasty
Antihistamines
Apgar score
Arrhythmias
Arteriosclerosis
Biofeedback
Bleeding
Blood and blood disorders
Blood testing
Blue baby syndrome
Bypass surgery
Cardiac arrest
Cardiac rehabilitation
Cardiology
Cardiology, pediatric
Cardiopulmonary resuscitation (CPR)
Catheterization
Chest
Cholesterol
Circulation
Claudication
Congenital heart disease
Decongestants
Dehydration
Diabetes mellitus
Dialysis
Disseminated intravascular coagulation (DIC)
Dizziness and fainting
Ebola virus
Echocardiography
Edema
Electrocardiography (ECG or EKG)
Electrocauterization
Embolism
Endarterectomy
Endocarditis
Ergogenic aids
Exercise physiology
Facial transplantation
Heart
Heart attack
Heart disease
Heart failure
Heart transplantation
Heart valve replacement
Heat exhaustion and heat stroke
Hematology
Hematology, pediatric
Hemorrhoid banding and removal
Hemorrhoids
Hormones
Hyperbaric oxygen therapy
Hypercholesterolemia
Hypertension
Hypotension
Ischemia
Juvenile rheumatoid arthritis
Kidneys
Kinesiology
Klippel-Trenaunay syndrome
Liver
Lymphatic system
Marburg virus
Marijuana
Mitral valve prolapse
Motor skill development
Nosebleeds
Obesity
Obesity, childhood
Osteochondritis juvenilis
Pacemaker implantation
Palpitations
Phlebitis
Phlebotomy
Placenta
Preeclampsia and eclampsia
Resuscitation
Reye's syndrome
Rheumatic fever
Scleroderma
Septicemia
Shock
Shunts
Smoking
Sports medicine
Stents
Steroid abuse
Strokes
Sturge-Weber syndrome
Systems and organs
Testicular torsion
Thrombocytopenia
Thrombolytic therapy and TPA
Thrombosis and thrombus
Transfusion
Transient ischemic attacks (TIAs)
Transplantation
Typhus
Varicose vein removal
Varicose veins
Vascular medicine
Vascular system
Venous insufficiency

EARS

Altitude sickness
Antihistamines
Audiology
Auras
Biophysics
Cornelia de Lange syndrome
Cytomegalovirus (CMV)
Deafness
Decongestants
Dyslexia
Ear infections and disorders
Ear surgery
Ears
Fragile X syndrome
Hearing aids
Hearing loss
Hearing tests
Histiocytosis
Leukodystrophy
Ménière's disease
Motion sickness
Myringotomy
Nervous system
Neurology
Neurology, pediatric
Osteogenesis imperfecta
Otoplasty
Otorhinolaryngology
Plastic surgery
Quinsy
Rubinstein-Taybi syndrome
Sense organs
Speech disorders
Wiskott-Aldrich syndrome

ENDOCRINE SYSTEM

EYES

FEET

GALLBLADDER

GASTROINTESTINAL SYSTEM

GENITALS

GLANDS

GUMS

HAIR

HANDS
Amputation
Arthritis
Bones and the skeleton
Bursitis
Carpal tunnel syndrome
Cerebral palsy
Cornelia de Lange syndrome
Corns and calluses
Cysts
Fracture and dislocation
Fracture repair
Fragile X syndrome
Frostbite
Ganglion removal
Nail removal
Nails
Neurology
Neurology, pediatric
Orthopedic surgery
Orthopedics
Orthopedics, pediatric
Osteoarthritis
Rheumatoid arthritis
Rheumatology
Rubinstein-Taybi syndrome
Scleroderma
Skin lesion removal
Sports medicine
Tendinitis
Tendon disorders
Tendon repair
Thalidomide
Upper extremities
Warts

HEAD
Altitude sickness
Aneurysmectomy
Aneurysms
Angiography
Antihistamines
Botox
Brain
Brain disorders
Brain tumors
Cluster headaches
Coma
Computed tomography (CT) scanning
Concussion
Cornelia de Lange syndrome
Craniosynostosis
Craniotomy
Dizziness and fainting
Electroencephalography (EEG)
Embolism
Epilepsy
Facial transplantation
Fetal tissue transplantation
Fibromyalgia
Hair loss and baldness
Hair transplantation
Head and neck disorders
Headaches
Hydrocephalus
Lice, mites, and ticks
Meningitis
Migraine headaches
Nasal polyp removal
Nasopharyngeal disorders
Neuroimaging
Neurology
Neurology, pediatric
Neurosurgery
Rhinoplasty and submucous resection
Rubinstein-Taybi syndrome
Seizures
Shunts
Sports medicine
Strokes
Sturge-Weber syndrome
Temporomandibular joint (TMJ) syndrome
Thrombosis and thrombus
Unconsciousness
Whiplash

HEART
Aneurysmectomy
Aneurysms
Angina
Angiography
Angioplasty
Anxiety
Apgar score
Arrhythmias
Arteriosclerosis
Biofeedback
Bites and stings
Blue baby syndrome
Bypass surgery
Caffeine
Cardiac arrest
Cardiac rehabilitation
Cardiology
Cardiology, pediatric
Cardiopulmonary resuscitation (CPR)
Catheterization
Circulation
Congenital heart disease
Cornelia de Lange syndrome
DiGeorge syndrome
Echocardiography
Electrical shock
Electrocardiography (ECG or EKG)
Embolism
Endocarditis
Exercise physiology
Fatty acid oxidation disorders
Glycogen storage diseases
Heart
Heart attack
Heart disease
Heart failure
Heart transplantation
Heart valve replacement
Hemochromatosis
Hypertension
Hypotension
Internal medicine
Juvenile rheumatoid arthritis
Kinesiology
Lyme disease
Marfan syndrome
Marijuana
Mitral valve prolapse
Nicotine
Obesity
Obesity, childhood
Pacemaker implantation
Palpitations
Prader-Willi syndrome
Respiratory distress syndrome
Resuscitation
Reye's syndrome
Rheumatic fever
Rubinstein-Taybi syndrome
Scleroderma
Shock
Sports medicine
Stents
Steroid abuse
Strokes
Thoracic surgery
Thrombolytic therapy and TPA
Thrombosis and thrombus
Toxoplasmosis
Transplantation
Ultrasonography
Yellow fever

LEGS

LIGAMENTS

LIVER

LUNGS

LYMPHATIC SYSTEM

MOUTH

MUSCLES

MUSCULOSKELETAL SYSTEM

NAILS

NECK

NERVES

Spinal cord disorders
Spine, vertebrae, and disks
Sturge-Weber syndrome
Sympathectomy
Tics
Touch
Tourette's syndrome
Upper extremities
Vagotomy

NERVOUS SYSTEM
Abscess drainage
Abscesses
Acupressure
Addiction
Alcoholism
Altitude sickness
Alzheimer's disease
Amnesia
Amputation
Amyotrophic lateral sclerosis
Anesthesia
Anesthesiology
Aneurysmectomy
Aneurysms
Antidepressants
Anxiety
Apgar score
Aphasia and dysphasia
Apnea
Aromatherapy
Ataxia
Attention-deficit disorder (ADD)
Auras
Autism
Back pain
Balance disorders
Batten's disease
Behçet's disease
Bell's palsy
Beriberi
Biofeedback
Botulism
Brain
Brain damage
Brain disorders
Brain tumors
Caffeine
Carpal tunnel syndrome
Cells
Cerebral palsy
Chagas' disease
Chiropractic
Chronic wasting disease (CWD)
Claudication
Cluster headaches
Cognitive development
Coma
Computed tomography (CT) scanning
Concussion
Craniotomy
Cretinism
Creutzfeldt-Jakob disease (CJD)
Cysts
Deafness
Dementias
Developmental stages
Diabetes mellitus
Diphtheria
Disk removal
Dizziness and fainting
Down syndrome
Dwarfism
Dyslexia
E. coli infection
Ear surgery
Ears
Electrical shock
Electroencephalography (EEG)
Emotions: Biomedical causes and effects
Encephalitis
Endocrinology
Endocrinology, pediatric
Epilepsy
Eye infections and disorders
Eyes
Facial transplantation
Fetal alcohol syndrome
Fetal tissue transplantation
Fibromyalgia
Gigantism
Glands
Guillain-Barré syndrome
Hallucinations
Hammertoe correction
Head and neck disorders
Headaches
Hearing aids
Hearing loss
Hearing tests
Heart transplantation
Hemiplegia
Histiocytosis
Huntington's disease
Hydrocephalus
Hypnosis
Insect-borne diseases
Intraventricular hemorrhage
Irritable bowel syndrome (IBS)
Kinesiology
Lead poisoning
Learning disabilities
Leprosy
Light therapy
Lower extremities
Lyme disease
Malaria
Maple syrup urine disease (MSUD)
Marijuana
Memory loss
Meningitis
Mental retardation
Mercury poisoning
Migraine headaches
Motor neuron diseases
Motor skill development
Multiple chemical sensitivity syndrome
Multiple sclerosis
Myasthenia gravis
Narcolepsy
Narcotics
Nausea and vomiting
Nervous system
Neuralgia, neuritis, and neuropathy
Neurofibromatosis
Neuroimaging
Neurology
Neurology, pediatric
Neurosurgery
Niemann-Pick disease
Nuclear radiology
Numbness and tingling
Orthopedic surgery
Orthopedics
Orthopedics, pediatric
Overtraining syndrome
Paget's disease
Palsy
Paralysis
Paraplegia
Parkinson's disease
Pharmacology
Pharmacy
Phenylketonuria (PKU)
Physical rehabilitation
Pick's disease
Poisoning
Poliomyelitis

NOSE

PANCREAS

PSYCHIC-EMOTIONAL SYSTEM

REPRODUCTIVE SYSTEM

RESPIRATORY SYSTEM

SKIN

Allergies
Amputation
Anesthesia
Anesthesiology
Anthrax
Anxiety
Athlete's foot
Auras
Bariatric surgery
Batten's disease
Behçet's disease
Biopsy
Birthmarks
Bites and stings
Blisters
Blood testing
Boils
Bruises
Burns and scalds
Candidiasis
Canker sores
Cells
Chagas' disease
Chickenpox
Cleft lip and palate repair
Cold sores
Corns and calluses
Corticosteroids
Cryotherapy and cryosurgery
Cyanosis
Cyst removal
Cysts
Dermatitis
Dermatology
Dermatology, pediatric
Dermatopathology
Diaper rash
Ebola virus
Eczema
Edema
Electrical shock
Electrocauterization
Face lift and blepharoplasty
Facial transplantation
Fifth disease
Frostbite
Fungal infections
Glands
Grafts and grafting
Gulf War syndrome
Hair
Hair loss and baldness
Hair transplantation
Hand-foot-and-mouth disease
Heat exhaustion and heat stroke
Hemolytic disease of the newborn
Histiocytosis
Hives
Host-defense mechanisms
Human papillomavirus (HPV)
Hyperhidrosis
Impetigo
Insect-borne diseases
Itching
Jaundice
Kaposi's sarcoma
Kawasaki disease
Laceration repair
Laser use in surgery
Leishmaniasis
Leprosy
Lice, mites, and ticks
Light therapy
Lower extremities
Lyme disease
Marburg virus
Measles
Melanoma
Moles
Monkeypox
Multiple chemical sensitivity syndrome
Nails
Necrotizing fasciitis
Neurofibromatosis
Nicotine
Numbness and tingling
Obesity
Obesity, childhood
Otoplasty
Pigmentation
Pinworm
Pityriasis alba
Pityriasis rosea
Plastic surgery
Poisonous plants
Porphyria
Psoriasis
Radiation sickness
Rashes
Reiter's syndrome
Ringworm
Rosacea
Roseola
Rubella
Scabies
Scarlet fever
Scurvy
Sense organs
Shingles
Skin
Skin cancer
Skin disorders
Skin lesion removal
Smallpox
Stretch marks
Sturge-Weber syndrome
Sunburn
Sweating
Systemic lupus erythematosus (SLE)
Tattoo removal
Tattoos and body piercing
Touch
Tularemia
Typhus
Umbilical cord
Upper extremities
Von Willebrand's disease
Warts
Wiskott-Aldrich syndrome
Wrinkles

SPINE

Anesthesia
Anesthesiology
Back pain
Bone cancer
Bone disorders
Bones and the skeleton
Cerebral palsy
Chiropractic
Disk removal
Fracture and dislocation
Head and neck disorders
Kinesiology
Laminectomy and spinal fusion
Lumbar puncture
Marfan syndrome
Meningitis
Motor neuron diseases
Multiple sclerosis
Muscle sprains, spasms, and disorders
Muscles
Muscular dystrophy
Nervous system
Neuralgia, neuritis, and neuropathy
Neurology
Neurology, pediatric
Neurosurgery
Numbness and tingling
Orthopedic surgery

Entries by Specialties and Related Fields

ALL
Accidents
African American health
American Indian health
Anatomy
Asian American health
Biostatistics
Clinical trials
Disease
Geriatrics and gerontology
Health maintenance organizations (HMOs)
Iatrogenic disorders
Imaging and radiology
Internet medicine
Invasive tests
Laboratory tests
Men's health
Neuroimaging
Noninvasive tests
Pediatrics
Physical examination
Physiology
Polypharmacy
Preventive medicine
Proteomics
Screening
Self-medication
Systems and organs
Telemedicine
Terminally ill: Extended care
Veterinary medicine
Women's health

ALTERNATIVE MEDICINE
Acupressure
Acupuncture
Allied health
Alternative medicine
Antioxidants
Aphrodisiacs
Aromatherapy
Biofeedback
Chronobiology
Club drugs
Colon therapy
Enzyme therapy
Healing
Herbal medicine
Holistic medicine
Hydrotherapy
Hypnosis
Magnetic field therapy
Marijuana
Massage
Meditation
Melatonin
Nutrition
Oxygen therapy
Pain management
Stress reduction
Supplements
Yoga

ANESTHESIOLOGY
Acupuncture
Anesthesia
Anesthesiology
Catheterization
Cesarean section
Critical care
Critical care, pediatric
Dentistry
Hyperbaric oxygen therapy
Hyperthermia and hypothermia
Hypnosis
Pain management
Pharmacology
Pharmacy
Surgery, general
Surgery, pediatric
Surgical procedures
Surgical technologists
Toxicology

AUDIOLOGY
Aging
Aging: Extended care
Audiology
Biophysics
Deafness
Dyslexia
Ear infections and disorders
Ear surgery
Ears
Hearing aids
Hearing loss
Hearing tests
Ménière's disease
Motion sickness
Neurology
Neurology, pediatric
Otoplasty
Otorhinolaryngology
Sense organs
Speech disorders

BACTERIOLOGY
Anthrax
Antibiotics
Bacterial infections
Bacteriology
Biological and chemical weapons
Blisters
Boils
Botulism
Cells
Childhood infectious diseases
Cholecystitis
Cholera
Cystitis
Cytology
Cytopathology
Diphtheria
Drug resistance
E. coli infection
Endocarditis
Fluoride treatments
Gangrene
Genomics
Gonorrhea
Gram staining
Impetigo
Infection
Laboratory tests
Legionnaires' disease
Leprosy
Lyme disease
Mastitis
Microbiology
Microscopy
Necrotizing fasciitis
Nephritis
Osteomyelitis
Pelvic inflammatory disease (PID)
Plague
Pneumonia
Salmonella infection
Scarlet fever
Serology

Shigellosis
Staphylococcal infections
Strep throat
Streptococcal infections
Syphilis
Tetanus
Tonsillitis
Tropical medicine
Tuberculosis
Tularemia
Typhoid fever
Typhus
Whooping cough

BIOCHEMISTRY
Acid-base chemistry
Antidepressants
Autopsy
Bacteriology
Caffeine
Cholesterol
Corticosteroids
Digestion
Endocrinology
Endocrinology, pediatric
Enzyme therapy
Enzymes
Ergogenic aids
Fatty acid oxidation disorders
Fluids and electrolytes
Fluoride treatments
Food biochemistry
Fructosemia
Gaucher's disease
Genetic engineering
Genomics
Glands
Glycogen storage diseases
Glycolysis
Gram staining
Histology
Hormones
Leptin
Leukodystrophy
Lipids
Malabsorption
Metabolism
Nephrology
Nephrology, pediatric
Niemann-Pick disease
Nutrition
Pathology
Pharmacology
Pharmacy
Respiration
Stem cells
Steroids
Toxicology
Urinalysis
Wilson's disease

BIOTECHNOLOGY
Assisted reproductive technologies
Bionics and biotechnology
Biophysics
Cloning
Computed tomography (CT) scanning
Dialysis
Echocardiography
Electrocardiography (ECG or EKG)
Electroencephalography (EEG)
Fatty acid oxidation disorders
Gene therapy
Genetic engineering
Genomics
Glycogen storage diseases
Huntington's disease
Hyperbaric oxygen therapy
In vitro fertilization
Magnetic resonance imaging (MRI)
Pacemaker implantation
Positron emission tomography (PET) scanning
Prostheses
Severe combined immunodeficiency syndrome (SCID)
Sperm banks
Stem cells
Xenotransplantation

CARDIOLOGY
Aging
Aging: Extended care
Aneurysmectomy
Aneurysms
Angina
Angiography
Angioplasty
Anxiety
Arrhythmias
Arteriosclerosis
Biofeedback
Blue baby syndrome
Bypass surgery
Cardiac arrest
Cardiac rehabilitation
Cardiology
Cardiology, pediatric
Cardiopulmonary resuscitation (CPR)
Catheterization
Chest
Cholesterol
Circulation
Congenital heart disease
Critical care
Critical care, pediatric
DiGeorge syndrome
Dizziness and fainting
Echocardiography
Electrocardiography (ECG or EKG)
Emergency medicine
Endocarditis
Exercise physiology
Fetal surgery
Geriatrics and gerontology
Heart
Heart attack
Heart disease
Heart failure
Heart transplantation
Heart valve replacement
Hematology
Hemochromatosis
Hypercholesterolemia
Hypertension
Hypotension
Internal medicine
Ischemia
Kinesiology
Leptin
Marfan syndrome
Metabolic syndrome
Mitral valve prolapse
Mucopolysaccharidosis (MPS)
Muscles
Neonatology
Nicotine
Noninvasive tests
Nuclear medicine
Pacemaker implantation
Palpitations
Paramedics
Physical examination
Polycystic kidney disease
Prader-Willi syndrome
Progeria
Prostheses
Pulmonary hypertension
Rheumatic fever

DERMATOLOGY
Abscess drainage
Abscesses
Acne
Age spots
Albinos
Anthrax
Anti-inflammatory drugs
Athlete's foot
Biopsy
Birthmarks
Blisters
Boils
Burns and scalds
Carcinoma
Chickenpox
Corns and calluses
Corticosteroids
Cryotherapy and cryosurgery
Cyst removal
Cysts
Dermatitis
Dermatology
Dermatology, pediatric
Dermatopathology
Eczema
Electrocauterization
Facial transplantation
Fungal infections
Ganglion removal
Glands
Grafts and grafting
Gray hair
Hair
Hair loss and baldness
Hair transplantation
Hand-foot-and-mouth disease
Healing
Histology
Hives
Hyperhidrosis
Impetigo
Itching
Laser use in surgery
Lice, mites, and ticks
Light therapy
Melanoma
Moles
Monkeypox
Multiple chemical sensitivity syndrome
Nail removal
Nails
Necrotizing fasciitis
Neurofibromatosis
Pigmentation
Pinworm
Pityriasis alba
Pityriasis rosea
Plastic surgery
Podiatry
Poisonous plants
Prostheses
Psoriasis
Puberty and adolescence
Rashes
Reiter's syndrome
Ringworm
Rosacea
Scabies
Scleroderma
Sense organs
Skin
Skin cancer
Skin disorders
Skin lesion removal
Stretch marks
Sturge-Weber syndrome
Sunburn
Sweating
Systemic lupus erythematosus (SLE)
Tattoo removal
Tattoos and body piercing
Touch
Von Willebrand's disease
Warts
Wiskott-Aldrich syndrome
Wrinkles

EMBRYOLOGY
Abortion
Amniocentesis
Assisted reproductive technologies
Birth defects
Blue baby syndrome
Brain damage
Brain disorders
Cerebral palsy
Chorionic villus sampling
Cloning
Conception
Down syndrome
Embryology
Fetal alcohol syndrome
Gamete intrafallopian transfer (GIFT)
Genetic counseling
Genetic diseases
Genetics and inheritance
Genomics
Growth
Hermaphroditism and pseudohermaphroditism
In vitro fertilization
Karyotyping
Klinefelter syndrome
Miscarriage
Mucopolysaccharidosis (MPS)
Multiple births
Nicotine
Obstetrics
Placenta
Pregnancy and gestation
Reproductive system
Rh factor
Rubella
Sexual differentiation
Spina bifida
Stem cells
Teratogens
Toxoplasmosis
Ultrasonography

EMERGENCY MEDICINE
Abdominal disorders
Abscess drainage
Accidents
Aging
Altitude sickness
Amputation
Anesthesia
Anesthesiology
Aneurysms
Angiography
Appendectomy
Appendicitis
Asphyxiation
Biological and chemical weapons
Bites and stings
Bleeding
Blurred vision
Botulism
Brain damage
Bruises
Burns and scalds
Cardiac arrest
Cardiology
Cardiology, pediatric
Cardiopulmonary resuscitation (CPR)
Catheterization
Cesarean section

ENDOCRINOLOGY

ENVIRONMENTAL HEALTH

EPIDEMIOLOGY

ETHICS

EXERCISE PHYSIOLOGY

FAMILY MEDICINE

FORENSIC MEDICINE

GASTROENTEROLOGY

GENERAL SURGERY

GENETICS

GERIATRICS AND GERONTOLOGY

GYNECOLOGY

HEMATOLOGY

HISTOLOGY

IMMUNOLOGY

INTERNAL MEDICINE

MICROBIOLOGY

NEONATOLOGY

NEPHROLOGY

NEUROLOGY

NUCLEAR MEDICINE

NURSING

Aging: Extended care
Allied health
Anesthesiology
Cardiac rehabilitation
Critical care
Critical care, pediatric
Emergency medicine
Emergency medicine, pediatric
Geriatrics and gerontology
Holistic medicine
Hospitals
Immunization and vaccination
Neonatology
Noninvasive tests
Nursing
Nutrition
Pediatrics
Physical examination
Physician assistants
Surgery, general
Surgery, pediatric
Surgical procedures
Surgical technologists
Well-baby examinations

NUTRITION

Aging: Extended care
Anorexia nervosa
Antioxidants
Appetite loss
Bariatric surgery
Beriberi
Breast-feeding
Bulimia
Cardiac rehabilitation
Cholesterol
Digestion
Eating disorders
Exercise physiology
Fatty acid oxidation disorders
Food biochemistry
Fructosemia
Galactosemia
Gastroenterology
Gastroenterology, pediatric
Gastrointestinal disorders
Gastrointestinal system
Geriatrics and gerontology
Gestational diabetes
Glycogen storage diseases
Hyperadiposis
Hypercholesterolemia
Irritable bowel syndrome (IBS)
Jaw wiring
Kwashiorkor
Lactose intolerance
Leptin
Leukodystrophy
Lipids
Malabsorption
Malnutrition
Metabolic disorders
Metabolic syndrome
Metabolism
Nursing
Nutrition
Obesity
Obesity, childhood
Osteoporosis
Phytochemicals
Scurvy
Sports medicine
Supplements
Taste
Tropical medicine
Ulcers
Vagotomy
Vitamins and minerals
Weaning
Weight loss and gain
Weight loss medications

OBSTETRICS

Amniocentesis
Apgar score
Assisted reproductive technologies
Birth defects
Breast-feeding
Breasts, female
Cervical, ovarian, and uterine cancers
Cesarean section
Childbirth
Childbirth complications
Chorionic villus sampling
Conception
Cytomegalovirus (CMV)
Disseminated intravascular coagulation (DIC)
Down syndrome
Ectopic pregnancy
Embryology
Emergency medicine
Episiotomy
Family medicine
Fetal alcohol syndrome
Fetal surgery
Gamete intrafallopian transfer (GIFT)
Genetic counseling
Genetic diseases
Genetics and inheritance
Genital disorders, female
Gestational diabetes
Gonorrhea
Growth
Gynecology
Hemolytic disease of the newborn
In vitro fertilization
Incontinence
Invasive tests
Karyotyping
Miscarriage
Multiple births
Neonatology
Nicotine
Noninvasive tests
Obstetrics
Perinatology
Placenta
Postpartum depression
Preeclampsia and eclampsia
Pregnancy and gestation
Premature birth
Pyelonephritis
Reproductive system
Rh factor
Rubella
Sexuality
Sperm banks
Spina bifida
Stillbirth
Teratogens
Toxemia
Toxoplasmosis
Trichomoniasis
Ultrasonography
Urology

OCCUPATIONAL HEALTH

Altitude sickness
Asbestos exposure
Asphyxiation
Back pain
Biofeedback
Blurred vision
Carcinogens
Cardiac rehabilitation
Carpal tunnel syndrome
Environmental diseases
Environmental health

Gulf War syndrome
Hearing aids
Hearing loss
Interstitial pulmonary fibrosis (IPF)
Lead poisoning
Leukodystrophy
Lung cancer
Lungs
Mercury poisoning
Multiple chemical sensitivity syndrome
Nasopharyngeal disorders
Occupational health
Pneumonia
Prostheses
Pulmonary diseases
Pulmonary medicine
Pulmonary medicine, pediatric
Radiation sickness
Skin cancer
Skin disorders
Stress
Stress reduction
Tendinitis
Tendon disorders
Tendon repair
Toxicology

ONCOLOGY

Aging
Aging: Extended care
Amputation
Antioxidants
Asbestos exposure
Biopsy
Bladder cancer
Bladder removal
Blood testing
Bone cancer
Bone disorders
Bone grafting
Bone marrow transplantation
Bones and the skeleton
Brain tumors
Breast biopsy
Breast cancer
Breasts, female
Burkitt's lymphoma
Cancer
Carcinogens
Carcinoma
Cells
Cervical, ovarian, and uterine cancers
Chemotherapy
Colon and rectal polyp removal
Colon cancer
Cryotherapy and cryosurgery
Cytology
Cytopathology
Dermatology
Dermatopathology
Disseminated intravascular coagulation (DIC)
Endometrial biopsy
Epstein-Barr virus
Ewing's sarcoma
Gallbladder cancer
Gastrectomy
Gastroenterology
Gastrointestinal disorders
Gastrointestinal system
Gastrostomy
Gene therapy
Genital disorders, female
Genital disorders, male
Gynecology
Hematology
Histology
Hodgkin's disease
Human papillomavirus (HPV)
Hysterectomy
Imaging and radiology
Immunology
Immunopathology
Kaposi's sarcoma
Karyotyping
Kidney cancer
Laboratory tests
Laryngectomy
Laser use in surgery
Liver cancer
Lung cancer
Lung surgery
Lungs
Lymphadenopathy and lymphoma
Malignancy and metastasis
Mammography
Massage
Mastectomy and lumpectomy
Melanoma
Mouth and throat cancer
Nephrectomy
Nicotine
Oncology
Pain management
Pap smear
Pathology
Pharmacology
Pharmacy
Plastic surgery
Proctology
Prostate cancer
Prostate gland
Prostate gland removal
Prostheses
Pulmonary diseases
Pulmonary medicine
Radiation sickness
Radiation therapy
Radiopharmaceuticals
Sarcoma
Serology
Skin
Skin cancer
Skin lesion removal
Smoking
Stem cells
Stomach, intestinal, and pancreatic cancers
Stress
Sunburn
Testicular cancer
Thalidomide
Toxicology
Transplantation
Tumor removal
Tumors
Wiskott-Aldrich syndrome

OPHTHALMOLOGY

Aging: Extended care
Albinos
Anti-inflammatory drugs
Astigmatism
Batten's disease
Behçet's disease
Biophysics
Blindness
Blurred vision
Botox
Cataract surgery
Cataracts
Color blindness
Conjunctivitis
Corneal transplantation
Eye infections and disorders
Eye surgery
Eyes
Geriatrics and gerontology
Glaucoma
Juvenile rheumatoid arthritis

OPTOMETRY

ORGANIZATIONS AND PROGRAMS

ORTHODONTICS

ORTHOPEDICS

OSTEOPATHIC MEDICINE
Alternative medicine
Back pain
Bones and the skeleton
Exercise physiology
Family medicine
Holistic medicine
Muscle sprains, spasms, and disorders
Muscles
Nutrition
Osteopathic medicine
Physical rehabilitation

OTORHINOLARYNGOLOGY
Anti-inflammatory drugs
Aromatherapy
Audiology
Cleft lip and palate
Cleft lip and palate repair
Common cold
Corticosteroids
Croup
Deafness
Decongestants
Ear infections and disorders
Ear surgery
Ears
Epiglottitis
Gastrointestinal system
Halitosis
Head and neck disorders
Hearing aids
Hearing loss
Hearing tests
Laryngectomy
Laryngitis
Ménière's disease
Motion sickness
Myringotomy
Nasal polyp removal
Nasopharyngeal disorders
Nausea and vomiting
Nicotine
Nosebleeds
Otorhinolaryngology
Pharyngitis
Pulmonary diseases
Pulmonary medicine
Pulmonary medicine, pediatric
Quinsy
Respiration
Rhinitis
Rhinoplasty and submucous resection
Sense organs
Sinusitis
Sleep apnea
Smell
Sore throat
Strep throat
Taste
Tonsillectomy and adenoid removal
Tonsillitis
Voice and vocal cord disorders

PATHOLOGY
Autopsy
Bacteriology
Biopsy
Blood testing
Cancer
Carcinogens
Corticosteroids
Cytology
Cytopathology
Dermatopathology
Disease
Electroencephalography (EEG)
Epidemiology
Forensic pathology
Hematology
Hematology, pediatric
Histology
Homeopathy
Immunopathology
Inflammation
Karyotyping
Laboratory tests
Malignancy and metastasis
Microbiology
Microscopy
Motor skill development
Mutation
Nicotine
Niemann-Pick disease
Noninvasive tests
Oncology
Pathology
Prion diseases
Serology
Toxicology

PEDIATRICS
Acne
Amenorrhea
Appendectomy
Appendicitis
Attention-deficit disorder (ADD)
Batten's disease
Bed-wetting
Birth defects
Birthmarks
Blurred vision
Bronchiolitis
Bulimia
Burkitt's lymphoma
Cardiology, pediatric
Chickenpox
Childhood infectious diseases
Cholera
Circumcision, female, and genital mutilation
Circumcision, male
Cleft lip and palate
Cleft lip and palate repair
Cognitive development
Colic
Congenital heart disease
Cornelia de Lange syndrome
Critical care, pediatric
Croup
Cystic fibrosis
Cytomegalovirus (CMV)
Dentistry, pediatric
Dermatology, pediatric
Diabetes mellitus
Diaper rash
Diarrhea and dysentery
DiGeorge syndrome
Domestic violence
Down syndrome
Dwarfism
Emergency medicine, pediatric
Endocrinology, pediatric
Enterocolitis
Epiglottitis
Ewing's sarcoma
Failure to thrive
Family medicine
Fatty acid oxidation disorders
Fetal surgery
Fever
Fifth disease
Fistula repair
Fructosemia
Gastroenterology, pediatric
Gaucher's disease
Genetic diseases
Genetics and inheritance
Giardiasis

PERINATOLOGY

PHARMACOLOGY

Digestion
Drug resistance
Emergency medicine
Emergency medicine, pediatric
Enzymes
Ergogenic aids
Fluids and electrolytes
Food biochemistry
Genetic engineering
Genomics
Geriatrics and gerontology
Glycolysis
Herbal medicine
Homeopathy
Hormones
Laboratory tests
Marijuana
Melatonin
Metabolism
Narcotics
Nicotine
Oncology
Over-the-counter medications
Pain management
Pharmacology
Pharmacy
Poisoning
Prader-Willi syndrome
Psychiatry
Psychiatry, child and adolescent
Psychiatry, geriatric
Rheumatology
Self-medication
Sports medicine
Steroid abuse
Steroids
Thrombolytic therapy and TPA
Toxicology
Tropical medicine

PHYSICAL THERAPY

Aging: Extended care
Amputation
Amyotrophic lateral sclerosis
Arthritis
Back pain
Bell's palsy
Biofeedback
Bowlegs
Burns and scalds
Cardiac rehabilitation
Cerebral palsy
Cornelia de Lange syndrome
Disk removal
Exercise physiology
Grafts and grafting
Hemiplegia
Hip fracture repair
Hip replacement
Hydrotherapy
Kinesiology
Knock-knees
Leukodystrophy
Lower extremities
Massage
Motor skill development
Muscle sprains, spasms, and disorders
Muscles
Muscular dystrophy
Neurology
Neurology, pediatric
Numbness and tingling
Orthopedic surgery
Orthopedics
Orthopedics, pediatric
Osteopathic medicine
Osteoporosis
Pain management
Palsy
Paralysis
Paraplegia
Parkinson's disease
Physical examination
Physical rehabilitation
Plastic surgery
Prostheses
Quadriplegia
Rickets
Scoliosis
Slipped disk
Spina bifida
Spinal cord disorders
Spine, vertebrae, and disks
Sports medicine
Tendinitis
Tendon disorders
Torticollis
Upper extremities
Whiplash

PLASTIC SURGERY

Aging
Amputation
Bariatric surgery
Birthmarks
Botox
Breast cancer
Breast disorders
Breast surgery
Breasts, female
Burns and scalds
Cancer
Carcinoma
Circumcision, female, and genital mutilation
Circumcision, male
Cleft lip and palate
Cleft lip and palate repair
Craniosynostosis
Cyst removal
Cysts
Dermatology
Dermatology, pediatric
DiGeorge syndrome
Face lift and blepharoplasty
Facial transplantation
Grafts and grafting
Hair loss and baldness
Hair transplantation
Healing
Jaw wiring
Laceration repair
Liposuction
Malignancy and metastasis
Moles
Necrotizing fasciitis
Neurofibromatosis
Obesity
Obesity, childhood
Otoplasty
Otorhinolaryngology
Plastic surgery
Prostheses
Ptosis
Rhinoplasty and submucous resection
Sex change surgery
Skin
Skin lesion removal
Sturge-Weber syndrome
Surgical procedures
Tattoo removal
Tattoos and body piercing
Varicose vein removal
Varicose veins
Wrinkles

PODIATRY

Athlete's foot
Bone disorders
Bones and the skeleton

PSYCHOLOGY

PUBLIC HEALTH

PULMONARY MEDICINE

Prader-Willi syndrome
Pulmonary diseases
Pulmonary hypertension
Pulmonary medicine
Pulmonary medicine, pediatric
Respiration
Respiratory distress syndrome
Severe acute respiratory syndrome (SARS)
Sleep apnea
Smoking
Thoracic surgery
Thrombolytic therapy and TPA
Tuberculosis
Tumor removal
Tumors
Wheezing

RADIOLOGY
Angiography
Biophysics
Biopsy
Bladder cancer
Bone cancer
Bone disorders
Bones and the skeleton
Brain tumors
Cancer
Catheterization
Computed tomography (CT) scanning
Critical care
Critical care, pediatric
Emergency medicine
Ewing's sarcoma
Gallbladder cancer
Imaging and radiology
Kidney cancer
Liver cancer
Lung cancer
Magnetic resonance imaging (MRI)
Mammography
Mouth and throat cancer
Noninvasive tests
Nuclear medicine
Nuclear radiology
Oncology
Positron emission tomography (PET) scanning
Prostate cancer
Radiation sickness
Radiation therapy
Radiopharmaceuticals
Sarcoma
Stents
Surgery, general
Testicular cancer
Ultrasonography

RHEUMATOLOGY
Aging
Aging: Extended care
Anti-inflammatory drugs
Arthritis
Arthroplasty
Arthroscopy
Autoimmune disorders
Behçet's disease
Bone disorders
Bones and the skeleton
Bursitis
Corticosteroids
Fibromyalgia
Geriatrics and gerontology
Gout
Hip replacement
Hydrotherapy
Inflammation
Lyme disease
Orthopedic surgery
Orthopedics
Orthopedics, pediatric
Osteoarthritis
Osteonecrosis
Physical examination
Rheumatic fever
Rheumatoid arthritis
Rheumatology
Rotator cuff surgery
Scleroderma
Sjögren's syndrome
Spondylitis
Sports medicine

SEROLOGY
Anemia
Blood and blood disorders
Blood testing
Cholesterol
Cytology
Cytopathology
Dialysis
Fluids and electrolytes
Forensic pathology
Hematology
Hematology, pediatric
Hemophilia
Hodgkin's disease
Host-defense mechanisms
Hyperbaric oxygen therapy
Hypercholesterolemia
Hyperlipidemia
Hypoglycemia
Immune system
Immunology
Immunopathology
Jaundice
Laboratory tests
Leukemia
Malaria
Pathology
Rh factor
Septicemia
Serology
Sickle cell disease
Thalassemia
Transfusion

SPEECH PATHOLOGY
Alzheimer's disease
Amyotrophic lateral sclerosis
Aphasia and dysphasia
Audiology
Autism
Cerebral palsy
Cleft lip and palate
Cleft lip and palate repair
Deafness
Dyslexia
Ear infections and disorders
Ear surgery
Ears
Electroencephalography (EEG)
Hearing loss
Hearing tests
Jaw wiring
Laryngitis
Learning disabilities
Lisping
Paralysis
Rubinstein-Taybi syndrome
Speech disorders
Strokes
Stuttering
Thumb sucking
Voice and vocal cord disorders

SPORTS MEDICINE
Acupressure
Anorexia nervosa
Arthroplasty
Arthroscopy

TOXICOLOGY

UROLOGY

VASCULAR MEDICINE

VIROLOGY